ANTIMICROBIAL RESISTANCE IN BACTERIA OF ANIMAL ORIGIN

ANTIMICROBIAL RESISTANCE
IN BACTERIA OF ANIMAL ORIGIN

EDITED BY

FRANK M. AARESTRUP

Danish Institute for Food and Veterinary Research
Copenhagen, Denmark

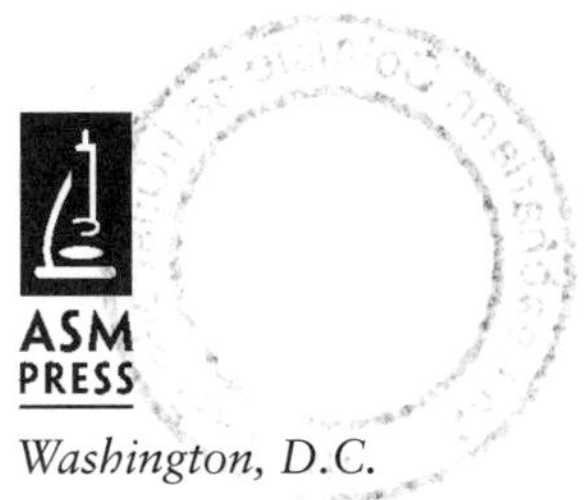

Washington, D.C.

Address editorial correspondence to ASM Press, 1752 N St. NW, Washington, DC 20036-2904, USA

Send orders to ASM Press, P.O. Box 605, Herndon, VA 20172, USA
Phone: (800) 546-2416 or (703) 661-1593
Fax: (703) 661-1501
E-mail: books@asmusa.org
Online: estore.asm.org

Library of Congress Cataloging-in-Publication Data

Antimicrobial resistance in bacteria of animal origin / edited by Frank M. Aarestrup.
p. ; cm.
Includes bibliographical references and index.
ISBN-13: 978-1-55581-306-2 (hardcover)
ISBN-10: 1-55581-306-2 (hardcover)
1. Veterinary drugs. 2. Drug resistance in microorganisms. 3. Antibiotics in veterinary medicine. 4. Zoonoses.
[DNLM: 1. Drug Resistance, Microbial. 2. Disease Transmission—veterinary. 3. Zoonoses—microbiology. QW 45 A6308 2006] I. Aarestrup, Frank M., 1966–

SF917.A58 2006
636.089'51—dc22 2005015924

10 9 8 7 6 5 4 3 2 1

Cover image: Cattle threshing grain, from the tomb of Menna in Egypt. Courtesy of the Carsten Niebuhr Institute, University of Copenhagen.

CONTENTS

CONTRIBUTORS

Frank M. Aarestrup
Danish Institute for Food and Veterinary Research, Bülowsvej 27, DK-1790 Copenhagen V, Denmark

Henk J. M. Aarts
RIKILT, Institute of Food Safety, Wageningen-UR, 6708 PD Wageningen, The Netherlands

Fariborz Shojaee Aliabadi
Khatam Co., 72 Shaghayeh St., Abdollahzadeh St., Keshavarz Blvd., 14156-33341 Tehran, Iran

Christopher Boland
Agricultural Chemicals and Veterinary Medicines, New Zealand Food Safety Authority, P.O. Box 2835, Wellington, New Zealand

Axel Cloeckaert
Unité BioAgresseurs, Santé, Environnement, Institut National de la Recherche Agronomique, 37380 Nouzilly, France

Didier Concordet
École Nationale Vétérinaire de Toulouse, UMR 181 de Physiopathologie et Toxicologie Expérimentales, 23 chemin des Capelles, 31076 Toulouse Cedex 03, France

Patrice Courvalin
Unité des Agents Antibacteriens, Institut Pasteur, 75015 Paris, France

Susan M. Donabedian
Division of Infectious Diseases, William Beaumont Hospital, Royal Oak, MI 40873

Jørgen Engberg
Unit of Gastrointestinal Infections, Statens Serum Institut, Artillerivej 5, DK-2300 Copenhagen S, Denmark

Sylvia Franke
Department of Soil, Water and Environmental Science, University of Arizona, Shantz Bldg. 38, Tucson, AZ 85721

Anders Franklin
Department of Antibiotics, National Veterinary Institute, SE-751 89 Uppsala, Sweden

Peter Gerner-Smidt
Unit of Gastrointestinal Infections, Statens Serum Institut, Artillerivej 5, DK-2300 Copenhagen S, Denmark

Kari Grave
Department of Food Hygiene and Infection Biology, Norwegian School of Veterinary Science, N 0033 Oslo, Norway

Luca Guardabassi
Department of Veterinary Pathobiology, The Royal Veterinary and Agricultural University, 1870 Frederiksberg C, Denmark

Beatriz Guerra
Federal Institute for Risk Assessment, National Salmonella Reference Laboratory, 12277 Berlin, Germany

David J. Hampson
School of Veterinary and Biomedical Sciences, Murdoch University, Murdoch, Western Australia, 6150, Australia

Henrik Hasman
Danish Institute for Food and Veterinary Research, Bülowsvej 27, DK-1790 Copenhagen V, Denmark

Lars B. Jensen
Danish Institute for Food and Veterinary Research, Bülowsvej 27, DK-1790 Copenhagen V, Denmark

Vibeke Frøkjær Jensen
Department of Epidemiology and Risk Assessment, Danish Institute for Food and Veterinary Research, DK-2860 Søborg, Denmark

David Jordan
New South Wales Department of Primary Industries, 1243 Bruxner Highway, Wollongbar, New South Wales 2477, Australia

Jack Kay
Veterinary Medicines Directorate, Department for Environment, Food and Rural Affairs, Woodham Ln., New Haw, Addlestone, Surrey KT15 3LS, United Kingdom

Monika Keelan
Laboratory for Foodborne Zoonoses, Public Health Agency of Canada, and Department of Laboratory Medicine and Pathology, University of Alberta, Edmonton, Alberta T6G 2G3, Canada

Corinna Kehrenberg
Institut für Tierzucht, Bundesforschungsanstalt für Landwirtschaft, D-31535 Neustadt-Mariensee, Germany

Isabelle Kempf
Mycoplasmology Bacteriology Unit, French Agency for Food Safety (AFSSA), BP53, F-22440 Ploufragan, France

Hilde Kruse
The Norwegian Zoonosis Center, National Veterinary Institute, N-0033 Oslo, Norway

Peter Lees
Department of Veterinary Basic Sciences, The Royal Veterinary College, Hawkshead Campus, North Mymms, Hatfield, Herts AL9 7TA, United Kingdom

Cynthia J. Lindeman
Pfizer Animal Health, Veterinary Medicine Research and Development, Kalamazoo, MI 49009

Burkhard Malorny
Federal Institute for Risk Assessment, National Salmonella Reference Laboratory, 12277 Berlin, Germany

Patrick F. McDermott
U.S. Food and Drug Administration, Center for Veterinary Medicine, Office of Research, Division of Animal and Food Microbiology, 8401 Muirkirk Road, Laurel, MD 20708

Scott A. McEwen
Department of Population Medicine, Ontario Veterinary College, University of Guelph, Guelph, Ontario N1G 2W1, Canada

Kåre Mølbak
Department of Epidemiology, Statens Serum Institut, Artillerivej 5, DK-2300 Copenhagen S, Denmark

Deborah Morris
Agricultural Chemicals and Veterinary Medicines, New Zealand Food Safety Authority, P.O. Box 2835, Wellington, New Zealand

Laura J. V. Piddock
Antimicrobial Agents Research Group, Division of Immunity and Infection, University of Birmingham, Edgbaston, Birmingham B15 2TT, United Kingdom

John F. Prescott
Department of Pathobiology, University of Guelph, Guelph, Ontario N1G 2W1, Canada

Märit Pringle
Department of Antibiotics, National Veterinary Institute, SE-751 89 Uppsala, Sweden

Christopher Rensing
Department of Soil, Water and Environmental Science, University of Arizona, Shantz Bldg. 38, Tucson, AZ 85721

Marilyn C. Roberts
Department of Pathobiology, School of Public Health and Community Medicine, University of Washington, Seattle, WA 98195-7238

Stefan Schwarz
Institut für Tierzucht, Bundesforschungsanstalt für Landwirtschaft, D-31535 Neustadt-Mariensee, Germany

Shabbir Simjee
Center for Veterinary Medicine, U.S. Food and Drug Administration, Laurel, MD 20708

Henning Sørum
Department of Food Hygiene and Infection Biology, Norwegian School of Veterinary Science, Oslo, Norway

Diane E. Taylor
Department of Medical Microbiology and Immunology, University of Alberta, Edmonton, Alberta T6G 2H7, Canada

Linda Tollefson
Center for Veterinary Medicine, U.S. Food and Drug Administration, 7519 Standish Pl., Rockville, MD 20878

Pierre-Louis Toutain
École Nationale Vétérinaire de Toulouse, UMR 181 de Physiopathologie et Toxicologie Expérimentales, 23 chemin des Capelles, 31076 Toulouse Cedex 03, France

David Vose
Vose Consulting, Le Bourg, 24400 Les Lèches, France

Robert D. Walker
Office of Research, Center for Veterinary Medicine, U.S. Food and Drug Administration, Laurel, MD 20708

Jeffrey L. Watts
Pfizer Animal Health, Veterinary Medicine Research and Development, Kalamazoo, MI 49009

Mark A. Webber
Antimicrobial Agents Research Group, Division of Immunity and Infection, University of Birmingham, Edgbaston, Birmingham B15 2TT, United Kingdom

David G. White
Division of Animal and Food Microbiology, Office of Research, Center for Veterinary Medicine, U.S. Food and Drug Administration, Laurel, MD 20708

Martin J. Woodward
Department of Food and Environmental Safety, Veterinary Laboratories Agency (Weybridge), New Haw, Addlestone, Surrey KT15 3NB, United Kingdom

Ching Ching Wu
Animal Disease Diagnostic Laboratory, Department of Veterinary Pathobiology, Purdue University School of Veterinary Medicine, West Lafayette, IN 47907-2065

Marcus J. Zervos
Division of Infectious Diseases, William Beaumont Hospital, Royal Oak, MI 40873, and Wayne State University School of Medicine, Detroit, MI 48202

PREFACE

In ancient Greece, it was considered a basic fact that there was a link between infections in animals and in humans, and veterinary medicine became a relatively advanced science. During the time of the Roman Empire, the importance society placed on veterinary medicine gradually diminished, and it was virtually a forgotten science for many centuries. It was not until the 19th century that the link between animals and humans was rediscovered. In the second half of that century, it was proven that tuberculosis could transfer between animals (6), and Robert Koch identified the causative agent of anthrax. Rudolf Virchow introduced the term "zoonosis" in 1855 (3). In 1888, August Gaertner isolated a bacterium *(Bacterium enteritidis)* from a cow with diarrhea. Forty-nine people died after having eaten the cow's meat (5). Since then it has become a well-established fact that a large number of bacteria are capable of spreading from animals to humans and causing infections.

The first written evidence of the use of antibacterial substances to cure bacterial infections dates back to the Bible (2 Kings 20:7 and Isaiah 38:21). In the Bible, figs are mentioned as a treatment for cutaneous anthrax. Later, a number of different remedies and medicines were used with more or less efficacy in European medicine. However, it was not until the 20th century with the discovery of antibiotics that more sophisticated and targeted usage became possible (4, 8). Antimicrobial agents also became widely used in the production of food animals. In the United States, the use of antimicrobial agents increased tremendously from the 1950s to the 1970s. In 1951, a total of 110 tons was produced for addition to animal feed and other applications, whereas 580 tons was produced for medical use in humans and animals (2). In 1978, 5,580 tons was produced as feed additives, whereas 6,080 tons was produced for medical use in humans and animals—50- and 10-fold increases since 1951, respectively. In 2001, the Union of Concerned Scientists (7) estimated the total amount of antimicrobial agents used for food animals in the United States to be 24.6 million lb, while the amount used for humans was estimated to be 3 million lb.

After the introduction of antimicrobial agents in veterinary medicine, bacteria resistant to antibiotics rapidly emerged, and the importance of the spread of antimicrobial-resistant bacteria from food animals to humans became gradually more and more recognized during the 1950s and 1960s. This resulted in a number of restrictions on the usage of antimicrobial agents in some countries, such as a ban on certain antimicrobial agents for growth promotion in Europe following the recommendations of the Swann report (9).

During the last few decades, major changes have occurred in the production of animals for human consumption. Animals are raised in ever larger units and are transported over long distances both for slaughter and afterwards as fresh food products. This is exemplified by the changes that have occurred in Danish production of pigs and cattle (Fig. 1). Since 1982, the number of farms has decreased considerably, whereas the number of cattle (mainly dairy) has remained almost constant and the number of pigs has increased. This increased concentration of livestock facilitates the spread of infections in animals, resulting in an increased need for antimicrobial agents and thereby selection of resistance, and it also facilitates the spread of the selected resistant bacteria. It also provides new and interesting possibilities for the bacteria to evolve. These new problems also require new solutions and national and international collaboration on a scale that we have not experienced previously.

The purpose of *Antimicrobial Resistance in Bacteria of Animal Origin* is to present an update on the current situation with regard to the veterinary and public health aspects of antimicrobial resistance in bacteria of animal origin. In addition, suggestions for intervention and research needs for the future are

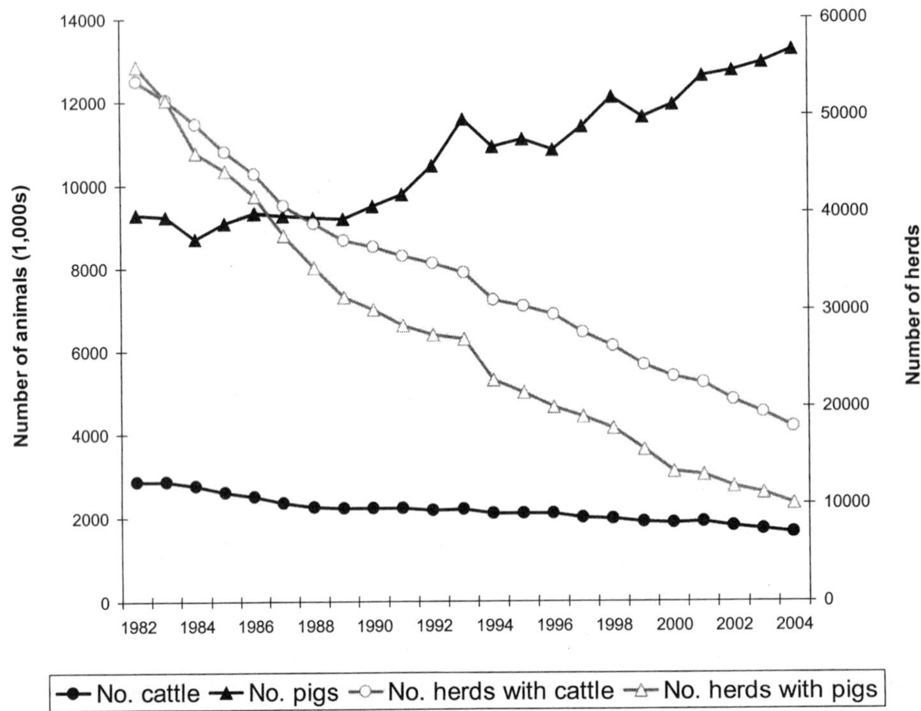

Figure 1. Changes in the number of farms with cattle and pigs and in the number of cattle and pigs in Denmark from 1982 to 2004 (1).

provided. We have tried to cover the most important topics. However, considering the complexity of the subject, this has not always been possible. Thus, although this book provides a large amount of useful information, anyone who wants to get a more thorough overview of the multiple aspects of antimicrobial resistance in bacteria from animals may wish to consult additional sources as well.

The book ends with some personal remarks and suggestions for future interventions and research needs that might enable better control of antimicrobial resistance among bacteria in animals in the future.

This book has been the combined work of a large number of people, and I thank everyone who has participated in or supported the work. Personally, I am especially grateful to my wife, Julie, and our little daughter, Amalie.

In conclusion, I hope that a large number of people will find useful knowledge in this book. I have certainly learned much from editing it, and I have perhaps most importantly also been inspired to further research.

REFERENCES

1. **Anonymous.** 2005. Statistics Denmark. http://www.statistikbanken.dk/statbank5a/default.asp?w=1024, accessed March 2005.
2. **Black, W. D.** 1984. The use of antimicrobial drugs in agriculture. *Can. J. Physiol. Pharmacol.* **62:**1044–1048.
3. **Brown, C.** 2004. Emerging zoonoses and pathogens of public health significance—an overview. *Rev. Sci. Tech.* **23:**435–442.
4. **Brown, J. M.** 2001. Wonder drugs: a history of antibiotics. *J. S. C. Med. Assoc.* **97:**38–39.
5. **Dewberry, E. B.** 1959. *Food Poisoning: Food-Borne Infection and Intoxications,* 4th ed. Leonard Hill, London, United Kingdom.
6. **Fleming, G.** 1874. The transmissibility of tuberculosis. *Br. Foreign Med.-Chir. Rev.* **54:**461–486.
7. **Mellon, M., C. Benbrook, and K. L. Benbrook.** 2001. *Hogging It: Estimates of Antimicrobial Abuse in Livestock.* Union of Concerned Scientists, Cambridge, Mass.
8. **Spink, W. W.** 1973. History of medicine. The drama of sulfanilamide, penicillin and other antibiotics 1936–1972. *Minn. Med.* **56:**551–556.
9. **Swann, M. M.** 1969. Report of the Joint Committee on the Use of Antibiotics in Animal Husbandry and Veterinary Medicine. HMSO, London, United Kingdom.

Antimicrobial Resistance in Bacteria of Animal Origin
Edited by Frank M. Aarestrup

Chapter 1

Modes of Antimicrobial Action and Mechanisms of Bacterial Resistance

LUCA GUARDABASSI AND PATRICE COURVALIN

Antimicrobial resistance is a very complex phenomenon involving a large variety of antimicrobial agents, bacterial species, resistance genes, and mechanisms of resistance. The complexity of the phenomenon has led to the genesis of many designations, definitions, and classifications, whose meaning may in some cases be controversial. Comprehensive understanding of the veterinary and public health aspects of antimicrobial resistance in bacteria of animal origin requires knowledge of the modes by which antimicrobial agents act on the bacterial cell as well as of the mechanisms by which bacteria become resistant. This introductory chapter is an overview of targets for antimicrobial action and mechanisms of resistance combined with information on the nature of antibacterial drugs, their classification, and their usage in animals. Above all, the chapter introduces concepts and definitions necessary for the understanding of the following chapters, with the challenge of making the book readable and hopefully even enjoyable to a broad audience of veterinarians, physicians, scientists, and students in various fields.

BASIC CONCEPTS AND DEFINITIONS

Definition of "Antimicrobial Agent" and "Antibiotic"

According to the etymology of the word "antimicrobial" (from the Greek *anti*, meaning "against," *mikros*, meaning "little," and *bios*, meaning "life"), antimicrobial agents are substances against life of microorganisms. Compounds used for treatment of bacterial diseases in humans and animals are commonly referred to by both professionals and laypeople as antibiotics. However, according to their definitions, the terms "antimicrobial agent" and "antibiotic" are not interchangeable. The adjective "antibiotic" (from the Greek *anti* and *biotikos*, "concerning life") was first used in 1889 by the French biologist P. Vuillemin to describe destruction of one organism by another. As a noun, the term "antibiotic" was introduced in 1941 by the Nobel laureate microbiologist S. A. Waksman, who defined antibiotics as "chemical substances that are produced by microorganisms and that have the capacity, in dilute solution, to selectively inhibit the growth of and even to destroy other microorganisms." Thus, according to its definition, the term "antibiotic" only refers to substances of microbial origin acting on microorganisms. It should not be used to indicate synthetic (e.g., sulfonamides and quinolones) or semisynthetic compounds (e.g., amoxicillin and amikacin), substances of plant (e.g., quinine and alkaloids) or animal origin (e.g., lysozyme), and substances active against animal cells (e.g., anticancer drugs).

Only drugs affecting pathogenic microorganisms more adversely than the host (selective toxicity) can be administered systemically to humans and animals. The mechanism of action of a drug accounts for its degree of selective toxicity. The most selectively toxic antimicrobial agents are those affecting microbial structures (e.g., the cell wall) and metabolic pathways (e.g., folic acid biosynthesis) that are not present in eukaryotic cells. On the contrary, antimicrobial agents acting on DNA (nitrofurans, nitroimidazoles, and quinoxalines) are more likely to induce toxic effects in humans or animals. Some agents are toxic to both prokaryotic and eukaryotic cells and can be applied only on inanimate objects (disinfectants) or on the surface of living tissues (antiseptics). Disinfectants and antiseptics are generally referred to as biocides. Most biocides (e.g., quaternary ammonium compounds)

Luca Guardabassi • Department of Veterinary Pathobiology, The Royal Veterinary and Agricultural University, 1870 Frederiksberg C, Denmark. **Patrice Courvalin** • Unité des Agents Antibacteriens, Institut Pasteur, 75015 Paris, France.

can be used for both disinfection and antisepsis depending on the concentration of active compound. However, some classes of biocides (e.g., aldehydes and phenols) can only be used as disinfectants due to their toxicity to eukaryotic cells.

Classification of Antibacterial Agents

Antimicrobial agents can be classified according to various criteria. On the basis of the target microorganism, drugs are classified as antiviral, antibacterial, antifungal, and antiparasitic. However, it should be noted that bacteria and protozoa can be susceptible to the same drug. For example, ionophores used for the control of coccidiosis in food animals (monensin and salinomycin) have antibacterial activity, in particular against gram-positive organisms. Some drugs generally referred to as antibacterial agents, namely sulfonamides, tetracyclines, furazolidone, and metronidazole, are active against protozoa and can be used for treatment of protozoal infestations of both humans and animals. On the contrary, all antibacterial agents are inactive against viruses and fungi at normal therapeutic concentrations and their chemical structures differ from those of antiviral and antifungal drugs.

Antibacterial agents include a wide array of substances that differ in both chemical structure and mode of action. Classification is therefore based on chemical structure. Each antibacterial class is characterized by a typical molecular core structure, which is responsible for drug activity. Addition or subtraction of chemical groups from the core structure leads to the various members of the class and influences their spectrum of activity, pharmacodynamics, and toxicology. The alphabet of antibacterial classes used in humans and/or in animals is reported in Table 1. Detailed information on the chemical structure and activity of antimicrobial drugs can be found elsewhere (28).

Based on the range of susceptible bacterial groups, antibacterial agents can be classified as broad-, intermediate-, or narrow-spectrum drugs. Tetracyclines, phenicols, fluoroquinolones, "third-generation" and "fourth-generation" cephalosporins, and carbapenems are generally considered as broad-spectrum drugs since their spectra of activity cover a wide variety of bacterial species, including gram-positive organisms, gram-negative organisms, aerobes, and anaerobes. Drugs with narrower spectra are mainly active against a specific bacterial group like gram-positive organisms (natural penicillins, glycopeptides, and bacitracin), gram-negative organisms (polymyxins), aerobes (aminoglycosides and sulfonamides), or anaerobes (nitroimidazoles). The spectrum of activity of a drug can be reduced by acquisition and spread of resistance across the bacterial population. For example, although tetracyclines are generally considered as broad-spectrum drugs, their range of activity has been substantially narrowed by the emergence of resistance in both gram-positive and gram-negative bacteria, with a consequent decrease in the clinical importance of these drugs. The potency of antibacterial agents is extremely variable and depends on the target bacterium. When considering a given species, some drugs are active at concentrations below 1 g/ml (e.g., fluoroquinolones) while others are active at 100-fold higher concentrations (e.g., sulfonamides). This should be taken into account when comparing the use of different drugs in animals based on total amounts of active drug.

Drugs that kill bacteria are defined as bactericidal, in contrast to drugs that inhibit or delay bacterial growth, which are defined as bacteriostatic (Table 1). The type of antibacterial activity of a drug depends mainly on how the drug binds to its target. Usually, bactericidal drugs bind to their targets irreversibly or with high affinity, whereas bacteriostatic drugs form unstable bonds. This classification, like most classifications, is quite arbitrary since the same drug may have either bactericidal or bacteriostatic effect depending on its concentration and the type, quantity, and growth state of the bacterium, as well as on the experimental conditions under which its activity is evaluated. For example, aminoglycosides are bactericidal but are poorly active against bacteria growing anaerobically. However, it is an important distinction in clinical practice since bacteriostatic drugs have a slower effect and their efficacy depends on the ability of the host immune response to kill and effectively eliminate bacteria. As a consequence, the use of bacteriostatic drugs is not indicated in immunosuppressed patients and for the treatment of life-threatening acute infections such as endocarditis and meningitis.

Definition of "Resistance"

Antimicrobial resistance is a relative term. There are numerous definitions of bacterial resistance, which are based on different criteria (genetic, biochemical, microbiological, and clinical) and do not necessarily overlap. The two most commonly used definitions are based on microbiological (in vitro resistance) and clinical (in vivo resistance) criteria. According to the microbiological definition, a strain is defined as resistant if it grows in the presence of higher concentrations of the drug compared with phylogenetically related strains. Resistance is therefore not a property that can be determined by studying a single strain but can only be assessed by comparison of two or

Table 1. The antibacterial alphabet

Class	Origin	Type of activity	Target
Aminoglycosides[a]	*Streptomyces*, *Micromonospora* spp.	Bactericidal	30S ribosomal subunit
Cephalosporins[a]	*Cephalosporium* spp.	Bactericidal	Transpeptidase
Carbapenems[a,b]	*Streptomyces* spp.	Bactericidal	Transpeptidase
Coumarins[c]	*Streptomyces niveus* or *Streptomyces spheroides*	Bacteriostatic	DNA gyrase
Cycloserine[d]	*Streptomyces* spp.	Bactericidal	Racemase
Diaminopyrimidines	Synthetic	Bacteriostatic	Dihydrofolate reductase
Ethambutol[d]	Synthetic	Bacteriostatic	Unknown
Everninomycins[c]	*Streptomyces viridochromogenes*	Bactericidal	50S ribosomal subunit
Fosfomycins	*Streptomyces* spp. or *Pseudomonas syringae*[e]	Bactericidal	Pyruvyl transferase
Fusidanes	*Microsporum* spp. or *Epidermophyton* spp.	Bacteriostatic	Elongation factor G
Glycopeptides	Various actinomycetes	Bactericidal	Acyl–D-alanyl–D-alanine
Isoniazid[d]	Synthetic	Bactericidal	Mycolic acides synthesis
Lincosamides[a]	*Streptomyces lincolnensis*	Bactericidal	50S ribosomal subunit
Macrolides[a]	Various actinomycetes	Bacteriostatic	50S ribosomal subunit
Monobactams	*Streptomyces* or synthetic	Bactericidal	Transpeptidase
Mupirocin	*Pseudomonas fluorescens*	Bactericidal	DNA gyrase
Nitrofurans[c]	Synthetic	Bactericidal	DNA
Nitroimidazoles	*Streptomyces* spp.	Bactericidal	DNA
Oxazolidones[b]	Synthetic	Bacteriostatic	30S ribosomal subunit
Penicillins[a]	*Penicillium* spp.	Bactericidal	Transpeptidase
Phenicols[a]	*Streptomyces venezuelae*[e]	Bacteriostatic	Peptidyl transferase
Phosphoglycolipids	*Streptomyces* spp.	Bactericidal	Transglycolase
Pleuromutilins[a,c]	Basidiomycetes	Bactericidal	50S ribosomal subunit
Polypeptides	*Bacillus polymyxa* (polymyxins A and B)	Bactericidal	Membrane phospholipids
	Bacillus licheniformis (bacitracin)	Bactericidal	Isoprenylphosphate
Pyrazinamide[d]	Synthetic	Variable	Mycolic acid synthesis
Quinolones	Synthetic	Bactericidal	Type II topoisomerases
Quinoxalines[c]	Synthetic	Bactericidal	DNA
Rifamycins[a,b]	*Amycolatopsis mediterranei*	Bactericidal	RNA polymerase
Streptogramins[a]	*Streptomyces* spp.	Bacteriostatic	50S ribosomal subunit
Sulfonamides	Synthetic	Bacteriostatic	Pteroate synthetase
Tetracyclines[a]	*Streptomyces* spp.	Bacteriostatic	30S ribosomal subunit

[a]Include semisynthetic compounds.
[b]Drugs used only in humans.
[c]Drugs used only in animals.
[d]Drugs used against *Mycobacterium tuberculosis*.
[e]Currently produced by chemical synthesis.

more strains under identical conditions. Since the natural levels of susceptibility to a drug can vary notably between bacterial species, resistance can only be assessed by comparing strains of the same species or genus. According to the clinical definition, a strain is defined as resistant when it survives antimicrobial therapy. Under in vivo conditions, a strain may be either resistant or sensitive to treatment depending on its location, the dosage and mode of drug administration, tissue distribution of the drug, and the state of the immune system of the individual under treatment. In some cases, the drug may not be able to penetrate the site where the pathogen is located (e.g., fibrotic abscesses) or is not active under the physicochemical conditions at the infection site (e.g., high pH or low oxygen content).

Resistance can be quantified under laboratory conditions by determining the MIC of a given drug, which is the lowest drug concentration that completely inhibits growth of the bacterial isolate under test. A strain is defined as resistant, intermediate, or susceptible based on either microbiological or clinical breakpoints. Microbiological breakpoints are based on MIC distribution for a bacterial species, with resistance occurring when higher MICs are observed in comparison with the wild-type population. These breakpoints are appropriate for surveillance studies, when the purpose is to track the occurrence of resistance in a bacterial population and identify the emergence of new resistant phenotypes. Clinical (or pharmacological) breakpoints are set up not only considering the MIC distribution for a species but also in vivo parameters such as bacterial distribution in the host, pharmacokinetics and pharmacodynamics of the drug, and correlation of MICs with clinical outcome. Clinical breakpoints are used when antimicrobial susceptibility testing is performed in clinical laboratories for providing information to physicians on the choice of an appropriate drug.

Intrinsic and Acquired Resistance

Intrinsic resistance is due to a structural or functional trait allowing tolerance of a particular drug or antimicrobial class by all members of a bacterial group (species, genus, or even a larger group). More accurately, this should be referred to as insensitivity since it occurs in bacteria that have never been susceptible to the drug. Insensitivity or reduced sensitivity can be due to scarce affinity of the drug for the bacterial target (e.g., low affinity of nalidixic acid for enterococcal gyrase), inaccessibility of the drug into the bacterial cell (e.g., impermeability to glycopeptides of the outer membrane in gram-negative species), extrusion of the drug by chromosomally encoded active exporters (resistance to tetracyclines, chloramphenicol, and quinolones in *Pseudomonas aeruginosa*), or innate production of enzymes inactivating the drug (e.g., AmpC beta-lactamase in some members of the family *Enterobacteriaceae*). Some bacteria are considered insensitive to a drug even if they are susceptible under in vivo conditions. For example, *Enterobacteriaceae* are considered insensitive to erythromycin in view of the MICs of the drug (2 to 256 μg/ml), although higher concentrations of erythromycin can be obtained in the intestinal lumen after oral administration of recommended doses (2). Intrinsic resistance represents a clinical problem in dealing with bacterial species that are insensitive to a large number of antimicrobial classes, for example *Mycobacterium tuberculosis* or *P. aeruginosa*, since it limits the range of drugs available for treatment and consequently increases the risk associated with emergence of acquired resistance.

Acquired resistance is a major threat to animal and human health because it causes the emergence and spread of resistance in normally susceptible bacterial populations and consequently may lead to therapeutic failure. Unlike intrinsic resistance, acquired resistance is a trait associated with only some strains of a particular bacterial genus or species. Acquisition is due to a genetic change in the bacterial genome, which can be the consequence of a mutation (endogenous resistance) or of horizontal acquisition of foreign genetic information (exogenous resistance). Resistance can also result from a combination of mutational and gene transfer events, like in the case of mutations that expand the spectrum of beta-lactamases or confer on them resistance to beta-lactamase inhibitors. Endogenous resistance plays an essential role in bacteria that are not known to acquire foreign DNA under natural conditions (e.g., *Mycobacterium* spp.). For all bacteria, it represents the main mode of acquiring resistance when high-level resistance is not conferred by mobile genetic elements (e.g., fluoroquinolone resistance).

Exogenous resistance can be secondary to acquisition of free DNA by transformation, bacteriophages by transduction, and cell-to-cell transfer by conjugation (43). Transformation and transduction do not require viability of the donor cell nor linkage in time and space between the donor and the recipient. However, the consequences of transformation and transduction in the spread of antimicrobial resistance are limited to closely related bacteria belonging to the same species or genus since transformation requires homology between donor and recipient DNA for recombination to occur, and the host range of transduction is limited by the high host specificity of bacteriophages. Transformation accounts for the buildup of mosaic genes responsible for penicillin resistance by production of hybrid penicillin-binding proteins (PBPs) in both gram-positive (*Streptococcus pneumoniae*) and gram-negative species (*Neisseria* spp.) (19). Transduction could have played an important role in the dissemination of the macrolide resistance gene *mefA* among group A streptococci, as indicated by the association of *mefA* with a transposon inserted into a prophage (4). Bacteriophages could also have been implicated in the spread of beta-lactamase genes (31) and in the evolution of the multiple resistance phenotype in the zoonotic pathogen *Salmonella enterica* serovar Typhimurium phage type DT104 (38). Conjugation is likely to play a more important role in the spread of antimicrobial resistance since resistance genes are often located on conjugative genetic elements such as plasmids or transposons (see chapter 6).

Mutations occur spontaneously in any gene of the bacterial genome but the frequency of mutation may differ between genes. Consequently, the frequencies of mutations leading to antimicrobial resistance may vary depending on the specific antimicrobial agent. For example, mutations leading to streptomycin, nalidixic acid, and rifampin resistance are a relatively common event (10^{-8} to 10^{-10} cells per generation), whereas mutations leading to resistance to other antimicrobial agents (e.g., vancomycin and polymyxin B) are rare genetic events. A single mutation can determine a 1,000-fold increase in the levels of resistance to a drug (e.g., streptomycin). In contrast, for other drugs (e.g., fluoroquinolones) the acquisition of resistance by mutation is a gradual, stepwise process in which different mutations are involved. The frequencies of mutations conferring drug resistance also differ between species as well as between strains of the same species. For example, the rate of mutations leading to rifampin resistance in *Staphylococcus aureus* is approximately 100-fold higher than in *Escherichia coli*, making the use of this antibiotic as a single agent not appropriate for the treatment of staphylococcal infections. Mutational resistance to drugs targeting the ribosome is more common in slow-growing bacteria with one (e.g., *Mycobacterium*) or two copies (e.g., *Helicobacter* and *Mycoplasma*) of rRNA than in bacteria with four copies (e.g., *S. pneumoniae*). Multiresistant clinical strains of *P. aeruginosa*, *E. coli*, *Salmonella enterica* serovar Enteritidis, and *S. aureus* display in vivo mutation rates that are 1,000-fold higher than in other members of these species. Such strains are generally referred as hypermutators and their increased mutation rate, due to deficiency in the mismatch repair system, a DNA repair system that identifies and corrects DNA mismatches during DNA replication, likely enhances the emergence of resistance in these strains (26, 33).

Cross-Resistance, Coresistance, and Antimicrobial Selection

The situation in which resistance to one drug is associated with resistance to another drug and due to a single biochemical mechanism is defined as cross-resistance. Cross-resistance can occur between all members of a given antimicrobial class (e.g., sulfonamides), be limited to some of them (e.g., aminoglycosides), or involve antimicrobials belonging to different classes. Either target overlapping or unspecific drug efflux can cause the latter phenomenon. For example, macrolides, lincosamides, B streptogramins (MLS) act on bacterial ribosomes, and methylation of a single adenine residue in 50S rRNA confers high-level resistance to the three antimicrobial classes despite the difference in their chemical structure. Unspecific drug efflux is an energy-dependent mechanism by which a broad range of substrates, including drugs with different chemical structures, is actively exported from the bacterial cell (see "Drug Efflux Pumps" below). Cross-resistance should be distinguished from coresistance, also designated associated resistance, which is due to the coexistence of genes or mutations in the same strain, each conferring resistance to a different class of drug.

Acquisition of antimicrobial resistance by gene transfer can in some cases be enhanced by the presence of antimicrobial agents in the environment. Subinhibitory concentrations of penicillins are known to enhance interspecies conjugal transfer of plasmid DNA, most likely by increasing cell permeability and by facilitating formation of effective mating aggregates (13). Low concentrations of tetracycline have been shown to increase the transfer frequencies of conjugative transposons mediating resistance to tetracycline and other antibiotics in gram-positive cocci (15) and in *Bacteroides* spp. (48). Independent of the effect of antimicrobial agents on gene transfer, exposure of bacteria to antimicrobial agents selects resistant genotypes arising by either mutation or gene transfer, allowing them to become predominant in the bacterial population. This situation, commonly referred to as antimicrobial selective pressure, occurs in the human or animal body during antimicrobial therapy as well as in populations or environments (hospitals, animal farms, and aquaculture sites) as a result of intensive antimicrobial use.

As a consequence of cross-resistance or coresistance, bacteria resistant to a certain antimicrobial agent can be selected by exposure to another agent (cross-selection and coselection, respectively). An example of coselection in animals is provided by the persistence of glycopeptide-resistant enterococci (GRE) after the ban of glycopeptides. This could be accounted for by the genetic link on self-transferable plasmids of the *ermB* macrolide resistance gene and of the *vanA* glycopeptide resistance operon, with consequent coselection of glycopeptide resistance by the use of macrolides (1). Even biocides and heavy metals have the potential to select for resistance to antimicrobial agents used in chemotherapy due to the fact that the genes encoding resistance to the various groups of molecules often coexist on the same genetic structure (see chapters 7 and 8).

ANTIBACTERIAL USAGE IN ANIMALS

There are important differences in the use of antibacterial agents in humans and animals, in particular food animals. In human medicine, and also in small-animal and equine veterinary medicine, antimicrobials are administered individually to patients after occurrence of infection (therapy) or, in rare cases, to prevent emergence of infection (prophylaxis). In animal production, antibacterial drugs are usually administered to groups of animals (herds, flocks, etc.) for prophylaxis, as therapy for sick individuals combined with prophylaxis in healthy ones (metaphylaxis), or for increasing animal growth rate (growth promotion). In the latter case, the drugs are used as feed supplement and administered at subtherapeutic concentrations for long periods of time without the need for veterinary prescription.

Antibacterial drugs used for animal health (therapy, prophylaxis, and metaphylaxis) generally belong to the same classes as those used in human

Table 2. Human health importance and clinical use of antibacterial drugs licensed for animal use in European Union countries and/or the United States[a]

Antibacterial class	Licensed drugs (uses)[b]	Human health importance[c] and clinical use in human medicine
Aminoglycosides	Gentamicin (A, B, C, F, P) Amikacin (C)[d]	High importance. Mainly used for treatment of hospital infections. In combination with penicillins in enterococcal, streptococcal, or *Listeria monocytogenes* infections; with antistaphylococcal penicillins in severe infections by *S. aureus*; with broad-spectrum beta-lactams or quinolones in systemic acute gram-negative infections.
	Streptomycin (A, B, C, F, P)	Low importance. Second-choice drug in the treatment of tuberculosis and enterococcal endocarditis. Does not select for resistance to other aminoglycosides.
	Kanamycin (A, B, C, F, P)	Medium importance. Limited use but can select for resistance to other aminoglycosides.
	Neomycin (A, B, C, F, P) Apramycin (A,[e] B,[e] P) Paromomycin (A, B, C, F, P)[e]	Kanamycin and neomycin are rarely used. Paromomycin is used for visceral leishmaniasis. Apramycin is not used in humans.
Aminocyclitols	Spectinomycin (A, B, C, P)	Low importance. It is used only for treatment of gonorrhea.
Cephalosporins	Narrow spectrum[f] (B, C, P, F)	Medium importance. Limited use, mainly for surgical wound prophylaxis, rarely for treatment of uncomplicated community-acquired infections in penicillin-allergic patients. Select for resistance to expanded-spectrum cephalosporins and other beta-lactams.
	Expanded spectrum[g] (A, B, C, P)	Very high importance. Used in nosocomial infections by gram-negative bacteria, in severe community-acquired infections (e.g., pneumonia and meningitis), and in case of failure of treatment with other beta-lactams.
Lincosamides	Lincomycin (B, P, A, C, F) Clindamycin (C, F) Pirlimycin (B)[d]	High importance. Drugs of choice for the treatment of anaerobic infections and osteomyelitis caused by *S. aureus*. Topical use for acne (clindamycin). Reserve drugs for penicillin-allergic patients. Pirlimycin is not used in humans.
Macrolides	Erythromycin (A, B, C, F, P) Tylosin (B, P, A) Tilmicosin (P, A) Spiramycin (A, B, C, F, P)[e] Kitasamycin (A, B, P)[e] Josamycin (A, B, P)[e] Tulathromycin (B, P)[e] Oleandomycin (B) Aivlosin (P)[e]	High importance. Drugs of choice in *Mycoplasma* and *Chlamydia* respiratory infections and legionellosis. Also used against *Bordetella pertussis* and *Campylobacter* enteric infections. Alternative to penicillins in mild to moderate skin infections and upper respiratory infections caused by susceptible gram-positive bacteria. Tylosin, tilmicosin, tulathromycin, aivlosin (acetylisovaleryltylosintartrate), and kitasamycin are not used in humans. The use of oleandomycin and josamycin is rare. Can coselect for GRE in animals.
Nitrofurans	Furazolidone (C)[d]	Low importance. Furantoin and other nitrofurans can be used only for treatment of cystitis.
Nitroimidazoles	Metronidazole (A,C, F)[e]	High importance. Drugs of choice in infections by anaerobes and in combination therapy against *Helicobacter pylori*.
Penicillins	Penicillins G and V (B, P, A, C, F)	Low importance. Limited use due to narrow spectrum. Penicillin V is used in streptococcal pharyngitis and other nonsevere streptococcal infections. Penicillin G can be used in streptococcal endocarditis and bacteremia by *S. pneumoniae* or *Clostridium perfringens*. Limited contribution to selection for resistance to other beta-lactams.
	Ampicillin, amoxicillin (all)[h]	Medium importance. Drugs of choice in upper respiratory infections, otitis media, streptococcal endocarditis, and other gram-positive infections.
	Cloxacillin, dicloxacillin (B, C) Nafcillin (B)[e]	High importance. Antistaphylococcal penicillins used for the treatment of methicillin-susceptible *S. aureus* infections.
Phenicols	Chloramphenicol (C, F) Florfenicol (AQ,[e] B, P)[d] Thiamphenicol (B, P, A)[e]	Low importance in developed countries, where they are used only as topical eye preparations or for treatment of brain abscesses. Higher importance in developing countries, where chloramphenicol is the first choice in typhoid fever and still used for treatment of meningitis. Florfenicol is not licensed for human use.
Pleuromutilins	Tiamulin, valnemulin (P, A)	Not used
Polypeptides	Bacitracin (A,[d] B,[d] C, F, P[d])	Very low importance. Topical use with gram-positive activity.
	Polymyxin B (B,[d] C, F)	Very low importance. Topical use with gram-negative activity.
	Colistin (A, B,[e] C,[e] F,[e] P[e])	Low importance. Rarely used as a reserve agent for infections caused by multiresistant *P. aeruginosa* and other gram-negative species.
Quinolones	Narrow spectrum,[e,i] (AQ)	Medium importance. Although their use is limited to urinary tract infections, select for resistance to fluoroquinolones.
Quinoxalines	Cardabox (P, A)	Not used

Continued on following page

Table 2. *Continued*

Antibacterial class	Licensed drugs (uses)[b]	Human health importance[c] and clinical use in human medicine
	Second generation[j] (B, P, A, C, F)	Very high importance. Drug of choice in lower respiratory, urinary, and skin gram-negative infections. Also used in acute sinusitis, intra-abdominal infections, bone and joint infections, typhoid fever, and syphilis.
Rifamycins	Rifampin (B)[e] Rifaximin (B, P)[e]	Very high importance. Rifampin is a drug of choice for treatment of tuberculosis and brucellosis in combination with other drugs.
Streptogramins	Virginiamycin (P, A)[d]	High importance. Streptogramins are used for the treatment of infections by MRSA and GRE.
Sulfonamides[k]	Many compounds (all)	Medium importance. Frequently used in urinary tract infections, less frequently in upper respiratory infections and in otitis media (associated with erythromycin).
Tetracyclines	Oxytetracycline, chlortetracycline, tetracycline (all) Doxycycline (C, F)	Medium importance. Drug of choice for treatment of infections caused by rickettsiae and other intracellular organisms with scarce ability to develop resistance. Can be used in *Mycoplasma* and *Chlamydia* respiratory infections and severe chronic acne vulgaris.
Miscellaneous	Fusidic acid (C)[e]	Low importance. Mainly used for topical treatment. Can be used in combination with other drugs for the treatment of MRSA infections.
	Mupirocin (C)[d]	Very low importance. Only topical use for eradication of MRSA carriage.
	Avilamycin (P)	Not used. An analog drug (everninomycin) is under evaluation as a human therapeutic agent.
	Novobiocin (B, C)	Not used
	Bambermycin (A, B, P)[d]	Not used

[a]The list of drugs licensed for animal use is based on data from the European Agency for the Evaluation of Medicinal Products, the U.S. Food and Drug Administration, the British Veterinary Medicine Directorate, and the International Veterinary Information Service.
[b]A, avian; B, bovine; C, canine; F, feline; P, porcine; AQ, aquaculture.
[c]The human health importance of a drug is defined on the basis of (i) clinical use of the drug in life-threatening infections, (ii) lack of alternative drugs, (iii) selection of resistance to important drugs, and (iv) frequency of use. Drugs are ranked in five categories: very high importance, last-choice drugs for the treatment of life-threatening infections for which limited or no alternatives exist; high importance, first-choice drugs used for treating life-threatening infections for which there are valid alternatives; medium importance, drugs frequently used for treatment of uncomplicated infections, drugs of limited use that can select for resistance to important drugs; low importance, drugs of limited use that cannot select for resistance to important drugs; and very low importance, drugs only used for topical treatment.
[d]Licensed only in the United States.
[e]Licensed only in the European Union.
[f]Cefadroxil (C, F), cefalexin (B, C, F, P), cefazolin (B), cefalonium (B), cefacetrile (B), and cephapirin (B). Cefazolin, cefalonium, and cefacetrile are licensed only in the European Union.
[g]Ceftiofur (A, B, C, P), cefquinone (B, P), and cefoperazone (B). Avian and canine use of ceftiofur is licensed only in the United States. Cefquinone is licensed only in the European Union.
[h]With or without the beta-lactamase inhibitor clavulanic acid.
[i]Narrow-spectrum quinolones: oxolinic acid (A, AQ, P) and flumequine (A, B, P).
[j]Second-generation quinolones: enrofloxacin (A, B, C, F, P), danofloxacin (B, P), difloxacin, (A, B, C), ibafloxacin (C, F), orbifloxacin (C, F), marbofloxacin (B, C, F, P), and sarafloxacin (A, AQ). Ibofloxacin, sarafloxacin, porcine use of danofloxacin, avian and bovine use of difloxacin, and bovine and porcine use of marbofloxacin are licensed only in the European Union.
[k]Cross-resistance between all sulfonamides. Often associated with diaminopyrimidines (trimethoprim, baquiloprim, or ormethoprim).

medicine. Tetracyclines constitute the antibacterial class used most often in animals, followed by macrolides, pleuromutilins, lincosamides, penicillins, potentiated sulfonamides (sulfonamides associated with diaminopyrimidines), aminoglycosides, fluoroquinolones, cephalosporins, and phenicols (41). Other drugs used for animal health purposes in the Western hemisphere include novobiocin, bacitracin, polymyxins, rifamycins, and, limited to companion animals, fusidic acid, mupirocin, nitrofurans, and nitroimidazoles. Pleuromutilins (tiamulin and valnemulin) are only used for food animals, mainly in the treatment of swine dysentery and respiratory diseases in swine and poultry. Bacitracin is widely used as a growth promoter in animal production outside Europe, but the use of this drug in human and veterinary therapy is confined to topical applications due to nephrotoxicity. Chloramphenicol, nitrofurans, and nitroimidazoles are prohibited in food-producing animals in the European Union and in the United States due to the risks associated with the presence of drug residues in food.

Antibacterial drugs previously used for growth promotion in the European Union include macrolides (tylosin and spiramycin), polypeptides (bacitracin), glycolipids (bambermycin), streptogramins (virginiamycin), glycopeptides (avoparcin), quinoxalines (carbadox and olaquindox), everninomycins (avilamycin), and ionophores (monensin and salinomycin). The distinction between growth promoters and drugs used for animal health is not always clear. Drugs such as tylosin and tetracyclines could be used for growth promotion, prophylaxis, or therapy depending on the dose. Quinoxalines are here regarded as growth promoters because they increase the rate of weight gain and improve feed efficiency, according to the manufacturers' indications. However, the inclusion of quinoxaline among growth promoters is questionable since these drugs, mainly carbadox, are usually employed for prevention of swine dysentery. Most growth promoters (avoparcin, bacitracin, virginiamycin, spiramycin, and tylosin) were banned in the European Union at the end of the 1990s because their use in animal feed was liable to select for resistance to clinically important drugs in human medicine or alternatively they were shown to have carcinogenic effects (quinoxalines). The only growth promoters currently in use are avilamycin, bambermycin, and ionophores, but the European Union has announced a total ban on growth promoters starting in 2006. Except avoparcin, the growth promoters banned in the European Union are still intensively used in other parts of the world, including the United States and Australia.

The antibacterial drugs currently registered for animal use in European Union countries and/or the United States are listed in Table 2, with specifications on human health importance and clinical use of individual drugs in human medicine. Worldwide, there are great differences in the regulatory control of antimicrobials for animal health and growth-promoting purposes. For example, furazolidones and chloramphenicol are still intensively used in Southeast Asia for fish and shrimp production. In some countries, such as the United States, penicillins and tetracyclines are still used as feed additives for prophylaxis and growth promotion without veterinary prescription. Fosfomycin, a synthetic drug that can be used for treating urinary tract infections or in combination for treatment of systemic infections in humans, is approved for animal use in Japan and other Eastern countries but not in Europe. Even between European countries, there are substantial differences in the numbers and types of drugs licensed for animal use. In many countries, drugs licensed for human use are administered to animals and veterinary products are used in animal species that are not indicated on the label (extralabel use).

TARGETS FOR ANTIBACTERIAL ACTION

Antibacterial activity is due to inhibition of biochemical pathways that are involved in the biosynthesis of essential components of the bacterial cell. The three main bacterial targets of antimicrobial agents are cell wall, protein, and nucleic acid biosynthesis. The following sections describe how various classes of antimicrobial agents interfere with these biological processes and other less common targets. The mechanisms of action of biocides are not covered due to the fact that these substances usually act on multiple targets (29).

Inhibition of Cell Wall Synthesis

The cell wall is an essential component of bacteria since it confers mechanical protection and provides a solid surface for proteins and appendages necessary for cell adhesion, motility, host infection, and horizontal gene transfer. The cell wall is a porous barrier that is not selectively permeable, allowing passage of substances through the pores. The cell wall of gram-positive bacteria has a thick peptidoglycan layer composed of multiple layers of cross-linked glycan and peptide strands crossed by molecules of teichoic and teichuronic acids. In gram-negative bacteria, the peptidoglycan layer is thinner and surrounded by a lipopolysaccharide layer (outer membrane). This structure confers lower permeability in comparison with gram-positive bacteria and prevents penetration of antimicrobials like glycopeptides that do not fit the size of the pores in the outer membrane, called porins.

There are three main phases in cell wall synthesis: (i) the structural unit of peptidoglycan layers, muramyl pentapeptide, is synthesized in the cytoplasm (cytoplasmic phase); (ii) muramyl pentapeptide is bound to the cytoplasmic surface of the cell membrane and translocated to its external face through formation of two lipid intermediates (membrane-associated phase); and (iii) glycan and peptide strands of muramyl pentapeptide are cross-linked by membrane-bound transglycolases and transpeptidases, respectively (extracytoplasmic phase) (46). Cell wall synthesis may be inhibited during any of these three phases, but the most important drugs, beta-lactams and glycopeptides, target the extracytoplasmic phase (Fig. 1).

Beta-lactams (penicillins, cephalosporins, and other subclasses used in human medicine, i.e., carbapenems and monobactams) block transpeptidation of peptidoglycan strands by covalently binding to one or more of the cell wall transpeptidases, better known as PBPs. PBPs catalyze formation of Lys–D-Ala or DAP–D-Ala isopeptide bonds and cleavage of the D-Ala–D-Ala termini of pentapeptide peptidoglycan precursors, with release of free D-Ala (47). Glycopeptides (vancomycin, teicoplanin, and the growth promoter avoparcin) do not act by inhibiting transglycosylation or transpeptidation, but rather by forming a tight noncovalent bond to the D-Ala–D-Ala termini of the pentapeptide precursor, making it no longer accessible to the transpeptidases (35). The growth promoter bambermycin inhibits peptidoglycan synthesis through impairment of the transglycosidase activities of PBPs (9).

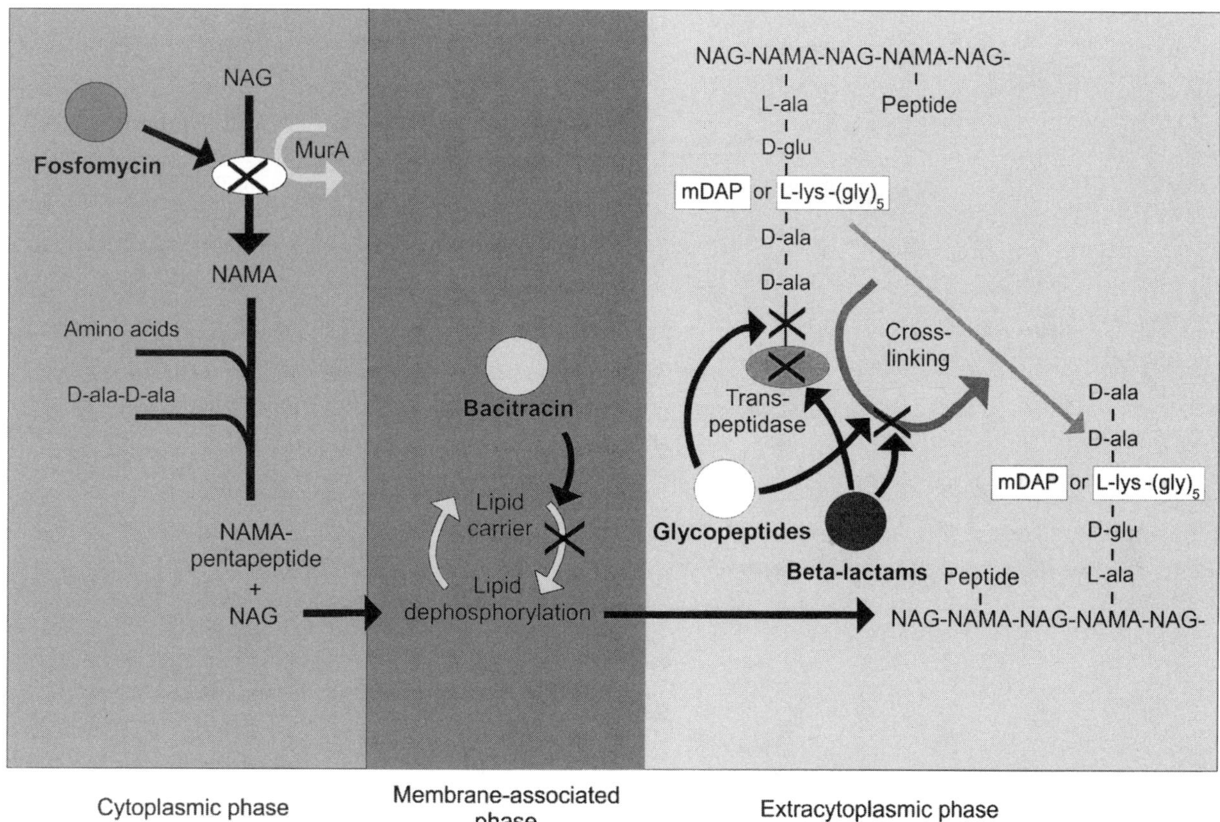

Figure 1. Modes of action of antibacterial drugs inhibiting cell wall synthesis. NAG, *N*-acetylglucosamine; NAMA, *N*-acetylmuramic acid; ala, alanine; glu, glutamic acid; lys, lysine; gly, glycine; mDAP, mesodiaminopimelic acid.

There are only two drugs currently used in animals that affect the cytoplasmic phase (fosfomycin) or the membrane-associated phase (bacitracin) of cell wall synthesis. Bacitracin blocks the membrane-associated cycle by complexation with the undecaprenylpyrophosphate lipid carrier, thus preventing formation of the first lipid intermediate (44). Fosfomycin blocks the formation of muramyl pentapeptide by inhibition of MurA, one of the enzymes (MurA to F) converting the nucleotide diphosphosugar UDP-*N*-acetylglucosamine to UDP-muramylpentapeptide. Fosfomycin is an analog of the substrate of MurA (phosphoenolpyruvate) and inhibits the enzyme by binding to its active-site cysteine (40).

Inhibition of Protein Synthesis

Proteins play an essential role in bacterial life since enzymes and cellular structures are generally proteins. Protein synthesis is a complex set of biological processes that starts with transcription of DNA into mRNA and concludes with mRNA translation and translocation. Of these biological processes, translation is most frequently targeted by antibacterial drugs (Fig. 2). In this step, the bacterial ribosome reads the mRNA and translates it into amino acid sequences. Most drugs act as translational inhibitors by binding to specific sites on the ribosome, with consequent loss of its functionality.

Bacterial ribosomes are composed of two subunits, a small 30S subunit containing 21 proteins (S1 to S21) and 16S rRNA, and a large 50S subunit containing 31 proteins (L1 to L31) and 23S and 5S rRNA. Some molecules targeting the bacterial ribosome bind to the 30S subunit (aminoglycosides, spectinomycin, and tetracyclines), whereas others bind to the 50S subunit (chloramphenicol, MLS, pleuromutilins, and oxazolidones). The two ribosomal subunits normally exist separately in the bacterial cell and have distinct functions during translation. Translation starts when mRNA binds to the 30S subunit and a special tRNA, formylmethionyl-tRNA (fMet-tRNA), is attached to the P (peptidyl donor) site vis-à-vis the AUG initiator codon (Fig. 2). The initiation complex is then completed by the addition of the 50S subunit, and the aminoacyl-tRNA carrying the amino acid corresponding to the second codon enters the A (aminoacyl receptor) site, which is adjacent to the P site. Finally, the first peptide bond is formed between the first (*N*-formylmethionine)

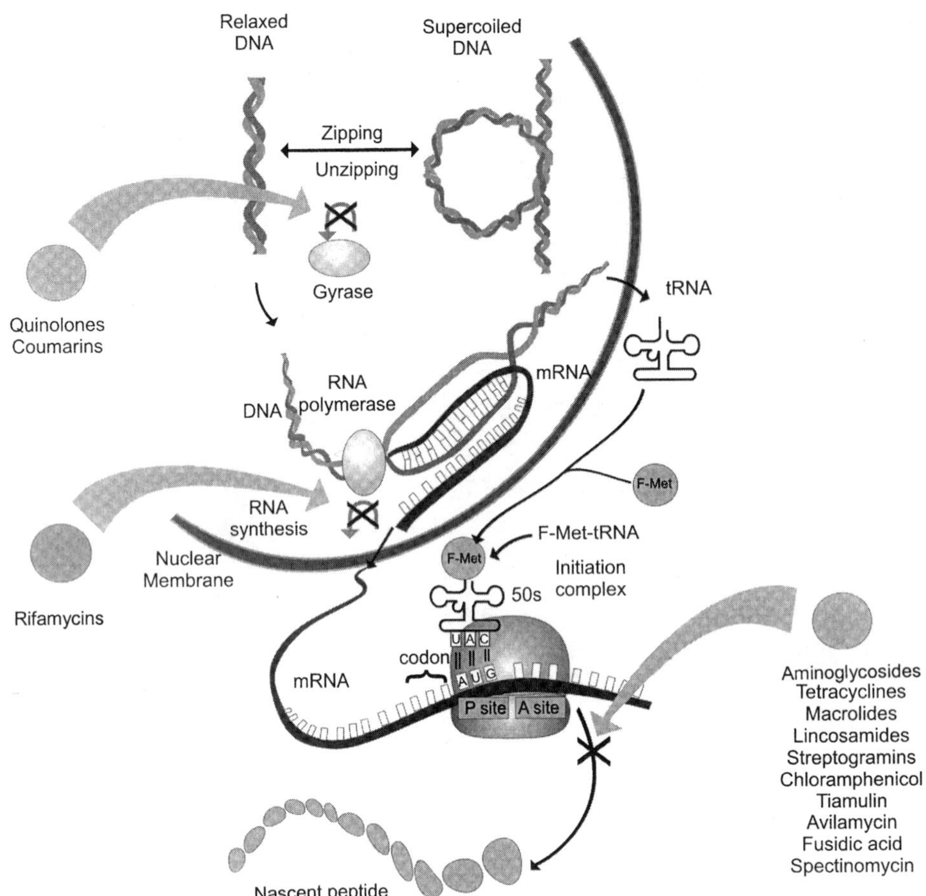

Figure 2. Modes of action of antibacterial drugs inhibiting nucleic acid or protein synthesis.

and the second amino acid by a specific peptidyl transferase on the 50S subunit (43).

Aminoglycosides are the only bactericidal drugs targeting the ribosome. All members of this class irreversibly bind to the A site on 16S rRNA, but differences exist in the number and location of specific target sites. Streptomycin tightly binds to the phosphate backbone of 16S rRNA (10). This unique binding site does not overlap with that of other aminoglycosides, which generally have multiple binding sites. As a consequence, a single amino acid change at protein S12 confers high-level resistance to this antibiotic but not to other aminoglycosides. Binding of aminoglycosides to the 30S subunit causes incorporation of incorrect amino acids (the so-called misreading), formation of nonfunctional initiation complexes, and rapid cell death. Tetracycline binds to various sites on the 30S subunit, but only binding to the primary target site in the vicinity of the A site has been shown to have a clear effect on protein synthesis. Biochemical studies indicate that tetracycline does not prevent binding of aminoacetylated tRNA to the A site but rather suppresses the movement of the tRNA along the ribosome, with consequent inhibition of the first peptide bond (22).

High-resolution X-ray structures of 50S ribosomal subunits complexed with chloramphenicol, lincosamides, and macrolides have shown that these drugs exclusively bind to domain V of 23S rRNA, where the so-called peptidyl transferase center is located, and do not interact with ribosomal proteins (37). The close location of drug targets explains why mutation or modification of a single base in the 23S rRNA can lead to resistance to structurally unrelated drugs. For example, lincosamides and macrolides have three overlapping target nucleotides, and this explains why RNA alterations leading to macrolide resistance often confer resistance to lincosamides. Chloramphenicol and clindamycin also have two overlapping target nucleotides. Although mutations at these sites do not confer cross-resistance, binding overlaps determine antagonism between the two drugs and preclude their use in combination therapy.

Chloramphenicol directly blocks peptide bond formation by binding to the A site, thus preventing binding by tRNA. Clindamycin interacts with both the A and the P site but also physically hinders the path of the growing peptide chain. The position of the streptogramin A dalfopristin on the ribosome largely overlaps that of chloramphenicol. The drug interferes with the delivery of amino acid substrates by tRNA, in particular at the P site. In contrast to chloramphenicol, lincosamides, and dalfopristin, 14-membered macrolides like erythromycin and the streptogramin B quinupristin do not interfere with peptidyl transferase activity but rather block the entrance of the ribosomal tunnel by which the nascent peptides exit the peptidyl transferase center. Thus, in the case of macrolides and quinupristin, the bacterial ribosome can still synthesize a short peptide chain but its elongation is stopped at either the entrance or the end of the exit tunnel (23).

Among the drugs used exclusively in animal production, tiamulin and avilamycin interact with the A site. Tiamulin stalls the ribosome by occupation of the peptidyl transferase center of the 50S ribosomal subunit and interferes with the correct positioning of substrates at both the A and the B site (36). A mutation in the gene encoding protein L3 has been shown to confer resistance to tiamulin, most likely by altering the drug-binding site either directly, by eliminating a specific interaction with tiamulin, or indirectly, by influencing the RNA structure of the peptidyl transferase center (7). The binding site of avilamycin is associated with domain V of 23S rRNA and probably protein L16 (25). It has been inferred that the drug interacts with the ribosomes at the A site and interferes with initiation factor IF2, which stimulates binding of fMet-tRNA to the 30S subunit at the beginning of translation (25).

As the peptide chain grows, the ribosome moves along the mRNA in a process known as translocation. RNA translocation is a step less involved in antibiotic activity. Fusidic acid blocks protein synthesis at this level by interacting with elongation factor G, which catalyzes transfer of the growing polypeptide chain from the A site to the P site (22). Another drug blocking peptide elongation is spectinomycin. Spectinomycin has a chemical structure similar to that of aminoglycosides but reversibly binds to 16S rRNA helix 34 and has only bacteriostatic activity. Biochemical studies show that spectinomycin inhibits translocation of peptidyl-tRNA from the A site to the P site (10).

Inhibition of DNA Synthesis

Nucleic acid synthesis is a vital function for the bacterial cell. DNA synthesis allows replication of the bacterial chromosome during the cell division cycle, and RNA synthesis allows gene expression and protein synthesis by transcription of DNA into RNA. There are three classes of antibacterial agents that inhibit nucleic acid synthesis: quinolones and coumarins, which act on DNA synthesis; and rifamycins, which act on RNA synthesis (Fig. 2).

In order to fit within the bacterial cell, DNA is negatively supercoiled and arranged around an RNA core. During replication and transcription, double-stranded DNA is unzipped; i.e., the negative supercoils are removed to allow synthesis of a new DNA strand or of mRNA, respectively. Quinolones target two enzymes that are essential for DNA unzipping: topoisomerase II, also known as DNA gyrase; and topoisomerase IV. DNA gyrase removes negative supercoils in front of the replication fork, whereas topoisomerase IV removes the interlinking of daughter chromosomes (decatenation), allowing their separation into two daughter cells at the end of the DNA replication (43). Gyrase is composed of two A (GyrA) and two B (GyrB) subunits encoded by the *gyrA* and *gyrB* genes, respectively. Topoisomerase IV has the same tetrameric structure, with the two A and the two B subunits being encoded by *parC* and *parE*, respectively. Based on the mutations conferring quinolone resistance, it appears that the main target of quinolones depends on the specific compound as well as on the type of organism. DNA gyrase is the main target in gram-negative bacteria, as indicated by the usual occurrence of mutations in *gyrA*. In contrast, topoisomerase IV is the main target in gram-positive bacteria since resistance to these drugs is usually associated with mutations in *parC* (39). Quinolones do not directly inhibit topoisomerase activity but rather interact with enzyme-bound DNA complex, determining conformational changes and accumulation of cleaved quinolone-topoisomerase-DNA. The mechanism leading to accumulation of these complexes and their consequence on rapid killing of the cell remains unclear. It is likely that progression of the replication fork is blocked by tripartite complexes.

Novobiocin is a coumarin drug used in animals. Like quinolones, novobiocin and other coumarins target primarily DNA gyrase and secondarily topoisomerase IV. However, the mechanism of action is extremely different between the two groups of drugs. Coumarins are competitive inhibitors of ATP and bind to the ATP binding sites in DNA GyrB and ParE (21). Rifamycins inhibit protein transcription of DNA into mRNA. Rifampin is the most famous representative of this class, employed as therapy for tuberculosis and other mycobacterial diseases. Rifampin blocks mRNA synthesis initiation by binding to the beta subunit of RNA polymerase; in other words, it renders bacterial DNA unable to transfer its information to RNA, with secondary inhibition of protein synthesis.

Other Targets for Antibacterial Action

Sulfonamides and diaminopyrimidines (trimethoprim and similar compounds) have an indirect inhibitory effect on nucleic acid synthesis by blocking folic acid synthesis. Folic acid is an essential precursor in nucleic acid synthesis, and bacteria, as opposed to eukaryotes, cannot utilize exogenous folic acid and thus have to produce it ex novo. Sulfonamides and trimethopim act on two successive biochemical steps in the synthesis of folic acid and are usually employed in combination because they display a synergic therapeutic effect. Sulfonamides are *p*-aminobenzoate (PABA) analogs that competitively inhibit the modification of PABA into dihydrofolate. Diaminopyrimidines are structural analogs of dihydrofolic acid that competitively inhibit the activity of dihydrofolate reductase, the enzyme that catalyzes the reduction of dihydrofolic acid into tetrahydrofolic acid.

Some antibacterial agents such as metronidazole and nitrofurans act directly on bacterial DNA, causing strand breakage. Metronidazole is a nitroimidazole derivative used in human medicine for treatment of infections caused by anaerobic bacteria and protozoan infestations. Under anaerobic conditions, the nitro group of the drug is reduced intracellularly to cytoxic nitroradicals that bind nonspecifically to the host DNA and induce strand breaks (42). Similarly, nitrofurans have been shown to undergo metabolic transformation in the cytoplasm and to induce DNA cross-linking (5). Quinoxalines are known to be genotoxic compounds, but their specific activity on DNA has not been clarified.

The target of polypeptides is the cell membrane of gram-negative organisms. Polymyxins act like some disinfectants by increasing the permeability of the cell membrane. These drugs interact with the phospholipids of the cell membrane of gram-negative bacteria and increase its permeability. Bacitracin affects the integrity of the cell membrane, but the mechanism is still unclear. Aminoglycosides also have a secondary effect on membrane permeability, resulting in leakage of small molecules and bacterial death. This effect has been associated with the bactericidal activity of aminoglycosides; in contrast, no other protein synthesis inhibitors are bactericidal.

MECHANISMS OF RESISTANCE

Bacteria have developed various mechanisms to neutralize the action of antibacterial agents (Fig. 3). The most widespread are enzymatic drug inactivation, modification or replacement of the drug target, active drug efflux, and reduced drug uptake. Other mechanisms such as protection and overproduction of the drug target are less common, and their importance is limited to certain classes.

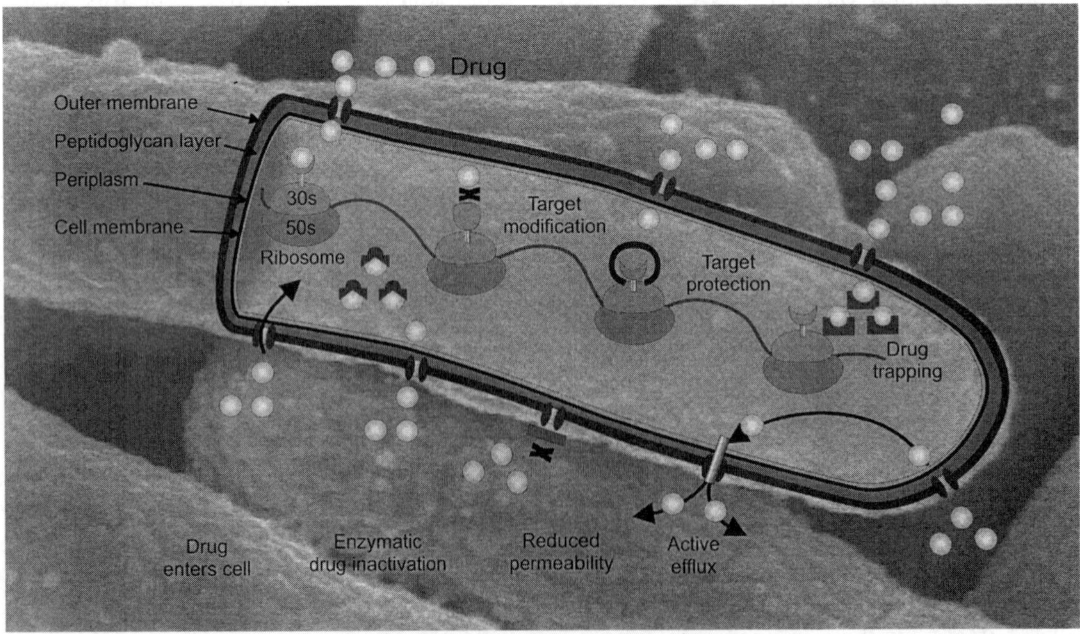

Figure 3. Mechanisms of resistance to antibacterial drugs.

Enzymatic Drug Inactivation

Enzymatic inactivation is the main mechanism of resistance to beta-lactams, aminoglycosides, and phenicols. Drug-inactivating enzymes are also known to confer resistance to MLS, tetracyclines, and fosfomycin, although drug inactivation is not the prevalent mechanism of resistance to these drugs. The enzymes modify the active nucleus of the drug, resulting in the drug's inability to bind to its target site and loss of antibacterial activity. Modification may consist of either cleavage of the molecule or addition of a chemical group. The biochemical reactions catalyzed by bacterial enzymes inactivating the various antibacterial classes are listed in Table 3.

Drug-inactivating enzymes are generally associated with mobile genetic elements. The most widespread and clinically important enzymes are the beta-lactamases and the aminoglycoside-modifying enzymes. The beta-lactamases hydrolyze the beta-lactam ring of penicillins, cephalosporins, and/or carbapenems, which are no longer able to bind the active serine site of PBPs and impede cross-linking of peptidoglycan during cell wall synthesis (47). The aminoglycoside-modifying enzymes catalyze transfer of an acetyl group (*N*-acetyltransferases) to amino groups or of a phosphoryl group (*O*-phosphotransferases) or a nucleotide (*O*-nucleotidyltransferases) to amino or hydroxyl groups in the aminoglycoside molecule, leading to a chemically modified drug that binds poorly to ribosomes and is less rapidly taken up by the cell (49).

Modification or Replacement of the Drug Target

A target can be structurally modified or replaced so that the drug can no longer bind and exert its activity on the cell. Target modification can be associated with resistance to nearly any antibacterial agent. However, from a clinical point of view, this mechanism is particularly important for resistance to penicillins, glycopeptides, and MLS in gram-positive bacteria and for resistance to quinolones in both gram-positive and gram-negative bacteria. For drugs targeting the bacterial ribosome (MLS and aminoglycosides), structural changes of the binding sites are usually due to methylation by genetically acquired methylases, more rarely to mutation of the target nucleotide sequence. For drugs targeting bacterial enzymes, the sequence of the target enzyme can be modified as a consequence of either gene mutation (quinolone resistance) or homologous recombination between housekeeping genes (penicillin resistance in streptococci and enterococci) (see chapter 6).

Two phenotypes of high clinical relevance, glycopeptide resistance in enterococci and more recently in staphylococci and methicillin resistance in *S. aureus*, are due to drug target replacement. In both

Table 3. Modes of enzymatic inactivation of antibacterial drugs

Drug class	Mode of inactivation	Enzymes	Bacterial host
Beta-lactams	Hydrolysis	Beta-lactamases, four classes (A to D)	Gram-negative species. Limited to class A, also gram-positive species
Aminoglycosides	Acetylation	Acetyltransferases	Gram-negative and -positive species
	Phosphorylation	Phosphotransferases	Gram-negative and -positive species
	Nucleotidylation	Nucleotidylases	Gram-negative and -positive species
Macrolides	Esterification	Ere(A) and Ere(B)	*Enterobacteriaceae*
	Phosphorylation	Mph(A) and Mph(B)	*Escherichia coli*
		Mph(C)	*Staphylococcus*
Lincosamides	Acetylation	Lnu(A)	*Staphylococcus*
		Lnu(B)	*Enterococcus*
Streptogramin A drugs	Acetylation	Vat(A), Vat(B), Vat(C)	*Staphylococcus*
		Vat(D) and Vat(E)	*Enterococcus*
Streptogramin B drugs	Hydrolysis	Vgb(A)	*Enterococcus*, *Staphylococcus*
		Vgb(B)	*Staphylococcus*
Chloramphenicol	Acetylation	Cat(A)	Gram-negative and -positive species
		Cat(B)	Only gram-negative species
	Phosphorylation	Not designated	*Streptomyces venezuelae*[a]
Tetracyclines	Reduction	Tet(X)	*Bacteroides*
	Reduction	Tet(34)	*Vibrio cholerae*
Fosfomycin	Glutathione addition	Fos(A)	Gram-negative species
		Fos(B)	Gram-positive species
		Fos(c)	*Pseudomonas syringae*
	Phosphorylation	Fom(A)	*Streptomyces wedmorensis*[a]

[a]Antibiotic producer.

cases, following the acquisition of exogenous genes, the bacteria are able to produce a new functional target with low affinity for the drug. GRE containing the *vanA* or *vanB* operon synthesize peptidoglycan precursors terminating by D-Ala–D-Lac with very low affinity for glycopeptides and remove the normal D-Ala–D-Ala precursors by a complex and coordinated mechanism of cell wall reprogramming (3). Methicillin-resistant *S. aureus* (MRSA) containing the *mecA* gene synthesizes a new PBP (PBP2A) with low affinity for methicillin that partially replaces normal transpeptidase PBP2 (47). Target replacement is also the main mechanism of acquired resistance to sulfonamides and trimethoprim (see chapter 6).

Drug Efflux Pumps

Active efflux is an energy-dependent mechanism used by bacteria as well as by eukaryotic cells and protozoa for extruding metabolites and foreign toxic compounds, including drugs. Transmembrane proteins, known as efflux pumps or active transporters, mediate active efflux. Such proteins generally have broad substrate specificity, and only some of them confer resistance to antimicrobial agents. Resistance is determined by reduction in the concentration of the drug in the cytoplasm, thus preventing or limiting access of the drug to its target. Efflux pumps can be classified based on substrate specificity, energy source, and phylogenic relationship. Substrate specificity of efflux pumps is extremely variable. Some pumps act on specific drugs (specific-drug-resistance [SDR] pumps), whereas others are active on multiple drugs (multiple-drug-resistance [MDR] pumps). SDR pumps are the most important mechanism of resistance to tetracyclines, especially in gram-negative bacteria. SDR pumps also confer resistance to MLS and phenicols. These pumps generally confer high-level resistance and are associated with mobile genetic elements (8).

The substrate of MDR pumps may include various antibacterial agents of medical importance (Table 4). These pumps generally confer low-level resistance and are frequently encoded by the chromosome. Depending on the source of energy used for active efflux, MDR pumps are divided into two main groups: ATP-binding cassette (ABC) transporters and secondary drug transporters (34). ABC transporters utilize ATP hydrolysis as a source of energy, have broad physiological functions in both eukaryotic and prokaryotic cells, and usually mediate the export of specific antimicrobial classes such as MLS. Secondary drug transporters utilize the transmembrane electrochemical gradient of protons or sodium ions to extrude drugs from the cell. This group accounts for most pumps mediating resistance to multiple antimicrobial agents. On the basis of their size and structure, secondary drug transporters can be classified in four families: the major facilitator superfamily (MFS), the small multidrug resistance (SMR) family, the resistance-nodulation-cell division (RND) family, and the multidrug and toxic compound extrusion (MATE) family. Evidence suggests that substrates are transported outward from the inner leaflet of the membrane rather than from the cytoplasmic aqueous phase (32). According to this model, substrates accumulate at high-affinity binding sites in the inner leaflet of the phospholipid bilayer and are subsequently transferred to low-affinity outward-facing binding sites at the expense of ATP or proton translocation (34).

Reduced Drug Uptake

In gram-negative bacteria, hydrophilic drugs enter the bacterial cell through porins and hydrophobic drugs diffuse through the phospholipid layer. The outer membrane of some bacterial species such as *P. aeruginosa* is less permeable than those of other species (approximately 10% of that of *E. coli*) (20), and this confers to these organisms lower levels of antimicrobial susceptibility. Mutations leading to loss, reduced size, or decreased expression of porins have been shown to confer acquired, generally low-level resistance to various antibacterial agents. For example, reduction in the expression of the OmpF porin has been shown to decrease the susceptibility of *E. coli* to quinolones, beta-lactams, tetracyclines, and chloramphenicol (11).

Reduced uptake is a clinically important mechanism of resistance to beta-lactams and fluoroquinolones in gram-negative bacteria, especially in *P. aeruginosa* and in *Enterobacteriaceae*. This mechanism generally confers low-level resistance but contributes to the resistant phenotype of multiresistant clinical strains in association with other mechanisms of resistance. Among zoonotic bacteria, expression of altered OmpC and OmpF porins in *E. coli* O157:H7 has been associated with reduced permeability to antibacterial drugs (27). Aminoglycoside resistance in anaerobes provides another example of resistance due to reduced drug uptake. Anaerobes are resistant to aminoglycosides because these drugs gain access to the bacterial cell via a transport mechanism that relies on aerobic metabolism.

Target Protection

Resistance by protection of the drug target has been reported for tetracyclines and more recently also for quinolones. There are eight distinct ribosomal protection proteins (RPPs) that are known to mediate

Table 4. Antibacterial substrate ranges of MDR efflux pumps in bacterial species that can be isolated from animals[a]

Pump	Family	Antimicrobial substrate range[b]	Bacterial host
EmrB	MFS	QUI, RIF	*Escherichia coli*
Lde	MFS	QUI	*Listeria monocytogenes*
LfrA	MFS	CHL, QUI, TET	*Mycobacterium smegmatis*
LmrP	MFS	LIN, MAC, TET, STR	*Lactococcus lactis*
MdfA	MFS	AMG, CHL, MAC, QUI, RIF, TET	*Escherichia coli*
MdtA	MFS	MAC, TET	*Lactococcus lactis*
NorA	MFS	CHL, QUI	*Staphylococcus aureus*
VceB	MFS	CHL, MAC, QUI, RIF	*Vibrio cholerae*
EmrE	SMR	MAC, TET	*Escherichia coli*
AcrB	RND	PEN, CHL, MAC, NOV, TRI, TET, QUI, FUS	*Escherichia coli*[c]
AdeB	RND	AMG, CHL, MAC, QUI, TET, TRI, CEP	*Acinetobacter baumannii*
AmrB	RND	AMG, MAC, NOV	*Burkholderia pseudomallei*
CmeB	RND	QUI, MAC, PEN, RIF, TET, CHL, AMG	*Campylobacter jejuni*
MexB	RND	PEN, CEP, CHL, MAC, QUI, TET, NOV, SUL, TRI	*Pseudomonas aeruginosa*
MexD	RND	CHL, MAC, QUI, TET, NOV, SUL, TRI, PEN, CEP	*Pseudomonas aeruginosa*
MexF	RND	CHL, QUI, TET, TRI	*Pseudomonas aeruginosa*
Mex I	RND	QUI	*Pseudomonas aeruginosa*
MexK	RND	MAC, TET, QUI	*Pseudomonas aeruginosa*
MexY	RND	AMG, MAC, QUI, CAR, CEP, PEN, TET	*Pseudomonas aeruginosa*
MexW	RND	QUI, CHL, TET, MAC	*Pseudomonas aeruginosa*
OqxB	RND	QXA, CHL	*Escherichia coli*
SdeY	RND	MAC, QUI, TET	*Serratia marcescens*
NorM	MATE	AMG, QUI	*Vibrio parahaemolyticus*[c]
YdhE	MATE	AMG, QUI	*Escherichia coli*
EfrAB	ABC	QUI, TET	*Enterococcus faecalis*
LmrA	ABC	AMG, CEP, PEN, CHL, LIN, MAC, QUI, TET	*Lactococcus lactis*
VcaM		QUI, TET	*Vibrio cholerae*

[a]Modified from reference 33. Abbreviations: AMG, aminoglycosides; CAR, carbapenems; CEP, cephalosporins; CHL, chloramphenicol; FUS, fusidic acid; LIN, lincosamides; MAC, macrolides; NOV, novobiocin; PEN, penicillins; QUI, quinolones; QXA, quinoxalines; RIF, rifampin; SUL, sulfonamides; TET, tetracyclines; TRI, trimethoprim.
[b]The table includes only antibacterial compounds of medical interest.
[c]Efflux pump also found in other gram-negative species. The substrate range varies depending on the species.

resistance to tetracyclines: Tet(M), Tet(O), Tet(Q), TetB(P), Tet(S), Tet(T), Tet(W), and OtrA (12). Tet(M) and Tet(O) are the most widespread and well-studied RPPs. These proteins bind to the ribosome in proximity to the binding site of elongation factor G and dislodge the tetracyclines from their binding site, the A site. Resistance cannot be attributed to occupation of the A site since there is no overlap with the binding site of RPPs. Most likely, dislodgment of tetracycline is due to a conformational change in helix 34, which forms an integral part of the A site. The conformation of helix 44 is also changed by binding of Tet(O) to the ribosome, but it is unclear how this can lead to dislodgment of tetracycline since helix 44 is not structurally related to the A site nor to the Tet(O) binding site (12).

Plasmid-mediated, low-level quinolone resistance attributable to DNA gyrase protection has been recently reported in *Enterobacteriaceae*. The proteins responsible for this mechanism of low-level fluoroquinolone resistance (QnrA and B) belong to the pentapeptide repeat family, a functionally diverse group of proteins. Qnr does not have any protective effect on topoisomerase IV, the secondary target of fluoroquinolones (45). The actual mode by which Qnr protects DNA gyrase has not been established. In particular, it remains to be determined whether the Qnr proteins interfere with binding of quinolone to DNA gyrase or destabilize the formation of complexes between quinolone, DNA gyrase, and double-stranded DNA.

Drug Trapping or Titration

Bacteria may trap a drug by increasing the production of the drug target or another molecule with affinity for the drug. In both cases, the consequence is a reduction of free drug at the target site (titration). Chromosomal mutations responsible for overproduction of the targets of sulfonamides (PABA) and diaminopyrimidines (dihydrofolate reductase) have been reported in various bacterial species. Drug trapping is also implicated in low-level glycopeptide resistance in staphylococci. Overproduction of peptidoglycan by glycopeptide intermediate-resistant *S. aureus* results in the formation of a thickened cell wall with low reticulation and increased levels of nonamidated muramyl pentapeptides with high affinity for vancomycin. This contributes to glycopeptide resistance through trapping of vancomycin molecules by the cell wall and clogging of the outer layers of peptidoglycan by bound vancomycin molecules (14). In *E. coli*, resistance to low levels of tobramycin can be due to formation of complexes between the drug and a 3′-aminoglycoside phosphotransferase type I, an enzyme that phosphorylates kanamycin but not tobramycin. Although tobramycin lacks the 3′-hydroxyl group and cannot be modified at this position, the enzyme has affinity for the drug and its overproduction can lead to trapping of the drug (30).

Combinatorial Resistance

Various determinants conferring resistance to the same antimicrobial class are frequently found in the same host. Bacteria may benefit in different ways from the association of genes encoding resistance to the same drug or drug class. First of all, combination of resistance mechanisms allows bacteria to survive the high drug concentrations achieved in the human or animal body during therapy. Combination of two resistance mechanisms may lead to resistance levels that are equal to the sum of the levels conferred by each mechanism individually (additive resistance). For example, *S. aureus* frequently carries two tetracycline resistance determinants: *tetK*, which encodes resistance by active efflux; and *tetM* or *tetO*, which confer resistance by ribosomal protection. As a result, tetracycline MICs for strains carrying two genes are equal to the sum of the MICs for strains harboring one of the two genes (6). In other cases, the resistance phenotype of the bacterial host quantitatively exceeds the mere addition of resistance levels conferred by each individual resistance gene (synergistic resistance). The increase in the resistance phenotype may result from combination of genes conferring resistance by either the same mechanism or different mechanisms. Combination of genes conferring resistance by the same mechanism occurs, for example, in the case of staphylococci encoding multiple aminoglycoside-modifying enzymes with overlapping substrate ranges or fluroquinolone-resistant bacteria carrying multiple mutations in the genes coding for DNA gyrase and topoisomerase IV. Combination of multiple genes conferring resistance by distinct mechanisms is common among gram-negative pathogens resistant to beta-lactams (drug inactivation combined with drug efflux and/or reduced uptake) and fluoroquinolones (target mutation combined with reduced drug uptake and/or target protection).

Bacteria also benefit from the combination of resistance mechanisms with nonoverlapping substrate ranges. The *aac6′-aph2″* gene in gram-positive cocci results from the fusion of two genes encoding distinct aminoglycoside-modifying enzymes (17). The two portions of the fused protein are complementary in substrate specificity and confer resistance to all aminoglycosides that can be used to treat systemic infections, with the exception of streptomycin. Similarly, clustering of genes can enable the bacterium to become resistant to synergic antibiotic combinations. Genes conferring resistance to type A and type B streptogramins in staphylococci (16) and in enterococci (24) are often adjacent on the same genetic structure, allowing the host to become resistant to each member of the antibiotic combination. This is particularly beneficial to the bacterial cell since no single mechanism confers cross-resistance to the two groups of molecules. More generally, gene clustering has important implications for the spread of antimicrobial resistance as well as for the emergence of multiple-resistant phenotypes (coresistance). Integrons are the best evidence of how bacteria are able to cluster and coexpress genes conferring resistance to various antimicrobial classes (18).

Clustering of genes encoding enzymes with different functions is a necessary step to achieve resistance and to reduce its cost for the host. This is the case for the *van* operons that confer resistance to glycopeptides in enterococci and other gram-positive bacteria, including *S. aureus*. These genetic elements contain a cluster of three genes encoding a D-lactate dehydrogenase (VanH), a D-Ala:D-Lac ligase (VanA, VanB, or VanD), and a D-Ala:D-Ala dipeptidase (VanX) (3). The three enzymes act synergistically to achieve a double goal: synthesis of (resistant) peptidoglycan precursors with low affinity for glycopeptides and elimination of the native (susceptible) precursors encoded by chromosomal genes. Coordinated expression of the gene cluster is regulated by a two-component regulatory system that activates this complex machinery exclusively in the presence of glycopeptides, thus avoiding useless energetic burden to the host when resistance is not needed. In a like manner, expression of MDR pumps capable of recognizing the presence of structurally diverse drug substrates is regulated positively or negatively (34).

In conclusion, bacteria display an extraordinary ability to cluster genes and combine resistance mechanisms. Antimicrobial use, in humans as well as in animals, favors dissemination of resistance not only by providing resistant bacteria with an ecological advantage but also by promoting gene transfer, shuffling, clustering, and expression of resistance genes.

Acknowledgments. L. Guardabassi was supported by grant no. 23-01-0170 from the Danish Agricultural and Veterinary Research Council.

We thank T. Evison for the preparation of the figures.

REFERENCES

1. **Aarestrup, F. M.** 2000. Characterization of glycopeptide-resistant *Enterococcus faecium* (GRE) from broilers and pigs in Denmark: genetic evidence that persistence of GRE in pig herds is associated with coselection by resistance to macrolides. *J. Clin. Microbiol.* **38:**2774–2777.
2. **Andremont, A., and C. Tancrede.** 1981. Reduction of the aerobic Gram negative bacterial flora of the gastro-intestinal tract and prevention of traveller's diarrhea using oral erythromycin. *Ann. Microbiol.* (Paris) **132 B:**419–427.
3. **Arthur, M., P. Reynolds, and P. Courvalin.** 1996. Glycopeptide resistance in enterococci. *Trends Microbiol.* **4:**401–407.
4. **Banks, D. J., S. F. Porcella, K. D. Barbian, J. M. Martin, and J. M. Musser.** 2003. Structure and distribution of an unusual chimeric genetic element encoding macrolide resistance in phylogenetically diverse clones of group A *Streptococcus. J. Infect. Dis.* **188:**1898–1908.
5. **Basak, J.** 1995. Inter-strand cross-linking of *Vibrio cholerae* DNA induced by furazolidone: a quantitative assay by four simple methods. *Mutat. Res.* **327:**5–15.
6. **Bismuth, R., R. Zilhao, H. Sakamoto, J. L. Guesdon, and P. Courvalin.** 1990. Gene heterogeneity for tetracycline resistance in *Staphylococcus* spp. *Antimicrob. Agents Chemother.* **34:**1611–1614.
7. **Bosling, J., S. M. Poulsen, B. Vester, and K. S. Long.** 2003. Resistance to the peptidyl transferase inhibitor tiamulin caused by mutation of ribosomal protein l3. *Antimicrob. Agents Chemother.* **47:**2892–2896.
8. **Butaye, P., A. Cloeckaert, and S. Schwarz.** 2003. Mobile genes coding for efflux-mediated antimicrobial resistance in Gram-positive and Gram-negative bacteria. *Int. J. Antimicrob. Agents* **22:**205–210.
9. **Butaye, P., L. A. Devriese, and F. Haesebrouck.** 2003. Antimicrobial growth promoters used in animal feed: effects of less well known antibiotics on gram-positive bacteria. *Clin. Microbiol. Rev.* **16:**175–188.
10. **Carter, A. P., W. M. Clemons, D. E. Brodersen, R. J. Morgan-Warren, B. T. Wimberly, and V. Ramakrishnan.** 2000. Functional insights from the structure of the 30S ribosomal subunit and its interactions with antibiotics. *Nature* **407:**340–348.
11. **Cohen, S. P., L. M. McMurry, D. C. Hooper, J. S. Wolfson, and S. B. Levy.** 1989. Cross-resistance to fluoroquinolones in multiple-antibiotic-resistant (Mar*) Escherichia coli* selected by tetracycline or chloramphenicol: decreased drug accumulation associated with membrane changes in addition to OmpF reduction. *Antimicrob. Agents Chemother.* **33:**1318–1325.
12. **Connell, S. R., D. M. Tracz, K. H. Nierhaus, and D. E. Taylor.** 2003. Ribosomal protection proteins and their mechanism of tetracycline resistance. *Antimicrob. Agents Chemother.* **47:**3675–3681.
13. **Courvalin, P., and P. Trieu-Cuot.** 2001. Minimizing potential resistance: the molecular view. *Clin. Infect. Dis.* **33** (Suppl. 3):S138–S146.
14. **Cui, L., H. Murakami, K. Kuwahara-Arai, H. Hanaki, and K. Hiramatsu.** 2000. Contribution of a thickened cell wall and its glutamine nonamidated component to the vancomycin resistance expressed by *Staphylococcus aureus* Mu50. *Antimicrob. Agents Chemother.* **44:**2276–2285.
15. **Doucet-Populaire, F., P. Trieu-Cuot, I. Dosbaa, A. Andremont, and P. Courvalin.** 1991. Inducible transfer of conjugative transposon Tn*1545* from *Enterococcus faecalis* to *Listeria monocytogenes* in the digestive tracts of gnotobiotic mice. *Antimicrob. Agents Chemother.* **35:**185–187.
16. **El Solh, N., and J. Allignet.** 1998. Staphylococcal resistance to streptogramins and related antibiotics. *Drug Resis. Updates* **1:**169–175.
17. **Ferretti, J. J., K. S. Gilmore, and P. Courvalin.** 1986. Nucleotide sequence analysis of the gene specifying the bifunctional 6'-aminoglycoside acetyltransferase 2"-aminoglycoside phosphotransferase enzyme in *Streptococcus faecalis* and identification and cloning of gene regions specifying the two activities. *J. Bacteriol.* **167:**631–638.
18. **Fluit, A. C., and F. J. Schmitz.** 1999. Class 1 integrons, gene cassettes, mobility, and epidemiology. *Eur. J. Clin. Microbiol. Infect. Dis.* **18:**761–770.
19. **Hakenbeck, R., and J. Coyette.** 1998. Resistant penicillin-binding proteins. *Cell Mol. Life Sci.* **54:**332–340.
20. **Hancock, R. E., and F. S. Brinkman.** 2002. Function of *Pseudomonas* porins in uptake and efflux. *Annu. Rev. Microbiol.* **56:**17–38.
21. **Hardy, C. D., and N. R. Cozzarelli.** 2003. Alteration of *Escherichia coli* topoisomerase IV to novobiocin resistance. *Antimicrob. Agents Chemother.* **47:**941–947.
22. **Harms, J. M., H. Bartels, F. Schlunzen, and A. Yonath.** 2003. Antibiotics acting on the translational machinery. *J. Cell Sci.* **116:**1391–1393.
23. **Harms, J. M., F. Schlunzen, P. Fucini, H. Bartels, and A. Yonath.** 2004. Alterations at the peptidyl transferase centre of the ribosome induced by the synergistic action of the streptogramins dalfopristin and quinupristin. *BMC Biol.* **2:**4.
24. **Jensen, L. B., A. M. Hammerum, F. Bager, and F. M. Aarestrup.** 2002. Streptogramin resistance among *Enterococcus faecium* isolated from production animals in Denmark in 1997. *Microb. Drug Resist.* **8:**369–374.
25. **Kofoed, C. B., and B. Vester.** 2002. Interaction of avilamycin with ribosomes and resistance caused by mutations in 23S rRNA. *Antimicrob. Agents Chemother.* **46:**3339–3342.
26. **LeClerc, J. E., B. Li, W. L. Payne, and T. A. Cebula.** 1996. High mutation frequencies among *Escherichia coli* and *Salmonella* pathogens. *Science* **274:**1208–1211.
27. **Martinez, M. B., M. Flickinger, L. Higgins, T. Krick, and G. L. Nelsestuen.** 2001. Reduced outer membrane permeability of *Escherichia coli* O157:H7: suggested role of modified outer membrane porins and theoretical function in resistance to antimicrobial agents. *Biochemistry* **40:**11965–11974.
28. **Mascaretti, O.** 2003. *Bacteria versus Antibacterial Agents: an Integrated Approach.* ASM Press, Washington, D.C.
29. **McDonnell, G., and A. D. Russell.** 1999. Antiseptics and disinfectants: activity, action, and resistance. *Clin. Microbiol. Rev.* **12:**147–179.
30. **Menard, R., C. Molinas, M. Arthur, J. Duval, P. Courvalin, and R. Leclercq.** 1993. Overproduction of 3′-aminoglycoside phosphotransferase type I confers resistance to tobramycin in *Escherichia coli. Antimicrob. Agents Chemother.* **37:**78–83.
31. **Muniesa, M., A. Garcia, E. Miro, B. Mirelis, G. Prats, J. Jofre, and F. Navarro.** 2004. Bacteriophages and diffusion of beta-lactamase genes. *Emerg. Infect. Dis.* **10:**1134–1137.
32. **Neyfakh, A. A.** 2002. Mystery of multidrug transporters: the answer can be simple. *Mol. Microbiol.* **44:**1123–1130.
33. **Oliver, A., R. Canton, P. Campo, F. Baquero, and J. Blazquez.** 2000. High frequency of hypermutable *Pseudomonas aeruginosa* in cystic fibrosis lung infection. *Science* **288:**1251–1254.

34. **Putman, M., H. W. van Veen, and W. N. Konings.** 2000. Molecular properties of bacterial multidrug transporters. *Microbiol. Mol. Biol. Rev.* **64:**672–693.
35. **Reynolds, P. E.** 1989. Structure, biochemistry and mechanism of action of glycopeptide antibiotics. *Eur. J. Clin. Microbiol. Infect. Dis.* **8:**943–950.
36. **Schlunzen, F., E. Pyetan, P. Fucini, A. Yonath, and J. M. Harms.** 2004. Inhibition of peptide bond formation by pleuromutilins: the structure of the 50S ribosomal subunit from *Deinococcus radiodurans* in complex with tiamulin. *Mol. Microbiol.* 54:1287–1294.
37. **Schlunzen, F., R. Zarivach, J. Harms, A. Bashan, A. Tocilj, R. Albrecht, A. Yonath, and F. Franceschi.** 2001. Structural basis for the interaction of antibiotics with the peptidyl transferase centre in eubacteria. *Nature* **413:**814–821.
38. **Schmieger, H., and P. Schicklmaier.** 1999. Transduction of multiple drug resistance of *Salmonella enterica* serovar Typhimurium DT104. *FEMS Microbiol. Lett.* **170:** 251–256.
39. **Schmitz, F. J., P. G. Higgins, S. Mayer, A. C. Fluit, and A. Dalhoff.** 2002. Activity of quinolones against gram-positive cocci: mechanisms of drug action and bacterial resistance. *Eur. J. Clin. Microbiol. Infect. Dis.* **21:**647–659.
40. **Schonbrunn, E., S. Eschenburg, F. Krekel, K. Luger, and N. Amrhein.** 2000. Role of the loop containing residue 115 in the induced-fit mechanism of the bacterial cell wall biosynthetic enzyme MurA. *Biochemistry* **39:**2164–2173.
41. **Schwarz, S., and E. Chaslus-Dancla.** 2001. Use of antimicrobials in veterinary medicine and mechanisms of resistance. *Vet. Res.* **32:**201–225.
42. **Sigeti, J. S., D. G. Guiney, Jr., and C. E. Davis.** 1983. Mechanism of action of metronidazole on *Bacteroides fragilis*. *J. Infect. Dis.* **148:**1083–1089.
43. **Snyder, L., and W. Champness.** 1997. *Molecular Genetics of Bacteria*. ASM Press, Washington, D.C.
44. **Toscano, W. A., Jr., and D. R. Storm.** 1982. Bacitracin. *Pharmacol. Ther.* **16:**199–210.
45. **Tran, J. H., and G. A. Jacoby.** 2002. Mechanism of plasmid-mediated quinolone resistance. *Proc. Natl. Acad. Sci. USA* **99:** 5638–5642.
46. **van Heijenoort, J.** 2001. Formation of the glycan chains in the synthesis of bacterial peptidoglycan. *Glycobiology* **11:** 25R–36R.
47. **Walsh, C.** 2003. *Antibiotics: Actions, Origins, Resistance.* ASM Press, Washington, D.C.
48. **Whittle, G., N. B. Shoemaker, and A. A. Salyers.** 2002. The role of *Bacteroides* conjugative transposons in the dissemination of antibiotic resistance genes. *Cell. Mol. Life Sci.* **59:** 2044–2054.
49. **Wright, G. D.** 1999. Aminoglycoside-modifying enzymes. *Curr. Opin. Microbiol.* **2:**499–503.

Antimicrobial Resistance in Bacteria of Animal Origin
Edited by Frank M. Aarestrup

Chapter 2

History of Antimicrobial Usage in Agriculture: an Overview

JOHN F. PRESCOTT

The introduction of antimicrobial drugs into agriculture shortly after the Second World War caused a revolution in the treatment of many diseases of food animals. In the "wonder drug era" of the late 1940s and early 1950s, the effective treatment of many infections that were previously considered incurable astonished veterinarians, such that some even feared for their livelihoods.

A broad overview of key features of the history of antimicrobial drug use in food animals is given in Table 1, which traces developments from the preantibiotic era to the present day, where there are highly arguable fears that we are moving into the "postantibiotic" era. Table 1 illustrates many important features in the history of agricultural use of antimicrobials:

1. The development of resistance to antimicrobial drugs followed soon after their introduction.

2. Resistance was usually dealt with by the development of new classes of antimicrobials, by isolation from nature of novel antibiotics within a particular class, or by development of synthetic analogs of an existing class.

3. The antimicrobial drugs used in food animals were the same as those in human medicine, although a number of antimicrobial drugs rejected by human medicine because of toxicity problems (e.g., streptogramins) became growth-promoting feed antimicrobials in food animals.

4. Antimicrobials were used by agriculture in feed as growth promoters or for subtherapeutic purposes almost as soon as they were discovered.

5. The majority of antimicrobial drugs used in animals belong to a small number of major classes, and only one new class of antimicrobial drugs, fluoroquinolones (pleuromutilins are an exception, but have very restricted use), has been introduced for food animal use in the last 30 years.

6. Significant contamination in carcasses or selected tissues was detected in the 1970s and 1980s, leading either to the banning of potentially toxic (e.g., carcinogenic or idiosyncratic effects) drugs or to rigorous, ongoing programs of detection in carcasses after slaughter as the major focus of regulating antimicrobial use in food animals.

7. The public health impact, because of the development of resistance and especially because of transmissible resistance, has been a major battleground between agriculture and medicine for over 30 years.

8. The science supporting optimal antimicrobial drug use in food animals has developed relatively slowly and is not complete.

DISCOVERY OF ANTIBIOTICS AND EARLY USAGE

Antimicrobial drugs were introduced for food animal use with a minimum of controlled experimental studies, so that from the start there were frequent calls to move from the wonder to the science. As in human medicine, the early dosing was largely empirical and based on inadequately controlled small-scale trials (14, 17), so that there was a "confusing hodgepodge of widely divergent optimum dose-ranges for the many livestock diseases allegedly amenable to the activity of penicillin" (6). In the United States such empiricism led to a licensed dosage of penicillin G in cattle that was clearly inadequate. It took 4 or 5 decades before the licensed drug dosage was more scientifically determined, based on quantitative understanding of the interaction of drug with the target microorganism (dosage, pharmacokinetic and pharmacodynamic parameters, in vitro susceptibility) as well as clinical data (Table 1). Clinical evaluation is

John F. Prescott • Department of Pathobiology, University of Guelph, Guelph, Ontario N1G 2W1, Canada.

Table 1. Historical timeline of important events and trends in use of antimicrobial drugs in food animals

Dates	Feature of period	Antimicrobial drug development	Important events
1925–1930	Antiseptic era	Discovery of penicillin, first beta-lactam, by Alexander Fleming	
1931–1935	Antiseptic era	Discovery of sulfonamides	
1936–1940	Antiseptic, sulfonamide period	Penicillin efficacy in humans is shown	Sulfonamides introduced into food animal use
1941–1945	Dawn of "wonder drug era"	Streptomycin, first aminoglycoside, discovered	Second World War is impetus for antimicrobial drug discovery for treatment of war wounds
1946–1950	"Wonder drug era"	Discovery of bacitracin, chloramphenicol, neomycin, polymyxin, streptogramins, and tetracycline antibiotics, all natural products of microorganisms, usually fungi	Penicillin and streptomycin released from military use for civilian population and animal use; widespread use in animals by 1950, largely empirical
1951–1955	"Wonder drug era": more wonder than science	Discovery of erythromycin, the first macrolide. Introduction of neomycin, an aminoglycoside, for topical or intestinal infections in animals. Introduction of nitrofurans into clinical use, especially for intestinal infections	Tetracyclines and chloramphenicol used therapeutically in animals; widespread, largely empirical, use. Intramammary use of antibiotics for mastitis treatment widespread. Discovery of and extensive use of antibiotics for growth promotion in food animals, pioneered in the United States.
1956–1960	"Wonder drug era"	Discovery of vancomycin, the first glycopeptide, and tylosin, a novel macrolide. Virginiamycin, a streptogramin, used as growth promoter.	More science and less wonder, but drug dose selection still largely empirical. Early studies of drug excretion in Denmark.
1961–1965	Emerging resistance period	Discovery of methicillin and other penicillinase-resistant penicillins. Introduction of spiramycin, a macrolide, into animal use. Discovery of gentamicin, an antipseudomonal aminoglycoside.	Discovery of transmissible, plasmid- or "R" factor-based, multiple-drug resistance in *Enterobacteriaceae*. Studies of drug residues and withdrawal periods.
1966–1970	New drug analog period	Discovery of cephalothin, a narrow-spectrum cephalosporin. Ampicillin, first broad-spectrum penicillin, used in food animals, example of a successful synthetic alteration of side chains of basic beta-lactam ring to expand activity. Introduction of amikacin, for gentamicin-resistant infections. Flavomycin introduced as growth promoter.	New drug analogs successfully address resistance problem. Multiple-drug-resistant, serious *Salmonella* infections found to be transmissible from calves to humans in United Kingdom. Because of transmissible resistance, Swann report in United Kingdom removes drugs important in human medicine as feed antibiotics and allows their use therapeutically in food animals by veterinary prescription only.
1971–1975	New drug analog period	Discovery of carbenicillin, an antipseudomonal penicillin.Other narrow-spectrum cephalosporins introduced. Introduction of trimethoprim-sulfonamide combination.	New drug analogs successfully address resistance problem. U.S. FDA report (1972) suggests stopping use of subtherapeutic penicillin and tetracyclines in feed; not implemented.
1976–1980	Tissue drug residues are problems in food animals; early pharmacokinetic period	Discovery of cefoxitin, first extended-spectrum cephalosporin, and moxalactam, an unusual beta-lactam. Introduction in Europe of avoparcin, a glycopeptide, for growth promotion in food animals.	Chloramphenicol use in food animals banned in United States and Denmark because of potential human toxicity through residues, followed by other countries. Transmissible, multiple-drug-resistant *S. enterica* serovar Typhimurium phage type 204 spreads from calves to humans. *Journal of Veterinary Pharmacology and Therapeutics* started, to improve drug use in animals. Focus on pharmacokinetics and drug metabolism in food animals by J. D. Baggot (Ireland, United States), L. E. Davis (United States), and P. Nielsen and F. Rasmussen (Denmark).
1981–1985	Pharmacokinetic and drug dosage prediction period	Discovery of cefotaxime, an antipseudomonal cephalosporin, and other broad-spectrum cephalosporins. Broad-spectrum beta-lactamase	Antimicrobial drug dosage prediction based on pioneering pharmacokinetic approach in food animals developed by Ziv in Israel, Hjerpe in United States, and others. Changes in sulfamethazine use in swine to

		inhibitors combined with aminopenicillins, e.g., sulbactam-ampicillin, used in food animals. Discovery of imipenem-cilastatin, an unusual broad-spectrum beta-lactam.	address residue issue. Ban on nitrofuran and nitroimidazole drugs for food animals in United States because of mutagenicity.
1986–1990	Increasing resistance problems in humans: methicillin-resistant *Staphylococcus aureus* emerges	Quinolones and fluoroquinolones introduced into human medicine. Ceftiofur, an expanded-spectrum cephalosporin, introduced for food animals.	Development of Food Animal Residue Avoidance Database in United States. Moratorium on sulfamethazine use in dairy cows in United States. Moratorium on most use of aminoglycosides in food animals in United States because of kidney residues.
1991–1995	Increasing resistance problems in humans: VRE emerge	Azithromycin and other improved macrolides introduced into human medicine. Tilmicosin (macrolide), tiamulin (pleuromutilin), and florfenicol (nontoxic) introduced for selective food animal use. Fluoroquinolones introduced for selective use in food animals in Europe.	First fluoroquinolone, enrofloxacin, introduced into food animal (poultry) use in United States, with severe restrictions; includes resistance monitoring through National Antimicrobial Resistance Monitoring System, which integrates food-animal and medical data. National Committee for Clinical Laboratory Standards (NCCLS) in United States establishes veterinary subcommittee to develop susceptibility testing methods and interpretations. Animal Medicines Use Clarification Act in United States allows extralabel use of certain approved drugs by veterinary prescription.
1996–2000	Resistance crisis in medicine; now includes penicillin-resistant *Streptococcus pneumoniae*	Oral, broad-spectrum cephalosporins introduced into human medicine; may partially drive resistance crisis. Effective antivirals introduced into human medicine. Fluoroquinolones introduced for treatment of acute pneumonia in cattle in United States.	VRE emergence linked to avoparcin use in food animals in Europe. Ban of avoparcin and four other growth promoters in Europe. World Health Organization (1998) recommends withdrawal of growth-promoting antimicrobials if significant for human medicine. Global emergence of multidrug-resistant *S. enterica* serovar Typhimurium DT104. Japanese Veterinary Antimicrobial Resistance Monitoring Program started. NCCLS guidelines for veterinary bacterial susceptibility testing published. U.S. FDA's CVM proposes "An approach for establishing thresholds in association with the use of antimicrobial drugs in food-producing animals" ("Framework Document"). CVM proposes withdrawal of fluoroquinolones in poultry because of resistance in *Campylobacter*.
2001–2005	Resistance crisis in medicine continues and expands	No new antimicrobial drugs introduced for food animals	World Health Organization's Global Strategy for Containment of Antimicrobial Resistance calls for prescription-only use of antimicrobials in food animals, national usage and resistance monitoring, and phasing out of growth promoters if the drugs are important for humans. Withdrawal of fluoroquinolones for use in poultry in United States because of emerging resistance in *C. jejuni*. Spread of multidrug resistance including cephalosporinase (Cmy2) genes among certain *Salmonella* serovars. Development of prudent-use guidelines by practitioner speciality groups at national levels.
2006–	"Postantibiotic" or new drug discovery period?	Have pathogens been "educated" over 50 years to become more rapidly resistant through various means? Will genomic, proteomic, combinatorial chemistry era revolutionize antimicrobial drug discovery and produce new drugs?	Resistance crisis in medicine focuses intense effort on improved infection and antimicrobial drug use control by physicians. Some benefits observed.

still an important component of the licensing of antimicrobial drugs, in part because the predictive science is imperfect.

In retrospect, for drugs the use of which "has advanced the practice of medicine farther than any other single factor of any of the previous centuries" (10), the time taken to establish the science of the clinical use of antimicrobial drugs seems astonishing. As human medicine's poor cousin, veterinary medicine lagged in the development of the science of optimal antimicrobial drug use, but the lag was only relative since the same delay was clearly visible in medicine. In general, the science of antimicrobial usage in animals largely paralleled that in human medicine, in the same way that most of the antimicrobial drugs used were the same or at least in the same drug class. There have been, however, a number of features unique to animal agriculture.

PRACTICES IN ANTIMICROBIAL DRUG USAGE UNIQUE TO ANIMAL HUSBANDRY

The greatest differences between animal husbandry and human medicine in the use of antimicrobial drugs were, and in many countries still are, their uses for growth promotion and for disease prophylaxis in agriculture.

The growth-promotional benefits of adding low concentrations of antibacterial drugs to feed was recognized almost as soon as antibiotics were introduced. The enhancement of growth rates and improved efficiency of use of feed were noted when pigs and poultry were fed the fungal waste derived from antibiotic production, originally intended as a source of vitamins and protein but mostly as an efficient way to use the waste. The effect was originally attributed to the presence of vitamin B_{12} ("animal protein factor") in the mycelial mass, but with time it was recognized to be a direct effect of residual antibiotic. Interestingly, how antimicrobial drugs improve growth rate and efficiency of feed utilization is still unknown, although it is thought to be through an inhibitory or metabolic effect of some kind on the gram-positive intestinal microflora. Curiously, until about the mid-1950s, prolonged low-dose oral tetracycline was even used to improve the growth of underweight human infants and children, but this practice was dropped because of both resistance and discoloration of teeth. In animals, the growth-promotional and disease-prophylactic benefits of this practice appear to have remained constant over the years (18), supporting the idea that these effects result from metabolic rather than antibacterial activities.

Not only have antimicrobial drugs been used for growth promotion, but some drugs were and in some countries still are administered in feed for prolonged periods at somewhat higher concentrations, known as "subtherapeutic levels" (defined in the United States as less than 200 g per ton of feed), which are lower concentrations than those approved for therapeutic purposes. The historical origin of subtherapeutic usage and even the meaning of the term are obscure, but it seems to have both beneficial growth-promotional and disease-prophylactic effects, particularly against pathogens that do not readily develop or acquire resistance. Drugs are administered "subtherapeutically" for many defined, licensed purposes at a range of concentrations varying with the drug, the animal species, and the purpose. Such use, which can often be prolonged, has been particularly widespread in the swine industry in countries in which the drugs are still allowed for this purpose (8). As noted earlier, a number of antimicrobial drugs (such as the streptogramins) that were too toxic for parenteral use in humans were relegated to growth-promotional and disease-prophylactic use in food animals.

Another practice that has historically been far more common in food animal use than in human medicine is mass medication with therapeutic concentrations of drugs immediately before an outbreak of disease is anticipated or immediately at the onset of disease in a population (4). This type of prophylaxis has been commonly practiced in the beef feedlot and in swine medicine and is most akin to the prophylactic use of antimicrobial drugs to prevent *Haemophilus* or *Neisseria* meningitis in humans. Prophylactic use of intramammary antimicrobial drugs to prevent development of new infections and to treat existing infections has become a standard practice in dairy cows in the 2 months before they calve and reenter the milking herd ("dry cow treatment"), with no apparent adverse effect on resistance development, perhaps in part because the very high concentrations of drugs achieved in the udder result in rapid killing of the target bacteria.

PUBLIC HEALTH ASPECTS OF USE OF ANTIMICROBIAL DRUGS IN FOOD ANIMALS

The effect of antimicrobial drug use in food animals on the development of resistance in bacteria that can cause disease in humans has been the subject of prolonged, acrimonious, and still ongoing debate. The major and most accessible reviews of this issue are summarized in Table 2. Table 2 shows that the intensity of the criticism of agricultural usage of antimicrobial drugs has reached a crescendo, particularly since the mid-1990s, coinciding with the antimicrobial resistance crisis in human medicine (Table 1).

The first major review of the effect of antimicrobial drug use on resistance in human and animal pathogens was carried out in the United Kingdom under the chairmanship of M. M. Swann (Table 2). The impetus for the review was a combination of recognition of the increasing importance of the phenomenon of "infectious," transferable drug resistance associated in part with the pioneering work of the distinguished British veterinary microbiologist H. Williams Smith, the emergence and dissemination in calves in Britain of multidrug-resistant *Salmonella enterica* serovar Typhimurium and its spread to humans (2), and experiences around this time of a difficult-to-control epidemic of chloramphenicol-resistant *Salmonella enterica* serovar Typhi in Central America. Chloramphenicol was then the drug of last resort for typhoid fever in humans (16). The 1969 Swann report to the British government gave a careful analysis of how different usage of antimicrobial drugs in animals might lead to selection of resistant bacteria and resistance plasmids, and how such resistant bacteria, or their transmissible resistance traits, could lead to difficult-to-treat infections in humans. The major recommendations of the committee were: (i) "Feed" antimicrobial drugs should only be used for growth promotion without prescription if they have little or no implication as therapeutic agents in humans, will not impair the value of prescribed drugs, and produce an economic benefit. Since penicillin and tetracyclines did not meet these criteria, they were withdrawn from growth-promotional use and could only be used therapeutically by veterinary prescription. (ii) The "therapeutic" antimicrobials (those other than growth-promotional antimicrobials) tylosin, sulfonamides, and nitrofurans should no longer be used without veterinary prescription. The spirit of the Swann report was to restrict therapeutically effective antibiotics only to therapeutic use on a veterinary prescription basis. Withdrawal of penicillin and tetracyclines for growth-promotional and subtherapeutic purposes was, however, soon followed by their substitution by bacitracin, virginiamycin, nitrovin, and flavomycin for similar purposes (22).

It was perhaps unfortunate that little effort was made in Britain following the Swann report to improve the scientific understanding of the effect of antimicrobial drug use in animals on human health, nor to document the effect of implementation of the report (22). Nevertheless, the sustained work of A. H. Linton (13) and his colleagues led to an important conceptual understanding of the routes of movement of resistant bacteria between animals and humans and the factors that enhanced the movement, although the scale of the movement had considerable uncertainty (Fig. 1).

In the United States, the response to the issues raised in the Swann report was largely unenthusiastic and critical (Table 2). Resistance to the report's recommendations was based on the estimates of the considerable economic contribution that growth-promoting and subtherapeutic ("feed") antimicrobial drugs made to agriculture in comparison to what was criticized as the inadequate evidence, the dubious and slender risk, and the "special case pleading" on which the recommendations of the Swann report were regarded as based. The strong lobby of antimicrobial drug manufacturers and the absence in the United States of a national health system (i.e., the patient pays for illness, whereas in Europe it is the nation that bears the cost) may have helped to fuel the criticism. The data were regarded as inadequate to make clear judgments, but the scale of the problem was also thought to be minor. For example, the 1989 Institute of Medicine study (Table 2) suggested that the use of subtherapeutic or growth-promoting drugs might contribute to perhaps 26 human deaths a year from antimicrobial drug-resistant *Salmonella*. To put this number in perspective, there were about 40,000 automobile-accident and 10,000 gunshot fatalities in the United States in the same year.

Despite the inconclusive nature of many of the reports in the United States in the period between 1972 and 1995, the issue refused to die. There were occasional highly publicized reports throughout this period of serious human illness caused by *Salmonella* carrying resistance genes thought to be acquired from subtherapeutic, or even therapeutic, use of antimicrobials in animals. One of several examples was the report by Spika et al. (20) on chloramphenicol-resistant *Salmonella enterica* serovar Newport traced from hamburger to dairy farms. Such reports led to apparently carefully orchestrated media and even major science journal frenzies about the discovery of the "smoking gun," with consequent fervent denials by the animal antimicrobial drug industry. Given the existing well-established understanding of the epidemiology of the movement of resistant intestinal bacteria (Fig. 1), these periodic frenzies seemed at the time both astonishing and somehow hysterical. The periodic surges in public interest, however, produced no political will within the United States to reexamine the problem.

The reason for the extensive reexamination of the issue beginning in the mid-1990s related to several factors. The most important of these was the antimicrobial resistance crisis in medicine, in which

Table 2. Historical timeline of major reports and their conclusions or recommendations relating to the public health aspects of antimicrobial drug use in food animals

Date	Report (source)	Major conclusions or recommendations
1962	Netherthorpe Committee (Joint Committee, Agricultural and Medical Research Councils, United Kingdom)	Recognized economic benefit of antimicrobials as growth promoters; saw no reason to discontinue. However, recommended continuing to examine situation and phasing out penicillin and tetracycline use if alternative nontherapeutic growth promoters become available.
1969	Committee on Antibiotic Uses in Animal Husbandry and Veterinary Medicine, "Swann report" (Report to Parliament, United Kingdom)	Recommended restricting use of antimicrobials to prescription-only therapeutic use and nonprescription feed additives. Growth-promotional and subtherapeutic use of drugs important in human medicine were banned.
1972	*The Use of Antibiotics in Animal Feeds* (FDA task force, United States)	Concluded that use of antimicrobial drugs in food animals may promote resistance in *Salmonella*; manufacturers to show this is not a problem. Found sufficient evidence to stop use of penicillin and chlortetracycline as growth promoters.
1979	*Drugs in Livestock Feed* (Office of Technology Assessment, United States)	Recommended discontinuing use of penicillin and tetracyclines as growth promoters, even though this would have short-term economic cost
1980	*The Effects on Human Health of Subtherapeutic Use of Antimicrobials in Animals* (National Research Council, United States)	Could not conclude from data available that there was a direct relationship between subtherapeutic drug use in animal feed and human health. Insufficient data from United Kingdom that implementation of Swann report had reduced postulated hazards to human health.
1981	*Antibiotics in Animal Feeds* (Council for Agricultural Sciences and Technology, United States)	Concluded it was irrational to ban subtherapeutic dosage without also banning therapeutic use. Calculated cost of a ban on feed antimicrobials at about $3.5 billion.
1989	*Human Health Risks with the Subtherapeutic Use of Penicillin or Tetracyclines in Animal Feed* (Institute of Medicine, United States)	Unable to find substantial direct evidence of definite human health hazard in the use of subtherapeutic concentrations of penicillins and tetracyclines in animal feeds
1995	*Impacts of Antibiotic-Resistant Bacteria* (Office of Technology Assessment, United States)	Cited need to collect more data to resolve the issue of the effect of feed antimicrobials in animals on human health, stating that a further report would not resolve the issue
1997	*Antimicrobial Feed Additives* (Ministry of Agriculture, Commission on Antimicrobial Feed Additives, Sweden)	As part of negotiations leading to European Union membership, Sweden, which had banned use of antimicrobial growth promoters in 1985, re-reviewed the benefits of antibacterial feed additives and again concluded that the benefit did not outweigh the risks.
1997	*The Medical Impact of the Use of Antimicrobials in Food Animals* (World Health Organization)	Recommended discontinuing use of antimicrobials for growth promotion or subtherapeutic purposes in animals if they are used in human therapeutics or if they select for cross-resistance to antimicrobials used in human medicine
1998	*A Review of Antimicrobial Resistance in the Food Chain* (Ministry of Agriculture, Fisheries and Food, United Kingdom)	Concluded that resistance in animal pathogens and commensal bacteria is selected for by antimicrobial drug use and can reach people through food chain, that these pathogens may cause disease or colonize people and can transfer resistance to human pathogens, and that *Campylobacter* and *Salmonella* and certain antimicrobials are especially problematic
1999	*The Use of Drugs in Food Animals: Benefits and Risks* (Committee on Drug Use in Food Animals: Panel on Animal Health, Food Safety and Public Health, National Research Council and Institute of Medicine, United States)	Concluded that use of drugs in food animals does not appear to constitute an immediate public health concern; additional data may alter conclusion but data are lacking. Recommended integrated national databases to support rational, visible, science-driven decision making and policy development for regulatory approval and use of antimicrobials in food animals. Estimated cost of ban on nontherapeutic use in animals between $5 and $10 per person per year in United States.
2000	*The Use of Antibiotics in Food-Producing Animals: Antibiotic-Resistant Bacteria in Animals and Humans* (Joint Expert Advisory Committee on Antibiotic Resistance, Australia)	Recommended discontinuing use of growth promoters if same drugs important in human medicine, making all antimicrobials for animals prescription only, predetermining "resistance thresholds" for animal antimicrobials that trigger investigation, developing a comprehensive and integrated resistance surveillance system, monitoring antimicrobial usage, and finding alternatives to antimicrobials for food animals

Continued on following page

Table 2. *Continued*

Date	Report (source)	Major conclusions or recommendations
2001	*Risk Assessment on the Human Health Impact of Fluoroquinolone Resistant* Campylobacter *Associated with the Consumption of Chicken* (Center for Veterinary Medicine, United States)	Risk assessment by highly detailed mathematical model with numerous explicit assumptions suggested that in 1998 an estimated 8,678 U.S. citizens acquired fluoroquinolone-resistant *Campylobacter* illnesses from chickens and received fluoroquinolones for treatment.
2002	*The Need to Improve Antimicrobial Use in Agriculture: Ecological and Human Health Consequences* (Alliance for the Prudent Use of Antibiotics. *Clinical Infectious Diseases*, vol. 34, supplement 3)	Concluded that elimination of nontherapeutic use of antimicrobials in food animals will lower burden of antimicrobial resistance in the environment, with benefits to human and animal health
2002	*Uses of Antimicrobials in Food Animals in Canada: Impact on Resistance and Human Health* (Health Canada Advisory Committee on Animal Uses of Antimicrobials and Impact on Resistance and Human Health, Canada)	Recommended making all antimicrobials for disease control available by prescription only, developing an extralabel drug use policy, closing a drug importation loophole, stringently reassessing growth-promotional use of drugs, and developing national surveillance of resistance and use
2002	*Food Safety and Pig Production in Denmark: Controls on Antibiotics, Veterinary Medicines and* Salmonella (Verner Wheelock Associates Limited; Danish Bacon and Meat Council)	Control of antimicrobial-resistant bacteria by banning of antimicrobial growth promoters and by *Salmonella* control programs has made Denmark a model and given the Danish pig industry competitive economic advantage.
2003	*Joint FAO/OIE/WHO Expert Workshop on Non-Human Antimicrobial Usage and Antimicrobial Resistance: Scientific Assessment* (World Health Organization)	Found clear evidence of adverse human health consequences due to resistant organisms resulting from nonhuman usage. Concluded that surveillance of usage and resistance is important to identify problems and choose interventions and that determining magnitude of impact is difficult.
2003	*Impacts of Antimicrobial Growth Promotion Termination in Denmark* (World Health Organization)	Review of the "Danish experiment" of terminating use of growth promoters concluded that there have been no serious negative effects on efficiency of food animal production, animal health, food safety, and consumer prices and that the approach has been very beneficial in reducing total quantity of antimicrobials used and reducing antimicrobial resistance in important food animal reservoirs.

for the first time resistant bacteria moved out of the hospital and into the community. The very serious nature of the crisis led to a reexamination within human medicine of all aspects of antimicrobial use and even to the apparent rediscovery of the importance of basic infection-control procedures such as hand washing. The antimicrobial resistance crisis in medicine once again focused the medical establishment on agricultural use of antimicrobials, in some cases almost to the extent of using it as the scapegoat for the crisis in medicine.

Improvements in understanding of the microbiology of infectious diseases acquired from animals were less important, but also critical, forces in the reexamination of antimicrobial usage in agriculture. For example, at the time of the Swann report, *Campylobacter jejuni* was not recognized as a human pathogen, although it subsequently became identified as the most common cause of bacterial gastroenteritis in humans. The emergence of fluoroquinolone resistance in *C. jejuni* of poultry origin in the United States because of the use of fluoroquinolones to treat *Escherichia coli* infections in chickens (19) subsequently led to the ban of all use of this class of drug in chickens in the United States (Table 2). A subsequent risk analysis in the United States suggested that 8,678 citizens treated for this illness with fluoroquinolones had fluoroquinolone-resistant *C. jejuni* illnesses acquired from chickens (Table 2), a huge number compared to the "26 possible deaths because of resistant *Salmonella*" identified in the 1989 Institute of Medicine report (Table 2). Similarly, at the time of the Swann report, vancomycin-resistant enterococci (VRE) were also unknown, although subsequently enterococcal infections emerged as major nosocomial infections in humans, with vancomycin as the drug of last resort in such infections. Acquisition of transmissible vancomycin resistance genes by these hospital-associated bacteria made them essentially untreatable, again raising the specter of the "postantibiotic" era (Table 1). Work by Bager and colleagues in Denmark was important in identifying avoparcin, a glycopeptide antimicrobial related to vancomycin, as selecting for the massive presence of VRE in the intestines of poultry and swine fed this drug as a growth promoter (3). For the first time, there was convincing large-scale evidence that eliminating use of antimicrobial drugs in food animals could dramatically reverse the rise of resistant bacteria

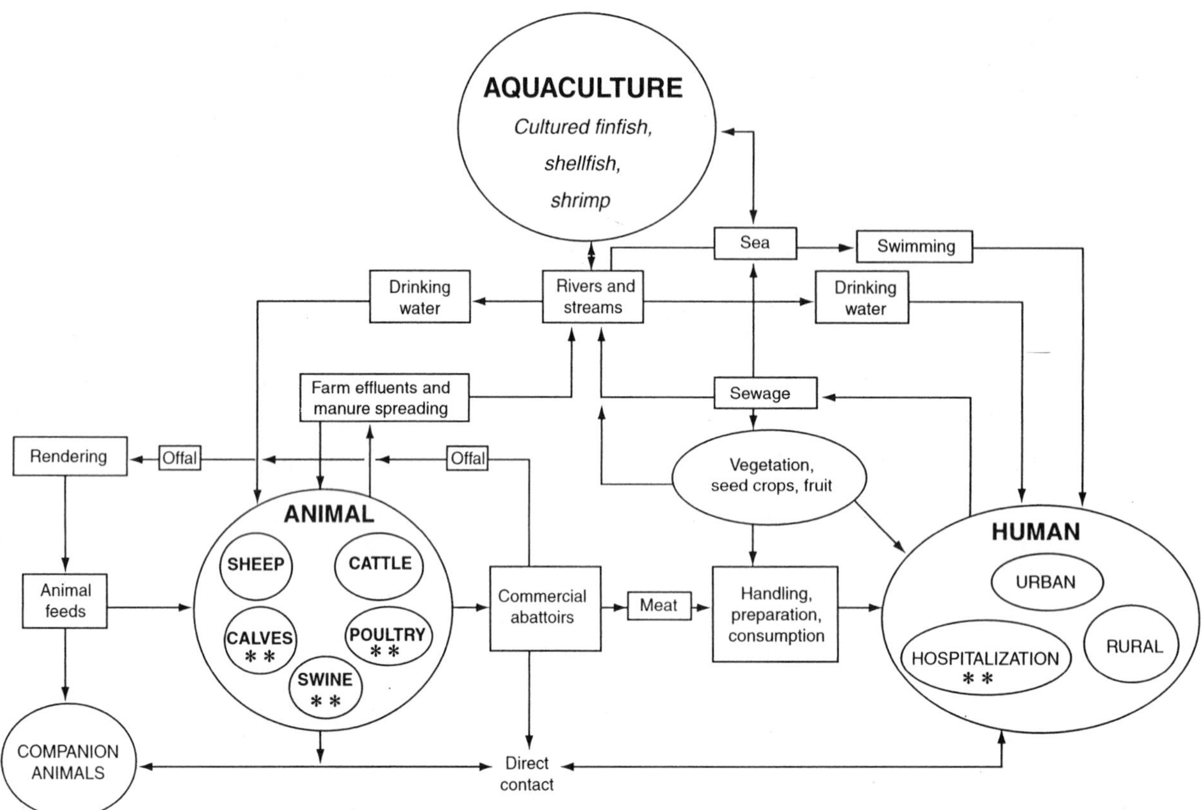

Figure 1. Routes of exchange of *E. coli* between animals and humans. Note the areas where antimicrobial drug selection for resistance is most likely. The size of the circles or boxes does not indicate the extent of the scale of the movement. **, high antibiotic selection pressure. Adapted from reference 13, as modified by R. Irwin; reproduced with permission.

in these animals (1). Convincing molecular genetic typing evidence showed that VRE from animals colonized humans (11), and most dramatically, the marked decline in human intestinal colonization by VRE in Europe following the withdrawal of avoparcin as a growth promoter (12) suggested that the scale of the movement of resistant intestinal bacteria from animals to humans, which had always been a matter of great uncertainty, was far larger than had been generally suspected. Molecular genetic typing and DNA sequencing of resistance genes and gene regions were unavailable at the time of the Swann report but were subsequently used extensively to characterize the relatedness (and therefore sometimes the source) of both bacteria and genes obtained from animals and humans (5, 15).

EUROPEAN AND NORTH AMERICAN RESPONSES TO PUBLIC HEALTH ISSUES RAISED BY USE OF ANTIMICROBIAL DRUGS IN FOOD ANIMALS

A marked contrast has developed between Europe and North America in the use of antimicrobial drugs in food animals for growth promotion and subtherapeutic applications. Such use was banned in Europe in 2000 (Table 1), whereas it continues in North America. The approach used by the U.S. Food and Drug Administration's (FDA's) Center for Veterinary Medicine (CVM) has been the collection of national data on antimicrobial resistance in food-borne pathogens through the National Antimicrobial Resistance Monitoring System (Table 1), providing a logical framework for evaluating the value of specific antimicrobial drug classes based on their importance in human medicine and the chance that resistance genes will reach specific types of human bacterial pathogens from animals and that resistant pathogens will reach humans, as well as defining when resistance in human pathogens derived from animals becomes so important (i.e., reaches a threshold) that some action needs to be taken to mitigate this resistance. This approach was captured in the CVM's "Framework Document" (Table 1) and was used as the basis for banning the use of fluoroquinolones in poultry in the United States. The careful and logical "science-based" approach in the United States was based on the need by the CVM to anticipate and to fight any court challenges successfully, although the

European ban was successfully upheld in a legal challenge in the European court. The economic effect of the removal of the growth promoters from European agriculture on animal health and productivity was found to have been minor (7, 21), important evidence in the continuing battles over the costs and benefits of antimicrobial drug use for growth promotion and disease prophylaxis.

CONCLUSIONS

The rise of antimicrobial resistance in animal and human pathogens in some ways represents a further example of the "tragedy of the commons" (9). Ready access to the "miracle drugs" by medicine and agriculture, coupled with the ability of chemists to alter existing drugs or develop new ones to counter resistance, led to the expectation that the preantibiotic era was to become a folk memory marked only on mossy gravestones. This has been proven wrong. The new technologies of recombinant DNA, diagnostic DNA microarrays, genomics, proteomics, and combinatorial chemistry hold considerable promise for the development of new, possibly pathogen-targeted, antimicrobial drugs. However, the question for the future is how to preserve existing and new drugs in the face of bacterial pathogens, some of which appear to have become particularly adept at developing or acquiring resistance over the last 60 years. Everyone using antimicrobial drugs, including those in agriculture, shares the blame for the rise of resistance and the burden to use these drugs responsibly.

REFERENCES

1. **Aarestrup, F. M., A. M. Seyfarth, H. D. Emborg, K. Pedersen, R. S. Hendriksen, and F. Bager.** 2001. Effect of abolishment of the use of antimicrobial agents for growth promotion on occurrence of antimicrobial resistance in fecal enterococci from food animals in Denmark. *Antimicrob. Agents Chemother.* **45:**2054–2059.
2. **Anderson, E. S.** 1968. Drug resistance in *Salmonella typhimurium* and its implications. *Br. Med. J.* **3:**333–339.
3. **Bager, F., M. Madsen, J. Christensen, and F. M. Aarestrup.** 1997. Avoparcin used as a growth promoter is associated with the occurrence of vancomycin-resistant *Enterococcus faecium* on Danish poultry and pig farms. *Prev. Vet. Med.* **31:**95–112.
4. **Bateman, K. G.** 2000. Antimicrobial drug use in cattle, p. 576–590. *In* J. F. Prescott, J. D. Baggot, and R. D. Walker (ed.), *Antimicrobial Therapy in Veterinary Medicine*, 3rd ed. Iowa State University Press, Ames.
5. **Boyd, D., G. A. Peters, A. Cloeckaert, K. S. Boumedine, E. Chaslus-Dancla, H. Imberechts, and M. R. Mulvey.** 2001. Complete nucleotide sequence of a 43-kilobase genomic island associated with the multidrug resistance region of *Salmonella enterica* serovar Typhimurium DT104 and its identification in phage type DT120 and serovar Agona. *J. Bacteriol.* **183:**5725–5732.
6. **Collins, J. H.** 1948. The present status of penicillin in veterinary medicine. *J. Am. Vet. Med. Assoc.* **113:**330–333.
7. **Emborg, H., A. K. Ersboll, O. E. Heuer, and H. C. Wegener.** 2001. The effect of discontinuing the use of antimicrobial growth promoters on the productivity in the Danish broiler production. *Prev. Vet. Med.* **50:**53–70.
8. **Friendship, R. M.** 2000. Antimicrobial drug use in swine. p. 602–611. *In* J. F. Prescott, J. D. Baggot, and R. D. Walker (ed.), *Antimicrobial Therapy in Veterinary Medicine*, 3rd ed. Iowa State University Press, Ames.
9. **Hardin, G.** 1968. The tragedy of the commons. *Science* **162:**1243–1248.
10. **Hussar, A. E., and H. W. Holley.** 1954. *Antibiotics and Antibiotic Therapy*. MacMillan, New York, N. Y.
11. **Jensen, L. B., A. M. Hammerum, R. L. Poulsen, and H. Westh.** 1999. Vancomycin-resistant *Enterococcus faecium* strains with highly similar pulsed-field gel electrophoresis patterns containing similar Tn*1546*-like elements isolated from a hospitalized patient and pigs in Denmark. *Antimicrob. Agents Chemother.* **43:**724–725.
12. **Klare, I., D. Badstubner, C. Konstabel, G. Bohme, H. Claus, and W. Witte.** 1999. Decreased incidence of VanA-type vancomycin-resistant enterococci isolated from poultry meat and from fecal samples of humans in the community after discontinuation of avoparcin usage in animal husbandry. *Microb. Drug Resist.* **5:**45–52.
13. **Linton, A. H.** 1977. Antibiotic resistance: the present situation reviewed. *Vet. Rec.* **100:**354–360.
14. **Little, R. B., C. S. Bryan, W. E. Petersen, W. N. Plastridge, and O. W. Schalm.** 1946. The intramammary therapy of bovine mastitis. *J. Am. Vet. Med. Assoc.* **108:**127–135.
15. **Piddock, L. J., V. Ricci, L. Pumbwe, M. J. Everett, and D. J. Griggs.** 2003. Fluoroquinolone resistance in *Campylobacter* species from man and animals: detection of mutations in topoisomerase genes. *J. Antimicrob. Chemother.* **51:**19–26.
16. **Randall, C. J.** 1969. The Swann Committee. *Vet. Rec.* **85:**616–621.
17. **Roberts, S. J.** 1953. Antibiotic therapy in large animals, p. 39–48. *In Conference Proceedings, American Veterinary Medical Association.*
18. **Shryock, T.** 2000. Growth promotion and feed antibiotics, p. 735–743. *In* J. F. Prescott, J. D. Baggot, and R. D. Walker (ed.), *Antimicrobial Therapy in Veterinary Medicine*, 3rd ed. Iowa State University Press, Ames.
19. **Smith, K. E., J. M. Besser, C. W. Hedberg, F. T. Leano, J. B. Bender, J. H. Wicklund, B. P. Johnson, K. A. Moore, and M. T. Osterholm.** 1999. Quinolone-resistant *Campylobacter jejuni* infections in Minnesota, 1992–1998. *N. Engl. J. Med.* **340:**1525–1532.
20. **Spika, J. S., S. H. Waterman, G. W. Hoo, M. E. St. Louis, R. E. Pacer, S. M. James, M. L. Bissett, L. W. Mayer, J. Y. Chiu, B. Hall, et al.** 1987. Chloramphenicol-resistant *Salmonella newport* traced through hamburger to dairy farms. A major persisting source of human salmonellosis in California. *N. Engl. J. Med.* **316:**565–570.
21. **Wierup, M.** 2001. The Swedish experience of the 1986 year ban of antimicrobial growth promoters, with special reference to animal health, disease prevention, productivity, and usage of antimicrobials. *Microb. Drug Resist.* **7:**183–190.
22. **Williams Smith, H.** 1977. Antibiotic resistance in bacteria and associated problems in farm animals before and after the 1969 Swann Report, p. 344–357. *In* M. Woodbine (ed.), *Antibiotics and Antibiosis in Agriculture.* Butterworths, London, United Kingdom.

Antimicrobial Resistance in Bacteria of Animal Origin
Edited by Frank M. Aarestrup

Chapter 3

Antimicrobial Susceptibility Testing of Bacteria of Veterinary Origin

JEFFREY L. WATTS AND CYNTHIA J. LINDEMAN

The judicious use of antimicrobial agents requires that the most efficacious agent be selected for use in the treatment of animal diseases. This is particularly true in this current era of increased antimicrobial resistance in human pathogens and concerns over the potential contribution of veterinary antimicrobial usage to overall resistance levels (5, 9, 12, 21, 22, 27). Antimicrobial susceptibility tests (ASTs) provide essential information that guides the veterinarian in selecting the most appropriate agent. A foundational characteristic of the AST is the relationship between the test outcome and clinical outcome following treatment of the animal (8, 15, 17). That is, an isolate yielding a susceptible AST result would be expected to clinically respond to the agent at the appropriate dosage. In contrast, an AST result of "resistant" would imply that treatment with that agent would fail. While ASTs meeting these criteria have been available in human medicine for many years, this has not been the case in veterinary medicine. This is not surprising given the variety of host species (companion animals, food animals, or exotics) and the differences in application of test results. AST results for a pathogen from a dog, for example, would be used to select treatment for that animal, while the same information for a pig might be used to devise therapy for the entire herd. This diversity in host animals and in the application of test results has made the development of ASTs that provide accurate, reproducible, clinically relevant results for veterinary pathogens daunting, with substantial progress only occurring in the past decade. However, the increasing availability of standardized AST methods for veterinary pathogens with veterinary-specific interpretive criteria has increased the importance of ASTs in veterinary medicine.

HISTORICAL PERSPECTIVE

The use of ASTs in veterinary medicine closely paralleled the development of ASTs in human medicine (as reviewed in reference 25). As the test methods used for human pathogens such as *Staphylococcus aureus* or *Escherichia coli* provided equivalent values for the same organisms isolated from animal diseases, veterinary application seemed to be a logical extension of the human methodologies. However, the use of these methods for the more fastidious veterinary pathogens as well as the use of human interpretive criteria were problematic. For example, four different media were recommended by various authors for susceptibility testing of *Histophilus somni* (formerly known as *Haemophilus somnus*), and five were recommended for testing of *Actinobacillus pleuropneumoniae* (as reviewed in reference 25). This not only made comparison of AST results from different laboratories difficult, but no single medium would reliably support the growth of all strains. Moreover, the only interpretive criteria available for categorizing isolates as susceptible or resistant were those developed for use with human pathogens, and veterinary laboratories routinely used these breakpoints for similar animal pathogens regardless of the host species. By the early 1980s, it had become apparent that the use of human interpretive criteria did not reliably predict clinical outcomes when applied to veterinary pathogens. This led some authors to question the use of ASTs in veterinary medicine, while other workers attempted to develop veterinary-specific interpretive criteria (as reviewed in references 25 and 28). It was apparent by the late 1980s that there was a need for the development of veterinary-specific AST methods and interpretive criteria.

In 1993 the National Committee for Clinical Laboratory Standards (NCCLS) formed the

Jeffrey L. Watts and Cynthia J. Lindeman • Pfizer Animal Health, Veterinary Medicine Research and Development, Kalamazoo, MI 49009.

Subcommittee on Veterinary Antimicrobial Susceptibility Testing (V-AST) with the task of developing veterinary-specific AST standards (16). This group decided that rather than attempt to address all uses of antimicrobial agents in veterinary medicine, such as growth promotion, prophylaxis, and extralabel usage, it would limit its efforts to therapeutic uses in systemic diseases. This allowed the V-AST to use the experience developed with human pathogens in the development of veterinary-specific methods and interpretive criteria. The group also decided that it would limit the development of interpretive criteria to the approved indication and pathogens for a specific agent. This eliminated the problems associated with establishing interpretive criteria for extralabel antimicrobial uses and allowed the development of host-, pathogen-, and antimicrobial-specific interpretive criteria (16).

By 1999 the V-AST had published the first standard for the performance of ASTs with veterinary pathogens, NCCLS document M31, as well the first guideline on the data requirements for susceptibility test development, NCCLS document M37 (16, 17). The first version of M31 included a standardized test method for *H. somni* and *A. pleuropneumoniae* that utilized a common test medium, veterinary fastidious medium (VFM), as well as quality control organisms for use when testing these organisms (13, 16). The document also included the first publication of veterinary-specific interpretive criteria for several veterinary-use antimicrobial agents such as ceftiofur and tilmicosin. The current version of document M31 adds a standardized method for testing of *Campylobacter* spp., as well as veterinary-specific interpretive criteria for antimicrobial agents in each of the major antimicrobial classes (16). The Food and Drug Administration (FDA)-approved antimicrobial agents in the United States with veterinary-specific interpretive criteria included in M31 are summarized in Table 1. NCCLS document M31 is the accepted standard for susceptibility testing of veterinary pathogens in the United States and is used by laboratories accredited by the American Association of Veterinary Laboratory Diagnosticians (4). The V-AST has recently issued a report on antimicrobial susceptibility testing of pathogens causing diseases of fish and other aquatic animals (19). In January 2005 the NCCLS officially changed its name to the Clinical and Laboratory Standards Institute (CLSI).

In Europe and Japan, the situation has developed differently, as no agencies have directly addressed the development of veterinary-specific methods and interpretive criteria. However, there has been a great deal of interest in antimicrobial susceptibility testing of veterinary pathogens with zoonotic potential, such as *Salmonella enterica* serovar Typhimurium or *Campylobacter* species (5, 9, 21, 22). As a result, laboratories have used one of the methods developed by their respective national standards organizations for testing of human pathogens (2). In 1996 the European Society for Clinical Microbiology and Infectious Diseases established the European Committee on Antimicrobial Susceptibility Testing (EUCAST) to harmonize antimicrobial breakpoints across Europe (6, 7). At present, EUCAST has addressed susceptibility testing of human pathogens. Clinical breakpoints have been harmonized for a large number of agents, and epidemiological cutoff values have been defined (10, 11). This latter approach may lend itself to the development of veterinary methods in the future. The Office International des Épizooties (OIE) has recently issued a guideline for the susceptibility testing of human and veterinary pathogens which should also promote the harmonization of the various AST methods in the future (20). The calibrated dichotomous sensitivity (CDS) method is widely used in Australia, and veterinary-specific methods and interpretive criteria have been developed for this method (3). A summary of selected AST standards organizations is presented in Table 2.

Table 1. Summary of antimicrobial agents with veterinary-specific interpretive criteria published in NCCLS document M31[a]

Antimicrobial agent or combination	Host species or disease with approved interpretive criteria
Cefpodoxime	Dogs
Ceftiofur	Cattle, swine, horses, bovine mastitis
Clindamycin	Dogs
Danofloxacin	Cattle
Difloxacin	Dogs
Enrofloxacin	Cattle, dogs, cats, chickens, turkeys
Florfenicol	Cattle, swine
Gentamicin	Horses, dogs
Marbofloxacin	Dogs, cats
Orbifloxacin	Dogs, cats
Penicillin-novobiocin	Bovine mastitis
Pirlimycin	Bovine mastitis
Spectinomycin	Cattle
Tilmicosin	Cattle, swine
Tiamulin	Swine

[a]Adapted from reference 12.

TEST METHODS

The veterinary diagnostic laboratory can select from several different methodologies for antimicrobial susceptibility testing of veterinary pathogens, with most laboratories using either the agar disk diffusion

Table 2. Summary of selected organizations that publish AST standards

Country	Organization	Website	AST methods	Interpretive criteria
United States	CLSI	www.clsi.org	Human, veterinary	Human, veterinary
European Union	EUCAST	www.eucast.org	Human	Human
European Union	OIE	www.oie.int	Human, veterinary	
United Kingdom	British Society for Antimicrobial Chemotherapy	www.bsac.org.uk	Human	Human
Germany	Deutsches Institut für Normung	www.beuth.de	Human	Human
France	Société Française de Microbiologie	www.sfm.assoc.fr	Human	Human
Sweden	Swedish Reference Group for Antibiotics	www.srga.org	Human	Human
Australia	CDS disk diffusion method	www.med.unsw.edu.au/pathology-cds	Human, veterinary	Human, veterinary

(ADD) method or the broth microdilution MIC method (4). In order to ensure the generation of accurate, reproducible results, laboratories should adhere to a standard, well-defined method that includes the appropriate quality control information. It should be kept in mind that the purpose is not to mimic in vivo conditions but to establish a method that provides reproducible results. In the United States, the majority of labs use either an NCCLS reference method or a commercial method that adheres to this standard (4, 23). The method selected by a laboratory depends upon a variety of factors including the cost per test; the availability of appropriate antimicrobial agents, as veterinary-specific agents are not available in all test systems; and the volume of samples to be handled by the laboratory. In general, smaller laboratories with relatively low test volumes tend to prefer the ADD method and larger laboratories prefer the more automated MIC methods.

The ADD method remains a flexible, low-cost means of conducting ASTs and is widely used in many veterinary laboratories. The test provides qualitative results that categorize isolates as susceptible, intermediate, or resistant rather than the quantitative values obtained using the MIC methodologies. Additionally, almost all veterinary-specific agents, such as ceftiofur, pirlimycin, enrofloxacin, and tilmicosin, are available in the antimicrobial-impregnated disks (or tablets) used in the ADD method. However, low-volume disks for veterinary-specific agents may only be available from the pharmaceutical manufacturer. Smaller veterinary laboratories, particularly those run by veterinarians, may have difficulties in standardizing the inoculum used in this method, but commercial systems are available for this purpose (24).

The MIC method may be performed using a variety of methods ranging from the agar dilution method to a commercially available gradient strip method (23). This method provides a quantitative value expressed in micrograms per milliliter, as well as a categorization of the organism as susceptible or resistant. Standardized methods for testing more-fastidious organisms such as anaerobes and *Campylobacter* spp. have been developed for the MIC methodology. The MIC method is preferred for use in surveillance or epidemiological programs as it allows calculation of summary statistics. Of the various MIC formats, the broth microdilution method is the most widely used and is available in a variety of commercial systems as either dry or frozen panels. Automated systems are also available that provide rapid results and full walk-away capabilities. The disadvantages of these systems are that MIC panel formats are inflexible unless the lab is willing to bear the cost of custom panels and not all veterinary-specific agents are available on all systems. The number of dilutions tested in the MIC method may vary from laboratory to laboratory depending on the final use of the results. Laboratories involved in surveillance programs or epidemiological studies usually prefer to test a smaller number of antimicrobial agents for an extended number of dilutions, while many diagnostic laboratories choose to use a "breakpoint" panel. Breakpoint panels allow the laboratory to test a larger number of compounds with dilution ranges spanning the interpretive criteria or breakpoints for each agent. Care should be taken in selecting a breakpoint panel that allows in-range values for at least one quality control strain to allow for validated test results.

Table 3. Culture collection numbers for selected organisms used for QC of antimicrobial susceptibility tests[a]

Organism	Strain no. for indicated culture collection					
	ATCC[b]	DSM[c]	NCTC[d]	JCM[e]	CIP[f]	CCUG[g]
Escherichia coli	25922	1103	12241	5491	7624	17620
Escherichia coli	35218	5923	11954		102181	30600
Pseudomonas aeruginosa	27853	1117	10896		76110	17619
Staphylococcus aureus	29213	2569		2874	103429	15915
Staphylococcus aureus	25923	1104	12702	2413	7625	17621
Enterococcus faecalis	29212	2570	12697	2875	103214	9997
Streptococcus pneumoniae	49619					
Actinobacillus pleuropneumoniae	27090					
Histophilus somni	700025					

[a]Adapted from reference 16.
[b]ATCC, American Type Culture Collection (www.atcc.org).
[c]DSM, Deutsche Sammlung von Mikroorganismen and Zellkulturen (www.dsmz.de).
[d]NCTC, National Collection of Type Cultures; included in the United Kingdom National Culture Collections (www.ukncc.co.uk).
[e]JCM, Japan Collection of Microorganisms (www.jcm.riken.go.jp).
[f]CIP, Collection of Bacterial Strains of Institut Pasteur.
[g]CCUG, Culture Collection, University of Göteborg; see the website of the Swedish Reference Group for Antibiotics (www.srga.org).

Regardless of the test method selected, the routine conduct of quality control (QC) testing is an essential component of the AST. The routine testing of QC strains allows the laboratory to verify that laboratory personnel, incubation conditions, test media, and antimicrobial agents are performing at an acceptable level. QC strains have been defined by the various standards organizations for use in their systems (1, 2, 3, 6, 16). The QC ranges should be developed using a multilaboratory study that examines both inter- and intralaboratory reproducibility such as those defined by the NCCLS (6, 16) or uses an external quality assurance system (1). A summary of selected quality control strains defined in NCCLS document M31, with the cross-reference numbers for other national culture collections, is provided in Table 3. Several of these strains are also used in other test methods. The interval at which quality control strains are tested varies between laboratories. While inclusion of QC strains on each day of testing is preferred, this is too costly and time-consuming for many smaller veterinary laboratories and these laboratories may choose to run these strains on a weekly basis. A procedure for conversion from daily to weekly QC testing is described in document M31 (16).

A primary responsibility of the veterinary laboratory is to select the appropriate agents for routine testing and reporting of AST results. Testing veterinary pathogens is more complicated than testing their human counterparts due to the differences in approved antimicrobial agents in the various host species. For this reason, most veterinary laboratories have predefined batteries or panels of compounds specifically used for testing pathogens from specific hosts, e.g., a cattle panel, a bovine mastitis panel, or a companion animal panel. The laboratory should not report specific agents in certain host animals. For example, the FDA prohibits use of chloramphenicol and aminoglycosides in cattle, and AST results for these agents should not be reported. Preference in reporting should be given to those agents with veterinary-specific interpretive criteria as opposed to those approved for other species or with human interpretive criteria. The reporting of agents that do not have specific approvals in a host species (termed "extralabel use" in the United States) should be done with care and after consultation with a veterinarian. In the United States, most veterinary laboratories use the information provided in Table 1 of NCCLS document M31 as a guideline for developing their specific routine and reporting schemes (16).

ESTABLISHMENT OF VETERINARY-SPECIFIC INTERPRETIVE CRITERIA

As indicated above, the AST method provides a means of generating reproducible results that have adequate quality control. The interpretive criteria provide the means of correlating an AST result (susceptible or resistant) with a clinical outcome (cure or failure). The development of veterinary-specific interpretive criteria requires a tripartite database that includes microbiological data, pharmacokinetic and pharmacodynamic information, and outcome data from clinical efficacy trials (8, 15, 17, 26). This information allows threshold values, or "breakpoints," to be established for categorizing isolates as susceptible, intermediate, or resistant. Organisms falling into the "susceptible" category are those that are likely to respond when treated with that agent at the approved dosages. In contrast, organisms falling into the "resistant" category would be expected to fail therapy with that agent. The "intermediate" category is used either as a technical buffer zone or for those situations where the agent is concentrated or increased dosages are defined.

Microbiological data such as MIC distributions provide information on the range of microorganisms that lack known resistance mechanisms to a particular agent. In this situation, the MIC distribution will reflect the potency of a particular agent against a specific pathogen(s). This distribution may include strains for which drugs have significantly higher MICs, which may indicate the existence of a specific resistance mechanism. This distribution represents the "natural," or wild-type, population of that particular pathogen (23). If the agent is in a class already in therapeutic use, then the number of strains for which drugs have high MICs may represent a significant proportion of the population and the distribution may be bimodal. For example, the distribution of MICs of ampicillin for bovine isolates of *Mannheimia haemolytica* is bimodal due to a large percentage of β-lactamase-positive strains (26). Other microbiological characteristics of a compound such as sub-MIC effects, postantibiotic effects, effects on toxin production, and time-kill kinetics are important and should be determined as well.

Pharmacokinetics provides essential information on the absorption, distribution, metabolism, and excretion of an antimicrobial agent in the target host. This provides information on the overall exposure of the pathogen to the antimicrobial agent in the target host. Due to differences in host species, the pharmacokinetics of an antimicrobial agent may differ dramatically from host to host, which should be reflected in differences in interpretive criteria (as reviewed in reference 25). Pharmacokinetics also provides insight into those situations where the antimicrobial agent may be concentrated, such as fluoroquinolones or β-lactams in urinary tract infections. In the past 15 years the use of pharmacodynamics has become important in establishing interpretive criteria, as these data provide the link between specific pharmacokinetic components and efficacy (8, 14, 23). Pharmacodynamic parameters have been established for the majority of antimicrobial classes. For example, the essential pharmacodynamic parameter for fluoroquinolones is the area under the curve divided by the MIC for the pathogen, while the key pharmacodynamic parameter for β-lactam agents is the time the antimicrobial concentration exceeds the MIC for the target pathogen. The pharmacodynamic parameters should be considered general characteristics of a class, as new agents may provide exceptions to these rules.

During the conduct of clinical trials, the microbiological eradication rates for the target pathogens should be established (8, 23; as reviewed in reference 25). This is most accurately done by obtaining an isolate prior to therapy, obtaining a posttherapy culture, and establishing that the organism was, in fact, eliminated. Once these data are obtained, the eradication rates can be stratified by the MIC for the target pathogen and the correlation between clinical outcome and a susceptible test result established. The use of pre- and postculturing to establish microbiological eradication rates is, in practice, most useful in the simplest of infections, such as urinary tract infections. This method has also been used to establish interpretive criteria for agents used to treat bovine mastitis, as this is a requirement in the current efficacy protocols in both the United States and Europe. In more complicated infections or those for which culturing is problematic, such as bovine respiratory disease, clinical response rates rather than microbiological eradication rates are used to establish cure rates (as reviewed in reference 25). Response rates of at least 80% at a specific MIC must be established for organisms to be categorized as susceptible.

Once breakpoints for the target pathogens have been established for the MIC test, the interpretive criteria for the ADD test can be selected. This is performed by plotting the MIC (in micrograms per milliliter) against the zone of inhibition (in millimeters) for a large number of organisms representing the target species. Lines representing the MIC breakpoints are then superimposed over the scattergram of plotted values. Finally, lines representing the ADD breakpoints are drawn in a manner that provides optimal separation of the susceptible and resistant populations. Statistical methods such as error-rate bounding or discrepancy rates are then calculated to determine the error rates. The ADD breakpoint lines may then be adjusted to minimize very-major-error (false-susceptible) and major-error (false-resistant) rates (15, 17). It should be noted that the "resistant" category may not be defined for new agents where no resistant populations exist at the time of introduction. In this case, only a "susceptible" category is defined.

In the United States, the NCCLS has chosen to establish interpretive criteria using this tripartite database approach for the indicated hosts and target pathogens. Thus, NCCLS document M31 lists those agents with veterinary-specific interpretive criteria by the FDA-approved hosts, disease conditions, and target pathogens. These interpretive criteria are only valid for the listed indication and may not be accurate when applied to other hosts or organisms (16, 25). It should be noted that not all standards organizations agree with this approach, and they may apply different weight to the various components to establish interpretive criteria (23). For example, microbiological distributions and clinical efficacy may be used as the primary datasets for setting breakpoints, with minor consideration given to pharmacokinetic information. Also, other organizations may prefer not to provide bacterial species-specific breakpoints but may prefer to set interpretive criteria at the disease or bacterial genus level. As the various standards organizations begin to establish veterinary-specific interpretive criteria, it will be interesting to observe the different approaches used for this purpose.

REPORTING OF AST RESULTS

In order for AST to be clinically relevant to the clinician, individual test results must be reported in an accurate, timely fashion. Each laboratory bears the responsibility for developing specific reporting cascades for the various host animals and pathogens to be tested. However, preference in reporting should be given to those agents with veterinary-specific interpretive criteria for the host-pathogen combination being tested, as these are the most clinically relevant values. The use of breakpoints developed for a specific disease in one host for categorizing isolates from another host as susceptible or resistant should be minimized whenever possible. If agents are to be reported using interpretive criteria developed for other animals or humans, then this should be indicated to the veterinarian. For example, if an *S. aureus* strain from a case of bovine mastitis is tested against enrofloxacin, it is inaccurate to report this isolate as susceptible to enrofloxacin; rather, it should be reported as susceptible to enrofloxacin based on the canine breakpoint. This allows the clinician to interpret the clinical relevance (or lack thereof) of the test result.

The preferred method for reporting MIC results is to present all data in a distribution table or graph, as this allows the user to understand the activity of a specific agent against a given population of target organisms. When large numbers of agents and pathogens need to be reported in a succinct manner, summary statistics are often the most practical method for reporting MIC data (18). The most common summary statistics are the MIC_{50}, the MIC_{90}, and the MIC range. The MIC at which 50% of the isolates are inhibited is defined as the MIC_{50}, while the MIC at which 90% of the isolates are inhibited is defined as the MIC_{90}. The use of calculated MIC_{90}s should be avoided, and only on-scale dilution values should be reported. The MIC_{50}s and MIC_{90}s may also be indicated when MIC distribution data are presented. If data for a single interpretive category are to be summarized, the percent susceptible is preferred, as it avoids the issue of handling the "intermediate" and resistant categories. Additional analyses can be performed, but direct comparison of MIC data across antimicrobial classes should be done only with great care due to the differences in activity. For example, ceftiofur has an MIC_{90} of ≤0.06 μg/ml for *M. haemolytica*, compared to an MIC_{90} of 64.0 μg/ml for spectinomycin. However, the efficacy of these two compounds is comparable when used to treat bovine respiratory disease. The differences in the MICs are due to the relative in vitro activity of these two classes on a per-weight basis and are further reflected in the substantially higher dose required for spectinomycin to achieve the same efficacy as ceftiofur. In this situation, it is more appropriate to use the percent-susceptible data for comparisons.

FUTURE DIRECTIONS AND TRENDS

Much progress has been made in the past decade in the development of veterinary-specific testing methods and interpretive criteria. However, much work remains to be done. The development of test methods for additional veterinary pathogens such as *Haemophilus parasuis* from swine needs to be addressed, as well as the continued development of veterinary-specific interpretive criteria for older, generic agents. At present, a standardized method for susceptibility testing of *Campylobacter* spp. has been developed, but no interpretive criteria for these organisms or other enteric pathogens are available. Additionally, the relevance of AST results to antimicrobial agents used in control (prophylaxis) or growth promotion has not been established. The continued development of veterinary-specific interpretive criteria will play an increasingly important role in the prudent use of antimicrobial agents, and the pharmaceutical industry must be encouraged to participate in this process. While much of the interpretive criteria to date have been developed by the NCCLS for agents approved in the United States, this work needs to be expanded to include agents approved in Europe and elsewhere. As other organizations such as EUCAST and OIE begin to address veterinary AST methods and interpretive criteria, the need for collaboration and harmonization among the various standards organizations will become critical.

Acknowledgments. We thank Tom Shryock and Gunnar Kahlmeter for their reviews of the manuscript and helpful suggestions.

REFERENCES

1. **Aarestrup, F.** 2004. Antibiotic resistance in bacteria of animal origin-II (ARBAO-II), external quality assurance systems. Danish Institute for Food and Veterinary Research, Copenhagen, Denmark.
2. **Andrews, J. M.** 2001. BSAC standardized disk susceptibility test method. *J. Antimicrob. Chemother.* **48:**S43–S57.
3. **Bell, S. M., B. J. Gatus, J. N. Pham, and D. L. Rafferty.** 2002. *Antibiotic Susceptibility Testing by the CDS Method.* The Antibiotic Reference Laboratory, Department of Microbiology, The Prince of Wales Hospital, Randwick, New South Wales, Australia.
4. **Brooks, M. B., P. S. Morley, D. A. Dargatz, D. R. Hyatt, and M. D. Salman.** 2003. Antimicrobial susceptibility testing practices of veterinary diagnostic laboratories in the U.S.: findings from a survey. *J. Am. Vet. Med. Assoc.* **222:**168–173.
5. **Danish Institute for Food and Veterinary Research.** 2004. *DANMAP 2003—Use of Antimicrobial Agents and Occurrence of Antimicrobial Resistance in Bacteria from Food Animals and Humans in Denmark.* Danish Institute for Food and Veterinary Research, Copenhagen, Denmark.
6. **European Committee for Antimicrobial Susceptibility Testing.** 2000. Determination of minimum inhibitory concentrations (MICs) of antibacterial agents by agar dilution. *Clin. Microbiol. Infect.* **6:**509–515.
7. **European Committee for Antimicrobial Susceptibility Testing.** 2000. Determination of antimicrobial susceptibility test breakpoints. *Clin. Microbiol. Infect.* **6:**570–572.
8. **Ferraro. M. J.** 2001. Should we reevaluate antibiotic breakpoints? *Clin. Infect. Dis.* **33:**S227–S229.
9. **Hidetake, E., A. Morioka, K. Ishihara, A. Kojima, S. Shiroki, Y. Tamura, and T. Takahashi.** 2004. Antimicrobial susceptibility of *Salmonella* isolated from cattle, swine and poultry (2001–2002): report from the Japanese Veterinary Antimicrobial Resistance Monitoring Program. *J. Antimicrob. Chemother.* **53:**266–270.
10. **Kahlmeter, G., D. F. J. Brown, F. W. Goldstein, A. P. MacGowan, J. W. Mouton, A. Osterlund, A. Rodloff, M. Steinbakk, P. Urbaskova, and A. Vatopoulos.** 2003. European harmonization of MIC breakpoints for antimicrobial susceptibility testing of bacteria. *J. Antimicrob. Chemother.* **52:**145–148.
11. **Kahlmeter, G., and D. Brown.** 2004. Harmonisation of European breakpoints—can it be achieved? *Clin. Microbiol. Newsl.* **26:**187–192.
12. **Levy, S.** 2001. Antibiotic resistance: consequences of inaction. *Clin. Infect. Dis.* **33:**S124–S129.
13. **McDermott, P. F., A. L. Barry, R. N. Jones, G. E. Stein, C. Thornsberry, C. C. Wu, and R. D. Walker.** 2001. Standardization of broth microdilution and disk diffusion susceptibility tests for *Actinobacillus pleuropneumoniae* and *Haemophilus somnus*: quality control standards for ceftiofur, enrofloxacin, florfenicol, gentamicin, penicillin, tetracycline, tilmicosin, and trimethoprim-sulfamethoxazole. *J. Clin. Microbiol.* **39:**4283–4287.
14. **McKellar, Q. A., S. F. Sanchez-Bruni, and D. G. Jones.** 2004. Pharmacokinetic/pharmacodynamic relationships of antimicrobial drugs used in veterinary medicine. *J. Vet. Pharmacol. Ther.* **27:**503–514.
15. **National Committee for Clinical Laboratory Standards.** 2001. Development of *in vitro* susceptibility testing criteria and quality control parameters. Approved guideline, 2nd ed. NCCLS document M23-A2. National Committee for Clinical Laboratory Standards, Wayne, Pa.
16. **National Committee for Clinical Laboratory Standards.** 2002. Performance standards for antimicrobial disk and dilution susceptibility tests for bacteria isolated from animals. Approved standard, 2nd ed. NCCLS document M31-A2. National Committee for Clinical Laboratory Standards, Wayne, Pa.
17. **National Committee for Clinical Laboratory Standards.** 2002. Development of *in vitro* susceptibility testing criteria and quality control parameters for veterinary antimicrobial agents. Approved guideline, 2nd ed. NCCLS document M37-A2. National Committee for Clinical Laboratory Standards, Wayne, Pa.
18. **National Committee for Clinical Laboratory Standards.** 2002. Analysis and presentation of cumulative antimicrobial susceptibility test data. Approved guideline. NCCLS document M39-A. National Committee for Clinical Laboratory Standards, Wayne, Pa.
19. **National Committee for Clinical Laboratory Standards.** 2003. Methods for antimicrobial disk susceptibility testing of bacteria isolated from aquatic animals: a report. NCCLS document M42-R. National Committee for Clinical Laboratory Standards, Wayne, Pa.
20. **Office International des Épizooties.** 2004. Laboratory methodologies for bacterial antimicrobial susceptibility testing. *In Manual of Diagnostic Tests and Vaccines for Terrestrial Animals.* Office International des Épizooties, Paris, France.
21. **Phillips, I., M. Casewell, T. Cox, B. De Groot, C. Friis, R. Jones, C. Nightingale, R. Preston, and J. Waddell.** 2004. Does the use of antibiotics in food animals pose a risk to human health? A critical review of published data. *J. Antimicrob. Chemother.* **53:**28–52.
22. **Seyfarth, A. M., H. C. Wegener, and N. Frimodt-Moller.** 1997. Antimicrobial resistance in *Salmonella enterica* subsp. *enterica* serovar Typhimurium from humans and production animals. *J. Antimicrob. Chemother.* **40:**67–75.
23. **Turnidge, J. D., M. J. Ferraro, and J. H. Jorgensen.** 2003. Susceptibility test methods: general considerations, p. 1102–1107. *In* P. R. Murray, E. J. Baron, J. H. Jorgensen, M. A. Pfaller, and R. H. Yolken (ed.), *Manual of Clinical Microbiology*, 8th ed. ASM Press, Washington, D.C.
24. **Watts, J. L., and S. C. Nickerson.** 1986. Evaluation of a rapid inoculum standardization system of antibiotic susceptibility testing of bovine mammary gland isolates. *Vet. Microbiol.* **12:**269–276.
25. **Watts, J. L., and R. J. Yancey, Jr.** 1994. Identification of veterinary pathogens by use of commercial systems and new trends in antimicrobial susceptibility testing of veterinary pathogens. *Clin. Microbiol. Rev.* **7:**346–356.
26. **Watts, J. L., R. J. Yancey, Jr., S. A. Salmon, and C. A. Case.** 1994. A four-year survey of antimicrobial susceptibility trends for isolates from cattle with bovine respiratory disease cases in North America. *J. Clin. Microbiol.* **32:**725–731.
27. **Witte, W.** 2004. International dissemination of antibiotic resistant strains of bacterial pathogens. *Infect. Genet. Evol.* **4:**187–191.
28. **Woolcock, J. B., and M. D. Mutimer.** 1983. Antimicrobial susceptibility testing: caeci caecos ducentes? *Vet. Rec.* **113:** 125–128.

Antimicrobial Resistance in Bacteria of Animal Origin
Edited by Frank M. Aarestrup

Chapter 4

Molecular Methods for Detection of Antibiotic Resistance

HENK J. M. AARTS, BEATRIZ GUERRA, AND BURKHARD MALORNY

The emergence of drug-resistant microorganisms is a serious problem worldwide. One of the strategies to combat this problem is to use rapid and informative diagnostic tests. From a clinical point of view, phenotypic methods for susceptibility testing usually provide all the necessary information; i.e., does the isolate grow in the presence of a specific antibiotic at a certain concentration or not? However, there are several reasons why genetic detection methods should be considered when antibiotic resistance is determined. Phenotypic methods, such as disk diffusion or dilution tests, may be time-consuming and less suitable as a rapid diagnostic tool, especially when slow-growing bacteria must be investigated. The direct detection of resistance genes in clinical specimens allows early antibiotic therapy before phenotypic results are available. Genetic methods can be also useful to estimate the resistance risk of strains for which MICs are near the breakpoints for resistance. In addition, genotypic methods are indispensable to better understand the diversity, distribution, and underlying molecular pathways, as well as to locate important reservoirs of antibiotic resistance genes. The combination of molecular characterization of resistant strains with precise identification of the antibiotic resistance gene(s) or mutation(s) and the genetic elements involved in the dissemination of these genes is an effective approach in the control of the spread of antibiotic resistance. Molecular methods also help to determine the location of the gene (chromosomal or extrachromosomal) and to differentiate between horizontal gene transfer and clonal spread. DNA testing is part of a completely different concept (6). Instead of testing for susceptibility, DNA tests indicate whether an antibiotic resistance gene is present or not. The presence or absence of a certain gene corresponding to a particular phenotype, however, does not necessarily imply that the particular strain is resistant or susceptible.

In past years, a large number of genes and mutations responsible for or contributing to resistance were identified and characterized. As a result of these molecular investigations, molecular assays were developed that are currently used in the genetic characterization of resistant strains. Two decades ago, hybridization techniques using radioactive-labeled DNA probes were the only techniques available for the identification of resistance genes. Since its introduction in the mid-1980s, the PCR has become very popular, and it is now a widely used molecular method due to its rapidity and simplicity. However, the molecular mechanisms underlying antibiotic resistance are numerous and complex, and in the future new genes, mutations, and pathways will certainly be discovered. This will lead to a situation where the number of targets is too large for an efficient characterization of the isolate by PCR. A more suitable method would be microarray analysis, a novel molecular tool. Microarray analysis enables screening for a large number of targets simultaneously. This technique was initially used in transcriptomics to study the expression level of many genes simultaneously and is increasingly used in molecular diagnostics. With microarray analysis, it is possible to detect a large number of single genes, mutations, and elements like plasmids, transposons, insertion elements, etc., and it is even possible to simultaneously characterize the strain at the molecular level. For this technology, hybridization of test nucleic acids to DNA probes has become significant. Both PCR and microarray analysis will be described in more detail in this chapter, and applications of these methods in the investigation of antibiotic-resistant strains will be specified. The detection of antibiotic resistance genes using traditional hybridization probes has been previously reviewed (60).

Henk J. M. Aarts • RIKILT, Institute of Food Safety, Wageningen-UR, 6708 PD Wageningen, The Netherlands. **Beatriz Guerra and Burkhard Malorny** • Federal Institute for Risk Assessment, National Salmonella Reference Laboratory, 12277 Berlin, Germany.

The most important molecular technique in unraveling genetic information is sequencing, and it provides the nucleotide sequences of genes and elements and helps to determine the precise location of mutations. Molecular biology has changed enormously in recent years with the advent of the era of genomics; sequencing remains a very important tool, and its speed has increased dramatically. No longer are single genes studied, but the whole genome is now seen as an entity. The number of complete microbial genome sequences is vastly increasing, and with the help of bioinformatics, this enormous amount of sequence data stored in the various public databases is being explored. Genomics and bioinformatics are two new weapons in the battle against antibiotic resistance, and they will improve our understanding of the evolutionary relationship between strains and the various molecular pathways behind antibiotic resistance and provide scientists with essential tools for the discovery of new drug targets or vaccines.

MOLECULAR METHODS TO DETECT RESISTANCE GENES

PCR

The introduction of PCR in the mid-1980s by Kary Mullis has revolutionized molecular diagnostics. Because of its speed, accuracy, and automation, PCR has in the last two decades increasingly been applied to identify and characterize various genetic targets, including a tremendous number of antibiotic resistance genes.

PCR is a three-step cyclic in vitro procedure based on the ability of DNA polymerase to copy a strand of DNA. When two primers bind to complementary strands of target DNA, the sequence in between is amplified exponentially with each cycle, making the technique a very sensitive tool. The choice of the primer sequences determines specificity and, consequently, the success of the PCR. A reaction requires, on average, 1.5 to 2 h of thermal cycling followed by detection of the PCR products. PCR products can be detected according to size or sequence or a combination of both. Commonly, agarose gel electrophoresis, which separates the PCR products in an electric field by size, is used. The products are visualized after separation by staining of the DNA with an intercalating double-stranded DNA (dsDNA) dye, such as ethidium bromide or SYBR Green. Size-dependent detection methods can lead to false interpretation of the result if a potential nonspecific product is the same size as the target product. Therefore, when applying electrophoretic methods, the product should be confirmed by a sequence-dependent detection method, such as restriction fragment analysis, sequencing, or solid-support hybridization technologies, using nylon membranes or microtiter plate-based colorimetric methods. In addition, when solid-support hybridization techniques are used, the sensitivity often increases by a factor of 20 to 100 in comparison to gel electrophoresis (3). Many detecting and genotyping methods have been developed based on the PCR technology and used to identify antibiotic resistance genes, such as restriction fragment length polymorphism-PCR (RFLP-PCR), PCR–single-strand conformation polymorphism (PCR-SSCP), or mismatch amplification mutation assay-PCR (MAMA-PCR) to detect single-nucleotide variations; nested PCR to increase sensitivity; and multiplex PCR to enable the amplification of multiple targets.

Real-time PCR

In the early 1990s, the second generation of PCR technology was introduced by the use of fluorescent dsDNA dyes or DNA probes where the PCR reaction and the detection occurs in a one-step, closed-tube procedure. This new technology is called real-time PCR, since it is possible to record the increase of PCR product online without opening the reaction tube. Data are therefore collected throughout the PCR process, rather than at the end of the PCR. Consequently, real-time PCR can be used for qualitative and quantitative analysis of DNA. The principle relies on fluorescence measurement. There are two main categories, those employing intercalating dsDNA dyes and those using FRET (fluorescence resonance energy transfer) sequence-specific hybridization probes (Fig. 1). The most commonly used intercalating dsDNA dye is SYBR Green. This cyanine dye has essentially no fluorescence of its own, but when it binds the minor groove of DNA it becomes intensely fluorescent following irradiation by light (73). SYBR Green binds nonspecifically to dsDNA, thereby detecting all types of dsDNA. However, the use of a melting curve analysis after amplification can discriminate between the specific and nonspecific PCR products. If highly specific PCR assays are necessary, FRET probe-based formats must be employed. FRET is used in a number of formats to provide specific homogeneous detection of PCR amplification products. The most common FRET probes are hydrolysis probes, or TaqMan probes (39), and hybridization FRET probes (73).

Hydrolysis probes (TaqMan) use a short oligonucleotide of 20 to 30 bases coupled with two

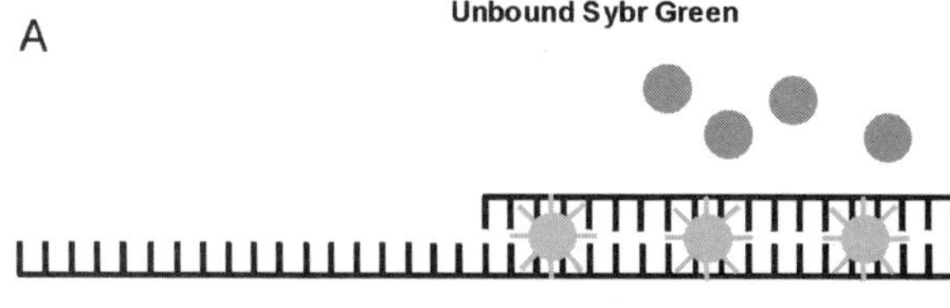

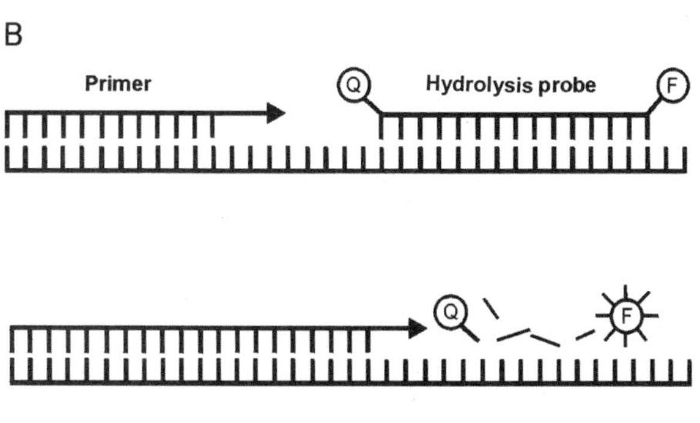

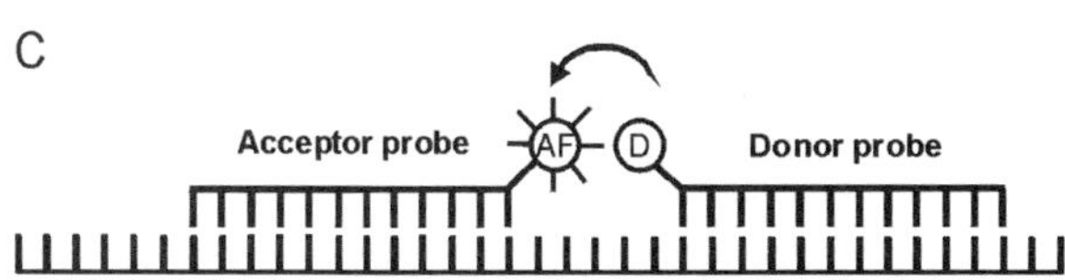

Figure 1. Detection methods in real-time PCR. (A) SYBR Green emits a fluorescent signal when it binds to dsDNA. (B) Specific binding of a double-labeled hydrolysis, or TaqMan, probe. Q indicates the quencher dye and F the fluorescent (reporter) dye. (C) Specific binding of the hybridization FRET probes (acceptor and donor). The donor fluorescence (D) is transmitted to the acceptor fluorescence (AF) only when it is in close proximity, generating a fluorescence signal. See the text for further explanation.

fluorescent dyes: a reporter dye on the 5′ end and a quencher dye attached to the 3′ end. The quencher dye adsorbs the fluorescence from the reporter, preventing the light signal from reaching the detector. During amplification, the 5′ nuclease activity of the DNA polymerase hydrolyzes the probe bound to the target amplification product. The released reporter dye is no longer quenched and can be detected. FRET probes hybridize close to each other (1- to 5-bp spacing) so that the donor and acceptor dye get into sterical conformation. In this conformation FRET can occur, resulting in an enhanced fluorescence signal of the acceptor dye, which serves as the reporter dye in this system. A number of other FRET probes have been described, such as molecular beacons and scorpions.

In the future there will be a demand for early and accurate detection of clinically important drug-resistant pathogens, such as methicillin-resistant *Staphylococcus aureus* (MRSA) strains and vancomycin-resistant enterococci, from carriers, patients, and other biological specimens. Real-time PCR has the potential to meet all diagnostic criteria, and well-validated PCR assays should be implemented routinely in hospital diagnosis.

Applications of PCR to detect resistance genes

Numerous PCR assays in different formats have been developed to detect genes that encode resistance to β-lactams, aminoglycosides, macrolides, glycopeptides, chloramphenicol, florfenicol, tetracyclines, quinolones and fluoroquinolones, sulfonamides, trimethroprim, rifampin, isoniazid, and mupirocin (19, 61). Table 1 shows examples of the detection of antibiotic resistance genes using real-time-based PCR technologies. The ideal target nucleic acid sequences should be located within the open reading frame of the resistance gene, avoiding sequences located outside of the gene.

β-Lactam resistance in gram-negative bacteria. β-Lactamases continue to be the leading cause of resistance to β-lactam antibiotics among gram-negative organisms. In particular, extended-spectrum β-lactamases (ESBLs) are increasingly spreading among gram-negative organisms (47). Genes encoding β-lactamases can be located on either plasmids or the bacterial chromosome and are found among both gram-negative and gram-positive bacteria. They can be discriminated based on their nucleotide sequence homologies and differ in their ability to hydrolyze the various β-lactam antibiotics. The easiest method for detecting the presence of a β-lactamase-encoding gene is PCR with primers that anneal in a highly homologous region of the β-lactamase gene family. However, using these kinds of primers will not discriminate variants within the family. For the identification of specific gene variants of the β-lactamase families AmpC, TEM, SHV, OXA, and CTX-M in gram-negative bacteria, methods using oligonucleotide probes, RFLP-PCR, PCR-SSCP, or a combination of these are necessary. For the determination of novel β-lactamase genes, nucleotide sequencing remains the "gold standard" because of the various point mutations found within the families. Molecular ESBL detection techniques have been summarized previously (8).

Methicillin-resistant staphylococcal strains have emerged worldwide as important nosocomial pathogens, and the use of rapid PCR may play an important role in infection control efforts. Methicillin resistance is mediated primarily by the expression of

Table 1. Real-time PCR assays for the detection of antibiotic resistance genes

Antibiotic agent(s) and gene(s)	Organism	Instrument	Probe format	Identification from:	Reference(s)
Quinolone					
gyrA	*S. enterica*	LightCycler	GAMA[a]	Isolates	70
gyrA	*Campylobacter coli*	LightCycler	Hybridization FRET probe	Isolates	12
grlA	*S. aureus*	SmartCycler	Molecular beacon	Isolates	36
β-Lactams					
mecA	*S. aureus*	LightCycler	TaqMan probe	Isolates	59
mecA	*S. aureus*	SmartCycler	Molecular beacon	Clinical specimens	32
mecA	*S. aureus*	LightCycler	Hybridization FRET probe	Isolates	26
mecA	*S. aureus*	LightCycler	SYBR Green	Isolates	18
ampC	*Enterobacteriaceae*	ABIPrism 7000 and 7700	TaqMan probe	Isolates	67
Glycopeptide					
vanA, *vanB*	Enterococci	LightCycler	Hybridization FRET probe	Isolates, clinical specimens	48, 49
Tetracycline					
tet(R)	*E. coli*	Opticon	SYBR Green	Isolates	43
Rifampin and isoniazid					
rpoB, *katG*	*M. tuberculosis*	LightCycler	Hybridization FRET probe	Clinical specimens	40
rpoB, *inhA*	*M. tuberculosis*	LightCycler	Hybridization FRET probe	Isolates	22, 63
rpoB, *inhA*, *katG*	*M. tuberculosis*	LightCycler	Hybridization FRET probe	Isolates	22
rpoB, *katG*, *erm*(B)	*M. tuberculosis*	ABIPrism 7700	TaqMan minor groove binder	Clinical specimens	69
Clarithromycin and erythromycin					
mefA, *erm*(B)	*Streptococcus pyogenes* and *S. pneumoniae*	LightCycler	SYBR Green	Isolates	52
Penicillin-binding protein					
pbp5	*Enterococcus faecium*	ABIPrism 7700	TaqMan probe	Isolates	42

[a]GAMA, *gyrA* mutation assay.

a unique penicillin-binding protein (PBP), PBP2a, encoded by the *mecA* gene. Numerous molecular approaches have been described for the rapid identification of MRSA based on the *mecA* gene. Recently, a real-time PCR assay was developed for screening and identification of MSRA from clinical samples after enrichment (18) and directly from specimens (32).

Resistance to vancomycin. Resistance to vancomycin is mediated by several gene clusters, including *vanA*, *vanB*, *vanC*, *vanD*, *vanE*, and *vanG*, and is of special interest in enterococci that play a major role in hospital infections. Acquired vancomycin resistances are associated with the *vanA* and *vanB* genotypes and are epidemiologically and clinically the most important types. In contrast, *vanC* causes intrinsic resistance. For the detection of vancomycin resistance, several multiplex PCRs have been described for the simultaneous detection of the *vanA*, *vanB*, *vanC1*, *vanC2*, and *vanC3* types (17). However, the different primer sets may vary in their specificity and sensitivity compared to a singleplex PCR. Therefore, it is recommended to use multiplex PCR assays followed by an additional hybridization step and the use of an internal probe, as routinely performed in the Danish surveillance program for clinical vancomycin-resistant enterococci (51).

Resistance to tetracyclines. There are 24 known tetracycline resistance determinants (*tet*), which encode genes for either efflux pumps or ribosomal protection occurring in many gram-negative and gram-positive genera. Several studies describe the successful use of *tet*-specific DNA probes (21), singleplex PCR in combination with *tet*-specific DNA probes (34), and multiplex PCR to detect specific *tet* genes in different clinical samples and genera (4, 27, 45, 64).

Resistance to fluoroquinolones. Resistance to fluoroquinolones is mediated mainly by point mutations within the QRDR region of the *gyrA* and *gyrB* genes (encoding DNA gyrase) and/or *parC* and *parE* genes (DNA topoisomerase IV) (*grlA* and *grlB* in *S. aureus*). Detection and identification of these point mutations has usually been done by RFLP-PCR, PCR-SSCP, MAMA-PCR, and sequencing (1). Recently, the use of real-time PCR probes (12) and oligonucleotide arrays (72) has been reported. Fluoroquinolone resistance may also be associated with active efflux. Due to the complex active efflux mechanisms in many species, controlled by several regulatory genes, it is complicated to identify potential determinants responsible for resistance. Consequently, the detection of active efflux involves a determination of many parameters and not necessarily a simple molecular test system.

Resistance to rifampin. Rifampin resistance is mainly caused by mutations in the *rpoB* gene of *Mycobacterium tuberculosis* (23). Although sequencing is one of the most frequently applied methods for identifying point mutations within the *rpoB* gene, real-time-based PCR assays are increasingly described for the detection of rifampin resistance (22), including the direct detection in specimens (53).

Resistance to aminoglycosides. Resistance to aminoglycosides is widespread, mediated by more than 50 aminoglycoside-modifying enzymes that are classified as aminoglycoside acetyltransferases (AAC), aminoglycoside adenyltransferases (AAD or ANT), and aminoglycoside phosphotransferases (APH). Probes for specific monitoring of aminoglycoside resistance genes have been previously described (27, 38, 55). Due to the molecular diversity between and within the aminoglycoside resistance families, multiplex PCR has been developed for the detection of aminoglycoside resistance in *Acinetobacter baumannii*, combining three primer sets in order to amplify the genes encoding AAC(6′)-Ih, AAC(3)-I, and AAC(3)-II; three primer pairs for the genes encoding ANT(2″)-I and APH(3′)-VI; and two primer pairs for the genes encoding AAC(6′)-Ib and APH(3′)-I (46). PCRs for the most important aminoglycoside resistance genes, *aac(6′)-Ie*, *aph(2″)*, *aph(3′)-IIIa*, and *ant(4′)-Ia*, in MSRA were developed by Vanhoof et al. (65).

Resistance to chloramphenicol and florfenicol. Genes for chloramphenicol resistance, especially those encoding acetyltransferases (*cat*), are widespread among most genera of gram-positive and -negative bacteria. Although a variety of *cat* determinants have been described, only a few detection methods have been published, probably because chloramphenicol plays a minor role in the treatment of severe infections. Three types of CAT (I to III) in gram-negative bacteria have been described, but type I has been encountered mainly in *Enterobacteriaceae* and is generally plasmid encoded. Genes involving nonenzymatic chloramphenicol and florfenicol resistance have also been described, i.e., *cmlA* from transposon Tn*1696* of *Pseudomonas aeruginosa*, *pp-flo* from *Pasteurella piscicida*, and *floR* from *Salmonella enterica* serovar Typhimurium phage type DT104 and *Escherichia coli*. PCR detection of the genes *catA1*, *cmlA1*-like, and *floR* has been used for the characterisation of multidrug-resistant *S. enterica* serovar Typhimurium strains (29).

Resistance to macrolides, lincosamides, and streptogramins. Macrolide, lincosamide, and streptogramin resistance is mediated by a number of different mechanisms. Many of the genes conferring resistance have been detected by PCR, including (i) the *erm* (erythromycin ribosome methylation) genes coding for methylases modifying the 23S rRNA posttranscriptionally (56); (ii) efflux-mediated genes *mef*, *msr* and *vga* (58); (iii) genes encoding enzymes that hydrolyze streptogramin B [*vgb*(A) and *vgb*(B)] (33); (iv) genes encoding phosphotransferases [*mph*(A) and *mph*(B)] (58); (v) genes encoding acetyltransferases [*vat*, *vat*(B), *vat*(C), *sat*(A), and *sat*(G)] (2, 71); and (vi) genes encoding enzymes that hydrolyze the lactone ring of the macrocyclic nucleus [*ere*(A) and *ere*(B)] (57).

Resistance to trimethoprim and sulfonamides. Trimethoprim resistance is mediated mainly by the acquisition of a *dfr* gene encoding a resistant dihydrofolate reductase. PCR detection assays have been described for some subtypes, such as *dfrA1*-like (28), *dfrA12* (29), *dfrA5-14*, and *dfrA7-dfrA17* (20). The *dfrA1* gene is one of the most frequently detected determinants, probably caused by the successful spread of its carrier transposon, Tn*7*.

Acquired resistance to sulfonamides can result from mutations in the chromosomal dihydropteroate synthase (DHPS) gene (*folP*) or by acquisition of resistant DHPS genes (*sul* genes), whose products have a lower affinity for sulfonamides. Three genes encoding resistance to DHPS in gram-negative bacteria are known (*sul1*, *sul2*, and *sul3*). They show low

DNA homology to each other and are often plasmid borne. PCR primers have been developed to detect them (13, 38, 50).

Detection and characterization of genetic elements involved in the dissemination of resistance genes. Mobile genetic elements such as plasmids, phages, transposons, and integrons and gene cassettes are usually implicated in the horizontal spread of resistance determinants between bacteria (11). The genotypic characterization of the antimicrobial resistance also implies the detection and characterization of some of these elements. For the detection of class 1 and class 2 integrons (the most common found among *Enterobacteriaceae*), primers that allow the amplification of their variable regions (binding to the conserved segments) have been used (38). The genes or gene cassettes forming part of these variable regions were characterized mainly by sequencing, RFLP-PCR, or PCR amplification combining primers of known genes (27). Additional information is given by the amplification of genes commonly associated with the integrons (i.e., integrase genes, *sul1*, *qacE*Δ1, etc.) and transposons (i.e., genes encoding transposases and resolvases, *merA*) (27, 41). Since resistance determinants are often located on plasmids, the characterization of these plasmids (i.e., self-transferability and incompatibility group) is an important tool for epidemiological purposes (27, 29). However, for *S. enterica* serovars it has been described that many drug resistance genes can be clustered within a specific 43-kb chromosomal region, called *Salmonella* genomic island 1 (SGI1) (7, 15). This region harbors many mobile genetic elements that are used for the rapid exchange of antibiotic resistance genes. Specific efflux systems have been identified with resistances mainly to macrolides, lincosamides, and/or streptogramins; tetracyclines; and chloramphenicol and florfenicol, in gram-positive and gram-negative bacteria. It has been shown that genes coding for specific efflux systems are often associated with mobile genetic elements that can be easily interchanged between bacteria (9).

Microarray Analysis

DNA microarray analysis is a promising alternative to PCR. Microarray analysis enables the screening of a large set of targets simultaneously. Although microarrays have been used mainly for gene expression studies in transcriptomics, they are becoming increasingly popular in diagnostic microbiology, including the detection of antibiotic resistance genes. A variety of platforms have been developed. The solid supports can be glass microscope slides, silicon chips, nylon membranes, three-dimensional chips, or even electrochips. Microarrays can be spotted or printed, or the probes can be synthesized directly onto the support (for example, one manufactured by Affymetrix), and spots can be DNA, cDNA, or oligonucleotides. The web pages found at http://genome-www5.stanford.edu give an overview of the available microarray resources and general microarray information.

The basic principle of microarray analysis is the same as in Southern blotting (probe hybridization), namely that complementary nucleotide sequences of DNA (or RNA) will match up. A DNA microarray consists of an orderly arrangement of spotted probes on a solid support. Due to the use of highly accurate robotic spotters, the density of spots on an array can be very high. This high density of probes makes it possible to analyze the expression of a large set of genes or to screen for the presence of a large set of targets (genes or mutations) simultaneously. In expression studies, RNA is converted to cDNA, fluorescently labeled, and laid atop the array. At least for highly expressed genes, the number of RNA copies is high, resulting in strong hybridization signals. If microarray analysis is used for detection purposes, the number of target molecules can be too low. In these cases the number of target DNA molecules is amplified by PCR methods prior to hybridization. For the detection of the β-lactam antibiotic resistance families PSE, OXA, FOX, MEN, CMY, TEM, SHV, OXY, and AmpC, Lee et al. (37) developed a microarray to analyze PCR-amplified target DNA. The probes spotted on the array consisted of DNA sequences that were generated by PCR with a primer set specific for each gene. The authors used primers that were modified at the 5′ ends with a $(CH_2)_6$ linker and an amine group. The amine group on the DNA was coupled with the aldehyde group on the slide by the Schiff's base reaction. Target plasmid DNA was isolated from *E. coli* and *Klebsiella pneumoniae* cells and amplified in a multiplex PCR reaction. It was demonstrated that *oxy* genes could be specifically detected even from a single bacterium.

Volokhov et al. (68) described the use of asymmetric multiplex PCR using three pairs of primers to synthesize Cy5-labeled single-stranded DNA samples. These fluorescently labeled PCR products were hybridized to an oligonucleotide microarray containing seven oligonucleotide probes for each of the six macrolide-lincosamide-streptogramin B (MLS) genes, namely *erm*(A), *erm*(B), *erm*(C), *ere*(A), *ere*(B), and *msr*(A/B). These genes account for more than 98% of MLS resistance in *S. aureus*. The length of the oligonucleotides used varied between 19 and 31 nucleotides, with a basic melting temperature varying between 47 and 61°C. Besides the correct identification of the MLS resistance genes in a set of reference strains, this microarray was also used to successfully screen clinical isolates.

Oligonucleotide microarray analysis was also used by Yue et al. (75) to detect single-nucleotide polymorphisms and other rearrangements in the *rpoB* gene region determining rifampin resistance. The target in the genetic material of rifampin-resistant and -susceptible *M. tuberculosis* strains was amplified, labeled, and used to overlay a 50-mer oligonucleotide probe array. With this approach, these authors were able to identify the 1% of the strains that were resistant in a background of 99% susceptible bacteria. It was shown that the oligonucleotide microarray technique can be used as a rapid method for the detection of rifampin resistance to complement standard culture-based methods. A similar approach was followed to detect single-nucleotide polymorphisms in TEM β-lactamase variants related to the ESBL or inhibitor-resistant TEM (IRT) phenotype (25) and to detect single-base mutations in quinolone-resistant *E. coli* (74). Grimm et al. (25) conducted experiments to reduce the time of analysis. The time-consuming hybridization step could be reduced to 30 min, resulting in a total assay time (PCR, hybridization, and image analysis) of less than 3.5 h, and still retained sufficient discriminatory power. As already mentioned, amplification methods are often used to increase the number of targets in order to reach an appropriate hybridization signal on the array. However, due to the small size of the bacterial genome, Call et al. (10) were able to correctly identify the *tet* genes present in, for instance, *Actinobacter* spp., *E. coli*, and *Pseudomonas fluorescens* by directly labeling the total DNA of the tested strains. The isolated DNA was labeled by nick translation prior to hybridization to an array containing PCR products varying in length between 494 and 571 bp. Results obtained by van Hoek et al. (64a) and Malorny et al. (B. Malorny et al., unpublished data) showed that a combination of direct labeling (random prime labeling) and the use of oligonucleotides having a length of 40 to 60 nucleotides is still feasible for the detection of antibiotic resistance genes in bacteria.

GENOMICS AND BIOINFORMATICS TO COMBAT ANTIBIOTIC RESISTANCE

In the pregenomic era, single genes and the mechanisms underlying the resistant phenotypes of microorganisms were detected and studied by standard molecular techniques. Probably the most important technique was and is still sequencing, and since its development in 1977 it has become a standard procedure in all molecular biology laboratories. In principle, the technique has not changed, but its speed, due to automation, has increased significantly. This has led to the current situation, in which the amount of DNA sequenced has expanded enormously. Sequencing and storage of the sequence information in databases is one of the first steps in genomics. Genomics does not deal with the investigation of individual genes but involves the discovery and identification of all the genes in a particular genome. The whole genome is seen as the unit of investigation. A genome is considered as the DNA that encompasses the entire genetic information of an organism, including extrachromosomal DNA, such as plasmids.

The effort put into sequencing has vastly increased the number of whole genomes that are being sequenced. For instance, Coenye and Vandamme (14) retrieved in total 323 bacterial genomes from a large number of databases. This overwhelming amount of sequence information will greatly contribute to a better understanding of the pathways involved in antibiotic resistance, through the detection of orthologs in different bacteria and paralogs within the same genome; furthermore, it can play a role in determining the evolutionary relationships of antibiotic resistance genes and the genomes of resistant bacteria. The availability of sequence information on such a large number of microorganisms and related technologies will also contribute to the discovery of new drugs and vaccines to combat antibiotic-resistant microorganisms.

The tremendous amount of information has necessitated the creation and maintenance of databases and the development of bioinformatics tools to carry out computational biology. Bioinformatics involves, besides the recording, annotation, and storage of sequences, the analytical approach of comparing sequence data to find shared characteristics. It also involves the prediction of the possible secondary and tertiary structure of proteins and accordingly the prediction of their possible function. A third approach in bioinformatics is the generation of phylogenetic trees to examine evolutionary relationships between strains or genes.

The Internet is becoming an essential aid for sequence retrieval and analysis. On the Internet, search engines are available to explore the huge amount of stored data. A very popular tool to compare the information in the databases with a query sequence is the Basic Local Alignment Search Tool (BLAST). This tool can be found on the National Center for Biotechnology Information web pages (http://www.ncbi.nlm.nih.gov/). These pages also contain tutorials for new and experienced users in employing BLAST and PSI-BLAST in their research. Searches end in the retrieval of related sequences. This is also the first step in the development of specific PCR primers and oligonucleotides that can be used for PCR detection or as probes on a microarray. After retrieval, the related sequences are aligned by using software that has been specifically designed for this purpose, such as CLUSTAL X, developed by Thompson et al. (62). Alignment will indicate those regions within a sequence with the highest or lowest level of variation and hence the preferred sequence regions for the development of the needed primers and probes. Another straightforward strategy for the development of primers and probes is first to design a number of possible candidates based on the whole sequence of the target gene and subsequently to check for their specificity by alignment with related sequences. In both cases, however, the developed oligonucleotides need to be checked for potential interference with other sequences, by alignment of the oligonucleotide sequences using BLAST with all sequences present in the databases. Despite this effort, the specificity and selectivity of the primers still have to be proven in the laboratory in all cases.

Aminov et al. (4) demonstrated the applicability of molecular ecology techniques by using bioinformatics in the development of appropriate PCR tests to estimate the gene pool and the flux of antibiotic resistance genes in production animals. Phylogenetic analysis was performed with 25 complete nucleotide sequences encoding ribosomal protection proteins, which revealed the monophyletic origin of these genes. On the basis of this phylogenetic analysis, these authors designed PCR primers that were used to detect antibiotic resistance genes in the microbiota of the rumina of cows, in swine feed and feces, and in swine fecal streptococci. It was observed, for instance, that *tet*(O) and *tet*(W) circulated in the microbiota of the rumina and the gastrointestinal tracts of pigs, despite the difference in animal host and antibiotic use regimens. Additionally, the authors demonstrated that the fecal streptococci (enterococci) are one of the main reservoirs of the *tet*(O) and *tet*(M) genes in the pig gastrointestinal tract.

Bioinformatics mostly precedes the "wet" science carried out in the laboratory, but bioinformatics tools are also used to confirm earlier observations, like the study carried out by Kim et al. (35). Using the information present in sequence databases, these authors carried out a binary alignment of the extended region of the LmrA multidrug resistance (MDR) efflux pump (a member of the ABC superfamily) with a portion of the MexB MDR efflux pump of the RND superfamily and showed a similarity between the two proteins. Statistical analyses indicated that this similarity could not have arisen by chance, but was most likely due to functional and evolutionary connection. Here bioinformatics confirmed the observations made by Saier (54), who had already suggested that the primary active transporter, LmrA, was derived from a secondary active transporter by superimposition of the ATP-hydrolyzing subunit.

QUALITY ASPECTS OF MOLECULAR ASSAYS

It should never be assumed that published probes and PCR primers were sufficiently tested or designed according to the state of the art in bioinformatics software and databases. Consequently, there must be a critical review of each assay with respect to the availability of validated data. Their often inherent complexity requires that special attention be paid to the design and use of controls and standards. Specifically, the detection of antibiotic resistance genes, with their often highly homologous gene sequences and localization in the genome of the bacterium, and the detection of the genes directly in the biological specimens requires a full range of validation before use. Fortunately, experts are increasingly focusing on validation of test systems and assays. Methods for validation are published by the National Committee for Clinical Laboratory Standards (44), and a protocol for the validation of alternative methods recently became an international standard document (5).

When an assay for the detection of antibiotic resistance genes is to be designed, the following steps should be strongly considered. (i) Primer and probe design should be based on sequence alignments and other bioinformatics aspects, for example, BLAST searches, in order to confirm their specificity. (ii) The selectivity should be tested empirically using appropriate reference material (e.g., target and nontarget pure cultures) with a sufficient number of samples. (iii) Assessment of the detection probability is necessary. (iv) The construction of an internal control is mandatory (30). (v) If diagnostic tests are desired, the accuracy should be investigated by using a variety and sufficient number of biological specimens and samples in comparison to another standard method. (vi) Ring trials have to be organized to document the interlaboratory performance of the assay.

Controls and Standards

Amplification assays should always be used with a set of controls that consists of at least a positive and negative assay control and, if necessary, a positive and negative process control. In addition, diagnostic nucleic acid amplification assays need an internal control to avoid false-negative results. The construction of internal controls for diagnostic PCR assays has been reviewed recently (31).

Standards are defined as well-characterized reference material used for assay validation, interlaboratory comparisons, and proficiency testing (16). Reference material should be always delivered and stored in a stabilized condition and tested regularly according to its characteristics. For nucleic acid-based detection methods, nucleic acids isolated from biological material can serve as a primary standard. Unfortunately, there is no organization providing the scientific community with DNA and RNA isolated from antibiotic-resistant strains. Therefore, strains and nucleic acids are exchanged between laboratories. The risk of this practice is that resistance determinants and other characteristics can be lost or modified due to inappropriate handling and storing. Personnel of laboratories receiving reference material should therefore be trained in handling and storage of such material. Laboratories sending out reference material should regularly confirm the properties of the material.

Quality Assurance of Laboratories

Besides validating applied test systems, the diagnostic laboratory should have an established quality assurance program. It should include regular participation in interlaboratory studies (ring trials) and proficiency tests as well as appropriate laboratory design and work flow in order to prevent false-positive results due to contamination with exogenous nucleic acids, in addition to other external quality assurance assessments (66). Laboratory controls and appropriate assay controls and standards are necessary to document the reliability of the results.

CONCLUDING REMARKS

As shown in this chapter, numerous PCR assays for the detection of antibiotic resistance genes have been developed and the development of microarrays for the simultaneous detection of a large number of these genes and the genetic elements involved in their dissemination is in progress. This development will eventually meet the demand for early and accurate detection and characterization of clinically important drug-resistant pathogens. PCR technologies are moving from conventional assays to real-time-based PCR assays, opening the possibility of quantitating antimicrobial resistance genes of pathogens directly in clinical samples.

The implementation of molecular methods in routine analysis can be achieved only when it is supported by the proper validation of the methods and the availability of the necessary controls, reference strains, and educated personnel.

The developments described above will probably lead to a situation in which antibiotic-resistant strains can be more easily characterized, not only as to their antibiotic properties but also their pathogenic and biochemical properties. The molecular characterization of antibiotic-resistant strains will help to identify atypical resistant strains, describe new outbreak strains at an early stage, elucidate the epidemiology of resistant strains at a genotypic level, and explain the processes leading to the selection of resistant and virulent strains. In addition, molecular methods will allow proper risk assessment with respect to the use of antimicrobial substances.

Phenotypic susceptibility testing is currently necessary for the determination of MICs. If the transcriptional and translational expression of antibiotic resistance genes becomes better understood, molecular methods may replace phenotypic measurements.

REFERENCES

1. **Aarts, H. J. M., K. S. Boumedine, X. Nesme, and A. Cloeckaert.** 2001. Molecular tools for the characterisation of antibiotic-resistant bacteria. *Vet. Res.* **32:**363–380.
2. **Allignet, J., S. Aubert, A. Morvan, and N. El Solh.** 1996. Distribution of genes encoding resistance to streptogramin A and related compounds among staphylococci resistant to these antibiotics. *Antimicrob. Agents Chemother.* **40:**2523–2528.
3. **Altweg, M.** 1995. General problems associated with diagnostic applications of amplification methods. *J. Microbiol. Methods* **23:**21–30.
4. **Aminov, R. I., N. Garrigues-Jeanjean, and R. I. Mackie.** 2001. Molecular ecology of tetracycline resistance: development and validation of primers for detection of tetracycline resistance genes encoding ribosomal protection proteins. *Appl. Environ. Microbiol.* **67:**22–32.
5. **Anonymous.** 2003. Microbiology of food and animal feeding stuffs—protocol for the validation of alternative methods (ISO 16140:2003). European Committee for Standardization, AFNOR, Paris, France.
6. **Bergeron, M. G., and M. Ouellette.** 1998. Preventing antibiotic resistance using rapid DNA-based diagnostic tests. *Infect. Control Hosp. Epidemiol.* **19:**560–564.
7. **Boyd, D., A. Cloeckaert, E. Chaslus-Dancla, and M. R. Mulvey.** 2002. Characterization of variant *Salmonella* genomic island 1 multidrug resistance regions from serovars Typhimurium DT104 and Agona. *Antimicrob. Agents Chemother.* **46:**1714–1722.
8. **Bradford, P. A.** 2001. Extended-spectrum beta-lactamases in the 21st century: characterization, epidemiology, and detection of this important resistance threat. *Clin. Microbiol. Rev.* **14:**933–951.
9. **Butaye, P., A. Cloeckaert, and S. Schwarz.** 2003. Mobile genes coding for efflux-mediated antimicrobial resistance in Gram-positive and Gram-negative bacteria. *Int. J. Antimicrob. Agents* **22:**205–210.

10. **Call, D. R., M. K. Bakko, M. J. Krug, and M. C. Roberts.** 2003. Identifying antimicrobial resistance genes with DNA microarrays. *Antimicrob. Agents Chemother.* **47:**3290–3295.
11. **Carattoli, A.** 2001. Importance of integrons in the diffusion of resistance. *Vet Res.* **32:**243–259.
12. **Carattoli, A., A. Dionisi, and I. Luzzi.** 2002. Use of a LightCycler *gyrA* mutation assay for identification of ciprofloxacin-resistant *Campylobacter coli. FEMS Microbiol. Lett.* **214:** 87–93.
13. **Chu, C., C. H. Chiu, W. Y. Wu, C. H. Chu, T. P. Liu, and J. T. Ou.** 2001. Large drug resistance virulence plasmids of clinical isolates of *Salmonella enterica* serovar Choleraesuis. *Antimicrob. Agents Chemother.* **45:**2299–2303.
14. **Coenye, T., and P. Vandamme.** 2004. Bacterial whole-genome sequences: minimal information and strain availability. *Microbiology* **150:**2017–2018.
15. **Doublet, B., R. Lailler, D. Meunier, A. Brisabois, D. Boyd, M. R. Mulvey, E. Chaslus-Dancla, and A. Cloeckaert.** 2003. Variant *Salmonella* genomic island 1 antibiotic resistance gene cluster in *Salmonella enterica* serovar Albany. *Emerg. Infect. Dis.* **9:**585–591.
16. **DuBois, D. B., and J. T. Brown.** 2004. Laboratory controls and standards, p. 697–703. *In* D. H. Persing, F. C. Tenover, J. Versalovic, Y.-W. Tang, E. R. Unger, D. A. Relman, and T. J. White (ed.), *Molecular Microbiology: Diagnostic Principles and Practice*. American Society for Microbiology, Washington, D.C.
17. **Dutka-Malen, S., S. Evers, and P. Courvalin.** 1995. Detection of glycopeptide resistance genotypes and identification to the species level of clinically relevant enterococci by PCR. *J. Clin. Microbiol.* **33:**24–27.
18. **Fang, H., and G. Hedin.** 2003. Rapid screening and identification of methicillin-resistant *Staphylococcus aureus* from clinical samples by selective-broth and real-time PCR assay. *J. Clin. Microbiol.* **41:**2894–2899.
19. **Fluit, A. C., M. R. Visser, and F. J. Schmitz.** 2001. Molecular detection of antimicrobial resistance. *Clin. Microbiol. Rev.* **14:**836–871.
20. **Frech, G., C. Kehrenberg, and S. Schwarz.** 2003. Resistance phenotypes and genotypes of multiresistant *Salmonella enterica* subsp. *enterica* serovar Typhimurium var. Copenhagen isolates from animal sources. *J. Antimicrob. Chemother.* **51:** 180–182.
21. **Frech, G., and S. Schwarz.** 2000. Molecular analysis of tetracycline resistance in *Salmonella enterica* subsp. *enterica* serovars Typhimurium, Enteritidis, Dublin, Choleraesuis, Hadar and Saintpaul: construction and application of specific gene probes. *J. Appl. Microbiol.* **89:**633–641.
22. **García de Viedma, D., M. D. S. Díaz Infantes, F. Lasala, F. Chaves, L. Alcalá, and E. Bouza.** 2002. New real-time PCR able to detect in a single tube multiple rifampin resistance mutations and high-level isoniazid resistance mutations in *Mycobacterium tuberculosis. J. Clin. Microbiol.* **40:**988–995.
23. **Garcia de Viedma, D. G.** 2002. Rapid detection of resistance in *Mycobacterium tuberculosis*: a review discussing molecular approaches. *Clin. Microbiol. Infect.* **9:**349–359.
24. Reference deleted.
25. **Grimm, V., S. Ezaki, M. Susa, C. Knabbe, R. D. Schmid, and T. T. Bachmann.** 2004. Use of DNA microarrays for rapid genotyping of TEM beta-lactamases that confer resistance. *J. Clin. Microbiol.* **42:**3766–3774.
26. **Grisold, A. J., E. Leitner, G. Muhlbauer, E. Marth, and H. H. Kessler.** 2002. Detection of methicillin-resistant *Staphylococcus aureus* and simultaneous confirmation by automated nucleic acid extraction and real-time PCR. *J. Clin. Microbiol.* **40:**2392–2397.
27. **Guerra, B., E. Junker, A. Miko, R. Helmuth, and M. C. Mendoza.** 2004. Characterization and localization of drug resistance determinants in multidrug-resistant, integron-carrying *Salmonella enterica* serotype Typhimurium strains. *Microb. Drug Resist.* **10:**83–91.
28. **Guerra, B., S. Soto, S. Cal, and M. C. Mendoza.** 2000. Antimicrobial resistance and spread of class 1 integrons among *Salmonella* serotypes. *Antimicrob. Agents Chemother.* **44:** 2166–2169.
29. **Guerra, B., S. M. Soto, J. M. Arguelles, and M. C. Mendoza.** 2001. Multidrug resistance is mediated by large plasmids carrying a class 1 integron in the emergent *Salmonella enterica* serotype [4,5,12:i:-]. *Antimicrob. Agents Chemother.* **45:**1305–1308.
30. **Hoorfar, J., N. Cook, B. Malorny, M. Wagner, D. De Medici, A. Abdulmawjood, and P. Fach.** 2003. Making internal amplification control mandatory for diagnostic PCR. *J. Clin. Microbiol.* **41:**5835.
31. **Hoorfar, J., B. Malorny, A. Abdulmawjood, N. Cook, and P. Fach.** 2003. Practical considerations when designing internal amplification control for diagnostic PCR assays. *J. Clin. Microbiol.* **42:**1863–1868.
32. **Huletsky, A., R. Giroux, V. Rossbach, M. Gagnon, M. Vaillancourt, M. Bernier, F. Gagnon, K. Truchon, M. Bastien, F. J. Picard, A. van Belkum, M. Ouellette, P. H. Roy, and M. G. Bergeron.** 2004. New real-time PCR assay for rapid detection of methicillin-resistant *Staphylococcus aureus* directly from specimens containing a mixture of staphylococci. *J. Clin. Microbiol.* **42:**1875–1884.
33. **Jensen, L. B., A. M. Hammerum, F. M. Aarestrup, A. E. van den Bogaard, and E. E. Stobberingh.** 1998. Occurrence of *satA* and *vgb* genes in streptogramin-resistant *Enterococcus faecium* isolates of animal and human origins in The Netherlands. *Antimicrob. Agents Chemother.* **42:**3330–3331.
34. **Kehrenberg, C., S. A. Salmon, J. L. Watts, and S. Schwarz.** 2001. Tetracycline resistance genes in isolates of *Pasteurella multocida*, *Mannheimia haemolytica*, *Mannheimia glucosida* and *Mannheimia varigena* from bovine and swine respiratory disease: intergeneric spread of the *tet*(H) plasmid pMHT1. *J. Antimicrob. Chemother.* **48:**631–640.
35. **Kim, S. H., A. B. Chang, and M. H. Saier, Jr.** 2004. Sequence similarity between multidrug resistance efflux pumps of the ABC and RND superfamilies. *Microbiology* **150:**2493–2495.
36. **Lapierre, P., A. Huletsky, V. Fortin, F. J. Picard, P. H. Roy, M. Ouellette, and M. G. Bergeron.** 2003. Real-time PCR assay for detection of fluoroquinolone resistance associated with *grlA* mutations in *Staphylococcus aureus*. *J. Clin. Microbiol.* **41:**3246–3251.
37. **Lee, Y., C. S. Lee, Y. J. Kim, S. Chun, S. Park, Y. S. Kim, and B. D. Han.** 2002. Development of DNA chip for the simultaneous detection of various beta-lactam antibiotic-resistant genes. *Mol. Cell* **14:**192–197.
38. **Levesque, C., L. Piche, C. Larose, and P. H. Roy.** 1995. PCR mapping of integrons reveals several novel combinations of resistance genes. *Antimicrob. Agents Chemother.* **39:**185–191.
39. **Livak, K. J., S. J. Flood, J. Marmaro, W. Giusti, and K. Deetz.** 1995. Oligonucleotides with fluorescent dyes at opposite ends provide a quenched probe system useful for detecting PCR product and nucleic acid hybridization. *PCR Methods Appl.* **4:**357–362.
40. **Marín, M., D. García de Viedma, M. J. Ruiz-Serrano, and E. Bouza.** 2004. Rapid direct detection of multiple rifampin and isoniazid resistance mutations in *Mycobacterium tuberculosis*

in respiratory samples by real-time PCR. *Antimicrob. Agents Chemother.* 48:4293–4300.

41. **Miko, A., K. Pries, A. Schroeter, and R. Helmuth.** 2003. Multiple-drug resistance in D-tartrate-positive *Salmonella enterica* serovar Paratyphi B isolates from poultry is mediated by class 2 integrons inserted into the bacterial chromosome. *Antimicrob. Agents Chemother.* 47:3640–3643.
42. **Mohn, S. C., A. Ulvik, R. Jureen, R. J. Willems, J. Top, H. Leavis, S. Harthug, and N. Langeland.** 2004. Duplex real-time PCR assay for rapid detection of ampicillin-resistant *Enterococcus faecium. Antimicrob. Agents Chemother.* 48: 556–560.
43. **Morsczeck, C., D. Langendorfer, and J. M. Schierholz.** 2004. A quantitative real-time PCR assay for the detection of *tetR* of Tn10 in *Escherichia coli* using SYBR Green and the Opticon. *J. Biochem. Biophys. Methods* 59:217–227.
44. **National Committee for Clinical Laboratory Standards.** 1995. Molecular diagnostics methods for infectious diseases. Approved guideline MM3-A, vol. 15, no. 22. National Committee for Clinical Laboratory Standards, Wayne, Pa.
45. **Ng, L. K., I. Martin, M. Alfa, and M. Mulvey.** 2001. Multiplex PCR for the detection of tetracycline resistant genes. *Mol. Cell Probes* 15:209–215.
46. **Noppe-Leclercq, I., F. Wallet, S. Haentjens, R. Courcol, and M. Simonet.** 1999. PCR detection of aminoglycoside resistance genes: a rapid molecular typing method for *Acinetobacter baumannii. Res. Microbiol.* 150:317–322.
47. **Nordmann, P.** 1998. Trends in beta-lactam resistance among Enterobacteriaceae. *Clin. Infect. Dis.* 27(Suppl. 1):S100–S106.
48. **Palladino, S., I. D. Kay, A. M. Costa, E. J. Lambert, and J. P. Flexman.** 2003. Real-time PCR for the rapid detection of *vanA* and *vanB* genes. *Diagn. Microbiol. Infect. Dis.* 45:81–84.
49. **Palladino, S., I. D. Kay, J. P. Flexman, I. Boehm, A. M. Costa, E. J. Lambert, and K. J. Christiansen.** 2003. Rapid detection of *vanA* and *vanB* genes directly from clinical specimens and enrichment broths by real-time multiplex PCR assay. *J. Clin. Microbiol.* 41:2483–2486.
50. **Perreten, V., and P. Boerlin.** 2003. A new sulfonamide resistance gene (*sul3*) in *Escherichia coli* is widespread in the pig population of Switzerland. *Antimicrob. Agents Chemother.* 47:1169–1172.
51. **Poulsen, R. L., L. V. Pallesen, N. Frimodt-Moller, and F. Espersen.** 1999. Detection of clinical vancomycin-resistant enterococci in Denmark by multiplex PCR and sandwich hybridization. *APMIS* 107:404–412.
52. **Reinert, R. R., C. Franken, L. M. van der, R. Lutticken, M. Cil, and A. Al Lahham.** 2004. Molecular characterisation of macrolide resistance mechanisms of *Streptococcus pneumoniae* and *Streptococcus pyogenes* isolated in Germany, 2002–2003. *Int. J. Antimicrob. Agents* 24:43–47.
53. **Ruiz, M., M. J. Torres, A. C. Llanos, A. Arroyo, J. C. Palomares, and J. Aznar.** 2004. Direct detection of rifampin- and isoniazid-resistant *Mycobacterium tuberculosis* in auramine-rhodamine-positive sputum specimens by real-time PCR. *J. Clin. Microbiol.* 42:1585–1589.
54. **Saier, M. H., Jr.** 2000. Vectorial metabolism and the evolution of transport systems. *J. Bacteriol.* 182:5029–5035.
55. **Sandvang, D., and F. M. Aarestrup.** 2000. Characterization of aminoglycoside resistance genes and class 1 integrons in porcine and bovine gentamicin-resistant *Escherichia coli. Microb. Drug Resist.* 6:19–27.
56. **Schmitz, F. J., R. Sadurski, A. Kray, M. Boos, R. Geisel, K. Kohrer, J. Verhoef, and A. C. Fluit.** 2000. Prevalence of macrolide-resistance genes in *Staphylococcus aureus* and *Enterococcus faecium* isolates from 24 European university hospitals. *J. Antimicrob. Chemother.* 45:891–894.
57. **Shortridge, V. D., R. K. Flamm, N. Ramer, J. Beyer, and S. K. Tanaka.** 1996. Novel mechanism of macrolide resistance in *Streptococcus pneumoniae. Diagn. Microbiol. Infect. Dis.* 26:73–78.
58. **Sutcliffe, J., T. Grebe, A. Tait-Kamradt, and L. Wondrack.** 1996. Detection of erythromycin-resistant determinants by PCR. *Antimicrob Agents Chemother.* 40:2562–2566.
59. **Tan, T. Y., S. Corden, R. Barnes, and B. Cookson.** 2001. Rapid identification of methicillin-resistant *Staphylococcus aureus* from positive blood cultures by real-time fluorescence PCR. *J. Clin. Microbiol.* 39:4529–4531.
60. **Tenover, F. C., and J. K. Rasheed.** 1999. Genetic methods for detecting antibacterial and antiviral resistance genes, p. 1578–1592. *In* P. R. Murray, E. J. Baron, M. A. Pfaller, F. C. Tenover, and R. H. Yolken (ed.), *Manual of Clinical Microbiology*, 7th ed. American Society for Microbiology, Washington, D.C.
61. **Tenover, F. C., and J. K. Rasheed.** 2004. Detection of antimicrobial resistance genes and mutations associated with antimicrobial resistance in microorganisms, p. 391–406. *In* D. H. Persing, F. C. Tenover, J. Versalovic, Y.-W. Tang, E. R. Unger, D. A. Relman, and T. J. White (ed.), *Molecular Microbiology: Diagnostic Principles and Practice.* American Society for Microbiology, Washington, D.C.
62. **Thompson, J. D., T. J. Gibson, F. Plewniak, F. Jeanmougin, and D. G. Higgins.** 1997. The CLUSTAL_X windows interface: flexible strategies for multiple sequence alignment aided by quality analysis tools. *Nucleic Acids Res.* 25: 4876–4882.
63. **Torres, M. J., A. Criado, M. Ruiz, A. C. Llanos, J. C. Palomares, and J. Aznar.** 2003. Improved real-time PCR for rapid detection of rifampin and isoniazid resistance in *Mycobacterium tuberculosis* clinical isolates. *Diagn. Microbiol. Infect. Dis.* 45:207–212.
64. **Trzcinski, K., B. S. Cooper, W. Hryniewicz, and C. G. Dowson.** 2000. Expression of resistance to tetracyclines in strains of methicillin-resistant *Staphylococcus aureus. J. Antimicrob. Chemother.* 45:763–770.

64a. **van Hoek, A. H. A. M., I. M. J. Scholtens, A. Cloeckaert, and H. J. M. Aarts.** 2005. Detection of antibiotic resistance genes in different *Salmonella* serovars by oligonucleotide microarray analysis. *J. Microbiol. Methods* 62:13–23.

65. **Vanhoof, R., C. Godard, J. Content, H. J. Nyssen, and E. Hannecart-Pokorni.** 1994. Detection by polymerase chain reaction of genes encoding aminoglycoside-modifying enzymes in methicillin-resistant *Staphylococcus aureus* isolates of epidemic phage types. *J. Med. Microbiol.* 41:282–290.
66. **Versalovic, J., and E. R. Unger.** 2004. External quality assessment and proficiency testing in diagnostic molecular microbiology, p. 691–696. *In* D. H. Persing, F. C. Tenover, J. Versalovic, Y.-W. Tang, E. R. Unger, D. A. Relman, and T. J. White (eds.), *Molecular Microbiology: Diagnostic Principles and Practice.* American Society for Microbiology, Washington, D.C.
67. **Volkmann, H., T. Schwartz, P. Bischoff, S. Kirchen, and U. Obst.** 2004. Detection of clinically relevant antibiotic-resistance genes in municipal wastewater using real-time PCR (TaqMan). *J. Microbiol. Methods* 56:277–286.
68. **Volokhov, D., V. Chizhikov, K. Chumakov, and A. Rasooly.** 2003. Microarray analysis of erythromycin resistance determinants. *J. Appl. Microbiol.* 95:787–798.
69. **Wada, T., S. Maeda, A. Tamaru, S. Imai, A. Hase, and K. Kobayashi.** 2004. Dual-probe assay for rapid detection of drug-resistant *Mycobacterium tuberculosis* by real-time PCR. *J. Clin. Microbiol.* 42:5277–5285.
70. **Walker, R. A., N. Saunders, A. J. Lawson, E. A. Lindsay, M. Dassama, L. R. Ward, M. J. Woodward, R. H. Davies,**

E. Liebana, and E. J. Threlfall. 2001. Use of a LightCycler *gyrA* mutation assay for rapid identification of mutations conferring decreased susceptibility to ciprofloxacin in multiresistant *Salmonella enterica* serotype Typhimurium DT104 isolates. *J. Clin. Microbiol.* **39:**1443–1448.

71. **Werner, G., and W. Witte.** 1999. Characterization of a new enterococcal gene, *satG*, encoding a putative acetyltransferase conferring resistance to streptogramin A compounds. *Antimicrob. Agents Chemother.* **43:**1813–1814.

72. **Westin, L., C. Miller, D. Vollmer, D. Canter, R. Radtkey, M. Nerenberg, and J. P. O'Connell.** 2001. Antimicrobial resistance and bacterial identification utilizing a microelectronic chip array. *J. Clin. Microbiol.* **39:**1097–1104.

73. **Wittwer, C. T., M. G. Herrmann, A. A. Moss, and R. P. Rasmussen.** 1997. Continuous fluorescence monitoring of rapid cycle DNA amplification. *Biotechniques* **22:**130–138.

74. **Yu, X., M. Susa, C. Knabbe, R. D. Schmid, and T. T. Bachmann.** 2004. Development and validation of a diagnostic DNA microarray to detect quinolone-resistant *Escherichia coli* among clinical isolates. *J. Clin. Microbiol.* **42:** 4083–4091.

75. **Yue, J., W. Shi, J. Xie, Y. Li, E. Zeng, L. Liang, and H. Wang.** 2004. Detection of rifampin-resistant *Mycobacterium tuberculosis* strains by using a specialized oligonucleotide microarray. *Diagn. Microbiol. Infect. Dis.* **48:** 47–54.

Antimicrobial Resistance in Bacteria of Animal Origin
Edited by Frank M. Aarestrup

Chapter 5

Drug Selection and Optimization of Dosage Schedules To Minimize Antimicrobial Resistance

Peter Lees, Didier Concordet, Fariborz Shojaee Aliabadi, and Pierre-Louis Toutain

The first effective and relatively safe antimicrobial agents to be introduced into human medicine in 1935, and shortly thereafter into veterinary medicine, were the sulfonamides, rapidly followed in the 1940s and 1950s by the major groups of antimicrobial drugs derived from soil-dwelling and other microorganisms (penicillins, aminoglycosides, tetracyclines, etc.). For individual drugs within each group, differences in potency and in antimicrobial spectrum of activity were quickly established. Therefore, over the last 60 to 70 years the fundamental therapeutic principle underlying the use of antimicrobial drugs has been to select an effective drug substance and administer it in a product and with a dosage regimen that ensure efficacy. To achieve this aim, the drug should be present at the site of infection for a sufficient time in sufficient concentration to achieve optimal bacteriological and clinical outcomes, namely complete bacteriological and clinical cures. This involves applying knowledge of the drug's pharmacokinetic and pharmacodynamic properties in the formulated product (43). The former comprises the absorption into, distribution within, and elimination from the body. Pharmacokinetics is used both to describe and predict drug concentration-time profiles in plasma and other biological fluids, including the putative biophase. Pharmacodynamics encompasses the spectrum of antimicrobial activity and quantitative measures of the potency, efficacy, sensitivity, and kill rate of bacteria.

Pharmacokinetics is in part determined by intrinsic drug parameters, of which clearance is particularly important because it controls drug exposure. However, pharmacokinetic variables are also dependent on the formulation used (incorporation of drug substance into a drug product) as well as on administered dose. For example, for use in veterinary (particularly in farm-animal) medicine, some drugs (e.g., most penicillins and cephalosporins) are rapidly cleared and have short elimination half-lives, so that it is generally not possible to maintain therapeutic concentrations for more than a few hours with single intravenous doses. The consequence is a requirement to repeat the intravenous dosage several times daily or to infuse the drug intravenously at a rate that precisely balances elimination rate. Neither dosage protocol is practicable under most clinical conditions in veterinary medicine. However, drug administration by an alternative route (e.g., intramuscularly or subcutaneously) may provide a longer terminal half-life (flip-flop pharmacokinetics), enabling a longer dosing interval to be used. It is common to formulate drugs in organic solvents or as aqueous or oily suspensions, particularly for use in farm-animal medicine. When such depot products are injected by a nonvascular (usually intramuscular) route, they are slowly taken up into solution at the injection site to achieve more-persistent concentrations in plasma and other biological fluids. Such products have the advantage of prolonged duration of plasma and tissue fluid levels, providing therapeutic efficacy with one or two doses. They also avoid the stress associated with repeated injections, reduce the costs of therapy, and avoid the peaks and troughs of concentration, which for some drug classes may be particularly likely to lead to resistance development.

To the fundamental aim of using a drug with the required spectrum of activity and adequate efficacy in a suitable formulation and with a dosage regimen designed to achieve bacteriological cure, an equally important aim has been recognized in recent years—the crucial need to use effective drugs in formulations and

Peter Lees • Department of Veterinary Basic Sciences, The Royal Veterinary College, Hawkshead Campus, North Mymms, Hatfield, Herts AL9 7TA, United Kingdom. **Didier Concordet and Pierre-Louis Toutain** • École Nationale Vétérinaire de Toulouse, UMR 181 de Physiopathologie et Toxicologie Expérimentales, 23 chemin des Capelles, 31076 Toulouse Cedex 03, France. **Fariborz Shojaee Aliabadi** • Khatam Co., 72 Shaghayeh St., Abdollahzadeh St., Keshavarz Blvd., 14156-33341 Tehran, Iran.

at dosage rates that minimize opportunities for the selection and spread of resistance. Optimal dosages for these two aims are not necessarily the same. In veterinary medicine antimicrobial drug therapy and prophylaxis have contributed to maintenance of the health of animals under intensified production systems for farm animals and in confined water spaces for fish. However, as one consequence of such usage it is now widely recognized that suboptimal drug concentrations both in the biophase and at other sites, e.g., within the gastrointestinal tract or on skin, resulting from suboptimal dosing and/or from the use of an inappropriate formulation, is an important determinant of resistance selection by both pathogenic and commensal bacteria. Hence, the theme of this chapter will be to review current concepts of dosage optimization to achieve optimal therapeutic effect with minimal resistance.

A given population of mixed microorganisms may comprise many subpopulations with different levels of susceptibility to antibiotics. In addition, for a given bacterial species genetic variation can confer resistance to one or more antimicrobial drugs of a given class, e.g., aminoglycosides, penicillins, or fluoroquinolones. When a mixed population that is sensitive to the inhibitory actions of a drug is exposed to adequate concentrations of that drug for an adequate period, the vast majority of sensitive organisms will either be killed (bactericidal action) or have their growth inhibited (bacteriostasis), leading to flora disruption. This typically occurs in gut flora with the use of some drug classes such as quinolones, including after parenteral administration, because quinolones are directly excreted in the digestive tract by intestinal efflux pumps. A similar phenomenon may occur in a pathogen inoculum after antibiotic administration, i.e., when a preexisting mutated subpopulation having a lower susceptibility to that antibiotic emerges during treatment: under this drug-imposed selection pressure, less-sensitive mutants may survive and multiply to establish a resistant colony. This is a classical example of natural selection. Thus, resistance is genetic in origin and at the molecular level may be due to several mechanisms, including alternative metabolic pathways, efflux pumps, and altered drug penetration into the bacterial cell. As Schentag (78) and Schentag et al. (77) have emphasized, the most important contribution of the pharmacologist to the resistance debate will be to design dosage schedules that minimize opportunities for its development.

This chapter briefly reviews categories of antimicrobial drugs and their pharmacokinetic and pharmacodynamic properties. It then deals with the classification of antimicrobial drugs by killing mechanism as concentration dependent, time dependent, codependent, or none of these. The use and limitations of surrogate markers predictive of clinical efficacy, such as C_{max}/MIC (ratio of maximum concentration in plasma to MIC), AUC/MIC (ratio of area under plasma concentration-time curve to MIC), and T > MIC (time for which plasma concentration exceeds MIC expressed as a percentage of interdosage interval), in in vitro, ex vivo, and in vivo studies, as a basis for optimizing efficacy and minimizing resistance, are discussed. This includes an appraisal of the contribution of population pharmacokinetic-pharmacodynamic (PK-PD) modeling in disease models and veterinary clinical trials to optimizing dosage schedules. In summary, the contribution of the pharmacologist to the resistance problem is to optimize dosage by linking the pharmacokinetic and pharmacodynamic properties of drugs. Unfortunately, this is no simple matter, as there are innumerable sources of variability, and these combine to make it difficult to formulate simple rules to guide dosing strategies.

DRUG PHARMACODYNAMICS

Antimicrobial drugs possess, at the molecular level, several mechanisms for inhibiting the growth of or killing target pathogens. These include inhibition of bacterial protein synthesis, inhibition of cell wall synthesis, enzyme inhibition, alteration of cell membrane permeability, and blockade of specific biochemical pathways. Examples are summarized in Table 1. Classically, antimicrobial drugs have been classified as bactericides, which kill bacteria, or bacteriostats, which only inhibit cell growth and therefore are more dependent than bactericides on the body's immune mechanisms for combating infection. In fact, this classification, although still retained, oversimplifies drug action, in that all drugs at low concentrations are only bacteriostatic and many drugs at higher concentrations, including those usually classified as bacteriostats, will kill microorganisms. A newer approach has been to classify drugs according to the type of killing action as concentration dependent, time dependent, or codependent (Table 2). However, this classification also oversimplifies the actions of antimicrobial drugs. For example, for a given drug the killing action may be time-, concentration-, or codependent, depending on the specific microorganism.

As well as knowledge of the killing mechanism, the rational use of antimicrobial drugs requires knowledge of (i) the spectrum of activity (which defines the range of organisms susceptible to the drug), (ii) whether significant levels of resistance have developed as a consequence of extensive use of the drug, and (iii) whether the drug action at concentrations achievable in vivo with therapeutic dose rates is

Table 1. Summary of mechanisms and types of action of antibacterial drugs

Mechanism of action	Drugs	Type of action
Binding to 50S ribosomal subunit, producing reversible inhibition of protein synthesis	Chloramphenicol,[a] florfenicol,[a] macrolides,[a] ketolides,[a] lincosamides,[a] fusidic acid	Bacteriostatic
Binding to 30S ribosomal subunit, causing misreading of the mRNA code or inhibition of the initiation step of protein synthesis	Aminoglycosides, aminocyclitols, tetracyclines	Bactericidal (aminoglycosides and aminocyclitols) or bacteriostatic (tetracyclines)
Inhibition of cell wall synthesis or activation of enzymes, disrupting cell walls	Penicillins, cephalosporins, bacitracin, glycopeptides, novobiocin	Bactericidal
Inhibition of enzymes involved in DNA metabolism: e.g., DNA gyrase and DNA-dependent RNA	Fluoroquinolones, novobiocin, rifamycins, nitrofurans, nitroimidazoles	Bactericidal
Action on cell membrane to alter cell permeability, leading to loss of intracellular molecules	Polymyxins	Bactericidal
Inhibition of nucleic acid synthesis by antimetabolites	Sulfonamides, dihydrofolate reductase inhibitors	Separately bacteriostatic but bactericidal in combination

[a]Bactericidal against some bacterial species.

primarily bacteriostatic or bactericidal. It may be particularly important to select a drug that will kill bacteria when there is immune deficiency in the host, in life-threatening infections, and in infections at sites where immune defenses are minimal, for example, in cerebrospinal fluid (CSF). Having selected an antimicrobial drug on the basis of these considerations, it is then usual to adopt a dosage schedule and formulation based on whether the killing action is time dependent, concentration dependent, or codependent.

The standard parameter for determining the susceptibility of bacterial species and strains to a given drug is the MIC, which provides a measure of potency. It is equivalent to a pharmacodynamic parameter, the 50% effective concentration, and is normally determined in vitro and is defined as the lowest concentration, usually measured in broth as an artificial medium, that completely inhibits bacterial growth. It is usually assessed experimentally by using doubling dilutions and therefore is subject to approaching 100% error! However, MIC has been shown to provide a reasonably reproducible measure of drug efficacy and potency. When many strains of the same bacterial species are studied, MIC varies

Table 2. Killing actions of antimicrobial drugs (tentative classification)

Action	Group	Examples	PK-PD variable
Predominantly time-dependent killing action with short or no postantibiotic effect	Penicillins	Benzylpenicillin, amoxicillin, cloxacillin, carbenicillin	T > MIC
	Cephalosporins	Cephalexin, ceftiofur, cephapirin	T > MIC
	Phenicols	Florphenicol, chloramphenicol	
	Macrolides	Erythromycin, tilmicosin, tulathromycin, aivlosin	T > MIC
	Lincosamides	Clindamycin	T > MIC
	Sulfonamides	Sulfadiazine, sulfadoxine	T > MIC
	Diaminopyrimidines	Trimethoprim	T > MIC
Predominantly concentration-dependent killing action with significant postantibiotic effect	Aminoglycosides	Streptomycin, gentamicin, amikacin, tobramycin	AUC/MIC, C_{max}/MIC
	Fluoroquinolones	Danofloxacin, enrofloxacin, marbofloxacin, difloxacin, sarafloxacin	AUC/MIC, C_{max}/MIC
	Nitroimidazoles	Metronidazole	AUC/MIC, C_{max}/MIC
	Polymyxins	Colistin	AUC/MIC
Codependent killing action, requiring both maintained concentration and long exposure	Tetracyclines	Oxytetracycline, chlortetracycline, doxycycline	AUC/MIC
	Ketolides	Azithromycin, clarithromycin	AUC/MIC
	Glycopeptides	Vancomycin	AUC/MIC

widely. The distribution of MICs may be normal, log-normal, or even bimodal, and it is therefore common practice to express activity in terms of MIC_{50} and MIC_{90} (MICs at which 50 and 90%, respectively, of strains are inhibited). Current European guidelines from the European Medicines Evaluation Agency/Committee for Veterinary Medicinal Products (EMEA/CVMP) on antimicrobial drug efficacy require that MIC_{50} should be based on all organisms tested and MIC_{90} should be based only on susceptible bacteria.

The MBC is also used occasionally as a measure of potency; it is defined as the concentration which, under defined conditions, produces a 3-$\log_{10}$-unit reduction in bacterial count (99.9% decrease). A third important term in relation to resistance is mutant prevention concentration (MPC); it measures the capacity of a microorganism to select drug-resistant mutants and is defined as the concentration that allows no mutant to be recovered from a population of more than 10^{10} microorganisms (11, 27, 71).

The limitations in applying MIC determined in vitro to the design of dosing schedules for clinical use are as follows:

1. The error associated with the doubling-dilution technique, which involves overestimation of MIC.

2. The exposure of organisms to a fixed drug concentration for a fixed time (18 to 24 h), whereas in vivo (unless intravenous infusions are administered at a rate to maintain a constant plasma concentration) in clinical subjects, concentrations in plasma either fall (after intravenous bolus dosing) or first rise to a peak and then fall (after any nonvascular administration route). Moreover, organisms are exposed for much longer periods than 24 h with most dosing regimens. As well as MIC, this limitation applies to MPC determination.

3. The differences in growth conditions in artificial media (pH and nutrient and electrolyte concentrations) from those in biological fluids, so that MICs determined in biological fluids and artificial media may or may not be the same. Differences in MIC are likely if drug binding to plasma proteins is high, as only the free (non-protein-bound) fraction is active.

4. The absence of the body's normal defense (immune) mechanisms, which normally play a significant role in combating infection. In addition, for some drugs (notably those with a concentration-dependent killing mechanism) MIC determined in vitro is likely to underestimate efficacy in vivo because of postantibiotic effect, postantibiotic sub-MIC effect, and postantibiotic leukocyte enhancement mechanisms.

An approach which attempts to overcome points 1 and 3 (but not points 2 and 4) has been to measure MIC directly in body fluids (serum, exudate, and transudate) and, by using five overlapping sets of doubling dilutions, to thereby considerably improve the accuracy of MIC determination (2, 3, 5). Other approaches to address point 2 have included more-complex in vitro models, in which drug concentration first rises and then falls by steady infusion of drug, followed by infusion of drug-free growth medium (42).

Methods of efficacy assessment for antimicrobial drugs depend on whether the studies are carried out in vitro, ex vivo, or in vivo. For the former the outcome is determined as some measure of growth inhibition or killing of bacteria, for example, by the determination of MIC and MBC or by time-kill curves. In in vivo studies using disease models or in clinical trials, main or sole reliance is sometimes placed on clinical end points and this can be misleading. As discussed in detail by Toutain et al. (89), there exists the Pollyanna phenomenon, according to which drugs that give a complete bacteriological cure may demonstrate less than complete resolution of clinical signs, while agents that are poorly effective in removing bacteria may show a good clinical response. A veterinary example is the efficacy of ceftiofur in colibacillosis in neonatal pigs (93). In this study there was little difference in mortality between dosage groups, but a relationship between dose and bacterial shedding over the dosage range of 0.5 to 64 mg/kg was established. Therefore, when possible, it is desirable to adopt bacteriological cure as the "gold standard," even though this can sometimes be difficult to determine, and this criterion is likely to be particularly important when a major consideration is avoidance of emergence of pathogen-resistant organisms. If organisms are not eradicated through the combined effects of body defenses and administered antimicrobial drug, less-susceptible bacteria will head the recolonization process when therapy is discontinued, leading to a population with greater resistance (24).

The Pollyanna phenomenon expresses the fact that, when different antimicrobial drugs (or different dose levels of the same drug) are compared, the use of end points based on clinical signs often fails to discern major differences between the drugs (or between dose levels of the same drug), as determined by antibacterial efficacy. The Pollyanna phenomenon further explains the common difficulty of veterinary drug companies in demonstrating superiority of new agents against established drugs (a fact that is seldom published in the scientific literature but frequently reported in registration submission dossiers). This difficulty is especially true in conditions for which the spontaneous resolution rate is high (placebo effect) or for drugs having other pharmacodynamic effects contributing to the clinical outcome independently of their direct antibacterial actions. This is the case for some macrolides, tetracyclines, and quinolones that possess anti-inflammatory and immunomodulatory properties (25, 39, 40). Therefore, a bacteriologic diagnostic outcome is always preferred to a clinical diagnostic outcome to establish a dose-effect relationship, because a bacteriological end point is more relevant as a means of distinguishing between two dose levels than a clinical end point (49).

Although antimicrobial drug action on bacterial cells cannot readily be defined quantitatively in terms of drug receptor or drug enzyme interaction, it is nevertheless possible to model data in silico relating bacterial cell count (determined as CFU per milliliter) to a surrogate of antimicrobial activity (usually AUC/MIC ratio; see below). The sigmoid AUC/MIC-log CFU per milliliter relationship has been determined by a number of groups, including some initial studies in veterinary medicine (1–5). The advantage of this approach is that it establishes the three key pharmacodynamic parameters of drug response, namely efficacy (E_{max}), potency (20, 50, 90%, etc. of E_{max}), and sensitivity (n, the slope of the relationship), in a single investigation (87, 88).

DRUG PHARMACOKINETICS

The pharmacokinetics of antimicrobial drugs has been extensively studied in veterinary as well as human medicine, and no more than a fraction of the available data can be considered here. For further discussion, see reference 44. The pharmacokinetics of an antimicrobial drug is determined both by parameters such as clearance that are a property of the drug substance and by other pharmacokinetic properties that are modified by route of administration and/or formulation, e.g., rate and extent of drug absorption. Drug absorption into, distribution within, and elimination from the body are thus determined both by the formulation and intrinsic drug properties. For the latter, it is generally simple physicochemical drug properties, such as water solubility, lipid solubility, and molecular size, that are important. However, for some antibiotics having a peptidomimetic structure (ampicillin, amoxicillin, cephalosporins, etc.), specific intestinal transporters for peptides (PEPT1) exist and may make an important contribution to drug absorption, explaining possible saturability and nonlinearity of drug disposition. Antimicrobial drugs may be classified into those compounds that are water soluble (polar) and usually lipid insoluble on the one hand and those that are nonpolar and lipid soluble on the other (Table 3). The differences are not absolute, and many antimicrobial drugs have intermediate properties between these extremes.

The importance of water solubility lies in the fact that the drug must be in aqueous solution (i) before it can be absorbed from the gastrointestinal tract or nonvascular injection sites and (ii) in order to gain access to the bacterial biophase, which is most often tissue extracellular fluid. Most drugs have high potency (effective in low microgram-per-milliliter

Table 3. Lipid solubility of antibacterial drugs and effects on tissue distribution

Drugs	Effects on tissue distribution
Drugs of low lipophilicity Strong acids Beta-lactams (penicillins, cephalosporins, beta-lactamase inhibitors [e.g., clavulanate]) Strong bases or polar bases Aminoglycosides, aminocyclitols, polymyxins	Do not readily penetrate cell membranes or "natural body barriers," so that effective concentrations in intracellular fluid and in CSF, milk, and other transcellular fluids are not always achieved, although effective concentrations may be obtained in synovial, pleural, and peritoneal fluids.
Drugs of moderate to high lipophilicity Weak acids Sulfonamides Weak bases Macrolides, lincosamides, ketolides, diaminopyrimidines Amphoteric Most tetracyclines (e.g., oxytetracycline, chlortetracycline)	Generally cross cell membranes readily to penetrate intracellular and transcellular fluids. Penetration into CSF and ocular fluids determined by plasma protein binding as well as lipophilicity; sulfonamides and diaminopyrimidines penetrate effectively, but macrolides, lincosamides, and tetracyclines generally do not. Weak bases are ion trapped in fluids that are more acidic than plasma (e.g., prostatic fluid, milk, intracellular fluid, carnivore urine). Weak acids are ion trapped in fluids that are more basic than plasma (e.g., herbivore urine).
Drugs of high lipophilicity Fluoroquinolones, lipophilic tetracyclines (e.g., minocycline, doxycycline), nitroimidazoles, rifamycins, phenicols	Penetrate intracellular fluids. Cross cell membranes very readily. Penetrate into all transcellular fluids including prostatic fluid and bronchial secretions. Penetrate CSF readily (except tetracyclines and rifampin).

or nanogram-per-milliliter concentrations), a property often associated with a high lipophilicity and low water solubility. The importance of lipid solubility derives from the fact that most drugs are too large to penetrate the pores in the cell membranes (except for the large pores in vascular endothelium) and thus to traverse the membranes by ultrafiltration through the pores. Their passage is therefore normally dependent on lipid solubility, which ensures that drugs can cross cell membranes (to enter intracellular and transcellular fluids, e.g., peritoneal fluid, synovial fluid, aqueous humor, and CSF) by passive diffusion. Their lipid solubility enables them to cross cell membranes down electrochemical or concentration gradients.

Distribution in the body is an important consideration in relation to exposure of microorganisms, as infections are most commonly confined to extracellular fluids. Therefore, limited ability to cross cell membranes does not negatively influence the passage of lipid-insoluble molecules to sites of infection. On the other hand, if passage to such potential sites of infection as synovial or prostatic fluids, CNS, or epithelial-lining fluid in the lungs is required, lipid-soluble drugs are likely to attain the highest concentrations (Table 3). A further consideration is that many antimicrobial drugs are either weak acids or weak bases; these are usually lipid soluble but only in the nonionized form, and if pH differs on two sides of a cell membrane, it is only the nonionized form that will penetrate. This gives rise to the phenomenon of diffusion/ion trapping, whereby weak acids are trapped in alkaline environments, e.g., urine of herbivores, while weak bases are trapped in acid environments, e.g., urine of carnivores, milk, and prostatic fluid. These factors have an important bearing on drug penetration to site of infection. When the site of infection is the kidney or bladder, it is lipid-insoluble drugs which are poorly reabsorbed and which achieve very high concentrations in urine.

Thus, for the majority of infections, the free (non-protein-bound) concentration in plasma is the best predictor of concentration in the biophase, as most infections are extracellular (76, 89). Penetration to such sites is generally rapidly achieved, irrespective of a drug's lipid solubility. However, when an anatomical (e.g., passage into CSF or into transcellular fluids) or pathological (e.g., abscess or shock) barrier exists, lipid solubility is an important determinant of penetration of drug to the infection site. In addition, there are for some drugs (e.g., macrolides and ketolides) and some situations (e.g., biofilms) additional complications (see below). Finally, it should be noted that for the majority of antimicrobial drugs biotransformation is of importance in that it usually leads to reduction or abolition of activity, but occasionally a drug metabolite has similar or even greater activity than the parent compound. An example is the conversion of enrofloxacin to ciprofloxacin.

CONCENTRATION-TIME-EFFECT RELATIONSHIPS AND EFFICACY BREAKPOINTS

Despite the limitations of using MIC determined in vitro as the pharmacodynamic measure for use in PK-PD integration approaches, effective use of this parameter has been made in practice. Three PK-PD surrogates of efficacy have been widely used (53, 58, 89). These are AUC/MIC and C_{max}/MIC ratios and T > MIC, the last of which is expressed as a percentage of the interdose interval, where AUC is area under the plasma concentration-time curve, usually over a 24-h period; C_{max} is the maximum concentration in plasma; and T > MIC is the time for which the concentration in plasma exceeds the MIC (Fig. 1). This approach has been described as dual dosage optimization, as it takes account of both factors, pharmacokinetics and pharmacodynamics, that influence the outcome of therapy. It should be noted that AUC, for a given dose, is determined solely by bioavailability and plasma clearance; C_{max} is a hybrid parameter dependent on plasma clearance, bioavailability, and rate constants of absorption and elimination; while T > MIC is kinetically complicated, determined mainly by terminal half-life, which is itself a hybrid process involving plasma clearance and drug distribution. For flip-flop pharmacokinetics, terminal half-life also depends on the absorption rate constant.

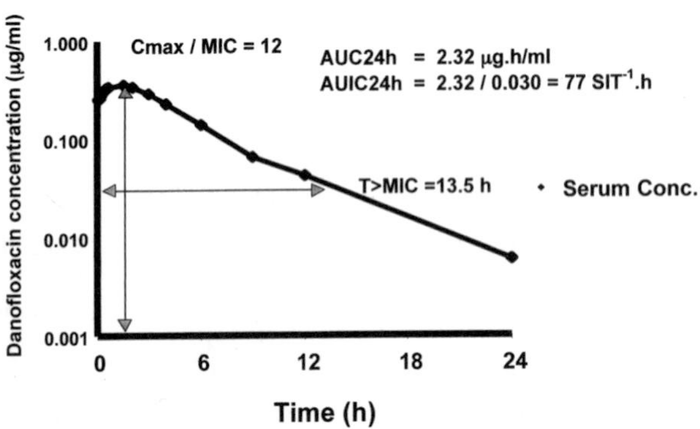

Figure 1. Illustration of PK-PD integration for danofloxacin in a goat receiving danofloxacin intramuscularly, showing values of C_{max}/MIC, AUC/MIC (AUIC), and T > MIC against a pathogen for which the drug's MIC (in serum) is 0.03 µg/ml. The serum sample was collected 9 h after intramuscular dosing with 1.25 mg of danofloxacin/kg. Reproduced with permission from AliAbadi and Lees (1).

Based on the use of these surrogates, derived from many human clinical trials, from a few veterinary trials, and from animal infection models, the killing actions of antimicrobial drugs have been classified as (i) concentration dependent, (ii) time dependent (concentration independent), or (iii) codependent (Table 2). For example, murine thigh and lung infection models in neutropenic mice, using a wide range of dosage regimens, have allowed discrimination between the three surrogate pharmacodynamic parameters: T > MIC, AUC/MIC, and C_{max}/MIC (23, 47, 92). For concentration-dependent-killing drugs of the fluoroquinolone and aminoglycoside groups, it has been widely recommended that the ratio of AUC from 0 to 24 h to MIC (AUC_{0-24}/MIC) should exceed 125 h (which is equivalent to saying that the average daily plasma concentration should be fivefold the MIC) and that C_{max}/MIC should be at least 10 (23, 29, 79). The former correlates well with bacteriological cure for fluoroquinolones. The latter has been suggested as a breakpoint value for minimizing resistance to aminoglycosides. For beta-lactam drugs, on the other hand, optimal efficacy is generally achieved when T > MIC exceeds 40 to 50% of the dosage interval, and increasing the concentration above four times the MIC usually fails to provide greater bacterial killing. However, for optimal antimicrobial effect it may be best to aim for a dosage that provides T > MIC of 80 to 100% (89), especially for gram-negative pathogens, whereas T > MIC of 40% may be appropriate for gram-positive pathogens.

As general guidelines, these numerical values of AUC/MIC, C_{max}/MIC, and T > MIC are very useful, but there are many examples that demonstrate the inapplicability of the quoted numerical values. As indicated by McKellar et al. (53), they are "drug and bug" specific. For example, beta-lactams generally have a longer postantibiotic effect against gram-positive organisms than against gram-negative bacteria, accounting for the fact that a shorter T > MIC (40 to 50% of dosing interval) may be optimal for inhibiting bacterial growth for the former, compared to 80% of dosing interval for the latter. There are also strain differences in PK-PD indices required to achieve a given level of antimicrobial activity. Thus, Guyonnet et al. (36) reported AUC_{0-5}/MIC values of 7.9, 6.2, 6.8, and 29.2 h for the bactericidal action of colistin against four strains of porcine *Escherichia coli*, suggesting that one strain was an outlier. These values correspond to 1.6, 1.2, 1.4, and 5.9 multiples of MIC. Moreover, for many drugs information correlating surrogate markers and bacteriological outcome is not available. Even when breakpoint values have been determined in experimental animal (usually mouse) infection models and/or in human clinical trials, the numerical values must be extrapolated to veterinary clinical circumstances with caution. It should be noted that PK-PD indices should also be based on free (non-protein-bound) concentrations in plasma, especially when the degree of protein binding is high, as only free concentration is microbiologically active and concentrations in interstitial fluid in steady-state conditions are theoretically equal to the free plasma concentration (17, 89).

Determining the relative importance of the three surrogate markers is complicated by the covariance between them, as all three increase with increased dosage. To deal with this problem, Corvaisier et al. (22) proposed a weighted AUC based on both AUC and T > MIC. Nevertheless, in a study of the efficacy of danofloxacin in a model of calf pneumonia, Sarasola et al. (73) were able to achieve similar AUC/MIC ratios but differing T > MIC and C_{max}/MIC ratio values comparing bolus intravenous injection and slow intravenous infusion. The former provided greater clinical and bacteriological cure responses than the latter.

As a general approach to dosage schedule design, Lees et al. (45) have proposed that preclinical studies should adopt a stepwise procedure as follows:

- Measurement of bacterial kill curves in vitro in broth to determine the killing mechanism of action of new drugs (time- vs. concentration-dependent killing, etc.). While such studies usually involve exposure of the test organism at a constant concentration for a fixed period, more-sophisticated models, simulating the variable concentrations that occur in vivo, have been used (42) (step 1).
- PK-PD modeling in vitro using bacterial kill curves in relevant biological matrices (serum, urine, milk, inflammatory exudate, etc.) to establish approximate breakpoint values for the new drug (step 2).
- PK-PD modeling ex vivo in target animal species using bacterial kill curves in relevant biological matrices (serum, exudate, transudate, etc.) to determine breakpoint values that allow first for possible matrix effects and second for the possibility of the combined action of parent drug and active metabolites (step 3).
- An in vivo pharmacokinetic trial in the target animal species using healthy animals or in a disease model, if available (e.g., calf pneumonia), during the dose-confirmation study (step 4).

It is of course inevitable that optimal dosage will vary with the pathogen, and for most drugs there will be several target organisms. These recommendations are made in light of the fact that, while no PK-PD indices have been firmly validated in veterinary medicine, data from animal infection models and human clinical trials are useful starting points for designing dosage schedules (89). This sequential procedure is recommended in preference to conventional dose-titration studies in animal disease models for determination of dosage for further evaluation in clinical trials. In dose-titration studies the body is a black box, providing information only on clinical and/or bacteriological outcome, and there are no data on the plasma or biophase concentrations required to achieve that outcome. Moreover, dose-titration studies for antimicrobial drugs conducted in disease models are necessarily undertaken using parallel (as opposed to crossover) designs, from which interpolation and extrapolation of data are not possible (86, 90). Furthermore, dose-titration studies commonly rely solely on suppression of clinical signs rather than bacteriological cure. Such studies commonly overestimate the efficacy of drugs giving a poor bacteriological response and underestimate efficacy when the bacteriological response is excellent (49, 89). The consequence is that an effective dose schedule is selected, but it is rarely the optimal dosage. The problem is compounded when this dose rate is then evaluated in clinical trials, leading to final selection of an effective (in terms of clinical cure), but not necessarily optimal, dose. PK-PD modeling, on the other hand, addresses the two principal sources (pharmacokinetics and pharmacodynamics) of inter- and intrasubject variability in treatment outcome. It therefore permits dual adaptation of the dosage regimen (75, 89). In principle, PK-PD modeling can be used to provide a dosing schedule that achieves eradication of bacteria.

Another limitation of the dose-titration approach using a parallel design is its implementation in association with an experimental infection model. Models of infection are generally developed to be severe to guarantee the statistical power of the design (no placebo effect), and their relevance to prophylactic, metaphylactic, and even therapeutic drug use is at best not validated and at worst very dubious. Moreover, dose-titration studies may be questionable from an ethical perspective, especially when it is recognized that the PK-PD approach offers an alternative to exploring the issue of dosage regimen selection in healthy subjects, allowing the pharmacodynamic component of the treatment to be explored in vitro or ex vivo. Hence, on several grounds, the PK-PD approach is the preferred preclinical approach to determination of a dosage regimen in human medicine (Table 4).

The advantages of the PK-PD approach over dose titration are based not only on their desirable metrological properties (sensitivity, reliability, continuity, etc.) but also on their direct mechanistic link with the ultimate objectives of therapy (i.e., a bacteriological cure and prevention of resistance amplification of a

Table 4. Comparison of PK/PD approach with dose titration or clinical trials[a]

Feature	Approach	
	PK/PD modeling	Dose titration or clinical trials
Subjects	Healthy	Infection models, clinical cases
End points	Surrogates: T > MIC, C_{max}/MIC, and AUC/MIC	Clinical outcome (cure, failure), bacteriological outcome (eradication, resistance)
Validity (clinical relevance)	Needs to be validated (prospectively or retrospectively)	"Gold standard," but many possible drawbacks and Pollyanna phenomenon
Sensitivity to dose ranging	Yes	No (difficult to perform dose ranging in ill animals)
Reliability	High	Low
Application to drug discovery and development	Early screening	Later confirmatory
Extrapolation (from in vitro models or between species)	Easy	Difficult
Dual dosage individualization	Yes	No
Prediction of the emergence of resistance	Possible	Possible
Breakpoint setting	To be explored (promising)	Yes
Population studies: pharmacokinetic or pharmacodynamic origin of variability allowed for	Yes	No, if only clinical outcomes are measured
Regulatory acceptance	In progress	Pivotal; designed to satisfy authorities but not to optimize treatments
Cost	Low	High
Independent evaluation, objectivity	Independent investigations possible	Requires commercial funding

[a]Reprinted from reference 89.

resistant subpopulation). This is explained by the fact that all PK-PD indices (AUC/MIC, C_{max}/MIC, and T > MIC) utilize the MIC for the pathogen. Intrinsically, therefore, they provide direct biological information on the susceptibility of the pathogen to be eradicated. This is not the case with clinical end points, which may be confounded by many nonbacterial factors. The advantages and disadvantages of the two approaches, dose titration and PK-PD modeling, are summarized in Table 4.

PK-PD MODELING AND PK-PD INTEGRATION OF FLUOROQUINOLONES IN RUMINANTS AND HUMANS

For four ruminant species, the ex vivo AUC/MIC ratios for danofloxacin, determined by PK-PD modeling against pathogenic isolates of three pathogenic strains of *Mannheimia haemolytica* (obtained from a calf, a sheep, and a goat) and a strain of *E. coli* (camel), are reported in Table 5. These data were obtained by PK-PD modeling, using the sigmoid E_{max} relationship between AUC/MIC in hours and bacterial count in CFU per milliliter, as illustrated in Fig. 2 for danofloxacin in goats (1). This approach defines the whole sweep of the AUC/MIC-effect relationship and allows any given level of inhibition of bacterial cell numbers from bacteriostasis to eradication to be determined, under the given experimental circumstances.

Accepting the limitation that the plasma concentration-time profile in a clinical subject resulting from intramuscular dosing with danofloxacin is not constant, but rises to a peak and then decreases, it is nevertheless possible to obtain an approximate indication of required daily maintenance dosage from the formula

$$\text{Dose} = \frac{\text{Cl} \times \text{AUC/MIC} \times \text{MIC}_{90}}{\text{fu} \times \text{F} \times 24\ \text{h}} \qquad (1)$$

where Dose is the daily dose, Cl is the plasma daily clearance, AUC/MIC is the PK/PD surrogate breakpoint value to be achieved (e.g., 125 h for a quinolone), MIC_{90} is the MIC at which 90% of the target pathogen population is eradicated (for an empirical antibiotherapy; but the actual MIC should be incorporated if known for a targeted antibiotherapy), F is bioavailability (from 0 to 1), and fu is the free drug fraction. The term "24 h" in equation 1 allows transformation of the AUC/MIC breakpoint value (expressed in hours) to a scaling factor (e.g., about 5 for a quinolone if AUC/MIC is 125 h) (89). Equation 1 may be simplified to equation 2 if protein binding is low and if the drug is administered intravenously.

$$\text{Dose} = \text{Cl} \times \text{MIC}_{90} \times \text{AUC/MIC} \qquad (2)$$

where Cl is the plasma clearance per hour (not per day as in equation 1), and dose, MIC_{90}, and AUC/MIC are as for equation 1.

In the studies of AliAbadi and Lees (1–3) and Aliabadi et al. (4, 5), danofloxacin and marbofloxacin were administered both intramuscularly and intravenously and, as MIC was determined in natural body fluids (serum, exudate, and transudate), no correction was required for protein binding.

There is no universal agreement on the level of antibacterial effect appropriate for a given drug against a particular organism. However, solving this equation for the AUC required to provide a bactericidal response or eradication of bacteria indicated

Table 5. Critical ex vivo AUC_{0-24}/MIC values for danofloxacin and marbofloxacin in serum to achieve bacteriostasis, bactericidal action, or bacterial eradication in four ruminant species[a]

Status	AUC_{0-24}/MIC ratio (h)				
	Marbofloxacin (calf)	Danofloxacin			
		Calf	Sheep	Goat	Camel
Bacteriostatic	37.3 ± 6.9	15.9 ± 2.0	17.8 ± 1.7	22.6 ± 1.7	17.2 ± 3.6
Bactericidal	46.5 ± 6.8	18.1 ± 1.9	20.2 ± 1.7	29.6 ± 2.5	21.2 ± 3.7
Eradication	119.0 ± 11.0	33.5 ± 3.5	28.7 ± 1.8	52.4 ± 8.1	68.7 ± 15.6

[a]Data are from references 1 to 5. Danofloxacin was administered intramuscularly to each species at a dose rate of 1.25 mg/kg. Marbofloxacin was administered intramuscularly at a dose rate of 2.5 mg/kg. Ex vivo antibacterial activity was evaluated by bacterial count after 24 h of incubation. The tested pathogens were strains of *M. haemolytica* (of calf, sheep, and goat origin) and *E. coli* (of camel origin). The relationship between ex vivo AUC_{0-24}/MIC in serum and the $\log_{10}$ difference in bacterial count (CFU per milliliter) was modeled by a Hill model; the AUC_{0-24}/MIC values for bacteriostasis and bactericidal activity were defined as values that resulted in no change in bacterial count and the value that resulted in 99.9% reduction in bacterial count, respectively. The AUC_{0-24}/MIC for bacterial eradication was defined as the lowest value that resulted in the maximum possible antibacterial effect (decrease in count to the limit of detection of 10 CFU/ml). Values are given as the mean ± standard error of the mean ($n = 6$).

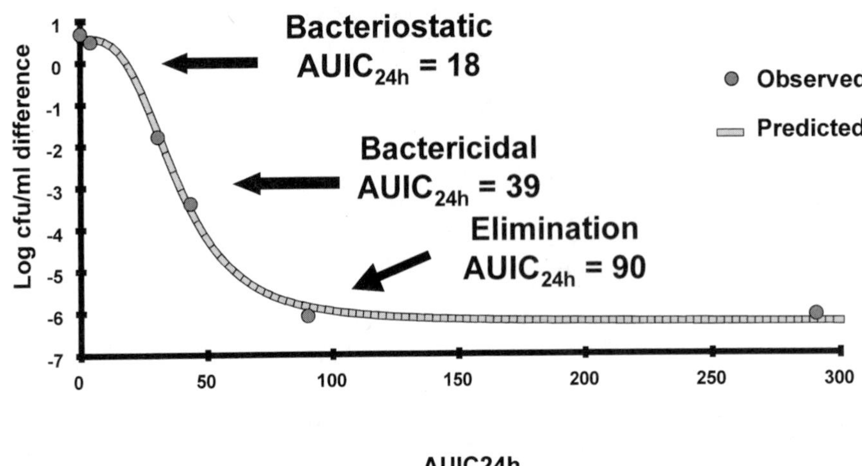

Figure 2. Sigmoidal E_{max} relationship for bacterial count versus ex vivo AUC_{0-24}/MIC ($AUIC_{24h}$) in a representative goat for a pathogenic strain of *M. haemolytica*, illustrating values required for bacteriostatic and bactericidal effects and eradication of bacteria. Reproduced with permission from AliAbadi and Lees (1).

danafloxacin doses of 4.06 and 7.50 mg/kg, respectively, in calves. If an effect level intermediate between 99.9% kill and eradication of bacteria is appropriate, this is supported by the clinically recommended dose of 6 mg/kg, which was established subsequently in clinical trials in pneumonic calves.

This effect level is similar to that proposed by Scaglione et al. (74) and Mouton (60) and Mouton et al. (58). The latter author proposed for fluoroquinolones that an AUC/MIC ratio based on 90% of E_{max} might be generally appropriate, but he further indicated that in immunocompetent subjects and when infections are not severe, the AUC/MIC ratio providing 50% of E_{max} is probably as acceptable as 90% of E_{max}. From the data of Scaglione et al. (74), 50% and 90% of E_{max} correspond approximately to reductions in bacterial count of 90% and 99.9%, respectively. Note that this consideration relates to efficacy but not necessarily to resistance development.

Most authors have suggested that MIC_{90} is the most appropriate pharmacodynamic index to use in predicting appropriate dosage, but this may be unnecessarily stringent and MIC_{50} (79) has been suggested as more precisely computable than MIC_{90}. There is for fluoroquinolones evidence from many studies based on in vitro data, animal models of disease, and clinical findings in human subjects that AUC/MIC ratio is the PK-PD surrogate that best correlates with efficacy. There is some agreement that the dosage should provide a ratio of at least 125 h, but lower values are proposed when the initial inoculum size is low, especially in patients with normal defense mechanisms, a situation that is likely to occur when antibiotics are used for prophylactic or metaphylactic treatments in food-producing animals. This may be consistent with the fact that a dosage regimen selected for danofloxacin against individual bacterial species provided AUC/MIC values that were numerically lower than 125 h in experimental ex vivo studies in four ruminant species (Table 5).

Mouton (60) has suggested that AUC/MIC values for several fluoroquinolones for a given outcome are generally similar. However, ex vivo studies in our laboratory suggest two potentially important differences between marbofloxacin and danofloxacin investigated against a calf pathogen. Against the same strain of *M. haemolytica*, AUC/MIC values for marbofloxacin and danofloxacin measured ex vivo in calf serum differed (Table 5). The differences between these two drugs of the same class could represent true differences in potency and sensitivity. The calculated average 24-h serum concentrations, expressed as multiples of MIC, required to eradicate a pathogenic strain of *M. haemolytica* isolated from calves were 1.40 and 4.96 for danofloxacin and marbofloxacin, respectively (Table 6). However, it should be noted that the differences were observed in separate studies in different groups of calves. This is unavoidable in ex vivo studies. Hence, more data are now required to confirm these initial findings; the ex vivo data require confirmation in a single within-study in vitro investigation. In the meantime, it should be noted that there is a general assumption that a single targeted AUC/MIC can be used for all drugs of a given class (89), i.e., that an optimal dosing regimen can be obtained for all antibiotics of the same class when achieving the same breakpoint value (e.g., 125 h, or five times the MIC for the targeted pathogen for all quinolones).

The dependence of antimicrobial drug dosage on both pharmacokinetic and pharmacodynamic

Table 6. Average 24-h concentrations of danofloxacin and marbofloxacin in serum[a]

Drug	Avg 24-h concn of drug in serum of indicated species			
	Calf	Sheep	Goat	Camel
Danofloxacin	1.40	1.20	2.18	2.86
Marbofloxacin	4.96			

[a]Data are expressed as multiples of the MIC required for eradication of organisms in four ruminant species (1–5). See Table 5, footnote *a*, for more details.

parameters is indicated by equations 1 and 2. For a given bacterial strain, the MIC is constant, so that the clinical breakpoint for that strain depends wholly on dosage. This is illustrated for a drug of the time-dependent-killing class, amoxicillin (57). These authors determined the relationship between T > MIC for amoxicillin-clavulanic acid and MIC for four different dosage regimens. It was assumed that T > MIC should be 40% of the interdose interval for a given effect, so that the MIC breakpoint for a dose of 875 mg every 12 h was 2 μg/ml, while a dosage of 500 mg every 6 h gave a breakpoint of 8 μg/ml. This illustrates the dependency of the breakpoint MIC on dosage regimen.

PK-PD INTEGRATION OF MACROLIDES AND KETOLIDES

Most macrolides have been classified as time-dependent-killing drugs, as T > MIC is normally the best surrogate marker of drug therapy. On the other hand, some newer macrolide-like drugs (azithromycin and clarithromycin) against some organisms possess a significant postantibiotic effect, and the best correlate with successful outcome is the surrogate AUC/MIC ratio (52). However, this correlation is based on the plasma concentration-time profile, which may not reflect concentration in the biophase.

A veterinary example is provided by tulathromycin, a recently developed novel macrolide for use in the treatment of respiratory disease in bovine and porcine medicine. Tulathromycin resembles other macrolides in that there is both a high level of tissue binding and associated high intracellular concentrations. Benchaoui et al. (9) and Nowakowski et al. (63) compared lung tissue and plasma concentrations after intramuscular or subcutaneous administration of tulathromycin in cattle and pigs. Plasma concentrations of tulathromycin were low, whereas lung concentrations were much higher. In the pig, the lung/plasma AUC ratio was 61 and the terminal half-life of elimination from lung was 142 h. The corresponding values in cattle were 74 and 184 h. The porcine pharmacokinetic data may be compared with MIC for important respiratory tract pathogens: 2 μg/ml for *Pasteurella multocida* (porcine isolate) and 16 μg/ml for *Actinobacillus*. Calculating for plasma concentration each of the conventional PK-PD surrogate indices, values are C_{max}/MIC, 0.32 for *P. multocida* and 0.04 for *A. pleuropneumoniae*; T > MIC, 0 h for both pathogens; and AUC/MIC, 7.6 h for *P. multocida* and 0.95 h for *A. pleuropneumoniae*. Comparing these indices with values quoted for aminoglycosides, fluoroquinolones, and beta-lactams, it is clear that they fall well short of those required for efficacy with these other drug classes. Nevertheless, the recommended dosage (2.5 mg/kg) and the resulting plasma concentration of tulathromycin have been shown to be effective clinically and in disease models. This example confirms the earlier reports of Nightingale (61) and Nightingale and Mattoes (62), who studied the actions of ketolides in murine models of infection. They reported efficacy of azithromycin and clarithromycin, with C_{max}/MIC values of 0.25 to 0.48 and AUC/MIC of 5 to 12 h, corresponding to average plasma concentrations over 24 h of only 0.2 to 0.5 of MICs. This suggests that for this group of drugs the in vitro and the in vivo situations are very different and that the in vitro MIC is not appropriate to predict drug efficacy, which results from a complex interaction between the pathogen, the neighboring cells, and the antimicrobial drug.

For other macrolides used in therapy for respiratory infections in farm-animal medicine, such as tilmicosin, it is well recognized that clinical and bacteriological efficacy are achieved with single-dose administration, despite the fact that the drug is rapidly cleared from plasma but is known to concentrate in lung tissue. Therefore, there clearly are factors that enable macrolides as a group to act effectively in vivo in clinical subjects at plasma concentrations well below those that would be predicted from correlating plasma concentration to the MIC determined in vitro. In reviewing possible explanations for the inability to correlate clinical and bacteriological success with the surrogates C_{max}/MIC, AUC/MIC, and T > MIC, Benchaoui et al. (9) and Nowakowski et al. (63) considered several possible factors. Macrolides possess several potentially beneficial nonantimicrobial actions, including stimulation of cytokine pathways and enhancement of programmed cell death (apoptosis). The studies of Chin et al. (20, 21) have emphasized the role of the acute inflammatory response, involving the local accumulation of neutrophils, that the body mounts in cases of infectious lung disease. When neutrophils undergo necrosis in large numbers at the site of lung inflammation under the influence of leukotaxin, they release a wide range of tissue-damaging agents, including free radicals, eicosanoids, and proteolytic enzymes (46). However, such release does not occur when neutrophils undergo apoptosis with cell fragments removed by macrophages; apoptosis is "an injury limiting disposal mechanism." Chin et al. (20, 21) showed that the macrolide tilmicosin effectively controlled, in calves, *M. haemolytica* infection, induced neutrophil apoptosis, and reduced pulmonary inflammation, concluding that the induction of apoptosis contributed to clinical efficacy. Other workers have demonstrated that erythromycin also enhances apoptosis, so this is likely to be a general property of macrolide drugs (7).

Other studies have indicated that macrolides exert potential anti-inflammatory effects by a range of other mechanisms, including reduced leukocyte accumulation, decreased secretory functions of airway cells, increased airway epithelial cell ciliary motility, and decreased epithelial synthesis of proinflammatory cytokines such as interleukin-6 (35, 56, 70, 81–83, 91). In summary, there are many potential mechanisms by which macrolides may exert beneficial effects in infectious lung diseases, in addition to their direct actions on microorganisms, and these may interact additively or synergistically with the direct antimicrobial actions. Benchaoui et al. (9) have discussed several other mechanisms as a possible basis for explaining the lack of the expected correlation between pharmacokinetic and pharmacodynamic data for macrolides. The use of total lung concentrations may be irrelevant (15, 76). However, others have argued that drug concentrations in the biophase (e.g., epithelial cell lining fluid) may exceed by severalfold concentrations predicted from plasma free drug concentrations (16, 19, 62, 72, 94).

MICROORGANISMS AND BIOFILMS

Bacteria growing as biofilms are less susceptible to antimicrobial agents than free-living cells, and in this circumstance predictions of biophase concentrations and dosages required to kill bacteria cannot be made by the conventional means of integrating drug concentrations and MICs or other susceptibility tests (26). Moreover, biofilm-associated infections are becoming more common (51). For example, it has long been recognized that *Pseudomonas aeruginosa* infections are among the most difficult to treat effectively. It is now known that it is a biofilm-producing organism; however, of 162 human clinical isolates, 14 and 8% produced biofilms after 8- and 24-h incubation periods, respectively. As well as the protection against antimicrobial drugs that organisms acquire by growth in a biofilm, human clinical isolates have accumulated more resistance phenotypes (26, 28), thus involving two mechanisms of bacterial cell protection against drug exposure.

The processes underlying this bacterial dual-protection mechanism are still poorly understood. In biofilms, bacteria are present in consortia rather than as nonaggregated (or planktonic) cells. The aggregative biopolymers that hold the biofilm together impose a permeability barrier to drug penetration. In addition, organisms forming biofilms exhibit slow growth and division rates, and most antibacterial drugs are effective only against growing organisms. A third proposed mechanism is reduced apoptosis (34). In addition, a hypermutability state causing antibiotic resistance has been reported in *P. aeruginosa* associated with infected human cystic fibrosis patients (65). Moreover, horizontal gene transfer has been demonstrated in in vitro biofilms (37). Thus, the processes seem to be complex and multiple, and the consequence is the possible inapplicability of the usual integrated PK-PD approach to dosage determination. Most biofilm studies have been performed in vitro, and the relevance to the clinical use of drugs against biofilm producers remains to be elucidated. An interesting development is the observation that a novel agent, ranbezolid, possesses significant activity against slime-producing staphylococci (requiring only two to four times the MIC for total clearance of methicillin-resistant *Staphylococcus aureus* and methicillin-resistant *Staphylococcus epidermidis*), and this drug inhibits biofilm formation at sub-MIC and MIC concentrations (51).

CONCENTRATION-TIME-EFFECT RELATIONSHIPS AND RESISTANCE BREAKPOINTS

Bacterial populations are not homogeneous; they comprise subpopulations with differing susceptibilities to a given antimicrobial drug. Organisms of lower susceptibility can arise as the consequence of a single point mutation. Antimicrobial drug exposure exerts selection pressure on the population and leads to the overgrowth of a subpopulation of organisms of low-level susceptibility, in classical Darwinian fashion. Exposure, particularly repeated exposure, to suboptimal drug concentrations is therefore the most important single factor for resistance emergence (14). It is important to note that this consideration applies to commensals as well as pathogens. Therefore, adequate exposure of pathogens may still leave commensals underexposed, and this may lead subsequently to the transfer of their resistance genes to pathogenic organisms (8).

When an antimicrobial drug is administered in bacteriologically effective concentrations, there will normally be a period in which all bacteria in the population are susceptible. However, eventually concentrations will decrease to a point where no organisms in the population are inhibited. The former concentration is the MPC, and the concentration between these two extremes is described as the selection window (11, 18). Therefore, the aim of antimicrobial therapy must be twofold: (i) to achieve eradication of bacteria before concentrations decrease below the MPC and, as this can never be guaranteed in all circumstances, (ii) to keep the selection window as short as possible. In principle, it is possible to achieve both aims by drug dosage and product formulation selection. For fluoroquinolones it is recognized that two successive mutations, first on gyrase and then on topoisomerase IV, lead to mutant strains of high resistance (38). A concentration window exists between the MIC of wild-type bacteria and the MPC, the concentration that prevents the growth of first-step mutants, with a selection advantage for first-step mutants within this window. At concentrations greater than the MPC, the probability that a wild-type subpopulation will undergo the two mutations is very low (95).

It cannot be assumed that values of the surrogate PK-PD indices, AUC/MIC, C_{max}/MIC, and T > MIC, required to avoid or reduce selection pressure for resistance will be the same as those required for a given level of efficacy, for example, to achieve a bactericidal response. Data in this field are currently limited. Nevertheless, several examples will be used to illustrate potential requirements for optimal resistance avoidance.

1. Firsov et al. (32) demonstrated, in vitro, a relationship between AUC/MIC for fluoroquinolones and the emergence of resistance. This was represented by a bell-shaped curve for four strains of *S. aureus* when resistance frequency was plotted against the AUC_{0-24}/MIC ratio. When values were either less than 10 h or greater than 200 h, no resistance occurred, and the peak of the bell-shaped curve was obtained for an AUC/MIC value of 43 h. The AUC/MIC commonly quoted for fluoroquinolones for optimal efficacy is 125 h (though some estimates are higher), which is only slightly more than half the 200-h value reported by Firsov et al. (32) for resistance avoidance.

2. A study in human pneumococcal patients demonstrated that the probability of emergence of resistance to fluoroquinolones after 5 days of therapy was 50% when AUC/MIC values were less than 100 h, and the corresponding value after 3 weeks of treatment was 93% (84). When AUC/MIC exceeded 100 h, the probability of organisms remaining susceptible was greater than 90%. For fluoroquinolones, the numerical value of this surrogate marker may need to be as high or higher to avoid resistance development than to achieve bacteriological cure. In an earlier study, Forrest et al. (33) suggested that for fluoroquinolones resistance selection is greater when C_{max}/MIC is less than 8. However, both studies were conducted with seriously ill and possibly immunocompromised human patients, and lower values of AUC/MIC and C_{max}/MIC may be sufficient to avoid resistance in animals and humans with normal immune status.

3. In a study with levofloxacin, Preston et al. (66) reported that, for prediction of clinical outcome, none of the indices, C_{max}/MIC, AUC/MIC, nor T > MIC, provided a distinction, whereas in those patients with C_{max}/MIC of ≥12.2 there was 100% microbiological eradication. In in vitro studies with ciprofloxacin and sparfloxacin, it was confirmed that high C_{max}/MIC ratios were linked to lower incidence of resistance (85). Likewise, for ciprofloxacin in a mouse peritonitis model, resistance was lower for *P. aeruginosa* when C_{max}/MIC was 20 compared to a value of 10 (54).

4. In an *E. coli* model in chickens, Toutain et al. (89) computed for a fluoroquinolone a 50% effective dose of 8 mg/kg for reduction in mortality and a 50% effective dose of 13 mg/kg for bacteriological cure. While the higher dose does not guarantee lack of emergence of resistance, resistance will be much less likely, being based on bacteriological cure, than with the lower dose.

5. In an early study, Blaser et al. (10) established a correlation between C_{max}/MIC ratio and resistance to the aminoglycoside netilmicin by *E. coli* and *S. aureus*. Regrowth was prevented when C_{max}/MIC was greater than 8. Likewise, for other drugs of the aminoglycoside group, a C_{max}/MIC of 8 to 10 was required to prevent the emergence of resistance (55).

6. The regrowth of *E. coli* occurred when four strains of this organism isolated from pigs were cultured in vitro in broth for 5 h, when AUC/MIC for colistin was <8 or 16 h; with lower ratios, the inhibition of growth was almost complete at 5 h, with regrowth by 24 h. However, when AUC/MIC was ≥8 or 16 h, there was no regrowth at 24 h (36).

7. In an experimental in vivo study, Stearne et al. (80) reported data for ceftizoxime, a cephalosporin with time-dependent-killing properties. Using a mixed infection model in the mouse, they measured resistant clones, plotting mutation frequency against T > MIC, expressed as a percentage of dosing interval. For T > MIC values of less than 40 and equal to 100%, no resistance occurred, whereas peak mutation frequency was obtained when T > MIC was 70%. Values for mutation were very low when T > MIC was 87% or greater. In contrast, both experimental animal and human clinical data have frequently indicated that the optimal T > MIC for efficacy against susceptible pathogens is of the order of 40 to 50% for beta-lactam drugs, although more-prolonged exposure can be required for some organisms.

These findings suggest that a higher T > MIC, perhaps ideally 90 or even 100%, should be the objective for minimizing resistance development for time-dependent-killing cephalosporins. Odenholt et al. (64) investigated whether certain concentrations of benzylpenicillin were critical for the selection of resistant subpopulations. They exposed a mixed culture of *Streptococcus pneumoniae* (containing susceptible, intermediate, and resistant bacteria) to the antibiotic, at concentrations above its MICs for the respective strains, for different times; they showed that selection of resistant bacteria occurs if dosing regimens are targeted only against fully susceptible strains.

Finally, it should be noted that an optimal dosing strategy for minimizing resistance may achieve this objective in two ways: (i) by eradicating all disease-causing pathogenic bacteria and (ii) by exerting minimal selection pressure on commensals. Of course, these two aims may often conflict.

VARIABILITY IN PHARMACODYNAMIC AND PHARMACOKINETIC PARAMETERS, VARIABLES, AND SURROGATE PK-PD INDICES

Any guidelines, formulae, or criteria designed to provide dosage schedules that optimize efficacy and minimize opportunity for resistance development must take account of the limitations and the variability of pharmacodynamic and pharmacokinetic data. The question arises as to how these should be taken into account in making predictions of outcome for both efficacy and avoidance of resistance. Initially, it is the mean values of surrogate markers that are used to select dosage regimens. However, if the distribution is close to normal, approximately half the animal population is likely to have an index lower than the calculated value and the other half will have a higher value. For example, in a study by Mouton (59), with a 1-g dose of ceftazidime, a T > MIC of 50% of the dosing interval was obtained in some human subjects, but in others T > MIC was greater than 80%. From a resistance perspective, the concern will be with those subjects or animals that fail to achieve the desired breakpoint. To meet this consideration, Toutain et al. (89) have proposed an integrated approach of population pharmacokinetics and microbiological susceptibility applying Monte Carlo simulations. This takes into account the variability in the input variables and therefore generates PK-PD indices not only for the population mean but for all individuals in the population. This subject is a crucial consideration for minimizing resistance and is further discussed by Mouton (59) and below.

Rationale for Undertaking Population Pharmacokinetics

Population pharmacokinetics is a key element in establishing optimal dosage regimens for antimicrobial drugs, i.e., dosage regimens that are both clinically effective and optimal in preventing or delaying the emergence of resistance. Population PK-PD analysis establishes in clinical subjects interrelationships between pharmacokinetics and pharmacodynamics and their variability in subjects representing the target animal population (patients) when standard dosage regimens are administered. Moreover, it aims to explain the origin of the variability with different demographic, physiological, or other covariables such as breed, age, sex, health status, and level of production. The ultimate goal is to design dosage regimens that take account of animal or group characteristics. The conceptual framework and methodological aspects of population pharmacokinetics in veterinary medicine have been described by Martin-Jimenez and Riviere (50) and Riviere (69).

The first justification for performing population studies on antimicrobial drugs developed according to the PK-PD paradigm is that PK-PD indices are normally established in homogeneous healthy animals kept in a well-controlled laboratory environment rather than in diseased animals under field conditions. These "laboratory" PK-PD values may be reasonably predictive of outcome when a drug is used prophylactically (in healthy animals) or administered on an individual basis (e.g., before surgery in companion animals or at drying off in dairy cattle). However, they may not be appropriate to determine a final dosage regimen for administration to diseased animals or healthy animals raised in a competitive environment (pigs, poultry) and dosed collectively for prophylactic and metaphylactic purposes. Population pharmacokinetics seeks to identify precisely the measurable factors (both physiological and pathophysiological) that may alter the dose-exposure relationship in the actual conditions of the target population. Generally, these investigations should be carried out during clinical trials conducted in a large number of animals but using a sparse sampling strategy. As an example, Fig. 3 shows the high interindividual dispersion of doxycycline exposure in a large sample of pigs under field conditions (del Castillo et al., unpublished data).

A second and even more cogent reason for performing population pharmacokinetic and pharmacodynamic investigations for antimicrobial drugs is to determine a dosage regimen suitable to the population paradigm. Although an "average" dosage regimen for a conventional drug may be satisfactory in terms of clinical efficacy, it is nevertheless unlikely to be an optimal regimen for an antimicrobial drug. An optimal dosage regimen should not only be clinically effective at the individual animal level but also be able to prevent, at the population level, the selection and propagation of resistant pathogens. For the emergence of resistance, interanimal variability in level of

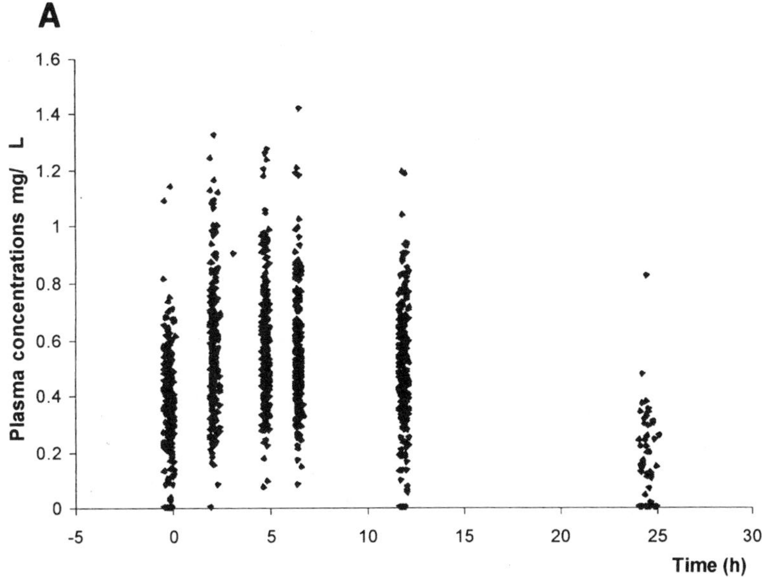

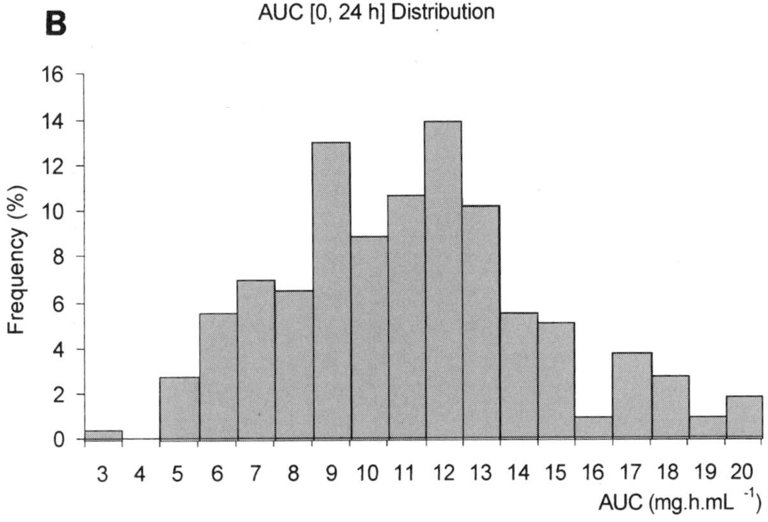

Figure 3. (A) Plasma concentration of doxycycline in 215 pigs under field conditions. Doxycycline was administered by the oral route as a metaphylactic treatment: the first dose (5 mg/kg, nominal dose) was given between 1800 and 1900 h (evening dose) and the second dose (5 mg/kg, nominal dose) was administered between 0800 and 0900 h (morning dose) on the following day. Blood samples were obtained approximately 30 min before, and approximately 1.8, 4.5, 6.7, and 11.5 h after, the second administration. For 25% of the pigs, a final blood sample was obtained 24 h after the second administration. Visual inspection of the raw data indicates the large variability of plasma doxycycline concentration. (B) Histogram of the area under the concentration-time curve (AUC from 0 to 24 h) for the 215 pigs. The range of exposure is approximately 4 to 5.

drug exposure is probably a major risk factor. Indeed, underexposure of the target pathogen in only a few animals within a flock or herd may lead to the establishment in these animals of a less susceptible subpopulation of the pathogen that subsequently may transmit resistance genes horizontally to the other members of the group. This may explain not only clinical failures or relapses in individual animals but also a progressive lack of efficacy of antimicrobial drugs in the population. In other words, an optimal dosage regimen for an antibiotic drug must take into account the population dimension because, in contrast to drugs of other classes, the efficacy of antimicrobial drugs may be subjected to a progressive resistance drift, the rate of which is a collective, rather than an individual, phenomenon.

Interindividual variability (and hence potential underexposure of some subjects) inevitably occurs during a prophylactic or metaphylactic group treatment in pigs and poultry. This is mainly due to the animals' feeding pattern, with competition between subjects for access to feed or variability in the consumption of medicated drinking water. In a field setting, therefore, the actual ingested dose becomes the first factor of exposure variability; the ingested dose is no longer the nominal dose, but a variable having a population distribution influenced by differing management procedures (size of the group, body weight heterogeneity within the group, modalities of food distribution, etc.). In addition, when the drug is given metaphylactically, i.e., administered or provided when a given percentage of the animals in the group display signs of infection, it may be hypothesized that fever, anorexia, and other factors in those animals displaying clinical signs are additional factors of interindividual variability. The possible underexposure of some animals with the largest bacterial burden (and thus the most prone to the highest pathogen mutational frequency) may be a major cause of the establishment of less susceptible pathogens, because it is clearly established that mutations are amplified with low antimicrobial drug concentrations (95). The consequence is that an optimal dosage regimen should be not an average dosage but a "population dosage regimen," with the objective of appropriately exposing most of the animals in a given population (e.g., at least 90% of animals) in order to limit as much as possible any individual underexposure to the drug and hence the risk of emergence of resistance.

PK-PD versus Dose-Titration Approach To Determine an Optimal Dosage Regimen

In terms of the crucial objective of minimizing the emergence of resistance, the PK-PD approach to dosage regimen determination offers several advantages over the current regulatory recommended (EMEA, CVMP) dose-titration approach (Fig. 4). The latter involves determining a dose that achieves a statistically significant effect, typically on a range of clinical end points (mortality, morbidity, necropsy scores, etc.). This allows selection of a clinically efficacious dose (over a placebo effect). However, this approach is flawed on several counts. First, the dose-effect relationships for antimicrobial drugs are generally very shallow, and it is often difficult, using only clinical end points, to distinguish between two different doses because the parallel design necessarily used in dose titration usually lacks sensitivity. Equally important, clinical end points do not unequivocally reflect the direct drug action on the target pathogen population. It should be the goal of all antimicrobial therapy to eradicate the targeted pathogen population, i.e., not only to obtain a good clinical outcome but also to prevent the emergence of a resistant pathogen subpopulation. This is because the emergence of resistance is linked to the mutational frequency in the pathogen population and hence is proportional to the pathogen burden (inoculum size) at the site of infection. When clinical end points are used alone to assess efficacy, there is no guarantee that "the best dose" to eradicate the pathogen population (or at least to drastically reduce it) has been selected.

PK/PD Indices and the Monte Carlo Approach To the Selection of Optimal Dosage

If both pharmacokinetic and pharmacodynamic (MIC) variabilities are known from relevant population investigations, the statistical distribution of the selected PK-PD index can readily be established using Monte Carlo simulations (30). "Monte Carlo" is a term applied to a numerical method with a built-in random process. It involves combining the variability of antimicrobial drug exposure with the variability in pathogen susceptibility according to their distribution. With Monte Carlo simulations, a large hypothetical population of animals (or outcomes) may be generated to determine the probability of attaining a given PK-PD breakpoint in a given proportion of the population (Fig. 5). This enables selection of a dosage regimen based on attaining the recommended PK-PD target breakpoint in a given quantile of animals. Thus, the goal of the Monte Carlo simulations is to ensure the clinical success of the treatment and to increase the likelihood of bacterial eradication. It may be also used to define a range of drug concentrations favoring the emergence of resistance and amplification of the resistant clone, as recently illustrated in human medicine by Jumbe et al. (41). In veterinary

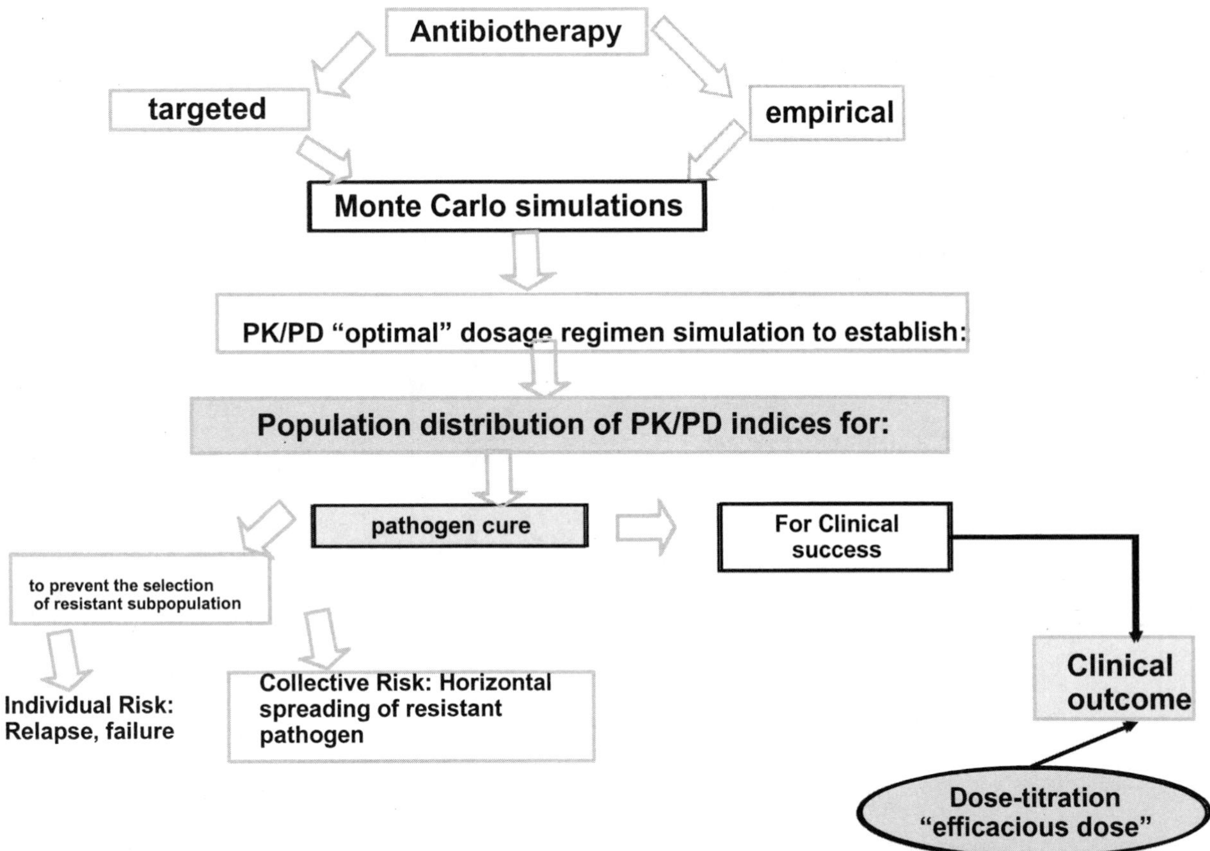

Figure 4. Dose-titration vs. PK-PD approach for the establishment of an optimal dosage regimen for antimicrobial drugs. Based on current regulatory policies (EMEA, U.S. Food and Drug Administration), dosage regimens for antimicrobial drugs are usually established by dose titration, generally in an experimental infection model. Dosage is determined taking account of clinical outcomes as pivotal criteria of efficacy (clinical cure). The dose-titration approach determines an efficacious dose, i.e., a dose significantly different from placebo (with respect to clinical outcomes), but it is unable to determine an "optimal dosage regimen" because clinical outcomes are not unequivocally related to bacteriological cure (an essential objective for a rational dosage therapy). The PK-PD approach offers a promising alternative to classical dose titration because it directly and mechanistically addresses antimicrobial efficacy. This approach also has the advantage of accounting for the two main sources of variability (pharmacokinetics and pharmacodynamics) influencing the response of the pathogen to the drug, and hence it is more able than a dose-titration study to determine an optimal dosage regimen. When using the PK-PD approach, two situations may be considered to determine a dosage regimen: the empirical vs. the targeted antibiotherapy approaches. For a company and for regulatory authorities, the dosage regimen selected and authorized is that which guarantees in a given percentage of the target population (e.g., 90% of animals) attainment of an "ideal" breakpoint value for the PK-PD index. This is the optimal dosage regimen for an empirical antibiotherapy, i.e., when the clinician undertakes an antibiotherapy with no knowledge of the pharmacokinetic characteristics in the treated animals and MIC for the involved pathogen. If the MIC is known (from epidemiological or laboratory data), variability is reduced solely to pharmacokinetic variability and a dosage regimen can be established using Monte Carlo simulation with the MIC in question, thus establishing a dosage regimen for a targeted antibiotherapy.

medicine, our group in Toulouse, France, has used Monte Carlo simulation to determine the dosage regimen of marbofloxacin in the dog to treat infection of the anterior segment of the eye (67). Figure 6 provides another veterinary example, of doxycycline in the pig. Pharmacokinetic variability was assessed in a population field study of 215 pigs (del Castillo et al., unpublished), and the MIC distribution for *P. multocida* was obtained from Intervet data files. By combining the pharmacokinetic and pharmacodynamic distributions, the authors computed the percentage of pigs attaining a given PK-PD index (AUC/MIC) value for different dosage rates of doxycycline (5, 10, and 20 mg/kg per 24 h). They concluded that a dose of at least 20 mg/kg was necessary to attain a PK-PD breakpoint value of 24 h (i.e., to achieve a mean total plasma concentration equal to the actual but unknown MIC over the dosage interval in 90% of pigs).

Monte Carlo simulations should take account of antimicrobial drug binding to plasma protein. This is because only the free concentration is active and a

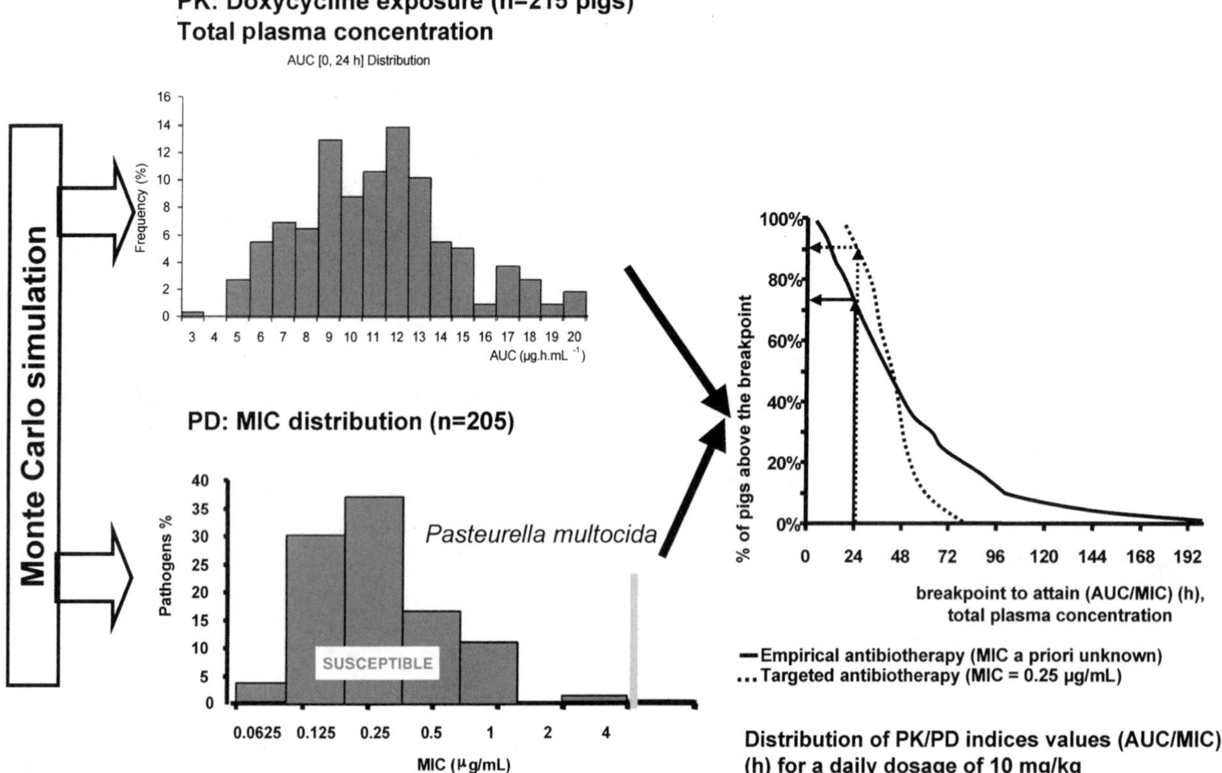

Figure 5. Monte Carlo simulation and the PK-PD index population distribution. The application of Monte Carlo simulation accounts in a balanced manner for variability in drug exposure (doxycycline AUC; upper left) as well as pathogen susceptibility data (MIC distribution for *P. multocida*; lower left) to establish the population distribution of the PK-PD index (AUC/MIC; right). The exposure distribution (AUC_{0-24}) is that obtained with a second doxycycline dose of 5 mg/kg administered approximately 14 h after an initial 5-mg/kg dose and is assumed to be representative of steady-state exposure. The curves at right give the percentage of pigs in a population attaining a given value of the PK-PD predictor (AUC/MIC). Two curves were generated, one for an empirical initial antibiotherapy (MIC distribution known, but the MIC for the involved pathogen unknown) and one for a targeted antibiotherapy (the MIC for the involved pathogen known to be 0.25 µg/ml). The administered dose of doxycycline was 10 mg/kg, i.e., the recommended daily dose regimen. Visual inspection of the curve indicates that 72% of pigs were able to attain a PK-PD index of 24 h (i.e., a daily mean plasma concentration equal to the corresponding MIC) for an empirical antibiotherapy. For a targeted antibiotherapy having a MIC of 0.25 µg/ml, a 10-mg/kg daily dosage regimen is able to cover 90% of the pig population. These simulations were performed using total plasma concentrations of doxycycline. If it is assumed that only free drug is active, the percentage of pigs above the breakpoint should be divided by approximately 10, as the extent of plasma protein binding for doxycycline is about 90% (D. Concordet et al., unpublished results).

correction for binding is required. For doxycycline in the pig, the extent of protein binding is high (approximately 90%) (68). This suggests that the current recommended dosage (10 mg/kg per day) is theoretically unable to attain a desirable breakpoint for an AUC/MIC of 24 h in terms of free plasma concentration (i.e., an average daily free plasma doxycycline concentration equal to the MIC). On the other hand, it was shown in a controlled clinical trial that a doxycycline dosage of 11 mg/kg per day in feed was effective in controlling pneumonia due to *P. multocida* in pigs (13). Further work is needed to explain this apparent discrepancy and especially to establish in a clinical setting the breakpoint values that are predictive of clinical success for prophylaxis and metaphylaxis in food-producing animals.

The contribution of Monte Carlo simulations to dosage selection is illustrated by comparing the dosage regimen calculated solely from typical parameter values (mean pharmacokinetic exposure and MIC_{50}) and also the mean pharmacokinetic exposure and the MIC_{90} (i.e., considering the worst-case scenario in terms of pathogen susceptibility) with the dosage regimen recommended to attain a mean daily plasma concentration equal to the MIC, i.e., a PK-PD breakpoint of 24 h for 90% of the pig population. Using a typical exposure value of 12 µg.h/ml over 24 h, as obtained after a doxycycline dose of 5 mg/kg, and

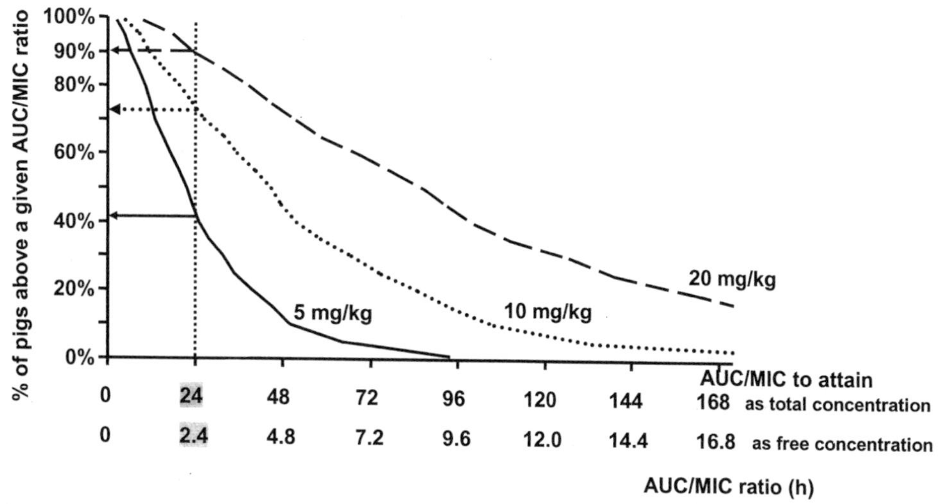

Figure 6. Dose-effect relationship for doxycycline in the pig using Monte Carlo simulation. The percentage of a pig population able to attain a given value of the PK-PD index (AUC/MIC) is given for three daily dose levels of doxycycline (5, 10, and 20 mg/kg) used against *P. multocida* (empirical antibiotherapy). For a PK-PD breakpoint value of 24 h, only the 20-mg/kg dose achieves the breakpoint in 90% of pigs; i.e., to guarantee a mean doxycycline plasma total concentration equal to the unknown MIC for the pathogen over 24 h, a dose of 20 mg/kg is required (Concordet et al., unpublished).

a modal MIC of 0.25 μg/ml for *P. multocida* (Fig. 7), a typical (average) dosage regimen for doxycycline in the pig would be 4.3 mg/kg per day. However, considering the MIC_{90} (1 μg/ml), the typical dosage regimen for doxycycline would be 17.4 mg/kg per day, i.e., almost twice the currently recommended dosage regimen. The Monte Carlo simulation thus takes into account variability in both pharmacokinetics and pharmacodynamics. It indicates that if the MIC is actually 0.25 μg/ml, the appropriate dose is 10 mg/kg (targeted antibiotherapy) to achieve a mean plasma concentration of 0.25 μg/ml over 24 h in 90% of pigs. The increase in dosage from 4.3 mg/kg (see above) to 10 mg/kg relates to the need to account for interindividual pharmacokinetic variability. The additional dose increase from 10 to 20 mg/kg for an empirical antibiotherapy is based on the necessity of accounting for pharmacodynamic variability. Such an approach in veterinary medicine could lead to a revision of dosage for some older antimicrobial drugs and to prolongation of their effective usage.

More generally, Monte Carlo simulations may be used to predict different dosing regimens that are impossible to determine for reasons of time or because of practical constraints. For example, they may

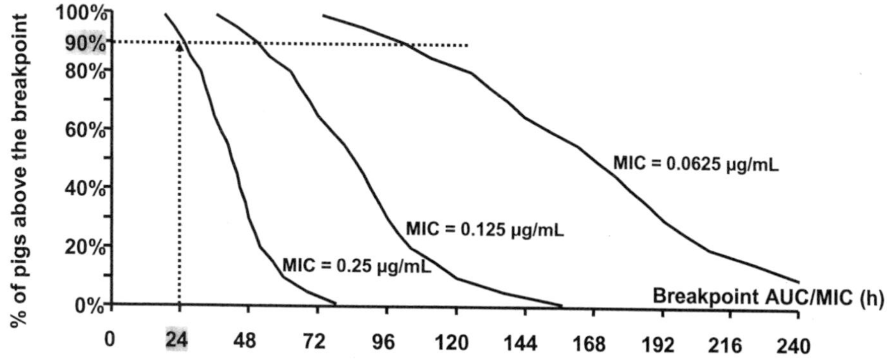

Figure 7. MIC breakpoint determination for *P. multocida* in the pig using Monte Carlo simulation. The distribution curves of the PK-PD indices (AUC/MIC) for doxycycline were generated by Monte Carlo simulations using a nominal daily dose of doxycycline of 10 mg/kg and a PK-PD breakpoint value to be achieved of 24 h. The critical MIC was 0.25 μg/ml (total doxycycline concentration) or 0.025 μg/ml (free plasma concentration). Pathogens for which the MIC is higher than 0.25 μg/ml (or 0.025 μg/ml if it is assumed that only the free doxycycline concentration is active) should be declared "clinically" resistant if the critical criterion is to maintain in 90% of a pig population a daily mean plasma concentration equal to the MIC with a daily 10-mg/kg dose of doxycycline.

be used to answer what-if questions concerning animal management, modalities of drug distribution (liquid versus solid formulation), duration of treatment, etc. However, it is not known to what extent regulatory agencies are willing to accept these simulated results in support of a new drug application (12).

Monte Carlo Simulation and the Establishment of MIC Breakpoints

Monte Carlo simulations may also be used to determine MIC breakpoints for antibiograms. The rationale is to first determine a dosage regimen based on multiple considerations, including not only bacteriological information but also other relevant drug properties (safety, withdrawal time, etc.). The question then becomes: what is the MIC above which the pathogen should be declared as "clinically" resistant? This can be defined as the critical MIC above which the proposed dosage regimen is unable to guarantee that 90% of the target animal population will be exposed to a daily mean concentration equal to one of the a priori MICs of the MIC distribution. An approach of this kind was used recently in human medicine to revise the breakpoint values of several cephalosporins for *Streptococcus pneumoniae* (6, 31). For example, for doxycycline in the pig, the MIC breakpoint value for *P. multocida* and for a doxycycline dose of 10 mg/kg per day would be 0.25 μg/ml, not 1 μg/ml, as would be recommended considering only the MIC distribution.

LIMITATIONS OF THE PK-PD APPROACH TO DETERMINATION OF AN OPTIMAL DOSAGE REGIMEN IN VETERINARY MEDICINE

Currently, the main limitation of the population PK-PD approach in veterinary medicine is the lack of firmly established PK-PD breakpoints; to fill this gap, the results of prospective multicenter trials are required. Normally the validation should be undertaken in clinical trials, and this is relatively straightforward in food animals when herd medication is used. Initially, the breakpoints used in humans can be adopted as starting values, because there are good reasons to believe that they are generally similar across species (23). However, there is an urgent need to determine breakpoint values of PK-PD indices in clinical settings that are specific to veterinary medicine, for example, in the prophylactic or metaphylactic use of antibiotics in groups of animals, especially when the ultimate goal is to prevent the emergence of resistance. Jumbe et al. (41) showed that the breakpoint AUC/MIC values for levofloxacin against *P. aeruginosa* in normal mice inoculated with either 10^7 or 10^8 injected bacteria per thigh were very different, 31 and 161 h, respectively. These data indicated that increasing by a factor of 10 the pathogen burden (inoculum size) led to a two- to sixfold increase in required drug exposure (AUC/MIC ratio) to obtain the same degree of antibacterial effect. This was explained by the increase in microbiological burden, which also increased the size of the resistant population. In contrast, for time-dependent-killing antibiotics, the size of T > MIC for optimal antibacterial effect is not influenced by bacterial inoculum or mechanism of resistance but is affected by host immune status (48). Transposing these results to a veterinary context, we can speculate whether or not the prophylactic and metaphylactic use of antibiotics requires the same breakpoint values as for therapeutic use. This question arises because it is reasonable to assume that prophylactic and metaphylactic conditions are usually characterized by a lower initial bacterial burden than that encountered under therapeutic conditions. Currently, prophylactic and metaphylactic uses of antimicrobial drugs are under scrutiny, because they expose large populations of animals to antimicrobial drugs. Conversely, prophylactic and metaphylactic strategies for disease control may be more desirable in terms of pathogen burden and also in terms of smaller interanimal variability. Thus, the question of the best strategy for using antibiotics in food-producing animals is one that can be considered in the context of risk analysis using Monte Carlo simulations.

Another limitation of currently available PK-PD approaches is the lack of consideration of impact on both zoonotic and commensal floras. In food-producing animals, antibiotics are generally given by the oral route. Due to their low systemic bioavailability (for example, less than 30% for tetracyclines and beta-lactams in pigs), the gut flora is extensively and, it may be argued, unnecessarily exposed to antibiotics. Such exposure may explain the shedding of zoonotic bacteria (salmonellae, chlamydiae, etc.) with a reduced susceptibility to drugs used in human medicine. Similarly, the gut flora may be the source of an increase in the gene pool of resistance factors transmissible to humans through the food chain. Moreover, exposure of the gut flora is also observed with some agents administered parenterally due to their active efflux by enterocytes, as shown for fluoroquinolones, for example.

In conclusion, the general framework of PK-PD concepts could be most useful in increasing our knowledge of antibiotic effects on the gut flora, but it should be recognized that refinements of available methods are required. Indeed, the situation differs between target pathogens and the commensal and zoonotic flora. First, the location of the target pathogen (for a systemic infection) is generally such that the free plasma concentration is a relevant surrogate for the biophase concentration. This is not the case for the gut flora located in the jejunum, cecum, and colon, where the organisms exist in a complex ecosystem with possible binding to cellulose and other digesta. In addition, the impact of antibiotics on the gut flora is exerted at multiple levels, with a direct influence on zoonotic bacteria and also on the global emergence of resistance genes in the commensal flora. Much more research in this area is needed before firm recommendations can be made in terms of dosage regimen. At this time we cannot conclude that an optimal dosage regimen against the target pathogen will also be the optimal dosage regimen to spare the gut flora. Furthermore, we can speculate that some antibiotics should be excluded from use in animal medicine as a consequence of an irreconcilable conflict between beneficial antimicrobial properties on target pathogens and negative effects on the gut flora.

REFERENCES

1. **AliAbadi, F. S., and P. Lees.** 2001. Pharmacokinetics and pharmacodynamics of danofloxacin in serum and tissue fluids of goats following intravenous and intramuscular administration. *Am. J. Vet. Res.* **62:**1979–1989.
2. **AliAbadi, F. S., and P. Lees.** 2002. Pharmacokinetics and pharmacokinetic/pharmacodynamic integration of marbofloxacin in calf serum, exudate and transudate. *J. Vet. Pharmacol. Ther.* **25:**161–174.
3. **AliAbadi, F. S., and P. Lees.** 2003. Pharmacokinetic-pharmacodynamic integration of danofloxacin in the calf. *Res. Vet. Sci.* **74:**247–259.
4. **Aliabadi, F. S., B. H. Ali, M. F. Landoni, and P. Lees.** 2003. Pharmacokinetics and PK-PD modelling of danofloxacin in camel serum and tissue cage fluids. *Vet. J.* **165:**104–118.
5. **Aliabadi, F. S., M. F. Landoni, and P. Lees.** 2003. Pharmacokinetics (PK), pharmacodynamics (PD), and PK-PD integration of danofloxacin in sheep biological fluids. *Antimicrob. Agents Chemother.* **47:**626–635.
6. **Ambrose, P. G., W. A. Craig, S. M. Bhavnani, and M. N. Dudley.** 2002. Pharmacodynamic comparisons of different dosing regimens of penicillin G against penicillin-susceptible and resistant pneumococci, abstr. A-635. *Abstr. 42nd Intersci. Conf. Antimicrob. Agents Chemother.* American Society for Microbiology, Washington, D.C.
7. **Aoshiba, K., A. Nagai, and K. Konno.** 1995. Erythromycin shortens neutrophil survival by accelerating apoptosis. *Antimicrob. Agents Chemother.* **39:**872–877.
8. **Baquero, F., M. C. Negri, M. I. Morosini, and J. Blazquez.** 1997. The antibiotic selective process: concentration-specific amplification of low-level resistant populations. *CIBA Found. Symp.* **207:**93–111.
9. **Benchaoui, H. A., M. Nowakowski, J. Sherington, T. G. Rowan, and S. J. Sunderland.** 2004. Pharmacokinetics and lung tissue concentrations of tulathromycin in swine. *J. Vet. Pharmacol. Ther.* **27:**203–210.
10. **Blaser, J., B. B. Stone, M. C. Groner, and S. H. Zinner.** 1987. Comparative study with enoxacin and netilmicin in a pharmacodynamic model to determine importance of ratio of antibiotic peak concentrations to MIC for bacterial activity and emergence of resistance. *Antimicrob. Agents Chemother.* **31:**1054–1060.
11. **Blondeau, J. M., X. Zhao, G. Hanson, and K. Drlica.** 2001. Mutant prevention concentrations of fluoroquinolones for clinical isolates of *Streptococcus pneumoniae*. *Antimicrob. Agents Chemother.* **45:**433–438.
12. **Bonate, P. L.** 2001. A brief introduction to Monte Carlo simulation. *Clin. Pharmacokin.* **40:**15–22.
13. **Bousquet, E., P. Pommier, S. Wessel-Robert, H. Morvan, H. Benoit-Valiergue, and A. Laval.** 1998. Efficacy of doxycycline in feed for the control of pneumonia caused by Pasteurella multocida and Mycoplasma hyopneumoniae in fattening pigs. *Vet. Rec.* **143:**269–272.
14. **Burgess, D. S.** 1999. Pharmacodynamic principles of antimicrobial therapy in the prevention of resistance. *Chest* **115:**195–233.
15. **Carbon, C.** 1990. Significance of tissue levels for prediction of antibiotic efficacy and determination of dosage. *Eur. J. Clin. Microbiol. Infect. Dis.* **9:**510–516.
16. **Carbon, C.** 1995. Clinical relevance of intracellular and extracellular concentrations of macrolides. *Infection* **23**(Suppl. 1): S10–S14.
17. **Cars, O.** 1997. Efficacy of beta-lactam antibiotics: integration of pharmacokinetics and pharmacodynamics. *Diagn. Microbiol. Infect. Dis.* **27:**29–33.
18. **Catry, B., H. Laevens, L. A. Devriese, G. Opsomer, and A. De Kruif.** 2003. Antimicrobial resistance in livestock. *J. Vet. Pharmacol. Ther.* **26:**81–93.
19. **Cazzola, M., F. Blasi, C. Terzano, M. G. Matera, and S. A. Marsico.** 2002. Delivering antibacterials to the lungs. *Am. J. Resp. Med.* **1:**261–272.
20. **Chin, A. C., W. D. Lee, K. A. Murrin, D. W. Morck, J. K. Merrill, P. Dick, and A. G. Buret.** 2000. Tilmicosin induces apoptosis in bovine peripheral neutrophils in the presence or in the absence of *Pasteurella haemolytica* and promotes neutrophil phagocytosis by macrophages. *Antimicrob. Agents Chemother.* **44:**2465–2470.
21. **Chin, A. C., D. W. Morch, J. K. Merrill, H. Ceri, M. E. Olson, R. R. Read, P. Dick, and A. G. Buret.** 1998. Anti-inflammatory benefits of tilmicosin in calves with *Pasteurella haemolytica*-infected lungs. *Am. J. Vet. Res.* **59:**765–771.
22. **Corvaisier, S., P. H. Maire, M. Y. Bouvier D'Yvoire, X. Barbaut, N. Bleyzac, and R. W. Jelliffe.** 1998. Comparisons between antimicrobial pharmacodynamic indices and bacterial killing as described by using the Zhi model. *Antimicrob. Agents Chemother.* **42:**1731–1737.
23. **Craig, W. A.** 1998. Pharmacokinetic/pharmacodynamic parameters: rationale for antibacterial dosing of mice and men. *Clin. Infect. Dis.* **26:**1–12.
24. **Dagan, R., K. P. Klugman, W. A. Craig, and F. Baquero.** 2001. Evidence to support the rationale that bacterial eradication in respiratory tract infection is an important aim of antimicrobial therapy. *J. Antimicrob. Chemother.* **47:**129–140.
25. **Dalhoff, A., and I. Shalit.** 2003. Immunomodulatory effects of quinolones. *Lancet Infect. Dis.* **3:**359–371.
26. **Delissalde, F., and C. F. Amabile-Cuevas.** 2004. Comparison of antibiotic susceptibility and plasmid content, between biofilm producing and non-producing clinical isolates of *Pseudomonas aeruginosa*. *Int. J. Antimicrob. Agents* **24:**405–408.
27. **Dong, Y., X. Zhao, B. N. Kreiswirth, K. Drlica, T. G. Evans, and L. Heifets.** 2000. Mutant prevention concentration as a measure of antibiotic potency: studies with clinical isolates of

Mycobacterium tuberculosis. Antimicrob. Agents Chemother. **44:**2581–2584.

28. **Drenkard, E., and F. M. Ausubel.** 2002. *Pseudomonas* biofilm formation and antibiotic resistance are linked to phenotypic variation. *Nature* **416:**740–743.
29. **Drusano, G. L., D. E. Johnson, M. Rosen, and H. C. Standiford.** 1993. Pharmacodynamics of a fluoroquinolone antimicrobial agent in a neutropenic rat model of *Pseudomonas sepsis. Antimicrob. Agents Chemother.* **37:**483–490.
30. **Drusano, G. L.** 2004. Antimicrobial pharmacodynamics: critical interactions of "bug and drug." *Nat. Rev. Microbiol.* **2:**289–300.
31. **Dudley, M. N., and P. G. Ambrose.** 2002. Monte Carlo PK-PD simulation and new cefotaxime (CTX), ceftriaxone (CRO), and cefepime (FEP) susceptibility breakpoints for *S. pneumoniae*, including strains with reduced susceptibility to penicillin, abstr. A-635. *Abstr. 42nd Intersci. Conf. Antimicrob. Agents Chemother.* American Society for Microbiology, Washington, D.C.
32. **Firsov, A. A., S. N. Vostrov, I. Y. Lubenko, K. Drlica, Y. A. Portnoy, and S. H. Zinner.** 2003. In vitro pharmacodynamic evaluation of the mutant selection window hypothesis using four fluoroquinolones against *Staphylococcus aureus. Antimicrob. Agents Chemother.* **47:**1604–1613.
33. **Forrest, A., D. E. Nix, C. H. Ballow, T. F. Goss, M. C. Birmingham, and J. J. Schentag.** 1993. Pharmacodynamics of intravenous ciprofloxacin in seriously ill patients. *Antimicrob. Agents Chemother.* **37:**1073–1081.
34. **Gilbert, P., A. McBain, and A. H. Rickard.** 2003. Biofilms and bacterial multi-resistance. *In* C. F. Amabile-Cuevas (ed.), *Multiple Drug Resistant Bacteria.* Horizon Scientific Press, Wymondham, United Kingdom.
35. **Goswami, S. K., S. Kivity, and Z. Marom.** 1990. Erythromycin inhibits respiratory glycoconjugate secretion from human airways *in vitro. Am. Rev. Respir. Dis.* **141:**72–78.
36. **Guyonnet, J., S. Monnoyer, B. Manco, F. S. Aliabadi, and P. Lees.** 2003. *In vivo* pharmacokinetics and *in vitro* pharmacodynamics as a basis for predicting dosage of colistin in piglet g.i.t. disease. *J. Vet. Pharmacol. Ther.* **26**(Suppl. 1)**:**148–149.
37. **Hausner, M., and S. Wuertz.** 1999. High rates of conjugation in bacterial biofilms as determined by quantitative in situ analysis. *Applied Environ. Microbiol.* **65:**3710–3713.
38. **Hooper, D. C., and J. S. Wolfson.** 1993. Mechanisms of bacterial resistance to quinolones, p. 97–118. *In* D. C. Hooper and J. S. Wolfson (ed.), *Quinolone Antimicrobial Agents*, 2nd ed. American Society for Microbiology, Washington, D.C.
39. **Hoyt, J. C., and R. A. Robbins.** 2001. Macrolide antibiotics and pulmonary inflammation. *FEMS Microbiol. Lett.* **205:**1–7.
40. **Ianaro, A., A. Ialenti, P. Maffia, L. Sautebin, L. Rombola, R. Carnuccio, T. Iuvone, F. D'Acquisto, and M. Di Rosa.** 2000. Anti-inflammatory activity of macrolide antibiotics. *J. Pharmacol. Exp. Ther.* **292:**156–163.
41. **Jumbe, N., A. Louie, R. Leary, W. Liu, M. R. Deziel, V. H. Tam, R. Bachhawat, C. Freeman, J. B. Kahn, K. Bush, M. N. Dudley, M. H. Miller, and G. L. Drusano.** 2003. Application of a mathematical model to prevent in vivo amplification of antibiotic-resistant bacterial populations during therapy. *J. Clin. Investig.* **112:**275–285.
42. **Koritz, G. D., C. R. Kilroy, and R. F. Bevill.** 1994. Pharmacokinetics-pharmacodynamic modelling of antibacterial therapy *in vitro*, p. 196–197. *In Proceedings of the 6th International Congress of the European Association for Veterinary Pharmacology and Therapeutics.* Blackwell Scientific Publications, Edinburgh, United Kingdom.
43. **Lees, P., and F. S. AliAbadi.** 2000. Rationalising dosage regimens of antimicrobial drugs; a pharmacological perspective. *J. Med. Microbiol.* **49:**943–945.
44. **Lees, P., and F. S. AliAbadi.** 2002. Rational dosing of antimicrobial drugs; animals versus humans. *Int. J. Antimicrob. Agents* **19:**269–284.
45. **Lees, P., F. S. Aliabadi, and P.-L. Toutain.** 2004. PK-PD modelling: an alternative to dose titration studies for antimicrobial drug dosage selection. *J. Regul. Affairs* **15:**175–180.
46. **Leff, J. A., and J. E. Repine.** 1993. Neutrophil-mediated tissue injury, p. 229–262. *In* J. S. Abramson and J. G. Wheeler (ed.), *The Neutrophil.* IRL Press/Oxford University Press, Oxford, United Kingdom.
47. **Leggett, J. E., S. Ebert, B. Fantin, and W. A. Craig.** 1991. Comparative dose-effect relations at several dosing intervals for beta-lactam, aminoglycoside and quinolone antibiotics against gram-negative bacilli in murine thigh-infection and pneumonitis models. *Scand. J. Infect. Dis.* **74**(Suppl.)**:**179–184.
48. **MacGowan, A. P.** 2004. Elements of design: the knowledge on which we build. *Clin. Microbiol. Infect.* **10**(Suppl. 2)**:**6–11.
49. **Marchant, C. D., S. A. Carlin, C. E. Johnson, and P. A. Shurin.** 1992. Measuring the comparative efficacy of antibacterial agents for acute otitis media: the "Pollyanna phenomenon." *J. Pediatr.* **120:**72–77.
50. **Martin-Jimenez, T., and J. E. Riviere.** 2001. Mixed effects modeling of the disposition of gentamicin across domestic animal species. *J. Vet. Pharmacol. Ther.* **24:**321–332.
51. **Mathur, T., P. Bhateja, M. Pandya, T. Fatma, and A. Rattan.** 2004. In vitro activity of RBx 7644 (ranbezolid) on biofilm producing bacteria. *Int. J. Antimicrob. Agents* **24:**369–373.
52. **Mazzei, T., and A. Novelli.** 1999. How macrolide pharmacodynamics affect bacterial killing. *Infect. Med.* **16:**22–28.
53. **McKellar, Q. A., S. F. Sanchez Bruni, and D. G. Jones.** 2004. Pharmacokinetic/pharmacodynamic relationships of antimicrobial drugs used in veterinary medicine. *J. Vet. Pharmacol. Ther.* **27:**503–514.
54. **Michae-Hamzehpour, M., R. Auckenthaler, P. Regamey, and J. C. Pechere.** 1987. Resistance occurring after fluoroquinolone therapy of experimental *Pseudomonas aeruginosa* peritonitis. *Antimicrob. Agents Chemother.* **31:**1803–1808.
55. **Moore, R. D., C. R. Smith, and P. S. Lietman.** 1984. Association of aminoglycoside plasma levels with therapeutic outcome in gram-negative pneumonia. *Am. J. Med.* **77:** 657–662.
56. **Morikawa, K., F. Oseko, S. Morikawa, and K. Iwamoto.** 1994. Immunomodulatory effects of three macrolides, midecamycin acetate, josamycin and clarithromycin, on human T-lymphocyte function *in vitro. Antimicrob. Agents Chemother.* **38:**2643–2647.
57. **Mouton, J. W., and N. Punt.** 2001. Use of the t>MIC to choose between different dosing regimens of beta-lactam antibiotics. *J. Antimicrob. Chemother.* **47:**500–501.
58. **Mouton, J. W., M. N. Dudley, O. Cars, H. Derendorf, and G. L. Drusano.** 2002. Standardization of pharmacokinetic/pharmacodynamic (PK/PD) terminology for anti-infective drugs. *Int. J. Antimicrob. Agents* **19:**355–358.
59. **Mouton, J. W.** 2003. Impact of pharmacodynamics on breakpoint selection for susceptibility testing. *Infect. Dis. Clin. N. Am.* **17:**579–598.
60. **Mouton, J. W.** 2005. Impact of pharmacodynamics on dosing schedules: optimising efficacy, reducing resistance, and detection of emergence of resistance, p. 387–407. *In* I. M. Gould and J. W. M. van der Meer (ed.), *Antibiotic Policies Theory and Practice.* Kluwer Academic/PTO Plenum Publishers, New York, N.Y.
61. **Nightingale, C. H.** 1997. Pharmacokinetics and pharmacodynamics of newer macrolides. *Pediatr. Infect. Dis. J.* **16:** 438–443.
62. **Nightingale, C. H., and H. M. Mattoes.** 2002. Macrolide, azalide and ketolide pharmacodynamics, p. 205–220. *In*

C. H. Nightingale, T. Murakawa, and P. G. Ambrose, (ed.), *Antimicrobial Pharmacodynamics in Theory and Clinical Practice.* Marcel Dekker, Inc., New York, N.Y.

63. **Nowakowski, M. A., P. B. Inskeep, J. E. Risk, T. L. Skogerboe, H. A. Benchaoui, T. R. Meinert, J. Sherington, and S. J. Sunderland.** 2004. Pharmacokinetics and lung tissue concentrations of tulathromycin, a new triamilide antibiotic, in cattle. *Vet. Ther.* **5**:60–74.
64. **Odenholt, I., I. Gustafsson, E. Lowdin, and O. Cars.** 2003. Suboptimal antibiotic dosage as a risk factor for selection of penicillin-resistant *Streptococcus pneumoniae:* in vitro kinetic model. *Antimicrob. Agents Chemother.* **47**:518–523.
65. **Oliver, A., R. Canton, P. Campo, F. Baquero, and J. Blazquez.** 2000. High frequency of hypermutable *Pseudomonas aeruginosa* in cystic fibrosis lung infection. *Science* **288**:1251–1253.
66. **Preston, S. L., G. L. Drusano, A. L. Berman, C. L. Fowler, A. T. Chow, B. Dornseif, V. Reichl, J. Natarajan, and M. Corrado.** 1998. Pharmacodynamics of levofloxacin: a new paradigm for early clinical trials. *JAMA* **279**:125–129.
67. **Regnier, A., D. Concordet, M. Schneider, B. Boisrame, and P. L. Toutain.** 2003. Population pharmacokinetics of marbofloxacin in the aqueous humour after intravenous administration in dogs. *Am. J. Vet. Res.* **64**:889–893.
68. **Riond, J. L., and J. E. Riviere.** 1989. Effects of tetracyclines on the kidney in cattle and dogs. *J. Am. Vet. Med. Assoc.* **195**:995–997.
69. **Riviere, J. E.** 1999. *Comparative Pharmacokinetics. Principles, Techniques and Applications.* Iowa State University Press, Ames.
70. **Roche, Y., M. A. Gougerot-Pocidalo, M. Fay, N. Forest, and J. J. Pocidalo.** 1986. Macrolides and immunity: effects of erythromycin and spiramycin on human mononuclear cell proliferation. *J. Antimicrob. Chemother.* **17**:195–203.
71. **Rodriguez, J. C., L. Cebrian, M. Lopez, M. Ruiz, and G. Royo.** 2004. Mutant prevention concentration: a new tool for choosing treatment in nontuberculous mycobacterial infections. *Antimicrob. Agents Chemother.* **24**:352–356.
72. **Rodvold, K. A., M. H. Gotfried, L. H. Danziger, and R. J. Servi.** 1997. Intrapulmonary steady-state concentrations of clarithromycin and azithromycin in healthy adult volunteers. *Antimicrob. Agents Chemother.* **41**:1399–1402.
73. **Sarasola, P., P. Lees, F. S. AliAbadi, Q. A. McKellar, W. Donachie, K. A. Marr, S. J. Sunderland, and T. G. Rowan.** 2002. Pharmacokinetic and pharmacodynamic profiles of danofloxacin administered by two dosing regimens in calves infected with *Mannheimia (Pasteurella) haemolytica. Antimicrob. Agents Chemother.* **46**:3013–3019.
74. **Scaglione, F., J. W. Mouton, R. Mattina, and F. Fraschina.** 2003. Pharmacodynamics of levofloxacin and ciprofloxacin in a murine pneumonia model: peak concentration/MIC versus area under the curve/MIC ratios. *Antimicrob. Agents Chemother.* **47**:2749–2755.
75. **Schentag, J. J., D. J. Swanson, and I. L. Smith.** 1985. Dual individualization: antibiotic dosage calculation from the integration of in vitro pharmacodynamics and in vivo pharmacokinetics. *J. Antimicrob. Chemother.* **15**:47–57.
76. **Schentag, J. J.** 1989. Clinical significance of antibiotic tissue penetration. *Clin. Pharmacokin.* **16**:25–31.
77. **Schentag J. J., D. E. Nix, A. Forrest, and M. M. Adelman.** 1996. AUIC—the universal parameter within the constraint of a reasonable dosing interval. *Ann. Pharmacother.* **30**:1029–1031.
78. **Schentag, J. J.** 1998. Pharmacodynamic evaluation of factors associated with the development of bacterial resistance in acutely ill patients during therapy. *Antimicrob. Agents Chemother.* **42**:521–527.
79. **Schentag, J. J.** 2000. Clinical pharmacology of the fluoroquinolones: studies in human dynamic/kinetic models. *Clin. Infect. Dis.* **31**(Suppl. 2):S40–S44.
80. **Stearne, L. E., N. Lemmens, W. H. F. Goessens, J. W. Mouton, and I. C. Gyssens.** 2002. Presented at the European Conference on Clinical Microbiology and Infectious Diseases, Milan, Italy.
81. **Takeyama, K., J. Tamaoki, A. Chiyotani, E. Tagaya, and K. Konno.** 1993. Effect of macrolide antibiotics on ciliary motility in rabbit airway epithelium *in vitro. J. Pharm. Pharmacol.* **45**:756–758.
82. **Takizawa, H., M. Desaki, T. Ohtoshi, T. Kikutani, H. Okazaki, M. Sato, N. Akiyama, S. Shoji, K. Hiramatsu, and K. Ito.** 1995. Erythromycin suppresses interleukin 6 expression by human bronchial epithelial cells: a potential mechanism of its anti-inflammatory action. *Biochem. Biophys. Res. Commun.* **210**:781–786.
83. **Tamaoki, J., S. Noritaka, E. Tagaya, and K. Konno.** 1994. Macrolide antibiotics protect against endotoxin-induced vascular leakage and neutrophil accumulation in rat trachea. *Antimicrob. Agents Chemother.* **38**:1641–1643.
84. **Thomas, J. K., A. Forrest, S. M. Bhaveni, J. M. Hyatt, A. Cheng, L. H. Ballow, and J. J. Schentag.** 1998. Pharmacodynamic evaluation of factors associated with the development of bacterial resistance in acutely ill patients during therapy. *Antimicrob. Agents Chemother.* **42**:521–527.
85. **Thorburn, C. E., and D. I. Edwards.** 2001. The effect of pharmacokinetics on the bactericidal activity of ciprofloxacin and sparfloxacin against *Streptococcus pneumoniae* and the emergence of resistance. *J. Antimicrob. Chemother.* **48**:15–22.
86. **Toutain, P. L.** 2002. Pharmacokinetics/pharmacodynamics integration in drug development and dosage regimen optimisation for veterinary medicine. *AAPS PharmSci.* **4**(4):E38.
87. **Toutain, P. L.** 2003a. Pharmacokinetics/pharmacodynamics integration in dosage regimen optimisation for veterinary medicine. *J. Vet. Pharmacol. Ther.* **26**(Suppl. 1):1–8.
88. **Toutain, P. L.** 2003b. Antibiotic treatment of animals—a different approach to rational dosing. *Vet. J.* **165**:98–100.
89. **Toutain, P. L., J. R. del Castillo, and A. Bousquet-Melou.** 2002. The pharmacokinetic-pharmacodynamic approach to a rational dosage regimen for antibiotics. *Res. Vet. Sci.* **73**:105–114.
90. **Toutain, P. L., and P. Lees.** 2004. Integration and modelling of pharmacokinetic and pharmacodynamic data to optimise dosage regimens in veterinary medicine. *J. Vet. Pharmacol. Ther.* **27**:467–477.
91. **Umeki, S.** 1993. Anti-inflammatory action of erythromycin: its inhibitory effect on neutrophil NADPH oxidase activity. *Chest* **104**:1191–1193.
92. **Vogelman, B., S. Gudmundsson, J. Leggett, J. Turnidge, S. Ebert, and W. A. Craig.** 1988. Correlation of antimicrobial pharmacokinetic parameters with therapeutic efficacy in an animal model. *J. Infect. Dis.* **158**:831–847.
93. **Yancey, R. J., Jr., R. A. Evans, D. D. Kratzer, J. B. Paulissen, and S. G. Carmer.** 1990. Efficacy of ceftiofur hydrochloride for treatment of experimentally induced colibacillosis in neonatal swine. *Am. J. Vet. Res.* **51**:831–847.
94. **Zhanel, G. G., M. Dueck, D. J. Hoban, L. M. Vercaigne, J. M. Embil, A. S. Gin, and J. A. Karlowsky.** 2001. Review of macrolides and ketolides. *Drugs* **61**:443–498.
95. **Zhao, X., and K. Drlica.** 2001. Restricting the selection of antibiotic-resistant mutants: a general strategy derived from fluoroquinolones studies. *Clin. Infect. Dis.* **33**(Suppl. 3):S147–S156.

Antimicrobial Resistance in Bacteria of Animal Origin
Edited by Frank M. Aarestrup

Chapter 6

Mechanisms and Spread of Bacterial Resistance to Antimicrobial Agents

Stefan Schwarz, Axel Cloeckaert, and Marilyn C. Roberts

With regard to their structures and functions, antimicrobial agents represent a highly diverse group of low-molecular-weight substances that interfere with bacterial growth, resulting in either time-limited growth inhibition (bacteriostatic effect) or the killing of the bacteria (bactericidal effect). For more than 50 years antimicrobial agents have been used to control bacterial infections in humans, animals, and plants. Nowadays, antimicrobial agents are among the most frequently used therapeutics in human and veterinary medicine (183, 186). In the early days of antimicrobial chemotherapy, antimicrobial resistance was not considered an important problem, since the numbers of resistant strains were low and a large number of new, highly effective antimicrobial agents of different classes were being discovered. These early antimicrobial agents were identified as products of metabolic pathways of soil bacteria (e.g., *Streptomyces* and *Bacillus* spp.) or fungi (e.g., *Penicillium*, *Cephalosporium*, and *Pleurotus* spp.) (Table 1) and rendered their producers a selective advantage in the struggle for resources and the colonization of ecological niches (188). This in turn forced the susceptible bacteria living in close contact with the antimicrobial producers to develop and/or refine mechanisms to circumvent the inhibitory effects of antimicrobial agents. As a consequence, the origins of bacterial resistance to antimicrobial agents can be assumed to have long preceded the clinical use of these substances. With the elucidation of the chemical structures of the antimicrobial agents, which commonly followed soon after their detection, it was possible not only to produce antimicrobial agents synthetically in larger amounts at lower costs but also to introduce modifications that altered the pharmacokinetic or pharmacodynamic properties of these substances and occasionally also extended their spectrum of activity.

The increased selective pressure as imposed by the widespread use of antimicrobial agents since the 1950s has distinctly accelerated the development and the spread of bacterial resistance to antimicrobial agents. In most cases it took not longer than 3 to 5 years after introduction of an antimicrobial agent into clinical use until the first resistant target bacteria occurred (183). This is in particular true for broad-spectrum antimicrobial agents, such as tetracyclines, aminoglycosides, and chloramphenicol, which have been used for multiple purposes in human and veterinary medicine, horticulture, and/or aquaculture. In contrast, this time span was extended to at least 15 years for narrow-spectrum agents, such as glycopeptides, which were used in distinctly lower quantities and only for specific applications. Multiple studies have also revealed that resistance to completely synthetic antimicrobial agents, such as sulfonamides, trimethoprim, and fluoroquinolones, can develop quickly. These observations underline the enormous flexibility of the bacteria to cope with less favorable environmental conditions by constantly exploring new ways to survive in the presence of antimicrobial agents.

RESISTANCE TO ANTIMICROBIAL AGENTS

Resistance to antimicrobial agents can be subdivided into two basic types of resistance, intrinsic resistance and acquired resistance (186; also see chapter 1). Intrinsic resistance, also known as primary resistance, describes a status of general insensitivity of

Stefan Schwarz • Institut für Tierzucht, Bundesforschungsanstalt für Landwirtschaft, D-31535 Neustadt-Mariensee, Germany. **Axel Cloeckaert** • Unité BioAgresseurs, Santé, Environnement, Institut National de la Recherche Agronomique, 37380 Nouzilly, France. **Marilyn C. Roberts** • Department of Pathobiology, School of Public Health and Community Medicine, University of Washington, Seattle, WA 98195-7238.

Table 1. Origins of antimicrobial agents

Class	Antimicrobial agent(s)	Producing organism(s)	Yr of isolation
β-Lactam antibiotics	Natural penicillins	*Penicillium notatum*, *Penicillium chrysogenum*	1929, 1940
	Cephalosporin C	*Cephalosporium acremonium*	1945, 1953
	Imipenem	*Streptomyces cattleya*	1976
	Aztreonam	*Gluconobacter* spp., *Chromobacterium violaceum*	1981
Glycopeptides	Vancomycin	*Amycolatopsis orientalis*	Mid-1950s
	Teicoplanin, avoparcin	*Amycolatopsis coloradensis* subsp. *labeda*	1975
Macrolides	Erythromycin	*Streptomyces erythraeus*	1952
	Spiramycin	*Streptomyces ambofaciens*	1955
Lincosamides	Lincomycin	*Streptomyces lincolnensis*	1963
Streptogramins	Streptogramins A and B	*Streptomyces diastaticus*	1953
	Virginiamycins A and B	*Streptomyces virginiae*	1955
Tetracyclines	Chlortetracycline	*Streptomyces aureofaciens*	1948
	Oxytetracycline	*Streptomyces rimosus*	
Phenicols	Chloramphenicol	*Streptomyces venezuelae*	1947
Aminoglycosides	Streptomycin	*Streptomyces griseus*	1943
	Neomycin	*Streptomyces fradiae*	1949
	Kanamycin	*Streptomyces kanamyceticus*	1957
	Gentamicin	*Micromonospora purpurea*	1963
	Tobramycin	*Streptomyces tenebrarius*	1967
Aminocyclitols	Spectinomycin	*Streptomyces spectabilis*	1961
Pleuromutilins	Tiamulin	*Pleurotus* spp.	
Polypeptide antibiotics	Polymyxin B	*Bacillus polymyxa (aerosporus)*	1947
	Polymyxin E (colistin)	*Bacillus polymyxa* subsp. *colistinus*	1949
	Bacitracin	*Bacillus licheniformis*	1943
Sulfonamides	Prontosil, sulfamethoxazole, etc.	Synthetic	1935
Trimethoprim	Trimethoprim	Synthetic	1956
Quinolones	Nalidixic acid	Synthetic	1962
Fluoroquinolones	Flumequine, enrofloxacin, etc.	Synthetic	1973
Oxazolidinones	Linezolid	Synthetic	1987, 1996

bacteria to a specific antimicrobial agent or class of agents. This is commonly due to the lack of target structures for certain antimicrobial agents (e.g., β-lactam resistance in cell wall-free bacteria) or their inaccessibility in specific bacteria. Intrinsic resistance is a genus- or species-specific property of bacteria. In contrast, acquired resistance is a strain-specific property which can be due to the acquisition of foreign resistance genes or mutational modification of chromosomal target genes. Mutations that upregulate the expression of multidrug transporter systems may also fall into the category of acquired resistance. Three basic types of resistance mechanisms can be differentiated: (i) reduced intracellular accumulation by decreased influx and/or increased efflux of antimicrobials (Table 2); (ii) enzymatic inactivation by either disintegration or chemical modification of the antimicrobials (Table 3); and (iii) modification of the cellular target sites by mutation, chemical modification, or protection of the target sites, but also overexpression of sensitive targets or the replacement of sensitive target structures by alternative resistant ones (Table 4) (186; also see chapter 1).

The following sections illustrate that bacterial resistance to antimicrobial agents varies depending on the agent, the bacterium, and the resistance mechanism. Resistance to the same antimicrobial agent can be mediated by up to six different mechanisms. In some cases the same resistance gene or mechanism is found in a wide variety of bacteria, whereas in other cases resistance genes or mechanisms appear to be limited to certain bacterial species or genera. The data presented in the following sections do not focus exclusively on the resistance genes and mechanisms so far detected in bacteria of animal origin, but also include resistance genes and mechanisms identified in bacteria from humans. For a better overview on the mechanisms and genes accounting for resistance to

Table 2. Examples of resistance to antimicrobials by decreased intracellular drug accumulation[a]

Resistance mechanism	Resistance gene(s)	Gene product	Resistance phenotype	Bacteria involved	Location of the resistance gene[b]
Efflux via specific exporters	*mef*(A)	Efflux system of the major facilitator superfamily	14-, 15-Membered macrolides	Gram-positive and -negative bacteria	T, P, C
	vga(A), *vga*(B)	Efflux system of the ABC transporter family	Streptogramin A compounds	*Staphylococcus*	P
	tet(A–E, G–L, Z), *tetA*(P), *tet*(30)	12-, 14-TMS efflux system of the major facilitator superfamily	Tetracyclines	Various gram-positive and -negative bacteria	P, T, C
	pp-flo, *floR*, *cmlA*-like	12-TMS efflux system of the major facilitator superfamily	Chloramphenicol, florfenicol	*Photobacterium*, *Vibrio*, *Salmonella*, *Escherichia*, *Klebsiella*, *Pasteurella*	T, P, C
	cmlA	12-TMS efflux system of the major facilitator superfamily	Chloramphenicol	*Pseudomonas*, *Salmonella*, *E. coli*	T, P, C
	fexA	14-TMS efflux system of the major facilitator superfamily	Chloramphenicol, florfenicol	*Staphylococcus*	T, P, C
	msr(A)	Efflux system of the ABC transporter family	Macrolides and perhaps streptogramin B compounds	*Staphylococcus*	P
Efflux via multidrug transporters	*emr*E	4-TMS multidrug efflux protein	Tetracyclines, nucleic acid-binding compounds	*E. coli*	C
	blt, *nor*A	12-TMS multidrug efflux protein of the major facilitator superfamily	Chloramphenicol, fluoroquinolones, nucleic acid-binding compounds	*Bacillus*, *Staphylococcus*	C
	mexB-mexA-oprM, *acrA-acrB-tolC*	Multidrug efflux in combination with specific outer membrane proteins	Chloramphenicol, β-lactams, macrolides, fluoroquinolones, tetracyclines, etc.	*Pseudomonas*, *E. coli*, *Salmonella*	C

[a]Modified from reference 183.
[b]P, plasmid; T, transposon; C, chromosomal DNA.

Table 3. Examples of resistance to antimicrobials by enzymatic inactivation[a]

Resistance mechanism	Resistance gene(s)	Gene product(s)	Resistance phenotype	Bacteria involved	Location of the resistance gene[b]
Hydrolytic degradation	*bla*	β-Lactamases	β-Lactam antibiotics	Various gram-positive and -negative, aerobic and anaerobic bacteria	P, T, GC, C
	ere(A), *ere*(B)	Esterases	Macrolides	Gram-negative bacteria	P, GC
	vgb(A), *vgb*(B)	Lactone hydrolases	Streptogramin B antibiotics	*Staphylococcus*	P
Chemical modification	*aac*, *aad* (*ant*), *aph*	Acetyl-, adenyl-, phosphotransferases	Aminoglycosides	Gram-positive and -negative, aerobic bacteria	T, GC, P, C
	aad (*ant*)	Adenyltransferases	Aminocyclitols	Gram-positive and -negative, aerobic bacteria	T, GC, P, C
	catA, *catB*	Acetyltransferases	Chloramphenicol	Gram-positive and -negative, aerobic and anaerobic bacteria	P, T, GC, C
	vat(A–F)	Acetyltransferases	Streptogramin A antibiotics	*Staphylococcus*, *Enterococcus*	P, C
	mph(A–D)	Phosphotransferases	Macrolides	*Escherichia*, *Shigella*, *Staphylococcus*	P, T, C
	lnu(A–C)	Nucleotidyl transferases	Lincosamides	*Staphylococcus*	P
	tet(X)	Oxidoreductase	Tetracyclines	*Bacteroides*	T, P

[a]Modified from reference 183.
[b]P, plasmid; T, transposon; GC, gene cassette; C, chromosomal DNA.

a specific class of antimicrobial agents, the information is arranged under the names of the nine classes of antimicrobial agents that play a major role as therapeutics in veterinary medicine or, as in the case of glycopeptides and streptogramins, are of relevance with regard to an animal-to-man transfer of resistance genes.

Resistance to β-Lactam Antibiotics

For use in veterinary medicine, a number of penicillins, alone or in combination with a β-lactamase inhibitor, as well as cephalosporins of all spectra of activity are licensed. No carbapenems or monobactams are currently approved for use in animals. Resistance to β-lactam antibiotics is mainly due to inactivation by β-lactamases (119) and decreased ability to bind to penicillin-binding proteins (PBPs) (73) in both gram-positive and gram-negative bacteria, but may also be based on decreased uptake of β-lactams due to permeability barriers or increased efflux via multidrug transporter systems (149, 164). Inactivation via β-lactamases is most commonly seen, with a wide range of β-lactamases involved. The evolution of β-lactamases that differ distinctly in their substrate spectra is believed to have occurred in response to the selective pressure imposed by the various β-lactam antibiotics that have been introduced into clinical use during the last 40 years (152).

Enzymatic inactivation

Enzymatic inactivation of β-lactam antibiotics is based on the cleavage of the amino bond in the β-lactam ring by β-lactamases (33, 34, 119, 223). At present, several hundred β-lactamases have been described, most of which are variants of known β-lactamases that, however, differ in their substrate spectra or their enzyme stability. The initial classification scheme based on the similarities in the amino acid sequences subdivided the β-lactamases into four classes, A to D (10). The currently used classification of β-lactamases is done on the basis of their substrate spectra and their susceptibility to β-lactamase inhibitors such as clavulanic acid (34). This system also subdivides the β-lactamases into four classes (1 to 4), with class 2 currently comprising eight subclasses (34, 223). Class 1 β-lactamases, such as AmpC, are widespread among gram-negative bacteria. The *ampC* genes are commonly located on the chromosome, but may also be found on plasmids. Some of these *ampC* genes are expressed inducibly, others constitutively (222). Point mutations in the promoter region may increase β-lactamase production. The substrate spectrum includes all β-lactams except carbapenems. These enzymes are not inhibited by clavulanic acid. Class 2 β-lactamases represent a diverse class of enzymes, most of which are sensitive to inhibition by clavulanic acid. Subclass 2a includes enzymes such as

Table 4. Examples of resistance to antimicrobials by target modification[a]

Resistance mechanism	Resistance gene(s)	Gene product(s)	Resistance phenotype	Bacteria involved	Location(s) of the resistance gene[b]
Methylation of the target site	*erm*	rRNA methylase	MLS_B	Various gram-positive bacteria, *Escherichia*, *Bacteroides*	P, T, C
Protection of the target site	*tet*(M, O, P, Q, S, T, W)	Ribosomal protection proteins	Tetracyclines	Various gram-positive and -negative bacteria	T, P, C
Replacement of a sensitive target by an alternative drug-resistant target	*sul1, sul2, sul3*	Sulfonamide-resistant dihydropteroate synthase	Sulfonamides	Various gram-negative bacteria	P, I
	dfr (dhfr)	Trimethoprim-resistant dihydrofolate reductase	Trimethoprim	Various gram-positive and -negative bacteria	P, GC, T, C
	mecA	PBP, with altered substrate specificity	Penicillins, cephalosporins, carbapenems, monobactams	*Staphylococcus*	C
	vanA–E	Alternative D-Ala–D-Lac or D-Ala–D-Ser peptidoglycan precursors	Glycopeptides	*Enterococcus*, *Staphylococcus*	T, P, C
Mutational modification of the target site		Mutation in the gene coding for ribosomal protein S12	Streptomycin	Several gram-positive and -negative bacteria	C
		Mutation in the 16S rRNA	Streptomycin	*Mycobacterium*	C
		Mutation in the 23S rRNA	Macrolides	*Mycobacterium*	C
		Mutation in the 16S rRNA	Tetracyclines	*Propionibacterium*	C
		Mutations in the genes for DNA gyrase and topoisomerase IV	Fluoroquinolones	Various gram-positive and -negative bacteria	C
		Mutation in the gene for the ribosomal protein L3	Tiamulin	*E. coli*	C
Mutational modification of regulatory elements		Mutations in the *marRAB*, *soxR*, or *acrR* genes	Fluoroquinolones	*E. coli*	C

[a]Modified from reference 183.
[b]P, plasmid; T, transposon; GC, gene cassette; C, chromosomal DNA 2; I, integron.

BlaZ from staphylococci that can inactivate only penicillins. Subclass 2b comprises broad-spectrum β-lactamases, such as TEM-1, SHV-1, and ROB-1, that can hydrolize penicillins and broad-spectrum cephalosporins. Subclass 2be represents extended-spectrum β-lactamases (ESBLs) (e.g., TEM-3 to TEM-20, SHV-2) that can also inactivate oxyimino cephalosporins and monobactams. Due to their wide spectrum of activity, ESBLs represent a serious cause of concern (29). Most ESBLs currently known belong to the TEM, SHV, CTX-M, or OXA families of β-lactamases. Details with regard to the structure and function of these ESBLs, their location on mobile elements, and their dissemination among bacteria of different species and genera, as well as information on ESBL detection methods, can be found in several recent reviews (25, 29). Moreover, a continuously updated database that lists the known ESBLs and inhibitor-resistant β-lactamases, including TEM, SHV, OXA, CTX-M, CMY, IMP, and VIM types, can be found at http://www.lahey.org/Studies/. The enzymes of subclass 2br are also broad-spectrum β-lactamases, such as TEM-30 to TEM-40 and SHV-10, which, however, cannot be inhibited by clavulanic acid. Analysis of the β-lactamases of subclasses 2b, 2be, and 2br, in particular those of the TEM or SHV types, revealed the presence of mutations that either extended the substrate spectrum or affected the enzyme stability (34, 119, 152). Subclass 2c includes inhibitor-sensitive carbenicillinases such as CARB-1 or BRO-1, whereas the β-lactamases of subclass 2d (e.g., OXA-1 to OXA-10) exhibit relative insensitivity to inhibitors and can hydrolyze oxacillin and cloxacillin. The β-lactamases of subclasses 2e and 2f represent cephalosporinases (e.g., CepA) or serine-carbapenemases (e.g., SME-1, IMI-1), both of which are inhibited by clavulanic acid. While the β-lactamases of classes 1 and 2 have a serine residue in the catalytic center, the β-lactamases of class 3 hydrolyze β-lactams by divalent cations (Zn^{2+}) and are referred to as metallo-β-lactamases (e.g., IMP-1, VIM-1). These enzymes can inactivate all β-lactams except monobactams and are insensitive to clavulanic acid. Finally, class 4 comprises all so far nonsequenced β-lactamases that cannot be assigned to any of the other groups. The location of many of the β-lactamase genes (*bla*) on either plasmids, transposons, or gene cassettes favors their dissemination (25, 217).

Altered PBPs

Altered PBPs are often associated with resistance due to decreased binding of β-lactam antibiotics (73). PBPs are transpeptidases that play an important role in cell wall synthesis. PBPs are present in most cell wall-containing bacteria, but they vary from species to species in number, size, amounts, and affinity for β-lactam antibiotics (73). The acquisition of a novel PBP2a that replaces the original β-lactam-sensitive PBP is the cause of methicillin resistance in *Staphylococcus aureus* and coagulase-negative staphylococci (74, 81). Methicillin-resistant staphylococci are resistant to virtually all β-lactam antibiotics. The *mecA* gene, which codes for the alternative PBP2a, is part of a 52-kb genetic element, designated Staphylococcus cassette chromosome *mec* (SCC*mec*) (98). So far, five different allotypes of SCC*mec* have been described (93). In addition to PBP2a, the Fem proteins are involved in expression of methicillin resistance. The FemAB proteins contribute to the formation of the pentaglycine cross bridge, which is a unique staphylococcal cell wall component (66). Inactivation of *femAB* has been found to completely restore susceptibility to β-lactams and other antimicrobial agents in methicillin-resistant *S. aureus* strains (118). PBPs with low affinity for β-lactams have also been detected in streptococci and enterococci (73). Homologous recombinations in the genes coding for PBP1a, -2a, and -2b are assumed to result in mosaic proteins with decreased affinity for β-lactams in *Streptococcus pneumoniae* and *Neisseria* spp. PBP3, which has a low affinity for β-lactams, has been reported to be overproduced in resistant strains of *Enterococcus faecium* and *Enterococcus faecalis*. It is noteworthy that alterations in PBPs do not necessarily result in complete resistance to all β-lactams, but can also lead to elevated MICs of selected β-lactam antibiotics. In this regard, several different PBPs, which show decreased binding of a more or less extended spectrum of β-lactams, have been identified in gram-negative bacteria (73).

Reduced β-lactam uptake

Reduced uptake of β-lactams due to decreased outer membrane permeability and/or the lack of certain outer membrane proteins, which serve as entry for β-lactams to the bacterial cell, has been described in various *Enterobacteriaceae*, *Pseudomonas* spp., and other bacteria (40, 89, 134). In *Escherichia coli* and *Klebsiella pneumoniae*, β-lactam resistance can be based on the decreased expression or the structural alteration of the porins OmpF (193) and OmpK38 (127), by which β-lactams cross the outer membrane. In *Pseudomonas aeruginosa*, resistance to imipenem has been shown to be based on the loss of the porin OprD (224).

Multidrug transporters

Several multidrug transporters such as the MexAB-OprM and the MexCD-OprJ systems in *P. aeruginosa*, the SmeAB-SmeC system in *Stenotrophomonas maltophilia*, and the AcrAB-TolC system in *Salmonella* and *E. coli* (159, 163) are known to mediate the export of β-lactam antibiotics.

Resistance to Tetracyclines

Among this family of antimicrobial agents, oxytetracycline, chlortetracycline, and tetracycline have been used since the 1950s in veterinary medicine. More recently, doxycycline has been approved for dogs, cats, and pigs. Up to now, minocycline and glycylcyclines have not been licensed for use in animals. A survey on the use of antimicrobial agents in 1997 in the European Union member states and Switzerland revealed that tetracyclines accounted for almost two-thirds of all antimicrobials used in 1997 for therapeutic applications in veterinary medicine (183). Therefore, it is not surprising that tetracycline resistance has become widespread among bacteria of veterinary importance, including in aquaculture (37, 56, 133). Tetracycline resistance is most often due to the acquisition of new genes (44). There have been 23 efflux genes, which code for energy-dependent efflux of tetracyclines; 11 ribosomal protection genes, which code for a protein that protects bacterial ribosomes; 3 genes that code for enzymes that modify and inactivate the tetracycline molecule; and 1 gene [*tet*(U)] that specifies tetracycline resistance by an unknown mechanism. The products of different *tet* genes share ≤79% amino acid identity (117). Though only the first two mechanisms are currently found in bacteria of veterinary importance, this is not a stagnant area and new acquired genes continue to be described, as do new species and genera with previously described *tet* genes. An updated database listing the currently known *tet* genes and their occurrence in different bacteria is at http://faculty.washington.edu/marilynr/. New *tet* gene names are approved by Stuart B. Levy, Tufts University, Boston, Mass.

Energy-dependent efflux

The energy-dependent efflux of tetracyclines is mediated by membrane-associated proteins that exchange a proton for a tetracycline-cation complex (44, 198). These tetracycline resistance efflux proteins are part of the major facilitator superfamily (MFS) and share amino acid and protein structure similarities with other efflux proteins (149). The Tn*10*-associated *tet*(B) gene codes for an efflux protein that confers resistance to both tetracycline and minocycline but not to the new glycylcyclines (38, 44). All the other efflux proteins confer resistance to tetracycline but not to minocycline or glycylcyclines. Laboratory-derived mutations in the *tet*(A) or *tet*(B) gene have led to glycylcycline resistance, suggesting that bacterial resistance to glycylcyclines may develop over time and with clinical use (44). The *tet* efflux genes code for an approximately 46-kDa membrane-bound efflux protein. The tetracycline efflux proteins present in gram-negative bacteria commonly exhibit 12 transmembrane segments (TMS), and upstream of the structural gene and read in the opposite direction is a specific *tet* repressor gene. Induction of the structural gene is based on the binding of a tetracycline-Mg^{2+} complex to the *tet* repressor protein, which, in the absence of tetracycline, blocks transcription of the *tet* structural gene (142). The *tet*(A), *tet*(B), *tet*(C), *tet*(D), and *tet*(H) genes are most widespread among gram-negative bacteria of human and veterinary origin, while *tet*(D) and *tet*(E) are often associated with aquaculture environments and fish (37, 56, 133). Their location on transposons, such as Tn*1721* [*tet*(A)] (8), Tn*10* [*tet*(B)] (38, 113), or Tn*5706* [*tet*(H)] (105), and plasmids facilitates the spread within the gram-negative bacterial gene pool. The *tet*(K) and *tet*(L) efflux genes of gram-positive bacteria are not regulated by repressors, and they confer resistance to tetracyclines but not minocycline. They code for proteins with 14 TMS and are regulated by translational attenuation, which requires the presence of tetracyclines as inducers for the translation of the *tet* gene transcripts (168). These genes are generally found on small transmissible plasmids, which on occasion become integrated into the chromosome and occasionally may undergo interplasmidic recombination with other resistance plasmids (162, 187, 218). They have primarily been found in gram-positive species, but both have been found in a few facultative and/or anaerobic gram-negative genera, where they appear to confer tetracycline resistance (44).

Ribosomal protection

The ribosomal protection genes code for cytoplasmic proteins that protect the ribosomes from the action of tetracycline both in vitro and in vivo and confer resistance to tetracycline, doxycycline, and minocycline (44, 204). These proteins have sequence similarity to the ribosomal elongation factors EF-G and EF-Tu and are grouped into the translation factor superfamily of GTPases (50). Their interaction with the ribosome causes an allosteric disruption of the primary tetracycline binding site(s), which then leads to the release of the tetracycline from the ribosome. This allows the ribosome to return to its functional normal posttranslocational conformational state, which was altered by the binding of tetracycline. A detailed review of the various experiments done to elucidate the mode of action of these proteins can be found in reference 50. The ribosomal protection genes are of gram-positive origin and found extensively among gram-positive cocci. However, they have also been found in a number of different gram-negative genera. The first gene of this group, the *tet*(M) gene, has the widest host range of all *tet* genes. This gene is located on the conjugative transposons, such as Tn*916* (44, 72, 176).

Enzymatic inactivation

Enzymatic inactivation of tetracycline is mediated by three genes. The first described was the *tet*(X) gene (197). This encodes an NADPH-requiring oxidoreductase, which modifies and inactivates the tetracycline molecule in the presence of oxygen but has been found only in a strict anaerobe, *Bacteroides*, where oxygen is excluded (197). More recently, a second gene, *tet*(37), has been identified from the oral cavity of humans; it also requires oxygen to function but is unrelated to the *tet*(X) gene (57). No bacterial host which carries this gene has been identified. A third gene, *tet*(34), with similarities to the xanthine-guanine phosphoribosyl transferase gene of *Vibrio cholerae*, has also been identified (140).

16S rRNA mutation

A mutation in the 16S rRNA consisting of a single base exchange (1058G→1058C) has been identified in tetracycline-resistant *Propionibacterium acnes* (171). Position 1058 is located in a region which plays an important role in the termination of peptide chain elongation as well as in the accuracy of translation.

Other mutations

Mutations which alter the permeability of the outer membrane porins and/or lipopolysaccharides in the outer membrane can also affect resistance to tetracycline. A permeability barrier due to the reduced production of the OmpF porin, by which tetracyclines cross the outer membrane, has been described in *E. coli*. Mutations in the *marRAB* operon, which also regulates OmpF expression, may play a role in this type of tetracycline resistance (164).

Multidrug transporters

Different types of multidrug transporters mediating resistance to tetracycline in addition to resistance to a number of structurally unrelated compounds have been described, for instance, in *E. coli* (EmrE), *Salmonella* (AcrAB/TolC), and *P. aeruginosa* (MexAB/OprM, MexCD/OprJ) (149, 159, 163).

Resistance to Macrolides, Lincosamides, and Streptogramins

Several macrolide antibiotics, such as erythromycin, spiramycin, tylosin, and tilmicosin, as well as lincosamide antibiotics, such as clindamycin, lincomycin, and pirlimycin, are approved for use in animals. Since the ban of growth promoters, no streptogramin antibiotics are licensed for veterinary use. The 16-membered macrolide antibiotics tylosin and spiramycin were previously used as feed additives for animal growth promotion, but remain as therapeutics for veterinary use for the control of bacterial dysentery, respiratory disease, and mastitis. Erythromycin, the first macrolide, was introduced into clinical use over 50 years ago and has good activity against gram-positive cocci and other gram-positive species and some activity against some gram-negative bacteria such as *Campylobacter*. *Enterobacteriaceae* and *Pseudomonas* spp. have been considered to be innately nonsusceptible to erythromycin due to innate multidrug transporters that have 14-membered macrolides as substrates (154). However, recent work illustrated that 78% of randomly selected gram-negative bacteria actually carry known genes (144), suggesting that this hypothesis needs to be reevaluated, because the data suggest that both gram-positive and gram-negative bacteria may become resistant by acquistion of resistance genes. Acquired resistance mechanisms include specific efflux pumps, rRNA methylases that alter the 50S and reduce the binding, and mechanisms that through a variety of genes inactivate the antibacterials. Macrolides, lincosamides, and streptogramins (MLS), though chemically distinct, are usually considered together because they share overlapping binding sites on the 50S ribosomal subunit and a number of resistance genes confer resistance to more than one class of antibiotics (169, 202).

Target site modification

Target site modification by rRNA methylases, encoded by *erm* genes, was the first identified mechanism of resistance to macrolides, lincosamides, and streptogramin B (MLS_B) antibiotics conferred by acquired genes (214, 215). These genes are found in gram-positive, gram-negative, aerobic, and anaerobic genera. Currently, 32 different rRNA methylases have been characterized and each adds one or two methyl groups to a single adenine (A2058 in *E. coli*) in the 23S rRNA moiety (94, 156, 169). Expression of the *erm* genes may be constitutive or inducible via translational attenuation (114, 185, 202, 219); the type of expression depends on a regulatory region upstream of the *erm* gene and which macrolide is used for induction (202, 215). In staphylococci, erythromycin and other 14- and 15-membered macrolides are able to induce *erm* gene expression whereas 16-membered MLS_B antibiotics are considered as noninducers (202). Recently, laboratory selection of *S. aureus* produced mutants that had structural alterations in the translational attenuator region due to deletions, tandem duplications, point mutations, and the insertion of IS*256* (180, 181). Similar mutations have also been detected in naturally occurring strains carrying the respective *erm* genes (215, 219).

Efflux genes

Efflux genes include 12 ATP transporters and 2 major facilitator transporters (MFS). These genes confer a variety of resistance patterns including resistance to lincomycin, oleandomycin, spiramycin, tylosin, streptogramin A, or both erythromycin and streptogramin B (115, 202). The *vga*(A) and *vga*(B) genes share 59% identical amino acids and have

G+C contents of 29 to 36%. The *msr*(A) gene confers inducible resistance to 14- and 15-membered macrolides and streptogramin B and is found in staphylococci. The hydrophilic protein made from the *msr*(A) gene contains two ATP-binding motifs characteristic of the ABC transporters (172). The *msr*(A) gene tends to confer lower levels of erythromycin resistance than the rRNA methylases (167). The two MFS transporters are *lmr*(A), which codes for a lincomycin-specific efflux pump, and the *mef*(A) gene, which is a specific efflux pump for 14- and 15-membered macrolides. The *mef*(A) gene was first described in the 1990s from *Streptococcus* spp. (45), but more recently it has been shown to be in old isolates of pathogenic *Neisseria* spp. (51) and was found to be the most common acquired macrolide resistance gene in a collection of 176 randomly collected commensal gram-negative bacteria (144). Downstream of the *mef*(A) gene is an ABC transporter that has now been shown to independently confer macrolide resistance and has been named *msr*(D) (53). Whether both genes function in the natural isolate or one is preferentially expressed has not been determined.

Inactivating enzymes

The 17 inactivating enzymes include two esterases, two lyases, three nucleotidyltransferases, six acetyltransferases, and four phosphotransferases (169). The esterases, Ere(A) and Ere(B), hydrolyze the lactone in the macrolide, creating an identical inactive product. The esterases have been found exclusively in gram-negative bacteria. These genes are often associated with plasmids, though recently the *ere*(A) gene has been associated with both class 1 and class 2 integrons. The transferases confer resistance by adding an acetyl group to streptogramin A, which inactivates the antibiotic. Five different genes have been found in gram-positive cocci, and one has been identified in gram-negative bacteria (169). Four macrolide phosphorylases have been identified. Each enzyme adds a phosphate group to the macrolide, inactivating it. Among the four phosphorylases, three of the genes, *mph*(A), *mph*(B), and *mph*(D), have been found exclusively in gram-negative species, while *mph*(C), which was originally found in *Staphylococcus* spp., has now been identified in gram-negative clinical *S. maltophilia* (http://faculty.washington.edu/marilynr/).

Mutational changes

Usually, mutational changes that affect the 23S rRNA, ribosomal proteins, and/or innate efflux pumps may lead to moderate changes in susceptibility. Various mutations have been identified in the 23S rRNA (208). Originally, mutations at either the A2058 or A2059 position (*E. coli* numbering) were found in pathogens that had one or two copies of the 23S rRNA, like *Mycobacterium* or *Helicobacter* (129). Resistance to tylosin, erythromycin, and clindamycin in *Brachyspira hyodysenteriae* was also associated with an A→T substitution at the nucleotide position homologous with position 2058 of the *E. coli* 23S rRNA gene (97). Variations at positions 2058 and 2059 in the 23S rRNA have also been described in erythromycin-resistant *Streptococcus pyogenes*, *S. pneumoniae*, *Campylobacter coli*, *Campylobacter jejuni*, and *Haemophilus influenzae* (80, 83). An A→G substitution at position 2075 of the 23S rRNA was detected in *C. coli* from poultry and pigs that exhibited high-level erythromycin resistance (150). Mutations in ribosomal proteins L4 and/or L22 have been identified that confer increasing resistance to the newer agent telithromycin and/or to the other members of the MLS group. Laboratory-created mutants and recent clinical gram-positive isolates have been found with the same mutations. Missense mutations, deletions, and/or insertions may alter expression of innate pumps, which then may alter resistance to the MLS antibiotics. A detailed discussion can be found in reference 202.

Resistance to Aminoglycosides and Aminocyclitols

Various aminoglycoside antibiotics, including gentamicin, kanamycin, neomycin, and streptomycin, are licensed for use in both human and veterinary medicine. Among the aminocyclitol antibiotics, spectinomycin is approved for use in humans and animals, whereas apramycin is used exclusively in veterinary medicine. The main mechanism of resistance to aminoglycosides and aminocyclitols is enzymatic inactivation (132, 190). In addition, reduced uptake of aminoglycosides and chromosomal mutations conferring high-level resistance to streptomycin have also been described (164).

Enzymatic inactivation

Enzymatic inactivation of aminoglycosides and aminocyclitols is conferred by any of the three types of modifying enzymes: *N*-acetyltransferases (AACs), *O*-nucleotidyltransferases (also referred to as *O*-adenyltransferases) (ANTs), and *O*-phosphotransferases (APHs) (132, 190). Acetyl coenzyme A serves as a donor of acetyl groups in acetylation reactions at amino groups, while ATP is used for the adenylation and phosphorylation reactions at hydroxyl groups. For each of these three classes of aminoglycoside-modifying enzymes, numerous members are known that differ more or less extensively in their structure. Most modifying enzymes exhibit a narrow substrate spectrum. Several reviews have listed the known enzymes involved in modification of aminoglycosides and aminocyclitols and their molecular relationships (54, 178, 190). However, new genes for aminoglycoside- or aminocyclitol-inactivating enzymes or variants of already known ones are constantly reported. Unfortunately, a continuously updated database for the currently known aminoglycoside- or aminocyclitol-inactivating enzymes is not available. Another problem is the lack of an unambiguous nomenclature. There are at least two alternatively used designations for genes coding for the same modifying enzyme: one designation, such as *aph(3″)-Ib*, refers to the type of modification (*aph*), the position where the modification is introduced (*3″*), and the subtype of the gene (*Ib*); whereas the other designation, such as *strA*, is easier to handle, refers only to the corresponding resistance phenotype (*str* for streptomycin resistance), and also indicates the subtype (*A*).

So far, four classes of AACs are known that acetylate the amino groups at positions 1, 3, 2′, and 6′ (54, 132, 190, 225). To date, at least 40 different AACs have been identified, most of which vary in their substrate spectra. The vast majority of the AAC enzymes were identified in gram-negative bacteria (178, 225). Combined resistance to apramycin and gentamicin is due to the enzyme AAC(3)-IV; the corresponding gene emerged after the introduction of apramycin into veterinary use (42). It was first detected in *E. coli* and *Salmonella* from animals and later on found in *E. coli* from humans as well (41, 43, 95). A bifunctional enzyme that codes for acetyltransferase AAC(6′) and phosphotransferase APH(2″) activities was found on transposon Tn*4001*, which is widely spread among staphylococci, streptococci, and enterococci (112, 122, 173). More than 20 ANTs, which act at positions 6, 9, 4′, 2″, and 3″, are differentiated (54, 132, 190, 225). The different ANT enzymes also vary considerably in their substrate spectra. Among the APHs, which modify the aminoglycosides at positions 4, 6, 3′, 2″, and 3″, more than 25 variants have been identified that confer distinctly different resistance phenotypes. Most *aac*, *ant*, and *aph* genes are located on mobile genetic elements, such as plasmids, transposons, or gene cassettes (54, 124, 132, 166, 178, 179, 190, 225).

Multidrug efflux systems

Multidrug efflux systems, such as MexXY in *Pseudomonas* and AmrAB in *Burkholderia pseudomallei* (159), or the multidrug transporter AcrD in *E. coli* (170), have been described to export aminoglycosides. The transporter MdfA from *E. coli* (65) has also been reported to mediate the efflux of the aminoglycosides kanamycin, neomycin, and hygromycin A.

Decreased uptake

Decreased uptake of aminoglycosides may be based on a mutation in lipopolysaccharide phosphates or on a change in the charge of the lipopolysaccharide in *E. coli* and *P. aeruginosa*, respectively (177). Since the entry of aminoglycosides across the cytoplasmic membrane is mainly based on the electron transport system, anaerobic bacteria and facultative anaerobic bacteria exhibit relatively high insensitivity to aminoglycosides (164).

16S rRNA methylation

Methylation of the 16S rRNA at position G-1405 or A-1408 results in high-level resistance to gentamicin and kanamycin or kanamycin and apramycin, respectively. Both rRNA methylases have been identified in aminoglycoside producers and are believed to represent self-defense systems (21).

Mutations

Mutations in the gene *rpsL* for the ribosomal protein S12 have been shown to result in high-level streptomycin resistance (130). Single-base-pair substitutions at different positions in the gene *rrs* encoding 16S rRNA in mycobacteria have been described to be involved in either streptomycin resistance (130) or resistance to amikacin, kanamycin, gentamicin, tobramycin, and neomycin, but not to streptomycin (160).

Resistance to Sulfonamides and Trimethoprim

Various sulfonamides, trimethoprim, and combinations of sulfonamides and trimethoprim are licensed for use in humans and animals. There are no restrictions for use of any of these compounds in food animals. Sulfonamides and trimethoprim are competitive inhibitors of different enzymatic steps in folate metabolism. In this regard, sulfonamides represent structural analogs of *p*-aminobenzoic acid and inhibit the enzyme dihydropteroic acid synthase (DHPS), whereas trimethoprim inhibits the enzyme dihydrofolate reductase (DHFR). Various mechanisms of intrinsic and acquired resistance to sulfonamides and trimethoprim have been described in bacterial pathogens (68, 91, 92, 194, 195).

Permeability barriers and efflux pumps

Permeability barriers and efflux pumps play a relevant role by either preventing the influx or promoting the efflux of both compounds. Intrinsic resistance to both compounds in *P. aeruginosa* was initially thought to be based on outer membrane impermeability. More recently, however, the multidrug exporter system MexAB/OprM was found to be mainly responsible for resistance to sulfonamides and trimethoprim in *P. aeruginosa* (110). For other bacteria, such as *K. pneumoniae* or *Serratia marcescens*, impaired membrane permeability is still considered to play a role in sulfonamide and trimethoprim resistance (91, 92).

DHFR and folate auxotrophy

Naturally insensitive DHFR enzymes and folate auxotrophy play an important role in intrinsic resistance to sulfonamides and trimethoprim. DHFR enzymes that exhibit low affinity for trimethoprim and thus render their hosts intrinsically resistant to trimethoprim are known to occur in several bacterial genera, including *Clostridium*, *Neisseria*, *Brucella*, *Bacteroides*, and *Moraxella* (164). Bacteria such as enterococci and lactobacilli which can utilize exogenous folates also show intrinsic resistance to trimethoprim and sulfonamides.

Changes in target enzymes

Mutational or recombinational changes in the target enzymes have been observed in a wide variety of bacteria. Mutations in the chromosomal *dhps* gene that lead to sulfonamide resistance by single amino acid substitutions can be generated under in vitro conditions but occur also in vivo. Such mutations have been identified in *E. coli*, *S. aureus*, *Staphylococcus haemolyticus*, *C. jejuni*, and *Helicobacter pylori* (91). In *S. pneumoniae*, two amino acid duplications that change the tertiary structure of the DHPS have been found to be responsible for sulfonamide resistance (147). Recombinational events between the naturally occurring gene coding for a susceptible DHPS and that of a horizontally acquired resistant DHPS are believed to account for sulfonamide resistance in *Neisseria meningitidis* (91). Trimethoprim resistance has also been shown to be due to a single amino acid substitution in the DHFR protein in *S. aureus* (52) and *S. pneumoniae* (153). Mutations in the promoter region of chromosomal *dhfr* genes have been described to occur in *E. coli* and resulted in overexpression of the trimethoprim-susceptible DHFR (91). Mutations in both the promoter region and the *dhfr* gene have been identified in trimethoprim-resistant *H. influenzae* (55).

Replacement of sensitive enzymes by resistant ones

The replacement of sensitive enzymes by resistant enzymes usually causes high-level resistance (68, 91, 92, 194, 195). To date, three different types of resistant DHPS enzymes encoded by the genes *sul1*, *sul2*, and *sul3* have been described to occur in gram-negative bacteria (165, 203). The gene *sul1* is part of the class 1 integrons and thus is often associated with other resistance genes. As part of the transposons, such as Tn*21*, and conjugative plasmids, it is spread into various gram-negative species and genera (201). The *sul2* gene often occurs together with the Tn*5393*-associated streptomycin resistance genes *strA-strB* on conjugative or nonconjugative plasmids (101, 165). The gene *sul3* was originally found on a conjugative plasmid from porcine *E. coli*, where it was flanked by copies of the insertion sequence IS*15Δ/26* (151). Meanwhile, it has also been identified in *E. coli* from humans and animals other than pigs, as well as in *Salmonella enterica* from animal and food sources (76, 78, 79).

Up to now, more than 25 different dihydrofolate reductase (*dfr*; also referred to as *dhfr*) genes have been identified. These are subdivided on the basis of their structure into two major groups, *dfrA* and *dfrB* (148). The *dfrA* genes code for DHFR enzymes of 152 to 189 amino acids, whereas the *dfrB*-encoded DHFR enzymes consist of only 78 amino acids. The *dfrA* genes have been detected more frequently than *dfrB* genes. Transferable trimethoprim resistance genes have been identified in a wide variety of gram-negative bacteria; several of these genes are part of plasmids, transposons, or gene cassettes (92, 166, 195) and thus are easily disseminated across species and genus borders. Several studies have shown the relationships between the different *dfr* genes (92, 101, 195). In staphylococci, the composite transposon Tn*4003* has been identified on various multiresistance plasmids (174). Tn*4003* is composed of a central *dfrA* gene bracketed by copies of the insertion sequence IS*257*. Related trimethoprim resistance genes have been found in other gram-positive bacteria, such as *S. haemolyticus*, *Staphylococcus epidermidis*, *Listeria monocytogenes*, and *Bacillus subtilis* (39, 101).

Resistance to Quinolones and Fluoroquinolones

Quinolones and fluoroquinolones are potent inhibitors of bacterial DNA replication. While early quinolones such as nalidixic acid and pipemidic acid have not been used in veterinary medicine, oxolinic acid and flumequine, the first fluorinated quinolone, have been used in food-producing animals including fish worldwide (183, 212). Since the first of the newer fluoroquinolones, enrofloxacin, was licensed for use in animals in the late 1980s (16), several other fluoroquinolones have been approved for veterinary use during recent years, including sarafloxacin, marbofloxacin, orbifloxacin, difloxacin, ibafloxacin, and danofloxacin. Two major mechanisms account for resistance to fluoroquinolones: mutations in the genes for DNA topoisomerases and decreased intracellular drug accumulation (63, 71, 87, 175). In addition, protection of DNA topoisomerases by the Qnr protein has also been described (205). So far, enzymatic inactivation has not been observed in clinically relevant bacteria. Several recent reviews dealt with the molecular basis and epidemiology of quinolone resistance in *E. coli* and *Salmonella* of animal origin (16, 48, 212).

Mutational alteration of target genes

Mutational alteration of the target genes *gyrA* and *gyrB* (coding for the A and B subunits of the DNA gyrase) as well as *parC* and *parE* (coding for the A and B subunits of the DNA topoisomerase IV) is frequently seen in quinolone- and fluoroquinolone-resistant bacteria. Both enzymes are tetramers consisting of two A and B units. The mutations in *gyrA* are commonly located within a region of ca. 130 bp which is referred to as the quinolone resistance-determining region (QRDR) (226). Mutations resulting in changes of Ser-83 (to Tyr, Phe, or Ala) and Asp-87 (to Gly, Asn, or Tyr) have been detected most frequently. In addition, double mutations at both positions and various other mutations in gram-positive and gram-negative bacteria of human and veterinary importance have been described (48, 71, 87, 175, 212). Stepwise mutations in *gyrA* and *parC* can result in an incremental increase in resistance to quinolones (212). Moreover, different mutations may also have different effects on resistance to the various fluoroquinolones (96). The complex interplay between individual mechanisms may also have different effects on fluoroquinolone resistance (70).

Multidrug efflux systems

Multidrug efflux systems also conferring fluoroquinolone resistance have been identified in various gram-positive and gram-negative bacteria, such as *P. aeruginosa* (MexAB/OprM, MexCD/OprJ), *S. aureus* (NorA), *S. pneumoniae* (PmrA), *B. subtilis* (Blt), and *E. coli* and *Salmonella* (AcrAB/TolC); for reviews, see references 157, 158, and 175. Since the basal level of expression of these efflux systems is low, upregulation of their expression is required to confer resistance to fluoroquinolones and other antimicrobials. In *E. coli* the level of production of the AcrAB-TolC efflux system is under the control of several regulatory genes, in particular the global regulatory systems *marRAB* and *soxRS* (6, 145), but also *acrR* (146). Mutations in these regulatory systems may lead to overproduction of the AcrAB-TolC efflux pump and expression of the multidrug resistance phenotype (142, 146). Besides overproduction of the AcrAB-TolC efflux pump, it has been recently shown using macroarrays that *E. coli* strains constitutively expressing *marA* showed altered expression of more than 60 chromosomal genes (18).

Interaction between resistance mechanisms

Interplay between several resistance mechanisms may lead to high-level resistance to quinolones and other antibiotics when multidrug efflux pumps and decreased outer membrane permeability are involved (70, 116). For in vitro-selected quinolone-resistant *E. coli* mutants it has been shown that first-step quinolone-resistant mutants acquire a *gyrA* mutation. Second-step mutants reproducibly acquire a multidrug resistance phenotype and show enhanced fluoroquinolone efflux. In some third-step mutants, fluoroquinolone efflux is further enhanced and additional topoisomerase mutations are acquired. In clinical *E. coli* isolates from humans and animals the situation appears to be the same, where high-level fluoroquinolone resistance is reached when mutations at several chromosomal loci are acquired (70, 141). It is noteworthy that inactivation of the AcrAB efflux pump renders resistant *E. coli* strains, including those with target gene mutations, hypersusceptible to fluoroquinolones and certain other unrelated drugs (141). Thus, in the absence of the AcrAB efflux pump, gyrase mutations fail to produce clinically relevant levels of fluoroquinolone resistance (141). The same observation has been made for *P. aeruginosa*, where deletion of the MexAB-OprM efflux pump, which is the homolog of the AcrAB-TolC efflux pump in this species, resulted in a significant decrease in resistance to fluoroquinolones even for strains carrying target gene mutations (120). In high-level fluoroquinolone-resistant *S. enterica* serovar Typhimurium DT204 strains carrying multiple target gene mutations in *gyrA*, *gyrB*, and *parC*, inactivation of AcrB or TolC resulted in a 16- to 32-fold decrease of resistance levels to fluoroquinolones (19, 20).

Decreased drug uptake

Decreased drug uptake in gram-negative bacteria is due to the MAR-mediated downregulation of OmpF porin production. OmpF is an important porin for the entry of quinolones and fluoroquinolones into the bacterial cell (49, 128). Moreover, mutations in different gene loci (*cfxB*, *norB*, *nfxB*, *norC*, or *nalB*) are also associated with decreased permeability (88).

DNA gyrase protection

Low-level quinolone resistance via protection of DNA gyrase from inhibition by quinolones is mediated by the *qnr* gene. This gene has been identified as part of the complex In4 family class 1 integrons on plasmids from *K. pneumoniae* and *E. coli* (205, 210, 211). The *qnr* gene codes for a protein of 218 amino acids belonging to the pentapeptide repeat family (175, 205).

Resistance to Phenicols

Two members of the phenicols, chloramphenicol and its fluorinated derivative, florfenicol, are currently admitted for use in animals. To protect consumers from potential side effects arising from chloramphenicol residues in food animal carcasses, the use of chloramphenicol is limited to pets and non-food-producing animals in the European Union and North America. Florfenicol is licensed for the control of respiratory diseases in cattle and pigs, infectious pododermatitis in cattle, as well as furunculosis in salmon. The predominant mechanism of chloramphenicol resistance in gram-positive and gram-negative bacteria is enzymatic inactivation (137, 184, 191). In addition, efflux systems that mediate either resistance to only chloramphenicol or combined resistance to chloramphenicol and florfenicol have been identified (184). Furthermore, permeability barriers and multidrug transporters play a role in certain gram-negative bacteria (7, 149, 184). A detailed review on the different genes and mechanisms accounting for bacterial resistance to chloramphenicol and florfenicol has recently been published (184).

Enzymatic inactivation

Enzymatic inactivation of chloramphenicol is commonly achieved by chloramphenicol acetyltransferases (CATs), which transfer acetyl groups from acetyl-coenzyme A to the C3 position of the chloramphenicol molecule. Subsequent transfer of the acetyl group to the C1 position and transfer of a second acetyl group to C3 result in mono- or diacetylated chloramphenicol derivatives, both of which are unable to inhibit bacterial protein biosynthesis (137, 184, 191). Two distinct types of CAT enzymes which differ in their structures are known: the classical CATs (type A) and a novel type of CATs (type B) (137, 184). All type A and type B CATs are of a trimeric structure composed of three identical monomers. The *cat* gene codes for a CAT monomer, the size of which varies between 207 and 238 amino acids (type A CATs) and 209 and 212 amino acids (type B CATs) (184). Using the cutoff as set for the classification of tetracycline and MLS resistance genes (117, 169), 16 different classes of *catA* determinants and another 5 classes of *catB* determinants can be differentiated. Among the *catA* genes, those formerly referred to as *catI*, *catII*, and *catIII* are most widespread among gram-negative bacteria (9, 135, 136). They are associated with either nonconjugative transposons, such as Tn*9*, or plasmids. Expression of these *catA* genes is constitutive. Various *catA* genes indistinguishable from or closely related to those present on the *S. aureus* plasmids pC221, pC223/pSCS7, and pC194 (30, 90, 162, 182) have been detected in coagulase-positive and -negative staphylococci, but also in members of the genera *Streptococcus*, *Bacillus*, and *Listeria*, respectively. Expression of these mostly plasmid-borne *catA* genes is inducible by chloramphenicol via translational attenuation (121), whereas the Tn*4451*-borne *catA* genes of *Clostridium* spp. are expressed constitutively (17). The *catB* genes—also referred to as *xat* (xenobiotic acetyltransferase) genes—differ distinctly from the *catA* genes but are related to acetyltransferase genes, such as *vat*(A) to *vat*(E), involved in streptogramin resistance (137). Some of the *catB* genes have been found exclusively on the chromosome of either *Agrobacterium tumefaciens*, *P. aeruginosa*, or *V. cholerae*, whereas others proved to be part of transposons (Tn*2424*, Tn*840*) or plasmid-borne integrons. Studies on the level of *catB*-mediated chloramphenicol resistance revealed a distinctly lower level of chloramphenicol resistance as compared to that conferred by type A CATs (137).

In addition to inactivation via CATs, enzymatic inactivation of chloramphenicol can also occur by O-phosphorylation or by hydrolytic degradation to *p*-nitrophenylserinol. Since these mechanisms have so far only been seen in the chloramphenicol producer *Streptomyces venezuelae*, they are believed to play a role as self-defense mechanisms (184).

Specific exporters

A total of eight different classes of specific exporters that mediate either chloramphenicol or chloramphenicol and florfenicol resistance have been identified. Among them, four classes are represented by 10- to 12-TMS chloramphenicol exporters of soil bacteria of the genera *Streptomyces*, *Rhodococcus*, and *Corynebacterium*, whereas three classes of 12-TMS exporters were found among gram-negative bacteria of medical importance (184). Among the latter classes, one class represents the *cmlA* subgroup and another represents the *floR* subgroup. The gene *cmlA*, coding for a chloramphenicol exporter, is a Tn*1696*-associated cassette-borne gene which, however, is inducibly expressed via translational attenuation (200). Genes related to *cmlA* are mainly found in *Enterobacteriaceae* and *Pseudomonas*. The gene *floR*, coding for a chloramphenicol and florfenicol exporter, has recently been shown to be associated with the small nonconjugative transposon Tn*floR* (61). Genes related to *floR* have been identified in *Photobacterium*, *Vibrio*, *Klebsiella*, *E. coli*, various *S. enterica* serovars, and recently also in *Pasteurella multocida* (46, 47, 86, 104, 106, 107, 221). In *Vibrio* and *Salmonella*, the gene *floR* has been detected as part of chromosomal multiresistance gene clusters (11, 31, 86) and in *E. coli* as part of conjugative and nonconjugative multiresistance plasmids (24, 47, 106, 221). The eighth class is represented by FexA, the first specific chloramphenicol and florfenicol exporter of gram-positive bacteria (102). The gene *fexA*, located on the transposon Tn*558* (103) from *Staphylococcus lentus*, codes for a 14-TMS exporter of the MFS and is expressed inducibly via translational attenuation.

Multidrug transporter systems

Multidrug transporter systems that export chloramphenicol have been described to occur in several gram-negative bacteria, including the systems MexAB/OprM and MexCD/OprJ in *P. aeruginosa*, AcrAB/TolC in *E. coli* and *Salmonella*, CeoAB/OpcM in *Burkholderia cepacia*, as well as ArpAB/ArpC and TtgAB/TtgC in *Pseudomonas putida* (128, 159).

Permeability barriers

Permeability barriers based on the reduced expression of the OmpF porin in *Salmonella* serovar Typhi or a major outer membrane protein in *H. influenzae* (184) have also been described to confer chloramphenicol resistance. The *mar* locus, which is found in various *Enterobacteriaceae*, can contribute to chloramphenicol resistance in two ways: (i) it can activate the AcrAB/TolC efflux system, thus leading to increased efflux of chloramphenicol; and (ii) MarA can activate the gene *micF*, whose transcripts represent an antisense RNA that effectively inhibits translation of *ompF* transcripts, which results in a decreased influx of chloramphenicol (49, 128).

Mutations

Mutations in the major ribosomal protein clusters of *E. coli* and *B. subtilis* as well as mutations in the 23S rRNA of *E. coli* have been described to mediate chloramphenicol resistance (69).

23S rRNA methylation

The *cfr* gene from *Staphylococcus sciuri* mediates combined resistance to chloramphenicol, florfenicol, and clindamycin (104a, 189). Cfr specifies a novel rRNA methyltransferase of the radical SAM superfamily. Cfr-mediated methylation occurs at A2503 in the 23S rRNA and results in a reduced binding of phenicols as well as clindamycin to the ribosome (104a).

Resistance to Glycopeptides

After the ban of the growth promoter avoparcin in 1996, there are no glycopeptide antibiotics currently approved for use in animals. Glycopeptide antibiotics, such as vancomycin and teicoplanin, act by binding to the D-alanine–D-alanine termini of peptidoglycan precursors, thereby preventing transglycosylation and transpeptidation of the bacterial cell wall (12, 13, 209).

Target site modification

Modification of the target site is the common mechanism of bacterial resistance to glycopeptides. So far, five different vancomycin resistance phenotypes are known, designated VanA through VanE, which differ in their levels of resistance to vancomycin and teicoplanin (209). In the types VanA, VanB, and VanD, the terminal dipeptide D-alanine–D-alanine is replaced by D-alanine–D-lactate, whereas in VanC and VanE it is replaced by D-alanine–D-serine. These replacements reduce the ability of glycopeptides to bind to the peptidoglycan precursors and result in the case of D-lactate in high-level and in the case of D-serine in low-level glycopeptide resistance. VanC is responsible for the intrinsic resistance of *Enterococcus gallinarum*, *Enterococcus casseliflavus*, and *Enterococcus flavescens* to glycopeptides (209). Like VanC, VanD and VanE, both from *E. faecalis*, have been reported to be not transferable. In contrast, VanA and VanB are associated with transposons that can be located on conjugative and nonconjugative plasmids in enterococci. The VanA phenotype is associated with the nonconjugative transposon Tn*1546*, which contains a total of nine reading frames, five of which are essential for high-level glycopeptide resistance (14). Among them, the two genes *vanR* and *vanS* code for a response regulator protein and a sensor protein, respectively, involved in regulatory processes. Three genes are directly involved in resistance: *vanH*, *vanA*, and *vanX*. The *vanH* gene codes for a cytoplasmatic dehydrogenase that produces D-lactate from pyruvate, whereas the gene *vanX* codes for a D,D-dipeptidase that cleaves the D-alanine–D-alanine, and the gene *vanA* codes for a ligase that joins the remaining D-alanine with D-lactate. There are genes with similar functions that account for the VanB–E phenotypes, with the exception that in the cases of VanC and VanE the gene *vanH* is replaced by a gene designated *vanT*. This gene codes for a membrane-associated serine racemase that produces D-serine. Moreover, the genes *vanA*, *vanB*, and *vanD*, specifying D-alanine–D-lactate ligases, as well as the genes *vanC* and *vanE*, specifying D-alanine–D-serine ligases, differ distinctly from one another. While glycopeptide resistance is often found in enterococci (1, 13, 108, 220), transfer studies showed that conjugative transfer of VanA-mediated vancomycin resistance from *E. faecalis* to *S. aureus* is possible under in vitro conditions (139). In 2002 the first patients infected with high-level vancomycin-resistant *S. aureus* isolates were detected in the United States (75, 213).

Impaired membrane permeability

Impaired membrane permeability renders gram-negative bacteria intrinsically resistant to glycopeptides. Glycopeptides are large molecules that can cross the outer membrane only poorly, if at all (209).

Resistance to Pleuromutilins

The pleuromutilins tiamulin and valnemulin are used in veterinary medicine exclusively for the control and specific therapy of gastrointestinal and respiratory tract infections in swine. The main target bacteria are *B. hyodysenteriae*, *Actinobacillus pleuropneumoniae*, and *Mycoplasma* spp. To date, relatively little is known about resistance to pleuromutilins. A mutation at position 445 (A$\rightarrow$G) in the gene coding for the ribosomal protein L3, resulting in an Asn149Asp alteration, was found to be responsible for tiamulin resistance in in vitro-selected *E. coli* (26). Footprinting experiments showed reduced binding of tiamulin to mutant ribosomes (26). In *Brachyspira* isolates with reduced susceptibility to tiamulin, mutations in the gene for the ribosomal protein L3 and at different positions in the 23S rRNA have also been identified to result in reduced drug binding (161).

Resistance to Substances with Antimicrobial Activity Formerly Used as Growth Promoters

A number of substances with antimicrobial activity have been licensed as growth promoters for livestock, and their conditions of use have been clearly defined with regard to the target animal, duration of use, and dosage of application. Since antimicrobial growth promoters belonging to the classes of macrolides (e.g., tylosin, spiramycin), streptogramins (e.g., virginiamycin), and glycopeptides (e.g., avoparcin) exhibit cross-resistance to antimicrobials of the same classes that are used for therapeutic purposes in human and veterinary medicine, they were banned or withdrawn in the European Union in 1997 and 1999, respectively. In 1999, approval of the polypeptide antibiotic Zn bacitracin as a growth promoter was also withdrawn to retain its efficacy for human therapy, while that of the quinoxalines carbadox and olaquindox was withdrawn because of toxicological reasons. The use of the remaining four growth promoters—flavophospholipol, avilamycin, and the ionophores salinomycin sodium and monensin sodium—is currently being phased out in the European Union.

The mechanisms of resistance to the macrolides tylosin and spiramycin, the streptogramin virginiamycin, and the glycopeptide avoparcin were described earlier in this chapter. Hence a brief summary on resistance to the remaining classes of growth promoters is given below. Two recent reviews (3, 35) provide detailed insight into the various aspects of the use of growth promoters.

Bacitracin resistance was first described in the producer organism *Bacillus licheniformis*, where an ABC transporter system, BcrABC, acts as a self-defense system by exporting the antibiotic from the producer cell (155). In *B. subtilis* two independent but complementary resistance mechanisms have been detected: an ABC transporter, YtsCD, that mediates the efflux of bacitracin; and a protein designated YwoA that is believed to compete with bacitracin for the dephosphorylation of the C55-isoprenyl pyrophosphate (23). In *E. coli* the gene *bacA*, coding for an undecaprenyl pyrophosphate phosphatase, may account for bacitracin resistance (67). Recently, an ABC transporter, termed BcrAB, that mediates bacitracin resistance was identified on a conjugative plasmid in *E. faecalis* (126). Avilamycin resistance in the producer organism *Streptomyces viridochromogenes* Tu57 is based on the activity of an ABC transporter and two rRNA methyltransferases (216). In

E. faecalis and *E. faecium* resistance to avilamycin was initially described to be based on variations in the ribosomal protein L16 (5). Later on, an rRNA methyltransferase, EmtA, conferring high-level resistance to avilamycin and evernimicin was identified (125). Another two methylases, AviRa, which methylates 23S rRNA at the guanosine 2535 base, and AviRb, which methylates the uridine 2479 ribose, have been shown to confer avilamycin resistance (206). In addition, mutations at specific positions in the 23S rRNA also give rise to avilamycin resistance (109). Flavophospholipol (also known as flavomycin or bambermycin) has been reported to have a "plasmid-curing effect" on multiresistant *E. coli* under experimental conditions in vitro and in vivo (207). Cross-resistance to other antimicrobials has not been observed (35). Moreover, no genes or mutations conferring flavophospholipol resistance have been observed to date. Ionophores, such as salinomycin sodium and monensin sodium, are mainly used for the prevention of infections with parasites such as *Eimeria* spp. (coccidiosis), *Plasmodium* spp., and *Giardia* spp. (35). Resistance or decreased susceptibility has been described in *Staphylococcus hyicus*, coagulase-negative staphylococci from cattle, but also *E. faecium* and *E. faecalis* from poultry and pigs. Genes or mutations accounting for acquired resistance to ionophores have not yet been described (35). Resistance to quinoxalines, such as carbadox and olaquindox, has been reported. An early study identified carbadox resistance to be associated with a conjugative multiresistance plasmid in *E. coli* (143). More than 20 years later the genes *oqxA* and *oqxB* responsible for olaquindox resistance were cloned from a conjugative plasmid in *E. coli* (82). The corresponding gene products are homologous to several resistance-nodulation-cell division family efflux systems and use TolC as the outer membrane component. Interestingly, the OqxAB-TolC system also mediates resistance to chloramphenicol and ethidium bromide (82).

SPREAD OF RESISTANCE

As described above, a large number of resistance genes have been identified in a wide variety of bacteria. In many cases, the same or closely related resistance genes are found in bacteria of different species or genera, suggesting the exchange of resistance genes by horizontal gene transfer. Such gene transfer events involve not only pathogenic bacteria but also harmless commensals constituting the normal flora (196). Usually, resistance genes were first present in the bacteria in which they evolved and were initially transmitted only vertically. However, when resistance genes were integrated into mobile genetic elements, such as plasmids or transposons, they were spread by horizontal transfer under the selective pressure imposed by the use of antimicrobial agents. While other chapters of this book will present more detailed information, the following paragraphs provide basic information for understanding the role of the mobile elements and their ways of spreading in the dissemination, coselection, and/or persistence of resistance genes.

Elements Involved in Horizontal Transfer of Resistance Genes

Plasmids, transposons, integrons and gene cassettes, and chromosomal genomic islands play a major role in horizontal transfer of antimicrobial resistance genes. These four types of elements are composed of double-stranded DNA, but differ distinctly in their sizes, structures, biological properties, and ways of spreading.

Plasmids

Plasmids are autonomously replicating extrachromosomal elements that vary in size between <2 and >100 kb. Plasmids can code for resistance to antimicrobial agents, disinfectants, heavy metal cations, anions, nucleic acid-binding substances, or bacteriocins, but also for metabolic or virulence properties (199). Resistance plasmids are known to carry one or more resistance genes, sometimes in addition to genes for other traits. Large plasmids can carry a *tra* gene complex that enables them to move from one host cell to another by conjugation. It is noteworthy that not every plasmid can replicate in every host bacterium. Therefore, when transferred into a new host cell, plasmids may stably replicate; form cointegrates with other plasmids; or integrate, either in part or completely, into the chromosomal DNA. Plasmids usually act as vectors for transposons and integrons/gene cassettes (22).

Transposons

Since transposons do not possess replication systems, for their stable maintenance they must integrate into the chromosomal DNA or plasmids. Transposons also vary in their structures and sizes. Insertion sequences represent the smallest type of transposons and usually carry only a transposase gene whose product mediates integration and excision of the element. Larger transposons often carry one or more additional genes, most of which are antibiotic resistance genes. Composite transposons, such as Tn*9* (9), Tn*10* (38, 113), and Tn*5706* (105), usually have one or more central antimicrobial resistance genes and insertion sequences at the termini. Complex transposons, such as Tn*1721* (8), commonly are characterized by terminal inverted repeats and occasionally also an internal repeat that separates the part carrying the resistance gene(s) from the part carrying the transposase genes. Some transposons integrate site-specifically, whereas others can insert at various positions in the chromosomal or plasmid DNA. Similar to the situation among plasmids, there are also nonconjugative and conjugative transposons (22, 176).

Gene cassettes

Gene cassettes represent small mobile elements of less than 2 kb that are present in gram-negative and gram-positive bacteria (138, 166). They commonly consist of only a specific recombination site and a single gene which most often is an antimicrobial resistance gene. Gene cassettes do not have replication systems or transposition systems, but move by site-specific recombination. They are usually present at specific sites within an integron. There are several known classes of integrons, with classes 1 and 2 being most frequently detected. Class 1 and 2 integrons represent intact or defective transposons and commonly consist of a 5′- and a 3′-conserved region. The 5′-conserved region harbors the integrase gene, whose product catalyzes the site-specific insertion of the gene cassettes, and also the promoter for the expression of the cassette-borne genes. The 3′-conserved region carries the *qacE*Δ*1* gene, a semifunctional derivative of the quaternary ammonium compounds resistance gene *qacE* (149), and the sulfonamide resistance gene *sul1* in class 1 integrons and transposition genes in class 2 integrons (36, 166). Integrons can carry several different gene cassettes and therefore play an important role in the dissemination of multiple antimicrobial resistance genes.

Mobile genomic islands

Since the 1990s, several mobile genomic islands carrying antibiotic resistance genes have been reported. These genomic islands integrate site-specifically into the chromosome; three well-studied examples are the SXT element of *V. cholerae* (86), the *Salmonella* genomic island 1 (SGI1) (28), and the SCC*mec* element of *S. aureus* (98). The 100-kb SXT element confers resistance to sulfonamides (*sul2*), trimethoprim (*dfrA1, dfrA18*), chloramphenicol/florfenicol (*floR*), and streptomycin (*strA, strB*) and contains all genes required for conjugative transfer and chromosomal integration and excision. SXT is transferable by conjugation between different *V. cholerae* strains and between *V. cholerae* and *E. coli* (86). SXT has been assigned to a novel group of mobile elements referred to as constins (conjugative, self-transmissible, integrating) or ICEs (integrative conjugative elements) (32).

The 43-kb SGI1 was first identified in epidemic multidrug-resistant strains of *S. enterica* serovar Typhimurium DT104 (28). SGI1 has also been identified in other *S. enterica* serovars, such as Agona, Albany, Newport, Meleagridis, and Paratyphi B (27, 59, 60, 62, 64, 131). Recently, SGI1 has been identified as an integrative mobilizable element (58). The 13-kb antibiotic resistance gene cluster within SGI1 (31) consists of a complex integron related to the In4 group of integrons. In most known cases, it mediates resistance to streptomycin and spectinomycin (*aadA2*), chloramphenicol and florfenicol (*floR*), tetracycline [*tet*(G)], ampicillin (bla_{PSE-1}), and sulfonamides (*sul1*). However, variant clusters have been identified containing additional or other resistance genes, such as *dfrA1* and *dfrA10*, conferring resistance to trimethoprim; *aadA7*, conferring resistance to streptomycin; and *aac*(3)*-Id*, conferring resistance to gentamicin (27, 59, 60, 62).

Five different types of SCC*mec* elements have been described in methicillin-resistant *S. aureus* (93, 98, 123). These elements differ in size between 21 and 66 kb and have been shown to carry the *mecA* gene for methicillin resistance and—except in SCC*mec* type IV—often other resistance genes as well, such as the Tn*554*-associated genes *erm*(A) for MLS resistance and *spc* for spectinomycin resistance. Occasionally, small resistance plasmids, such as the *tet*(K)-carrying tetracycline resistance plasmid pT181 or the *aadD*-carrying kanamycin-neomycin resistance plasmid pUB110, were found to be integrated via insertion sequences (93). The SCC*mec* elements are excised precisely from the donor chromosome and inserted into a specific site in the recipient chromosome.

Mechanims of Horizontal Gene Transfer

Plasmids, genomic islands, transposons, gene cassettes, and integrons are spread vertically during the division of the host cell, but can also be transferred horizontally between bacteria of the same or different species and genera via transduction, conjugation and mobilization, or transformation.

Transduction

Transduction describes a bacteriophage-mediated transfer process (22). Bacteriophages inject their

DNA into host cells, where it can direct the production of new phage particles. This includes expression of phage-borne genes, replication of the phage DNA, and packaging of this DNA into new phage particles, which are released from the bacterial cell (lytic cycle). However, phage DNA may also integrate as a "prophage" into the host cell chromosome and remain there for long periods in an inactive state (lysogenic cycle). External factors, such as UV irradiation, can activate the prophage and initiate a lytic cycle. Resistance plasmids may accidentally be packaged into phage heads during phage assembly. The resulting "pseudophages" are also able to infect new host cells, thereby injecting the plasmid DNA into the new host cells. The spread of resistance genes via transduction is limited by the amount of DNA that can be packaged into a phage head and the requirement of specific receptors for phage attachment on the surface of the new host cell. For staphylococci, it has been reported that 45 kb is the upper size limit of DNA that can be transduced. Since host cells that are phylogenetically closely related commonly carry the same receptors for phage attachment, transduction is mainly observed between bacteria of the same species, but rarely seen between bacteria of different species and genera. Transducing phages have been detected in a wide variety of bacteria (111).

Conjugation

Conjugation describes the self-transfer of a conjugative plasmid, transposon, and ICE from a donor cell to a recipient cell (22). Close contact between donor and recipient is one of the major requirements for efficient conjugation. The *tra* gene complex, whose gene products represent components of the transfer apparatus, is at least 15 kb in size. Small nonconjugative plasmids that coreside in the same host cell may use the transfer apparatus provided by the conjugative element, as long as they have an origin of transfer (*oriT* region) and mobilization proteins are present to start a strand separation at the *oriT*. This process is known as mobilization. Conjugation and mobilization are believed to be of major importance for the spread of resistance genes under in vivo conditions.

Transformation

Transformation describes the transfer of free DNA into competent recipient cells. Transformation is the major way of introducing plasmids into new host bacteria under in vitro conditions. Under in vivo conditions, transformation is considered to play only a limited role in the transfer of resistance genes (22). On the one hand, free DNA originating from lysed bacteria is usually rapidly degraded under most environmental conditions. On the other hand, only a few bacteria, such as *S. pneumoniae* or *Bacillus* spp., exhibit a natural ability to take up DNA from their environment.

Coselection and Persistence of Resistance Genes

During the last 20 years, a large number of resistance plasmids have been identified in a wide variety of bacteria. A continuously updated list of completely sequenced plasmids is available at http://www.ncbi.nih.gov/genomes/static/eub_p.html. Many of the known resistance plasmids carry not a single resistance gene but two or more resistance genes. These can be original plasmidic resistance genes, transposon-borne genes, cassette-borne genes, or a mixture of them. Multiresistance plasmids are often the result of interplasmidic recombination, integration of transposons, and/or insertion of gene cassettes. Acquisition of such a multiresistance plasmid is particularly problematic since the bacterial strain becomes simultaneously resistant to several different classes of antimicrobials. Concerning the linkage of the resistance genes within multiresistance plasmids, there are two different options: (i) the different resistance genes are located on the same plasmid but have their own promoter and terminator structures, or (ii) the resistance genes are physically linked and form a resistance gene cluster in which the resistance genes are transcribed from a common promoter. Gene cassettes located within an integron structure represent a specific form of resistance gene cluster which is variable due to the mobility of the different gene cassettes. Chromosomal multiresistance gene clusters, such as those located in the SXT constin or in SGI1 (described above), can also develop by individual integration events involving resistance genes originally located on plasmids, transposons, or integrons/gene cassettes.

All the resistance genes located on a multiresistance plasmid are usually transferred when this plasmid moves to a new host, independently of whether there is selective pressure for all the resistance genes or for just one of them. Such selective pressure can also lead to the persistence of resistance genes in the absence of selective pressure. Two examples from the veterinary field illustrate this situation. A study from Denmark showed that after the ban of the growth promoter avoparcin, a glycopeptide antibiotic similar to vancomycin, the percentage of glycopeptide-resistant *E. faecium* isolates from broilers dropped during a 30-month period from 81 to 12%, whereas virtually no reduction was seen during the same period among *E. faecium* isolates from pigs. Further analysis showed that the *vanA*-carrying glycopeptide resistance plasmids in the *E. faecium* isolates also harbored the MLS resistance gene *erm*(B) (2, 4). During that period (mid-1995 to the end of 1997) the macrolide antibiotic tylosin was still used in pigs as a growth promoter, but not in broilers (15). Thus, the use of tylosin provided the selective pressure for the porcine *E. faecium* to maintain the *vanA-erm*(B) plasmid, whereas it was lost in the absence of any selective pressure from the majority of the *E. faecium* strains from broilers (2). Another study from Germany, conducted in 2000, found that 60% of *Pasteurella* and *Mannheimia* isolates from pigs and cattle were chloramphenicol resistant but florfenicol susceptible. This was surprising since chloramphenicol was not allowed for use in food-producing animals after 1994. Analysis of these unrelated chloramphenicol-resistant isolates showed that they carried a resistance gene cluster—either on plasmids or in the chromosomal DNA—in which the chloramphenicol resistance gene *catA3* was bracketed by the sulfonamide resistance gene *sul2* and the streptomycin resistance gene *strA* (99, 100). Location of a resistance gene, such as *catA3*, within a resistance gene cluster ensures coselection and persistence of the resistance gene even in the absence of direct selective pressure.

Besides coselection of resistance genes in the presence of antibiotic selective pressure, coselection of antimicrobial resistance genes by either metals or disinfectants also needs to be taken into account. There are several examples of *S. aureus* plasmids harboring the β-lactamase gene *blaZ*, the *erm*(B)-carrying transposon Tn*551*, and/or the *aac(6′)-aph(2″)*-carrying transposon Tn*4001* in addition to genes for resistance to mercury, cadmium, and/or quaternary ammonium compounds (122). Recent papers described the linkage between copper (*tcrB*), glycopeptide (*vanA*), and macrolide [*erm*(B)] resistance among *E. faecium* strains isolated from pigs in Denmark (84, 85). In *E. faecium* strains from poultry in the United States, the copper resistance gene *tcrB* was found to be linked to the streptogramin resistance gene *vatE* (192). Surprisingly, the study from Denmark showed that the continued use of copper sulfate as a growth-promoting feed supplement for pigs from 1997 to 2003 obviously did not maintain high levels of macrolide and glycopeptide resistance (85). Whether the use of copper may contribute to the maintenance and selection of streptogramin resistance remains to be answered.

CONCLUSION

The development of antimicrobial resistance—by either mutations, generation of new resistance genes, or acquisition of resistance genes already present in other bacteria—is a complex process that involves different mechanisms. The speed of resistance development differs based on the bacteria involved, the selective pressure imposed by the use of antimicrobial agents, and the availability and transferability of resistance genes in the gene pools accessible to the respective bacteria. These basic facts apply to resistance development in bacteria from humans as well as in bacteria from animals. The loss of acquired resistance properties is often a cumbersome process that is influenced mainly by selective pressure but also by the colocation of the resistance genes on multiresistance plasmids or in the chromosome and the organization of the resistance genes in multiresistance gene clusters or integron structures. When resistance genes are organized in resistance gene clusters or integrons, their loss may not be expected even in the absence of direct selective pressure. Because the use of every antimicrobial substance can select for resistant bacteria, prudent use of these agents is strongly recommended in both human and veterinary medicine, as well as in food animal production, to retain the efficacy of antimicrobial agents for the control of bacterial infections in animals.

REFERENCES

1. **Aarestrup, F. M.** 1995. Occurrence of glycopeptide resistance among *Enterococcus faecium* from conventional and ecological poultry farms. *Microb. Drug Resist.* **1:**255–257.
2. **Aarestrup, F. M.** 2000. Characterization of glycopeptide-resistant *Enterococcus faecium* (GRE) from broilers and pigs in Denmark: genetic evidence that persistence of GRE in pig herds is associated with coselection by resistance to macrolides. *J. Clin. Microbiol.* **38:**2774–2777.
3. **Aarestrup, F. M.** 2000. Occurrence, selection and spread of resistance to antimicrobial agents used for growth promotion for food animals in Denmark. *APMIS Suppl.* **101:**1–48.
4. **Aarestrup, F. M., P. Ahrens, M. Madsen, L. V. Pallesen, R. L. Poulsen, and H. Westh.** 1996. Glycopeptide susceptibility among Danish *Enterococcus faecium* and *Enterococcus faecalis* isolates of animal and human origin and PCR identification of genes within the VanA cluster. *Antimicrob. Agents Chemother.* **40:**1938–1940.
5. **Aarestrup, F. M., and L. B. Jensen.** 2000. Presence of variations in ribosomal protein L16 corresponding to susceptibility of enterococci to oligosaccharides (avilamycin and evernimicin). *Antimicrob. Agents Chemother.* **44:**3425–3427.
6. **Alekshun, M. N., and S. B. Levy.** 1999. The *mar* regulon: multiple resistance to antibiotics and other toxic chemicals. *Trends Microbiol.* **7:**410–413.
7. **Alekshun, M. N., and S. B. Levy.** 2000. Bacterial drug resistance: response to survival threats, p. 323–366. *In* G. Storz and R. Hengge-Aronis (ed.), *Bacterial Stress Responses.* ASM Press, Washington, D.C.
8. **Allmeier, H., B. Cresnar, M. Greck, and R. Schmitt.** 1992. Complete nucleotide sequence of Tn*1721*: gene organization and a novel gene product with features of a chemotaxis protein. *Gene* **111:**11–20.

9. **Alton, N. K., and D. Vapnek.** 1979. Nucleotide sequence analysis of the chloramphenicol resistance transposon Tn9. *Nature* **282:**864–869.
10. **Ambler, R. P.** 1980. The structure of β-lactamases. *Philos. Trans. R. Soc. Lond. Biol.* **289:**321–331.
11. **Arcangioli, M. A., S. Leroy-Setrin, J. L. Martel, and E. Chaslus-Dancla.** 1999. A new chloramphenicol and florfenicol resistance gene linked to an integron structure in *Salmonella typhimurium* DT104. *FEMS Microbiol. Lett.* **174:**327–332.
12. **Arthur, M., and P. Courvalin.** 1993. Genetics and mechanisms of glycopeptide resistance in enterococci. *Antimicrob. Agents Chemother.* **37:**1563–1571.
13. **Arthur, M., P. Reynolds, and P. Courvalin.** 1996. Glycopeptide resistance in enterococci. *Trends Microbiol.* **4:**401–407.
14. **Arthur, M., C. Molinas, F. Depardieu, and P. Courvalin.** 1993. Characterization of Tn*1546*, a Tn*3*-related transposon conferring glycopeptide resistance by synthesis of depsipeptide peptidoglycan precursors in *Enterococcus faecium* BM4147. *J. Bacteriol.* **175:**117–127.
15. **Bager, F., F. M. Aarestrup, M. Madsen, and H. C. Wegener.** 1999. Glycopeptide resistance in *Enterococcus faecium* from broilers and pigs following discontinued use of avoparcin. *Microb. Drug Resist.* **5:**53–56.
16. **Bager, F., and R. Helmuth.** 2001. Epidemiology of quinolone resistance in *Salmonella*. *Vet. Res.* **32:**285–290.
17. **Bannam, T. L., and J. I. Rood.** 1991. The relationship between the *Clostridium perfringens catQ* gene product and chloramphenicol acetyltransferases from other bacteria. *Antimicrob. Agents Chemother.* **35:**471–476.
18. **Barbosa, T. M., and S. B. Levy.** 2000. Differential expression of over 60 chromosomal genes in *Escherichia coli* by constitutive expression of MarA. *J. Bacteriol.* **182:**3467–3474.
19. **Baucheron, S., E. Chaslus-Dancla, and A. Cloeckaert.** 2004. Role of TolC and *parC* mutation in high-level fluoroquinolone resistance in *Salmonella enterica* serotype Typhimurium DT204. *J. Antimicrob. Chemother.* **53:**657–659.
20. **Baucheron, S., H. Imberechts, E. Chaslus-Dancla, and A. Cloeckaert.** 2002. The AcrB multidrug transporter plays a major role in high-level fluoroquinolone resistance in *Salmonella enterica* serovar Typhimurium phage type DT204. *Microb. Drug Resist.* **8:**281–289.
21. **Beauclerk, A. A., and E. Cundliffe.** 1987. Sites of action of two ribosomal RNA methylases responsible for resistance to aminoglycosides. *J. Mol. Biol.* **20:**661–671.
22. **Bennett, P. M.** 1995. The spread of drug resistance, p. 317–344. *In* S. Baumberg, J. P. W. Young, E. M. H. Wellington, and J. R. Saunders (ed.), *Population Genetics in Bacteria*. Cambridge University Press, Cambridge, United Kingdom.
23. **Bernard. R., P. Joseph, A. Guiseppi, M. Chippaux, and F. Denizot.** 2003. YtsCD and YwoA, two independent systems that confer bacitracin resistance to *Bacillus subtilis*. *FEMS Microbiol. Lett.* **228:**93–97.
24. **Blickwede, M., and S. Schwarz.** 2004. Molecular analysis of florfenicol-resistant *Escherichia coli* isolates from pigs. *J. Antimicrob. Chemother.* **53:**58–64.
25. **Bonnet, R.** 2004. Growing group of extended-spectrum β-lactamases: the CTX-M enzymes. *Antimicrob. Agents Chemother.* **48:**1–14.
26. **Bosling, J., S. M. Poulsen, B. Vester, and K. S. Long.** 2003. Resistance to the peptidyl transferase inhibitor tiamulin caused by mutation of ribosomal protein l3. *Antimicrob. Agents Chemother.* **47:**2892–2896.
27. **Boyd, D., A. Cloeckaert, E. Chaslus-Dancla, and M. R. Mulvey.** 2002. Characterization of variant *Salmonella* genomic island 1 multidrug resistance regions from serovars Typhimurium DT104 and Agona. *Antimicrob. Agents Chemother.* **46:**1714–1722.
28. **Boyd, D., G. A. Peters, A. Cloeckaert, K. Sidi Boumedine, E. Chaslus-Dancla, H. Imberechts, and M. R. Mulvey.** 2001. Complete nucleotide sequence of a 43-kilobase genomic island associated with the multidrug resistance region of *Salmonella enterica* serovar Typhimurium DT104 and its identification in phage type DT120 and serovar Agona. *J. Bacteriol.* **183:**5725–5732.
29. **Bradford, P.** 2001. Extended-spectrum β-lactamases in the 21st century: characterization, epidemiology, and detection of this important resistance threat. *Clin. Microbiol. Rev.* **14:** 933–951.
30. **Brenner, D. G., and W. V. Shaw.** 1985. The use of synthetic oligonucleotides with universal templates for rapid DNA sequencing: results with staphylococcal replicon pC221. *EMBO J.* **4:**561–568.
31. **Briggs, C. E., and P. M. Fratamico.** 1999. Molecular characterization of an antibiotic resistance gene cluster of *Salmonella typhimurium* DT104. *Antimicrob. Agents Chemother.* **43:**846–849.
32. **Burrus, V., G. Pavlovic, B. Decaris, and G. Guedon.** 2002. Conjugative transposons: the tip of the iceberg. *Mol. Microbiol.* **46:**601–610.
33. **Bush, K.** 2001. New beta-lactamases in gram-negative bacteria: diversity and impact on the selection of antimicrobial therapy. *Clin. Infect. Dis.* **32:**1085–1089.
34. **Bush, K., G. A. Jacoby, and A. A. Medeiros.** 1995. A functional classification scheme for β-lactamases and its correlation with molecular structure. *Antimicrob. Agents Chemother.* **39:** 1211–1233.
35. **Butaye, P., L. A. Devriese, and F. Haesebrouck.** 2003. Antimicrobial growth promoters used in animal feed: effects of less known antibiotics on gram-positive bacteria. *Clin. Microbiol. Rev.* **16:**175–188.
36. **Carattoli, A.** 2001. Importance of integrons in the diffusion of resistance. *Vet. Res.* **32:**243–259.
37. **Casas, C., E. C. Anderson, K. K. Ojo, I. Keith, D. Whelan, D. Rainnie, and M. C. Roberts.** 2005. Characterization of pRAS1-like plasmids from atypical North American psychrophilic *Aeromonas salmonicida*. *FEMS Microbiol. Lett.* **242:**59–63.
38. **Chalmers, S., R. Sewitz, K. Lipkow, and P. Crellin.** 2000. Complete nucleotide sequence of Tn*10*. *J. Bacteriol.* **182:** 2970–2972.
39. **Charpentier, E., and P. Courvalin.** 1997. Emergence of the trimethoprim resistance gene *dfrD* in *Listeria monocytogenes* BM4293. *Antimicrob. Agents Chemother.* **41:**1124–1136.
40. **Charrel, R. N., J.-M. Pages, P. de Micco, and M. Mallea.** 1996. Prevalence of outer membrane porin alteration in β-lactam-antibiotic-resistant *Enterobacter aerogenes*. *Antimicrob. Agents Chemother.* **40:**2854–2858.
41. **Chaslus-Dancla, E., Y. Glupczynski, G. Gerbaud, M. Lagorce, and J. P. Lafont.** 1989. Detection of apramycin resistant *Enterobacteriaceae* in hospital isolates. *FEMS Microbiol. Lett.* **52:**261–265.
42. **Chaslus-Dancla, E., J.-L. Martel, C. Carlier, J.-P. Lafont, and P. Courvalin.** 1986. Emergence of aminoglycoside 3-*N*-acetyltransferase IV in *Escherichia coli* and *Salmonella typhimurium* isolated from animals in France. *Antimicrob. Agents Chemother.* **29:**239–243.
43. **Chaslus-Dancla, E., P. Pohl, M. Meurisse, M. Marin, and J. P. Lafont.** 1991. High genetic homology between plasmids of human and animal origins conferring resistance to the aminoglycosides gentamicin and apramycin. *Antimicrob. Agents Chemother.* **35:**590–593.

44. **Chopra, I., and M. C. Roberts.** 2001. Tetracycline antibiotics: mode of action, applications, molecular biology and epidemiology of bacterial resistance. *Microbiol. Mol. Biol. Rev.* **65:**232–260.
45. **Clancy, J., J. W. Petitpas, F. Dib-Hajj, W. Yuan, M. Cronan, A. Kamath, J. Bergeron, and J. Retsema.** 1996. Molecular cloning and functional analysis of a novel macrolide-resistance determinant *mefA* from *Streptococcus pyogenes. Mol. Microbiol.* **22:**867–879.
46. **Cloeckaert, A., S. Baucheron, and E. Chaslus-Dancla.** 2001. Nonenzymatic chloramphenicol resistance mediated by IncC plasmid R55 is encoded by a *floR* gene variant. *Antimicrob. Agents Chemother.* **45:**2381–2382.
47. **Cloeckaert, A., S. Baucheron, G. Flaujac, S. Schwarz, C. Kehrenberg, J. L. Martel, and E. Chaslus-Dancla.** 2000. Plasmid-mediated florfenicol resistance by the *floR* gene in *Escherichia coli* isolated from cattle. *Antimicrob. Agents Chemother.* **44:**2858–2860.
48. **Cloeckaert, A., and E. Chaslus-Dancla.** 2001. Mechanism of quinolone resistance in *Salmonella. Vet. Res.* **32:** 291–300.
49. **Cohen, S. P., L. M. McMurry, and S. B. Levy.** 1988. *marA* locus causes decreased expression of OmpF porin in multiple-antibiotic-resistant (Mar) mutants of *Escherichia coli. J. Bacteriol.* **170:**5416–5422.
50. **Connell, S. R., D. M. Tracz, K. H. Nierhaus, and D. E. Taylor.** 2003. Ribosomal protection proteins and their mechanism of tetracycline resistance. *Antimicrob. Agents Chemother.* **47:** 3675–3681.
51. **Cousin, S. L., Jr., W. L. Whittington, and M. C. Roberts.** 2003. Acquired macrolide resistance genes in pathogenic *Neisseria* spp. isolated between 1940 and 1987. *Antimicrob. Agents Chemother.* **47:**3877–3880.
52. **Dale, G. E., C. Broger, A. D'Arcy, P. G. Hartman, R. DeHoogt, S. Jolidon, I. Kompis, A. M. Labhardt, H. Langen, H. Locher, M. G. Page, D. Stuber, R. L. Then, B. Wipf, and C. Oefner.** 1997. A single amino acid substitution in *Staphylococcus aureus* dihydrofolate reductase determines trimethoprim resistance. *J. Mol. Biol.* **266:**23–30.
53. **Daly, M. M., S. Doktor, R. Flamm, and D. Shortridge.** 2004. Characterization and prevalence of MefA, MefE, and associated *msr*(D) gene in *Streptococcus pneumoniae* clinical isolates. *J. Clin. Microbiol.* **42:**3570–3574.
54. **Davies, J., and G. D. Wright.** 1997. Bacterial resistance to aminoglycoside antibiotics. *Trends Microbiol.* **5:**375–382.
55. **De Groot, R., M. Sluijter, A. de Bruyn, J. Campos, W. H. F. Goessens, A. L. Smith, and P. W. M. Hermans.** 1996. Genetic characterization of trimethoprim resistance in *Haemophilus influenzae. Antimicrob. Agents Chemother.* **40:**2131–2136.
56. **DePaola, A., and M. C. Roberts.** 1995. Class D and E tetracycline resistance determinants in gram-negative catfish pond bacteria. *Mol. Cell. Probes* **9:**311–313.
57. **Diaz-Torres, M. L., R. McNab, D. A. Spratt, A. Villedieu, N. Hunt, M. Wilson, and P. Mullany.** 2003. Characterization of a novel tetracycline resistance determinate from the oral metagenome. *Antimicrob. Agents Chemother.* **47:**1430–1432.
58. **Doublet, B., D. Boyd, M. R. Mulvey, and A. Cloeckaert.** 2005. The *Salmonella* genomic island 1 is an integrative mobilizable element. *Mol. Microbiol.* **55:**1911–1924.
59. **Doublet, B., P. Butaye, H. Imberechts, D. Boyd, M. R. Mulvey, E. Chaslus-Dancla, and A. Cloeckaert.** 2004. *Salmonella* genomic island 1 multidrug resistance gene clusters in *Salmonella enterica* serovar Agona isolated in Belgium in 1992 to 2002. *Antimicrob. Agents Chemother.* **48:** 2510–2517.
60. **Doublet, B., R. Lailler, D. Meunier, A. Brisabois, D. Boyd, M. R. Mulvey, E. Chaslus-Dancla, and A. Cloeckaert.** 2003. Variant *Salmonella* genomic island 1 antibiotic resistance gene cluster in *Salmonella enterica* serovar Albany. *Emerg. Infect. Dis.* **9:**585–591.
61. **Doublet, B., S. Schwarz, C. Kehrenberg, and A. Cloeckaert.** 2005. Florfenicol resistance gene *floR* is part of a novel transposon. *Antimicrob. Agents Chemother.* **49:**2106–2108.
62. **Doublet, B., F.-X. Weill, L. Fabre, E. Chaslus-Dancla, and A. Cloeckaert.** 2004. Variant *Salmonella* genomic island 1 antibiotic resistance gene cluster containing a novel 3′-*N*-aminoglycoside acetyltransferase gene cassette, *aac*(3)-*Id*, in *Salmonella enterica* serovar Newport. *Antimicrob. Agents Chemother.* **48:**3806–3812.
63. **Drlica, K., and X. L. Zhao.** 1997. DNA gyrase, topoisomerase IV, and the 4-quinolones. *Microbiol. Rev.* **61:**377–392.
64. **Ebner, P., K. Garner, and A. Mathew.** 2004. Class 1 integrons in various *Salmonella enterica* serovars isolated from animals and identification of genomic island SGI1 in *Salmonella enterica* var. Meleagridis. *J. Antimicrob. Chemother.* **53:** 1004–1009.
65. **Edgar, R., and E. Bibi.** 1997. MdfA, an *Escherichia coli* multidrug resistance protein with an extraordinarily broad spectrum of drug recognition. *J. Bacteriol.* **179:**2274–2280.
66. **Ehlert, K.** 1999. Methicillin resistance in *Staphylococcus aureus*—molecular basis, novel targets and antibiotic therapy. *Curr. Pharm. Des.* **5:** 45–55.
67. **El Ghachi, M., A. Bouhss, D. Blanot, and D. J. Mengin-Lecreulx.** 2004. The *bacA* gene of *Escherichia coli* encodes an undecaprenyl pyrophosphate phosphatase activity. *J. Biol. Chem.* **279:**30106–30113.
68. **Elwell, L. P., and M. E. Fling.** 1989. Resistance to trimethoprim, p. 249–290. *In* L. E. Bryan (ed.), *Microbial Resistance to Drugs.* Springer-Verlag, Berlin, Germany.
69. **Ettayebi, M., S. M. Prasad, and E. A. Morgan.** 1985. Chloramphenicol-erythromycin resistance mutations in a 23S rRNA gene of *Escherichia coli. J. Bacteriol.* **162:**551–557.
70. **Everett, M. J., Y. F. Jin, V. Ricci, and L. J. V. Piddock.** 1996. Contributions of individual mechanisms to fluoroquinolone resistance in 36 *Escherichia coli* strains isolated from humans and animals. *Antimicrob. Agents Chemother.* **40:**2380–2386.
71. **Everett, M. J., and L. J. V. Piddock.** 1998. Mechanisms of resistance to fluoroquinolones, p. 259–296. *In* J. Kuhlmann, A. Dalhoff, and H.-J. Zeiler (ed.), *Quinolone Antibacterials.* Springer-Verlag, Berlin, Germany.
72. **Flannagan, S. E., L. A. Zitzow, Y. A. Su, and D. B. Clewell.** Nucleotide sequence of the 18-kb conjugative transposon Tn*916* from *Enterococcus faecalis. Plasmid* **32:**350–354.
73. **Georgeopapadakou, N. H.** 1993. Penicillin-binding proteins and bacterial resistance to β-lactams. *Antimicrob. Agents Chemother.* **37:**2045–2053.
74. **Gilmore, K. S., M. S. Gilmore, and D. F. Sahm.** 2002. Methicillin resistance in *Staphylococcus aureus*, p. 331–354. *In* K. Lewis, A. A. Salyers, H. W. Taber, and R. G. Wax (ed.), *Bacterial Resistance to Antimicrobials.* Marcel Dekker, Inc., New York, N.Y.
75. **Gonzalez-Zorn, B., and P. Courvalin.** 2003. VanA-mediated high-level glycopeptide resistance in MRSA. *Lancet Infect. Dis.* **3:**67–68.
76. **Grape, M., L. Sundström, and G. Kronvall.** 2003. Sulphonamide resistance gene *sul3* found in *Escherichia coli* isolates from human sources. *J. Antimicrob. Chemother.* **52:** 1022–1024.
77. Reference deleted.
78. **Guerra, B., E. Junker, and R. Helmuth.** 2004. Incidence of the newly described sulfonamide resistance gene *sul3* among

German *Salmonella enterica* strains isolated from livestock and food. *Antimicrob. Agents Chemother.* **48**:2712–2715.

79. **Guerra, B., E. Junker, A. Schroeter, B. Malorny, S. Lehmann, and R. Helmuth.** 2003. Phenotypic and genotypic characterization of antimicrobial resistance in German *Escherichia coli* isolates from cattle, swine and poultry. *J. Antimicrob. Chemother.* **52**:489–492.
80. **Haanperä, M., P. Huovinen, and J. Jalava.** 2005. Detection and quantification of macrolide resistance mutations at positions 2058 and 2059 of the 23S rRNA gene by pyrosequencing. *Antimicrob. Agents Chemother.* **49**:457–460.
81. **Hackbarth, C. J., and H. F. Chambers.** 1989. Methicillin-resistant staphylococci: genetics and mechanism of resistance. *Antimicrob. Agents Chemother.* **33**:991–994.
82. **Hansen, L. H., E. Johannesen, M. Burmølle, A. H. Sørensen, and S. J. Sorensen.** 2004. Plasmid-encoded multidrug efflux pump conferring resistance to olaquindox in *Escherichia coli*. *Antimicrob. Agents Chemother.* **48**:3332–3337.
83. **Harrow, S. A., B. J. Gilpin, and J. D. Klena.** 2004. Characterization of erythromycin resistance in *Campylobacter coli* and *Campylobacter jejuni* isolated from pig offal in New Zealand. *J. Appl. Microbiol.* **97**:141–148.
84. **Hasman, H., and F. M. Aarestrup.** 2002. *tcrB*, a gene conferring transferable copper resistance in *Enterococcus faecium*: occurrence, transferability, and linkage to macrolide and glycopeptide resistance. *Antimicrob. Agents Chemother.* **46**: 1410–1416.
85. **Hasman, H., and F. M. Aarestrup.** 2005. Relationship between copper, glycopeptide, and macrolide resistance among *Enterococcus faecium* strains isolated from pigs in Denmark between 1997 and 2003. *Antimicrob. Agents Chemother.* **49**:454–456.
86. **Hochhut, B., Y. Lotfi, D. Mazel, S. M. Faruque, R. Woodgate, and M. K. Waldor.** 2001. Molecular analysis of antibiotic resistance gene clusters in *Vibrio cholerae* O139 and O1 SXT constins. *Antimicrob. Agents Chemother.* **45**:2991–3000.
87. **Hooper, D. C.** 1999. Mechanisms of fluoroquinolone resistance. *Drug Res. Updates* 2:38–55.
88. **Hooper, D. C., J. S. Wolfson, M. A. Bozza, and E. Y. Ng.** 1992. Genetics and regulation of outer protein expression by quinolone resistance loci *nfx*B, *nfx*C, and *cfx*B. *Antimicrob. Agents Chemother.* **36**:1151–1154.
89. **Hopkins, J. M., and K. J. Towner.** 1990. Enhanced resistance to cefotaxime and imipenem associated with outer membrane protein alterations in *Enterobacter aerogenes*. *J. Antimicrob. Chemother.* **25**:49–55.
90. **Horinouchi, S., and B. Weisblum.** 1982. Nucleotide sequence and functional map of pC194, a plasmid that specifies inducible chloramphenicol resistance. *J. Bacteriol.* **150**:815–825.
91. **Huovinen, P.** 2001. Resistance to trimethoprim-sulfamethoxazole. *Clin. Infect. Dis.* **32**:1608–1614.
92. **Huovinen, P., L. Sundström, G. Swedberg, and O. Sköld.** 1995. Trimethoprim and sulfonamide resistance. *Antimicrob. Agents Chemother.* **39**:279–289.
93. **Ito, T., X. X. Ma, F. Takaeuchi, K. Okuma, H. Yuzawa, and K. Hiramatsu.** 2004. Novel type V staphylococcal cassette chromosome *mec* driven by a novel cassette chromosome recombinase, *ccrC*. *Antimicrob. Agents Chemother.* **48**: 2637–2651.
94. **Jensen, L. B., N. Fimodt-Moller, and F. M. Aarestrup.** 1999. Presence of *erm* gene classes in gram-positive bacteria of animal and human origin in Denmark. *FEMS Microbiol. Lett.* **170**:151–158.
95. **Johnson, A. P., L. Burns, N. Woodford, E. J. Threlfall, J. Naidoo, E. M. Cooke, and R. C. George.** 1994. Gentamicin resistance in clinical isolates of *Escherichia coli* encoded by genes of veterinary origin. *J. Med. Microbiol.* **40**:221–226.
96. **Jones, M. E., D. F. Sahm, N. Martin, S. Scheuring, P. Heisig, C. Thornsberry, K. Köhrer, and F.-J. Schmitz.** 2000. Prevalence of *gyrA*, *gyrB*, *parC*, and *parE* mutations in clinical isolates of *Streptococcus pneumoniae* with decreased susceptibilities to different fluoroquinolones and originating from worldwide surveillance studies during the 1997–1998 respiratory season. *Antimicrob. Agents Chemother.* **44**:462–466.
97. **Karlsson, M., C. Fellstrom, M. U. Heldtander, K. E. Johansson, and A. Franklin.** 1999. Genetic basis of macrolide and lincosamide resistance in *Brachyspira* (*Serpulina*) *hyodysenteriae*. *FEMS Microbiol. Lett.* **15**:255–260.
98. **Katayama, Y., T. Ito, and K. Hiramatsu.** 2000. A new class of genetic element, Staphylococcus cassette chromosome *mec*, encodes methicillin resistance in *Staphylococcus aureus*. *Antimicrob. Agents Chemother.* **44**:1549–1555.
99. **Kehrenberg, C., and S. Schwarz.** 2002. Nucleotide sequence and organisation of plasmid pMVSCS1 from *Mannheimia varigena*: identification of a multiresistance gene cluster. *J. Antimicrob. Chemother.* **49**:383–386.
100. **Kehrenberg, C., and S. Schwarz.** 2001. Occurrence and linkage of genes coding for resistance to sulfonamides, streptomycin and chloramphenicol in bacteria of the genera *Pasteurella* and *Mannheimia*. *FEMS Microbiol. Lett.* **205**:283–290.
101. **Kehrenberg, C., and S. Schwarz.** 2004. Identification of *dfrA20*, a novel trimethoprim resistance gene from *Pasteurella multocida*. *Antimicrob. Agents Chemother.* **49**:414–417.
102. **Kehrenberg, C., and S. Schwarz.** 2004. *fexA*, a novel *Staphylococcus lentus* gene encoding resistance to florfenicol and chloramphenicol. *Antimicrob. Agents Chemother.* **48**:615–618.
103. **Kehrenberg, C., and S. Schwarz.** 2004. The florfenicol/chloramphenicol exporter gene *fexA* is part of the novel transposon Tn*558*. *Antimicrob. Agents Chemother.* **49**:813–815.
104. **Kehrenberg, C., and S. Schwarz.** 2005. Plasmid-borne florfenicol resistance in *Pasteurella multocida*. *J. Antimicrob. Chemother.* **55**:773–775.

104a. **Kehrenberg, C., S. Schwarz, L. Jacobsen, L. H. Hansen, and B. Vester.** 2005. A new mechanism for chloramphenicol, florfenicol and clindamycin resistance: methylation of 23S ribosomal RNA at A2503. *Mol. Microbiol.* **57**:1064–1073.

105. **Kehrenberg, C., C. Werckenthin, and S. Schwarz.** 1998. Tn*5706*, a transposon-like element from *Pasteurella multocida* mediating tetracycline resistance. *Antimicrob. Agents Chemother.* **42**:2116–2118.
106. **Keyes, K., C. Hudson, J. J. Maurer, S. Thaye, D. G. White, and M. D. Lee.** 2000. Detection of florfenicol resistance genes in *Escherichia coli* from sick chickens. *Antimicrob. Agents Chemother.* **44**:421–424.
107. **Kim, E., and T. Aoki.** 1996. Sequence analysis of the florfenicol resistance gene encoded in the transferable R plasmid from a fish pathogen *Pasteurella piscicida*. *Microbiol. Immunol.* **40**:665–669.
108. **Klare, I., H. Heier, H. Claus, R. Reissbrodt, and W. Witte.** 1995. *vanA*-mediated high-level glycopeptide resistance in *Enterococcus faecium* from animal husbandry. *FEMS Microbiol. Lett.* **125**:165–171.
109. **Kofoed, C. B., and B. Vester.** 2002. Interaction of avilamycin with ribosomes and resistance caused by mutations in 23S rRNA. *Antimicrob. Agents Chemother.* **46**:3339–3342.
110. **Köhler, T., M. Kok, M. Michea-Hamzehpour, P. Plesiat, N. Gotoh, T. Nishino, L. K. Curty, and J.-C. Pechere.** 1996. Multidrug efflux in intrinsic resistance to trimethoprim and sulfamethoxazole in *Pseudomonas aeruginosa*. *Antimicrob. Agents Chemother.* **40**:2288–2290.

111. **Kokjohn, T. A.** 1989. Transduction: mechanism and potential for gene transfer in the environment, p. 73–97. *In* S. B. Levy and R. V. Miller (ed.), *Gene Transfer in the Environment*. McGraw-Hill Book Co., New York, N.Y.
112. **Lange, C. C., C. Werckenthin, and S. Schwarz.** 2003. Molecular analysis of the plasmid-borne *aacA/aphD* resistance gene region of coagulase-negative staphylococci from chickens. *J. Antimicrob. Chemother.* **51:**1397–1401.
113. **Lawley, T. D., V. D. Burland, and D. E. Taylor.** 2000. Analysis of the complete nucleotide sequence of the tetracycline resistance transposon Tn*10*. *Plasmid* **43:**235–239.
114. **Leclercq, R., and P. Courvalin.** 1991. Bacterial resistance to macrolide, lincosamide, and streptogramin antibiotics by target modification. *Antimicrob. Agents Chemother.* **35:**1267–1272.
115. **Leclercq, R., and P. Courvalin.** 1991. Intrinsic and unusual resistance to macrolide, lincosamide, and streptogramin antibiotics in bacteria. *Antimicrob. Agents Chemother.* **35:** 1273–1276.
116. **Lee, A., W. Mao, M. S. Warren, A. Mistry, K. Hoshino, R. Okumura, H. Ishida, and O. Lomovskaya.** 2000. Interplay between efflux pumps may provide either additive or multiplicative effects on drug resistance. *J. Bacteriol.* **182:** 3142–3150.
117. **Levy, S. B., L. M. McMurry, T. M. Barbosa, V. Burdett, P. Courvalin, W. Hillen, M. C. Roberts, J. I. Rood, and D. E. Taylor.** 1999. Nomenclature for new tetracycline resistance determinants. *Antimicrob. Agents Chemother.* **43:**1523–1524.
118. **Ling, B., and B. Berger-Bächi.** 1998. Increased overall antibiotic susceptibility in *Staphylococcus aureus femAB* null mutants. *Antimicrob. Agents Chemother.* **42:**936–938.
119. **Livermore, D. M.** 1995. β-Lactamases in laboratory and clinical resistance. *Clin. Microbiol. Rev.* **8:**557–584.
120. **Lomovskaya, O., A. Lee, K. Hoshino, H. Ishida, A. Mistry, M. S. Warren, E. Boyer, S. Chamberland, and V. J. Lee.** 1999. Use of a genetic approach to evaluate the consequences of inhibition of efflux pumps in *Pseudomonas aeruginosa*. *Antimicrob. Agents Chemother.* **43:**1340–1346.
121. **Lovett, P. S.** 1990. Translational attenuation as the regulator of inducible *cat* genes. *J. Bacteriol.* **172:**1–6.
122. **Lyon, B. R., and R. Skurray.** 1987. Antimicrobial resistance in *Staphylococcus aureus*: genetic basis. *Microbiol. Rev.* **51:** 88–134.
123. **Ma, X. X., T. Ito, C. Tiensasitorn, M. Jamklang, P. Chongtrakool, S. Boyle-Vavra, R. S. Daum, and K. Hiramatsu.** 2002. Novel type of staphylococcal cassette chromosome *mec* identified in community-acquired methicillin-resistant *Staphylococcus aureus* strains. *Antimicrob. Agents Chemother.* **46:**1147–1152.
124. **Madsen, L., F. M. Aarestrup, and J. E. Olsen.** 2000. Characterisation of streptomcin resistance determinants in Danish isolates of *Salmonella* Typhimurium. *Vet. Microbiol.* **75:**73–82.
125. **Mann, P. A., L. Xiong, A. S. Mankin, A. S. Chau, C. A. Mendrick, D. J. Najarian, C. A. Cramer, D. Loebenberg, E. Coates, N. J. Murgolo, F. M. Aarestrup, R. V. Goering, T. A. Black, R. S. Hare, and P. M. McNicholas.** 2001. EmtA, a rRNA methyltransferase conferring high-level evernimicin resistance. *Mol. Microbiol.* **41:**1349–1356.
126. **Manson, J. M., S. Keis, J. M. Smith, and G. M. Cook.** 2004. Acquired bacitracin resistance in *Enterococcus faecalis* is mediated by an ABC transporter and a novel regulatory protein, BcrR. *Antimicrob. Agents Chemother.* **48:** 3743–3748.
127. **Martinez-Marzinez, L., S. Hernandez-Alles, S. Alberti, J. M. Tomas, V. J. Benedi, and G. A. Jacoby.** 1996. In vivo selection of porin-deficient mutants of *Klebsiella pneumoniae* with increased resistance to cefoxitin and expanded-spectrum cephalosporins. *Antimicrob. Agents Chemother.* **40:**342–348.
128. **McMurray, L. M., A. M. George, and S. B. Levy.** 1994. Active efflux of chloramphenicol in susceptible *Escherichia coli* strains and in multiple-antibiotic-resistant (Mar) mutants. *Antimicrob. Agents Chemother.* **38:**542–546.
129. **Meier, A., P. Kirschner, S. Burkhardt, V. A. Steingrube, B. A. Brown, R. J. Wallace, Jr., and E. C. Böttger.** 1994. Identification of mutations in 23S rRNA gene of clarithromycin-resistant *Mycobacterium intracellulare*. *Antimicrob. Agents Chemother.* **38:**381–384.
130. **Meier, A., P. Sander, K. J. Schaper, M. Scholz, and E. C. Böttger.** 1996. Correlation of molecular resistance mechanisms and phenotypic resistance levels in streptomycin-resistant *Mycobacterium tuberculosis*. *Antimicrob. Agents Chemother.* **40:**2452–2454.
131. **Meunier, D., D. Boyd, M. R. Mulvey, S. Baucheron, C. Mammina, A. Nastasi, E. Chaslus-Dancla, and A. Cloeckaert.** 2002. *Salmonella enterica* serotype Typhimurium DT 104 antibiotic resistance genomic island I in serotype Paratyphi B. *Emerg. Infect. Dis.* **8:**430–433.
132. **Mingeot-Leclercq, M.-P., Y. Glupczynski, and P. M. Tulkens.** 1999. Aminoglycosides: activity and resistance. *Antimicrob. Agents Chemother.* 43:727–737.
133. **Miranda, C. D., C. Kehrenberg, C. Ulep, S. Schwarz, and M. C. Roberts.** 2003. Diversity of tetracycline resistance genes in bacteria from Chilean salmon farms. *Antimicrob. Agents Chemother.* **47:**883–888.
134. **Mitsuyama, J. R., R. Hiruma, A. Yamaguchi, and T. Sawai.** 1987. Identification of porins in outer membrane of *Proteus*, *Morganella*, and *Providencia* spp. and their role in outer membrane permeation of β-lactams. *Antimicrob. Agents Chemother.* **31:**379–384.
135. **Murray, I. A., J. Hawkins, J. W. Keyte, and W. V. Shaw.** 1988. Nucleotide sequence analysis and overexpression of the gene encoding a type III chloramphenicol acetyltransferase. *Biochem. J.* **252:**173–179.
136. **Murray, I. A., J. V. Martinez-Suarez, T. J. Close, and W. V. Shaw.** 1990. Nucleotide sequences of genes encoding the type II chloramphenicol acetyltransferases of *Escherichia coli* and *Haemophilus influenzae*, which are sensitive to inhibition by thiol-reactive reagents. *Biochem. J.* **272:**505–510.
137. **Murray, I. A., and W. V. Shaw.** 1997. *O*-acetyltransferases for chloramphenicol and other natural products. *Antimicrob. Agents Chemother.* **41:**1–6.
138. **Nandi, S., J. J. Maurer, C. Hofacre, and A. O. Summers.** 2004. Gram-positive bacteria are a major reservoir of class 1 antibiotic resistance integrons in poultry litter. *Proc. Natl. Acad. Sci. USA.* **101:**7118–7122.
139. **Noble, W. C., Z. Virani, and R. G. Cree.** 1992. Co-transfer of vancomycin and other resistance genes from *Enterococcus faecalis* NCTC12201 to *Staphylococcus aureus*. *FEMS Microbiol. Lett.* **72:**195–198.
140. **Nonaka, L., and S. Suzuki.** 2002. New Mg^{2+}-dependent oxytetracycline resistance determinant Tet34 in *Vibrio* isolates from marine fish intestinal contents. *Antimicrob. Agents Chemother.* **46:**1550–1552.
141. **Oethinger, M., W. V. Kern, A. S. Jellen-Ritter, L. M. McMurry, and S. B. Levy.** 2000. Ineffectiveness of topoisomerase mutations in mediating clinically significant fluoroquinolone resistance in *Escherichia coli* in the absence of the AcrAB efflux pump. *Antimicrob. Agents Chemother.* **44:**10–13.
142. **Oethinger, M., I. Podglajen, W. V. Kern, and S. B. Levy.** 1998. Overexpression of the *marA* or *soxS* regulatory gene in clinical topoisomerase mutants of *Escherichia coli*. *Antimicrob. Agents Chemother.* **42:**2089–2094.

143. **Ohmae, K., S. Yonezawa, and N. Terakado.** 1981. R plasmid with carbadox resistance from *Escherichia coli* of porcine origin. *Antimicrob. Agents Chemother.* **19:**86–90.
144. **Ojo, K. K., C. Ulep, N. Van Kirk, H. Luis, M. Bernardo, J. Leitao, and M. C. Roberts.** 2004. The *mef*(A) gene predominates among seven macrolide resistant genes identified in 13 gram-negative genera from healthy Portuguese children. *Antimicrob. Agents Chemother.* **48:**3451–3456.
145. **Okusu, H., and H. Nikaido.** 1996. AcrAB efflux pump plays a major role in the antibiotic resistance phenotype of *Escherichia coli* multiple-antibiotic-resistance (Mar) mutants. *J. Bacteriol.* **178:**306–308.
146. **Olliver, A., M. Vallé, E. Chaslus-Dancla, and A. Cloeckaert.** 2004. Role of an *acrR* mutation in multidrug resistance of *in vitro*-selected fluoroquinolone-resistant mutants of *Salmonella enterica* serovar Typhimurium. *FEMS Microbiol. Lett.* **238:**267–272.
147. **Padayachee, T., and K. P. Klugman.** 1999. Novel expansions of the gene encoding dihydropteroate synthase in trimethoprim-sulfamethoxazole-resistant *Streptococcus pneumoniae. Antimicrob. Agents Chemother.* **43:**2225–2230.
148. **Pattishall, K. H., J. Acar, J. J. Burchall, F. W. Goldstein, and R. J. Harvey.** 1977. Two distinct types of trimethoprim-resistant dihydrofolate reductase specified by R-plasmids of different incompatibility groups. *J. Biol. Chem.* **252:** 2319–2323.
149. **Paulsen, I. T., M. H. Brown, and R. A. Skurray.** 1996. Proton-dependent multidrug efflux systems. *Microbiol. Rev.* **60:**575–608.
150. **Payot, S., L. Avrain, C. Magras, K. Praud, A. Cloeckaert, and E. Chaslus-Dancla.** 2004. Relative contribution of target gene mutation and efflux to fluoroquinolone and erythromycin resistance in French poultry and pig isolates of *Campylobacter coli. Int. J. Antimicrob. Agents* **23:**468–472.
151. **Perreten, V., and P. Boerlin.** 2003. A new sulfonamide resistance gene (*sul3*) in *Escherichia coli* is widespread in the pig population in Switzerland. *Antimicrob. Agents Chemother.* **47:**1169–1172.
152. **Petrosino, J., C. Cantu III, and T. Palzkill.** 1998. β-Lactamases: protein evolution in real time. *Trends Microbiol.* **6:**323–327.
153. **Pikis, A., J. A. Donkersloot, W. J. Rodriquez, and J. M. Keith.** 1998. A conservative amino acid mutation in the chromosome-encoded dihydrofolate reductase confers trimethoprim resistance in *Streptococcus pneumoniae. J. Infect. Dis.* **178:**700–706.
154. **Plante, I., D. Centron, and P. H. Roy.** 2003. An integron cassette encoding erythromycin esterase, *ere*(A), from *Providencia stuartii. Antimicrob. Agents Chemother.* **51:**787–790.
155. **Podlesek, Z., A. Comino, B. Herzog-Velikonja, D. Zgur-Bertok, R. Komel, and M. Grabnar.** 1995. *Bacillus licheniformis* bacitracin-resistance ABC transporter: relationship to mammalian multidrug resistance. *Mol. Microbiol.* **16:** 969–976.
156. **Poehlsgaard, J., and S. Douthwaite.** 2003. Macrolide antibiotic interaction and resistance on the bacterial ribosome. *Curr. Opin. Invest. Drugs* **4:**140–148.
157. **Poole, K.** 2000. Efflux-mediated resistance to fluoroquinolones in gram-negative bacteria. *Antimicrob. Agents Chemother.* **44:**2233–2241.
158. **Poole, K.** 2000. Efflux-mediated resistance to fluoroquinolones in gram-positive bacteria and the mycobacteria. *Antimicrob. Agents Chemother.* **44:**2595–2599.
159. **Poole, K.** 2002. Multidrug efflux pumps and antimicrobial resistance in *Pseudomonas aeruginosa* and related organisms, p. 273–298. *In* I. T. Paulsen and K. Lewis (ed.), *Microbial Multidrug Efflux*. Horizon Scientific Press, Wymondham, United Kingdom.
160. **Prammanaman, T., P. Sander, B. A. Brown, K. Frischkorn, G. O. Onyi, Y. Zhang, E. C. Böttger, and R. J. Wallace, Jr.** 1998. A single 16S ribosomal RNA substitution is responsible for resistance to amikacin and other 2-deoxystreptamine aminoglycosides in *Mycobacterium abscessus* and *Mycobacterium chelonae. J. Infect. Dis.* **177:**1573–1581.
161. **Pringle, M., J. Poehlsgaard, B. Vester, and K. S. Long.** 2004. Mutations in ribosomal protein L3 and 23S ribosomal RNA at the peptidyl transferase centre are associated with reduced susceptibility to tiamulin in *Brachyspira* spp. isolates. *Mol. Microbiol.* **54:**1295–1306.
162. **Projan, S. J., J. Kornblum, S. L. Moghazeh, I. Edelman, M. L. Gennaro, and R. P. Novick.** 1985. Comparative sequence and functional analysis of pT181 and pC221, cognate plasmid replicons from *Staphylococcus aureus. Mol. Gen. Genet.* **199:**452–464.
163. **Putman, M., H. W. van Veen, and W. N. Konings.** 2000. Molecular properties of bacterial multidrug transporters. *Microbiol. Mol. Biol. Rev.* **64:**672–693.
164. **Quintiliani, R., Jr., D. F. Sahm, and P. Courvalin.** 1999. Mechanisms of resistance to antimicrobial agents, p. 1505–1525. *In* P. R. Murray, E. J. Baron, M. A. Pfaller, F. C. Tenover, and R. H. Yolken (ed.), *Manual of Clinical Microbiology*, 7th ed. ASM Press, Washington, D.C.
165. **Radström, P., and G. Swedberg.** 1988. RSF1010 and a conjugative plasmid contain *sul*II, one of two known genes for plasmid-borne sulfonamide resistance dihydropteroate synthase. *Antimicrob. Agents Chemother.* **32:**1684–1692.
166. **Recchia, G. D., and R. M. Hall.** 1995. Gene cassettes: a new class of mobile element. *Microbiology* **141:**3015–3027.
167. **Reynolds, E., J. I. Ross, and J. H. Cove.** 2003. *msr*(A) and related macrolide/streptogramin resistance determinants: incomplete transporters? *Int. J. Antimicrob. Agents* **22:** 228–236.
168. **Roberts, M. C.** 1996. Tetracycline resistance determinants: mechanisms of action, regulation of expression, genetic mobility, and distribution. *FEMS Microbiol. Rev.* **19:**1–24.
169. **Roberts, M. C., J. Sutcliffe, P. Courvalin, L. B. Jensen, J. I. Rood, and H. Seppala.** 1999. Nomenclature for macrolide and macrolide-lincosamide streptogramin B antibiotic resistance determinants. *Antimicrob. Agents Chemother.* **43:**2823–2830.
170. **Rosenberg, E., D. Ma, and H. Nikaido.** 2000. AcrD of *Escherichia coli* is an aminoglycoside efflux pump. *J. Bacteriol.* **182:**1754–1756.
171. **Ross, J. I., E. A. Eady, J. H. Cove, and W. J. Cunliffe.** 1998. 16S rRNA mutation associated with tetracycline resistance in a gram-positive bacterium. *Antimicrob. Agents Chemother.* **42:**1702–1705.
172. **Ross, J. I., E. A. Eady, J. H. Cove, W. J. Cunliffe, S. Baumberg, and J. C. Wootton.** 1990. Inducible erythromycin resistance in staphylococci is encoded by a member of the ATP-binding transport super gene family. *Mol. Microbiol.* **4:**1207–1214.
173. **Rouch, D. A., M. E. Byrne, Y. C. Kong, and R. A. Skurray.** 1987. The *aac*A-*aph*D gentamicin and kanamycin resistance determinant of Tn*4001* from *Staphylococcus aureus*: expression and nucleotide sequence analysis. *J. Gen. Microbiol.* **133:**3039–3052.
174. **Rouch, D. A., L. J. Masserotti, L. S. L. Loo, C. A. Jackson, and R. A. Skurray.** 1989. Trimethoprim resistance transposon Tn*4003* from *Staphylococcus aureus* encodes genes for a dihydrofolate reductase and thymidylate synthetase flanked by three copies of IS*257*. *Mol. Microbiol.* **3:**161–175.

175. **Ruiz, J.** 2003. Mechanisms of resistance to quinolones: target alterations, decreased accumulation and DNA gyrase protection. *J. Antimicrob. Chemother.* **51:**1109–1117.
176. **Salyers, A. A., N. B. Shoemaker, A. M. Stevens, and L.-Y. Li.** 1995. Conjugative transposons: an unusual and diverse set of integrated gene transfer elements. *Microbiol. Rev.* **59:** 579–590.
177. **Salyers, A. A., and D. D. Whitt.** 1994. *Bacterial Pathogenesis: a Molecular Approach.* ASM Press, Washington, D.C.
178. **Sandvang, D.** 2001. Aminoglycoside resistance genes and their mobility in gram-negative bacteria from production animals. Ph.D. thesis. The Royal Veterinary and Agricultural University, Copenhagen, Denmark.
179. **Sandvang, D., and F. M. Aarestrup.** 2000. Characterization of aminoglycoside resistance genes and class 1 integrons in porcine and bovine gentamicin-resistant *Escherichia coli. Microb. Drug Resist.* **6:**19–27.
180. **Schmitz, F.-J., J. Petridou, H. Jagusch, N. Astfalk, S. Scheuring, and S. Schwarz.** 2002. Molecular characterization of ketolide-resistant *erm*(A)-carrying *Staphylococcus aureus* isolates selected in vitro by telithromycin, ABT-773, quinupristin and clindamycin. *J. Antimicrob. Chemother.* **49:**611–617.
181. **Schmitz, F.-J., J. Petridou, N. Astfalk, S. Scheuring, K. Köhrer, and S. Schwarz.** 2002. Molecular analysis of constitutively expressed *erm*(C) genes selected in-vitro by incubation in the presence of the non-inducers quinupristin, telithromycin or ABT-773. *Microb. Drug Resist.* **8:**171–177.
182. **Schwarz, S., and M. Cardoso.** 1991. Nucleotide sequence and phylogeny of a chloramphenicol acetyltransferase encoded by the plasmid pSCS7 from *Staphylococcus aureus. Antimicrob. Agents Chemother.* **35:**1551–1556.
183. **Schwarz, S., and E. Chaslus-Dancla.** 2001. Use of antimicrobials in veterinary medicine and mechanisms of resistance. *Vet. Res.* **32:**201–225.
184. **Schwarz, S., C. Kehrenberg, B. Doublet, and A. Cloeckaert.** 2004. Molecular basis of bacterial resistance to chloramphenicol and florfenicol. *FEMS Microbiol. Rev.* **28:**519–542.
185. **Schwarz, S., C. Kehrenberg, and K. K. Ojo.** 2002. *Staphylococcus sciuri* gene *erm*(33), encoding inducible resistance to macrolides, lincosamides, and streptogramin B antibiotics, is a product of recombination between *erm*(C) and *erm*(A). *Antimicrob. Agents Chemother.* **46:**3621–3623.
186. **Schwarz, S., C. Kehrenberg, and T. R. Walsh.** 2001. Use of antimicrobial agents in veterinary medicine and food animal production. *Int. J. Antimicrob. Agents* **17:**431–437.
187. **Schwarz, S., and W. C. Noble.** 1994. Tetracycline resistance genes in staphylococci from the skin of pigs. *J. Appl. Bacteriol.* **76:**320–326.
188. **Schwarz, S., and W. C. Noble.** 1999. Aspects of bacterial resistance to antimicrobial agents used in veterinary dermatological practice. *Vet. Dermatol.* **10:**163–176.
189. **Schwarz, S., C. Werckenthin, and C. Kehrenberg.** 2000. Identification of a plasmid-borne chloramphenicol/florfenicol resistance gene in *Staphylococcus sciuri. Antimicrob. Agents Chemother.* **44:**2530–2533.
190. **Shaw, K. J., P. N. Rather, S. R. Hare, and G. H. Miller.** 1993. Molecular genetics of aminoglycoside resistance genes and familial relationships of the aminoglycoside-modifying enzymes. *Microbol. Rev.* **57:**138–163.
191. **Shaw, W. V.** 1983. Chloramphenicol acetyltransferase: enzymology and molecular biology. *Crit. Rev. Biochem.* **14:**1–46.
192. **Simjee, S., S. M. Donabedian, and M. J. Zervos.** 2004. Linkage of the streptogramin resistance gene, *vatE*, to the copper resistance gene, *tcrB*, on a 10kb plasmid recovered from *Enterococcus faecium* isolated from poultry farms in the USA, abstr. C2–649, p. 91. Abstracts of the 44th Interscience Conference on Antimicrobial Agents and Chemotherapy, ASM Press, Washington, D.C.
193. **Simonet, V., M. Mallea, and J.-M. Pages.** 2000. Substitutions in the eyelet region disrupt cefepime diffusion through the *Escherichia coli* OmpF channel. *Antimicrob. Agents Chemother.* **44:**311–315.
194. **Sköld, O.** 2000. Sulfonamide resistance: mechanisms and trends. *Drug Resist. Updates.* **3:**155–160.
195. **Sköld, O.** 2001. Resistance to trimethoprim and sulfonamides. *Vet. Res.* **32:**261–273.
196. **Sorum, H., and M. Sunde.** 2001. Resistance to antibiotics in the normal flora of animals. *Vet. Res.* **32:**227–241.
197. **Speer, B. S., L. Bedzyk, and A. A. Salyers.** 1991. Evidence that a novel tetracycline resistance gene found on two *Bacteroides* transposons encodes an NADP-requiring oxidoreductase. *J. Bacteriol.* **173:**176–183.
198. **Speer, B. S., N. B. Shoemaker, and A. A. Salyers.** 1992. Bacterial resistance to tetracyclines: mechanisms, transfer, and clinical significance. *Clin. Microbiol. Rev.* **5:**387–399.
199. **Stanisich, V. A.** 1988. Identification and analysis of plasmids at the genetic level, p. 11–48. *In* J. Grinsted and P. M. Bennett (ed.), *Plasmid Technology.* Academic Press, London, United Kingdom.
200. **Stokes, H. W., and R. M. Hall.** 1991. Sequence analysis of the inducible chloramphenicol resistance determinant in the Tn*1696* integron suggests regulation by translational attenuation. *Plasmid* **26:**10–19.
201. **Sundström, L., P. Radström, G. Swedberg, and O. Sköld.** 1988. Site-specific recombination promotes linkage between trimethoprim- and sulfonamide resistance genes. Sequence characterization of *dhfrV* and *sulI* and a recombination active locus of Tn*21*. *Mol. Gen. Genet.* **213:**191–201.
202. **Sutcliffe, J. A., and R. Leclercq.** 2003. Mechanisms of resistance to macrolides, lincosamides and ketolides, p. 281–317. *In* W. Schonfeld and H. A. Kirst (ed.), *Macrolide Antibiotics.* Birkhauser Verlag, Basel, Switzerland.
203. **Swedberg, G., and O. Sköld.** 1980. Characterization of different plasmid-borne dihydropteroate synthases mediating bacterial resistance to sulfonamides. *J. Bacteriol.* **142:**1–7.
204. **Taylor, D. E., and A. Chau.** 1996. Tetracycline resistance mediated by ribosomal protection. *Antimicrob. Agents Chemother.* **40:**1–5.
205. **Tran, J. H., and G. A. Jacoby.** 2002. Mechanism of plasmid-mediated quinolone resistance. *Proc. Natl. Acad. Sci. USA* **99:**5638–5642.
206. **Treede, I., L. Jakobsen, F. Kirpekar, B. Vester, G. Weitnauer, A. Bechthold, and S. Douthwaite.** 2003. The avilamycin resistance determinants AviRa and AviRb methylate 23S rRNA at the guanosine 2535 base and the uridine 2479 ribose. *Mol. Microbiol.* **49:**309–318.
207. **van den Bogaard, A. E., M. Hazen, M. Hoyer, P. Oostenbach, and E. E. Stobberingh.** 2002. Effects of flavophospholipol on resistance in fecal *Escherichia coli* and enterococci of fattening pigs. *Antimicrob. Agents Chemother.* **46:**110–118.
208. **Vester, B., and S. Douthwaite.** 2001. Macrolide resistance conferred by base substitutions in 23S rRNA. *Antimicrob. Agents Chemother.* **45:**1–12.
209. **Walsh, C.** 2003. *Antibiotics: Actions, Origins, Resistance.* ASM Press, Washington, D.C.
210. **Wang, M., D. F. Sahm, G. A. Jacoby, and D. C. Hooper.** 2004. Emerging plasmid-mediated quinolone resistance associated with the *qnr* gene in *Klebsiella pneumoniae* clinical isolates in the United States. *Antimicrob. Agents Chemother.* **48:**1295–1299.
211. **Wang, M., J. H. Tran, G. A. Jacoby, Y. Zhang, F. Wang, and D. C. Hooper.** 2003. Plasmid-mediated quinolone resistance

in clinical isolates of *Escherichia coli* from Shanghai, China. *Antimicrob. Agents Chemother.* **47**:2242–2248.

212. **Webber, M., and L. J. V. Piddock.** 2001. Quinolone resistance in *Escherichia coli. Vet. Res.* **32**:275–284.
213. **Weigel, L. M., D. B. Clewell, S. R. Gill, N. C. Clark, L. K. McDougal, S. E. Flannagan, J. F. Kolonay, J. Shetty, G. E. Kilgore, and F. C. Tenover.** 2003. Genetic analysis of a high-level vancomycin-resistant isolate of *Staphylococcus aureus. Science* **302**:1569–1571.
214. **Weisblum, B.** 1995. Erythromycin resistance by ribosome modification. *Antimicrob. Agents Chemother.* **39**: 577–585.
215. **Weisblum, B.** 1995. Insights into erythromycin action from studies of its activity as inducer of resistance. *Antimicrob. Agents Chemother.* **39**:797–805.
216. **Weitnauer, G., S. Gaisser, A. Trefzer, S. Stockert, L. Westrich, L. M. Quiros, C. Mendez, J. A. Salas, and A. Bechthold.** 2001. An ATP-binding cassette transporter and two rRNA methyltransferases are involved in resistance to avilamycin in the producer organism *Streptomyces viridochromogenes* Tu57. *Antimicrob. Agents Chemother.* **45**:690–695.
217. **Weldenhagen, G. F.** 2004. Integrons and β-lactamases—a novel perspective on resistance. *Int. J. Antimicrob. Chemother.* **23**:556–562.
218. **Werckenthin, C., S. Schwarz, and M. C. Roberts.** 1996. Integration of pT181-like tetracycline resistance plasmids into large staphylococcal plasmids involves IS257. *Antimicrob. Agents Chemother.* **40**:2542–2544.
219. **Werckenthin, C., S. Schwarz, and H. Westh.** 1999. Structural alterations in the translational attenuators of constitutively expressed *erm*(C) genes. *Antimicrob. Agents Chemother.* **43**:1681–1685.
220. **Werner, G., I. Klare, and W. Witte.** 1999. Large conjugative plasmids in vancomycin-resistant *Enterococcus faecium. J. Clin. Microbiol.* **37**:2383–2384.
221. **White, D. G., C. Hudson, J. J. Maurer, S. Ayers, S. Zhao, M. D. Lee, L. Bolton, T. Foley, and J. Sherwood.** 2000. Characterization of chloramphenicol and florfenicol resistance in *Escherichia coli* associated with bovine diarrhea. *J. Clin. Microbiol.* **38**:4593–4598.
222. **Wiedemann, B., D. Pfeifle, I. Wiegand, and E. Janas.** 1998. β-Lactamase induction and cell wall recycling in gram-negative bacteria. *Drug Resist. Updates* **1**:223–226.
223. **Wiegand, I.** 2003. Molecular and biochemical elements of β-lactam resistance by β-lactamases. *Chemother. J.* **12**: 151–167.
224. **Wolter, D. J., N. D. Hanson, and P. D. Lister.** 2004. Insertional inactivation of *oprD* in clinical isolates of *Pseudomonas aeruginosa* leading to carbapenem resistance. *FEMS Microbiol. Lett.* **236**:137–143.
225. **Wright, G. D.** 1999. Aminoglycoside-modifying enzymes. *Curr. Opin. Microbiol.* **2**:499–503.
226. **Yoshida, H., M. Bogaki, M. Nakamura, and S. Nakamura.** 1990. Quinolone resistance determining region in the DNA gyrase *gyrA* gene of *Escherichia coli. Antimicrobial Agents Chemother.* **34**:1271–1272.

Antimicrobial Resistance in Bacteria of Animal Origin
Edited by Frank M. Aarestrup

Chapter 7

Resistance to Metals Used in Agricultural Production

HENRIK HASMAN, SYLVIA FRANKE, AND CHRISTOPHER RENSING

INTRODUCTION

A large number of metals play a vital role as trace elements in the physiology of production animals and must be present in adequate quantities in feed in order to maintain a normal healthy state. Two of these metals, however, are added to the feed in larger quantities than can be explained by the physiological needs of the animals. Copper and zinc are essential trace metals, but in addition to their role in the normal growth of the animal, they also seem to have additional effects when used in high doses. In addition to copper and zinc, livestock producers in the United States, but not in Europe, also use the nonessential metal arsenic as a feed supplement to chickens, turkeys, and pigs.

Requirements and Recommendations for Copper and Zinc Supplementation to Livestock Animals

The minimal nutritional requirements for copper and zinc depend on the animal species, on the age of the animal, and especially on the presence of other substances in the feed. A level of 6 ppm of copper in the diet is adequate for normal growth of the neonatal pig (68, 102). The zinc requirement for young pigs consuming a nonphytate diet is 15 to 18 ppm (119, 129). However, diet-related factors can interfere with uptake of copper and zinc in the gut. Such factors include the presence of high levels of zinc (in the case of copper uptake); high levels of copper (in the case of zinc uptake); high concentrations of calcium (Ca), nickel (Ni), molybdenum (Mo), magnesium (Mg), and iron (Fe); and the presence of plant phytates (83, 86, 119). Therefore, the actual nutritional recommendations of zinc and copper are inflated in order to avoid malnutrition due to reduced absorption of the metals caused by diet-related factors. The requirements and general recommendations of copper and zinc supplementation for selected animal groups are listed in Tables 1 and 2.

Supplements of Copper, Zinc, and Arsenicals

In addition to the minimum amounts given to ensure normal growth, most pig producers use additional supplements of copper (often as copper sulfate) and zinc (often as zinc chloride, oxide, or sulfate), as well as different arsenicals in the form of *p*-arsenilic acid and 4-nitro-3-hydroxyphenylarsonate (Roxarsone). These perform a dual purpose, as they seem to increase the daily growth rate and feed conversion rate in the animals as well as limit and control the cases of postweaning scouring. However, it is unlikely that the growth-promoting effect is due to the high levels of dietary zinc or copper improving the nutrient status of the piglets.

In most of the European Community, the maximum amount of copper allowed for pig feedstuff is 170 mg/kg (170 ppm) for piglets (up to 12 weeks of age) and 25 ppm thereafter. Zinc is allowed as a supplement for pigs in quantities of 250 ppm. In contrast to this, copper and zinc supplements are not restricted in the United States. Typical amounts range from 125 to 250 ppm of copper independent of the age of the pigs and 2,500 to 3,000 ppm of zinc immediately postweaning, which decreases to 1,500 ppm at the end of the nursing phase. Thereafter, zinc does not seem to have growth-promoting effects and much lower amounts of zinc are normally used (G. Willis, Primary Nutrition LLC, personal communication). For production of chickens, 25 ppm of copper is allowed in the European Community. In addition, arsenilic acid is allowed in the United States for use in pigs (100 ppm) and broilers and turkeys (both 90 ppm), but it is normally used at levels between 20 and 40 ppm (71).

Henrik Hasman • Danish Institute for Food and Veterinary Research, Bülowsvej 27, DK-1790 Copenhagen V, Denmark. **Sylvia Franke and Christopher Rensing** • Department of Soil, Water and Environmental Science, University of Arizona, Shantz Bldg. 38, Tucson, AZ 85721.

Table 1. Requirements of copper and zinc supplements for production animals[a]

Metal	Required supplement (mg/kg of feedstuff) for:			
	Piglets (<20 kg)	Growing pigs	Poultry	Cattle
Copper	5–6	4–5	2.5–8	9–10
Zinc	80–100	50–60	29–40	14.8–63

[a]Data from references 41 and 42.

A recent report by the European Commission (41) analyzed a large number of dose-response studies with copper supplements given to pigs of different ages, ranging from the postweaning period (up to 20 kg in body weight) to growing pigs (20 to 60 kg in body weight) and to finishing pigs (above 60 kg in body weight). The conclusion from this analysis was that the presence of high amounts of copper (from approximately 63 to 73 ppm up to 280 ppm) does improve the growth rate of the youngest age group significantly, but no significant effect was observed for growing and finishing pigs (41). Prolonged use of copper in high doses (250 ppm and above) has been reported to affect animal growth negatively, therefore resulting in toxic effects. High levels of copper (125 and 250 mg/kg of feedstuff) also have a growth-promoting effect in broilers (43, 76, 108, 126).

The growth-promoting effect of pharmaceutical levels of zinc (2,000 to 6,000 ppm) has been reported in piglets shortly after weaning (18, 27, 67, 75, 127). However, not all studies show beneficial effects of high doses of zinc (151). The growth-promoting effect seems to be most pronounced for the first 2 weeks after weaning (75), and copper does not seem to have an additive effect together with zinc on growth promotion of pigs (67, 127).

The mechanism behind the effect of zinc and copper in the treatment of postweaning scouring is not well understood. Zinc oxide has been suggested to prevent diarrhea by helping to maintain the stability of the intestinal flora in weaned pigs, thus preserving its protective ability, which would otherwise be lost due to weaning (75). This stability then renders the gut less susceptible to the establishment of pathogens, either indirectly, by competing for the same niche, or directly, by the growth inhibition of pathogenic organisms by the metals (73). Zinc oxide did not have any effect on the normal fecal flora of weaned pigs when the number of excreted *Escherichia coli* and enterococci per gram of feces of pigs supplemented with 2,500 ppm of ZnO were compared to a control group of pigs not fed ZnO (73). However, the diversity of the coliform bacteria does increase within the population, at least within the first 2 weeks after weaning (75). This, however, does not exclude changes in the remaining bacterial community of the gut, as only coliforms were examined.

Table 2. Recommendations of copper and zinc supplements for production animals[a]

Metal	Recommended supplement (mg/kg of feedstuff) for:			
	Piglets (<20 kg)	Growing pigs	Poultry	Cattle
Copper	6–10	4–10	7	10
Zinc	80–100	50–100	39–44	40–50

[a]Data from references 41 and 42.

Estimated Annual Consumption

The annual production of pigs is approximately 200 million animals in the European Community and almost 100 million in the United States. On average, approximately 220 kg of feedstuff is needed from postweaning to slaughter, with around 50 kg used for piglets (below 25 kg in body weight) and 170 kg to get from piglets to finishing pigs. Adhering to the maximal allowances in the European Community and the common usage in the United States for copper and zinc supplements to pigs, this amounts to a total of 5,200 tons of copper and 21,000 tons of zinc used every year in these two regions. According to estimates from the Union of Concerned Scientists (www.ucsusa.org), approximately 10 tons and 170 tons of arsenilic acid are used annually for pig and poultry production in the United States, respectively.

METAL HOMEOSTASIS AND METAL RESISTANCE

Detection of Metal Resistance

Metal resistance measurements of bacteria in the laboratory are calculated either in milligrams of metal per liter of medium or in millimolar units (millimoles per liter). The conversion factors between these for the three metals are as follows: 1 mM metal equals 63.5 mg of copper per liter, 65.39 mg of zinc per liter, and 74.92 mg of arsenic per liter. Most often, the MIC of the metal is determined, but some data are reported in maximal tolerable concentration (MTC).

Metal resistance measurements for bacteria involving copper and zinc in complex media typically range from <1 to 35 mM copper sulfate (pH 7) and <1 to 30 mM zinc sulfate (pH 5.5), but MIC of zinc sulfate up to 1 M have been reported in the bacterium *Acidocella* (52). At pH values above 5.5, the low solubility of zinc sulfate in complex media causes precipitation of the metal (1). This precipitation has been suggested to be caused by the presence of phosphates in the complex media and can in some cases be circumvented by using TRIS-buffered minimal media (90). Resistance to arsenic depends on the speciation of the oxyanion. Resistance to arsenates (As^{5+}) typically ranges from <1 to 100 mM and to arsenites (As^{3+}) from <1 to 10 mM (117).

Two factors have great influence on the detection of metal resistance levels. These are choice of growth media and pH of the media. The choice of media obviously depends on the bacteria to be tested. All complex media will have an increased potential to bind the supplied metal compared to minimal medium, thus rendering most of the metal unavailable to the bacteria. Therefore, metal resistance data are difficult to compare between studies, unless the same medium is used. Also, most complex media are not standardized, which reduces the reproducibility of the testing. An exception to this is Mueller-Hinton medium, which is commonly used to determine resistance to antibiotics (2). Minimal media has been reported to increase the sensitivity of the tested isolates to the metals by 20-fold or more (16).

As Cu(II) and Zn(II) are weak acids, the supplementation of these to media in millimolar concentrations lowers the pH of the media. Standard brain heart infusion (BHI) (pH = 7.4) broth supplemented with 2 mM copper sulfate has a pH of 6.8, while the same media has a pH of 6 with 7.5 mM copper sulfate and a pH of 4.6 when supplemented with 20 mM copper sulfate (H. Hasman, unpublished data). Similar results have been described for other media (138). Therefore, the pH of the media has to be adjusted in order to ensure optimal growth of the bacteria and to avoid misleading results based on acid instead of metal resistance. In addition, the fraction of unbound Cu(II) ions available for the bacteria increase by a factor of 5 when the pH of Mueller-Hinton broth is changed from 7 to 6 (M. Bjerrum, Royal Veterinary and Agricultural University, Frederiksberg, Denmark, personal communication). Finally, pH values above 7 favor the formation of insoluble copper hydroxides, which again reduce the amount of active metal available to the bacteria.

Zinc (chloride, sulfate, and acetate) has a similar effect on the pH of BHI media. However, zinc solutions of BHI media with concentrations above 3 mM (zinc chloride and zinc acetate) and 10 mM (zinc sulfate) are turbid, and here the pH has to be lowered in order to dissolve the metal completely.

Metal Tolerance Assays

Typically, three different assays are used to detect increased tolerance (resistance) to metals. These are (i) gradient agar plates (39, 136, 152), (ii) agar dilution assay based on National Committee for Clinical Laboratory Standards recommendations (1, 16, 95, 98, 140, 147), and (iii) liquid media dilution assay (74). Rarely, disc diffusion with discs impregnated with salt solutions have been used for screening purposes (3, 80). Gradient agar plates are made of two different solid agar layers, one containing a high metal concentration (pH adjusted) and the other containing no metal. The first layer is poured into 10-cm-square petri dishes and allowed to set, with the dishes inclined at an angle of approximately 4°. This layer is allowed to solidify, after which the second layer is added, this time with the petri dishes in a horizontal position. Bacterial suspensions of standardized densities (e.g., McFarland Standard = 0.5) are applied across the metal gradient shortly after the second layer has solidified, using an inoculating wire. In this assay, the plates have to be used the same day they are made, to avoid diffusion of metal between the two layers. After inoculation, the plates are incubated according to the requirement of the organism, and subsequently the length of bacterial growth into the high metal concentration is measured. However, variation between plates often makes it necessary to include a positive and a negative control on each plate.

The other two methods are both based on metal dilution, dissolved in either agar or liquid broth. Here, dilution series of the metals are made, as is common in detection of antibiotic resistance, and the MIC or the MTC is determined. Frequently, linear instead of exponential serial dilutions are made, but as these dilution steps are not standardized, an MTC is often more meaningful than an MIC. Again, pH of the metal-supplemented media has to be adjusted and bacterial densities have to be normalized before inoculation.

Metal Tolerance Levels in Bacteria

Unlike with antibiotic resistance, there are no universally acceptable metal ion concentrations that are used to designate microbial tolerance. As mentioned above, the detection of metal tolerance levels is extremely dependent on the chosen bacteria, media, and growth conditions. Little has been done to determine MIC distributions of metals for bacterial populations under standardized conditions. One study tested populations of *Salmonella*, *E. coli*, *Staphylococcus aureus*, *Staphylococcus hyicus*, *Enterococcus faecalis*, and *Enterococcus faecium* isolated from Danish food animals for their tolerance to copper sulfate and zinc chloride in Mueller-Hinton media at either pH 7 (copper sulfate) or pH 5.5 (zinc

Table 3. Susceptibility of 569 bacterial isolates from livestock in Denmark to copper sulfate[a]

Bacterium	No. of isolates	No. of isolates for which the MIC of copper sulfate (mM) is:								
		1	2	4	8	12	16	20	24	28
Salmonella	156							26	84	46
E. coli	202				1	5	26	169	1	
S. aureus	43		22	3	8	10				
S. hyicus	38				24	14				
E. faecalis	52		19	2		3	25	1	2	
E. faecium	78			5	8		20	3	16	

[a]Adapted from reference 1.

chloride) (1). The enterococcal isolates formed a bimodal distribution for copper sulfate, but not zinc chloride, indicative of a specific resistance mechanism in these two species (see below). Each of the other species tested formed one large population of susceptibilities to both zinc and copper (Tables 3 and 4). In this study the *Salmonella* isolates had the highest tolerance to copper sulfate, with the MICs for all 156 isolates ranging between 20 and 28 mM (Table 3). A second study has suggested the cutoff value between susceptible and resistant *E. coli* for copper sulfate to be 4 mM for media, which was not adjusted for the ΔpH effect, and 6 mM when the adjustment was done. Here, the MIC for resistant bacteria was 8 mM in unadjusted media and between 12 and 20 mM in pH-adjusted media, but only a few isolates were tested (140). Adhering to the result of this last study but using a cutoff value of 7.5 mM copper sulfate, Jayasheela et al. found 68 (out of 330) *Salmonella* isolates from India to be copper resistant (72). However, the Danish study shows that *Salmonella* in general seem to have slightly higher tolerance to copper than *E. coli*, which could indicate that the cutoff value should be set slightly higher (Table 3).

Resistance to copper (MIC ≥7.5 mM $CuSO_4$) and arsenite (MIC ≥0.04 mM arsenite) has also been reported among populations of several different *Enterobacteriaceae* isolated between 1917 and 1954 (the so-called Murray collection), thus isolated within the "pre-antibiotic" era (70). In this study, the resistance determinants were not mobilizable, indicating chromosomal localization of these determinants.

Most other bacterial species that have been tested and found positive for increased tolerance to copper and zinc are environmental isolates from locations with high exposure to metals (Tables 5 and 6). In most of these studies, cutoff values for the metals examined have not been determined in the context of a large bacterial population, as only a single or very few isolates have been tested in each case. An exception is a study regarding copper resistance among *Pseudomonas syringae* pv. tomato, where 20 isolates were tested and could be divided into three groups, depending on their copper resistance levels. MICs for susceptible strains were 0.4 to 0.6 mM copper sulfate, for moderately resistant strains were 1.2 mM, and for very resistant strains were between 1.6 and 2.0 mM. Here, copper resistance could be transferred by conjugation to susceptible recipients, showing plasmid localization of the resistance determinant (10). Plasmid-borne copper resistance has also been described in other *Pseudomonas* spp. (53, 134), *Acidocella* spp. (52), *Staphylococcus* spp. (147), *E. faecium* (64), *E. coli* (14, 140), *Desulfovibrio*

Table 4. Susceptibility of 177 bacterial isolates from livestock in Denmark to zinc chloride[a]

Bacterium	No. of isolates	No. of isolates for which the MIC of zinc chloride (mM)[b] is:							
		0.25	0.5	1	2	4	8	12	16
Salmonella	26				26				
E. coli	51				1	50			
S. aureus	26	2	3	10	11				
S. hyicus	22	22							
E. faecalis	26				2		11	13	
E. faecium	26				1	11	14		

[a]Adapted from reference 1.
[b]Determined on Mueller-Hinton II agar adjusted to pH 5.5.

Table 5. Organisms which have been tested for copper tolerance and in which resistance to copper has been suggested to occur

Organism	Reference(s)
Acidiphilium	87
Acidocella	52
Acinetobacter	16, 98
Desulfovibrio	74
Enterobacter	16
E. faecalis	1
E. faecium	1
E. coli	1, 70, 118
Flavobacterium	98
Halomonas	98
K. pneumoniae	26, 28, 70
Lactobacillus	38
Micrococcus	16, 98
Microcystis aeruginosa	50
M. scrofulaceum	40
Proteus	70
Pseudomonas pickettii	53
Pseudomonas putida	29
P. syringae pv. tomato	10
Salmonella	1, 70, 118
Shigella	70
S. aureus	1, 98, 147
S. hyicus	1
Streptococcus pyrogenes	118
V. fluvialis	118
X. campestris pv. vesicatoria	51

spp. (74), *Citrobacter freundii* and *Salmonella* spp. (152), *Klebsiella pneumoniae* (26, 149), *Xanthomonas campestris* pv. vesicatoria (51), *Mycobacterium scrofulaceum* (40), *Vagococcus fluvialis* (118), and *Lactococcus lactis* (84). The genetic determinants responsible for the resistance have only been identified in some of these cases (see below).

Table 6. Organisms which have been tested for zinc tolerance and in which resistance to zinc has been suggested to occur

Organism	Reference(s)
Acidiphilium	87
Acidocella	52
Acinetobacter	16, 98
Arthrobacter	16
Enterobacter	16
E. faecalis	1
E. faecium	1
E. coli	1
Flavobacterium	98
K. pneumoniae	26, 28
Lactobacillus	38
Micrococcus	16
R. metallidurans CH34	31, 59, 82, 90
Salmonella	1
S. aureus	1, 147, 155
S. hyicus	1

Studies have reported isolates with increased zinc tolerance (resistance) for many of the same organisms described in the copper studies mentioned above (Table 6) and also among the hydrogen-oxidizing bacterium *Ralstonia metallidurans* CH34 (renamed from *Alicaligenes eutrophus* CH34 and recently renamed *Wausteria metallidurans* CH34) (32, 59, 82, 90). Plasmid-associated zinc resistance has been reported among *S. aureus* (80, 145, 155), *K. pneumoniae* (149), *Salmonella* spp. (4, 140), and *Acidocella* spp. (52), but a specific mechanism has been identified only for *S. aureus* (the CadA transporter described below).

Transferable arsenate and arsenite resistance has only been reported in *S. aureus* (13, 123), *Staphylococcus xylosus* (37), *Pseudomonas aeruginosa* (19, 93), *Yersinia enterocolitica* (35, 96), *E. coli* (66, 115), *Acidiphilium multivorum* (135), and *Rhodococcus* spp. (36).

METAL HOMEOSTASIS VERSUS METAL RESISTANCE

Heavy metal homeostasis versus resistance is a complicated balancing act between maintaining a full supply of cells with essential trace elements on one hand and protection against accumulation of toxic metal concentrations on the other. There is some confusion in the literature as to what constitutes zinc and copper (and other heavy metal) resistance, in contrast to intrinsic homeostasis mechanisms.

Genes in any given organism can be subdivided into core, operational, and accessory genetic elements. Since most of the earlier studies on heavy metal resistance were carried out with plasmid-encoded systems, there is the misconception that there is a difference between resistance and homeostasis mechanisms. Basically, all organisms have some mechanism of controlling metal uptake and efflux, and these determinants are often necessary for the functional expression and phenotype of additional metal resistance determinants (81). However, there are great differences among organisms. For example, analysis of the genome of the obligate symbiont *Buchnera* in comparison with those of related enteric bacteria suggests that extensive changes, including large deletions, repetitive element proliferation, and chromosomal rearrangements, occurred initially, followed by extreme stasis in gene order and the slow decay of additional genes (137, 148). *Buchnera aphidicola* does not seem to contain any metal efflux systems, whereas the extremely metal-resistant bacterium *R. metallidurans* CH34 contains a vast number of transporters (89, 97, 147). In addition, genes homologous to the plasmid-encoded *cadA* determinant are present on many chromosomes, e.g., *E. coli*, *Bacillus subtilis*, and *P. aeruginosa*. The same is true for the plasmid-encoded *pco* determinant from *E. coli* since an almost exact copy is present on the chromosome of *K. pneunomiae*. In addition, genes encoding homologues of the multicopper oxidase PcoA are present on many bacterial chromosomes. On the other hand, not all bacteria, such as *B. aphidicola*, encode genes specifically needed to combat heavy metal toxicity. It therefore seems conclusive that the presence or absence of genetic determinants conferring resistance to certain metals is dependent on the natural environment of an organism. If these microorganisms are routinely exposed to metals, they will contain genes on the chromosome that are capable of protecting them. If these conditions change dramatically, as when pigs are fed with copper, these same organisms will acquire additional genetic determinants, typically on mobile genetic elements, capable of conferring increased resistance. On the other hand, if they live in an environment devoid of metals, as in the case of the obligate symbiont *B. aphidicola*, the chromosome will lose these genes over time.

MECHANISMS OF METAL HOMEOSTASIS AND RESISTANCE

Zinc Homeostasis and Resistance

Zinc uptake

One of the best-characterized systems of zinc homeostasis is in *E. coli* (Fig. 1). Zinc is taken up by at least three systems of differing specificity and efficiency. Under zinc deficiency the ZnuABC system, an ABC (ATB-binding cassette) transporter, is expressed (106). ZnuA is a periplasmic zinc-binding protein, ZnuB the membrane-spanning pump, and ZnuC the ATPase catalytic subunit. If zinc is in excess, expression of *znuA znuBC* is repressed by Zur (105).

Another uptake system is ZupT (58), the first identified bacterial member of the ZIP (ZRT-, IRT-like protein [ZRT, zinc-regulated transporter; IRT, iron-regulated transporter]) family of transporters, previously only described in eukaryotes (48, 61). They were initially identified as transporters of zinc and ferrous iron. Further studies showed that they are also responsible for manganese and cadmium uptake. In *E. coli*, ZupT was also shown to have a broad

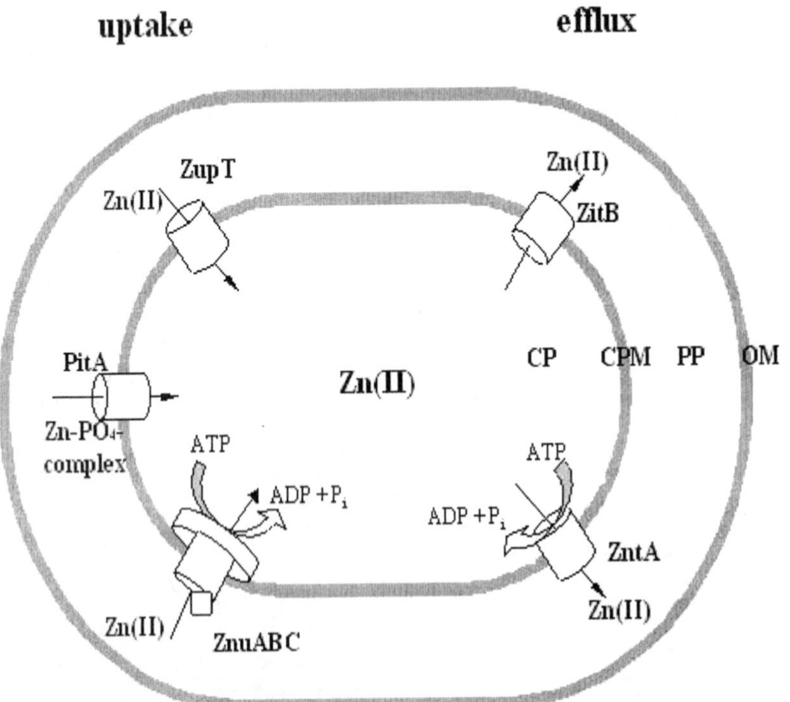

Figure 1. Zn(II) transport systems in *E. coli*. This model shows the known Zn^{2+} transport systems of *E. coli*. Under conditions of zinc deficiency Zn^{2+} is taken up by ZupT and ZnuABC (58, 106). ZupT belongs to the ZIP family of metal transporters (61), and ZnuABC is an ABC transport system. Zn^{2+} can also be taken up as inorganic Zn-PO_4 complex via PitA (9). Zinc-translocating efflux pumps are the P-type ATPase ZntA and the CDF protein ZitB (56, 112). ZnuABC and ZntA (both ATP dependent) are probably more powerful transporters than ZitB or ZupT, which might be responsible for zinc homeostasis under physiological conditions. CP, cytoplasm; CPM, cytoplasmic membrane; PP, periplasm; OM, outer membrane.

substrate spectrum (G. Grass and C. Rensing, unpublished data). However, specificity and affinity to different metals are specific for each ZIP transporter (61). The *zupT* gene is expressed at a low constitutive level and not affected by the availability of zinc in *E. coli* (Grass and Rensing, unpublished). The mechanism of metal uptake by ZIP transporters is still not solved. They could function as a channel, where cations move along their gradient and membrane potential, or as a symporter, as indicated by preliminary results of cotransport of Zn^{2+} and HCO_3^+ by human ZIP2 (49).

There are other ways for *E. coli* to take up zinc under nonlimiting conditions. For example, zinc can be taken up as metal-phosphate complexes via the inorganic phosphate uptake system (PitA) (9). In addition, it has been shown that different magnesium uptake systems exhibit a wide substrate spectrum and might also be able to take up zinc, as members of the Nramp superfamily can do.

How other bacteria take up zinc is not known in much detail. In many organisms, e.g., *Haemophilus influenzae*, *Neisseria gonorrhoeae*, *Salmonella enterica* serovar Typhimurium, and *B. subtilis*, genes encoding ZnuABC homologues can be identified (17, 24, 30, 46, 47, 85). Members of the ZIP family can be identified as hypothetical zinc transporters in many prokaryotic genome sequences, indicating a wide occurrence of this family not only in eukaryotes but also in bacteria and archaea. As mentioned above, there are other metal transporters with broad substrate specificity. Examples include the magnesium uptake systems of *S. enterica* serovar Typhimurium (MgtA) and *Bacillus firmus* OF4 (MgtE), which are able to take up Zn^{2+} in addition to Mg^{2+} (11, 128, 130).

Zinc efflux

Several mechanisms are in place to protect cells against toxic metal cation concentrations. In the case of zinc, bacterial resistance is mainly mediated by efflux. Presently, at least three different systems are known to be involved in the handling of excessive zinc in different bacteria. These systems can be encoded on the chromosome or on a plasmid.

Proteins of the cation diffusion facilitator (CDF) family form the first line of defense against excess cytoplasmic zinc concentrations. Found in all kingdoms of life, genes encoding CDF proteins can be located both on the chromosome or on a plasmid in bacteria. If plasmid encoded, an additional gene encoding a CDF protein is usually found on the bacterial chromosome.

Most bacterial CDF proteins have common structural characteristics. They contain six transmembrane helices; an N-terminal, cytoplasmic, histidine-rich domain; and a large C terminus, also located in the cytoplasm (5). The mechanism of Zn(II) transport across the cytoplasmic membrane was shown to be metal cation/proton antiport (22, 62). In gram-positive bacteria zinc is directly expelled into the environment; in gram-negative bacteria into the periplasmic space. However, the maximum capacity of zinc transport by a CDF protein is less than for a P-type ATPase.

In *E. coli* two genes encoding CDF proteins have been identified. ZitB (formerly YbgR) was shown to be necessary to handle elevated zinc (and cadmium) concentrations in the absence of the other export system, the P-type ATPase ZntA (see next paragraph) (56). Expression of *zitB* is regulated by zinc, but the mechanism of regulation is unknown. The second CDF protein in *E. coli*, YiiP, has no influence on zinc tolerance. However, it has been demonstrated that YiiP binds Zn(II) [and Cd(II)] (23) and is able to transport zinc into everted membrane vesicles (G. Grass et al., unpublished results).

S. aureus has a chromosomally encoded determinant of two open reading frames conferring resistance against Zn(II) and Co(II) (154). The *zntA* gene encodes a protein of the CDF family, whereas *zntR* encodes a regulator of the ArsR family (15, 125, 154). Disruption of *zntA* leads to higher sensitivity against Zn(II) and Co(II), suggesting involvement of ZntA in the handling of zinc and cobalt.

Analysis of genomic sequences (http://www.ncbi.nlm.nih.gov/sutils/genom_table.cgi) indicates the presence of CDF protein-encoding genes in a wide variety of microorganisms. It seems that this is an almost ubiquitous element in bacteria for handling heavy metals.

The second, and more powerful, line of defense against excess intracellular zinc concentrations is the soft metal ion-translocating P-type ATPases. They constitute one subgroup of P-type ATPases and can be further separated into Cu(I)/Ag(I)-translocating (see below) and Zn(II)/Cd(II)/Pb(II)-translocating P-type ATPases (11, 110). Soft metal ion-translocating P-type ATPases are proteins located in the cytoplasmic membrane that use the energy of ATP hydrolysis to translocate metal cations across the membrane. Also called CPx-type or P1-type ATPases, they are predicted to contain 8 to 10 transmembrane helices with conserved sequence motifs in the amino-terminal region and phosphatase and aspartyl kinase domains as well as the CPx motif in transmembrane helix 6 (however, exceptions to this CPx motif are known to occur) (11, 110, 131).

One of the first identified members of the Zn(II)/Cd(II)/Pb(II)-translocating P-type ATPases was CadA of *S. aureus* (99, 141, 142, 144, 146). The *cadA* gene is plasmid encoded and forms an operon with *cadC*, encoding a metalloregulatory repressor of the ArsR family (144, 146, 155). CadA was first shown to confer Cd(II) resistance and subsequently Zn(II) and Pb(II) resistance (113, 143).

Whereas *cadA* of *S. aureus* is plasmid encoded, a gene encoding a Zn(II)/Cd(II)/Pb(II)-translocating P-type ATPase could be identified on the chromosome of *E. coli* (112). Expression of *zntA* is regulated by the activator ZntR (12, 103). ZntA uses the energy of ATP hydrolysis to transport Zn(II), Cd(II), and Pb(II) across the cytoplasmic membrane into the periplasmic space of *E. coli* (112, 113, 120).

Members of the subfamily of Zn(II)/Cd(II)/Pb(II)-translocating P-type ATPases could be identified in many bacteria, gram positive as well as gram negative, and are thought to be involved in handling elevated zinc, lead, and cadmium. Genes encoding CPx-type ATPases could be located on plasmids as well as on the bacterial chromosome (11).

Efflux complexes of the CBA type (CBA-efflux complexes) are involved in the handling of heavy metals [monovalent Cu(I)/Ag(I) or divalent Co(II)/Zn(II)/Cd(II)/Ni(II), respectively], as well as organic compounds. In this section we only mention their influence in zinc tolerance, but we will come back to them in the section on copper resistance.

CBA-efflux complexes are composed of a central transporter of the resistance-nodulation-cell division (RND) family, a membrane fusion protein, and an outer membrane factor (OMF). RND proteins are the central transporter of the CBA complex and form a homotrimer located in the cytoplasmic membrane (92). The RND proteins can be divided into the integral membrane part and a periplasmic part, the latter generated by the two large periplasmic loops of each of the monomers (45, 54, 55, 60, 92). The periplasmic part of the RND trimer forms a pore that is connected to the OMF. As shown for TolC, a member of the family of OMFs, the OMF is also present as a homotrimer (78, 79). TolC is located in the outer membrane and spans through the periplasm to the RND protein. In the current model the RND protein and the OMF form a channel spanning the whole periplasmic space to the external medium (92). Little is known of how the membrane fusion protein functions in this transport complex. At the moment its role is thought of as stabilizing the RND-OMF channel.

Genes encoding a CBA complex involved in handling excessive zinc were first identified and characterized on (mega)plasmids (90). Recently, a CBA-encoding determinant located on the chromosome of *Pseudomonas* was shown to be involved in zinc resistance (65). Subsequent screening of bacterial genomic sequences identified many chromosomal genes encoding hypothetical RND transporters that might be involved in zinc and cadmium resistance.

Additional zinc transporters

In *S. enterica* serovar Typhimurium an additional transporter, ZntB, was shown to be involved in zinc tolerance. Even though ZntB belongs to the CorA family of transporters, unlike the other family members, ZntB does not appear to function as a magnesium uptake system. Instead, ZntB was described as a novel system mediating Zn^{2+} and Cd^{2+} tolerance (153).

Copper Homeostasis and Resistance

Mechanisms of copper homeostasis are almost ubiquitously distributed in bacteria. In mammals the concentration of copper is highest in the digestive tract, particularly in the stomach and duodenum. The particular concentrations are highly dependent on the diet. In addition, copper becomes much more toxic under acidic anaerobic conditions, which prevail in that part of the digestive tract. Thus, intestinal flora have evolved elaborate mechanisms for copper homeostasis as an adaptation to their specific ecological niche, the animal gut.

Chromosomally encoded systems of defense against toxic levels of copper

The main line of defense in both gram-positive and gram-negative bacteria is a copper-transporting P-type ATPase located in the cytoplasmic membrane. The P-type ATPases belong to a superfamily of proteins involved in transport of charged substrates across biological membranes (6). The copper-translocating P-type ATPases are members of a phylogenetically related subgroup of P-type ATPases that catalyze transport of transition or heavy metal ions. Well-studied prokaryotic copper transport systems are the copper ATPases of *Enterococcus hirae*, CopA and CopB (100, 101), and CopA from *Helicobacter pylori* (8), *B. subtilis* (7), and *E. coli* (44, 109). Eukaryotes possess similar copper ATPases (63). These P-type ATPases transport reduced cuprous ion (Cu^{+}) across the cytoplasmic membrane to keep the cytoplasmic level of free copper at extremely low levels (21, 44).

Copper not only exerts its toxic effects inside the cytoplasm, but cuprous ions can generate reactive oxygen species near the cytoplasmic and outer membranes, disturbing vital processes. Bacteria have therefore developed methods to minimize the presence of the prooxidant Cu^{+} in the periplasm and the immediate vicinity of the cell. One way to minimize Cu^{+}-mediated toxicity is to shift the balance toward Cu^{2+} by oxidizing Cu^{+}. Multicopper oxidases such as CueO in *E. coli* and Fet3 in yeast have recently been shown to possess this activity (121, 124, 133). Multicopper oxidases couple the one-electron oxidation of substrate(s) to full reduction of molecular oxygen to water by employing a functional unit formed by three types of copper binding sites with different spectroscopic and functional properties (132). Type 1 blue copper (T1) is the primary electron acceptor from the substrate, while a trinuclear cluster formed by type 2 copper and binuclear type 3 copper (T2/T3) is the oxygen binding and reduction site.

Many gram-negative and gram-positive bacteria appear to contain homologues of *E. coli* CueO. In gram-negative bacteria, these multicopper oxidases are located in the periplasm. The mechanism of protection from copper-mediated toxicity by CueO was postulated to be the oxidation of cuprous copper. This hypothesis was recently strengthened by the ability of CueO and the related multicopper oxidases, Fet3 from yeast and human ceruloplasmin, to oxidize Cu^{+} to Cu^{2+} (111, 124). Related multicopper oxidases are found not only on the chromosomes of many bacteria but also on plasmids conferring copper resistance in both gram-positive (84) and gram-negative (14, 33) bacteria.

Some gram-negative bacteria, such as *E. coli*, also contain a three- or four-part system that presumably transports Cu^{+} ions from the periplasm across the outer membrane. In *E. coli* the *cus* determinant is induced by copper and both the genetic and phenotypical analyses strongly suggest that the protein encoded by the *cusCFBA* structural genes form a copper-extruding complex (57, 91, 104). This system is particularly important under anaerobic conditions since CueO is not active without oxygen. The *cusCBA* genes are homologous to a family of proton/cation antiporter complexes involved in export of metal ions, xenobiotics, and drugs (described above). CusF is a putative periplasmic copper-binding protein with two potential copper-binding sites, one for Cu^{2+} and one for Cu^{+}. The physiological significance of these two sites is not yet known.

Plasmid-encoded copper resistance

In gram-negative bacteria, plasmid-encoded copper resistance determinants can often be found in environments with exceptionally high levels of copper. Examples include the *pco* determinant on plasmid pRJ1004 in *E. coli* and the *cop* determinant on plasmid pPT23D in *P. syringae* pv. tomato. In all cases, these proteins are involved in elaborate periplasmic copper handling and give additional copper resistance. However, they are dependent on the presence of other copper homeostasis mechanisms, such as a copper-translocating P-type ATPase (81). The copper resistance specified by plasmid pRJ1004 involves the *pco* gene cluster, which contains seven genes, *pcoABCDRSE* (14). Copper resistance in *P. syringae* pv. tomato is specified by the *cop* determinant, which contains six genes, *copABCDRS*, arranged in a single operon, homologous to the equivalent *pco* genes (14, 34, 122). In all cases, copper resistance has been shown to be inducible (88, 116). Our current model for the resistance mechanism of the *pco* determinant is illustrated in Fig. 2. PcoA is the central protein of the *pco* determinant. The *pcoA* gene encodes a 605-amino-acid protein homologous to multicopper oxidases. Periplasmic extract containing PcoA showed copper-inducible oxidase activity (69). In addition, PcoA could functionally substitute for CueO in *E. coli*, indicating they might have a similar function. PcoB is a 296-amino-acid protein that has been predicted to be localized in the outer membrane. In a copper-sensitive *E. coli* strain, *pcoA* and *pcoB* could confer copper resistance at a much lower expression level compared to *pcoA* alone, indicating that they might interact. It is possible that PcoB translocates the prooxidant Cu^{+} across the outer membrane into the periplasm to be immediately oxidized by PcoA. In *P. syringae*, CopA and CopB alone were also able to confer copper resistance and needed CopC and CopD only for maximal resistance. These observations are reflected when looking at genomic sequences. Often, only homologues of PcoA (CopA) and PcoB (CopB) are encoded in a genome, but not PcoC (CopC) and PcoD (CopD). However, in both the Cop and Pco systems, PcoC and PcoD are required for full resistance. In *P. syringae*, studies indicated that CopC and CopD may function together in copper uptake (20). The homologous PcoC and PcoD might have a similar function. PcoC, containing 126 amino acids, was shown to bind one copper atom per molecule and might act as a dimer (69, 81). PcoC might regulate copper uptake by PcoD. PcoD is a 309-amino-acid integral membrane protein with eight putative membrane-spanning domains (77). The *pco* determinant also possesses another gene, *pcoE*, involved in binding of copper in the periplasm. The *pcoE* gene is not part of the *pcoABCD* operon but is located downstream on plasmid pRJ1004. Expression of *pcoE* is regulated by its own copper-regulated promoter and is under the control of the two-component systems PcoRS and CusRS (116). PcoE is required to confer full resistance and is

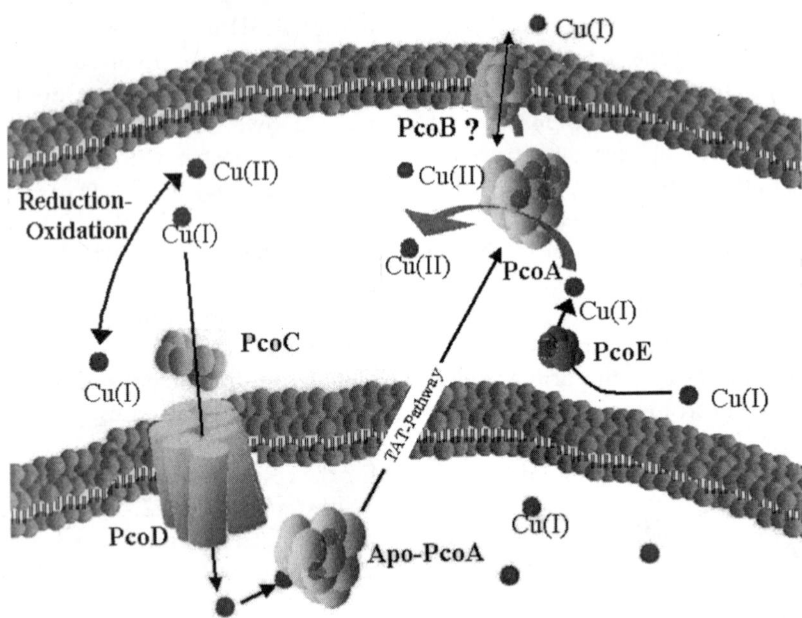

Figure 2. Proposed mechanism of Pco-mediated copper detoxification. The function of the outer membrane protein PcoB has not been elucidated, but it could transport Cu(II) from the periplasm across the outer membrane or transport Cu(I) from the outside to PcoA. Cu(I) could be oxidized to the less toxic Cu(II) by the multicopper oxidase PcoA. In order to load copper into catalytic sites within PcoA, PcoC and PcoD might transport it across the cytoplasmic membrane, with PcoC delivering copper to PcoD. PcoE binds copper in the periplasm and possibly shuttles it to PcoA.

homologous to SilE. In addition to these well-known copper resistance determinants, there are other putative periplasmic copper-binding proteins that are induced under copper stress in various microorganisms. Examples include a putative azurin/rusticyanine-like protein in *Pseudomonas fluorescens* (139).

In gram-positive bacteria there are some recent reports of additional, plasmid-encoded copper resistance. One example is the *lco* operon of *L. lactis* (84). The *lco* operon contains two regulatory genes, *lcoRS*, encoding a two-component system and three structural genes. The *lcoA* gene probably encodes a prolipoprotein diacylglycerol transferase and *lcoC* a multicopper oxidase. The function of *lcoB* is not apparent from the sequence information. Since there is no periplasmic space in gram-positive bacteria, the multicopper oxidase LcoC, involved in copper resistance in the gram-positive bacterium *L. lactis*, has to be anchored to the outer leaflet of the cytoplasmic membrane as a lipoprotein.

Another plasmid-encoded determinant conferring additional copper resistance is the *tcrB* gene in *E. faecium*. The *tcrB* gene encodes a putative Cu(I)-translocating ATPase (64). Interestingly, a putative copper-translocating P-type ATPase and a multicopper oxidase appear to form an operon on the chromosome of *Staphylococcus epidermidis* and other staphylococci.

Bacterial Arsenic Resistance

The most commonly occurring forms of inorganic arsenic in the natural aqueous environment are arsenate, As^{5+}, encountered under aerobic conditions, and the more toxic arsenite, As^{3+}, encountered under anaerobic conditions. The most common arsenic resistance mechanism is arsenite efflux. However, oxidation or methylation of arsenic can also change the mobility and toxicity of this oxyanion. Since very little is known about the molecular aspects of arsenic resistance through oxidation or methylation, the well-characterized *ars* operons, conferring arsenic and antimonite resistance through efflux, will be briefly discussed.

The *ars* operons of gram-negative and gram-positive bacteria are frequently present on both plasmids and chromosomes, and most of these determinants are three-gene *arsRBC* operons (114). The *arsR* gene encodes the As^{3+}- and Sb^{3+}-responsive regulator that acts as a repressor in the absence of these oxyanions. The actual transporter responsible for proton-gradient-dependent extrusion of As^{3+} and Sb^{3+} is encoded by *arsB*. Additional resistance to arsenate As^{5+} is mediated by an arsenate reductase encoded by *arsC*. A few operons contain two additional genes, *arsA* and *arsD*, conferring increased resistance. ArsA is an ATPase that is activated by As^{3+} or Sb^{3+}. ArsA binds to ArsB and converts the arsenite permease into a primary ATP-driven arsenite pump. ArsD is an additional transcriptional repressor, unrelated in primary sequence, but binding to the same regulatory region as ArsR (25). ArsD has been shown to regulate the maximal expression of the ATP-requiring pump, which itself can be toxic to the cell if overexpressed (114). Other operons also contain genes of unknown function such as *arsH*.

RELATIONSHIP BETWEEN COPPER, ZINC, AND ARSENIC RESISTANCE AND ANTIBIOTIC RESISTANCE

An important implication of the selection of metal tolerance among bacteria is that it may contribute to the selection of pathogenic bacteria that are intrinsically resistant to metals or have acquired metal resistance from other organisms. For instance, the establishment of an arsenic-resistant clone of *Y. enterocolitica* among pigs in the United States might have been favored by the use of arsenicals in pig production (96). Also, *E. coli* and especially *Salmonella* seem to be highly resistant to copper (1). The use of copper as a feed supplement to poultry and pigs could therefore shift the bacterial populations toward increased levels of these potential pathogens in the guts of the animals. A more critical issue is the maintenance of antibiotic resistance genes by increasing the selective pressure of the bacterial populations through coselection by metals. This is of particular concern when the resistance determinants are located on transferable elements (e.g., plasmids or transposons), as these are able to accumulate antibiotic resistance genes and have the potential to spread between species (94). Still, resistance levels of pathogens to metals are rarely tested in parallel with resistance to antibiotics. Therefore, it is difficult to estimate the role that metals play in coselecting for antibiotic resistance.

The relationship between copper, zinc, and arsenic resistance and resistance to antibiotics has occasionally been reported in the literature. However, most studies fail to establish a definitive link between a given metal and antibiotic resistance. This requires localization of these resistance phenotypes on the same plasmid, or at least identification of a statistically significant correlation between the metal and antibiotic resistance within a population of the same organism. For instance, several studies have examined the relationship between metal and antibiotic resistance among mixed populations of bacteria isolated from the same geographical site but different habitants. However, these kinds of studies are difficult to evaluate, as it is virtually impossible to determine if the bacterial communities are comparable or not. This is exemplified in a study of unspecified bacterial isolates from drinking water systems of an Oregon coastal community that showed a relationship between tolerances to high levels of copper, lead, and zinc and multiple-antibiotic resistance in isolates from raw water (16). Other studies examined the relationship between metal and antibiotic resistance but often did not compare the result to the metal-susceptible bacterial population. This was the case in two studies from India, which found 73 to 77% of copper-resistant *Salmonella* to be multidrug resistant but did not examine the same relationship for the copper-sensitive isolates (30, 72).

Some studies do establish a direct link between copper, zinc, and arsenic resistance and resistance to antibiotics. In these cases, the metal resistance mechanism has the potential to select for resistance to antibiotics through coselection, when the bacterial host is exposed to selective concentrations of the metal, for instance, copper and streptomycin resistance transferred together in a conjugation study on *P. syringae* pv. syringae. This cotransfer was associated with a single plasmid of either 68, 190, or 220 kbp (134). Here, the streptomycin resistance determinants were identified to be homologous to *strA* and *strB* from the broad-host-range plasmid RSF1010. However, the authors were not able to identify the copper resistance determinant, as Southern blot analysis with the *copABCD* from *P. syringae* pv. tomato, described above, was unsuccessful. Inducible zinc resistance in *P. aeruginosa* (*czcCBA*) has been shown to be associated with carbapenem resistance caused by reduced expression of the porin and the carbapenem transporter *oprD* through the two-component regulator genes *czcR-czcS* (107).

The *E. coli* strain RJ92, carrying the plasmid pRJ1004, from which the *pco* resistance determinant responsible for transferable copper resistance in *E. coli* was first identified, was also resistant to tetracycline and sulfonamides. However, these resistances did not consistently cotransfer with the copper resistance, indicating their localization on a different mobile element than the *pco* genes (140). The *pco* determinant has also been identified on a large 219-kb plasmid, called pLVPK, from *K. pneumoniae* CG4. Even though this plasmid is presumed to be associated with virulence, it does not seem to carry antibiotic resistance genes (28).

The *cadA* gene from *S. aureus*, conferring zinc as well as cadmium resistance, is located on pI258, which also carries the *blaZ* gene, responsible for beta-lactamase resistance in this organism (99, 150). The *arsRBC* genes, conferring resistance to arsenic in

S. aureus, are also located on plasmid pI258, further linking metal and antibiotic resistance in this organism (13). Arsenic resistance (*arsHRBC*) has also been associated with resistance to tetracycline, chloramphenicol, and kanamycin on the IncHI2 plasmid R478 from *Serratia marcescens* (117). Finally, the copper resistance determinant *tcrB* from glycopeptide-resistant *E. faecium* isolated from pigs in Denmark has been associated with resistance to macrolides [*erm*(B)] and vancomycin (*vanA*) (64).

Even though all these studies suggest a possibility for metal-associated coselection of certain pathogens or multiple-antibiotic-resistant bacteria, direct evidence of such a mechanism outside the laboratory is still lacking. However, the existence of a metal-associated coselective mechanism could be a potential threat to human health and should be examined further.

REFERENCES

1. **Aarestrup, F. M., and H. Hasman.** 2004. Susceptibility of different bacterial species isolated from food animals to copper sulphate, zinc chloride and antimicrobial substances used for disinfection. *Vet. Microbiol.* **100:**83–89.
2. **Acar, J. F., and F. W. Goldstein.** 2004. Disc susceptibility test, p. 1–51. *In* V. Lorian (ed.), *Antibiotics in Laboratory Medicine*. Williams & Wilkins, New York, N.Y.
3. **Aguiar, J. M., E. Guzman, and J. L. Martinez.** 1990. Heavy metals, chlorine and antibiotic resistance in *Escherichia coli* isolates from ambulatory patients. *J. Chemother.* **2:**238–240.
4. **Alonso, G., G. Vilchez, I. Bruzual, and V. Rodriguez-Lemoine.** 2002. Characterization of plasmid MIP233 (IncHI3) of the H complex. *Res. Microbiol.* **153:**149–153.
5. **Anton, A., C. Grosse, J. Reissmann, T. Pribyl, and D. H. Nies.** 1999. CzcD is a heavy metal ion transporter involved in regulation of heavy metal resistance in *Ralstonia* sp. strain CH34. *J. Bacteriol.* **181:**6876–6881.
6. **Axelsen, K. B., and M. G. Palmgren.** 1998. Evolution of substrate specificities in the P-type ATPase superfamily. *J. Mol. Evol.* **46:**84–101.
7. **Banci, L., I. Bertini, S. Ciofi-Baffoni, L. Gonnelli, and X. C. Su.** 2003. Structural basis for the function of the N-terminal domain of the ATPase CopA from *Bacillus subtilis*. *J. Biol. Chem.* **278:**50506–50513.
8. **Bayle, D., S. Wangler, T. Weitzenegger, W. Steinhilber, J. Volz, M. Przybylski, K. P. Schafer, G. Sachs, and K. Melchers.** 1998. Properties of the P-type ATPases encoded by the *copAP* operons of *Helicobacter pylori* and *Helicobacter felis*. *J. Bacteriol.* **180:**317–329.
9. **Beard, S. J., R. Hashim, G. Wu, M. R. Binet, M. N. Hughes, and R. K. Poole.** 2000. Evidence for the transport of zinc(II) ions via the pit inorganic phosphate transport system in *Escherichia coli*. *FEMS Microbiol. Lett.* **184:**231–235.
10. **Bender, C. L., and D. A. Cooksey.** 1986. Indigenous plasmids in *Pseudomonas syringae* pv. *tomato*: conjugative transfer and role in copper resistance. *J. Bacteriol.* **165:**534–541.
11. **Blencowe, K. R., and A. P. Morby.** 2003. Zn(II) metabolism in procaryotes. *FEMS Microbiol. Rev.* **27:**291–311.
12. **Brocklehurst, K. R., J. L. Hobman, B. Lawley, L. Blank, S. J. Marshall, N. L. Brown, and A. P. Morby.** 1999. ZntR is a Zn(II)-responsive MerR-like transcriptional regulator of *zntA* in *Escherichia coli*. *Mol. Microbiol.* **31:**893–902.
13. **Broer, S., G. Ji, A. Broer, and S. Silver.** 1993. Arsenic efflux governed by the arsenic resistance determinant of *Staphylococcus aureus* plasmid pI258. *J. Bacteriol.* **175:**3480–3485.
14. **Brown, N. L., S. R. Barrett, J. Camakaris, B. T. Lee, and D. A. Rouch.** 1995. Molecular genetics and transport analysis of the copper-resistance determinant (*pco*) from *Escherichia coli* plasmid pRJ1004. *Mol. Microbiol.* **17:**1153–1166.
15. **Busenlehner, L. S., M. A. Pennella, and D. P. Giedroc.** 2003. The SmtB/ArsR family of metalloregulatory transcriptional repressors: structural insights into prokaryotic metal resistance. *FEMS Microbiol. Rev.* **27:**131–143.
16. **Calomiris, J. J., J. L. Armstrong, and R. J. Seidler.** 1984. Association of metal tolerance with multiple antibiotic resistance of bacteria isolated from drinking water. *Appl. Environ. Microbiol.* **47:**1238–1242.
17. **Campoy, S., M. Jara, N. Busquets, A. M. Perez De Rozas, I. Badiola, and J. Barbe.** 2002. Role of the high-affinity zinc uptake *znuABC* system in *Salmonella enterica* serovar Typhimurium virulence. *Infect. Immun.* **70:**4721–4725.
18. **Carlson, M. S., G. M. Hill, and J. E. Link.** 1999. Early- and traditionally weaned nursery pigs benefit from phase-feeding pharmacological concentrations of zinc oxide: effect on metallothionein and mineral concentrations. *J. Anim. Sci.* **77:**1199–1207.
19. **Cervantes, C., and J. Chavez.** 1992. Plasmid-determined resistance to arsenic and antimony in *Pseudomonas aeruginosa*. *Antonie Leeuwenhoek* **61:**333–337.
20. **Cha, J.-S., and D. A. Cooksey.** 1993. Copper hypersensitivity and uptake in *Pseudomonas syringae* containing cloned components of the copper resistance operon. *Appl. Environ. Microbiol.* **59:**1671–1674.
21. **Changela, A., K. Chen, Y. Xue, J. Holschen, C. E. Outten, T. V. O'Halloran, and A. Mondragon.** 2003. Molecular basis of metal-ion selectivity and zeptomolar sensitivity by CueR. *Science* **301:**1383–1387.
22. **Chao, Y., and D. Fu.** 2004. Kinetic study of the antiport mechanism of an *Escherichia coli* zinc transporter, ZitB. *J. Biol. Chem.* **279:**12043–12050.
23. **Chao, Y., and D. Fu.** 2004. Thermodynamic studies of the mechanism of metal binding to the *Escherichia coli* zinc transporter YiiP. *J. Biol. Chem.* **279:**17173–17180.
24. **Chen, C. Y., and S. A. Morse.** 2001. Identification and characterization of a high-affinity zinc uptake system in *Neisseria gonorrhoeae*. *FEMS Microbiol. Lett.* **202:**67–71.
25. **Chen, Y., and B. P. Rosen.** 1997. Metalloregulatory properties of the ArsD repressor. *J. Biol. Chem.* **272:**14257–14262.
26. **Chen, Y. T., H. Y. Chang, Y. C. Lai, C. C. Pan, S. F. Tsai, and H. L. Peng.** 2004. Sequencing and analysis of the large virulence plasmid pLVPK of *Klebsiella pneumoniae* CG43. *Gene* **337:**189–198.
27. **Cheng, J., E. T. Kornegay, and T. Schell.** 1998. Influence of dietary lysine on the utilization of zinc from zinc sulphate and a zinc-lysine complex by young pigs. *J. Anim. Sci.* **76:**1064–1074.
28. **Choudhury, P., and R. Kumar.** 1998. Multidrug- and metal-resistant strains of *Klebsiella pneumoniae* isolated from Penaeus monodon of the coastal waters of deltaic Sundarban. *Can. J. Microbiol.* **44:**186–189.
29. **Choudhury, R., and S. Srivastava.** 2001. Mutational analysis of zinc resistance in *Pseudomonas putida* strain S4. *Curr. Microbiol.* **43:**316–321.
30. **Ciraj, A. M., M. Mohammed, K. G. Bhat, and P. G. Shivananda.** 1999. Copper resistance & its correlation to multiple drug resistance in *Salmonella typhi* isolates from south Karnataka. *Indian J. Med. Res.* **110:**181–182.

31. **Claverys, J. P.** 2001. A new family of high-affinity ABC manganese and zinc permeases. *Res. Microbiol.* **152:**231–243.
32. **Collard, J. M., A. Provoost, S. Taghavi, and M. Mergeay.** 1993. A new type of *Alcaligenes eutrophus* CH34 zinc resistance generated by mutations affecting regulation of the *cnr* cobalt-nickel resistance system. *J. Bacteriol.* **175:**779–784.
33. **Cooksey, D. A.** 1993. Copper uptake and resistance in bacteria. *Mol. Microbiol.* **7:**1–5.
34. **Cooksey, D. A.** 1994. Molecular mechanisms of copper resistance and accumulation in bacteria. *FEMS Microbiol. Rev.* **14:**381–386.
35. **Cornelis, G. R., A. Boland, A. P. Boyd, C. Geuijen, M. Iriarte, C. Neyt, M. P. Sory, and I. Stainier.** 1998. The virulence plasmid of *Yersinia*, an antihost genome. *Microbiol. Mol. Biol. Rev.* **62:**1315–1352.
36. **Dabbs, E. R., and G. J. Sole.** 1988. Plasmid-borne resistance to arsenate, arsenite, cadmium, and chloramphenicol in a *Rhodococcus* species. *Mol. Gen. Genet.* **211:**148–154.
37. **Datta, N., and V. M. Hughes.** 1983. Plasmids of the same Inc groups in enterobacteria before and after the medical use of antibiotics. *Nature* **306:**616–617.
38. **Dutta, G. N., and L. A. Devriese.** 1981. Sensitivity and resistance to growth promoting agents in animal lactobacilli. *J. Appl. Bacteriol.* **51:**283–288.
39. **Elek, S. D., and L. Higney.** 1970. Resistogram typing—a new epidemiological tool: application to *Escherichia coli*. *J. Med. Microbiol.* **3:**103–110.
40. **Erardi, F. X., M. L. Failla, and J. O. Falkinham III.** 1987. Plasmid-encoded copper resistance and precipitation by *Mycobacterium scrofulaceum*. *Appl. Environ. Microbiol.* **53:** 1951–1954.
41. **European Commission's Scientific Committee for Animal Nutrition (SCAN).** 2003. *Opinion of the Scientific Committee for Animal Nutrition on the Use of Copper in Feedingstuffs*, p. 1–47.
42. **European Commission's Scientific Committee for Animal Nutrition (SCAN).** 2003. *Opinion of the Scientific Committee for Animal Nutrition on the Use of Zinc in Feedingstuffs*, p. 1–33.
43. **Ewing, H. P., G. M. Pesti, R. I. Bakalli, and J. F. Menten.** 1998. Studies on the feeding of cupric sulphate pentahydrate, cupric citrate, and copper oxychloride to broiler chickens. *Poult. Sci.* **77:**445–448.
44. **Fan, B., and B. P. Rosen.** 2002. Biochemical characterization of CopA, the *Escherichia coli* Cu(I)-translocating P-type ATPase. *J. Biol. Chem.* **277:**46987–46992.
45. **Fujihira, E., N. Tamura, and A. Yamaguchi.** 2002. Membrane topology of a multidrug efflux transporter, AcrB, in *Escherichia coli*. *J. Biochem. (Tokyo)* **131:**145–151.
46. **Gaballa, A., and J. D. Helmann.** 1998. Identification of a zinc-specific metalloregulatory protein, Zur, controlling zinc transport operons in *Bacillus subtilis*. *J. Bacteriol.* **180:**5815–5821.
47. **Gaballa, A., T. Wang, R. W. Ye, and J. D. Helmann.** 2002. Functional analysis of the *Bacillus subtilis* Zur regulon. *J. Bacteriol.* **184:**6508–6514.
48. **Gaither, L. A., and D. J. Eide.** 2001. Eukaryotic zinc transporters and their regulation. *Biometals* **14:**251–270.
49. **Gaither, L. A., and D. J. Eide.** 2000. Functional expression of the human hZIP2 zinc transporter. *J. Biol. Chem.* **275:** 5560–5564.
50. **Garcia-Villada, L., M. Rico, M. M. Altamirano, L. Sanchez-Martin, V. Lopez-Rodas, and E. Costas.** 2004. Occurrence of copper resistant mutants in the toxic cyanobacteria *Microcystis aeruginosa*: characterisation and future implications in the use of copper sulphate as algaecide. *Water Res.* **38:**2207–2213.
51. **Garde, S., and C. L. Bender.** 1991. DNA probes for detection of copper resistance genes in *Xanthomonas campestris* pv. *vesicatoria*. *Appl. Environ. Microbiol.* **57:**2435–2439.
52. **Ghosh, S., N. R. Mahapatra, and P. C. Banerjee.** 1997. Metal resistance in *Acidocella* strains and plasmid-mediated transfer of this characteristic to *Acidiphilium multivorum* and *Escherichia coli*. *Appl. Environ. Microbiol.* **63:**4523–4527.
53. **Gilotra, U., and S. Srivastava.** 1997. Plasmid-encoded sequestration of copper by *Pseudomonas pickettii* strain US321. *Curr. Microbiol.* **34:**378–381.
54. **Goldberg, M., T. Pribyl, S. Juhnke, and D. H. Nies.** 1999. Energetics and topology of CzcA, a cation/proton antiporter of the resistance-nodulation-cell division protein family. *J. Biol. Chem.* **274:**26065–26070.
55. **Gotoh, N., T. Kusumi, H. Tsujimoto, T. Wada, and T. Nishino.** 1999. Topological analysis of an RND family transporter, MexD of *Pseudomonas aeruginosa*. *FEBS Lett.* **458:**32–36.
56. **Grass, G., B. Fan, B. P. Rosen, S. Franke, D. H. Nies, and C. Rensing.** 2001. ZitB (YbgR), a member of the cation diffusion facilitator family, is an additional zinc transporter in *Escherichia coli*. *J. Bacteriol.* **183:**4664–4667.
57. **Grass, G., and C. Rensing.** 2001. Genes involved in copper homeostasis in *Escherichia coli*. *J. Bacteriol.* **183:**2145–2147.
58. **Grass, G., M. D. Wong, B. P. Rosen, R. L. Smith, and C. Rensing.** 2002. ZupT is a Zn(II) uptake system in *Escherichia coli*. *J. Bacteriol.* **184:**864–866.
59. **Grosse, C., G. Grass, A. Anton, S. Franke, A. N. Santos, B. Lawley, N. L. Brown, and D. H. Nies.** 1999. Transcriptional organization of the *czc* heavy-metal homeostasis determinant from *Alcaligenes eutrophus*. *J. Bacteriol.* **181:**2385–2393.
60. **Guan, L., M. Ehrmann, H. Yoneyama, and T. Nakae.** 1999. Membrane topology of the xenobiotic-exporting subunit, MexB, of the MexA,B-OprM extrusion pump in *Pseudomonas aeruginosa*. *J. Biol. Chem.* **274:**10517–10522.
61. **Guerinot, M. L.** 2000. The ZIP family of metal transporters. *Biochim. Biophys. Acta* **1465:**190–198.
62. **Guffanti, A. A., Y. Wei, S. V. Rood, and T. A. Krulwich.** 2002. An antiport mechanism for a member of the cation diffusion facilitator family: divalent cations efflux in exchange for K^+ and H^+. *Mol. Microbiol.* **45:**145–153.
63. **Hall, J. L., and L. E. Williams.** 2003. Transition metal transporters in plants. *J. Exp. Bot.* **54:**2601–2613.
64. **Hasman, H., and F. M. Aarestrup.** 2002. *tcrB*, a gene conferring transferable copper resistance in *Enterococcus faecium*: occurrence, transferability, and linkage to macrolide and glycopeptide resistance. *Antimicrob. Agents Chemother.* **46:** 1410–1416.
65. **Hassan, M. T., D. van der Lelie, D. Springael, U. Romling, N. Ahmed, and M. Mergeay.** 1999. Identification of a gene cluster, *czr*, involved in cadmium and zinc resistance in *Pseudomonas aeruginosa*. *Gene* **238:**417–425.
66. **Hedges, R. W., and S. Baumberg.** 1973. Resistance to arsenic compounds conferred by a plasmid transmissible between strains of *Escherichia coli*. *J. Bacteriol.* **115:**459–460.
67. **Hill, G. M., G. L. Cromwell, T. D. Crenshaw, C. R. Dove, R. C. Ewan, D. A. Knabe, A. J. Lewis, G. W. Libal, D. C. Mahan, G. C. Shurson, L. L. Southern, and T. L. Veum.** 2000. Growth promotion effects and plasma changes from feeding high dietary concentrations of zinc and copper to weanling pigs (regional study). *J. Anim. Sci.* **78:**1010–1016.
68. **Hill, G. M., P. K. Ku, E. R. Miller, D. E. Ullrey, T. A. Losty, and B. L. O'Dell.** 1983. A copper deficiency in neonatal pigs induced by a high zinc maternal diet. *J. Nutr.* **113:** 867–872.

69. **Huffman, D. L., J. Huyett, F. W. Outten, P. E. Doan, L. A. Finney, B. M. Hoffman, and T. V. O'Halloran.** 2002. Spectroscopy of Cu(II)-PcoC and the multicopper oxidase function of PcoA, two essential components of *Escherichia coli pco* copper resistance operon. *Biochemistry* **41:**10046–10055.
70. **Hughes, V. M., and N. Datta.** 1983. Conjugative plasmids in bacteria of the "pre-antibiotic" era. *Nature* **302:**725–726.
71. **Jackson, B. P., and P. M. Bertsch.** 2001. Determination of arsenic speciation in poultry wastes by IC-ICP-MS. *Environ. Sci. Technol.* **35:**4868–4873.
72. **Jayasheela, M., P. Kaur, R. Bhatia, P. C. John, and H. Singh.** 1993. Prevalence of copper resistant salmonellae in India. *Indian J. Med. Res.* **97:**60–63.
73. **Jensen-Waern, M., L. Melin, R. Lindberg, A. Johannisson, L. Petersson, and P. Wallgren.** 1998. Dietary zinc oxide in weaned pigs—effects on performance, tissue concentrations, morphology, neutrophil functions and faecal microflora. *Res. Vet. Sci.* **64:**225–231.
74. **Karnachuk, O. V., S. Y. Kurochkina, D. Nicomrat, Y. A. Frank, D. A. Ivasenko, E. A. Phyllipenko, and O. H. Tuovinen.** 2003. Copper resistance in *Desulfovibrio* strain R2. *Antonie Leeuwenhoek* **83:**99–106.
75. **Katouli, M., L. Melin, M. Jensen-Waern, P. Wallgren, and R. Mollby.** 1999. The effect of zinc oxide supplementation on the stability of the intestinal flora with special reference to composition of coliforms in weaned pigs. *J. Appl. Microbiol.* **87:**564–573.
76. **Kaukas, A., M. Hinton, and A. H. Linton.** 1988. The effect of growth-promoting antibiotics on the faecal enterococci of healthy young chickens. *J. Appl. Bacteriol.* **64:**57–64.
77. **Klein, P., M. Kanehisa, and C. DeLisi.** 1985. The detection and classification of membrane-spanning proteins. *Biochim. Biophys. Acta* **815:**468–476.
78. **Koronakis, V., J. Li, E. Koronakis, and K. Stauffer.** 1997. Structure of TolC, the outer membrane component of the bacterial type I efflux system, derived from two-dimensional crystals. *Mol. Microbiol.* **23:**617–626.
79. **Koronakis, V., A. Sharff, E. Koronakis, B. Luisi, and C. Hughes.** 2000. Crystal structure of the bacterial membrane protein TolC central to multidrug efflux and protein export. *Nature* **405:**914–919.
80. **Laddaga, R. A., L. Chu, T. K. Misra, and S. Silver.** 1987. Nucleotide sequence and expression of the mercurial-resistance operon from *Staphylococcus aureus* plasmid pI258. *Proc. Natl. Acad. Sci. USA* **84:**5106–5110.
81. **Lee, S. M., G. Grass, C. Rensing, S. R. Barrett, C. J. Yates, J. V. Stoyanov, and N. L. Brown.** 2002. The Pco proteins are involved in periplasmic copper handling in *Escherichia coli*. *Biochem. Biophys. Res. Commun.* **295:**616–620.
82. **Legatzki, A., G. Grass, A. Anton, C. Rensing, and D. H. Nies.** 2003. Interplay of the Czc system and two P-type ATPases in conferring metal resistance to *Ralstonia metallidurans*. *J. Bacteriol.* **185:**4354–4361.
83. **Lewis, P. K., Jr., W. C. Hoekstra, R. H. Grummer, and P. H. Phillips.** 1956. The effects of certain nutritional factors including calcium, phosphorus and zinc on parakeratosis. *J. Anim. Sci.* **15:**741–751.
84. **Liu, C. Q., P. Charoechai, N. Khunajakr, Y. M. Deng, Widodo, and N. W. Dunn.** 2002. Genetic and transcriptional analysis of a novel plasmid-encoded copper resistance operon from *Lactococcus lactis*. *Gene* **297:**241–247.
85. **Lu, D., B. Boyd, and C. A. Lingwood.** 1997. Identification of the key protein for zinc uptake in *Hemophilus influenzae*. *J. Biol. Chem.* **272:**29033–29038.
86. **Luecke, R. W., J. A. Hoefer, W. G. Brammell, and F. Thorp, Jr.** 1956. Mineral interrelationships in parakeratosis of swine. *J. Anim. Sci.* **15:**247–251.
87. **Mahapatra, N. R., and P. C. Banerjee.** 1996. Extreme tolerance to cadmium and high resistance to copper, nickel and zinc in different *Acidiphilium* strains. *Lett. Appl. Microbiol.* **23:**393–397.
88. **Mellano, M. A., and D. A. Cooksey.** 1988. Nucleotide sequence and organization of copper resistance genes from *Pseudomonas syringae* pv. *tomato*. *J. Bacteriol.* **170:**2879–2883.
89. **Mergeay, M., S. Monchy, T. Vallaeys, V. Auquier, A. Benotmane, P. Bertin, S. Taghavi, J. Dunn, D. van der Lelie, and R. Wattiez.** 2003. *Ralstonia metallidurans*, a bacterium specifically adapted to toxic metals: towards a catalogue of metal-responsive genes. *FEMS Microbiol. Rev.* **27:**385–410.
90. **Mergeay, M., D. Nies, H. G. Schlegel, J. Gerits, P. Charles, and F. Van Gijsegem.** 1985. *Alcaligenes eutrophus* CH34 is a facultative chemolithotroph with plasmid-bound resistance to heavy metals. *J. Bacteriol.* **162:**328–334.
91. **Munson, G. P., D. L. Lam, F. W. Outten, and T. V. O'Halloran.** 2000. Identification of a copper-responsive two-component system on the chromosome of *Escherichia coli* K-12. *J. Bacteriol.* **182:**5864–5871.
92. **Murakami, S., R. Nakashima, E. Yamashita, and A. Yamaguchi.** 2002. Crystal structure of bacterial multidrug efflux transporter AcrB. *Nature* **419:**587–593.
93. **Nakahara, H., T. Ishikawa, Y. Sarai, I. Kondo, H. Kozukue, and S. Silver.** 1977. Linkage of mercury, cadmium, and arsenate and drug resistance in clinical isolates of *Pseudomonas aeruginosa*. *Appl. Environ. Microbiol.* **33:**975–976.
94. **Nandi, S., J. J. Maurer, C. Hofacre, and A. O. Summers.** 2004. Gram-positive bacteria are a major reservoir of class 1 antibiotic resistance integrons in poultry litter. *Proc. Natl. Acad. Sci. USA* **101:**7118–7122.
95. **National Committee for Clinical Laboratory Standards.** 2003. *Methods for Dilution Antimicrobial Susceptibility Tests for Bacteria That Grow Aerobically*. Approved standard M7-A4. National Committee for Clinical Laboratory Standards, Villanova, Pa.
96. **Neyt, C., M. Iriarte, V. H. Thi, and G. R. Cornelis.** 1997. Virulence and arsenic resistance in Yersiniae. *J. Bacteriol.* **179:**612–619.
97. **Nies, D. H.** 2003. Efflux-mediated heavy metal resistance in prokaryotes. *FEMS Microbiol. Rev.* **27:**313–339.
98. **Nieto, J. J., R. Fernandez-Castillo, M. C. Marquez, A. Ventosa, E. Quesada, and F. Ruiz-Berraquero.** 1989. Survey of metal tolerance in moderately halophilic eubacteria. *Appl. Environ. Microbiol.* **55:**2385–2390.
99. **Nucifora, G., L. Chu, T. K. Misra, and S. Silver.** 1989. Cadmium resistance from *Staphylococcus aureus* plasmid pI258 cadA gene results from a cadmium-efflux ATPase. *Proc. Natl. Acad. Sci. USA* **86:**3544–3548.
100. **Odermatt, A., H. Suter, R. Krapf, and M. Solioz.** 1992. An ATPase operon involved in copper resistance by *Enterococcus hirae*. *Ann. N. Y. Acad. Sci.* **671:**484–486.
101. **Odermatt, A., H. Suter, R. Krapf, and M. Solioz.** 1993. Primary structure of two P-type ATPases involved in copper homeostasis in *Enterococcus hirae*. *J. Biol. Chem.* **268:**12775–12779.
102. **Okonkwo, A. C., P. K. Ku, E. R. Miller, K. K. Keahey, and D. E. Ullrey.** 1979. Copper requirement of baby pigs fed purified diets. *J. Nutr.* **109:**939–948.
103. **Outten, C. E., F. W. Outten, and T. V. O'Halloran.** 1999. DNA distortion mechanism for transcriptional activation by

ZntR, a Zn(II)-responsive MerR homologue in *Escherichia coli*. *J. Biol. Chem.* **274**:37517–37524.

104. **Outten, F. W., D. L. Huffman, J. A. Hale, and T. V. O'Halloran.** 2001. The independent *cue* and *cus* systems confer copper tolerance during aerobic and anaerobic growth in *Escherichia coli*. *J. Biol. Chem.* **276**:30670–30677.

105. **Patzer, S. I., and K. Hantke.** 2000. The zinc-responsive regulator Zur and its control of the *znu* gene cluster encoding the ZnuABC zinc uptake system in *Escherichia coli*. *J. Biol. Chem.* **275**:24321–24332.

106. **Patzer, S. I., and K. Hantke.** 1998. The ZnuABC high-affinity zinc uptake system and its regulator Zur in *Escherichia coli*. *Mol. Microbiol.* **28**:1199–1210.

107. **Perron, K., O. Caille, C. Rossier, C. Van Delden, J. L. Dumas, and T. Kohler.** 2004. CzcR-CzcS, a two-component system involved in heavy metal and carbapenem resistance in *Pseudomonas aeruginosa*. *J. Biol. Chem.* **279**:8761–8768.

108. **Pesti, G. M., and R. I. Bakalli.** 1996. Studies on the feeding of cupric sulphate pentahydrate and cupric citrate to broiler chickens. *Poult. Sci.* **75**:1086–1091.

109. **Rensing, C., B. Fan, R. Sharma, B. Mitra, and B. P. Rosen.** 2000. CopA: an *Escherichia coli* Cu(I)-translocating P-type ATPase. *Proc. Natl. Acad. Sci. USA* **97**:652–656.

110. **Rensing, C., M. Ghosh, and B. P. Rosen.** 1999. Families of soft-metal-ion-transporting ATPases. *J. Bacteriol.* **181**:5891–5897.

111. **Rensing, C., and G. Grass.** 2003. *Escherichia coli* mechanisms of copper homeostasis in a changing environment. *FEMS Microbiol. Rev.* **27**:197–213.

112. **Rensing, C., B. Mitra, and B. P. Rosen.** 1997. The *zntA* gene of *Escherichia coli* encodes a Zn(II)-translocating P-type ATPase. *Proc. Natl. Acad. Sci. USA* **94**:14326–14331.

113. **Rensing, C., Y. Sun, B. Mitra, and B. P. Rosen.** 1998. Pb(II)-translocating P-type ATPases. *J. Biol. Chem.* **273**:32614–32617.

114. **Rosen, B. P.** 1999. Families of arsenic transporters. *Trends Microbiol.* **7**:207–212.

115. **Rosen, B. P., and M. G. Borbolla.** 1984. A plasmid-encoded arsenite pump produces arsenite resistance in *Escherichia coli*. *Biochem. Biophys. Res. Commun.* **124**:760–765.

116. **Rouch, D. A., and N. L. Brown.** 1997. Copper-inducible transcriptional regulation at two promoters in the *Escherichia coli* copper resistance determinant *pco*. *Microbiology* **143**:1191–1202.

117. **Ryan, D., and E. Colleran.** 2002. Arsenical resistance in the IncHI2 plasmids. *Plasmid* **47**:234–240.

118. **Shakoori, A. R., and B. Muneer.** 2002. Copper-resistant bacteria from industrial effluents and their role in remediation of heavy metals in wastewater. *Folia Microbiol. (Praha)* **47**:43–50.

119. **Shanklin, S. H., E. R. Miller, D. E. Ullrey, J. A. Hoefer, and R. W. Luecke.** 1968. Zinc requirements of baby pigs on casein diets. *J. Nutr.* **96**:101–108.

120. **Sharma, R., C. Rensing, B. P. Rosen, and B. Mitra.** 2000. The ATP hydrolytic activity of purified ZntA, a Pb(II)/Cd(II)/Zn(II)-translocating ATPase from *Escherichia coli*. *J. Biol. Chem.* **275**:3873–3878.

121. **Shi, X., C. Stoj, A. Romeo, D. J. Kosman, and Z. Zhu.** 2003. Frelp Cu^{2+} reduction and Fet3p Cu^{1+} oxidation modulate copper toxicity in *Saccharomyces cerevisiae*. *J. Biol. Chem.* **278**:50309–50315.

122. **Silver, S., and L. T. Phung.** 1996. Bacterial heavy metal resistance: new surprises. *Annu. Rev. Microbiol.* **50**: 753–789.

123. **Silver, S., K. Budd, K. M. Leahy, W. V. Shaw, D. Hammond, R. P. Novick, G. R. Willsky, M. H. Malamy, and H. Rosenberg.** 1981. Inducible plasmid-determined resistance to arsenate, arsenite, and antimony (III) in *Escherichia coli* and *Staphylococcus aureus*. *J. Bacteriol.* **146**:983–996.

124. **Singh, S. K., G. Grass, C. Rensing, and W. R. Montfort.** 2004. Cuprous oxidase activity of CueO from *Escherichia coli*. *J. Bacteriol.* **186**:7815–7817.

125. **Singh, V. K., A. Xiong, T. R. Usgaard, S. Chakrabarti, R. Deora, T. K. Misra, and R. K. Jayaswal.** 1999. ZntR is an autoregulatory protein and negatively regulates the chromosomal zinc resistance operon *znt* of *Staphylococcus aureus*. *Mol. Microbiol.* **33**:200–207.

126. **Skrivan, M., V. Skrivanova, M. Marounek, E. Tumova, and J. Wolf.** 2000. Influence of dietary fat source and copper supplementation on broiler performance, fatty acid profile of meat and depot fat, and on cholesterol content in meat. *Br. Poult. Sci.* **41**:608–614.

127. **Smith, J. W., M. D. Tokach, R. D. Goodband, J. L. Nelssen, and B. T. Richert.** 1997. Effects of the interrelationship between zinc oxide and copper sulphate on growth performance of early-weaned pigs. *J. Anim. Sci.* **75**:1861–1866.

128. **Smith, R. L., L. J. Thompson, and M. E. Maguire.** 1995. Cloning and characterization of MgtE, a putative new class of Mg^{2+} transporter from *Bacillus firmus* OF4. *J. Bacteriol.* **177**:1233–1238.

129. **Smith, W. H., M. P. Plumlee, and W. M. Beeson.** 1962. Effect of source of protein on zinc requirement of the growing pig. *J. Anim. Sci.* **21**:399–405.

130. **Snavely, M. D., J. B. Florer, C. G. Miller, and M. E. Maguire.** 1989. Magnesium transport in *Salmonella typhimurium*: $28Mg^{2+}$ transport by the CorA, MgtA, and MgtB systems. *J. Bacteriol.* **171**:4761–4766.

131. **Solioz, M., and C. Vulpe.** 1996. CPx-type ATPases: a class of P-type ATPases that pump heavy metals. *Trends Biochem. Sci.* **21**:237–241.

132. **Solomon, E. I., U. M. Sundaram, and T. E. Machonkin.** 1996. Multicopper oxidases and oxygenases. *Chem. Rev.* **96**:2563–2606.

133. **Stoj, C., and D. J. Kosman.** 2003. Cuprous oxidase activity of yeast Fet3p and human ceruloplasmin: implication for function. *FEBS Lett.* **554**:422–426.

134. **Sundin, G. W., and C. L. Bender.** 1993. Ecological and genetic analysis of copper and streptomycin resistance in *Pseudomonas syringae* pv. syringae. *Appl. Environ. Microbiol.* **59**:1018–1024.

135. **Suzuki, K., N. Wakao, Y. Sakurai, T. Kimura, K. Sakka, and K. Ohmiya.** 1997. Transformation of *Escherichia coli* with a large plasmid of *Acidiphilium multivorum* AIU 301 encoding arsenic resistance. *Appl. Environ. Microbiol.* **63**:2089–2091.

136. **Szybalski, W., and V. Bryson.** 1952. Genetic studies on microbial cross resistance to toxic agents. I. Cross resistance of *Escherichia coli* to fifteen antibiotics. *J. Bacteriol.* **64**:489–499.

137. **Tamas, I., L. Klasson, B. Canback, A. K. Naslund, A. S. Eriksson, J. J. Wernegreen, J. P. Sandstrom, N. A. Moran, and S. G. Andersson.** 2002. 50 million years of genomic stasis in endosymbiotic bacteria. *Science* **296**:2376–2379.

138. **Tetaz, T. J., and R. K. Luke.** 1983. Plasmid-controlled resistance to copper in *Escherichia coli*. *J. Bacteriol.* **154**:1263–1268.

139. **Tom-Petersen, A., C. Hosbond, and O. Nybroe.** 2001. Identification of copper-induced genes in *Pseudomonas fluorescens* and use of a reporter strain to monitor bioavailable copper in soil. *FEMS Microbiol. Ecol.* **38**:59–67.

140. **Top, E., M. Mergeay, D. Springael, and W. Verstraete.** 1990. Gene escape model: transfer of heavy metal resistance genes from *Escherichia coli* to *Alcaligenes eutrophus* on agar plates and in soil samples. *Appl. Environ. Microbiol.* 56:2471–2479.

141. **Tsai, K. J., Y. F. Lin, M. D. Wong, H. H. Yang, H. L. Fu, and B. P. Rosen.** 2002. Membrane topology of the p1258 CadA Cd(II)/Pb(II)/Zn(II)-translocating P-type ATPase. *J. Bioenerg. Biomembr.* **34**:147–156.

142. **Tsai, K. J., and A. L. Linet.** 1993. Formation of a phosphorylated enzyme intermediate by the *cadA* Cd^{2+}-ATPase. *Arch. Biochem. Biophys.* **305**:267–270.

143. **Tsai, K. J., K. P. Yoon, and A. R. Lynn.** 1992. ATP-dependent cadmium transport by the *cadA* cadmium resistance determinant in everted membrane vesicles of *Bacillus subtilis*. *J. Bacteriol.* **174**:116–121.

144. **Tynecka, Z., and Z. Gos.** 1974. Cadmium resistance of *Staphylococcus aureus* determined by penicillinase plasmids. *Ann. Univ. Mariae Curie Sklodowska* **29**:17–26.

145. **Tynecka, Z., and W. Zylinska.** 1974. Plasmid borne resistance to some inorganic ions in *Staphylococcus aureus*. *Acta Microbiol. Pol. A* **6**:83–92.

146. **Tynecka, Z., Z. Gos, and J. Zajac.** 1981. Energy-dependent efflux of cadmium coded by a plasmid resistance determinant in *Staphylococcus aureus*. *J. Bacteriol.* **147**:313–319.

147. **Ug, A., and O. Ceylan.** 2003. Occurrence of resistance to antibiotics, metals, and plasmids in clinical strains of *Staphylococcus* spp. *Arch. Med. Res.* **34**:130–136.

148. **van Ham, R. C., J. Kamerbeek, C. Palacios, C. Rausell, F. Abascal, U. Bastolla, J. M. Fernandez, L. Jimenez, M. Postigo, F. J. Silva, J. Tamames, E. Viguera, A. Latorre, A. Valencia, F. Moran, and A. Moya.** 2003. Reductive genome evolution in *Buchnera aphidicola*. *Proc. Natl. Acad. Sci. USA* **100**:581–586.

149. **Walia, S. K., D. R. Arora, T. D. Chugh, and K. B. Sharma.** 1986. Plasmid linked mercury & zinc resistance in *Klebsiella pneumoniae*. *Indian J. Med. Res.* **83**:369–373.

150. **Wang, P. Z., and R. P. Novick.** 1987. Nucleotide sequence and expression of the beta-lactamase gene from *Staphylococcus aureus* plasmid pI258 in *Escherichia coli*, *Bacillus subtilis*, and *Staphylococcus aureus*. *J. Bacteriol.* **169**: 1763–1766.

151. **Wedekind, K. J., A. J. Lewis, M. A. Giesemann, and P. S. Miller.** 1994. Bioavailability of zinc from inorganic and organic sources for pigs fed corn-soybean meal diets. *J. Anim. Sci.* **72**:2681–2689.

152. **Williams, J. R., A. G. Morgan, D. A. Rouch, N. L. Brown, and B. T. Lee.** 1993. Copper-resistant enteric bacteria from United Kingdom and Australian piggeries. *Appl. Environ. Microbiol.* **59**:2531–2537.

153. **Worlock, A. J., and R. L. Smith.** 2002. ZntB is a novel Zn^{2+} transporter in *Salmonella enterica* serovar Typhimurium. *J. Bacteriol.* **184**:4369–4373.

154. **Xiong, A., and R. K. Jayaswal.** 1998. Molecular characterization of a chromosomal determinant conferring resistance to zinc and cobalt ions in *Staphylococcus aureus*. *J. Bacteriol.* **180**:4024–4029.

155. **Yoon, K. P., and S. Silver.** 1991. A second gene in the *Staphylococcus aureus cadA* cadmium resistance determinant of plasmid pI258. *J. Bacteriol.* **173**:7636–7642.

Antimicrobial Resistance in Bacteria of Animal Origin
Edited by Frank M. Aarestrup

Chapter 8

Disinfectant Resistance in Bacteria

Mark A. Webber, Martin J. Woodward, and Laura J. V. Piddock

Effective hygiene is crucial to preventing the spread of infectious diseases (1, 19, 63); this often involves measures to eradicate pathogens from a particular environment (64). Disinfectants are diverse compounds used for eradication or inhibition of microorganisms in a wide range of applications (27). Perhaps the earliest formal study of disinfection was Pringle's work on the inhibition of putrefaction in the mid-18th century. Later studies by Bucholtz, Baxter, Lister, and then Koch established methods to determine the "germicidal" properties of substances and their application. Today, disinfectants are widely used in all areas of life. Animal production requires disinfectants to prevent outbreaks of disease on farms as well as to prevent contamination of produce with potential pathogens during food processing (7, 59). In human medicine, applications include decolonization of the skin, decontamination of surgical instruments, and eradication of microorganisms from surfaces to prevent transmission (63, 64). Disinfectants are also used increasingly in the home environment to improve hygiene as well as being incorporated into many different commercially available products, which are consequently advertised as being antimicrobial (32). Recently, concern has been voiced about the possible consequences of increased disinfectant use, in particular, the potential for inappropriate use of disinfectants to select for bacteria with reduced susceptibilities to disinfectants and possible cross-resistance to therapeutically important antibiotics (28, 31, 60).

WHY DO WE USE DISINFECTANTS?

Disinfection in Livestock Production

Disinfectants are used extensively in animal husbandry to prevent infection of livestock, to control outbreaks of disease, and to clean animal houses during periods of inactivity (22, 59, 66, 75). Strategies to prevent disease on the farm and prevent transmission of bacteria and other microorganisms from one animal house to another commonly limit the movement of vehicles and people onto the farm and include the use of disinfectants to spray vehicles on entry and exit, as well as providing disinfectant foot dips outside animal houses and in anterooms. Decontamination of animal houses is complicated by the large amounts of organic material present (feces, urine, litter, etc.); extensive cleaning is required to remove this material before disinfection, as the presence of organic material can greatly reduce the efficacy of some disinfectants (including quaternary ammonium compounds [QACs], iodophors, peracetic acid, and hydrogen peroxide). Recent legislation in the European Union on the removal from use of certain antibiotics, and the consequent sensitivity in the farming industry toward a general reduction of antibiotic use in animal husbandry, has prompted the wider use of alternative measures to protect animals from infections. Additionally, the heightened awareness, particularly in Western nations, of food-borne infections of humans has stimulated renewed interest in intervention strategies such as pre-, pro- and synbiotics, vaccines, and physicochemical controls to provide improved biosecurity of food-producing animals on farms. Cleansing and disinfection regimens are considered important and are used widely as part of biosecurity measures. Failure to clean properly prior to disinfection, infrequent changing of disinfectants in foot dips, or dilution of disinfectants by rainfall can all lead to situations where the activity of the disinfectant is lost (59).

Davies and Wray (21) showed that commonly used cleansing and disinfection regimens are not uniformly successful in eliminating *Salmonella* from

Mark A. Webber and Laura J. V. Piddock • Antimicrobial Agents Research Group, Division of Immunity and Infection, University of Birmingham, Edgbaston, Birmingham B15 2TT, United Kingdom. **Martin J. Woodward** • Department of Food and Environmental Safety, Veterinary Laboratories Agency (Weybridge), New Haw, Addlestone, Surrey KT15 3NB, United Kingdom.

contaminated farm premises. In their study, 20 *Salmonella enterica* serotype Enteritidis-infected poultry farms (broiler, breeder, and layer) were assessed for persistence of this serotype after disinfection. On all premises three phases of cleansing were used that included a prewash (with detergent, QAC, or water), spray (with tar oil mixture, peroxides, phenolics, or formaldehyde), and fogging (with peroxides and formaldehyde). Of the farms examined, about two-thirds used contract cleaners. Bacteriological examination was performed on between 79 and 300 samples collected immediately after cleansing and disinfection. Only four farms achieved complete clearance of *Salmonella*; for two farms, up to 36% of samples were still positive for these bacteria, indicating minimal reduction of contamination. This study concluded that of the many widely used disinfectants, formaldehyde application was associated with the greatest reductions in contamination but highest risk to the operatives. There were many factors that militated against efficacy, such as the presence of rodents that enabled rapid reinfection of a cleaned area, operator error in the administration or dilution of the disinfectant, and the type of cleansing and the disinfecting regimen used. Disinfectants are also used in veterinary medicine when animals require surgical operations; disinfectants are used as antiseptics for the prevention and treatment of skin infections (11).

Disinfectant Use in Hospitals

Use of disinfectants in human medicine (in hospitals) is crucial in the prevention of hospital-acquired infections (19, 63). There are many risk factors for infection in hospitals; patients may be unusually susceptible to infection by being immunocompromised or may have invasive devices that provide an unnatural route of entry for a pathogen. Spread of bacteria within the hospital environment is facilitated by the movement of medical personnel, patients, and visitors, and pathogenic bacteria encountered within the hospital may be multiply resistant to antibiotics. Consequently, the use of disinfectants to reduce transmission and prevent infection is important. In 1968 Spaulding classified different hospital areas and instruments into three classes with differing disinfection requirements: critical, semicritical, and noncritical. Critical items are those which will be in direct contact with sterile parts of the body, where the risk of infection is high. These include surgical instruments, implants, indwelling devices, and intimate probes. These items require sterilization, and as such, chemical disinfection is only used for heat-sensitive, repeat-use instruments where glutaraldehyde, hydrogen peroxide, or peracetic acid can be used (63). Semicritical items are those which come into contact with mucous membranes or damaged skin; these require high-level disinfection to remove all viable bacteria. Noncritical items are those that may have contact with intact skin; these include furniture, blood pressure cuffs, floors and walls, etc. Current opinion assesses the risk of transmission from such items to be low, so their disinfection is not treated with the same urgency as for more high-risk items. The role of the environment in perpetuating infections has recently come under more scrutiny, and some studies have shown extensive environmental cleaning using disinfectants to be necessary for the eradication of *Acinetobacter* and *Staphylococcus aureus* strains that cause outbreaks (24, 29, 55).

Home Hygiene

Many cases of food poisoning originate from inadequately cooked food in the home; especially common are cases caused by *S. enterica* and *Campylobacter* bacteria, which commonly contaminate poultry (35, 77). It has been shown that use of a disinfectant (5,000 ppm of hypochlorite) as part of a kitchen cleaning regimen can greatly assist in reducing the risks of cross-contamination with infected meat (9). There has been a great increase in the incorporation of antimicrobial products into a variety of household products (32), including hand washes, cutting boards, shower gels, and toothpaste. Many of these products contain triclosan. Whilst good home hygiene is clearly desirable, the extra value of this bombardment of antimicrobial products is questionable—thorough cleaning of surfaces and utensils allied with adequate cooking of food should prove sufficient to prevent infection.

Use of Disinfectants in the Food Industry

Disinfectants are widely used in the food industry to prevent contamination of foodstuffs during processing. Any surface, utensil, or container that may come into contact with food is likely to be subjected to disinfection. This disinfection is crucial to preventing cross-contamination between different foodstuffs. Particularly important in the food industry is the inactivation of bacteria attached to surfaces and at low temperatures, both conditions where bacterial tolerance to disinfectants can be enhanced (34, 74). In some circumstances in the food industry, disinfectants may be applied continuously (e.g., to conveyor belts) or left on surfaces without rinsing, both practices which can result in exposure of bacteria to sublethal concentrations of disinfectants (74).

FACTORS AFFECTING THE CHOICE OF A DISINFECTANT

Different disinfectants have different properties (Table 1), which dictate their suitability for a particular purpose (27). Generally, disinfectants inhibit or kill a wide range of bacteria (39). Laboratory tests to determine the efficacy of a disinfectant are performed on planktonic cells in suspension or against bacteria attached to a surface (carrier tests). Other factors to consider when choosing a disinfectant include safety; certain disinfectants can have irritant effects or can be toxic following exposure to high concentrations. Some materials to be treated can be adversely affected by disinfectants; for instance, chlorine-containing compounds cannot not be used on metal due to their corrosive effect. Disposal of disinfectants into the environment is also an issue. Therefore, the final concentrations to be released into the water system need to be calculated and any adverse environmental impacts, including potential toxicity to wildlife, determined. Cost is also a consideration in choosing a disinfectant.

Whilst there are many factors that influence the efficacy of disinfectants, some are particularly pertinent. Disinfectants are nonselective antimicrobials that act following single-step kinetics. Thus, the exposure of the organisms to the disinfectant for an appropriate time and effective concentration is of prime importance. Disinfectants are only active when in contact and many need to accumulate within an organism; therefore, the state and number of the organisms present are significant factors. Some disinfectants, notably chlorine-releasing agents and QACs, are largely inactivated by binding to organic materials, e.g., blood, urine, or feces (59). Therefore, the complexity of the environment to be treated, be it a farmyard, animal pen, abattoir, hospital floor, or kitchen table, will have a significant influence on efficacy due to organic matter content. Another issue is the innate resistance susceptibility of the specific organism to be treated. Recent studies have indicated that there are intrinsic differences in the susceptibility of *Salmonella* strains to disinfectants (48, 66, 76). Ramesh and others (54) showed that five different serovars of *S. enterica* that

Table 1. Classes of disinfectant and their advantages, disadvantages, and applications

Class	Mechanism of action	Advantages	Disadvantages	Applications
Alcohols	Denature proteins	Broad spectrum, rapid action, quick to dry	Flammable	Skin cleansing, hand washes, environmental cleaning
Aldehydes (formaldehyde, glutaraldehyde)	Interact with proteins and nucleic acids	Broad spectrum of activity, cheap	Toxic to humans, limited shelf life (glutaraldehyde), slow killing	Fumigation, fogging; used less than in the past due to toxicity. Instrument cleansing.
Chlorhexidine (bisguanidine)	Damages membrane	Persistent residual activity	Not sporicidal	Popular hand wash and skin antiseptic
Chlorine-releasing agents (hypochlorite, etc.)	Hypochlorous acid denatures proteins	Broad activity spectrum	Corrosive to metals, bind well to organic material so unsuitable on "dirty" surfaces	Surface and environmental cleaning, foot dips, animal house cleaning
Hydrogen peroxide	Produces radicals, denatures cell wall and enzymes		Unstable, irritant	Farm foot dips, vehicle disinfectants
Iodine-releasing agents (iodophors, povidone iodine)	Disrupt DNA and protein synthesis		Not sporicidal	Hand washes, skin antiseptics, vehicle disinfectants
Peracetic acid	Strong oxidizing agent	Rapid action	Corrosive to brass and copper	Vehicle disinfectants, foot dips, instrument cleaning
Phenolics (carbolic acid derivatives)	Inhibit enzyme activity		Toxic, not sporicidal or virucidal, *mar* inducer?	Farm foot dips
QACs		Good antibacterial action	Easily inactivated by organic materials and resistance mechanisms	Farm foot dips, animal house cleaning, domestic products
Triclosan	Inhibits fatty acid biosynthesis and others?	Very safe, rapid killing, cheap	Potential to select resistance? Inactivated by soap.	Hand washes, environmental cleaning, domestic products

readily formed biofilms on simulated poultry and egg carriage trays were significantly less sensitive when treated with 13 commercially available disinfectants. The ultrastructural detail of the biofilm identified "fibrils" and exopolysaccharide as two factors that contributed to reducing the penetration of the disinfectants. Given these factors, there is obvious potential for sublethal doses of disinfectant being administered.

CLASSES OF COMMONLY USED DISINFECTANTS

Many compounds have disinfectant properties; these agents include inorganic acids and alkalis, as well as salts and fatty acids that are incorporated in soaps. Several nonchemical methods are also used to kill bacteria, including treatment with UV light, ozone, or exposure to heat. These are not considered in this section.

Alcohols

Alcohols are commonly used in hand washes (50) and to clean certain instruments and surfaces. They have a rapid killing effect against a broad spectrum of microorganisms, including bacteria, viruses, and fungi. As alcohols are volatile, they dry quickly; this has made them especially suitable for use in hand washes and gels where frequent hand cleansing is necessary, e.g., in hospitals, where staff may move frequently from patient to patient. The alcohols most commonly used as disinfectants are ethyl alcohol and isopropyl alcohol at formulations of between 60 and 90% (vol/vol). Benzyl alcohol has also been used as a teat sanitizer to prevent mastitis in cows but is not as active as iodophors (25). The main disadvantage of alcohols is their flammability, which is an issue in locations where they may be likely to pool (for example, on an uneven surface such as a rough floor in an animal house), thus creating a fire risk.

Aldehydes

Aldehydes kill a broad range of microorganisms by altering host proteins and nucleic acids. The most commonly used agents are formaldehyde and glutaraldehyde. Formaldehyde is used to decontaminate rooms by fumigation, particularly where there is a high microbial load. Toxicity concerns have led to a fall in its use in recent years. Glutaraldehyde is less active than formaldehyde and is used as an instrument disinfectant for semicritical items (27). Aldehydes are used in agriculture as fumigants in fogging of animal houses postproduction (normally formaldehyde) (20) and as vehicle disinfectants (glutaraldehyde) (23).

Chlorhexidine

Chlorhexidine is used to disinfect the skin of animals before surgery, to treat skin infections, and to prevent mastitis in cows (13, 18, 46, 51). Chlorhexidine is also commonly used in human medicine as a skin disinfectant in hand washes and in preparing skin for surgery (6, 27). Chlorhexidine damages bacterial cell membranes, leading to cell death, and is notable for its residual activity, making it an attractive option as a surgical scrub. Chlorhexidine is antibacterial and antiviral but is not sporicidal.

Halogenated Compounds

These compounds act by releasing free chlorine, forming hypochlorous acid, and are rapidly active against a broad range of microorganisms. They are commonly used surface cleaners but are readily inactivated by organic material and should not be used in a "dirty" environment. Halogenated compounds have been used as teat antiseptics (14). They are also corrosive to metals and should not be used on many instruments.

Peroxygen Compounds

Release of free radicals accounts for the activity of hydrogen peroxide, which has a broad spectrum of antibacterial, antiviral, and fungicidal activity. Hydrogen peroxide is often used in combination with peracetic acid on farms for house cleaning and in foot dips (66). Concerns about toxicity to humans limit the use of this compound. Peracetic acid is widely used, as it has good antibacterial activity and acts rapidly due to its strong action as an oxidizing agent (36). Uses include decontamination of equipment and surfaces, although it is not suitable for use on some instruments due to its corrosive nature against brass and copper. Peracetic acid is commonly included in foot dips and as a vehicle disinfectant on farms, often in combination with hydrogen peroxide (e.g., Sorgene). Peracetic acid-producing compounds (such as Virkon) have increasingly been used instead of formaldehyde in animal house cleaning due to lower toxicity and faster turnaround times (30).

Iodophors

Iodine-releasing agents generate free iodine, which exhibits an antimicrobial effect; povidone iodine is commonly used as a skin disinfectant in hospitals prior to surgery. Iodophors have good antibacterial activity, but chlorhexidine is often considered a superior skin antiseptic. Iodophors are commonly used to prevent mastitis as the active ingredient in various teat dips (14, 46). They are also used in foot dips and as vehicle disinfectants on farms, although they are not stable and are inactivated by organic material (T. J. Humphrey, personal communication).

Phenolic Compounds

Phenolic compounds are halogenated derivatives of carbolic acid (made famous by Lister's observations of its antiseptic activity). They have good antibacterial activity but are poorly virucidal, which compromises their utility, as empirical use of disinfectants requires antiviral activity (27). Phenolics are also toxic and can prove to be irritants but are used in foot dips on farms.

QACs

QACs have good antibacterial activity at low concentrations and are cheap to use (40). Many QACs (benzalkonium chloride, for example) display poor activity against viruses and mycobacteria and are easily inactivated by organic materials (blood, serum, feces, etc.) and certain diluents (27), making them unsuitable for applications where organic material may be present (in animal houses, where feces may be present, or in slaughterhouses, where body fluids may be present). QACs are commonly incorporated in products sold for domestic use as adjuncts due to their surfactant activity (40), which enables them to lyse cells and induce cell death.

Triclosan

Triclosan is a broad-spectrum antimicrobial that has been in widespread use since the 1960s. It is used as a skin decontaminant, as a hand wash, in toothpaste, and in a very large array (>700) of other domestic products marketed as being antimicrobial (67). As triclosan is heat stable, it is often incorporated into plastics. Triclosan was historically thought to have multiple mechanisms of antimicrobial action, depending on concentration, but a defined biochemical target, FabI, involved in fatty acid biosynthesis has been described in *Escherichia coli* (42, 70).

MECHANISMS OF ACTION AND RESISTANCE

Constraints that often govern the use of antibiotics do not necessarily apply to the use of disinfectants; concentrations of disinfectants used are typically much higher than those possible for antibiotics (61). At recommended usage concentrations, disinfectants are thought to attack several targets at once, so it is hypothesized that resistance to disinfectants is difficult to achieve. However, bacteria with increased tolerance to disinfectants have been observed and selected in the laboratory (15, 17, 33, 42, 44, 58, 73). Even when not sufficient to allow a bacterium to survive treatment with an in-use concentration, it is conceivable that this may allow it to survive when the active concentration of disinfectant is reduced by dilution, inactivation by organic materials, or inadequate application over the target area. Concerns about possible antibiotic and disinfectant cross-resistance are discussed in "Potential for Selection of Resistant Strains" below.

Methods to Determine Disinfectant Activity

Methods for determining the efficacy of disinfectants differ from those used to analyze antibiotic activity. For disinfectants the D-value is a key parameter—the time taken to reduce a population of indicator organisms by 90%. This property is more relevant than the MIC, as the D-value gives practical information on contact times required at a specific concentration to achieve the desired reduction in microbial load (39). Laboratory tests to determine the efficacy of a disinfectant generally measure activity against an indicator organism(s) in suspension or attached to a surface (carrier test). Standard European suspension tests require a disinfectant to demonstrate a 5-log reduction of bacteria under the test conditions to illustrate efficacy. Carrier tests are particularly useful, as bacteria attached to a surface are commonly less susceptible to disinfectants than those in suspension, often after formation of a biofilm (38). Biofilms are less susceptible to antibiotics and detergents (41, 53), and this is thought to be due to physical properties of the biofilm itself as well as changes to the phenotype of the individual bacteria that constitute the biofilm. Cells at the surface of a biofilm are likely to be exposed to higher concentrations of disinfectant than those protected at its center. Similarly, there will be a concentration gradient of oxygen and nutrients, which will affect the physiology of the cells. Individual cells will be in different stages of growth, and biofilm cells tend to excrete large amounts of extracellular material, which further reduces permeability of the biofilm (32).

Mechanisms of Resistance to Disinfectants

Isolates with decreased susceptibility to various biocides have been described for a number of bacterial species, including *Pseudomonas* spp., staphylococci, *E. coli*, *S. enterica*, *Campylobacter* spp., and *Listeria monocytogenes* (8, 16, 56, 57, 71). Strains of *E. coli* and *S. aureus* with mutations within genes encoding target proteins have been described, notably with resistance to triclosan (mutations within *fabI*), but this mechanism appears to be uncommon for disinfectants, perhaps because these agents are thought to attack multiple targets, thereby necessitating mutations in several genes for resistance (32, 53). For some disinfectants development of resistance has not been observed; these compounds include ethanol and hydrogen peroxide.

Resistance mechanisms that affect the ability of the disinfectant to permeate the cell have been described (53). Gram-negative bacteria are generally less susceptible to disinfectants than gram-positive bacteria, presumably due to the reduced permeability of the double membrane. Mutants which exhibit changes to their cell membranes that reduce permeability and/or display enhanced efflux activity can be less susceptible to disinfectants. Disinfectant susceptibility can be determined by mobile genetic elements or by mutation of chromosomal genes (53).

Target site alterations

Mutants of various bacterial species (*S. enterica* serovar Typhimurium, *E. coli*, and *S. aureus*) with reduced susceptibility to triclosan can be selected in vitro after exposure to sublethal (0.2 to 2 times the MIC) concentrations of the compound (15, 16, 42, 58). McMurry et al. (42) demonstrated that mutant *E. coli* with reduced susceptibility to triclosan (approximately 3- to 12-fold increases in triclosan MIC, to 2.4 to 9.6 μg/ml) had missense mutations within *fabI*, conferring substitutions of Gly-93 to Val, Met-159 to Thr, or Phe-203 to Leu. FabI encodes enoyl-acyl carrier protein (ACP) reductase, an enzyme involved in fatty acid biosynthesis. The levels of triclosan resistance conferred by *fabI* mutations (MICs of 1 to 64 μg/ml) are well below the concentrations used in practice (variable, but between 2,000 and 20,000 μg/ml). It should be noted that a recent report described in vitro selection of a highly resistant (triclosan MIC of >1,024 μg/ml) mutant *E. coli* O157 (15), although the genetic mechanism underlying this phenotype was not defined. This paper also demonstrated that the ability to select mutants varies between different strains of one species (15). This is important, as in vitro tests used to predict the likelihood of such mutants being generated are usually performed with wild-type or "indicator" strains, which may not necessarily be indicative of a species as a whole.

Triclosan resistance (MICs of 1 to 4 μg/ml) in *S. aureus* from clinical isolates and laboratory mutants, including methicillin-resistant *S. aureus*, has also been described (16, 26). Some of these mutants possessed alterations within FabI, but others (with equal levels of resistance [triclosan MICs of 4 μg/ml]) did not, indicating that other mechanisms of triclosan resistance exist. In *Mycobacterium tuberculosis* and *Mycobacterium smegmatis*, the *inhA* gene is a common target for triclosan and the antibiotic isoniazid (43). This has led to concerns that triclosan could directly select for antibiotic resistance in mycobacteria, although there is no evidence that this has happened in practice (60).

Cell wall changes

The inherent resistance of gram-negative bacteria to antibacterial agents and disinfectants is often attributed to poor permeability of the cell to these agents. For antibiotics, data in the last decade have shown that resistance can be due to active efflux pumps, which can be coupled with slow or little uptake of antibiotic into the cell (e.g., carbenicillin resistance in *Pseudomonas aeruginosa* [53]). Studies with disinfectants investigating decreased uptake versus enhanced efflux are rare, so the role of decreased permeability is still to be defined. A role for permeability in disinfectant resistance has been proposed, as membrane changes (alterations in outer membrane proteins and lipopolysaccharides) have been observed among *Pseudomonas* isolates with decreased susceptibility to chlorhexidine and QACs (33, 72, 73).

Efflux pumps

Efflux pumps are transport proteins that actively extrude toxic substrates from the cell into the surrounding environment, thereby reducing their accumulation within the cell (37). Many efflux pumps have a very wide substrate range and as such are termed "multidrug resistance" pumps. Substrates commonly include antibiotics, dyes, disinfectants, detergents, and other toxic substances. Efflux pumps fall into five families: resistance–nodulation–cell division (RND), multidrug and toxic efflux (MATE), drug metabolite transporters (DMT), ATP-binding cassette family (ABC), and major facilitator superfamily (MFS) (65).

Gram-positive bacteria possess disinfectant transporters of the small multidrug resistance (SMR) and MFS families, which are commonly plasmid encoded. These include the *qac* genes (QacA and B are MFS; QacC, D, E, G, and H are SMR [52]), which are common among staphylococci (11, 52, 69). Gram-negative species (*E. coli* and *Pseudomonas* spp.) can carry transporters on plasmids (QacE and QacEΔ1) as well as on the chromosome (AcrAB-TolC and MexAB-OprM). The RND family of transporters are multidrug resistance pumps with a broad specificity and have been shown to mediate intrinsic tolerance to disinfectants, including triclosan (44; A. M. Buckley et al., unpublished data). The AcrAB system of *E. coli* has been shown to confer resistance to triclosan and pine oils when overexpressed (44). Similarly, the chromosomally encoded Mex pumps of *P. aeruginosa* can mediate intrinsic and acquired resistance to disinfectants, which can approach in-use concentrations for triclosan (52). This has been identified as a possible problem, as selection of a Mex or Acr efflux mutant by a disinfectant would generate a strain cross-resistant to antibiotics in clinical use, which are also typical substrates of these pumps. The MexCD-OprJ system of *P. aeruginosa* can be induced by disinfectants, including benzalkonium chloride and chlorhexidine, which results in cross-resistance to the antibiotic norfloxacin (45). Concern has been raised about the potential for phenolic compounds to select for antibiotic resistance, as several such chemicals have been shown to act as inducers of the multiple antibiotic resistance (*mar*) operon and pregrowth with phenolic compounds has been shown to increase the ability of *Salmonella* to develop antibiotic resistance (58).

Transferable resistance

The ability of antibiotic resistance genes to mobilize and spread within and between species has proved to be a major problem in human and veterinary medicine, as isolates resistant to multiple antibiotics have emerged after acquisition of a plasmid or other mobile resistance determinant (e.g., *S. enterica* serovar Typhimurium DT104). Disinfectant resistance determinants can also be mobile and are often found on plasmids associated with antibiotic resistance genes. Plasmids from staphylococci have been described that carry *qac* genes as well as antibiotic resistance genes conferring resistance to *β*-lactams, aminoglycosides, and trimethoprim (69). Linkage between disinfectant resistance and antibiotic resistance genes has been demonstrated for staphylococci, and it has been speculated that both contribute to a selective advantage for these strains (69).

POTENTIAL FOR SELECTION OF RESISTANT STRAINS

Selection of mutants fully resistant to in-use concentrations of disinfectants is thought to be impossible due to their toxicity at these concentrations (31, 32). The MICs of disinfectants for most bacteria are normally greatly below the concentrations used in practice. Mutants that cannot be eradicated by treatment with in-use concentrations of disinfectants have not been observed to date. However, the concentration of disinfectant encountered by a bacterium may fall below that intended due to factors such as inactivation by organic material, dilution, or the formation of a biofilm. In these situations, bacteria may be exposed to sublethal concentrations of disinfectants, which could select for mutants that display reduced susceptibility to these agents. Conditions where sublethal exposure may occur are likely to exist in inaccessible or contaminated locations where the desired concentration of disinfectant may not be achieved, where a disinfectant may be inactivated, or within a bacterial biofilm. Locations where these conditions may occur include food processing plants, hospitals, farms, and homes. It has been postulated that exposure to a disinfectant could generate mutants with decreased susceptibility to antibiotics and an inherent propensity to mutate to high-level antibiotic resistance upon antibiotic challenge (Fig. 1). Mutants with cross-resistance between disinfectants and antibiotics have been selected in the laboratory, and it has recently been demonstrated that exposure to sublethal doses of triclosan and phenolic compounds increases the propensity (by between 10- and 100-fold) of *S. enterica* to develop antibiotic resistance upon exposure to various antimicrobial agents (58). An association between resistance to disinfectants (QACs and chlorhexidine) and antibiotics (penicillin, cephalothin, imipenem, doxycycline, trimethoprim, oxacillin, gentamicin, and fusidic acid) in *S. aureus*, including methicillin-resistant *S. aureus* isolates, has also been observed (4, 68). Other studies, which have looked for an association between triclosan usage and cross-resistance to antibiotics, have not been able to demonstrate a link, despite the wide use of triclosan (3, 8). Overuse of antibiotics is widely accepted as a driving factor responsible for increasing antibiotic resistance, and it is possible that disinfectant use can also drive selection for bacteria with decreased susceptibility to disinfectants. An association between chlorhexidine use and sensitivity has been demonstrated within the hospital environment, where bacteria isolated from areas of highest use (e.g., the intensive care unit) required higher concentrations of the compound for inhibition than those from areas of the hospital with lower use (e.g., the psychiatric ward). This was not significant for any individual species, but rather for all bacteria as a whole; cross-resistance to antibiotics was not investigated (12). A recent study has also

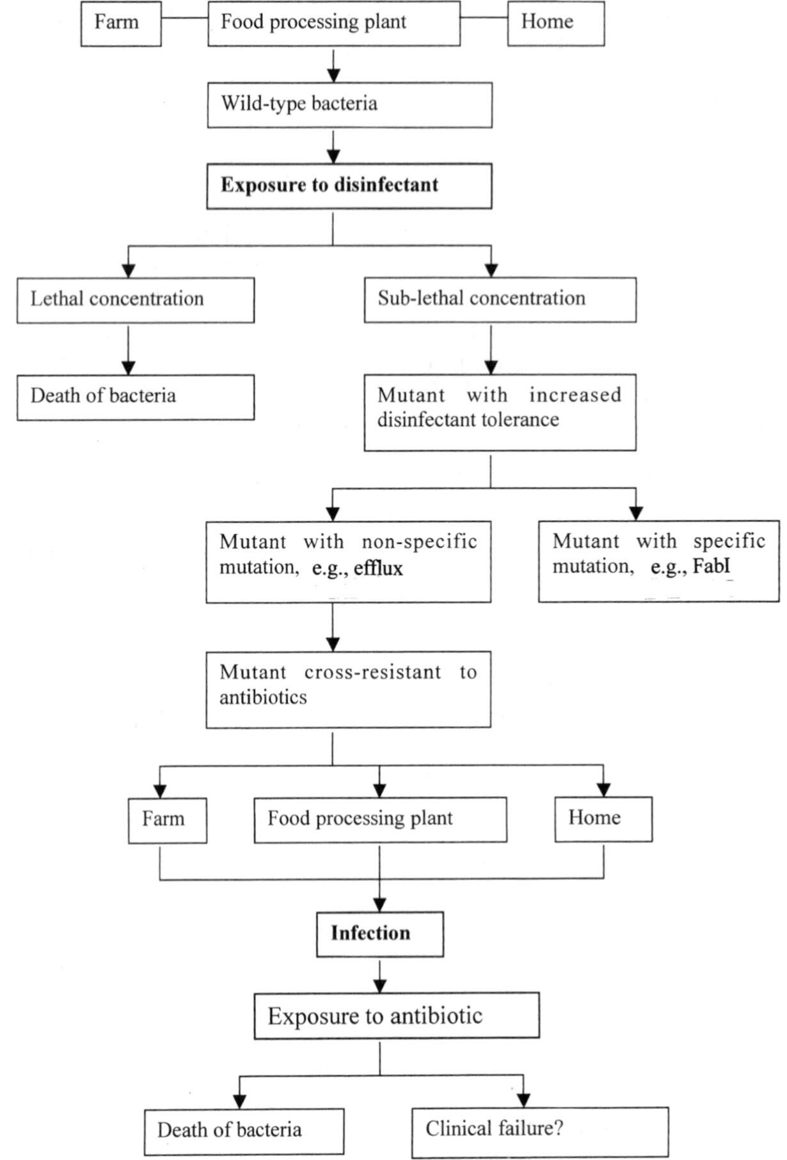

Figure 1. Potential outcomes of exposure to a disinfectant.

demonstrated differences between the hand flora isolated from "homemakers" and intensive care nurses. The nurses had fewer bacteria, but those present were more antibiotic resistant. A key difference between the two groups was the increased hand hygiene practiced by the nurses, and it is possible that disinfectant exposure has contributed to the differences in flora observed in this study (2).

Selection of disinfectant-resistant mutants is a potential concern if they entered the food chain or became endemic in the hospital environment—both situations where transfer to a human is possible, which could lead to infections caused by bacteria with reduced antibiotic susceptibility. It is difficult to evaluate the significance of this risk to human health (if any). Caution has been requested when translating laboratory data to the clinical environment (61). There is currently insufficient evidence to adequately assess the potential risks of disinfectant use and consequent cross-resistance to antibiotics. In particular, more work is required to determine the impact of disinfectant use during food production on bacteria in the food chain.

SUMMARY

Exposure to sublethal concentrations of disinfectants can select for bacteria with reduced susceptibility to them. Whilst resistance may not always allow bacteria to survive exposure to an in-use concentration of a disinfectant, low-level disinfectant resistance may be a problem if the mechanism of resistance selected is nonspecific, i.e., efflux, and confers cross-resistance to antibiotics as well as the potential to adapt readily to high-level antibiotic resistance. A challenge ahead is to investigate the potential risks posed by mutants with decreased susceptibility to disinfectants. Researchers need to conduct work with pathogenic strains, not just wild-type representative strains that clearly respond differently to challenge with disinfectants under certain circumstances than pathogenic strains of the same species. Subjecting relevant strains to realistic disinfectant challenges and then characterizing these strains in terms of their ability to develop both disinfectant and antibiotic resistance and determining whether this is achieved at a cost to the fitness of the bacterium will help identify the likely outcome of sublethal disinfectant challenge. The genetic mechanisms responsible for tolerance to disinfectants need to be identified, particularly the contribution of nonspecific mechanisms, such as efflux. Validation of genes involved will allow clinical isolates to be analyzed to ascertain whether the same mechanisms of resistance can be found in relevant isolates, which would further support a link between disinfectant resistance, antibiotic resistance, and pathogenicity.

CONCLUDING REMARKS

The use of disinfectants is crucial in a wide variety of situations where microbial decontamination is necessary. Just as important is making sure that disinfectants are used appropriately, i.e., that correct dilutions, concentrations, and contact times are used and that the agent used is appropriate for the task. Cleaning prior to disinfection is important in order to remove organic material and other contaminants that might interfere with disinfectant activity. The rotation of disinfectants is commonly carried out in hospitals, but it has been questioned whether this is necessary if correct use procedures are followed (47). Thorough analysis of the link between antibiotic and disinfectant resistance will help to inform policies designed to eradicate microorganisms while minimizing the likelihood of selecting resistant strains. While there is evidence that the use of disinfection in the home (9, 19) prevents infections, it is likely that many of the products available for domestic use containing triclosan, QACs, or other antimicrobial substances are not contributing to improved hygiene, and frivolous use of antimicrobial compounds should be discontinued; there should be a clear benefit associated with the use of such products.

Acknowledgments. M.A.W. is supported by the Bristol-Myers Squibb Unrestricted Award in Infectious Diseases awarded to L.J.V.P., and M.J.W. is supported by Defra (United Kingdom).

We are grateful to Tom Humphrey for helpful comments made in the preparation of the manuscript.

REFERENCES

1. **Aiello, A. E., and E. L. Larson.** 2002. Causal inference: the case of hygiene and health. *Am. J. Infect. Control* **30:** 503–511.
2. **Aiello, A. E., J. Cimiotti, P. Della-Latta, and E. L. Larson.** 2003. A comparison of the bacteria found on the hands of "homemakers" and neonatal intensive care unit nurses. *J. Hosp. Infect.* **54:**310–315.
3. **Aiello, A. E., B. Marshall, S. B. Levy, P. Della-Latta, and E. Larson.** 2004. Relationship between triclosan and susceptibilities of bacteria isolated from hands in the community. *Antimicrob. Agents Chemother.* **48:**2973–2979.
4. **Akimitsu, N., H. Hamamoto, R. Inoue, M. Shoji, A. Akamine, K. Takemori, N. Hamasaki, and K. Sekimizu.** 1999. Increase in resistance of methicillin-resistant *Staphylococcus aureus* to beta-lactams caused by mutations conferring resistance to benzalkonium chloride, a disinfectant widely used in hospitals. *Antimicrob. Agents Chemother.* **43:**3042–3043.
5. **Association of Official Analytical Chemists.** 1990. *Official Methods of the Association of Official Analytical Chemists*, 15th ed. Association of Official Analytical Chemists, Inc., Arlington, Va.
6. **Ayliffe, G. A., J. R. Babb, J. G. Davies, and H. A. Lilly.** 1988. Hand disinfection: a comparison of various agents in laboratory and ward studies. *J. Hosp. Infect.* **11:**226–243.
7. **Bailey, J. S., R. J. Buhr, N. A. Cox, and M. E. Berrang.** 1996. Effect of hatching cabinet sanitation treatments on Salmonella cross-contamination and hatchability of broiler eggs. *Poult. Sci.* **75:**191–196.
8. **Bamber, A. I., and T. J. Neal.** 1999. An assessment of triclosan susceptibility in methicillin-resistant and methicillin-sensitive *Staphylococcus aureus*. *J. Hosp. Infect.* **41:**107–109.
9. **Barker, J., M. Naeeni, and S. F. Bloomfield.** 2003. The effects of cleaning and disinfection in reducing *Salmonella* contamination in a laboratory model kitchen. *J. Appl. Microbiol.* **95:**1351–1360.
10. **Bierer, B., B. D. Barnett, and H. D. Valentine.** 1961. Experimentally killing *Salmonella typhimurium* on egg shells by washing. *Poult. Sci.* **40:**1009–1014.
11. **Bjorland, J., T. Steinum, M. Sunde, S. Waage, and E. Heir.** 2003. Novel plasmid-borne gene *qacJ* mediates resistance to quaternary ammonium compounds in equine *Staphylococcus aureus*, *Staphylococcus simulans*, and *Staphylococcus intermedius*. *Antimicrob. Agents Chemother.* **47:**3046–3052.
12. **Block, C., and M. Furman.** 2002. Association between intensity of chlorhexidine use and micro-organisms of reduced susceptibility in a hospital environment. *J. Hosp. Infect.* **51:** 201–206.
13. **Boddie, R. L., and S. C. Nickerson.** 2002. Reduction of mastitis caused by experimental challenge with *Staphylococcus aureus* and *Streptococcus agalactiae* by use of a quaternary ammonium and halogen-mixture teat dip. *J. Dairy Sci.* **85:**258–262.
14. **Boddie, R. L., W. E. Owens, C. H. Ray, S. C. Nickerson, and N. T. Boddie.** 2002. Germicidal activities of representatives of five different teat dip classes against three bovine mycoplasma species using a modified excised teat model. *J. Dairy Sci.* **85:** 1909–1912.

15. **Braoudaki, M., and A. C. Hilton.** 2004. Low level of cross-resistance between triclosan and antibiotics in *Escherichia coli* K-12 and *E. coli* O55 compared to *E. coli* O157. *FEMS Microbiol. Lett.* **235:**305–309.
16. **Brenwald, N. P., and A. P. Fraise.** 2003. Triclosan resistance in methicillin-resistant *Staphylococcus aureus* (MRSA). *J. Hosp. Infect.* **55:**141–144.
17. **Chaplin, C. E.** 1951. Observations on quaternary ammonium compound disinfectants. *Can. J. Bot.* **29:**373–382.
18. **Coolman, B. R., S. M. Marretta, I. Kakoma, M. A. Wallig, S. L. Coolman, and A. J. Paul.** 1998. Cutaneous antimicrobial preparation prior to intravenous catheterization in healthy dogs: clinical, microbiological, and histopathological evaluation. *Can. Vet. J.* **39:**757–763.
19. **Cozad, A., and R. D. Jones.** 2003. Disinfection and the prevention of infectious disease. *Am. J. Infect. Control* **31:** 243–254.
20. **Davies, R. H., and M. F. Breslin.** 2004. Observations on the distribution and control of Salmonella contamination in poultry hatcheries. *Br. Poult. Sci.* **45**(Suppl.1):S12–S14.
21. **Davies, R. H., and C. Wray.** 1995. Observations on disinfection regimens used on *Salmonella enteritidis* infected poultry units. *Poult. Sci.* **74:**638–647.
22. **Davison, S., C. E. Benson, D. S. Munro, S. C. Rankin, A. E. Ziegler, and R. J. Eckroade.** 2003. The role of disinfectant resistance of *Salmonella enterica* serotype enteritidis in recurring infections in Pennsylvania egg quality assurance program monitored flocks. *Avian Dis.* **47:**143–148.
23. **Dee, S., J. Deen, D. Burns, G. Douthit, and C. Pijoan.** 2004. An assessment of sanitation protocols for commercial transport vehicles contaminated with porcine reproductive and respiratory syndrome virus. *Can. J. Vet. Res.* **68:**208–214.
24. **Denton, M., M. H. Wilcox, P. Parnell, D. Green, V. Keer, P. M. Hawkey, I. Evans, and P. Murphy.** 2004. Role of environmental cleaning in controlling an outbreak of *Acinetobacter baumannii* on a neurosurgical intensive care unit. *J. Hosp. Infect.* **56:**106–110.
25. **Erskine, R. J., P. M. Sears, P. C. Bartlett, and C. R. Gage.** 1998. Efficacy of postmilking disinfection with benzyl alcohol versus iodophor in the prevention of new intramammary infections in lactating cows. *J. Dairy Sci.* **81:**116–120.
26. **Fan, F., K. Yan, N. G. Wallis, S. Reed, T. D. Moore, S. F. Rittenhouse, W. E. DeWolf, Jr., J. Huang, D. McDevitt, W. H. Miller, M. A. Seefeld, K. A. Newlander, D. R. Jakas, M. S. Head, and D. J. Payne.** 2002. Defining and combating the mechanisms of triclosan resistance in clinical isolates of *Staphylococcus aureus*. *Antimicrob. Agents Chemother.* **46:**3343–3347.
27. **Fraise, A. P.** 1999. Choosing disinfectants. *J. Hosp. Infect.* **43:**255–264.
28. **Fraise, A. P.** 2002. Biocide abuse and antimicrobial resistance—a cause for concern? *J. Antimicrob. Chemother.* **49:**11–12.
29. **French, G. L., J. A. Otter, K. P. Shannon, N. M. Adams, D. Watling, and M. J. Parks.** 2004. Tackling contamination of the hospital environment by methicillin-resistant *Staphylococcus aureus* (MRSA): a comparison between conventional terminal cleaning and hydrogen peroxide vapour decontamination. *J. Hosp. Infect.* **57:**31–37.
30. **Gasparini, R., T. Pozzi, R. Magnelli, D. Fatighenti, E. Giotti, G. Poliseno, M. Pratelli, R. Severini, P. Bonanni, and L. De Feo.** 1995. Evaluation of in vitro efficacy of the disinfectant Virkon. *Eur. J. Epidemiol.* **11:**193–197.
31. **Gilbert, P., A. J. McBain, and S. F. Bloomfield.** 2002. Biocide abuse and antimicrobial resistance: being clear about the issues. *J. Antimicrob. Chemother.* **50:**137–139.
32. **Gilbert, P., and A. J. McBain.** 2003. Potential impact of increased use of biocides in consumer products on prevalence of antibiotic resistance. *Clin. Microbiol. Rev.* **16:**189–208.
33. **Guerin-Mechin, L., J. Y. Leveau, and F. Dubois-Brissonnet.** 2004. Resistance of spheroplasts and whole cells of *Pseudomonas aeruginosa* to bactericidal activity of various biocides: evidence of the membrane implication. *Microbiol. Res.* **159:**51–57.
34. **Holah, J. T., J. H. Taylor, D. J. Dawson, and K. E. Hall.** 2002. Biocide use in the food industry and the disinfectant resistance of persistent strains of *Listeria monocytogenes* and *Escherichia coli*. *J. Appl. Microbiol.* **92:**111S–120S.
35. **Jorgensen, F., R. Bailey, S. Williams, P. Henderson, D. R. Wareing, F. J. Bolton, J. A. Frost, L. Ward, and T. J. Humphrey.** 2002. Prevalence and numbers of *Salmonella* and *Campylobacter* spp. on raw, whole chickens in relation to sampling methods. *Int. J. Food Microbiol.* **76:**151–164.
36. **Kitis, M.** 2004. Disinfection of wastewater with peracetic acid: a review. *Environ. Int.* **30:**47–55.
37. **Levy, S. B.** 2002. Active efflux, a common mechanism for biocide and antibiotic resistance. *J. Appl. Microbiol.* **92**(Suppl.): 65S–71S.
38. **Luppens, S. B., M. W. Reij, R. W. van der Heijden, F. M. Rombouts, and T. Abee.** 2002. Development of a standard test to assess the resistance of *Staphylococcus aureus* biofilm cells to disinfectants. *Appl. Environ. Microbiol.* **68:**4194–4200.
39. **Mazzola, P. G., T. C. Penna, and A. M. Martins.** 2003. Determination of decimal reduction time (D value) of chemical agents used in hospitals for disinfection purposes. *BMC Infect. Dis.* **3:**24.
40. **McBain, A. J., R. G. Ledder, L. E. Moore, C. E. Catrenich, and P. Gilbert.** 2004. Effects of quaternary-ammonium-based formulations on bacterial community dynamics and antimicrobial susceptibility. *Appl. Environ. Microbiol.* **70:** 3449–3456.
41. **McDonnell, G., and A. D. Russell.** 1999. Antiseptics and disinfectants: activity, action, and resistance. *Clin. Microbiol. Rev.* **12:**147–179. (Erratum, **14:**227, 2001.)
42. **McMurry, L. M., M. Oethinger, and S. B. Levy.** 1998. Triclosan targets lipid synthesis. *Nature* **394:**531–532.
43. **McMurry, L. M., P. F. McDermott, and S. B. Levy.** 1999. Genetic evidence that InhA of *Mycobacterium smegmatis* is a target for triclosan. *Antimicrob. Agents Chemother.* **43:** 711–713.
44. **Moken, M. C., L. M. McMurry, and S. B. Levy.** 1997. Selection of multiple-antibiotic-resistant (mar) mutants of *Escherichia coli* by using the disinfectant pine oil: roles of the *mar* and *acrAB* loci. *Antimicrob. Agents Chemother.* **41:** 2770–2772.
45. **Morita, Y., T. Murata, T. Mima, S. Shiota, T. Kuroda, T. Mizushima, N. Gotoh, T. Nishino, and T. Tsuchiya.** 2003. Induction of *mexCD-oprJ* operon for a multidrug efflux pump by disinfectants in wild-type *Pseudomonas aeruginosa* PAO1. *J. Antimicrob. Chemother.* **51:**991–994.
46. **Murdough, P. A., and J. W. Pankey.** 1993. Evaluation of 57 teat sanitizers using excised cow teats. *J. Dairy Sci.* **76:** 2033–2038.
47. **Murtough, S. M., S. J. Hiom, M. Palmer, and A. D. Russell.** 2002. A survey of rotational use of biocides in hospital pharmacy aseptic units. *J. Hosp. Infect.* **50:**228–231.
48. **Mostellar, T. M., and J. R. Bishop.** 1993. Sanitizer efficacy against attached bacteria in a milk biofilm. *J. Food Prot.* **56:** 34–41.
49. **Parkinson, E.** 1981. Testing of disinfectants for veterinary and agricultural use, p. 33–36. *In* C. H. Collins, M. C. Allwood,

S. F. Bloomfield, and A. Fox (ed.), *Disinfectants: Their Use and Evaluation of Effectiveness*. Academic Press, London, United Kingdom.

50. **Patel, S.** 2004. The efficacy of alcohol-based hand disinfectant products. *Nurs. Times* **100:**32–34.
51. **Paterson, S.** 1999. Miconazole/chlorhexidine shampoo as an adjunct to systemic therapy in controlling dermatophytosis in cats. *J. Small Anim. Pract.* **40:**163–166.
52. **Paulsen, I. T., M. H. Brown, T. G. Littlejohn, B. A. Mitchell, and R. A. Skurray.** 1996. Multidrug resistance proteins QacA and QacB from *Staphylococcus aureus*: membrane topology and identification of residues involved in substrate specificity. *Proc. Natl. Acad. Sci. USA* **93:**3630–3635.
53. **Poole, K.** 2002. Mechanisms of bacterial biocide and antibiotic resistance. *J. Appl. Microbiol.* **92**(Suppl.):55S–64S.
54. **Ramesh, N., S. W. Joseph, L. E. Carr, L. W. Douglass, and F. W. Wheaton.** 2002. Evaluation of chemical disinfectants for the elimination of *Salmonella* biofilms from poultry transport containers. *Poult. Sci.* **81:**904–910.
55. **Rampling, A., S. Wiseman, L. Davis, A. P. Hyett, A. N. Walbridge, G. C. Payne, and A. J. Cornaby.** 2001. Evidence that hospital hygiene is important in the control of methicillin-resistant *Staphylococcus aureus*. *J. Hosp. Infect.* **49:** 109–116.
56. **Randall, L. P., S. W. Cooles, A. R. Sayers, and M. J. Woodward.** 2001. Association between cyclohexane resistance in *Salmonella* of different serovars and increased resistance to multiple antibiotics, disinfectants and dyes. *J. Med. Microbiol.* **50:**919–924.
57. **Randall, L. P., A. M. Ridley, S. W. Cooles, M. Sharma, A. R. Sayers, L. Pumbwe, D. G. Newell, L. J. Piddock, and M. J. Woodward.** 2003. Prevalence of multiple antibiotic resistance in 443 *Campylobacter* spp. isolated from humans and animals. *J. Antimicrob. Chemother.* **52:**507–510.
58. **Randall, L. P., S. W. Cooles, L. J. Piddock, and M. J. Woodward.** 2004. Effect of triclosan or a phenolic farm disinfectant on the selection of antibiotic-resistant *Salmonella enterica*. *J. Antimicrob. Chemother.* **54:**621–627.
59. **Rodgers, J. D., J. J. McCullagh, P. T. McNamee, J. A. Smyth, and H. J. Ball.** 2001. An investigation into the efficacy of hatchery disinfectants against strains of *Staphylococcus aureus* associated with the poultry industry. *Vet. Microbiol.* **82:** 131–140.
60. **Russell, A. D.** 2000. Do biocides select for antibiotic resistance? *J. Pharm. Pharmacol.* **52:**227–233.
61. **Russell, A. D.** 2003. Biocide use and antibiotic resistance: the relevance of laboratory findings to clinical and environmental situations. *Lancet Infect. Dis.* **3:**794–803.
62. **Rutala, W. A., and D. J. Weber.** 2001. Surface disinfection: should we do it? *J. Hosp. Infect.* **48**(Suppl. A):S64–S68.
63. **Rutala, W. A., and D. J. Weber.** 2004. Disinfection and sterilization in health care facilities: what clinicians need to know. *Clin. Infect. Dis.* **39:**702–709.
64. **Rutala, W. A., and D. J. Weber.** 2004. The benefits of surface disinfection. *Am. J. Infect. Control* **32:**226–231.
65. **Saier, M. H., Jr., and I. T. Paulsen.** 2001. Phylogeny of multidrug transporters. *Semin. Cell Dev. Biol.* **12:**205–213.
66. **Sander, J. E., C. L. Hofacre, I. H. Cheng, and R. D. Wyatt.** 2002. Investigation of resistance of bacteria from commercial poultry sources to commercial disinfectants. *Avian Dis.* **46:** 997–1000.
67. **Schweizer, H. P.** 2001. Triclosan: a widely used biocide and its link to antibiotics. *FEMS Microbiol. Lett.* **202:**1–7.
68. **Sidhu, M. S., E. Heir, H. Sorum, and A. Holck.** 2001. Genetic linkage between resistance to quaternary ammonium compounds and beta-lactam antibiotics in food-related *Staphylococcus* spp. *Microb. Drug Resist.* **7:**363–371.
69. **Sidhu, M. S., E. Heir, T. Leegaard, K. Wiger, and A. Holck.** 2002. Frequency of disinfectant resistance genes and genetic linkage with beta-lactamase transposon Tn*552* among clinical staphylococci. *Antimicrob. Agents Chemother.* **46:**2797–2803.
70. **Sivaraman, S., J. Zwahlen, A. F. Bell, L. Hedstrom, and P. J. Tonge.** 2003. Structure-activity studies of the inhibition of FabI, the enoyl reductase from *Escherichia coli*, by triclosan: kinetic analysis of mutant FabIs. *Biochemistry* **42:**4406–4413.
71. **Suller, M. T., and A. D. Russell.** 2000. Triclosan and antibiotic resistance in *Staphylococcus aureus*. *J. Antimicrob. Chemother.* **46:**11–18.
72. **Tabata, A., H. Nagamune, T. Maeda, K. Murakami, Y. Miyake, and H. Kourai.** 2003. Correlation between resistance of *Pseudomonas aeruginosa* to quaternary ammonium compounds and expression of outer membrane protein OprR. *Antimicrob. Agents Chemother.* **47:**2093–2099.
73. **Tattawasart, U., J. Y. Maillard, J. R. Furr, and A. D. Russell.** 2000. Outer membrane changes in *Pseudomonas stutzeri* resistant to chlorhexidine diacetate and cetylpyridinium chloride. *Int. J. Antimicrob. Agents* **16:**233–238.
74. **Taylor, J. T., S. J. Rogers, and J. T. Holah.** 1999. A comparison of the bactericidal efficacy of 18 disinfectants used in the food industry aginst *Escherichia coli* O157:H7 and *Pseudomonas aeruginosa* at 10°C and 20°C. *J. Appl. Microbiol.* **87:**718–726.
75. **Walker, S. E., J. E. Sander, I. H. Cheng, and R. E. Wooley.** 2002. The in vitro efficacy of a quaternary ammonia disinfectant and/or ethylenediaminetetraacetic acid-Tris against commercial broiler hatchery isolates of *Pseudomonas aeruginosa*. *Avian Dis.* **46:**826–830.
76. **Willighan, E. M., J. E. Sander, S. G. Thayer, and J. L. Wilson.** 1996. Investigation of bacterial resistance to hatchery disinfectants. *Avian Dis.* **40:**510–515.
77. **Zhao, C., B. Ge, J. De Villena, R. Sudler, E. Yeh, S. Zhao, D. G. White, D. Wagner, and J. Meng.** 2001. Prevalence of *Campylobacter* spp., *Escherichia coli*, and *Salmonella* serovars in retail chicken, turkey, pork, and beef from the Greater Washington, D.C., area. *Appl. Environ. Microbiol.* **67:**5431–5436.

Antimicrobial Resistance in Bacteria of Animal Origin
Edited by Frank M. Aarestrup

Chapter 9

Antimicrobial Resistance in *Clostridium* and *Brachyspira* spp. and other Anaerobes

ANDERS FRANKLIN, MÄRIT PRINGLE, AND DAVID J. HAMPSON

Of the anaerobic bacterial species that colonize animals, many remain poorly studied and incompletely understood. This fact primarily results from difficulties in their isolation and identification, as well their tendency to be involved in complex polymicrobial interactions. Anaerobic bacteria of animals are an extremely diverse group, including various gram-positive and gram-negative members; they have a great range of genetic backgrounds and colonize many anatomical sites. Numerically, the anaerobic bacteria far outnumber other bacterial groups associated with animals, and they dominate the microbiota in the oral cavity, rumen, and lower intestinal tract. These anaerobic bacteria include a relatively small group of primary pathogens, and many others that are present as part of the rich and varied autochthonous microbiota associated with the mucosal surfaces of the mouth; the intestinal, upper respiratory, urinary, and genital tracts; and the skin. These autochthonous bacteria occasionally cause clinical problems; for example, they may cause necrotic and suppurative lesions such as abscesses and cellulitis when they translocate into other normally sterile tissues or are transmitted in bite wounds. They also are important as potential in situ reservoirs of both antimicrobial-resistant strains and of antimicrobial resistance genes that might be transmitted to other bacterial species, including pathogens (147, 158).

The main, commonly encountered, primary anaerobic bacterial pathogens of animals include certain species of the genera *Clostridia*, *Brachyspira*, *Bacteroides*, and *Fusobacterium*, as well as *Dichelobacter nodosus*. Other species that may be less frequently associated with disease include *Actinobaculum (Eubacterium) suis*, *Peptostreptococcus* spp., *Peptococcus* spp., *Prevotella* spp., and *Porphyromonas* spp. Disease production by these bacteria often requires predisposing factors, for example, local trauma, a sudden change of diet, or alterations in environmental factors that permit invasion and/or survival in normally sterile or damaged tissues, such as occurs in abscess formation in the liver or mammary gland.

Effective antimicrobial treatment of infections with anaerobic bacteria requires consideration of the need to target more than one of the various species that may be present. Unfortunately, there is a paucity of data both on laboratory diagnosis of anaerobic bacterial infections in animals and on effective treatment regimens. Nonstandardized susceptibility testing methods are sometimes used for anaerobic species, and this makes it difficult to evaluate and correlate the available in vitro antimicrobial susceptibility data with the outcomes of treatment.

Accurate antimicrobial susceptibility testing of anaerobic, fastidious bacteria can be difficult to achieve. For some species, there is a need for long incubation periods and high initial concentrations of bacteria to obtain satisfactory growth. Supplements to the media are also frequently required, and the requirements for growth differ between the anaerobic species. Hence, when susceptibility testing of anaerobic bacteria is performed, quality control is of the utmost importance. One obstacle to this is that few anaerobic control strains for antimicrobial susceptibility tests have been evaluated. For example, three strains are recommended by the Clinical and Laboratory Standards Institute (formerly the National Committee for Clinical Laboratory Standards) (117), and the list of antimicrobial agents with accepted ranges is limited. It would be desirable to have more internationally available and recommended anaerobic control strains that give reproducible results and have accepted ranges for drugs used in veterinary medicine.

Anders Franklin and Märit Pringle • Department of Antibiotics, National Veterinary Institute, SE-751 89 Uppsala, Sweden. **David J. Hampson** • School of Veterinary and Biomedical Sciences, Murdoch University, Murdoch, Western Australia 6150, Australia.

In human medicine, patterns of antimicrobial resistance among clinically important anaerobes have been shown to vary between hospitals, geographic regions, and antibiotic-prescribing regimens (5, 133). Similar comparative high-quality data are largely unavailable for anaerobic bacterial species recovered from animals, and there is relatively little information available about the mechanisms by which anaerobic isolates from animals may develop or acquire resistance to antimicrobial agents. As a general rule, anaerobic bacteria are inherently rather susceptible to most classes of antimicrobial agents, except to the aminoglycosides and the early fluoroquinolones. The aminoglycosides require oxygen-dependent transport into the bacterial cytoplasm, and consequently obligate anaerobic bacteria are resistant to their effects (28). *Clostridium* species usually are not susceptible to trimethoprim (TMP) because they have TMP-insensitive dihydrofolate reductases and also possess a permeability barrier for TMP (166, 167). Other anaerobes that appear susceptible to trimethoprim-sulfonamides in vitro may not respond to this combination in vivo, due to the presence of thymidine in necrotic tissue (71). Members of the *Bacteroides fragilis* group are frequently not sensitive to the penicillins and to some cephalosporins because they produce beta-lactamases. However, the activity of these antibiotics may be restored by their use in combination with clavulanic acid (7). As a general rule, the nitroimidazoles, such as metronidazole, are useful for treating infections with anaerobic bacteria, as their intracellular reduction to antimicrobial metabolites occurs under anaerobic conditions. Unfortunately, despite their potential value, they are not available for use in food-producing animals in many legislative areas, most notably in the European Union and the United States, because they are genotoxic. Similarly, a number of other antimicrobial drugs that have been shown to be effective against anaerobic infections in production animals are now not available in the European Union and in certain other countries. Hence, issues of resistance to these antimicrobial agents by bacterial pathogens of production animals are no longer of particular veterinary relevance. Examples of such drugs that are no longer widely available in the European Union include the quinoxalines carbadox and olaquindox, previously used for the control of swine dysentery, and bacitracin and virginiamycin, previously used for the control of necrotic enteritis in broiler chickens. The two latter antimicrobial agents were authorized as growth promoters in the European Union until 1999, when antimicrobial agents or derivatives thereof used for therapy in human or veterinary medicine were no longer allowed as feed additives.

This chapter focuses on issues relating to antimicrobial resistance in some of the more commonly encountered anaerobic bacterial pathogens of animals. Most of the available data on specific antimicrobial resistance relate to *Clostridium perfringens* type A, causing necrotic enteritis in broiler chickens, and to *Brachyspira hyodysenteriae*, causing swine dysentery.

CLOSTRIDIUM

The genus *Clostridium* encompasses a wide range of species, including members that are only distantly related (79). All are gram-positive, spore-forming anaerobic rods, and most form part of the normal intestinal microbiota of different animal species. Some *Clostridium* species are essentially nonpathogenic; others, such as *C. perfringens*, may act as opportunistic pathogens, occasionally causing disease; and others are classified as major pathogens. The pathogenic clostridia all produce powerful exotoxins and can be divided into four groups according to the types of disease they cause in animals (131).

1. Neurotoxic clostridia (*C. botulinum* and *C. tetani*). These species produce potent neurotoxins.

2. Enterotoxin-producing clostridia (*C. perfringens* types A to E). This species produces toxins in the intestinal lumen that may act locally and/or systemically.

3. Histotoxic clostridia (*C. chauvoei*, *C. septicum*, *C. haemolyticum*, *C. sordellii*, *C. perfringens*, and *C. colinum*). These bacteria produce histotoxins that are less inherently toxic than those in group 1.

4. Clostridia involved with antibiotic-associated diarrhea (*C. difficile* and *C. spiroforme*). These species produce locally acting cytotoxins in the intestinal lumen.

The neurotoxic clostridia are rarely, if ever, treated with antibiotics. Hence, data on their antimicrobial susceptibility are not reviewed here.

Enterotoxin-Producing Clostridia: *C. perfringens*

C. perfringens is a major causative agent of enteric diseases in many animal species (152); consequently, most of the data on antimicrobial susceptibility in animal isolates of clostridia concern this species. Furthermore, much of the published susceptibility data on *C. perfringens* concern isolates from broilers (37, 78, 107, 175). Diseases associated with *C. perfringens* in other species, such as horses, sheep, cattle, and pigs, are rarely treated with antimicrobial agents.

In broilers, *C. perfringens* type A causes necrotic enteritis (NE), a common and economically significant disease. NE can occur as an acute disease with high mortality in 2- to 4-week-old broiler chickens, but also as a subclinical enteric disease or as a *C. perfringens*-associated hepatitis (45). Turkeys may also be affected, but the pathogenesis in this species is relatively poorly understood (39, 56). Various antimicrobial agents are used as in-feed medication for the control of NE; avilamycin is authorized as a feed additive in the European Union until 2006 and used in the control of NE. Before the ban on avoparcin as a growth promoter in the European Union in December 1996, and of bacitracin and virginiamycin (among others) in July 1999, these antimicrobial agents were also used for the same purpose. In the United States, bacitracin, lincomycin, and virginiamycin are approved as in-feed medication for NE (175). Ionophoric antimicrobial agents, commonly used as coccidiostatic agents in broilers, are also active against gram-positive bacteria and are used in the control of NE (44).

Occurrence of antimicrobial resistance in *C. perfringens*

Quantitative data on antimicrobial susceptibility in animal isolates of *C. perfringens* are available using agar or broth microdilution. Both methods were compared for susceptibility testing of certain antimicrobial agents for *C. perfringens* strains isolated from pigs and poultry (18). There was a good correlation between the methods for virginiamycin, erythromycin, and tetracycline, whereas there was less agreement for bacitracin. Relatively recent data on antimicrobial susceptibilities obtained using either agar dilution or broth microdilution are available for poultry isolates of *C. perfringens* from different countries.

In a survey of antimicrobial susceptibility of 58 Swedish (2000 to 2001), 20 Danish (1997 to 2002), and 24 Norwegian (1996 to 2001) *C. perfringens* type A poultry isolates, recovered both from diseased and healthy birds, resistance to oxytetracycline (MIC >1 mg/liter) was most frequent and observed in samples from Sweden (76%), Denmark (10%), and Norway (29%) (78) (Table 1). A bimodal distribution of MICs was observed. Similarly, among *C. perfringens* isolates obtained from broilers in Belgium in 2002, 66% were designated as low-level resistant to oxytetracycline, with an MIC range of 1 to 8 mg/liter (107).

For other antimicrobial agents investigated, resistance has been relatively uncommon in broiler and turkey isolates. All recent broiler isolates from the Nordic countries, Belgium, and the United States have been susceptible to ampicillin and amoxicillin or penicillin (78, 107, 143, 175). Susceptibility to avilamycin, vancomycin, avoparcin, and the ionophores narasin, salinomycin, lasalocid, and monensin seems to be inherent in *C. perfringens* (37, 78, 107, 175).

The use of virginiamycin and bacitracin in broilers in many countries reflects the antimicrobial resistance situation in relation to these drugs. In susceptible poultry isolates, virginiamycin and bacitracin MICs are ≤1 mg/liter and 4 U/liter, respectively (78). Resistance to virginiamycin and bacitracin was not found in isolates from Sweden, where these substances have not been used for growth promotion since 1985. On the other hand, 18% of isolates from Denmark were resistant to bacitracin, while in Norway 16% were resistant to virginiamycin (78). In a study from the United States, 88% of broiler isolates were resistant to bacitracin and 31% to virginiamycin (175).

The resistance rates among *C. perfringens* isolates from poultry for the macrolides erythromycin and tylosin are generally low (37, 78, 107, 175), but a relatively high frequency of macrolide-resistant strains in turkeys in the United States has been reported (175). Resistance to lincomycin is common in isolates from certain countries, with a bimodal distribution of MICs. In Belgium 34% of *C. perfringens* poultry isolates were resistant to lincomycin (MIC ≥1 mg/liter) (107), and in the United States MICs for all broiler strains were ≥8 mg/liter (175).

There are only a few reports on antimicrobial susceptibility of *C. perfringens* from pigs. In an investigation in the United States from the 1970s, a comparison was made between strains from herds using in-feed medication and nonusers (143). Feed antimicrobial agents used included penicillin, sulfonamides, tetracyclines, streptomycin, and tylosin. Of 258 isolates from herds using in-feed medication, 78 and 22%, respectively, were resistant to tetracycline or erythromycin and clindamycin. Resistance to erythromycin, lincomycin, and clindamycin was always linked, and often associated with tetracycline resistance. Comparative figures for 240 strains from farms not using in-feed medication were 25 and 0.8%, respectively. All isolates were susceptible to penicillin and chloramphenicol (143). In a similar study in Australia, the susceptibility to tetracycline, erythromycin, and chloramphenicol among fecal *C. perfringens* isolates from weaned pigs given feed or water supplemented with antimicrobial agents was compared with the susceptibility of isolates from a nonmedicated herd (144). The strains were categorized as susceptible or resistant, and the percentage of strains resistant to

Table 1. Resistance to tetracycline and erythromycin or tylosin in *C. perfringens* of animal origin

Country	Animal species	No. of strains	% resistant to[a]:		Reference
			Tetracycline	Erythromycin[b]	
Sweden	Broilers	58	76 (>2)	0 (>16)	78
Denmark	Broilers	20	10 (>2)	0 (>16)	78
Norway	Broilers	24	29 (>2)	0 (>32)	78
Belgium	Broilers	47	66 (>2)	**0 (>1)**	107
United States	Broilers	26		**0 (>4)**	175
United States	Turkeys	22		**18 (>4)**	175
United States (medicated feed)	Pigs	258	78 (>8)	23 (>8)	143
United States (nonmedicated feed)	Pigs	131	21 (>8)	2 (>8)	143

[a]Breakpoints used (milligrams per liter) are indicated in parentheses.
[b]Data in boldface type are for tylosin.

tetracycline and macrolide-lincosamides was significantly higher in isolates from weaners on farms using antimicrobial-supplemented feed.

MICs obtained by agar dilution for *C. perfringens* isolates from 72 diarrheic and 59 nondiarrheic dogs in California have been reported (106). As with *C. perfringens* isolates from other animal species, tetracycline resistance was most frequently found. Two strains were highly resistant to erythromycin, and one strain was resistant to metronidazole.

Genetic basis of antimicrobial resistance in *C. perfringens*

Overall, the most common resistance trait in *C. perfringens* is to tetracyclines (100). Independent of origin, *C. perfringens* is reported to commonly carry the tetracycline resistance genes *tetA*(P), *tetB*(P), and *tet*(M) (30, 78, 99, 148). The *tet*(P) gene has been sequenced and shown to encode two tetracycline resistance genes, *tetA*(P) and *tetB*(P) (30, 150). Apparently, all tetracycline-resistant strains of *C. perfringens* carry *tetA*(P) with or without a second gene. The role of *tetB*(P) is unclear and seems not to affect the MIC of tetracycline in broiler *C. perfringens* isolates when *tetA*(P) is present (78). Cloning of *tetB*(P) into *Escherichia coli* or *C. perfringens* resulted in only low-level resistance to tetracycline (150).

The *tetA*(P) gene encodes a protein, TetA(P), that has been shown to mediate an active efflux of tetracycline in *E. coli*. The *tetB*(P) gene encodes a protein with similar amino acid sequence to the TetM-like proteins conferring ribosomal protection, and may thus function in a similar way (150). The *tetB*(P) gene in *C. perfringens*, however, does not hybridize with *tet*(M) from *Enterococcus faecalis* (100). Among *C. perfringens* isolates recovered from broilers in Belgium in 2002, 50% of the low-level-resistant strains carried *tetB*(P), whereas *tet*(Q) and *tet*(M) were found only in one strain each; *tet*(M) was found to confer high-level tetracycline resistance (107). Among broiler isolates from Sweden, Norway, and Denmark, both *tetA*(P) and *tetB*(P) were found in 80% of the tetracycline-resistant isolates, while only *tetA*(P) was present in the remainder; other *tet* genes were not detected (78).

Conjugative tetracycline resistance plasmids are relatively common, but most *C. perfringens* strains that are resistant to tetracycline cannot transfer the resistance (100). These conjugative plasmids are all closely related to the prototype conjugative *C. perfringens* R-plasmid pCW3 (1). The tetracycline resistance gene *tet*(P) was originally isolated from pCW3 and is found on all tetracycline resistance plasmids from *C. perfringens* (100). Large plasmids coding for tetracycline resistance and/or often for erythromycin and chloramphenicol resistance in *C. perfringens* have been characterized (149).

Chloramphenicol resistance in *C. perfringens* is mediated by chloramphenicol acetyltransferase (CAT) enzymes (143, 160, 182). The chloramphenicol resistance gene *cat*(P) in *C. perfringens* is borne on plasmids and located on a transposon, Tn*4451* (1, 26, 100). The nucleotide sequence of *cat*(P) is not very similar to other known *cat* genes, but the amino acid sequence of the gene product is significantly similar to those from other bacterial genera and most similar to CAT monomers from *Vibrio anguillarum* and *Campylobacter coli* (10).

Macrolide resistance is common in clostridia and is exclusively mediated by *erm* (erythromycin resistance methylase) genes, and to date *erm*(B), *erm*(F), and *erm*(Q) have been found in this genus (139). The Erm proteins methylate nucleotide position 2058 of the 23S rRNA and thereby inhibit the binding of the drug. As a rule, the *erm* genes confer cross-resistance to lincosamides and streptogramin B, the so-called macrolide-lincosamide-streptogramin B (MLS) phenotype, and in *C.*

perfringens this resistance has been shown to be plasmid mediated (26, 100).

The first *erm* gene described in clostridia was cloned from *C. perfringens*. It was designated *erm*(P) and shown to be identical to *erm*(B) (20). Another *erm* gene named *ermB*(P), which mostly did not hybridize with other *erm* genes in *C. perfringens*, has also been described (20, 100). The *ermB*(P) gene has been found to be common in bovine and ovine *C. perfringens* isolates (34), whereas it was detected only in one of four poultry and porcine isolates (37). A very close similarity between the *C. perfringens* *ermB*(P) gene and corresponding determinants commonly found on plasmids from *E. faecalis* and *Streptococcus agalactiae* has been revealed. These plasmids are conjugative with a broad host range (22). The *erm*(B) gene is often carried by transposon Tn*917* and is widely spread among human and animal isolates of enterococci and other bacteria (95, 141). The most common macrolide resistance determinant in *C. perfringens* is *erm*(Q), which has been found in porcine and human isolates from a wide geographic range (21).

The lincomycin resistance genes *lnu*(A) and *lnu*(B) have been found in Belgian broiler isolates of *C. perfringens* with low-level resistance to lincomycin (107).

Histotoxic Clostridia: *C. septicum* and *C. sordellii*

C. septicum is the causative agent of malignant edema in cattle and braxy in sheep, whereas *C. sordellii* is associated with gas gangrene in cattle, sheep, and horses. Penicillin and ampicillin had low MICs for Japanese isolates of *C. septicum* ($n = 23$) and *C. sordellii* ($n = 3$) from cattle with malignant edema that were tested by agar dilution. For oxytetracycline, 22% of the *C. septicum* isolates were designated as resistant, while all the *C. sordellii* isolates were resistant. The MICs of the other antimicrobial agents tested—enrofloxacin, erythromycin, vancomycin, and chloramphenicol—were all uniformly low (148).

Genetic basis of antimicrobial resistance in *C. septicum* and *C. sordellii*

Among the tetracycline-resistant bovine isolates, *tetA*(P) genes were found in four of five *C. septicum* isolates and in the three isolates of *C. sordellii*. This gene was about 90% homologous to *tetA*(P) of *C. perfringens*. The *C. sordellii* isolates also carried *tet*(B). One strain of *C. septicum* carried *tet*(B), and one carried *tet*(M) (148).

Clostridia Associated with Antibiotic-Associated Diarrhea: *Clostridium difficile*

In human medicine, *C. difficile* is a major nosocomial pathogen, commonly causing antibiotic-associated diarrhea (2, 120, 168). Prior treatment with antibiotics, and in particular clindamycin, erythromycin, cephalosporins, and ampicillin or amoxicillin, is an important risk factor for the disease in humans (8, 80, 90). Penicillin is associated with many cases, probably because it is the antibiotic most commonly used in humans (8). Pathogenic *C. difficile* strains from humans and animals produce two potent toxins, enterotoxin A and cytotoxin B, which are of major importance in clinical disease (13).

In recent years *C. difficile* has been implicated as a causative agent of colitis in mature horses, and, in common with humans, mostly in connection with and as a sequel to treatment with antimicrobial agents (12, 17, 38, 60, 101, 103, 177). The use of antimicrobial agents such as erythromycin, lincomycin, tetracyclines, and trimethoprim-sulfonamides has been associated with the occurrence of colitis in horses (6, 15, 33, 46, 60, 132, 155). With respect to colitis associated with *C. difficile* in horses, erythromycin has been identified as a particular risk factor (16, 60). Penicillin is the drug mostly associated with *C. difficile* and colitis in horses, and by analogy with the situation in human medicine, this is probably because it is the most widely used antibiotic (12). Foals are frequently asymptomatic carriers of *C. difficile* (14), but *C. difficile* also has been implicated as a causative agent of foal diarrhea (81, 104, 177).

C. difficile is also commonly isolated from mature dogs and cats (29, 102, 108, 135, 177) and puppies (121). The significance of *C. difficile* as a cause of disease in dogs and cats, however, is unclear and needs further study. In recent years *C. difficile* also has been identified as a causative agent of neonatal diarrhea in piglets (153, 174, 181).

Occurrence of antimicrobial resistance in *C. difficile*

Horses suspected to be suffering from colitis due to *C. difficile* are sometimes treated with antibiotics. In Europe, metronidazole is a first-line drug and has been shown to be effective in the treatment of horses suffering from colitis associated with *C. difficile* (110). In the United States, vancomycin and bacitracin have been used (75, 103, 177).

The antimicrobial susceptibility of *C. difficile* isolated from animals has not been systematically investigated, and there is a paucity of comparable data. Data on horse isolates have been based on studies using the Etest (14, 177), agar dilution (75), or broth microdilution (16). The Etest, basically an agar diffusion method, is a relatively simple and convenient method for determination of MICs for *C. difficile* isolates. A relatively good agreement between results for the Etest and agar dilution has been reported for human strains of *C. difficile* with a number of antimicrobial agents, except for metronidazole and clindamycin (11, 125, 146). The Etest has also been compared with agar dilution for various anaerobic bacteria of veterinary interest, including clostridia, and there was an agreement of 79% between the methods when accepting a difference corresponding to two doubling dilutions (122). In another study of *C. difficile* isolates from horses, the agreement between the Etest and broth microdilution results varied between 62 and 87% for different antimicrobial agents when a difference corresponding to one doubling dilution was accepted (16).

Isolates of *C. difficile* from horses appear to be more or less intrinsically resistant to bacitracin (36, 75, 177) and to the modern cephalosporins ceftiofur and cefotaxime (126, 176). As a possible consequence of the clinical use of metronidazole in horses, 19% of horse isolates of *C. difficile* in one study were reported to be resistant using a breakpoint of 8 mg/liter (75). In other studies all investigated isolates from horses and dogs were reported to be susceptible to both metronidazole and vancomycin (14, 106, 177) (Table 2). In isolates from humans, resistance to vancomycin and metronidazole is also reported to be rare (2, 11, 25, 40, 80, 178). As with *C. difficile* isolates from humans, the susceptibility of animal isolates to penicillin is relatively low (16, 177).

MLS resistance is a common resistance phenotype in *C. difficile* isolated from humans (2, 35, 50, 115). Recently, MLS resistance was found to be associated with fluoroquinolone resistance in *C. difficile*, and 12% of human isolates from Germany were reported as resistant to moxifloxacin (2). Of the 10 described serotypes of *C. difficile*, serotype C from humans frequently had a specific phenotype associated with resistance to chloramphenicol, clindamycin, erythromycin, rifampin, and tetracyclines (35). Other serogroups had variable patterns, except serogroup A, which was susceptible to most antimicrobial agents. A similar MLS and multiple resistance phenotype recently was found in *C. difficile* isolates from horses with colitis (16). In that study, all 36 clinical and 14 environmental isolates were susceptible to vancomycin and avilamycin, whereas 50% had the MLS phenotype with typical bimodal MIC distributions of erythromycin, virginiamycin, and oxytetracycline. All these isolates also were resistant to rifampin.

MIC_{90}s (MICs at which 90% of the strains are inhibited) for *C. difficile* isolated from diarrheic neonatal piglets in the United States have been determined by agar dilution for bacitracin (MIC_{90}, >256 mg/liter), ceftiofur (MIC_{90}, >256 mg/liter), erythromycin (MIC_{90}, >256 mg/liter), tetracycline (MIC_{90}, 32 mg/liter), tiamulin (MIC_{90}, 8 mg/liter), tylosin (MIC_{90}, 64 mg/liter), and virginiamycin (MIC_{90}, 2 mg/liter) (126). The high occurrence of resistance to bacitracin, erythromycin, and tetracycline concurs with the results reported for isolates of *C. difficile* from horses.

Genetic basis of antimicrobial resistance in *C. difficile*

As for other clostridia, MLS resistance in *C. difficile* is encoded by *erm* genes. Several *erm* genes are described in *C. difficile* of human origin, namely *erm*(B), *erm*(Q), and *erm*(F) (138). The *erm*(B) genes in *C. difficile* and *C. perfringens* are closely related (21, 50, 61, 62, 138, 139, 145, 154). The *erm*(B) gene in *C. difficile* has been shown to transfer easily within the species (180) and to and from *Bacillus subtilis* (115). Transfer of *erm*(B) to *Staphylococcus aureus* in the absence of plasmids also has been reported (61). A mobilizable element, Tn*5398*, has been shown to carry *erm*(B) in *C. difficile* (51, 115). Isolates from different geographic areas show heterogeneity in the genetic arrangement of this element, indicating frequent recombination between strains from various sources. The conjugative transposons Tn*916* and Tn*5397*, with a high similarity to Tn*5398*, were, however, transferred to *C. difficile* only at a low frequency in the laboratory (113, 114). A recent analysis of MLS resistance in *C. difficile* revealed that the majority of toxigenic strains carried one species-specific *erm*(B) gene copy, mediating a rather low MIC of erythromycin (16 to 24 mg/liter), whereas in some strains *erm*(B) was identical to the one found in *C. perfringens*. Some *C. difficile* strains had two copies of the *erm* gene, resulting in a high MIC of erythromycin (≥256 mg/liter) (154).

Tn*5398* also has been shown to encode tetracycline resistance of the *tet*(M) type (61, 113). Tetracycline resistance in *C. difficile* also has been associated with *tet*(P), *tet*(K), and *tet*(L) (138). Chloramphenicol resistance in *C. difficile* is encoded by the *cat*(D) gene, a gene that is closely related to *cat*(P) in *C. perfringens*. The *cat*(D) gene is located in multiple copies on the chromosome and is not transferable (179, 180).

BRACHYSPIRA

The genus *Brachyspira* is the only member in the spirochetal family *Brachyspiraceae*. *Brachyspira* spp. are weakly gram-negative, fastidious, anaerobic,

Table 2. Antimicrobial resistance in *C. difficile* isolates from horses, piglets, and dogs

Country	Animal species	No. of isolates	% of isolates with indicated drug resistance[a]											Reference
			Pc (4)	Am (2)	Em (8)	Ce (128)	Cl (4)	Tc (8)	Cm (8)	Va (1)	Ri (0.25)	Me (8)	Ba (128)	
Sweden	Horses	52	0	0	27				0		27	0	100	14
Sweden	Horses	50	0		36		100	40	56	0				16
United States	Horses	105							0	4	4	19	100	75
Canada	Horses	43	10–25		26	95		<10		0		0	95	177
United States	Piglets	80			<50	100		<50					100	126
United States	Dogs	70								0		0		106

[a]Breakpoints used (milligrams per liter) are indicated in parentheses; they were set in order to clearly separate microbiologically susceptible strains from strains with acquired resistance. Pc, penicillin; Am, ampicillin; Em, erythromycin; Ce, ceftiofur/cefotaxime; Cl, clindamycin; Tc, tetracycline; Cm, chloramphenicol; Va, vancomycin; Ri, rifampin; Me, metronidazole; Ba, bacitracin.

oxygen-tolerant spirochetes that colonize the large intestine. Currently, there are seven officially named species in the genus, of which *B. hyodysenteriae*, *B. intermedia*, *B. alvinipulli*, and *B. pilosicoli* are considered to be pathogenic or potentially pathogenic in various animal species; the other *Brachyspira* species are considered to be commensals. The most economically significant infections with these "intestinal spirochetes" occur in pigs, although infections in adult poultry are also common and are potentially important.

Brachyspira Infections in Pigs

Brachyspira spp. are associated with two diseases in pigs. Swine dysentery (SD) is a severe mucohemorrhagic colitis and results in diarrhea and dysentery in weaner and grower or finisher pigs that can be fatal if not treated (64). The essential etiological agent of SD is *B. hyodysenteriae*, and due to the great economic impact of the disease, this is the best studied of the *Brachyspira* species. A second species, *B. pilosicoli*, causes a milder colitis, called porcine colonic spirochetosis (PCS) or porcine intestinal spirochetosis (63). A recent study has shown that *B. pilosicoli* is commonly isolated from pigs in herds with diarrheal problems and poor performance (72).

Brachyspira Infections in Chickens

Infections with *Brachyspira* spp. have been associated with wet-litter problems and/or reduced egg production in laying hens and broiler breeder hens in different parts of the world. The potentially pathogenic species that may be involved are *B. intermedia*, *B. pilosicoli*, and *B. alvinipulli* (161). Broilers can be colonized with intestinal spirochetes, but this does not seem to be a clinical problem in the field. Experimental infection with *B. intermedia* caused reduced egg production and wet droppings (65), while *B. pilosicoli* caused reduced egg production (162). Besides the economic losses associated with reduced egg production, the wet droppings lead to downgrading of table eggs due to fecal staining of eggshells.

Brachyspira Infections in Other Animal Species

Brachyspira spp. have been recovered from the feces and intestines of a range of other animal species, including dogs, cats, cattle, and horses. *B. pilosicoli* is considered to be a potential cause of diarrhea in dogs.

Antimicrobial Resistance in *Brachyspira* spp.

Occurrence of antimicrobial resistance in *B. hyodysenteriae*

The drugs most commonly used for the treatment of SD are the pleuromutilins (tiamulin and valnemulin), as well as tylosin and lincomycin. Of these, the pleuromutilins are considered the most suitable antimicrobial agents available for the treatment of SD (23, 31, 87, 93, 111, 112, 142, 173, 176). For more than 20 years tiamulin has been an effective drug against SD, but recently in several countries, such as the United Kingdom (59), the Czech Republic (98), and Sweden (159), a decreased susceptibility to tiamulin among *B. hyodysenteriae* isolates has been reported. As illustrated in Fig. 1, isolates for which pleuromutilins have high MICs also have been reported from Germany (86, 140). In vitro studies indicate that development of tiamulin resistance is a slow and gradual process in *B. hyodysenteriae* (84).

High levels of resistance to tylosin and lincomycin have been reported in *B. hyodysenteriae*, and in many countries nearly all isolates tested are resistant, e.g., various studies have shown resistance rates of 100% (69), 97% (68), 95% (91), 100% (142), 87% (151), and 89% (159). The widespread tylosin resistance is not surprising considering the selective pressure exerted on the spirochetes from the frequent use of tylosin, both as a therapeutic agent and as a growth promoter in swine production. Furthermore, the resistance to tylosin is caused by a single point mutation, and tylosin resistance in *B. hyodysenteriae* can develop within two weeks in vitro (83).

Aivlosin (3-acetyl-4′-isovaleryltylosin), a chemically modified tylosin, is used for treatment of SD in some countries. There are a few reports on aivlosin susceptibility, but the mutation causing tylosin resistance also seems to be associated with a slightly increased aivlosin MIC. Isolates for which MICs are even higher also have been found, indicating that other resistance mechanisms may exist (88).

Because of the withdrawal of a number of drugs previously authorized for use in pigs and reduced susceptibility among *B. hyodysenteriae* isolates, the antibiotic arsenal available for treating SD is diminishing. Since the European Union's ban on all but four growth promoters in 1999, virginiamycin, olaquindox, carbadox, and the nitroimidazoles are no longer available for use in the control of SD. In other parts of the world some of these substances, as well as salinomycin, gentamicin, bacitracin, and isovaleryltylosin, are still used for treatment and/or growth promotion.

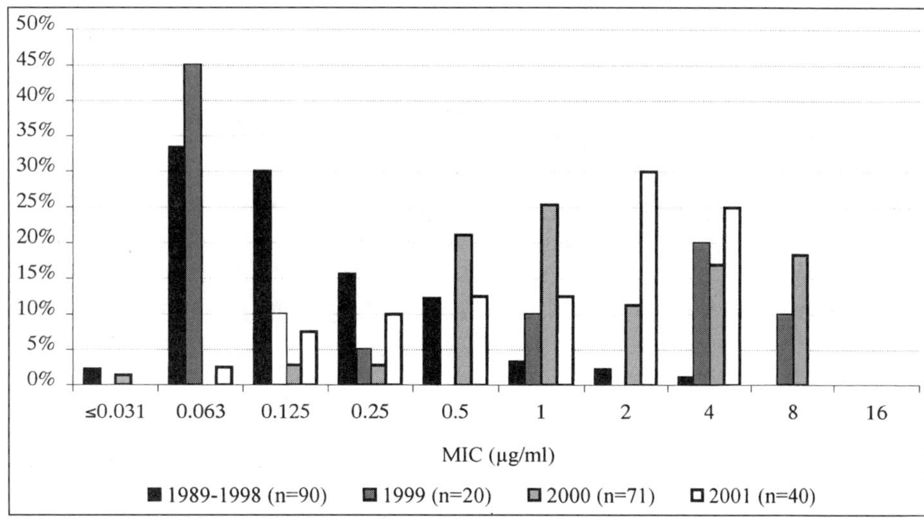

Figure 1. Distribution of MICs of tiamulin for 221 German field isolates of *B. hyodysenteriae* isolated between 1989 and 2001. Adapted from reference 86.

Occurrence of antimicrobial resistance in *B. pilosicoli*

A number of antimicrobial agents that are effective against *B. hyodysenteriae*, including tiamulin, valnemulin, carbadox, dimetridazole, and to a lesser extent lincomycin, have been shown to have low MICs when tested against collections of porcine *B. pilosicoli* isolates (27, 31, 41, 54, 68, 92, 171). Fewer isolates have been found to be susceptible to tylosin (31, 68, 92, 130). In many countries tiamulin is the drug of choice for treatment of PCS. Hence, of great concern is the recent emergence of *B. pilosicoli* strains resistant to tiamulin among field isolates obtained from pigs (54, 130). Treatment failure for PCS using tiamulin in a Swedish pig herd, where tiamulin-resistant *B. pilosicoli* isolates were found, was reported in 2002 (85).

Only a few isolates of *B. pilosicoli* from dogs and poultry have been studied for antimicrobial susceptibility (4, 53, 128, 170). Generally, these isolates were susceptible to more antimicrobial agents than the pig isolates. Treatment of infected layer hens is problematic, because of potential antimicrobial residues in the eggs; hence, antimicrobial susceptibility testing of intestinal spirochete isolates is rarely undertaken.

Antimicrobial susceptibility testing of *Brachyspira* spp.

Susceptibility testing of *Brachyspira* spp. has been performed predominantly by the agar dilution procedure. The most common medium used is Trypticase soy agar supplemented with 5% bovine or ovine blood (42, 68, 91, 94, 142, 151, 171). The MIC has been determined as the lowest concentration of the antimicrobial agent that prevents growth or hemolysis.

Broth dilution has been used for susceptibility testing of *B. hyodysenteriae* in a few studies. A broth dilution procedure with antimicrobial agents dried in tissue culture trays has been evaluated for different *Brachyspira* spp. (87). For pleuromutilins, these broth dilution panels have been compared with conventional agar dilution (140). Both methods gave reproducible results, but the broth method on average gave MICs lower by one twofold dilution.

Genetic basis of antimicrobial resistance in *Brachyspira* spp.

Point mutations. Resistance to macrolides in *B. hyodysenteriae* and *B. pilosicoli* has limited the usefulness of these drugs. Point mutations in nucleotide position 2058 of the 23S rRNA gene (*E. coli* numbering) cause macrolide and lincosamide resistance in *B. hyodysenteriae*, and mutations in positions 2058 and 2059 do the same in *B. pilosicoli* (83, 89). In vitro-selected tylosin-resistant isolates of *Brachyspira* spp. from dogs had a mutation in nucleotide position 2062 of the 23S rRNA gene (128). There is only one copy each of the rRNA genes in both *B. hyodysenteriae* and *B. pilosicoli* (183, 184), and single-step mutations in 23S rRNA consequently dominate.

Recently, in vitro development of resistance to coumermycin A_1 in *B. hyodysenteriae* was reported

(156). The resistance was associated with single-nucleotide mutations in the *gyr*(B) gene (encoding the GyrB subunit of DNA gyrase). Coumarins are not used for treatment of infections with *Brachyspira* spp., and this study was performed to evaluate this resistance as a selective marker for genetic studies.

Both tiamulin and valnemulin are used exclusively in veterinary medicine. During the 1970s and 1980s studies on the mode of action of the pleuromutilin derivatives showed that tiamulin inhibits prokaryotic protein biosynthesis by binding to the ribosome. It was concluded that either the binding of puromycin (to the A-site) was blocked or the peptidyltransferase was affected (67). No pleuromutilin derivative was successfully developed for human therapy, and the research concerning this group of antibiotics was discontinued. Subsequently, Poulsen and colleagues demonstrated that tiamulin and valnemulin are strong inhibitors of peptidyltransferase; they interact with domain V of 23S rRNA, giving chemical footprints at nucleotides 2506 and 2584–2585 (127).

The first mechanism described for tiamulin resistance was a mutation in ribosomal protein L3 (24). The mutation was selected for in *E. coli* in the laboratory. This finding led to further studies searching for the corresponding mutation in *Brachyspira* spp. Recently, three different mutations in the ribosomal protein L3 gene and six mutations in the 23S rRNA gene that are associated with tiamulin resistance in *B. hyodysenteriae* and *B. pilosicoli* were described (129). Only one of the L3 mutations was found in resistant field isolates, and the results suggest that other nonribosomal mechanisms of resistance may be present.

Transduction. An inducible prophage designated VSH-1 (virus of *Serpulina hyodysenteriae*) has been shown to transduce genes between *B. hyodysenteriae* strains in vitro (70). The DNA in VSH-1 is 7.5 kb, linear, double stranded, and seems to consist of random fragments from the host DNA. In the 1970s bacteriophages that appeared spontaneously in cultures of *B. hyodysenteriae* were demonstrated using the electron microscope (136, 137). Even though there is no direct evidence, there is a possibility that VSH-1 can transfer resistance genes between *B. hyodysenteriae* cells in vivo. The wide distribution of the bacteriophage was demonstrated in a recent study in which VSH-1 was found in 27 strains of six different *Brachyspira* spp. (157).

In the coumermycin A_1 study mentioned above, gene transfer occurred in broth culture after overnight incubation. No transfer was detected when antiserum to VSH-1 was added, but when the phage was induced, the transfer increased fivefold. Hence, it was concluded that VSH-1 was probably responsible for the gene transfer (156).

Transferable genes. The role of plasmids or other possible transferable genetic elements in the spread of antimicrobial resistance genes within and between *Brachyspira* spp. has not been clarified. The presence of plasmids in *B. hyodysenteriae* isolates has been reported (3, 77), but no plasmid has been characterized. When a physical and genetic map was constructed for the *B. hyodysenteriae* type strain, $B78^T$, no extrachromosomal DNA was found (183).

Some strains of *B. pilosicoli* from pigs (and humans) have been shown to be resistant to amoxicillin, with susceptibility being restored by clavulanic acid. This implies the presence of beta-lactamase enzyme(s) in these strains (27). Such beta-lactamase activity has been shown to be membrane bound and noninducible in human strains of intestinal spirochetes (169). Currently, it is unclear whether the genes encoding these enzymes have been acquired from other bacterial species, although this is being investigated.

Antimicrobial resistance epidemiology

Pulsed-field gel electrophoresis (PFGE) has been shown to be suitable for genotyping of *Brachyspira* spp. at a level that is sufficiently discriminatory for epidemiological studies (9, 52). To investigate whether the spread of tiamulin resistance is associated with one clone, or if it has emerged independently in different strains, PFGE was applied to a set of resistant *B. hyodysenteriae* isolates from northwestern Germany and the United Kingdom (88). The German isolates originated from a larger region and from a longer time period than the British isolates. Several PFGE types were found, suggesting different sources for development of resistance. On the other hand, the resistant British isolates all had the same PFGE type, while susceptible isolates from the same region were of a different PFGE type. This suggests that a single resistant strain (clone) had spread between British piggeries through trade with pigs. This clone had the ribosomal protein L3 mutation described above.

In another study, the relationship between 13 tiamulin-resistant *B. pilosicoli* isolates from Swedish pigs was analyzed by PFGE. The isolates had 10 different PFGE patterns, suggesting that resistance is developing independently in different strains (130).

BACTEROIDES

The genus *Bacteroides* includes a large number of species of anaerobic gram-negative rods and represents one of the major genera colonizing the large intestines of humans and animals (97, 163). The species that comprise the *B. fragilis* group are most commonly identified in diseased animals and humans and are associated with conditions such as intra-abdominal abscesses, soft tissue infections, and bacteremia. Strains of *B. fragilis* that produce enterotoxins also cause diarrhea in lambs, calves, piglets, foals, infant rabbits, and children.

Depending on their origin, strains of *Bacteroides* spp. recovered from humans are frequently resistant to one or more antimicrobial agents, particularly to the beta-lactams, tetracycline, and clindamycin (119). Resistance to penicillin and ciprofloxacin is almost universal (5). The prime mechanism for beta-lactam resistance is through production of beta-lactamases; resistance to tetracycline is mediated by ribosomal protection by the *tet*(Q) class; resistance to clindamycin is mediated by ribosomal modification (133). Resistance to metronidazole is associated with reduced uptake; altered reduction of the nitro group, mediated through the *nim* genes, is less commonly encountered (49, 55, 165). Quinolone resistance associated with *gyrA* mutations also has been recorded in *B. fragilis* group strains from humans (118).

Information about antimicrobial agent susceptibilities in animal strains of *Bacteroides* is far more limited than it is for human strains. In an early study of the susceptibility of 129 strains of *Bacteroides* spp. from swine abscesses, clindamycin, penicillin, ampicillin, minocycline, chloramphenicol, and cefoxitin all were highly active against most strains (19). In comparison, in another early study analyzing 702 clinical isolates of *Bacteroides* species from a number of animal species, 167 (24%) were resistant to penicillin, ampicillin, and cephalothin, and 64 (9% of the total) of the resistant strains also were resistant to tetracycline (66). Clindamycin, chloramphenicol, and metronidazole were active against all strains. In more recent studies, Cohen et al. found that all *Bacteroides* isolates from the uteri of dairy cows were susceptible to clindamycin, and all but two were susceptible to metronidazole (32). The MIC_{90} of tetracycline was >256 mg/liter. Among 113 *Bacteroides* clinical isolates from cats and dogs, 29% were resistant to ampicillin and 17% to clindamycin (74). All ampicillin-resistant strains had beta-lactamase activity. They were susceptible to amoxicillin-clavulanic acid and to chloramphenicol, and nearly all were susceptible to metronidazole. In another study of clinical anaerobic isolates from various animal species, resistant strains mainly belonged to the *B. fragilis* group, with 18% being resistant to penicillin and 20% to tetracycline (48). All were susceptible to metronidazole.

In summary, clinical isolates of *Bacteroides* spp. from various animal species tend to have a similar spectrum of resistance to those from humans, although in general, resistant strains occur less commonly. This is most obvious with penicillin resistance, which is almost universal in human isolates but which still only occurred in 20 to 30% of animal isolates in the late 1990s. More up-to-date data on animal *Bacteroides* isolates are clearly needed, to determine whether there has been an upward trend in these resistance figures, lagging behind a similar trend in human isolates. Mechanisms of antimicrobial resistance in animal isolates of *Bacteroides* species have not been investigated in detail but presumably are similar to those found in isolates from humans.

FUSOBACTERIUM

The genus *Fusobacterium* includes a number of species of gram-negative rods with tapering or fusiform ends, of which *F. necrophorum* is a major animal pathogen (73). In humans *F. nucleatum* is the most common species recovered from clinical isolates, and it is also common among isolates from cats and dogs (74). *F. necrophorum* is a normal inhabitant of the mouth and gastrointestinal and urogenital tracts and is present in soil. It is classified into subspecies *necrophorum* and *funduliforme* (formerly biotypes or biovars A and B), which have different morphology, growth patterns, and biochemical and biological characteristics (116). *F. necrophorum* causes a variety of necrotic infections ("necrobacillosis"), often with polymicrobial involvement, including necrotic stomatitis of calves, lambs, and pigs; foot rot in cattle and sheep; gangrenous dermatitis in horses and mules; pulmonary and hepatic abscesses in cattle and pigs; and jaw abscesses in wild ruminants and marsupials (164). The most economically important infections in cattle are hepatic necrobacillosis (liver abscesses), necrotic laryngitis (calf diphtheria), and interdigital necrobacillosis (foot rot).

There is a considerable amount of data on human infections with *Fusobacterium* species, sometimes associated with isolates from bite wounds. Goldstein et al. compared susceptibility amongst isolates from animal bite wounds with those from human bite wounds (57). Three of 12 animal isolates of *F. nucleatum* were beta-lactamase producers, while none of 14 human isolates were. In a contemporaneous large multicenter survey of infections involving anaerobic bacteria in the United States, only 2 of 22 human clinical isolates of *Fusobacterium* spp. were resistant to penicillin and clindamycin, and one to ciprofloxacin and trovafloxacin (5). The other isolates were susceptible to a range of beta-lactams and to metronidazole. In contrast, much higher levels of resistance were found among 19 clinical isolates from humans in Taiwan (165).

In an early study of the antimicrobial susceptibility of animal isolates of *Fusobacterium*, 86 isolates from various animal species were all found to be susceptible to penicillin, ampicillin, cephalothin, chloramphenicol, clindamycin, tetracycline, and metronidazole (66). Similarly, Jang et al. found that 25 *Fusobacterium* spp. isolates from cats and dogs were all susceptible to ampicillin, metronidazole, chloramphenicol, and clindamycin (74). In a contemporaneous study of 13 beta-lactam and 22 non-beta-lactam antimicrobial agents tested against 100 *Fusobacterium* spp. isolates from hepatic abscesses in cattle and sheep in Spain, only one of the beta-lactams (cefotetan) was not active against all the isolates (109). As expected, there was variable and often high in vitro resistance to aminoglycosides, while the macrolides generally had good activity. For clindamycin, 42% of isolates were resistant, and all were resistant to bacitracin. Among 37 U.S. isolates of *F. necrophorum* from hepatic abscesses, most were susceptible to penicillins, tetracyclines, lincosamides, and macrolides, whilst most were resistant to aminoglycosides, ionophores (except narasin), glycopeptides, and polymyxin (96). Continuous feeding of cattle with either tylosin or chloramphenicol did not increase the associated MICs among the clinical isolates. In a recent study, the susceptibilities to 25 antimicrobial agents of 108 *Fusobacterium* spp. isolates from cases of foot rot in sheep in Spain and Portugal were examined (76). Generally, the beta-lactam agents had good activity against most isolates, including *F. necrophorum*, although beta-lactam resistance occurred in other *Fusobacterium* spp. The aminoglycosides were ineffective against the majority of isolates. Among the macrolides, resistance to erythromycin and spiramycin was seen in 77% and 60% of isolates, respectively. Most isolates were susceptible to chloramphenicol, the lincosamides, and metronidazole, while the activity of different tetracyclines varied, with 68.5% of isolates being susceptible to oxytetracycline. In summary, animal isolates of *Fusobacterium* spp. generally remain susceptible to a wide range of antimicrobial agents.

DICHELOBACTER NODOSUS

Dichelobacter (*Bacteroides*) *nodosus* is a large gram-negative rod and is the primary etiologic agent of ovine foot rot, an economically important disease primarily affecting sheep and goats. Cattle, deer, and pigs may develop a mild form of foot rot. Lesions of foot rot commence in the epithelium of the interdigital space and then progress through the soft horn of the hoof, with the severity of underrunning of the hoof ranging from mild to severe. The infection is polymicrobial, usually involving *F. necrophorum*, *Arcanobacterium pyogenes*, and *Spirochaeta penortha*, but it does not develop into true foot rot without the presence of *D. nodosus*. Furthermore, severe (progressive) foot rot is only caused by virulent strains of *D. nodosus*, i.e., strains that characteristically produce heat-stable proteases. The clinical expression of foot rot is also influenced by host and environmental factors (36, 47).

In some legislative jurisdictions, such as the state of Western Australia, virulent foot rot is notifiable and subject to compulsory eradication; hence, antimicrobial treatment is not appropriate. Control of foot rot usually involves visual assessment of lesions, followed by either culling for severely affected individuals or treatment. The latter involves paring the hoof to remove necrotic debris and horn, then standing the animals in a footbath containing topical bactericidal agents, such as a 5% solution of copper sulfate or a 10% solution of zinc sulfate. The treated sheep then are moved to pastures that have not been contaminated with the bacteria (which survive no longer than 14 days on the pasture) and are checked after 3 to 4 weeks (105).

Antibiotic treatment is generally effective as a means for the control of foot rot, particularly if applied in dry conditions. The feet do not need to be pared, although treated sheep should be moved to clean pastures before being reinspected after 3 to 4 weeks. Antimicrobial agents that have proved effective in this setting include penicillin-streptomycin (43), erythromycin (134), long-acting oxytetracycline (82), and lincomycin-spectinomycin (172).

Early studies on the in vitro susceptibility of 18 U.S. strains of *D. nodosus* indicated that penicillin was the most effective antimicrobial, followed by cefamandole, clindamycin, tetracycline, chloramphenicol, erythromycin, cefoxitin, tylosin, nitrofurazone, tinidazole, and dihydrostreptomycin (58). Later studies on isolates from goats ($n = 37$) and sheep ($n = 68$) in Spain found more resistance to penicillin, to three aminoglycosides, and to tetracycline (123, 124). Chloramphenicol was found to be highly active in both studies, although its use in treating food-producing animals is now restricted worldwide. More recent in vitro MIC data for 69 strains of *D. nodosus* isolated from sheep with foot rot in Spain and Portugal have become available (76). The strains were tested against 25 antimicrobial agents, and 90% were susceptible at the MIC breakpoint to penicillin and ampicillin, kanamycin, streptomycin, erythromycin, spiramycin, tylosin, chloramphenicol, and enrofloxacin. The percentage of strains resistant to the remaining antimicrobial agents were as follows: gentamicin (40%), neomycin (60%), flumequine (31%), metronidazole (17.5%), oxytetracycline (42%), doxycycline (14%), and trimethoprim (10%). Generally, the levels of resistance remain relatively low, perhaps associated with the generally infrequent use of antibiotics in small ruminants. The presence of strains with reduced susceptibility to the beta-lactams and, in particular, the tetracyclines may reflect the selective pressure associated with their use to control foot rot. Mechanisms of antimicrobial resistance in *D. nodosus* to these drugs do not appear to have been studied.

CONCLUSIONS

One major theme emerges when antimicrobial susceptibilities of anaerobic bacteria from animals are considered: for many of these species, including the pathogenic ones, there is a comparative paucity of recent comprehensive and comparable data available. Most studies emanate from point prevalence studies and give little information about trends in the development of resistance. Where data are available, they suggest that the susceptibility of some of these species to different antimicrobial agents is decreasing, presumably in line with their continuing therapeutic usage. This development mirrors what is happening in the aerobic bacterial species and has important implications for treatment and control of the associated diseases in animals in the future. Furthermore, it suggests that some anaerobic species may increasingly act as reservoirs of resistance genes. Clearly, much additional work is required to increase our knowledge about these important issues.

REFERENCES

1. **Abraham, L. J., and J. I. Rood.** 1985. Molecular analysis of transferable tetracycline resistance plasmids from *Clostridium perfringens*. *J. Bacteriol.* **161:**636–640.
2. **Ackermann, G., A. Degner, S. H. Cohen, J. Silva, Jr., and A. C. Rodloff.** 2003. Prevalence and association of macrolide–lincosamide–streptogramin B (MLS_B) resistance with resistance to moxifloxacin in *Clostridium difficile*. *J. Antimicrob. Chemother.* **51:**599–603.
3. **Adachi, Y., M. Hara, K. Hirano, P. Poomvises, and P. Ingkaninun.** 1994. Biological properties of *Serpulina hyodysenteriae* and *Serpulina innocens* like organism with plasmid DNAs, p. 147. *In Proceedings of the 13th International Pig Veterinary Society Congress.*
4. **Adachi, Y., C. Tasu, T. Tanaka, K. Kajiwara, and T. Tanaka.** 2004. *Brachyspira pilosicoli* isolated from pigs and dogs in Japan and the susceptibility to 14 antibiotics, p. 268. *In Proceedings of the 18th International Pig Veterinary Society Congress.*
5. **Aldridge, K. E., D. Ashcraft, K. Cambre, C. L. Pierson, S. G. Jenkins, and J. E. Rosenblatt.** 2001. Multicenter survey of the changing in vitro antimicrobial susceptibilities of clinical isolates of *Bacteroides fragilis* group, *Prevotella, Fusobacterium, Porphyromonas,* and *Peptostreptococcus* species. *Antimicrob. Agents Chemother.* **45:**1238–1243.
6. **Andersson, G., L. Ekman, I. Månsson, S. Persson, S. Rubarth, and G. Tufvesson.** 1971. Lethal complications following administration of oxytetracycline in the horse. *Nord. Vet. Med.* **23:**9–22.
7. **Appelbaum P. C., S. K. Spangler, and M. R. Jacobs.** 1990. Beta-lactamase production and susceptibilities to amoxicillin, amoxicillin-clavulanate, ticarcillin, ticarcillin-clavulanate, cefoxitin, imipenem, and metronidazole of 320 non-*Bacteroides fragilis Bacteroides* isolates and 129 fusobacteria from 28 U.S. centers. *Antimicrob. Agents Chemother.* **34:**1546–1550.
8. **Aronsson, B., R. Möllby, and C. E. Nord.** 1985. Antimicrobial agents and *Clostridium difficile* in acute enteric disease: epidemiological data from Sweden, 1980–1982. *J. Infect. Dis.* **151:**476–481.
9. **Atyeo, R. F., S. L. Oxberry, and D. J. Hampson.** 1999. Analysis of *Serpulina hyodysenteriae* strain variation and its molecular epidemiology using pulsed-field gel electrophoresis. *Epidemiol. Infect.* **123:**133–138.
10. **Bannam, T. L., and J. I. Rood.** 1991. Relationship between the *Clostridium perfringens catQ* gene product and chloramphenicol acetyltransferases from other bacteria. *Antimicrob. Agents Chemother.* **35:**471–476.
11. **Barbut, F., D. Decre, B. Burghoffer, D. Lesage, F. Delisle, V. Lalande, M. Delmee, V. Avesani, N. Sano, C. Coudert, and J. C. Petit.** 1999. Antimicrobial susceptibilities and serogroups of clinical strains of *Clostridium difficile* isolated in France in 1991 and 1997. *Antimicrob. Agents Chemother.* **43:**2607–2611.
12. **Båverud, V., A. Gustafsson, A. Franklin, A. Lindholm, and A. Gunnarsson.** 1997. *Clostridium difficile* associated with acute colitis in mature horses treated with antibiotics. *Equine Vet. J.* **29:**279–284.
13. **Båverud, V.** 2002. *Clostridium difficile* infections in animals with special reference to the horse. A review. *Vet. Q.* **24:**203–219.
14. **Båverud, V., A. Gustafsson, A. Franklin, A. Aspán, and A. Gunnarsson.** 2003. *Clostridium difficile*: prevalence in horses and environment, and antimicrobial susceptibility. *Equine Vet. J.* **35:**465–471.
15. **Båverud, V.** 2004. *Clostridium difficile* diarrhea: infection control in horses. *Vet. Clin. N. Am. Equine Pract.* **20:** 615–630.
16. **Båverud, V., A. Gunnarsson, M. Karlsson, and A. Franklin.** 2004. Antimicrobial susceptibility of equine and environmental isolates of *Clostridium difficile*. *Microb. Drug Resist.* **10:** 57–63.
17. **Beier, R., G. Amtsberg, and M. Peters.** 1994. Bakteriologische Untersuchungen zum Vorkommen und zur Bedeutung von *Clostridium difficile* beim Pferd. *Pferdeheilkunde* **10:**3–8.

18. **Benning, V. R., and J. J. Mathers.** 1999. Comparison of agar dilution and broth microdilution methods of anaerobic antimicrobial susceptibility testing using several veterinary antibiotics against *Clostridium perfringens* strains originating from porcine and avian sources. *Anaerobe* **5**:561–569.
19. **Benno, Y., and T. Mitsuoka.** 1984. Susceptibility of *Bacteroides* from swine abscesses to 13 antibiotics. *Am. J. Vet. Res.* **45**:2631–2633.
20. **Berryman, D. I., and J. I. Rood.** 1989. Cloning and hybridization analysis of *ermP*, a macrolide-lincosamide-streptogramin B resistance determinant from *Clostridium perfringens*. *Antimicrob. Agents Chemother.* **33**:1346–1353.
21. **Berryman, D. I., M. Lyristis, and J. I. Rood.** 1994. Cloning and sequence analysis of *ermQ*, the predominant macrolide-lincosamide-streptogramin B resistance gene in *Clostridium perfringens*. *Antimicrob. Agents Chemother.* **38**:1041–1046.
22. **Berryman, D. I., and J. I. Rood.** 1995. The closely related *ermB-ermAM* genes from *Clostridium perfringens*, *Enterococcus faecalis* (pAMβ1), and *Streptococcus agalactiae* (pIP501) are flanked by variants of a directly repeated sequence. *Antimicrob. Agents Chemother.* **39**:1830–1834.
23. **Binek, M., U. Wojcik, Z. Synkiewicz, T. Jakubowski, P. Poomvises, and P. Ingkaninun.** 1994. Dynamics of susceptibility of *Serpulina hyodysenteriae* to different chemotherapeutics in-vitro, p. 203. *In Proceedings of the 13th International Pig Veterinary Society Congress.*
24. **Bøsling, J., S. M. Poulsen, B. Vester, and K. S. Long.** 2003. Resistance to the peptidyl transferase inhibitor tiamulin caused by mutation of ribosomal protein L3. *Antimicrob. Agents Chemother.* **47**:2892–2896.
25. **Brazier, J. S., P. N. Levett, A. J. Stannard, K. D. Phillips, and A. T. Willis.** 1985. Antibiotic susceptibility of clinical isolates of clostridia. *J. Antimicrob. Chemother.* **15**:181–185.
26. **Brefort, G., M. Magot, H. Ionesco, and M. Sebald.** 1977. Characterization and transferability of *Clostridium perfringens* plasmids. *Plasmid* **1**:52–66.
27. **Brooke, C. J., D. J. Hampson, and T. V. Riley.** 2003. In vitro antimicrobial susceptibility of *Brachyspira pilosicoli* isolates from humans. *Antimicrob. Agents Chemother.* **47**:2354–2357.
28. **Bryan, L. E., and S. Kwan.** 1981. Mechanisms of aminoglycoside resistance of anaerobic bacteria and facultative bacteria grown anaerobically. *J. Antimicrob. Chemother.* **8**(Suppl. D): 1–8.
29. **Buogo, C., A. P. Burnens, J. Perrin, and J. Nicolet.** 1995. Presence of *Campylobacter* spp., *Clostridium difficile*, *C. perfringens* and *Salmonella* in some litters and in a kennel population of adult dogs. *Schweiz. Arch. Tierheilkd.* **137**:165–171.
30. **Chopra, I., and M. Roberts.** 2001. Tetracycline antibiotics: mode of action, applications, molecular biology, and epidemiology of bacterial resistance. *Microbiol. Mol. Biol. Rev.* **65**: 232–260.
31. **Cizek, A., J. Smola, and P. Mádr.** 1998. *In vitro* activity of six anti-dysenteric drugs on *Serpulina hyodysenteriae* and *S. pilosicoli* strains isolated in the Czech Republic, p. 135. *In Proceedings of the 15th International Pig Veterinary Society Congress.*
32. **Cohen, R. O., R. Colodner, G. Ziv, and J. Keness.** 1996. Isolation and antimicrobial susceptibility of obligate anaerobic bacteria recovered from the uteri of dairy cows with retained fetal membranes and postparturient endometritis. *Zentbl. Veterinärmed. B* **43**:193–199.
33. **Cohen, N. D., and A. M. Woods.** 1999. Characteristics and risk factors for failure of horses with acute diarrhea to survive: 122 cases (1990–1996). *J. Am. Vet. Med. Assoc.* **214**: 382–390.
34. **Daube, G., J. Mainil, B. Limbourg, and A. Kaekenbeeck.** 1992. Etude de l'antibioresistence de *Clostridium perfringens* par l'emploi de sondes genetiques. *Ann. Med. Vet.* **136**:53–56.
35. **Delmee, M., and V. Avesani.** 1988. Correlation between serogroup and susceptibility to chloramphenicol, clindamycin, erythromycin, rifampicin and tetracycline among 308 isolates of *Clostridium difficile*. *J. Antimicrob. Chemother.* **22**:325–331.
36. **Depiazzi, L. J., W. D. Roberts, C. D. Hawkins, M. A. Palmer, D. R. Pitman, N. C. McQuade, P. D. Jelinek, D. J. Devereaux, and R. J. Rippon.** 1998. Severity and persistence of footrot in Merino sheep experimentally infected with a protease thermostable strain of *Dichelobacter nodosus* at five sites. *Aust. Vet. J.* **76**:32–38.
37. **Devriese, L. A., G. Daube, J. Hommez, and F. Haesebrouck.** 1993. In vitro susceptibility of *Clostridium perfringens* isolated from farm animals to growth-enhancing antibiotics. *J. Appl. Bacteriol.* **75**:55–57.
38. **Donaldson, M. T., and J. E. Palmer.** 1999. Prevalence of *Clostridium perfringens* enterotoxin and *Clostridium difficile* toxin A in feces of horses with diarrhea and colic. *J. Am. Vet. Med. Assoc.* **215**:358–361.
39. **Droual, R., H. L. Shivaprasad, and R. P. Chin.** 1994. Coccidiosis and necrotic enteritis in turkeys. *Avian Dis.* **38**: 177–183.
40. **Drummond, L. J., J. McCoubrey, D. G. Smith, J. M. Starr, and I. R. Poxton.** 2003. Changes in sensitivity patterns to selected antibiotics in *Clostridium difficile* in geriatric inpatients over an 18-month period. *J. Med. Microbiol.* **52**: 259–263.
41. **Duhamel, G. E., J. M. Kinyon, M. R. Mathiesen, D. P. Murphy, and D. Walter.** 1998. *In vitro* activity of four antimicrobial agents against North American isolates of porcine *Serpulina pilosicoli*. *J. Vet. Diagn. Investig.* **10**:350–356.
42. **Dünser, M., H. Schweighardt, R. Pangerl, M. Awad Masalmeh, and M. Schuh.** 1997. Swine dysentery and spirochaetal diarrhoea—a comparative study of enteritis cases caused by *Serpulina*. *Wien. Tierarztl. Monatsschr.* **84**: 151–161.
43. **Egerton, J. R., I. M. Parsonson, and N. P. Graham.** 1968. Parenteral chemotherapy of ovine foot-rot. *Aust. Vet. J.* **44**: 275–283.
44. **Elwinger, K., B. Engström, O. Fossum, S. Hassan, and B. Teglöf.** 1994. Effect of coccidiostats on necrotic enteritis and performance in broiler chickens. *Swedish J. Agric. Res.* **24**:39–44.
45. **Engström, B. E., C. Fermer, A. Lindberg, E. Saarinen, V. Båverud, and A. Gunnarsson.** 2003. Molecular typing of isolates of *Clostridium perfringens* from healthy and diseased poultry. *Vet. Microbiol.* **94**:225–235.
46. **Ensink, J. M., W. R. Klein, A. Barneveld, A. S. van Miert, and A. G. Vulto.** 1996. Side effects of oral antimicrobial agents in the horse: a comparison of pivampicillin and trimethoprim/sulphadiazine. *Vet. Rec.* **138**:253–256.
47. **Escayg, A. P., J. G. Hickford, and D. W. Bullock.** 1997. Association between alleles of the ovine major histocompatibility complex and resistance to footrot. *Res. Vet. Sci.* **63**:283–287.
48. **Even, H., J. Rohde, J. Verspohl, M. Ryll, and G. Amtsberg.** 1998. Investigations into the occurrence and the antibiotic susceptibility of gram negative anaerobes of the genera *Bacteroides*, *Prevotella*, *Porphyromonas* and *Fusobacterium* in specimens obtained from diseased animals. *Berl. Munch. Tierarztl. Wochenschr.* **111**:379–386.
49. **Fang, H., C. Edlund, M. Hedberg, and C. E. Nord.** 2002. New findings in beta-lactam and metronidazole resistant *Bacteroides fragilis* group. *Int. J. Antimicrob. Agents* **19**:361–370.

50. **Farrow, K. A., D. Lyras, and J. I. Rood.** 2000. The macrolide-lincosamide-streptogramin B resistance determinant from *Clostridium difficile* 630 contains two *erm*(B) genes. *Antimicrob. Agents Chemother.* **44:**411–413.
51. **Farrow, K. A., D. Lyras, and J. I. Rood.** 2001. Genomic analysis of the erythromycin resistance element Tn*5398* from *Clostridium difficile*. *Microbiology* **147:**2717–2728.
52. **Fellström, C., M. Karlsson, B. Pettersson, U. Zimmerman, A. Gunnarsson, and A. Aspan.** 1999. Emended descriptions of indole negative and indole positive isolates of *Brachyspira (Serpulina) hyodysenteriae*. *Vet. Microbiol.* **70:**225–238.
53. **Fellström, C., U. Zimmerman, D. Jansson, A. Gunnarsson, and M. Karlsson.** 2002. *In vitro* susceptibility of avian isolates of *Brachyspira* spp. to six antimicrobial agents, p. 356. *In Proceedings of the XII International Congress of the World Veterinary Poultry Association.*
54. **Fossi, M., T. Saranpää, and E. Rautiainen.** 1999. *In vitro* sensitivity of the swine *Brachyspira* species to tiamulin in Finland 1995–1997. *Acta Vet. Scand.* **40:**355–358.
55. **Gal, M., and J. S. Brazier.** 2004. Metronidazole resistance in *Bacteroides* spp. carrying nim genes and the selection of slow-growing metronidazole-resistant mutants. *J. Antimicrob. Chemother.* **54:**109–116.
56. **Gazdzinski, P., and R. J. Julian.** 1992. Necrotic enteritis in turkeys. *Avian Dis.* **36:**792–798.
57. **Goldstein, E. J., D. M. Citron, C. V. Merriam, Y. A. Warren, K. Tyrrell, and H. Fernandez.** 2001. Comparative in vitro activity of ertapenem and 11 other antimicrobial agents against aerobic and anaerobic pathogens isolated from skin and soft tissue animal and human bite wound infections. *J. Antimicrob. Chemother.* **48:**641–651.
58. **Gradin, J. L., and J. A. Schmitz.** 1983. Susceptibility of *Bacteroides nodosus* to various antimicrobial agents. *J. Am. Vet. Med. Assoc.* **183:**434–437.
59. **Gresham, A. C., B. W. Hunt, and R. W. Dalziel.** 1998. Treatment of swine dysentery—problems of antibiotic resistance and concurrent salmonellosis. *Vet. Rec.* **143:**619.
60. **Gustafsson, A., V. Båverud, A. Gunnarsson, M. H. Rantzien, A. Lindholm, and A. Franklin.** 1997. The association of erythromycin ethylsuccinate with acute colitis in horses in Sweden. *Equine Vet. J.* **29:**314–318.
61. **Hächler, H., B. Berger-Bächi, and F. H. Kayser.** 1987. Genetic characterization of a *Clostridium difficile* erythromycin-clindamycin resistance determinant that is transferable to *Staphylococcus aureus*. *Antimicrob. Agents Chemother.* **31:** 1039–1045.
62. **Hächler, H., and F. H. Kayser.** 1993. Genetics and molecular biology of antibiotic resistance in *Clostridium difficile*: general and specific overview, p. 156–173. *In* M. Sebald (ed.), *Genetics and Molecular Biology of Anaerobic Bacteria.* Springer-Verlag, New York, N.Y.
63. **Hampson, D. J., and G. E. Duhamel.** Porcine colonic spirochetosis/intestinal spirochetosis. *In* B. E. Straw et al. (ed.), *Diseases of Swine*, 9th ed., in press. Blackwell Publishing, Oxford, United Kingdom.
64. **Hampson, D. J., C. Fellström, and J. R. Thomson.** Swine dysentery. *In* B. E. Straw et al. (ed.), *Diseases of Swine*, 9th ed., in press. Blackwell Publishing, Oxford, United Kingdom.
65. **Hampson, D. J., and A. J. McLaren.** 1999. Experimental infection of laying hens with *Serpulina intermedia* causes reduced egg production and increased faecal water content. *Avian Pathol.* **28:**113–117.
66. **Hirsh, D. C., M. C. Indiveri, S. S. Jang, and E. L. Biberstein.** 1985. Changes in prevalence and susceptibility of obligate anaerobes in clinical veterinary practice. *J. Am. Vet. Med. Assoc.* **186:**1086–1089.
67. **Hodgin, L. A., and G. Högenauer.** 1974. The mode of action of pleuromutilin derivatives. Effect on cell-free polypeptide synthesis. *Eur. J. Biochem.* **47:**527–533.
68. **Hommez, J., F. Castryck, C. Miry, A. Lein, L. A. Devriese, and F. Haesebrouck.** 1998. Susceptibility of different *Serpulina* species in pigs to antimicrobial agents. *Vlaams Diergeneeskd. Tijdschr.* **67:**32–35.
69. **Honkanen-Buzalski, T., and P. Huovinen.** 1999. Bacterial resistance to antimicrobial agents in Finland: FINRES 1999, p. 32–33. Ministry of Agriculture and Forestry and Ministry of Social Affairs and Health, Helsinki, Finland.
70. **Humphrey, S. B., T. B. Stanton, N. S. Jensen, and R. L. Zuerner.** 1997. Purification and characterization of VSH-1, a generalized transducing bacteriophage of *Serpulina hyodysenteriae*. *J. Bacteriol.* **179:**323–329.
71. **Indiveri, M. C., and D. C. Hirsh.** 1992. Tissues and exudates contain sufficient thymidine for growth of anaerobic bacteria in the presence of inhibitory levels of trimethoprim-sulfamethoxazole. *Vet. Microbiol.* **31:**235–242.
72. **Jacobson, M., C. Hård af Segerstad, A. Gunnarsson, C. Fellström, K. de Verdier Klingenberg, P. Wallgren, and M. Jensen-Waern.** 2003. Diarrhoea in the growing pig—a comparison of clinical, morphological and microbial findings between animals from good and poor performance herds. *Res. Vet. Sci.* **74:**163–169.
73. **Jang, S. S., and D. C. Hirsh.** 1994. Characterization, distribution, and microbiological associations of *Fusobacterium* spp. in clinical specimens of animal origin. *J. Clin. Microbiol.* **32:**384–387.
74. **Jang, S. S., J. E. Breher, L. A. Dabaco, and D. C. Hirsh.** 1997. Organisms isolated from dogs and cats with anaerobic infections and susceptibility to selected antimicrobial agents. *J. Am. Vet. Med. Assoc.* **210:**1610–1614.
75. **Jang, S. S., L. M. Hansen, J. E. Breher, D. A. Riley, K. G. Magdesian, J. E. Madigan, Y. J. Tang, J. Silva, Jr., and D. C. Hirsh.** 1997. Antimicrobial susceptibilities of equine isolates of *Clostridium difficile* and molecular characterization of metronidazole-resistant strains. *Clin. Infect. Dis.* **25**(Suppl. 2):S266–S267.
76. **Jimenez, R., S. Piriz, E. Mateos, and S. Vadillo.** 2004. Minimum inhibitory concentrations for 25 selected antimicrobial agents against *Dichelobacter nodosus* and *Fusobacterium* strains isolated from footrot in sheep of Portugal and Spain. *J. Vet. Med. B Infect. Dis. Vet. Public Health* **51:**245–248.
77. **Joens, L. A., A. B. Margolin, and M. J. Hewlett.** 1986. The characterization of a plasmid isolated from *Treponema hyodysenteriae* and *Treponema innocens*, abstr. H-173, p. 156. *Abstr. 86th Annu. Meet. Am. Soc. Microbiol. 1986*. American Society for Microbiology, Washington, D.C.
78. **Johansson, A., C. Greko, B. E. Engström, and M. Karlsson.** 2004. Antimicrobial susceptibility of Swedish, Norwegian and Danish isolates of *Clostridium perfringens* from poultry, and distribution of tetracycline resistance genes. *Vet. Microbiol.* **99:**251–257.
79. **Johnson, J. L., and B. S. Francis.** 1975. Taxonomy of the Clostridia: ribosomal ribonucleic acid homologies among the species. *J. Gen. Microbiol.* **88:**229–244.
80. **Johnson, S., M. H. Samore, K. A. Farrow, G. E. Killgore, F. C. Tenover, D. Lyras, J. I. Rood, P. DeGirolami, A. L. Baltch, M. E. Rafferty, S. M. Pear, and D. N. Gerding.** 1999. Epidemics of diarrhea caused by a clindamycin-resistant strain of *Clostridium difficile* in four hospitals. *N. Engl. J. Med.* **341:**1645–1651.
81. **Jones, R. L., W. S. Adney, and R. K. Shideler.** 1987. Isolation of *Clostridium difficile* and detection of cytotoxin in the feces of diarrheic foals in the absence of antimicrobial treatment. *J. Clin. Microbiol.* **25:**1225–1227.

82. **Jordan, D., J. W. Plant, H. I. Nicol, T. M. Jessep, and C. J. Scrivener.** 1996. Factors associated with the effectiveness of antibiotic treatment for ovine virulent footrot. *Aust. Vet. J.* **73:**211–215.

83. **Karlsson, M., C. Fellström, M. U. Heldtander, K.-E. Johansson, and A. Franklin.** 1999. Genetic basis of macrolide and lincosamide resistance in *Brachyspira (Serpulina) hyodysenteriae. FEMS Microbiol. Lett.* **172:**255–260.

84. **Karlsson, M., A. Gunnarsson, and A. Franklin.** 2001. Susceptibility to pleuromutilins in *Brachyspira (Serpulina) hyodysenteriae. Anim. Health Res. Rev.* **2:**59–65.

85. **Karlsson, M., A. Franklin, M. Stampe, and C. Fellström.** 2002. Treatment failure in spirochaetal diarrhoea. *Sven. Veterinartidn.* **54:**245–247.

86. **Karlsson, M., J. Rohde, M. Kessler, and A. Franklin.** 2002. Decreased susceptibility to tiamulin in German isolates of *Brachyspira hyodysenteriae,* p. 189. *In Proceedings of the 17th International Pig Veterinary Society Congress.*

87. **Karlsson, M., C. Fellström, A. Gunnarsson, A. Landén, and A. Franklin.** 2003. Antimicrobial susceptibility testing of porcine *Brachyspira (Serpulina)* species isolates. *J. Clin. Microbiol.* **41:**2596–2604.

88. **Karlsson, M., A. Aspán, A. Landen, and A. Franklin.** 2004. Further characterization of porcine *Brachyspira hyodysenteriae* isolates with decreased susceptibility to tiamulin. *J. Med. Microbiol.* **53:**281–285.

89. **Karlsson, M., C. Fellström, K.-E. Johansson, and A. Franklin.** 2004. Antimicrobial resistance in *Brachyspira pilosicoli* with special reference to point mutations in the 23S rRNA gene associated with macrolide and lincosamide resistance. *Microb. Drug Resist.* **10:**204–208.

90. **Kelly, C. P., and J. T. LaMont.** 1998. *Clostridium difficile* infection. *Annu. Rev. Med.* **49:**375–390.

91. **Kinyon, J. M., and D. L. Harris.** 1980. In vitro susceptibility of *Treponema hyodysenteriae* and *Treponema innocens* by the agar dilution method, p. 1125–1128. *In Proceedings of the Second International Symposium of Veterinary Laboratory Diagnosticians.*

92. **Kinyon, J. M., D. Murphy, C. Stryker, V. Turner, J. T. Holck, and G. Duhamel.** 2002. Minimum inhibitory concentration for US swine isolates of *Brachyspira pilosicoli* to valnemulin and four other antibiotic, p. 50. *In Proceedings of the 17th International Pig Veterinary Society Congress.*

93. **Kitai, K., M. Kashiwazaki, Y. Adachi, T. Kume, and A. Akarawa.** 1979. *In vitro* activity of 39 antimicrobial agents against *Treponema hyodysenteriae. Antimicrob. Agents Chemother.* **15:**392–395.

94. **Kitai, K., M. Kashiwazaki, Y. Adachi, K. Kunugita, and A. Arakawa.** 1987. *In vitro* antimicrobial activity against reference strains and field isolates of *Treponema hyodysenteriae. Antimicrob. Agents Chemother.* **31:**1935–1938.

95. **LeBlanc, D. J., J. M. Inamine, and L. N. Lee.** 1986. Broad geographical distribution of homologous erythromycin, kanamycin, and streptomycin resistance determinants among group D streptococci of human and animal origin. *Antimicrob. Agents Chemother.* **29:**549–555.

96. **Lechtenberg, K. F., T. G. Nagaraja, and M. M. Chengappa.** 1998. Antimicrobial susceptibility of *Fusobacterium necrophorum* isolated from bovine hepatic abscesses. *Am. J. Vet. Res.* **59:**44–47.

97. **Leser, T. D., J. Z. Amenuvor, T. K. Jensen, R. H. Lindecrona, M. Boye, and K. Møller.** 2002. Culture-independent analysis of gut bacteria: the pig gastrointestinal tract microbiota revisited. *Appl. Environ. Microbiol.* **68:**673–690.

98. **Lobova, D., J. Smola, and A. Cizek.** 2004. Decreased susceptibility to tiamulin and valnemulin among Czech isolates of *Brachyspira hyodysenteriae. J. Med. Microbiol.* **53:**287–291.

99. **Lyras, D., and J. I. Rood.** 1996. Genetic organization and distribution of tetracycline resistance determinants in *Clostridium perfringens. Antimicrob. Agents Chemother.* **40:**2500–2504.

100. **Lyras, D., and J. L. Rood.** 1997. Transposable genetic elements and antibiotic resistance determinants from *Clostridium perfringens* and *Clostridium difficile*, p. 73–92. *In* J. I. Rood, B. A. McClane, J. G. Songer, and R. W. Titball (ed.), *The Clostridia, Molecular Biology and Pathogenesis.* Academic Press, San Diego, Calif.

101. **Madewell, B. R., Y. J. Tang, S. Jang, J. E. Madigan, D. C. Hirsh, P. H. Gumerlock, and J. Silva, Jr.** 1995. Apparent outbreaks of *Clostridium difficile*-associated diarrhea in horses in a veterinary medical teaching hospital. *J. Vet. Diagn. Investig.* **7:**343–346.

102. **Madewell, B. R., J. K. Bea, S. A. Kraegel, M. Winthrop, Y. J. Tang, and J. Silva, Jr.** 1999. *Clostridium difficile*: a survey of fecal carriage in cats in a veterinary medical teaching hospital. *J. Vet. Diagn. Investig.* **11:**50–54.

103. **Magdesian, K. G., J. E. Madigan, D. C. Hirsh, S. S. Jang, Y. J. Tang, T. E. Carpenter, L. M. Hansen, and J. Silva.** 1997. *Clostridium difficile* and horses: a review. *Rev. Med. Microbiol.* **8:**46–48.

104. **Magdesian, K. G., D. C. Hirsh, S. S. Jang, L. M. Hansen, and J. E. Madigan.** 2002. Characterization of *Clostridium difficile* isolates from foals with diarrhea: 28 cases (1993–1997). *J. Am. Vet. Med. Assoc.* **220:**67–73.

105. **Malecki, J. C., and L. Coffey.** 1987. Treatment of ovine virulent footrot with zinc sulphate/sodium lauryl sulphate footbathing. *Aust. Vet. J.* **64:**301–304.

106. **Marks, S. L., and E. J. Kather.** 2003. Antimicrobial susceptibilities of canine *Clostridium difficile* and *Clostridium perfringens* isolates to commonly utilized antimicrobial drugs. *Vet. Microbiol.* **94:**39–45.

107. **Martel, A., L. A. Devriese, K. Cauwerts, K. De Gussem, A. Decostere, and F. Haesebrouck.** 2004. Susceptibility of *Clostridium perfringens* strains from broiler chickens to antibiotics and anticoccidials. *Avian Pathol.* **33:**3–7.

108. **Martirossian, G., B. Sokol-Leszcynska, J. Mierzejewski, and F. Meisel-Mikolajczyk.** 1992. Occurrence of *Clostridium difficile* in the digestive system of dogs. *Med. Dosw. Mikrobiol.* **44:**49–54.

109. **Mateos, E., S. Piriz, J. Valle, M. Hurtado, and S. Vadillo.** 1997. Minimum inhibitory concentrations for selected antimicrobial agents against *Fusobacterium necrophorum* isolated from hepatic abscesses in cattle and sheep. *J. Vet. Pharmacol. Ther.* **20:**21–23.

110. **McGorum, B. C., P. M. Dixon, and D. G. Smith.** 1998. Use of metronidazole in equine acute idiopathic toxaemic colitis. *Vet. Rec.* **142:**635–638.

111. **Messier, S., R. Higgins, and C. Moore.** 1990. Minimal inhibitory concentrations of five antimicrobials against *Treponema hyodysenteriae* and *Treponema innocens. J. Vet. Diagn. Investig.* **2:**330–333.

112. **Molnar, L.** 1996. Sensitivity of strains of *Serpulina hyodysenteriae* isolated in Hungary to chemotherapeutic drugs. *Vet. Rec.* **138:**158–160.

113. **Mullany, P., M. Wilks, I. Lamb, C. Clayton, B. Wren, and S. Tabaqchali.** 1990. Genetic analysis of a tetracycline resistance element from *Clostridium difficile* and its conjugal transfer to and from *Bacillus subtilis. J. Gen. Microbiol.* **136:**1343–1349.

114. **Mullany, P., M. Wilks, and S. Tabaqchali.** 1991. Transfer of Tn*916* and Tn*916* delta E into *Clostridium difficile*:

demonstration of a hot-spot for these elements in the *C. difficile* genome. *FEMS Microbiol. Lett.* **63**:191–194.

115. **Mullany, P., M. Wilks, and S. Tabaqchali.** 1995. Transfer of macrolide-lincosamide-streptogramin B (MLS) resistance in *Clostridium difficile* is linked to a gene homologous with toxin A and is mediated by a conjugative transposon, Tn*5398*. *J. Antimicrob. Chemother.* **35**:305–315.
116. **Nagaraja, T. G., and M. M. Chengappa.** 1998. Liver abscesses in feedlot cattle: a review. *J. Anim. Sci.* **76**:287–298.
117. **National Committee for Clinical Laboratory Standards.** 2004. Methods for antimicrobial susceptibility testing of anaerobic bacteria, 5th ed. Approved standard M11-A6. National Committee for Clinical Laboratory Standards, Wayne, Pa.
118. **Oh, H., N. El Amin, T. Davies, P. C. Appelbaum, and C. Edlund.** 2001. *gyrA* mutations associated with quinolone resistance in *Bacteroides fragilis* group strains. *Antimicrob. Agents Chemother.* **45**:1977–1981.
119. **Paula, G. R., L. S. Falcao, E. N. Antunes, K. E. Avelar, F. N. Reis, M. A. Maluhy, M. C. Ferreira, and R. M. Domingues.** 2004. Determinants of resistance in *Bacteroides fragilis* strains according to recent Brazilian profiles of antimicrobial susceptibility. *Int. J. Antimicrob. Agents* **24**:53–58.
120. **Pelaez, T., L. Alcala, R. Alonso, M. Rodriguez-Creixems, J. M. Garcia-Lechuz, and E. Bouza.** 2002. Reassessment of *Clostridium difficile* susceptibility to metronidazole and vancomycin. *Antimicrob. Agents Chemother.* **46**:1647–1650.
121. **Perrin, J., C. Buogo, A. Gallusser, A. P. Burnens, and J. Nicolet.** 1993. Intestinal carriage of *Clostridium difficile* in neonate dogs. *Zentbl. Veterinärmed. B* **40**:222–226.
122. **Piriz, S., J. Valle, M. A. Hurtado, E. M. Mateos, P. Martin-Palomino, and S. Vadillo.** 1995. Efficacy of the E-test in evaluating the antimicrobial susceptibility of anaerobic bacteria of veterinary interest. *Lett. Appl. Microbiol.* **20**:345–348.
123. **Piriz Duran, S., J. Valle Manzano, R. Cuenca Valera, and S. Vadillo Machota.** 1990. In-vitro antimicrobial susceptibility of *Bacteroides* and *Fusobacterium* isolated from footrot in goats. *Br. Vet. J.* **146**:437–442.
124. **Piriz Duran, S., R. Cuenca Valera, J. Valle Manzano, and S. Vadillo Machota.** 1991. Comparative *in vitro* susceptibility of *Bacteroides* and *Fusobacterium* isolated from footrot in sheep to 28 antimicrobial agents. *J. Vet. Pharmacol. Ther.* **14**:185–192.
125. **Poilane, I., P. Cruaud, J. C. Torlotin, and A. Collignon.** 2000. Comparison of the E test to the reference agar dilution method for antibiotic susceptibility testing of *Clostridium difficile*. *Clin. Microbiol. Infect.* **6**:155–156.
126. **Post, K. W., and J. G. Songer.** 2004. Antimicrobial susceptibility of *Clostridium difficile* isolated from neonatal pigs with enteritis. *Anaerobe* **10**:47–50.
127. **Poulsen, S. M., M. Karlsson, L. B. Johansson, and B. Vester.** 2001. The pleuromutilin drugs tiamulin and valnemulin bind to the RNA at the peptidyl transferase centre on the ribosome. *Mol. Microbiol.* **41**:1091–1099.
128. **Prapasarakul, N., K. Ochi, and Y. Adachi.** 2003. *In vitro* susceptibility and a new point mutation associated with tylosin-resistance in Japanese canine intestinal spirochetes. *J. Vet. Med. Sci.* **65**:1275–1280.
129. **Pringle, M., J. Poehlsgaard, B. Vester, and K. S. Long.** 2004. Mutations in ribosomal protein L3 and 23S ribosomal RNA at the peptidyl transferase centre are associated with reduced susceptibility to tiamulin in *Brachyspira* spp. isolates. *Mol. Microbiol.* **54**:1295–1306.
130. **Pringle, M., A. Landén, and A. Franklin.** Tiamulin resistance in Swedish *Brachyspira pilosicoli* isolates. *Res. Vet. Sci.*, in press.
131. **Quinn, P. J., M. E. Carter, B. Markey, and G. R. Carter.** 1994. *Clostridium* species, p. 191–208. *In* J. I. Rood, B. A. McClane, J. G. Songer, and R. W. Titball (ed.), *Clinical Veterinary Microbiology*. Wolfe Publishing, Mosby-Year Book Europe Ltd., London, United Kingdom.
132. **Raisbeck, M. F., G. R. Holt, and G. D. Osweiler.** 1981. Lincomycin-associated colitis in horses. *J. Am. Vet. Med. Assoc.* **179**:362–363.
133. **Rasmussen, B. A., K. Bush, and F. P. Tally.** 1993. Antimicrobial resistance in Bacteroides. *Clin. Infect. Dis.* **16**(Suppl. 4):S390–S400.
134. **Rendell, D. K., and A. P. Callinan.** 1997. Comparison of erythromycin and oxytetracycline for the treatment of virulent footrot in grazing sheep. *Aust. Vet. J.* **75**:354.
135. **Riley, T. V., J. E. Adams, G. L. O'Neill, and R. A. Bowman.** 1991. Gastrointestinal carriage of *Clostridium difficile* in cats and dogs attending veterinary clinics. *Epidemiol. Infect.* **107**:659–665.
136. **Ritchie, A. E., and L. N. Brown.** 1971. An agent possibly associated with swine dysentery. *Vet. Rec.* **89**:608–609.
137. **Ritchie, A. E., I. M. Robinson, L. A. Joens, and J. M. Kinyon.** 1978. A bacteriophage for *Treponema hyodysenteriae*. *Vet. Rec.* **103**:34–35.
138. **Roberts, M. C., L. V. McFarland, P. Mullany, and M. E. Mulligan.** 1994. Characterization of the genetic basis of antibiotic resistance in *Clostridium difficile*. *J. Antimicrob. Chemother.* **33**:419–429.
139. **Roberts, M. C.** 2003. Acquired tetracycline and/or macrolide-lincosamides-streptogramin resistance in anaerobes. *Anaerobe* **9**:63–69.
140. **Rohde, J., M. Kessler, C. G. Baums, and G. Amtsberg.** 2004. Comparison of methods for antimicrobial susceptibility testing and MIC values for pleuromutilin drugs for *Brachyspira hyodysenteriae* isolated in Germany. *Vet. Microbiol.* **102:** 25–32.
141. **Rollins, L. D., L. N. Lee, and D. J. LeBlanc.** 1985. Evidence for a disseminated erythromycin resistance determinant mediated by Tn*917*-like sequences among group D streptococci isolated from pigs, chickens, and humans. *Antimicrob. Agents Chemother.* **27**:439–444.
142. **Rønne, H., and J. Szancer.** 1990. In vitro susceptibility of Danish field isolates of *Treponema hyodysenteriae* to chemotherapeutics in swine dysentery (SD) therapy. Interpretation of MIC results based on the pharmacokinetic properties of the antibacterial agents, p. 126. *In Proceedings of the 11th International Pig Veterinary Society Congress.*
143. **Rood, J. I., E. A. Maher, E. B. Somers, E. Campos, and C. L. Duncan.** 1978. Isolation and characterization of multiply antibiotic-resistant *Clostridium perfringens* strains from porcine feces. *Antimicrob. Agents Chemother.* **13**:871–880.
144. **Rood, J. I., J. R. Buddle, A. J. Wales, and R. Sidhu.** 1985. The occurrence of antibiotic resistance in *Clostridium perfringens* from pigs. *Aust. Vet. J.* **62**:276–279.
145. **Rood, J. I., and S. T. Cole.** 1991. Molecular genetics and pathogenesis of *Clostridium perfringens*. *Microbiol. Rev.* **55**:621–648.
146. **Rosenblatt, J. E., and D. R. Gustafson.** 1995. Evaluation of the Etest for susceptibility testing of anaerobic bacteria. *Diagn. Microbiol. Infect. Dis.* **22**:279–284.
147. **Salyers, A. A., A. Gupta, and Y. Wang.** 2004. Human intestinal bacteria as reservoirs for antibiotic resistance genes. *Trends Microbiol.* **12**:412–416.
148. **Sasaki, Y., K. Yamamoto, Y. Tamura, and T. Takahashi.** 2001. Tetracycline-resistance genes of *Clostridium perfringens*, *Clostridium septicum* and *Clostridium sordellii* isolated from cattle affected with malignant edema. *Vet. Microbiol.* **83**:61–69.
149. **Sebald, M.** 1994. Genetic basis for antibiotic resistance in anaerobes. *Clin. Infect. Dis.* **18**(Suppl. 4):297–304.

150. **Sloan, J., L. M. McMurry, D. Lyras, S. B. Levy, and J. I. Rood.** 1994. The *Clostridium perfringens* Tet P determinant comprises two overlapping genes: *tetA*(P), which mediates active tetracycline efflux, and *tetB*(P), which is related to the ribosomal protection family of tetracycline-resistance determinants. *Mol. Microbiol.* **11:**403–415.

151. **Smith, S. C., T. Muir, M. Holmes, and P. J. Coloe.** 1991. In vitro antimicrobial susceptibility of Australian isolates of *Treponema hyodysenteriae*. *Aust. Vet. J.* **68:**408–409.

152. **Songer, J. G.** 1996. Clostridial enteric diseases of domestic animals. *Clin. Microbiol. Rev.* **9:**216–234.

153. **Songer, J. G., K. W. Post, and D. J. Larson.** 2000. Infection of neonatal swine with *Clostridium difficile*. *J. Swine Health Prod.* **8:**185–189.

154. **Spigaglia, P., and P. Mastrantonio.** 2002. Analysis of macrolide-lincosamide-streptogramin B (MLS(B)) resistance determinant in strains of *Clostridium difficile*. *Microb. Drug Resist.* **8:**45–53.

155. **Staempfli, H. R., J. F. Prescott, and M. L. Brash.** 1992. Lincomycin-induced severe colitis in ponies: association with *Clostridium cadaveris*. *Can. J. Vet. Res.* **56:**168–169.

156. **Stanton, T. B., E. G. Matson, and S. B. Humphrey.** 2001. *Brachyspira* (*Serpulina*) *hyodysenteriae gyrB* mutants and interstrain transfer of coumermycin A_1 resistance. *Appl. Environ. Microbiol.* **67:**2037–2043.

157. **Stanton, T. B., M. G. Thompson, S. B. Humphrey, and R. L. Zuerner.** 2003. Detection of bacteriophage VSH-1 *svp38* gene in *Brachyspira* spirochetes. *FEMS Microbiol. Lett.* **224:**225–229.

158. **Stark, C. A., C. Edlund, S. Sjöstedt, G. Kristensen, and C. E. Nord.** 1993. Antimicrobial resistance in human oral and intestinal anaerobic microfloras. *Antimicrob. Agents Chemother.* **37:**1665–1669.

159. **Statens Veterinärmedicinska Anstalt.** 2004. *SVARM 2003: Swedish Veterinary Antimicrobial Resistance Monitoring.* National Veterinary Institute, Uppsala, Sweden.

160. **Steffen, C., and H. Matzura.** 1989. Nucleotide sequence analysis and expression studies of a chloramphenicol-acetyltransferase-coding gene from *Clostridium perfringens*. *Gene.* **75:**349–354.

161. **Stephens, C. P., and D. J. Hampson.** 2001. Intestinal spirochete infections of chickens: a review of disease associations, epidemiology and control. *Anim. Health Res. Rev.* **2:**83–91.

162. **Stephens, C. P., and D. J. Hampson.** 2002. Experimental infection of broiler breeder hens with the intestinal spirochaete *Brachyspira* (*Serpulina*) *pilosicoli* causes reduced egg production. *Avian Pathol.* **31:**169–175.

163. **Suau, A., R. Bonnet, M. Sutren, J. J. Godon, G. R. Gibson, M. D. Collins, and J. Dore.** 1999. Direct analysis of genes encoding 16S rRNA from complex communities reveals many novel molecular species within the human gut. *Appl. Environ. Microbiol.* **65:**4799–4807.

164. **Tan, Z. L., T. G. Nagaraja, and M. M. Chengappa.** 1996. *Fusobacterium necrophorum* infections: virulence factors, pathogenic mechanism and control measures. *Vet. Res. Commun.* **20:**113–140.

165. **Teng, L. J., P. R. Hsueh, J. C. Tsai, S. J. Liaw, S. W. Ho, and K. T. Luh.** 2002. High incidence of cefoxitin and clindamycin resistance among anaerobes in Taiwan. *Antimicrob. Agents Chemother.* **46:**2908–2913.

166. **Then, R. L., and P. Angehrn.** 1979. Low trimethoprim susceptibility of anaerobic bacteria due to insensitive dihydrofolate reductases. *Antimicrob. Agents Chemother.* **15:**1–6.

167. **Then, R. L.** 1982. Mechanisms of resistance to trimethoprim, the sulfonamides, and trimethoprim-sulfamethoxazole. *Rev. Infect. Dis.* **4:**261–269.

168. **Thomas, C., M. Stevenson, and T. V. Riley.** 2003. Antibiotics and hospital-acquired *Clostridium difficile*-associated diarrhoea: a systematic review. *J. Antimicrob. Chemother.* **51:**1339–1350.

169. **Tompkins, D. S., M. R. Millar, J. Heritage, and A. P. West.** 1987. Beta-lactamase production by intestinal spirochaetes. *J. Gen. Microbiol.* **133:**761–765.

170. **Trampel, D. W., J. M. Kinyon, and N. S. Jensen.** 1999. Minimum inhibitory concentration of selected antimicrobial agents for *Serpulina* isolated from chickens and rheas. *J. Vet. Diagn. Investig.* **11:**379–382.

171. **Trott, D. J., T. B. Stanton, N. S. Jensen, G. E. Duhamel, J. L. Johnson, and D. J. Hampson.** 1996. *Serpulina pilosicoli* sp. nov., the agent of porcine intestinal spirochetosis. *Int. J. Syst. Bacteriol.* **46:**206–215.

172. **Venning, C. M., M. A. Curtis, and J. R. Egerton.** 1990. Treatment of virulent footrot with lincomycin and spectinomycin. *Aust. Vet. J.* **67:**258–260.

173. **Walter, D. H., and J. M. Kinyon.** 1990. Recent MIC determination of six antimicrobials for *Treponema hyodysenteriae* in the United States; use of tiamulin to eliminate swine dysentery from two farrow to finish herds, p. 129. *In Proceedings of the 11th International Pig Veterinary Society Congress.*

174. **Waters, E. H., J. P. Orr, E. G. Clark, and C. M. Schaufele.** 1998. Typhlocolitis caused by *Clostridium difficile* in suckling piglets. *J. Vet. Diagn. Investig.* **10:**104–108.

175. **Watkins, K. L., T. R. Shryock, R. N. Dearth, and Y. M. Saif.** 1997. In-vitro antimicrobial susceptibility of *Clostridium perfringens* from commercial turkey and broiler chicken origin. *Vet. Microbiol.* **54:**195–200.

176. **Weber, F. H., and D. L. Earley.** 1991. Novel method for measuring growth of *Treponema hyodysenteriae* and its application for monitoring susceptibility of clinical isolates to antimicrobial agents. *Antimicrob. Agents Chemother.* **35:** 2012–2015.

177. **Weese, J. S., H. R. Staempfli, and J. F. Prescott.** 2001. A prospective study of the roles of *Clostridium difficile* and enterotoxigenic *Clostridium perfringens* in equine diarrhoea. *Equine Vet. J.* **33:**403–409.

178. **Wong, S. S., P. C. Woo, W. K. Luk, and K. Y. Yuen.** 1999. Susceptibility testing of *Clostridium difficile* against metronidazole and vancomycin by disk diffusion and Etest. *Diagn. Microbiol. Infect. Dis.* **34:**1–6.

179. **Wren, B. W., P. Mullany, C. Clayton, and S. Tabaqchali.** 1988. Molecular cloning and genetic analysis of a chloramphenicol acetyltransferase determinant from *Clostridium difficile*. *Antimicrob. Agents Chemother.* **32:**1213–1217.

180. **Wüst, J., and U. Hardegger.** 1983. Transferable resistance to clindamycin, erythromycin, and tetracycline in *Clostridium difficile*. *Antimicrob. Agents Chemother.* **23:**784–786.

181. **Yaeger, M., N. Funk, and L. Hoffman.** 2002. A survey of agents associated with neonatal diarrhea in Iowa swine including *Clostridium difficile* and porcine reproductive and respiratory syndrome virus. *J. Vet. Diagn. Investig.* **14:** 281–287.

182. **Zaidenzaig, Y., J. E. Fitton, L. C. Packman, and W. V. Shaw.** 1979. Characterization and comparison of chloramphenicol acetyltransferase variants. *Eur. J. Biochem.* **100:**609–618.

183. **Zuerner, R. L., and T. B. Stanton.** 1994. Physical and genetic map of the *Serpulina hyodysenteriae* B78^T chromosome. *J. Bacteriol.* **176:**1087–1092.

184. **Zuerner, R. L., T. B. Stanton, F. C. Minion, C. Li, N. W. Charon, D. J. Trott, and D. J. Hampson.** 2004. Genetic variation in *Brachyspira*: chromosomal rearrangements and sequence drift distinguish *B. pilosicoli* from *B. hyodysenteriae*. *Anaerobe* **10:**229–237.

Antimicrobial Resistance in Bacteria of Animal Origin
Edited by Frank M. Aarestrup

Chapter 10

Antimicrobial Resistance in Pathogenic *Escherichia coli* from Animals

David G. White

Escherichia coli, originally identified as *Bacterium coli* commune, was identified in 1885 by the German pediatrician Theodor Escherich (59). This bacterium was considered to be a ubiquitous organism for almost 50 years after its initial discovery, until it was first suspected to be the cause of an outbreak of neonatal diarrhea (54). Since then, *E. coli* has been shown to be widely distributed in the intestines of humans and warm-blooded animals and is considered the predominant facultative anaerobe in the bowel (39). Thus, *E. coli* was long considered as having low virulence and being generally beneficial to the host. There are many pathogenic *E. coli* strains, however, that can cause a variety of diseases in animals and humans. Particular pathogenic types of *E. coli* differ from those that predominate in the enteric flora of healthy animals and individuals in that they are more likely to express specific virulence factors (48).

Historically, serotyping, based on the O (somatic lipopolysaccharide), F (fimbrial), K (capsular), and H (flagellar) antigens, has been used to compare strains. Based on the 100 different K groups, 180 O groups, and 60 H antigens (and growing) described, nearly 700 different antigenic types can be determined (151). The plethora of research in this area, however, shows that a relatively small number of serogroups predominate in cases of both diarrheal and extraintestinal animal infections (140, 141). While useful for differentiating strains, serotyping alone does not indicate the presence of specific virulence factors. With the introduction of modern molecular technology, a range of specific virulence factors have been identified in distinct pathogenic strains associated with a spectrum of animal diseases, including diarrheal illness. Pathogenic types of *E. coli* are classified by their specific virulence mechanisms (e.g., toxins, adhesins, and invasiveness), serotypes, and pathogenesis. Currently, at least seven distinct classes of pathogenic *E. coli* are recognized: (i) enterotoxigenic *E. coli* (ETEC), (ii) enteropathogenic *E. coli*, (iii) enterohemorrhagic *E. coli*, (iv) enteroinvasive *E. coli*, (v) diffuse-adhering *E. coli*, (vi) necrotoxigenic *E. coli* (NTEC), and (vi) enteroaggregative *E. coli* (134, 186).

In veterinary medicine, *E. coli* infections usually manifest more frequently in young animals and are usually associated with enteritis and septicemia in a variety of domestic species including poultry, pigs, ruminants, dogs, cats, and horses. Clinical disease in these animals may be limited to the intestines (e.g., enteric colibacillosis and neonatal diarrhea) or may manifest as septicemia (e.g., colisepticemia and systemic colibacillosis) or toxemia (colibacillary toxemia) (196a). Additionally, nonenteric infections in adult animals can involve the uterus, urinary tract, and mammary glands (58, 110, 136, 137, 174). With regard to acute diarrheal disease in food animals, the cornerstone of therapy has traditionally been fluid and electrolyte replacement. However, broad-spectrum antimicrobials have also been used as primary therapeutic aids for infectious diarrheal diseases for years. Antimicrobial use in veterinary medicine is critical to the economic health of the food animal production industry. This use is focused primarily on the treatment and/or prevention of animal diseases. In veterinary medicine, diseases requiring the most extensive use of antimicrobial drugs for treatment or prophylaxis are respiratory and enteric diseases in pigs and cattle, mastitis in dairy cattle, and colibacillosis in poultry.

After several decades of successful antimicrobial use, we are seeing the emergence of multiresistant bacterial pathogens, which are less responsive to

David G. White • Division of Animal and Food Microbiology, Office of Research, Center for Veterinary Medicine, U.S. Food and Drug Administration, Laurel, MD 20708.

therapy. The emergence of antimicrobial resistance is increasing the overall mortality, morbidity, and economic costs associated with treating bacterial infections caused by resistant organisms worldwide (93, 195). Thus, addressing the issue of antimicrobial resistance is one of the most urgent priorities in the field of infectious disease today (157). The remainder of this chapter will focus on the prevalence of antimicrobial resistance phenotypes among *E. coli* isolates associated with enteric and systemic colibacillosis in minor species, cattle, pigs, and poultry, as well as bovine mastitis and uterine and urinary tract infections in companion animals.

AVIAN COLIBACILLOSIS

Colibacillosis is the primary cause of morbidity, mortality, and condemnation of carcasses in the poultry industry worldwide (18, 44, 46, 47, 69). It is an economically devastating disease for the poultry industry in the United States and many parts of the world (18, 46, 74, 113). In the past few years, both the incidence and severity of colibacillosis have increased rapidly, and current trends indicate that it is likely to continue and become an even greater problem in the poultry industry (7, 8, 17).

Although *E. coli* is present in the normal microflora of the intestinal tracts of chickens, a certain subset of extraintestinal pathogenic *E. coli*, termed avian pathogenic *E. coli* (APEC), possesses specific virulence attributes that have been associated with colibacillosis (44, 46, 47, 99, 113, 127, 197). Several of the more commonly reported virulence factors associated with APEC strains include increased serum survival (Iss), production of aerobactin and K1 capsule, presence of type 1 and P fimbriae, and temperature-sensitive hemagglutinin (Tsh) of the autotransporter group of proteins (18, 44, 46, 47, 51, 64, 99).

Approaches to prevent and control APEC infections in the poultry industry include improved hygienic methods, vaccination, use of competitive exclusion products, and the introduction of novel immunopotentiators. Each of these practices has had limited success (72, 108, 111, 112, 126). This has necessitated the use of antimicrobial chemotherapy to control outbreaks of colibacillosis. However, recent reports have described increased resistance to those antimicrobial agents commonly used for treatment (7, 8, 10, 11, 17, 41, 60, 70, 178, 192, 197).

Strains of *E. coli* displaying resistance to multiple antimicrobial agents have been recovered from the fecal flora of broiler chickens since the earliest reports in the 1960s and 1970s (27, 89, 117, 131, 164, 166, 175). One of the first studies to demonstrate resistance among *E. coli* isolates from poultry was published in 1961 in Great Britain (170). The authors noticed that from 1957 to 1960, the practice of feeding broiler fowls diets containing tetracyclines increased greatly and progressively. They further recorded the increasing incidence of tetracycline resistance among pathogenic avian *E. coli* isolates during this same time period, from 3.5% in 1957 to 20.5% in 1958, 40.9% in 1959, and 63.2% in 1960 (170). A later study reported by Smith in 1966 examined antimicrobial resistance among *E. coli* isolates obtained from cases of human neonatal diarrhea, swine diarrhea, calf scours, and avian colisepticemia (164). Among the avian *E. coli* isolates tested, resistance was most often observed to sulfonamides (17.1%), tetracyclines (17.1%), and to a lesser extent streptomycin (2.9%). Twenty-nine percent of avian isolates demonstrated resistance to one or more drugs, with the most common multidrug resistance patterns being streptomycin, tetracycline, and sulfonamides or tetracycline and sulfonamides (164).

The majority of publications from this time period echoed the same conclusions: that the antimicrobial resistance phenotypes observed reflected the wide use of antibiotics in the livestock industry and was primarily due to the presence of resistance plasmids (initially referred to as R factors) (89, 120, 131, 164, 175, 187). These experiments and others increased both the scientific and public scrutiny of the administration of therapeutic and subtherapeutic doses of antimicrobials to animals and ultimately led to the release of the Swann report in the United Kingdom in 1969, which recommended that antibiotics used to treat infections in humans not be used as animal-food additives (173). Despite implementing these recommendations, the United Kingdom and other countries have observed mixed results with regard to observing reductions in antimicrobial resistance phenotypes among pathogenic *E. coli* isolates. In fact, a survey conducted in 1980, 9 years after the banning of the use of tetracyclines as feed additives in the United Kindgdom, indicated that chickens and pigs were still a reservoir of tetracycline-resistant *E. coli* (168).

During this time, other nations were dealing with the same issues of antibiotic use in animals and development of resistance among *E. coli* and increasingly *Salmonella* (see chapter 17). For example, in the 1970s Kanai et al. in Japan examined over 2,000 *E. coli* isolates obtained from broilers for antimicrobial resistance patterns and the presence of conjugative R plasmids (104). The most common resistance pattern observed was to tetracycline, streptomycin, sulfonamides, and kanamycin and was attributed to the presence of conjugative R plasmids. Similarly, in 1980 Nazer reported a high prevalence of multiple-antibiotic resistance among *E. coli* isolated from fecal samples and the carcasses of poultry in a university farm in Iran (135). Almost all of the isolates were resistant to tetracycline, streptomycin, ampicillin, and sulfonamide. The authors noted an association between antibiotic use for prophylaxis or growth promotion and isolation of *E. coli* resistance phenotypes (135).

Data on the prevalence of antimicrobial-resistant veterinary pathogens from Asia and Africa are sparse. However, a recent report from China described the incidence of resistance among pathogenic *E. coli* isolates recovered from diseased chickens and swine (197). Seventy-one *E. coli* isolates recovered from the livers of chickens diagnosed with colibacillosis from poultry farms in Beijing and Hebei province from January to October 2000 were assayed for antimicrobial susceptibility and the presence of virulence factors. The majority of *E. coli* isolates recovered from diseased chickens were resistant to multiple classes of antimicrobials, including nalidixic acid (100%), tetracycline (100%), streptomycin (80%), sulfamethoxazole (79%), and ampicillin (77%). Surprisingly, 90% of these isolates were also resistant to the veterinary fluoroquinolone enrofloxacin (197). All the quinolone-resistant isolates possessed the typical mutations in the topoisomerase genes, *gyrA* and *parC*, reported previously (60, 87, 153). The authors concluded that a lack of restriction on antibiotic use in food animals in China has resulted in the dissemination of multidrug-resistant pathogenic *E. coli* isolates, including fluoroquinolone-resistant variants.

Africa is not exempt from the reports of antimicrobial resistance among avian *E. coli*. For example, in Morocco, Amara et al. reported on the prevalence of antimicrobial resistance among *E. coli* strains recovered from clinical cases of avian colibacillosis (8). Among 258 *E. coli* isolates tested, resistance was most often observed to sulfonamides (78%), oxytetracycline (65%), trimethoprim-sulfamethoxazole (61%), and chloramphenicol (41%). Resistance was also noted to streptomycin (32%), as well as the early quinolones nalidixic acid (25%) and oxolinic acid (24%) (8). A significant percentage of isolates (82.5%) were also resistant to at least 2 antimicrobial agents. Another study from Kenya documented resistance among 37 avian *E. coli* isolates to trimethoprim-sulfamethoxazole (Septrin) (100%), ampicillin (62.2%), tetracycline (51.4%), kanamycin (13.5%), and gentamicin (2.7%) (13). The authors further demonstrated genetic transfer of the trimethoprim resistance determinant to recipient susceptible strains and indicated a potential public health hazard, as trimethoprim was used extensively for treating diarrheal cases in children in Kenya (13). Lastly, a more recent study from South Africa examined antimicrobial susceptibilities among a collection of *E. coli* isolates obtained from a poultry abattoir (69). The majority of strains were resistant to tetracyclines (90%), and a smaller percentage (20%) were resistant to neomycin. All isolates were susceptible to the veterinary fluoroquinolone danofloxacin (for which the MIC at which 90% of the isolates were inhibited was ≤0.125 μg/ml); however, no information was provided as to the extent that fluoroquinolones are used in poultry production in South Africa (69).

Antimicrobial resistance phenotypes among avian pathogenic *E. coli* recovered from diseased turkeys are similar to those reported from chickens. For example, Dubel et al. reported in 1982 the presence of antibiotic-resistant strains of *E. coli* in the fecal microflora of commercial turkeys, in particular a common resistance pattern of gentamicin, kanamycin, and streptomycin (53). They further attributed the high incidence of gentamicin resistance (86%) to the common practice of dipping eggs in gentamicin and injecting newly hatched poults with gentamicin. van den Bogaard et al. reported antimicrobial resistance phenotypes among *E. coli* isolates recovered from both chickens and turkeys as well as poultry farmers and slaughterhouse workers in The Netherlands (179). The highest prevalence of resistance was detected in turkey fecal samples, followed closely by broiler samples. Resistance to ciprofloxacin, flumequine, and neomycin was significantly higher ($P<0.005$) in turkeys and broilers than in laying hens (179). Quinolone resistance was most likely associated with the therapeutic use of flumequine and enrofloxacin, which accounted for approximately 14% of all antibiotic use in poultry in The Netherlands at the time of the study (179). Similar observations were noted by Cormican et al. (41), who looked at 209 clinical *E. coli* isolates obtained from turkeys and chickens (broilers and layers). Resistance to sulfonamides, trimethoprim, and nalidixic acid were more common in *E. coli* originating from turkeys as compared to those from chickens.

A more recent study by Altekruse et al. examined 1,104 fecal and 105 clinical *E. coli* isolates recovered from turkeys in West Virginia and Virginia for antimicrobial susceptibilities (7). More fecal than clinical isolates were resistant to ampicillin (53 versus 14%); however, more clinical than fecal isolates were resistant to ciprofloxacin (8 versus 2%) and sulfamethoxazole (84 versus 58%) (7). Resistance to gentamicin was observed in most clinical isolates and fewer than a quarter of fecal isolates, a significant difference ($P < 0.001$) that, much like the earlier conclusions of Dubel et al. (53), was attributed to 1-day-old poults being routinely injected with gentamicin at the hatchery.

Due to numerous reports of resistance to traditional antimicrobials approved globally for use in treatment of avian *E. coli* infections (e.g., tetracyclines and sulfonamides), as well as an increased potency against poultry bacterial pathogens, fluoroquinolones have been approved in numerous countries for therapeutic treatment of animal diseases, including avian colibacillosis (56, 71, 188). However, the approval of fluoroquinolones in veterinary medicine has drawn increased scrutiny due to the possibility that these antimicrobials can select for resistant food-borne pathogens that can be transferred to humans via ingestion of contaminated food and/or water (3, 88, 146, 197). Additionally, there are an increasing number of reports describing quinolone and fluoroquinolone resistance among the target animal pathogens (e.g., avian pathogenic *E. coli*) (11, 17, 60, 70, 192).

Fluoroquinolone-resistant avian *E. coli* isolates were first identified in Saudi Arabia and were attributed to the introduction of the older quinolones oxolinic acid and flumequine for prophylaxis in 1987 (11). An approximate increase of 50% in the proportion of quinolone-resistant clinical avian *E. coli* isolates was observed in the following year. Resistance was most likely due to accumulation of mutations in the *E. coli* DNA gyrase gene; however, this was not confirmed (11). Another survey by Blanco et al. revealed that approximately 13 to 44% of 468 avian *E. coli* isolates surveyed displayed increased levels of resistance to ciprofloxacin and nalidixic acid, respectively (17). They attributed this high level of resistance to the over-the-counter use of antibiotics on Spanish poultry farms. Additionally, Everett et al. observed that the majority of veterinary *E. coli* isolates (6 of 8) resistant to fluoroquinolones isolated in the United Kingdom had mutations only in the quinolone resistance-determining region (QRDR) of the *gyrA* gene (60).

Similar reports from France have described fluoroquinolone resistance among *E. coli* O78:K80 isolates recovered from diseased turkeys in the mid-1990s (70). Among 170 clinical *E. coli* isolates tested for susceptibility, 84 (49%), 82 (48%), and 68 (40%) were resistant to nalidixic acid, flumequine, and enrofloxacin, respectively. The level of resistance to fluoroquinolones of the isolates appeared closely correlated with substitutions in GyrA and ParC, but not with the production of the AcrAB efflux pump. The authors suggested that the use of the veterinary fluoroquinolone enrofloxacin since 1992 led to the selection of resistant strains (70).

The first occurrence of fluoroquinolone resistance in veterinary *E. coli* isolates recovered from clinical cases of avian colibacillosis in the United States was reported in 2000 (192). A marked increase in sarafloxacin and enrofloxacin resistance was observed among pathogenic avian *E. coli* in north Georgia from 1996 to 1999. This trend coincided with the approval of these fluoroquinolones in 1995 and 1996 for treatment of *E. coli*-related poultry infections in the United States. In addition to quinolone resistance, the majority of avian *E. coli* isolates displayed multiple-antimicrobial resistance, as typified by resistance to as many as five different antimicrobial classes. Antimicrobial resistance percentages ranged from 93% resistance to sulfamethoxazole to 14% resistance to ceftiofur. *E. coli* exhibited decreased susceptibilities to gentamicin and ampicillin as well (62 and 55%, respectively). Thirty-one percent of the isolates were also resistant to chloramphenicol (MIC, ≥32 μg/ml).

Over time, with the advent of new molecular techniques (e.g., nucleic acid hybridization and PCR), experiments yielded information with regard to the genetics and evolution of antimicrobial resistance among *E. coli* isolates in animals. For example, Chaslus-Dancla et al. examined a set of avian *E. coli* isolates recovered from the intestinal tracts of broilers that demonstrated trimethoprim, ampicillin, and streptomycin resistance despite the absence of any antibiotic-selective pressures (27). They found that these isolates shared a 56-kb plasmid that contained genes conferring resistance to trimethoprim (*dfrI*) and ampicillin ($bla_{TEM\text{-}1}$) and that was further shown to be stable in their tested ecosystem (27). More recently, analysis of a plasmid isolated from an avian pathogenic *E. coli* isolate revealed a mosaic of virulence genes, insertion sequences, antimicrobial resistance cassettes, and their remnants (100). Many of the resistance genes found in this region were expressed under laboratory conditions, indicating that certain antimicrobial agents, including disinfectants, antibiotics, and heavy metals, could promote selection of *E. coli* containing such plasmids in the production environment (100).

A limited number of studies have focused on the association of antimicrobial resistance genes with extrachromosomal DNA elements, in particular transposons and integrons, among avian *E. coli* isolates (10, 79, 110, 197). These DNA mobile elements have been shown to encompass genetic determinants for several different antimicrobial resistance mechanisms and may be accountable for the rapid dissemination of resistance genes among different bacteria. Class 1 integrons, specifically, have been shown to be important in the dissemination of *intI*, *sulI*, and one or more antimicrobial resistance gene cassettes among gram-negative bacteria (10, 150, 154).

In one of the first studies to look at the prevalence of class 1 integrons among avian pathogenic *E. coli*, Bass et al. (10) showed that 63% of 100 clinical isolates were positive for the class 1 integron markers *intI1* and *qacEΔ1*. PCR analysis with the conserved class 1 integron primers yielded amplicons of approximately 1 kb and were shown to contain the spectinomycin-streptomycin resistance gene *aadA1* (10). Further characterization of the identified integrons revealed that many were part of the transposon Tn*21*, a genetic element that encodes resistance to both antibiotics and mercuric compounds. Fifty percent of the clinical isolates positive for the integron marker gene *intI1* as well as for the *qacEΔ1* and *aadA1* cassettes also contained the mercury reductase gene *merA*. The correlation between the presence of the *merA* gene and of the integrase and antibiotic resistance genes suggested that these integrons were located in Tn*21*.

Further data suggest similar integron prevalences among avian pathogenic *E. coli* (110, 197). As part of a larger study, Lanz et al. (110) characterized 122 pathogenic *E. coli* isolates from septicemia in laying hens collected in Switzerland between 1999 and 2001. A significant proportion of isolates resistant to sulfonamides or streptomycin carried the integrase gene *int1*. A more recent study in China in 2004 reported on the high incidence of class 1 integrons among a collection of pathogenic avian and porcine *E. coli* isolates (197). Fifty-nine percent of the Chinese avian *E. coli* isolates examined ($n = 71$) contained class 1 integrons ranging in size from 0.7 to 1.5 kb. Thirty-four of these isolates contained a 1.5-kb integron with *dhfr1* and *aadA1*, and one isolate contained a 1.5-kb integron with *dhfr17* and *aadA2*. Six isolates contained both the 1.5-kb integron (*dhfr1* and *aadA1*) and the 0.7-kb integron (*dhfr13*). Two isolates contained the 1.0-kb integron with the *aadA1* gene. No class 1 integrons were found that possessed the plasmid-mediated quinolone resistance gene, *qnr* (197).

Other studies have looked for the presence of resistance determinants associated with phenicol and β-lactam resistance among avian *E. coli* isolates (23, 107). Florfenicol-resistant avian pathogenic *E. coli* isolates were first detected from clinical cases in Georgia and North Carolina in the late 1990s, despite the fact that this drug is not used in poultry in the United States (107). Resistance was associated with the presence of the florfenicol resistance efflux gene, *flo*, and was shown to be plasmid encoded. A study from Spain examined the presence of β-lactamases among *E. coli* isolates recovered from healthy chickens between November 2000 and February 2001 (23). Genes encoding the CMY-2, CTX-M-14, and SHV-12 β-lactamases were detected in *E. coli* isolates that showed resistance or diminished susceptibility to extended-spectrum cephalosporins (23). However, the authors hinted that extended-spectrum cephalosporin use in poultry was unusual and that the discovery of resistance to this antimicrobial class may be due to cross-selection with other antimicrobials used in poultry (e.g., sulfonamides and tetracyclines) (23).

In summary, the use of antimicrobials in the poultry industry has played a significant role in controlling losses due to infectious diseases; however, the emergence of multidrug resistance among avian *E. coli* and other zoonotic food-borne pathogens is an undesired consequence that has been documented on a global basis (3, 88, 104, 146, 197). Resistance to commonly used antimicrobials (e.g., tetracyclines and sulfonamides) has been observed since the early studies in the 1960s, and few new antimicrobials have been introduced for use in the treatment of avian diseases, the notable exception being the fluoroquinolones. However, the increased public and scientific scrutiny of fluoroquinolones in the treatment of animal diseases, in particular avian colibacillosis, necessitates the development of other antimicrobial agents and the development and implementation of judicious antimicrobial use guidelines that emphasize proper animal husbandry and hygiene as well as discourage the inappropriate use of antimicrobials.

BOVINE SCOURS

Bovine scours is a severe form of diarrhea that causes more financial loss to cow and calf producers than any other disease-related problem (22, 98, 191). Scours is a clinical sign of disease that may have many causes, although *E. coli* has been frequently implicated as the primary bacterial cause in calves (22, 91, 98, 191). Numerous *E. coli* serotypes have been incriminated, but the majority are ETEC strains. These strains usually possess the F5 (K99) adhesin and produce heat-stable (STa or STb) and/or heat-labile (LT) enterotoxins (22, 98, 191). Several serotypes of enterohemorrhagic *E. coli*, such as O5, O26, and O111, have also been shown to be associated with diarrhea in calves and possess different virulence factors than the traditional ETEC isolates (e.g., intimin and Shiga toxins) (106). Additionally, certain fimbrial adhesins, such as F165 and other members of the P family of fimbriae, F17, and CS31A, as well as certain cytotoxic necrotizing toxins (type I and II), have been associated with bovine extraintestinal infections (14, 62). Regardless of the virulence potential of these isolates, the most important aspect of treating *E. coli*-related colibacillosis is to correct the accompanying electrolyte loss, dehydration, and acidosis. However, antimicrobial therapy is often initiated at the same time in an attempt to eliminate the pathogenic *E. coli* (22, 38, 191).

Early studies in the 1950s and 1960s documented the incidence of antimicrobial resistance among *E. coli* isolates from healthy and diseased cattle (5, 89, 165, 184). Transferable drug resistance was first reported in 1956 among *E. coli* isolated from calves (163, 167). Early work by Walton in the 1960s investigated the incidence of drug resistance among *E. coli* isolated from the feces of healthy calves in Great Britain (184). Multidrug-resistant *E. coli* isolates were recovered from 46% of fecal samples collected from calves, with the most common pattern being resistance to tetracycline, sulfonamide, and streptomycin (184). Resistance was also observed to ampicillin, neomycin, and chloramphenicol, but to a lesser extent. Walton attributed observed resistance phenotypes among *E. coli* isolates to the use of various antimicrobials, including tetracyclines, neomycin, ampicillin, and chloramphenicol, in feeds. In 1968 Smith also reported a high incidence of drug resistance, most of which was transferable, among *E. coli* strains isolated from animals suffering from diarrhea (165). Smith also discussed the effects of animal feeds that contained antimicrobials on the emergence of drug-resistant strains; however, reliable feeding records detailing the presence or absence of antimicrobials in feeds were not available.

Data from other European countries were slowly accumulating as well, and the reports were similar in nature to those described in Great Britain. In fact, the Nordic countries (Denmark, Finland, Norway, and Sweden) have a long tradition of infectious disease control in animal production, especially with regard to the use of antimicrobials (4, 194). Early work in the mid-1970s by Wierup in Sweden demonstrated that *E. coli* isolates from 5-day-old calves exhibited higher rates of resistance than those obtained from 30-day-old healthy calves (193). Resistance to sulfonamide and tetracycline was most often observed, with sulfonamide resistance being the most commonly transferred phenotype. A later study by Aalbaek et al. reported on antimicrobial resistance phenotypes among *E. coli* isolates from Danish piglets and calves in 1987 and 1988 and compared the results with those of similar investigations performed during the periods 1971–1972 and 1977–1978 (2). Rectal swabs from 78 calves were examined, and all animals yielded *E. coli* resistant to at least one antimicrobial. A significant incidence of resistance was noted in comparison to the previous investigations; however, the number of isolates displaying three or more resistance phenotypes did not differ appreciably from the previous findings. The most common multidrug resistance patterns observed were sulfonamide and streptomycin; sulfonamide, streptomycin, and tetracycline; and sulfonamide, streptomycin, tetracycline, and ampicillin (2). The spectrum of resistance markers among Danish piglets and calves had increased through all three investigations, and resistance to chloramphenicol was still found to be considerable 10 years after the withdrawal of chloramphenicol as a therapeutic drug for farm animals in Denmark in 1978.

In the late 1980s Gonzalez and Blanco examined antimicrobial resistance phenotypes among a collection of 51 verotoxigenic (VTEC) and 33 necrotizing (NTEC) bovine *E. coli* strains and compared the results with 205 non-VTEC, non-NTEC strains isolated from the same batch of calves in Spain (73). VTEC isolates were shown to exhibit higher rates of resistance than either NTEC or non-VTEC, non-NTEC isolates. Additionally, VTEC isolates possessed more multidrug resistance patterns than the other isolates tested (73). Later research from Spain demonstrated similar findings (138, 139). Orden et al. evaluated 195 *E. coli* strains isolated from diarrheic dairy calves for the presence of potential virulence factors and antimicrobial susceptibilities (138, 139). The overall percentage of strains resistant to streptomycin and tetracycline was very high (>65%). High levels of resistance were also observed to ampicillin, neomycin, kanamycin, spectinomycin, chloramphenicol, sulfadimethoxine, and trimethoprim (from 23 to 50%). Most of the strains exhibited multidrug resistance: 77% were resistant to at least two antibiotics and 50% were resistant to at least six (139). However, the majority of *E. coli* strains were susceptible to apramycin, gentamicin, polymyxin B, florfenicol, and nitrofurazone. The authors also reported resistance rates among the strains of between 11 and 18% to cephalothin, nalidixic acid, enoxacin, and enrofloxacin; however, no resistance was observed to either cefotaxime or cefquinome (138). The authors concluded that extended-spectrum cephalosporins are highly effective against bovine *E. coli* isolates.

During the winter of 1979–1980 in France, an epizootiological study of diarrheic calves revealed the presence of K99+ *E. coli* among 19% of diseased calves. Antimicrobial resistance was particularly high among recovered K99+ strains (121). Later work by Chaslus-Dancla et al. described apramycin and gentamicin resistance among both *Salmonella* and *E. coli* isolates from two outbreaks of calf salmonellosis in 1986 after the approval of apramycin and gentamicin into veterinary therapy in France in the early 1980s (30). *E. coli* isolates demonstrated resistance to apramycin and gentamicin, in addition to ampicillin, chloramphenicol, kanamycin, streptomycin, tetracycline, trimethoprim, and nalidixic acid. Apramycin and gentamicin resistance was associated with a common plasmid encoding a type IV aminoglycoside 3-*N*-acetyltransferase, which had been previously described in *E. coli* strains from animals in Great Britain and France (29, 84). A subsequent, second mechanism of plasmid-mediated resistance to gentamicin among *E. coli* isolates associated with bovine diarrhea was reported a year later and was associated with a type II aminoglycoside 3-*N*-acetyltransferase (28). Interestingly, the same plasmid carrying the resistance gene (aminoglycoside 3-*N*-acetyltransferase) was later isolated from patients in hospitals in Belgium (31).

Similar observations were also noted in Great Britain when apramycin was licensed for veterinary use in 1980 (196). The incidence of resistance in *E. coli* to apramycin increased from 0.6% in 1982 to 2.6% in 1984 and was associated with transferable plasmids possessing the aminoglycoside 3-*N*-acetyltransferase IV [ACC(3)-IV] gene (196). Comparable observations were made by Hunter et al., who followed an outbreak of salmonellosis in calves and monitored the subsequent effects of apramycin treatment (97). Prior to treatment, apramycin-resistant *E. coli* were present but all *Salmonella enterica* serovar Typhimurium isolates were susceptible. Following the treatment of six calves with apramycin, apramycin-resistant *Salmonella* serovar Typhimurium were isolated from two treated calves and one untreated calf. Plasmid profiles of *E. coli* and *Salmonella* serovar Typhimurium were compared and plasmids conferring resistance to apramycin and several other antibiotics were transferred by conjugation in vitro from calf *E. coli* and *Salmonella* serovar Typhimurium isolates to *E. coli* K-12 and from *E. coli* to *Salmonella* serovar Typhimurium. The plasmids conjugated with high frequency in vitro from *E. coli* to serovar Typhimurium and hybridized to a DNA probe specific for the gene encoding AAC(3)-IV, which confers resistance to apramycin, gentamicin, netilmicin, and tobramycin (97).

A more recent study by Werckenthin et al. examined resistance rates of *E. coli* populations from 67 hospitalized calves both before and after hospitalization (with or without antimicrobial therapy) from 1998 to 2000 in Bavaria (189). Resistance to tetracycline, ampicillin, sulfonamide-trimethoprim, and chloramphenicol was observed in more than 80% of all tested isolates. However, a significant increase or decrease in resistance over the years was not observed. Analysis of the data obtained from hospitalized calves showed that an increase of resistance to some antimicrobials correlated with the use of those drugs in the clinic (189).

The resistance situation among bovine *E. coli* isolates in North America appears similar to that seen in Europe. The first report describing the incidence of antimicrobial resistance among *Enterobacteriaceae* recovered from diseased domestic animals in the United States was not published until 1969 (5). In that study, Aden et al. demonstrated that transferable drug resistance was common among *Enterobacteriaceae* isolated from cases of neonatal diarrhea in calves and piglets from the state of Nebraska (5). Specifically, 92 *Enterobacteriaceae* isolates cultured from fecal specimens from cases of neonatal diarrhea among young calves and pigs were tested for susceptibility to a number of antimicrobial agents using a rudimentary agar dilution scheme. Fifty-one of these isolates were identified as *E. coli* and were resistant to one or more of the relevant antimicrobial agents. Resistance to tetracycline, streptomycin, and sulfamethizole (in 22 of 51 isolates) was most often observed. Another large study in the United States was published in 1971 by researchers at the U.S. Food and Drug Administration (128). Mercer et al. characterized 555 *E. coli* isolates from fecal specimens obtained from swine, dairy calves, and cattle for antimicrobial resistance and obtained antimicrobial drug use information from the farms enrolled in the study. The incidence of multiple-antibiotic resistance phenotypes in *E. coli* was higher in herds exposed to continuous feeding of antimicrobial agents (85%) than in herds not receiving antimicrobials (16%) (128). The most common multidrug resistance pattern observed among the *E. coli* isolates was to dihydrostreptomycin, sulfonamide, and tetracycline, followed by ampicillin, dihydrostreptomycin, sulfonamide, and tetracycline. These results mirrored similar data from Great Britain showing that associations exist between the types of drugs administered to animals and the isolation of fecal *E. coli* isolates exhibiting resistance to these same agents (89, 165, 184).

Other studies from North America presented similar findings. de Lopez et al. tested a select group of *E. coli* isolates associated with diarrhea in neonatal calves and pigs in 1982 in the United States (45). Fourteen of the 15 bovine strains tested produced ST toxin only, whereas 1 strain elaborated LT toxin only. All of the isolates were multidrug resistant, and the most common resistance phenotype was to sulfonamides. However, none of the isolates were resistant to nalidixic acid, nitrofurantoin, or gentamicin. Harnett and Gyles also examined a small collection of Canadian and American swine and bovine ETEC strains for resistance to antimicrobials and heavy metals (82). Multiple resistance to antimicrobial agents was common among the bovine ETEC isolates, with the highest rates of resistance to sulfamethoxazole, tetracycyline, streptomycin, and ampicillin. Resistance to chloramphenicol and kanamycin was infrequent and was attributed to the limited use of these drugs in calves and pigs (82). A later study by the same authors also documented genetic linkages among enterotoxin production, K99 antigen, and antimicrobial resistance phenotypes on large plasmids (83). A more recent Canadian study by Hariharan et al. evaluated resistance to eight antimicrobials among ETEC from piglets and calves over a 13-year period (81). The least resistance occurred against ceftiofur for all isolates, followed by apramycin and gentamicin for porcine and florfenicol for bovine isolates. No significant differences were found between the first 8 and last 5 years of the study (81).

Holland et al. compared virulence factors, serotypes, and antimicrobial susceptibilities among *eae*⁺ *E. coli* isolated from healthy and diarrheic calves (92). All *E. coli* isolates were susceptible to amikacin, enrofloxacin, and nalidixic acid. However, significantly more *eae*⁺ and *eae/stx*⁺ *E. coli* that exhibited single- and multiple-antimicrobial resistance phenotypes were isolated from diarrheic calves. Resistance to ceftiofur, chloramphenicol, and trimethoprim-sulfamethoxazole was only seen in *E. coli* isolates recovered from diarrheic calves. Ceftiofur is a veterinary extended-spectrum cephalosporin with activity against a variety of animal pathogens associated with bovine and swine respiratory diseases (22). Although this antimicrobial is not approved for treatment of bovine calf scours in the United States, it is often used to treat bacterial diarrheal diseases (22). Additionally, most multidrug resistance patterns included resistance to tetracycline, ampicillin, and gentamicin. The authors concluded that selection for resistance among the *E. coli* isolates from diarrheic calves may have been due to a greater use of antimicrobials among these animals as compared to healthy calves (92).

Comparable results were observed by Bradford et al., who examined a collection of *E. coli* isolates obtained from individual bovine calf scours cases in North Dakota during 1996 for expanded-spectrum cephalosporin resistance (22). Many of the isolates were multiply resistant to β-lactams, including expanded-spectrum cephalosporins, aminoglycosides, sulfonamides, tetracycline, and fluoroquinolones, and possessed virulence factors associated with both animal and human diarrheal diseases. Resistance to expanded-spectrum cephalosporins was initially thought to be due to the hyperproduction of the chromosomally encoded AmpC β-lactamase, which is found naturally in *E. coli* but usually not expressed at high levels. However, recent work in our laboratory demonstrated that this resistance phenotype among these isolates was actually due to the presence of the bla_{CMY} genes located on transferable plasmids (198).

More-recent work from Japan isolated *E. coli* strains producing CTX-M-2 β-lactamases from 6 (1.5%) of 396 cattle fecal samples and 2 (0.7%) of 270 surface swabs of cattle carcasses sampled from November 2000 to June 2001 (160). The $bla_{CTX\text{-}M\text{-}2}$ gene was encoded on transferable plasmids and was transferred to *E. coli* CSH2 with a very high frequency (2×10^{-4} to 6×10^{-1} per donor cell) by conjugation. Random amplified polymorphic DNA analysis of nine isolates showed at least five different patterns. These findings suggest that CTX-M-2 producers might have originated from cattle through the use of cephalosporins such as ceftiofur and that cattle could be a reservoir of CTX-M-2-producing *E. coli*.

Other antimicrobial agents for which resistance has been recently documented among bovine *E. coli* isolates are fluoroquinolones and florfenicol (52, 60, 125, 191). Fluoroquinolones are highly efficacious antimicrobial agents commonly used in human medicine (94, 192, 197). This class of drugs has also been approved for certain bacterial diseases in animals, including acute bovine respiratory disease and avian colibacillosis (94, 192, 197). Fluoroquinolone resistance does not appear to be as common in pathogenic bovine *E. coli* isolates as it is in avian *E. coli* isolates. For example, Everett et al. characterized a collection of nalidixic acid-resistant *E. coli* from animals and humans in 1996 (60). Eight veterinary isolates recovered from calves and chickens from the Central Veterinary Laboratory in the United Kingdom were part of the study; however, no further data were provided to indicate which strains were of bovine or avian origin. All isolates possessed mutations in *gyrA*, resulting in a substitution of leucine for serine at codon 83. Two other isolates had a further mutation in *gyrA* resulting in changes at the aspartate at codon 87, and three isolates also had a mutation in the topoisomerase IV A subunit gene, *parC* (60). Later work by McDermott et al. in the United States characterized 54 nalidixic acid-resistant isolates of bovine *E. coli* recovered from cases of calf scours over a 3-year period (1996 to 1998) (125). The majority of isolates displayed resistance to sarafloxacin (100%), difloxacin (96%), enrofloxacin (54%), and orbifloxacin (50%), followed by ciprofloxacin (48%), levofloxacin (31%), and gatifloxacin (30%). All isolates contained a mutation in serine 83 of the *gyrA* gene, whereas 32 isolates also had mutations at aspartate 87. Thirty-one of the 54 quinolone-resistant isolates (57%) demonstrated growth in cyclohexane, a marker phenotype for overexpression of the AcrAB multidrug efflux pump. Data from both these studies indicate that fluoroquinolone resistance among *E. coli* isolates incriminated in bovine diarrhea results from a combination of topoisomerase mutations and efflux mechanisms.

Other data from Europe indicate that fluoroquinolone resistance among bovine *E. coli* isolates increased between 1994 and 2001 (129). Meunier et al. evaluated 633 *E. coli* isolates from bovine intestinal infections for susceptibility to the newly approved fluoroquinolone marbofloxacin. Isolates were collected from eight European countries (Belgium, France, Ireland, Italy, Germany, The Netherlands, Spain, and the United Kingdom). From 1994 the distribution of MICs showed that the majority of isolates (65.9%) were very susceptible to marbofloxacin, with MICs between 0.004 and 0.06 μg/ml. However, a subpopulation of less susceptible bacteria was observed (marbofloxacin MICs of ≥16 μg/ml) at the start of the study in 1994, prior to marketing of this drug, and was attributed to cross-selection pressures from previously approved fluoroquinolones in cattle (enrofloxacin and danofloxacin) (129).

Florfenicol [*d*-threo-3-fluoro-2-dichloroacetamido-1-(4-methylsulfonylphenyl)-1-propanol] is a fluorinated structural analog of thiamphenicol and chloramphenicol approved by the U.S. Food and Drug Administration in 1996 for treatment of bovine respiratory pathogens such as *Pasteurella* spp. However, it is not currently approved for treatment of *E. coli*-related cattle enteric diseases in the United States (191). Florfenicol has been shown to have a spectrum of activity similar to that of chloramphenicol, except that it is active at lower concentrations than chloramphenicol against a variety of clinical bacterial isolates, including chloramphenicol-resistant bacteria (36, 162, 191). White et al. reported florfenicol resistance among 48 antimicrobial-resistant strains of *E. coli* isolated from diarrheic calves and submitted to the North Dakota Veterinary Diagnostic Laboratory from 1997 to 1998 (191). All 48 bovine isolates were resistant to at least four antimicrobials, and 37 (77%) isolates were resistant to at least nine antimicrobials. Ninety-two percent of *E. coli* isolates were considered florfenicol resistant; this resistance was associated with high-molecular-weight conjugative plasmids encoding the putative florfenicol efflux gene, *flo* (191). Florfenicol-resistant *E. coli* have also been recovered from dairy cattle in the United States and cattle in France and Germany, as well as from diarrheic calves in China (36, 50, 52, 162). The finding of florfenicol-resistant *E. coli* in France and Germany is not surprising considering the fact that this drug has been approved for use in cattle in Europe since 1995 (50). However, the finding of florfenicol-resistant *E. coli* in China cannot be as easily explained, as this drug was not licensed for use in China at the time of isolation. The authors attributed florfenicol resistance to prior chloramphenicol selection pressures in food animals (52). The emergence and dissemination of florfenicol resistance globally among pathogenic bovine *E. coli* isolates will limit the use of this antimicrobial as an extralabel alternative for treating calf diarrhea.

In summary, acute neonatal diarrhea can occur wherever farm animals are maintained and is a significant cause of morbidity and mortality. The etiology of neonatal diarrhea is most complex and can involve interactions between numerous pathogens, including *E. coli*, *Salmonella*, rota- and coronaviruses, *Cryptosporidium* spp., and others. As mentioned previously, if *E. coli* or *Salmonella* are suspect pathogens, antimicrobial therapy is often initiated, with mixed results (91). Since the earliest published data from the 1960s, resistance to front-line antimicrobials has been documented among *E. coli* strains incriminated in bovine calf scours. This combination of virulence coupled with multidrug resistance may pose an increasing threat to successful treatment of *E. coli*-related veterinary diseases in the near future.

BOVINE MASTITIS

Mastitis remains the most common cause of antibacterial use on dairy farms, as therapy is a major component and a primary tool for mastitis control in lactating and dry cows (57, 58, 149). Environmental bovine mastitis caused by coliform bacteria appears to have increased in many dairy herds and countries at the same time that contagious mastitis is being more successfully controlled (61, 103, 115, 147). Coliform mastitis is most often caused by fecal flora, usually *E. coli*, originating from the cow's environment, which infect the udder via the teat canal (103, 115). Unfortunately, it has not been possible to distinguish *E. coli* strains that cause mastitis from strains comprising the normal microflora, and no common virulence factor has yet to be identified (12, 103). Broad-spectrum antimicrobial agents are generally used to treat coliform mastitis (58, 103), although there is no convincing evidence that antimicrobials significantly affect the outcome (148, 156).

Resistance patterns among *E. coli* isolates associated with coliform mastitis vary between countries and may reflect differences in antimicrobial treatments and herd management techniques (3, 103). Early reports characterizing antimicrobial resistance among *E. coli* isolates from coliform mastitis showed that most isolates were susceptible to the majority of antimicrobials tested (118). For example, in 1973 Rollins et al. reported on the effects of antibiotic use in a dairy herd and subsequent resistance development among *E. coli* isolates from New York State (152). More than 50% of the 87 *E. coli* isolates tested during this study demonstrated susceptibility to all tested antibiotics. However, some resistance was observed to streptomycin, tetracycline, ampicillin, and sulfa drugs (152). Other reports from Great Britain and continental Europe showed similar observations (118, 169). In the mid-1970s Linton, Howe, and colleagues documented a low incidence of resistance among 279 *E. coli* isolates associated with clinical mastitis (118). Resistance was infrequently observed to sulfa drugs, streptomycin, and tetracycline. Sogaard tested 131 *E. coli* strains isolated from cases of coliform mastitis in Denmark for susceptibility to eight antibiotics in 1982. Resistance was most frequently observed to either tetracycline or dihydrostreptomycin, whereas all strains were susceptible to colistin, gentamicin, and polymyxin B (169).

More recent papers indicate that resistance among *E. coli* isolates associated with bovine mastitis does not appear to be increasing at a rapid rate. As part of the German national antibiotic resistance monitoring program, Wallmann et al. tested 214 *E. coli* isolates from mastitis milk samples for antimicrobial susceptibilities in 2001 (183). Resistance was most often observed to narrow-spectrum cephalosporins (cephalothin, 42%) and ampicillin (9%). One *E. coli* isolate demonstrated resistance to the broad-spectrum cephalosporin ceftiofur, whereas no resistance was observed to either nalidixic acid or the veterinary fluoroquinolone enrofloxacin (183).

Lehtolainen et al. reported in 2003 on the antimicrobial susceptibility profiles of 200 *E. coli* isolates recovered from bovine mastitis cases from either Finland or Israel (115). The majority of *E. coli* isolates demonstrated susceptibility to the tested antimicrobials, with only 27% exhibiting resistance to one or more agents. Fifteen percent of the Israeli isolates ($n = 100$) and 14% of the Finnish isolates ($n = 100$) were resistant to tetracycline, 13 and 9% to dihydrostreptomycin, 3 and 16% to cephalexin, 10 and 7% to ampicillin, and 4 and 2% to trimethoprim-sulfadiazine. Resistance to gentamicin, ceftazidime, or ciprofloxacin was not detected in any isolate. The authors concluded that antimicrobial resistance among *E. coli* isolates recovered from bovine mastitis from both countries was not a problem and that the low incidence was probably due to the controlled use of antimicrobial agents in the treatment of dairy herds in each country (115).

In Switzerland, Lanz et al. examined 211 *E. coli* isolates isolated from bovine mastitis for antimicrobial susceptibilities as part of a larger study focusing on resistance among different animal species (110). Seventy-eight percent of bovine isolates showed susceptibility to all tested antimicrobials. When resistance was observed, it was most often to streptomycin (22%), sulfonamide (22%), ampicillin (21%), tetracycline (20%), and kanamycin (16%) (110). A study by scientists in Switzerland echoed similar findings, as 79% of *E. coli* isolates ($n = 100$) recovered from bovine mastitis milk samples between November 2002 and April 2003 demonstrated susceptibility to all tested antimicrobials (42). The authors further concluded that no important changes in the resistance situation among mastitis pathogens have occurred during the last 20 years in Switzerland. Similar results with regard to *E. coli* antimicrobial susceptibilities were reported by Fang and Pyorala in the mid-1990s in Finland (61).

The situation appears to be similar in the United States. For example, from 1994 to 2000 Erskine et al. tested antimicrobial susceptibility in a total of 2,778 bacterial isolates recovered from milk samples from dairy cattle suspected of having mastitis (58). Among the 647 *E. coli* isolates tested, the proportion that was susceptible to ampicillin and cephalothin increased annually; however, the proportion of susceptible isolates did not change substantially over the 7-year period for the other antimicrobials tested (e.g., ceftiofur, gentamicin, tetracycline, and sulfamethoxazole-trimethoprim) (58). Overall, there was no indication of increased resistance of mastitis isolates to antimicrobials that are commonly used to treat Michigan dairy cattle.

A larger study by Makovec and Ruegg characterized 8,905 bacterial isolates obtained from milk samples submitted to the Wisconsin Veterinary Diagnostic Laboratory between January 1994 and June 2001 for antimicrobial susceptibilities using the disk diffusion method (119). Among the 1,939 *E. coli* isolates tested, resistance was most often observed to tetracycline (37%), cephalothin (28%), ampicillin (22%), and sulfisoxazole (16%). However, the percentage of isolates exhibiting resistance did not increase significantly over time; in fact, the percentage of *E. coli* isolates resistant to sulfisoxazole decreased significantly ($P < 0.001$), from 26 to 14% (119). Much like the conclusions reiterated by other mastitis researchers, the results did not indicate a trend toward increased antimicrobial resistance among mastitis pathogens isolated from milk samples from dairy cows between 1994 and 2001 (119).

Resistance to narrow-spectrum cephalosporins and tetracyclines among *E. coli* isolates may be due to their use for intramammary treatment for clinical mastitis in dairy cows. Cephapirin is a narrow-spectrum cephalosporin that is approved for treatment of mastitis and is the second most commonly prescribed intramammary treatment for clinical mastitis in dairy cows, whereas oxytetracycline is the most commonly prescribed nonapproved antimicrobial for parenteral treatment in lactating dairy cows (172). Additionally, unweaned dairy heifers are commonly fed milk replacers, many of which contain medications intended to decrease the incidence of common diseases often observed during the neonatal period (e.g., scours) (86, 177). A recent survey conducted by the National Animal Health Monitoring System in the United States showed that approximately 55% of dairy farms surveyed in 21 major dairy states during 2002 reported using calf milk replacer that contained antimicrobials, most often oxytetracycline and neomycin combined (177).

Despite global efforts, mastitis has remained the most economically important disease of dairy cattle (57, 115, 156, 161). Although systemic and intramammary antimicrobials are widely used in the treatment of coliform mastitis, resistance among *E. coli* isolates associated with bovine mastitis does not appear to be increasing on a global scale. However, in light of the concern about the use of antibiotics in food-producing animals, studies are needed to examine the dynamics of antimicrobial resistance in mastitis pathogens over time, particularly following exposure to antibacterial therapy. Additionally, the routine use of medicated milk replacer in young calves may need to be reassessed, as recent research indicates that the use of nonantimicrobial compounds such as oligosaccharides, allicin, and probiotics can obtain similar results in increasing weight gain and decreasing the incidence of scours (49, 85).

SWINE DIARRHEA

ETEC strains are one of the most important causes of diarrhea in neonatal and young pigs (133). Illness associated with ETEC usually occurs either the during the first week of life (neonatal diarrhea) or in 3- to 6-week-old piglets (postweaning diarrhea) (67, 142). Both of these disease syndromes are associated with certain *E. coli* serotypes, which produce a combination of specific LT and/or ST enterotoxins, in conjunction with fimbrial colonization factors (19, 122). Each of these toxin groups comprises at least two toxin variants: LTI and LTII, and STI and STII (67, 133). The LTI, STI, and STII enterotoxins have been found in ETEC recovered from both humans and pigs, whereas LTII is only sometimes reported from *E. coli* strains of pig origin (159). Additionally, the EAST1 toxin has been shown to be widely distributed among *E. coli* strains isolated from piglets with postweaning diarrhea, especially F4-positive ETEC isolates that mainly express LTI or LTI and STII enterotoxins (143). Most porcine ETEC isolates also possess one of the pilus adherence factors: F4 (K88), F5 (K99), F6 (987P), F18, or F41 (143); of these, F4 fimbriae appear to play a major role in the adherence of toxigenic *E. coli* bacteria to porcine intestinal epithelial cells (181). Some F18-positive ETEC also produce Shiga-like toxin IIe (SLTIIe) and can cause edema disease. It is also thought that F18-positive *E. coli* that only produce SLTIIe in the absence of enterotoxins cause only edema disease and not diarrhea (77).

Animal diseases due to ETEC typically result in severe watery diarrhea during the first few days of life (also a few days after weaning in pigs). ETEC adhere to the small intestinal microvilli and produce enterotoxins that act locally on enterocytes. This action results in hypersecretion (of water and electrolytes) and reduced absorption (133). Efforts to develop biological products aimed at protecting piglets from ETEC-associated diarrhea have yielded several commercial vaccines but have met with limited success under field conditions (77, 132, 144). Therefore, antimicrobial therapy is usually relied upon in an attempt to control morbidity and mortality associated with these bacterial pathogens (124).

Much like the situation in poultry and cattle, antimicrobial-resistant strains of *E. coli* recovered from both healthy and diseased swine have been documented since the earliest reports in the 1960s and 1970s (5, 120, 131, 184). One of the earliest reports, by Walton, examined antimicrobial-resistant *E. coli* obtained from healthy pigs 8 to 20 weeks old from farms in the northwest of England in the mid-1960s (184). Eighty-nine of the 105 swine fecal samples tested contained multiple-antibiotic-resistant strains of *E. coli*, with resistance being most often observed to tetracycline, streptomycin, and sulfonamide (184). Similar results with regard to the presence of multidrug resistance phenotypes among *E. coli* isolates from healthy and diseased swine were also reported by scientists froym both Japan and the United States in the late 1960s (5, 120, 131).

Numerous reports have accumulated over the past several decades describing antimicrobial resistance among pathogenic and commensal swine *E. coli* isolates (15, 24, 66, 102, 110, 124, 184). Early work reported by Franklin and Glatthard in Sweden showed increases in resistant phenotypes among *E. coli* isolates recovered from piglets between 1964 and 1968 and between 1974 and 1975 (66). The proportion of strains displaying resistance to one antimicrobial decreased from 50% in 1964 to 1968 to 27% in 1974 to 1975, while resistance to two or more agents increased from 13 to 22% over the same time period. Resistance was most often observed to sulfonamides, tetracycline, streptomycin, ampicillin, chloramphenicol, and neomycin; however, all strains were susceptible to trimethoprim (66). Later work by Franklin in the early 1980s showed higher rates of resistance among ETEC strains isolated from herds with piglet diarrhea to streptomycin, sulfonamides, tetracycline, ampicillin, neomycin, and trimethoprim (65, 66).

During this same time period, Jorgensen and Poulsen examined a collection of 359 hemolytic *E. coli* strains isolated from pigs with enteric disease in Denmark for transferable antimicrobial resistance (102). Transferable resistance to tetracycline, streptomycin, and/or sulfonamides was found in 47% of the total number of strains and 80% of the resistant ones. Though chloramphenicol resistance was seldom observed, a study by Jorgensen a few years later documented the emergence of plasmids conferring resistance to chloramphenicol among *E. coli* isolated from diseased piglets (101). Similar data from Austria showed high rates of resistance to tetracycline and streptomycin among hemolytic *E. coli* isolates recovered from diarrheic piglets in the late 1970s (6). More recently, Lanz et al. characterized antimicrobial susceptibilities and resistance determinants among 126 *E. coli* isolates recovered from swine diarrhea and enterotoxemia in Switzerland as part of a larger study (110). Resistance was most often observed to sulfonamide (81%), tetracycline (54%), streptomycin (37%), and ampicillin (16%). Ten percent of isolates also exhibited resistance to gentamicin, kanamycin, or chloramphenicol. Swine isolates also tended to display higher rates of resistance to gentamicin, streptomycin, sulfonamide, and tetracycline as compared with bovine, avian, and companion animal (dogs and cats) *E. coli* isolates (110). A significant proportion of isolates resistant to sulfonamides or streptomycin also carried the integrase gene *intI*.

Comparable results have been reported by veterinary scientists in North America. Early work by Miniats and Roe in the late 1960s showed that the majority of hemolytic *E. coli* isolates recovered from early weaned pigs in Canada demonstrated resistance to streptomycin, tetracycline, and sulfa drugs (130). Similar data were reported by Broes et al., who characterized antimicrobial resistance phenotypes among ETEC isolates of the O8 serogroup associated with piglet diarrhea in Quebec, Canada, in the late 1980s (24). All but 3 of the *E. coli* isolates demonstrated resistance to at least four antibiotics, and 11 strains were resistant to six or more antibiotics. Resistance to streptomycin, tetracycline, and sulfonamides was most common; however, all isolates were susceptible to gentamicin and trimethoprim-sulfamethoxazole (24). Amezcua characterized antimicrobial resistance phenotypes among 75 ETEC isolates implicated in postweaning diarrhea in pigs in Ontario, Canada (9). At least 40% of isolates demonstrated resistance to spectinomycin, tetracycline, ampicillin, or sulfamethoxazole. A later study by Maynard et al. focused on antimicrobial resistance phenotypes and genotypes among a collection of 112 *E. coli* O149:K91 isolates recovered from pigs with diarrhea in Quebec over a 23-year period (124). Resistance to tetracycline and sulfonamides was found to be the most common, and an increase in the number of isolates resistant to at least three antimicrobials was observed over time. Resistance to ampicillin, neomycin, kanamycin, chloramphenicol, and trimethoprim ranged from 21 to 38%, whereas only 14% of the isolates were gentamicin resistant (124). Sixty percent of the isolates were also shown to possess class 1 integrons. Overall, the data indicated that antimicrobial resistance gene distribution among *E. coli* O149:K91 isolates was dynamic and that the observed increases in resistance phenotypes correlated with an increase in multigene resistance over the 23-year study period (124).

Dunlop et al. compared antimicrobial use information and the occurrence of resistance in *E. coli* from 34 pig herds in Canada in the late 1990s (55). Treatment in grower-finisher rations was significantly associated with resistance to ampicillin, spectinomycin, sulfisoxazole, and tetracycline. However, there was little evidence that in-feed antimicrobials increased the risk of resistance to gentamicin, which was a drug used only for individual-pig treatment in this study population. These results suggested that certain antimicrobial medications of rations of postweaning pigs can select for and maintain antimicrobial resistance among *E. coli* recovered from finisher pigs.

Libal and Gates determined antimicrobial susceptibilities among 1,037 *E. coli* isolates cultured from the intestines of pigs with diarrhea in the

United States in the early 1980s (116). Isolates from suckling pigs were more often resistant to chloramphenicol than were those from weaned pigs. *E. coli* isolates from weaned pigs demonstrated greater rates of resistance to kanamycin and neomycin than those recovered from suckling pigs. *E. coli* isolates that were the primary cause of diarrhea (colibacillosis isolates) were more resistant to kanamycin, neomycin, and spectinomycin than noncolibacillosis isolates. However, ampicillin resistance was more often observed among the nonpathogenic isolates (116).

A later study by Bischoff et al. examined 90 beta-hemolytic *E. coli* isolates associated with diarrhea in neonatal pigs from multiple farms in Oklahoma for known associated disease serotypes, virulence factors, ribotypes, and antimicrobial susceptibility phenotypes (15). Fifteen different serotypes were observed, with 58% of isolates belonging to groups that produce one of three major enterotoxins: O149, O147, and O139. Seventy-three percent of the *E. coli* isolates were resistant to five or more antibiotics. Interestingly, 53% of swine *E. coli* isolates exhibited resistance to chloramphenicol, an antibiotic whose use in food animals has been prohibited in the United States since the mid-1980s. The *cmlA* gene, which encodes a putative chloramphenicol efflux pump, was detected by PCR in 47 of the 48 chloramphenicol-resistant isolates, and 4 of these also possessed the *cat2* gene, which encodes a chloramphenicol acetyltransferase. The one chloramphenicol-resistant isolate that did not contain either *cmlA* or *cat2* possessed the putative *flo* efflux gene, which confers resistance to both florfenicol and chloramphenicol (15). Florfenicol resistance in pathogenic swine *E. coli* isolates was also recently documented in Germany and was attributed to the *flo* efflux gene as well (20).

Similar observations have been reported by scientists from China and Korea with regard to the incidence of resistance among pathogenic *E. coli* isolates recovered from diseased swine (33, 197). Choi et al. determined in vitro susceptibilities of 285 isolates of *E. coli* obtained from pigs with diarrhea and edema disease in Korea (33). Resistance was most often observed to tetracycline (91%), trimethoprim-sulfamethoxazole (90%), spectinomycin and ampicillin (87%), gentamicin (67%), and enrofloxacin (31%). The only antimicrobial to which resistance was infrequent was ceftiofur (1%) (33). The majority of *E. coli* isolates recovered from diseased piglets from Chinese swine farms were resistant to more than 8 of the 19 antimicrobials tested, 86% were resistant to more than 11 antimicrobials, and 2% were resistant to 16 antimicrobials (197). Seventy-six percent of isolates were resistant to enrofloxacin and contained the typical mutations in the topoisomerase genes *gyrA* and *parC*, reported previously (60, 87, 153). Nineteen percent of swine *E. coli* isolates were also shown to possess class 1 integrons bearing gene cassettes conferring resistance primarily to trimethoprim and streptomycin (197).

A recent report also documented the first gene-encoded resistance mechanism to the swine growth enhancer olaquindox among an *E. coli* isolate recovered from swine manure in Denmark (80). The genetic elements (*oqxAB*) involved in resistance to olaquindox were identified as a multidrug efflux pump encoded on a conjugative plasmid. Plasmids containing the *oqxAB* genes yielded high (MIC, >128 μg/ml) resistance to olaquindox as well as chloramphenicol (MIC, >64 μg/ml) in *E. coli* (80). This raises some concern that the use of olaquindox could select for the proliferation of a conjugative plasmid that also carries resistance determinants for ampicillin and chloramphenicol.

The use of tetracyclines in swine production is considerable, and has been ever since the growth-promoting properties of tetracyclines were discovered in 1949, when it was observed that low levels of chlortetracycline in livestock rations beneficially affected growth rates and feed utilization by young chickens (34). These initial observations were confirmed and extended to swine and cattle, leading to the development of both chlortetracycline and oxytetracycline as animal growth promoters in the early 1950s (34). It should not be surprising, then, that tetracycline resistance is relatively common in both pathogenic and commensal *E. coli* isolates recovered from pigs (68, 89, 110, 114, 123, 124, 158, 171).

More than 30 different tetracycline resistance determinants have been described to date, with *tetA*, *tetB*, *tetC*, *tetD*, and *tetE* most frequently found in tetracycline-resistant *E. coli* isolates (34). The majority of these *tet* genes are associated with either conjugative or mobilizable DNA elements, which may partially explain their wide distribution among bacterial species. Differences in tetracycline resistance determinants have been observed among commensal and pathogenic swine *E. coli* isolates from various countries. For example, the *tetA* gene was most frequently observed among pathogenic swine *E. coli* isolates from Switzerland (110). Sengelov et al. showed that *tetA* also predominated among pathogenic swine *E. coli* isolates from Denmark (158). These results are in contrast with other investigations that have found that either *tetB* or *tetC* predominated among both pathogenic and commensal swine *E. coli* isolates from either Norway or North America (25, 114, 124, 171). The diversity of tetracycline resistance genes among swine *E. coli* from different countries may reflect dissimilarities in animal husbandry practices with regard to past or present use of tetracyclines and/or the presence of specific conjugative plasmids conferring distinct resistance determinants.

In summary, ETECs are important pathogens of swine, causing diarrhea in newborn and postweaning pigs worldwide. Various control methods have been investigated in an attempt to eliminate or reduce *E. coli*-related illness in pigs, from the introduction of good management practices and high hygiene standards to increased vaccination (77, 132, 144). However, antimicrobials have been used frequently during the last 5 decades as the immediate solution in trying to control *E. coli*-related disease (15, 33, 116, 123, 124, 197). Data from numerous studies indicate that antimicrobial use during swine production is associated with increased resistance to those antimicrobials among both pathogenic and commensal *E. coli*. However, there is also evidence that nonantimicrobial selection pressures may maintain antimicrobial resistance in populations of bacteria in the swine production environment. Regardless, the swine industry must continue to invest in the maintenance of high herd health production systems, which ultimately should lead to a reduction in the amount of antimicrobials used in swine production.

COMPANION ANIMALS

E. coli is also commonly isolated from both canine and feline urinary tract infections and pyometra (32, 63, 78, 190). Antimicrobial agents are frequently used in pet animals to treat these and other diseases and commonly include penicillins, cephalosporins, potentiated sulfonamides, phenicols, aminoglycosides, and fluoroquinolones (76). Early work by Hirsh in the 1970s in the United States documented multidrug resistance among *E. coli* isolates recovered from the urine of dogs and cats with cystitis (90). Though only 33 *E. coli* isolates were tested, resistance among canine isolates ($n = 13$) was most often observed to streptomycin, tetracycline, ampicillin, and sulfa drugs, whereas feline isolates ($n = 20$) demonstrated resistance primarily to streptomycin, tetracycline, ampicillin, and chloramphenicol (90). Since then, a number of longitudinal retrospective studies in Europe and the United States have reported an increase in the prevalence of antimicrobial-resistant bacteria from pet animals (37, 43, 76, 136).

National antimicrobial resistance monitoring programs generally do not include bacteria recovered from companion animals, with the exceptions of Sweden (SVARM), Norway (NORM-VET), and more recently Germany (BfT-GermVet) (76). SVARM has reported data on antimicrobial susceptibilities among *E. coli* isolates from canine and feline urinary tract infections since 1992 (134a). Resistance against ampicillin, streptomycin, tetracycline, and or trimethoprim-sulfamethoxazole occurred among 10 to 20% of canine and feline *E. coli* isolates from urinary tract infections (134a). However, the comparatively high resistance frequencies among canine and feline *E. coli* isolates probably reflect a high proportion of treatment failures and recurrent illness among the cases sampled.

Two of the largest retrospective investigations detailing prevalence of antimicrobial resistance among bacterial isolates from canine and feline clinical cases were reported by Normand et al. in the United Kingdom between 1989 and 1997 and Oluoch et al. in the United States between 1990 and 1998 (136, 137). Trends of increasing resistance over time among *E. coli* isolates in the United Kingdom were noted for streptomycin and amoxicillin-clavulanic acid as well as those isolates demonstrating multidrug resistance phenotypes (136). With the exception of tetracycline, no significant changes in susceptibility patterns were observed among American *E. coli* isolates (137). Resistance was noted, however, to amoxicillin, carbenicillin, and cephalothin. Similar resistance rates have been reported elsewhere. For example, Feria et al. characterized 72 *E. coli* isolates collected from canine urinary tract infections in Portugal for β-lactam resistance (63). Thirty-six percent of isolates exhibited resistance to amoxicillin; however, only 19% were resistant to the combination of amoxicillin-clavulanate. Resistance was more often observed to cephalothin (25%) than to either ceftazidime or ceftriaxone (1.4%). Almost three-quarters of the isolates (73%) produced a single β-lactamase, with the most common being TEM-1 (77%), followed by AmpC (31%), SHV (11.5%), and OXA-1 (7.7%) (63).

Lanz et al. characterized antimicrobial susceptibilities and resistance determinants among 122 *E. coli* isolates recovered from urinary tract infections in dogs and cats between 2000 and 2001 in Switzerland (110). Resistance was most often observed to sulfonamide (20%), ampicillin (18%), streptomycin (16%), and tetracycline (14%). One canine isolate demonstrated resistance to 13 antimicrobial agents, including amoxicillin-clavulanic acid, cefoperazone, streptomycin, kanamycin, enrofloxacin, and chloramphenicol (113). Sanchez et al. characterized 34 multidrug-resistant *E. coli* isolates associated with nosocomial infections in dogs from Georgia (155). Isolates were resistant to most cephalosporins, including cephalothin, ceftiofur, and ceftriaxone.

Extended-spectrum cephalosporin resistance was most often associated with the presence of the $bla_{CMY\text{-}2}$ cephamycinase gene (in 32 of 34 isolates). Interestingly, 97% of isolates also demonstrated resistance to chloramphenicol, which was most often associated with the putative chloramphenicol/florfenicol efflux pump, *flo* (155). Class 1 integrons were often identified among the nosocomial isolates and contained gene cassettes most often conferring resistance to spectinomycin and trimethoprim. The authors concluded that emergence of multidrug-resistant nosocomial pathogens in dogs, especially in intensive care units, most likely reflects the abundant use of broad-spectrum antimicrobials at veterinary hospitals.

In recent years, the dissemination of *E. coli* strains harboring extended-spectrum β-lactamases (ESBLs) in clinical settings has caused a great deal of concern. Most ESBLs are derived from the classical TEM-1, TEM-2, and SHV-1 enzymes by amino acid substitutions in their sequences (21). Teshager et al. isolated an SHV-12 β-lactamase-producing *E. coli* strain from a dog in Spain with recurrent urinary tract infections (174). This strain demonstrated multidrug resistance to cefotaxime, ceftazidime, and aztreonam as well as to ciprofloxacin, chloramphenicol, and sulfonamides. Costa et al. recently reported on the incidence of ESBLs among healthy pets in Portugal (43). They tested for the presence of ESBL-containing *E. coli* strains from feces of 75 healthy pets (39 dogs and 36 cats) that had not received previous antibiotic treatment. Five *E. coli* strains displayed broad-spectrum cephalosporin resistance and were further shown to possess either the $bla_{TEM\text{-}52b}$ gene (three strains) or the $bla_{CTX\text{-}M\text{-}1}$ gene (one strain) (43).

Approval of fluoroquinolones for use in small animals has also been associated with increasing rates of resistance to these antimicrobials among *E. coli* isolates from companion animals (37, 40, 76). Cooke et al. documented an increase in the occurrence of enrofloxacin resistance among uropathogenic *E. coli* isolates from dogs in California during the mid- to late 1990s (40). Enrofloxacin-resistant isolates also demonstrated resistance to other antimicrobials commonly used to treat urinary tract infections (e.g., ampicillin, trimethoprim-sulfamethoxazole, and cephalexin). The increased prevalence of enrofloxacin-resistant *E. coli* was attributable not to a resistant clone but rather to acquisition of resistance in genetically unrelated strains. Fluoroquinolone resistance was associated with increased use of enrofloxacin at the veterinary hospital. The presence of resistance to both fluoroquinolones and extended-spectrum cephalosporins has also been observed among *E. coli* isolates associated with clinical infections in dogs in Australia (185).

A more recent study by Cohn et al. examined fluoroquinolone susceptibility data from bacteria isolated from canine urinary tract infections between 1992 and 2001 in Missouri (37). MICs of either ciprofloxacin (1992 to 1998) or enrofloxacin (1998 to 2001) were determined for 1,478 bacterial isolates from the canine urinary tract, including 547 *E. coli* isolates. A significant increase in the overall proportion of resistant bacterial isolates was documented from 1992 to 2001 (Cochran-Armitage test for trend, $P < 0.0001$). The same increase in resistant isolates was documented when either ciprofloxacin or enrofloxacin was analyzed separately ($P < 0.0001$ and $P < 0.0002$, respectively). Although the overall efficacy of fluoroquinolones remained high (>80% susceptible), the data demonstrated an increase in the proportion of resistant bacteria isolated from the canine urinary tracts (37).

In summary, the effects of antimicrobial use and its subsequent impact on the development of antimicrobial-resistant bacterial pathogens in small-animal veterinary practice do not differ from those observed in food animal production. Resistance to broad-spectrum antimicrobials, such as the fluoroquinolones and cephalosporins, among pathogenic *E. coli* isolates from companion animals is not surprising since veterinarians commonly use these drugs as first-line therapeutics in the treatment of certain infections in pet animals (76, 110, 155). Thus, with increasing rates of resistance being documented to these and other antimicrobials among *E. coli* isolates associated with illness in companion animals, the need for culture and subsequent antimicrobial susceptibility testing as a basis for antimicrobial selection takes on added urgency.

MINOR SPECIES

Diarrhea associated with *E. coli* infection is responsible for high rates of morbidity and mortality in goat kids and lambs (16, 35). These infections are often treated with antimicrobial agents; however, therapy has been frequently ineffective due in part to the presence of drug-resistant strains. Blanco et al. examined 144 *E. coli* isolates recovered from diarrheic lambs in Spain for serogroups, toxins, and antimicrobial resistance phenotypes (16). Resistance was most often observed to tetracycline (76%), streptomycin (74%), sulfadiazine (69%), ampicillin (50%), and kanamycin (47%). The percentages of isolates with antibiotic resistance observed among *E. coli* recovered from goat kids with diarrhea were generally greater than those seen among lamb *E. coli* isolates (e.g., streptomycin, 93%; sulfadiazine, 89%; tetracycline, 84%; and ampicillin, 69%) (16, 35). The authors indicated that the highest rates of resistance were to antimicrobials generally used by Spanish veterinary clinics.

E. coli is also commonly found in outbreaks of diarrhea in mink during the production season, although its role as a primary causal organism has yet to be fully elucidated. Vulfson et al. characterized 210 *E. coli* isolates from healthy and diarrheic mink in Denmark for serogroups and antimicrobial susceptibilities (182). All isolates were susceptible to enrofloxacin, neomycin, and gentamicin; however, resistance was observed to tetracycline, ampicillin, spectinomycin, sulfamethoxazole, and trimethoprim (182). Research by Tibbetts et al. in the United States showed similar findings with regard to antimicrobial resistance phenotypes among *E. coli* associated with mink colisepticemia cases (176). The highest rates of resistance were to tetracycline (83%), sulfamethoxazole (63%), streptomycin (60%), ampicillin (38%), and kanamycin (28%). Resistance was also observed to a lesser extent to gentamicin (20%), trimethoprim-sulfamethoxazole (13%), and chloramphenicol (8%). All isolates were susceptible to amikacin, ciprofloxacin, ceftiofur, ceftriaxone, cefoxitin, amoxicillin-clavulanic acid, and imipenem. Multiple-drug resistance was frequently observed, with 20 of 40 (50%) isolates resistant to four or more antibiotics (176). Overall, these data show that the *E. coli* isolates implicated in mink colisepticemia possess similar antimicrobial resistance phenotypes to those associated with diarrheal diseases in food animals.

SUMMARY

Over the past 6 decades, the introduction of new classes or modifications of antimicrobials has been matched slowly but surely by the development of new bacterial resistance mechanisms. Since the first reports in the late 1950s and early 1960s, numerous retrospective and prospective studies have demonstrated that increases in antimicrobial resistance among both pathogenic and commensal bacteria can be observed after introduction of an antimicrobial (3, 11, 15, 20, 22, 29, 40, 53, 70, 75, 95, 96, 109, 110, 128, 145, 155, 164, 179, 180, 191, 192). Additionally, the widespread observation of a relationship between increasing use of broad-spectrum antimicrobials and increasing resistance to these agents suggests a continuous cycle of antibiotic use, bacterial resistance development, reduced efficacy of antibiotics, and the invariable need for newer antimicrobial agents.

The control of *E. coli*-related disease in food and companion animals involves numerous strategies that depend on the animal species, of which antimicrobials are but one aspect. Antimicrobials are essential tools of disease management regimens in food and companion animals worldwide. The most commonly used antimicrobial drugs in food and companion animals are from five major classes: β-lactams, tetracyclines, aminogylcosides, macrolides, and sulfonamides. In addition, fluoroquinolones have been available in some European countries for more than 20 years, with large-animal approval occurring in the United States in 1998. However, the use of antimicrobial agents in any venue, including therapeutically in human and veterinary medicine or as prophylaxis for growth promotion in animal husbandry, ultimately exerts selective pressure favorable for the propagation of antimicrobial-resistant bacteria. Thus, the basic rule in slowing the evolution of resistance is reducing the unnecessary use of antibiotics. Accordingly, efforts to maintain the effectiveness of these drugs in veterinary medicine must address the ecological and health consequences of their use. Intervention strategies aimed at ultimately reducing the use of antimicrobials, increased biosecurity, improved production methods in animal husbandry and disease eradication, and optimal use of existing vaccines and development of newer ones can all help in achieving the goal of minimizing antimicrobial resistance in the animal production environment.

REFERENCES

1. Reference deleted.
2. **Aalbaek, B., J. Rasmussen, B. Nielsen, and J. E. Olsen.** 1991. Prevalence of antibiotic-resistant *Escherichia coli* in Danish pigs and cattle. *APMIS* **99:**1103–1110.
3. **Aarestrup, F. M.** 1999. Association between the consumption of antimicrobial agents in animal husbandry and the occurrence of resistant bacteria among food animals. *Int. J. Antimicrob. Agents* **12:**279–285.
4. **Aarestrup, F. M., and A. M. Seyfarth.** 2000. Effect of intervention on the occurrence of antimicrobial resistance. *Acta Vet. Scand. Suppl.* **93:**99–102.
5. **Aden, D. P., N. D. Reed, N. R. Underdahl, and C. A. Mebus.** 1969. Transferable drug resistance among *Enterobacteriaceae* isolated from cases of neonatal diarrhea in calves and piglets. *Appl. Microbiol.* **18:**961–964.
6. **Adetosoye, A. I., and M. Awad-Masalmeh.** 1979. Drug resistance in *Escherichia coli* isolated from diarrhoeic piglets. *Vet. Rec.* **105:**306.
7. **Altekruse, S. F., F. Elvinger, K. Y. Lee, L. K. Tollefson, E. W. Pierson, J. Eifert, and N. Sriranganathan.** 2002. Antimicrobial susceptibilities of *Escherichia coli* strains from a turkey operation. *J. Am. Vet. Med. Assoc.* **221:**411–416.

8. **Amara, A., Z. Ziani, and K. Bouzoubaa.** 1995. Antibioresistance of *Escherichia coli* strains isolated in Morocco from chickens with colibacillosis. *Vet. Microbiol.* **43:**325–330.
9. **Amezcua, R., R. M. Friendship, C. E. Dewey, C. Gyles, and J. M. Fairbrother.** 2002. Presentation of postweaning *Escherichia coli* diarrhea in southern Ontario, prevalence of hemolytic *E. coli* serogroups involved, and their antimicrobial resistance patterns. *Can. J. Vet. Res.* **66:**73–78.
10. **Bass, L., C. A. Liebert, M. D. Lee, A. O. Summers, D. G. White, S. G. Thayer, and J. J. Maurer.** 1999. Incidence and characterization of integrons, genetic elements mediating multiple-drug resistance, in avian *Escherichia coli. Antimicrob. Agents Chemother.* **43:**2925–2929.
11. **Bazile-Pham-Khac, S., Q. C. Truong, J. P. Lafont, L. Gutmann, X. Y. Zhou, M. Osman, and N. J. Moreau.** 1996. Resistance to fluoroquinolones in *Escherichia coli* isolated from poultry. *Antimicrob. Agents Chemother.* **40:**1504–1507.
12. **Bean, A., J. Williamson, and R. T. Cursons.** 2004. Virulence genes of *Escherichia coli* strains isolated from mastitic milk. *J. Vet. Med. B Infect. Dis. Vet. Public Health* **51:**285–287.
13. **Bebora, L. C., J. O. Oundo, and H. Yamamoto.** 1994. Resistance of *E. coli* strains, recovered from chickens to antibiotics with particular reference to trimethoprim-sulfamethoxazole (Septrin). *East Afr. Med. J.* **71:**624–627.
14. **Bertin, Y., C. Martin, J. P. Girardeau, P. Pohl, and M. Contrepois.** 1998. Association of genes encoding P fimbriae, CS31A antigen and EAST 1 toxin among CNF1-producing *Escherichia coli* strains from cattle with septicemia and diarrhea. *FEMS Microbiol. Lett.* **162:**235–239.
15. **Bischoff, K. M., D. G. White, P. F. McDermott, S. Zhao, S. Gaines, J. J. Maurer, and D. J. Nisbet.** 2002. Characterization of chloramphenicol resistance in beta-hemolytic *Escherichia coli* associated with diarrhea in neonatal swine. *J. Clin. Microbiol.* **40:**389–394.
16. **Blanco, J., D. Cid, J. E. Blanco, M. Blanco, J. A. Ruiz Santa Quiteira, and R. de la Fuente.** 1996. Serogroups, toxins and antibiotic resistance of *Escherichia coli* strains isolated from diarrhoeic lambs in Spain. *Vet. Microbiol.* **49:**209–217.
17. **Blanco, J. E., M. Blanco, A. Mora, and J. Blanco.** 1997. Prevalence of bacterial resistance to quinolones and other antimicrobials among avian *Escherichia coli* strains isolated from septicemic and healthy chickens in Spain. *J. Clin. Microbiol.* **35:**2184–2185.
18. **Blanco, J. E., M. Blanco, A. Mora, and J. Blanco.** 1997. Production of toxins (enterotoxins, verotoxins, and necrotoxins) and colicins by *Escherichia coli* strains isolated from septicemic and healthy chickens: relationship with in vivo pathogenicity. *J. Clin. Microbiol.* **35:**2953–2957.
19. **Blanco, M., J. E. Blanco, E. A. Gonzalez, A. Mora, W. Jansen, T. A. Gomes, L. F. Zerbini, T. Yano, A. F. de Castro, and J. Blanco.** 1997. Genes coding for enterotoxins and verotoxins in porcine *Escherichia coli* strains belonging to different O:K:H serotypes: relationship with toxic phenotypes. *J. Clin. Microbiol.* **35:**2958–2963.
20. **Blickwede, M., and S. Schwarz.** 2004. Molecular analysis of florfenicol-resistant *Escherichia coli* isolates from pigs. *J. Antimicrob. Chemother.* **53:**58–64.
21. **Bradford, P. A.** 2001. Extended-spectrum β-lactamases in the 21st century: characterization, epidemiology, and detection of this important resistance threat. *Clin. Microbiol. Rev.* **14:**933–951.
22. **Bradford, P. A., P. J. Petersen, I. M. Fingerman, and D. G. White.** 1999. Characterization of expanded-spectrum cephalosporin resistance in *E. coli* isolates associated with bovine calf diarrhoeal disease. *J. Antimicrob. Chemother.* **44:**607–610.
23. **Brinas, L., M. A. Moreno, M. Zarazaga, C. Porrero, Y. Saenz, M. Garcia, L. Dominguez, and C. Torres.** 2003. Detection of CMY-2, CTX-M-14, and SHV-12 β-lactamases in *Escherichia coli* fecal-sample isolates from healthy chickens. *Antimicrob. Agents Chemother.* **47:**2056–2058.
24. **Broes, A., J. M. Fairbrother, J. Mainil, J. Harel, and S. Lariviere.** 1988. Phenotypic and genotypic characterization of enterotoxigenic *Escherichia coli* serotype O8:KX105 and O8:K"2829" strains isolated from piglets with diarrhea. *J. Clin. Microbiol.* **26:**2402–2409.
25. **Bryan, A., N. Shapir, and M. J. Sadowsky.** 2004. Frequency and distribution of tetracycline resistance genes in genetically diverse, nonselected, and nonclinical *Escherichia coli* strains isolated from diverse human and animal sources. *Appl. Environ. Microbiol.* **70:**2503–2507.
26. Reference deleted.
27. **Chaslus-Dancla, E., G. Gerbaud, M. Lagorce, J. P. Lafont, and P. Courvalin.** 1987. Persistence of an antibiotic resistance plasmid in intestinal *Escherichia coli* of chickens in the absence of selective pressure. *Antimicrob. Agents Chemother.* **31:**784–788.
28. **Chaslus-Dancla, E., G. Gerbaud, J. L. Martel, M. Lagorce, J. P. Lafont, and P. Courvalin.** 1987. Detection of a second mechanism of resistance to gentamicin in animal strains of *Escherichia coli. Antimicrob. Agents Chemother.* **31:**1274–1277.
29. **Chaslus-Dancla, E., and J. P. Lafont.** 1985. Resistance to gentamicin and apramycin in *Escherichia coli* from calves in France. *Vet. Rec.* **117:**90–91.
30. **Chaslus-Dancla, E., J. L. Martel, C. Carlier, J. P. Lafont, and P. Courvalin.** 1986. Emergence of aminoglycoside 3-*N*-acetyltransferase IV in *Escherichia coli* and *Salmonella typhimurium* isolated from animals in France. *Antimicrob. Agents Chemother.* **29:**239–243.
31. **Chaslus-Dancla, E., P. Pohl, M. Meurisse, M. Marin, and J. P. Lafont.** 1991. High genetic homology between plasmids of human and animal origins conferring resistance to the aminoglycosides gentamicin and apramycin. *Antimicrob. Agents Chemother.* **35:**590–593.
32. **Chen, Y. M., P. J. Wright, C. S. Lee, and G. F. Browning.** 2003. Uropathogenic virulence factors in isolates of *Escherichia coli* from clinical cases of canine pyometra and feces of healthy bitches. *Vet. Microbiol.* **94:**57–69.
33. **Choi, C., H. J. Ham, D. Kwon, J. Kim, D. S. Cheon, K. Min, W. S. Cho, H. K. Chung, T. Jung, K. Jung, and C. Chae.** 2002. Antimicrobial susceptibility of pathogenic *Escherichia coli* isolated from pigs in Korea. *J. Vet. Med. Sci.* **64:**71–73.
34. **Chopra, I., and M. Roberts.** 2001. Tetracycline antibiotics: mode of action, applications, molecular biology, and epidemiology of bacterial resistance. *Microbiol. Mol. Biol. Rev.* **65:**232–260.
35. **Cid, D., M. Blanco, J. E. Blanco, J. A. Ruiz Santa Quiteira, R. de la Fuente, and J. Blanco.** 1996. Serogroups, toxins and antibiotic resistance of *Escherichia coli* strains isolated from diarrhoeic goat kids in Spain. *Vet. Microbiol.* **53:**349–354.
36. **Cloeckaert, A., S. Baucheron, G. Flaujac, S. Schwarz, C. Kehrenberg, J. L. Martel, and E. Chaslus-Dancla.** 2000. Plasmid-mediated florfenicol resistance encoded by the *floR* gene in *Escherichia coli* isolated from cattle. *Antimicrob. Agents Chemother.* **44:**2858–2860.
37. **Cohn, L. A., A. T. Gary, W. H. Fales, and R. W. Madsen.** 2003. Trends in fluoroquinolone resistance of bacteria isolated from canine urinary tracts. *J. Vet. Diagn. Investig.* **15:**338–343.
38. **Constable, P. D.** 2004. Antimicrobial use in the treatment of calf diarrhea. *J. Vet. Intern. Med.* **18:**8–17.

39. **Conway, P. L.** 1995. Microbial ecology of the human large intestine, p. 1–24. *In* G. R. Gibson and G. T. Macfarlane (ed.), *Human Colonic Bacteria: Role in Nutrition, Physiology, and Pathology*. CRC Press, Inc., Boca Raton, Fla.

40. **Cooke, C. L., R. S. Singer, S. S. Jang, and D. C. Hirsh.** 2002. Enrofloxacin resistance in *Escherichia coli* isolated from dogs with urinary tract infections. *J. Am. Vet. Med. Assoc.* **220:**190–192.

41. **Cormican, M., V. Buckley, G. Corbett-Feeney, and F. Sheridan.** 2001. Antimicrobial resistance in *Escherichia coli* isolates from turkeys and hens in Ireland. *J. Antimicrob. Chemother.* **48:**587–588.

42. **Corti, S., D. Sicher, W. Regli, and R. Stephan.** 2003. Current data on antibiotic resistance of the most important bovine mastitis pathogens in Switzerland. *Schweiz. Arch. Tierheilkd.* **145:**571–575. (In German.)

43. **Costa, D., P. Poeta, L. Brinas, Y. Saenz, J. Rodrigues, and C. Torres.** 2004. Detection of CTX-M-1 and TEM-52 β-lactamases in *Escherichia coli* strains from healthy pets in Portugal. *J. Antimicrob. Chemother.* **54:**960–961.

44. **Delicato, E. R., B. G. de Brito, L. C. Gaziri, and M. C. Vidotto.** 2003. Virulence-associated genes in *Escherichia coli* isolates from poultry with colibacillosis. *Vet. Microbiol.* **94:**97–103.

45. **de Lopez, A. G., S. Kadis, and E. B. Shotts, Jr.** 1982. Enterotoxin production and resistance to antimicrobial agents in porcine and bovine *Escherichia coli* strains. *Am. J. Vet. Res.* **43:**1286–1287.

46. **Dho-Moulin, M., and J. M. Fairbrother.** 1999. Avian pathogenic *Escherichia coli* (APEC). *Vet. Res.* **30:**299–316.

47. **Dias de Silveira, W., A. Ferreira, M. Brocchi, L. M. de Hollanda, A. F. Pestana de Castro, A. T. Yamada, and M. Lancellotti.** 2002. Biological characteristics and pathogenicity of avian *Escherichia coli* strains. *Vet. Microbiol.* **85:**47–53.

48. **Donnenberg, M. S., and T. S. Whittam.** 2001. Pathogenesis and evolution of virulence in enteropathogenic and enterohemorrhagic *Escherichia coli. J. Clin. Investig.* **107:** 539–548.

49. **Donovan, D. C., S. T. Franklin, C. C. Chase, and A. R. Hippen.** 2002. Growth and health of Holstein calves fed milk replacers supplemented with antibiotics or Enteroguard. *J. Dairy Sci.* **85:**947–950.

50. **Doublet, B., S. Schwarz, E. Nussbeck, S. Baucheron, J. L. Martel, E. Chaslus-Dancla, and A. Cloeckaert.** 2002. Molecular analysis of chromosomally florfenicol-resistant *Escherichia coli* isolates from France and Germany. *J. Antimicrob. Chemother.* **49:**49–54.

51. **Dozois, C. M., J. M. Fairbrother, J. Harel, and M. Bosse.** 1992. *pap-* and *pil*-related DNA sequences and other virulence determinants associated with *Escherichia coli* isolated from septicemic chickens and turkeys. *Infect. Immun.* **60:**2648–2656.

52. **Du, X., C. Xia, J. Shen, B. Wu, and Z. Shen.** 2004. Characterization of florfenicol resistance among calf pathogenic *Escherichia coli. FEMS Microbiol. Lett.* **236:**183–189.

53. **Dubel, J. R., D. L. Zink, L. M. Kelley, S. A. Naqi, and H. W. Renshaw.** 1982. Bacterial antibiotic resistance: frequency of gentamicin-resistant strains of *Escherichia coli* in the fecal microflora of commercial turkeys. *Am. J. Vet. Res.* **43:**1786–1789.

54. **Dulaney, A. D., and I. D. Michelson.** 1935. A study of *B. coli* mutabile from an outbreak of diarrhea in the newborn. *Am. J. Public Health* **25:**1241–1251.

55. **Dunlop, R. H., S. A. McEwen, A. H. Meek, R. C. Clarke, W. D. Black, and R. M. Friendship.** 1998. Associations among antimicrobial drug treatments and antimicrobial resistance of fecal *Escherichia coli* of swine on 34 farrow-to-finish farms in Ontario, Canada. *Prev. Vet. Med.* **34:**283–305.

56. **Engberg, J., F. M. Aarestrup, D. E. Taylor, P. Gerner-Smidt, and I. Nachamkin.** 2001. Quinolone and macrolide resistance in *Campylobacter jejuni* and *C. coli*: resistance mechanisms and trends in human isolates. *Emerg. Infect. Dis.* **7:**24–34.

57. **Erskine, R. J., S. Wagner, and F. J. DeGraves.** 2003. Mastitis therapy and pharmacology. *Vet. Clin. N. Am. Food Anim. Pract.* **19:**109–138, vi.

58. **Erskine, R. J., R. D. Walker, C. A. Bolin, P. C. Bartlett, and D. G. White.** 2002. Trends in antibacterial susceptibility of mastitis pathogens during a seven-year period. *J. Dairy Sci.* **85:**1111–1118.

59. **Escherich, T.** 1989. The intestinal bacteria of the neonate and breast-fed infant. *Rev. Infect. Dis.* **11:**352–356.

60. **Everett, M. J., Y. F. Jin, V. Ricci, and L. J. Piddock.** 1996. Contributions of individual mechanisms to fluoroquinolone resistance in 36 *Escherichia coli* strains isolated from humans and animals. *Antimicrob. Agents Chemother.* **40:**2380–2386.

61. **Fang, W., and S. Pyorala.** 1996. Mastitis-causing *Escherichia coli*: serum sensitivity and susceptibility to selected antibacterials in milk. *J. Dairy Sci.* **79:**76–82.

62. **Fecteau, G., J. M. Fairbrother, R. Higgins, D. C. Van Metre, J. Pare, B. P. Smith, C. A. Holmberg, and S. Jang.** 2001. Virulence factors in *Escherichia coli* isolated from the blood of bacteremic neonatal calves. *Vet. Microbiol.* **78:**241–249.

63. **Feria, C., E. Ferreira, J. D. Correia, J. Goncalves, and M. Canica.** 2002. Patterns and mechanisms of resistance to β-lactams and β-lactamase inhibitors in uropathogenic *Escherichia coli* isolated from dogs in Portugal. *J. Antimicrob. Chemother.* **49:**77–85.

64. **Foley, S. L., S. M. Horne, C. W. Giddings, M. Robinson, and L. K. Nolan.** 2000. Iss from a virulent avian *Escherichia coli. Avian Dis.* **44:**185–191.

65. **Franklin, A.** 1984. Antimicrobial drug resistance in porcine enterotoxigenic *Escherichia coli* of O-group 149 and non-enterotoxigenic Escherichia coli. *Vet. Microbiol.* **9:**467–475.

66. **Franklin, A., and V. Glatthard.** 1977. R-factor-mediated antibiotic resistance in *E. coli* strains isolated from piglets in Sweden. *Zentbl. Bakteriol. Orig. A* **238:**208–215.

67. **Frydendahl, K.** 2002. Prevalence of serogroups and virulence genes in *Escherichia coli* associated with postweaning diarrhoea and edema disease in pigs and a comparison of diagnostic approaches. *Vet. Microbiol.* **85:**169–182.

68. **Gellin, G., B. E. Langlois, K. A. Dawson, and D. K. Aaron.** 1989. Antibiotic resistance of gram-negative enteric bacteria from pigs in three herds with different histories of antibiotic exposure. *Appl. Environ. Microbiol.* **55:**2287–2292.

69. **Geornaras, I., J. W. Hastings, and A. von Holy.** 2001. Genotypic analysis of *Escherichia coli* strains from poultry carcasses and their susceptibilities to antimicrobial agents. *Appl. Environ. Microbiol.* **67:**1940–1944.

70. **Giraud, E., S. Leroy-Setrin, G. Flaujac, A. Cloeckaert, M. Dho-Moulin, and E. Chaslus-Dancla.** 2001. Characterization of high-level fluoroquinolone resistance in *Escherichia coli* O78: K80 isolated from turkeys. *J. Antimicrob. Chemother.* **47:** 341–343.

71. **Glisson, J. R., C. L. Hofacre, and G. F. Mathis.** 2004. Comparative efficacy of enrofloxacin, oxytetracycline, and sulfadimethoxine for the control of morbidity and mortality caused by *Escherichia coli* in broiler chickens. *Avian Dis.* **48:**658–662.

72. **Gomis, S., L. Babiuk, D. L. Godson, B. Allan, T. Thrush, H. Townsend, P. Willson, E. Waters, R. Hecker, and A. Potter.** 2003. Protection of chickens against *Escherichia coli* infections by DNA containing CpG motifs. *Infect. Immun.* **71:**857–863.

73. **Gonzalez, E. A., and J. Blanco.** 1989. Serotypes and antibiotic resistance of verotoxigenic (VTEC) and necrotizing (NTEC) *Escherichia coli* strains isolated from calves with diarrhoea. *FEMS Microbiol. Lett.* **51:**31–36.
74. **Gross, W. G.** 1994. Diseases due to *Escherichia coli* in poultry, p. 237–259. *In* C. L. Gyles (ed.), Escherichia coli *in Domestic Animals and Humans*. CAB International, Wallingford, United Kingdom.
75. **Grugel, C., and J. Wallmann.** 2004. Antimicrobial resistance in bacteria from food-producing animals. Risk management tools and strategies. *J. Vet. Med. B* **51:**419–421.
76. **Guardabassi, L., S. Schwarz, and D. H. Lloyd.** 2004. Pet animals as reservoirs of antimicrobial-resistant bacteria. *J. Antimicrob. Chemother.* **54:**321–332.
77. **Haesebrouck, F., F. Pasmans, K. Chiers, D. Maes, R. Ducatelle, and A. Decostere.** 2004. Efficacy of vaccines against bacterial diseases in swine: what can we expect? *Vet. Microbiol.* **100:** 255–268.
78. **Hagman, R., and I. Kuhn.** 2002. *Escherichia coli* strains isolated from the uterus and urinary bladder of bitches suffering from pyometra: comparison by restriction enzyme digestion and pulsed-field gel electrophoresis. *Vet. Microbiol.* **84:**143–153.
79. **Hall, R. M., and H. W. Stokes.** 1993. Integrons: novel DNA elements which capture genes by site-specific recombination. *Genetica* **90:**115–132.
80. **Hansen, L. H., E. Johannesen, M. Burmolle, A. H. Sorensen, and S. J. Sorensen.** 2004. Plasmid-encoded multidrug efflux pump conferring resistance to olaquindox in *Escherichia coli*. *Antimicrob. Agents Chemother.* **48:**3332–3337.
81. **Hariharan, H., M. Coles, D. Poole, and R. Page.** 2004. Antibiotic resistance among enterotoxigenic *Escherichia coli* from piglets and calves with diarrhea. *Can. Vet. J.* **45:** 605–606.
82. **Harnett, N. M., and C. L. Gyles.** 1984. Resistance to drugs and heavy metals, colicin production, and biochemical characteristics of selected bovine and porcine *Escherichia coli* strains. *Appl. Environ. Microbiol.* **48:**930–935.
83. **Harnett, N. M., and C. L. Gyles.** 1985. Linkage of genes for heat-stable enterotoxin, drug resistance, K99 antigen, and colicin in bovine and porcine strains of enterotoxigenic *Escherichia coli*. *Am. J. Vet. Res.* **46:**428–433.
84. **Hedges, R. W., and K. P. Shannon.** 1984. Resistance to apramycin in *Escherichia coli* isolated from animals: detection of a novel aminoglycoside-modifying enzyme. *J. Gen. Microbiol.* **130**(Pt. 3)**:**473–482.
85. **Heinrichs, A. J., C. M. Jones, and B. S. Heinrichs.** 2003. Effects of mannan oligosaccharide or antibiotics in neonatal diets on health and growth of dairy calves. *J. Dairy Sci.* **86:**4064–4069.
86. **Heinrichs, A. J., S. J. Wells, and W. C. Losinger.** 1995. A study of the use of milk replacers for dairy calves in the United States. *J. Dairy Sci.* **78:**2831–2837.
87. **Heisig, P.** 1996. Genetic evidence for a role of *parC* mutations in development of high-level fluoroquinolone resistance in *Escherichia coli*. *Antimicrob. Agents Chemother.* **40:**879–885.
88. **Heisig, P., B. Kratz, E. Halle, Y. Graser, M. Altwegg, W. Rabsch, and J. P. Faber.** 1995. Identification of DNA gyrase A mutations in ciprofloxacin-resistant isolates of *Salmonella typhimurium* from men and cattle in Germany. *Microb. Drug Resist.* **1:**211–218.
89. **Hinton, M.** 1986. The ecology of *Escherichia coli* in animals including man with particular reference to drug resistance. *Vet. Rec.* **119:**420–426.
90. **Hirsh, D. C.** 1973. Multiple antimicrobial resistance in *Escherichia coli* isolated from the urine of dogs and cats with cystitis. *J. Am. Vet. Med. Assoc.* **162:**885–887.
91. **Holland, R. E.** 1990. Some infectious causes of diarrhea in young farm animals. *Clin. Microbiol. Rev.* **3:**345–375.
92. **Holland, R. E., R. A. Wilson, M. S. Holland, V. Yuzbasiyan-Gurkan, T. P. Mullaney, and D. G. White.** 1999. Characterization of eae+ *Escherichia coli* isolated from healthy and diarrheic calves. *Vet. Microbiol.* **66:**251–263.
93. **Holmberg, S. D., S. L. Solomon, and P. A. Blake.** 1987. Health and economic impacts of antimicrobial resistance. *Rev. Infect. Dis.* **9:**1065–1078.
94. **Hooper, D. C.** 2001. Emerging mechanisms of fluoroquinolone resistance. *Emerg. Infect. Dis.* **7:**337–341.
95. **Hummel, R., H. Tschape, and W. Witte.** 1986. Spread of plasmid-mediated nourseothricin resistance due to antibiotic use in animal husbandry. *J. Basic Microbiol.* **26:**461–466.
96. **Hunter, J. E., M. Bennett, C. A. Hart, J. C. Shelley, and J. R. Walton.** 1994. Apramycin-resistant *Escherichia coli* isolated from pigs and a stockman. *Epidemiol. Infect.* **112:** 473–480.
97. **Hunter, J. E., J. C. Shelley, J. R. Walton, C. A. Hart, and M. Bennett.** 1992. Apramycin resistance plasmids in *Escherichia coli*: possible transfer to *Salmonella typhimurium* in calves. *Epidemiol. Infect.* **108:**271–278.
98. **Jay, C. M., S. Bhaskaran, K. S. Rathore, and S. D. Waghela.** 2004. Enterotoxigenic K99+ *Escherichia coli* attachment to host cell receptors inhibited by recombinant pili protein. *Vet. Microbiol.* **101:**153–160.
99. **Jeffrey, J. S., L. K. Nolan, K. H. Tonooka, S. Wolfe, C. W. Giddings, S. M. Horne, S. L. Foley, A. M. Lynne, J. O. Ebert, L. M. Elijah, G. Bjorklund, S. J. Pfaff-McDonough, R. S. Singer, and C. Doetkott.** 2002. Virulence factors of *Escherichia coli* from cellulitis or colisepticemia lesions in chickens. *Avian Dis.* **46:**48–52.
100. **Johnson, T. J., J. Skyberg, and L. K. Nolan.** 2004. Multiple antimicrobial resistance region of a putative virulence plasmid from an *Escherichia coli* isolate incriminated in avian colibacillosis. *Avian Dis.* **48:**351–360.
101. **Jorgensen, S. T.** 1978. Chloramphenicol resistance plasmids in *Escherichia coli* isolated from diseased piglets. *Antimicrob. Agents Chemother.* **13:**710–715.
102. **Jorgensen, S. T., and A. L. Poulsen.** 1976. Antibiotic resistance and Hly plasmids in serotypes of *Escherichia coli* associated with porcine enteric disease. *Antimicrob. Agents Chemother.* **9:**6–10.
103. **Kaipainen, T., T. Pohjanvirta, N. Y. Shpigel, A. Shwimmer, S. Pyorala, and S. Pelkonen.** 2002. Virulence factors of *Escherichia coli* isolated from bovine clinical mastitis. *Vet. Microbiol.* **85:**37–46.
104. **Kanai, H., H. Hashimoto, and S. Mitsuhashi.** 1983. Drug resistance and R plasmids in *Escherichia coli* strains isolated from broilers. *Microbiol. Immunol.* **27:**471–478.
105. Reference deleted.
106. **Kang, S. J., S. J. Ryu, J. S. Chae, S. K. Eo, G. J. Woo, and J. H. Lee.** 2004. Occurrence and characteristics of enterohemorrhagic *Escherichia coli* O157 in calves associated with diarrhoea. *Vet. Microbiol.* **98:**323–328.
107. **Keyes, K., C. Hudson, J. J. Maurer, S. Thayer, D. G. White, and M. D. Lee.** 2000. Detection of florfenicol resistance genes in *Escherichia coli* isolated from sick chickens. *Antimicrob. Agents Chemother.* **44:**421–424.
108. **Kwaga, J. K., B. J. Allan, J. V. van der Hurk, H. Seida, and A. A. Potter.** 1994. A *carAB* mutant of avian pathogenic *Escherichia coli* serogroup O2 is attenuated and effective as a live oral vaccine against colibacillosis in turkeys. *Infect. Immun.* **62:**3766–3772.
109. **Langlois, B. E., G. L. Cromwell, T. S. Stahly, K. A. Dawson, and V. W. Hays.** 1983. Antibiotic resistance of fecal coliforms

after long-term withdrawal of therapeutic and subtherapeutic antibiotic use in a swine herd. *Appl. Environ. Microbiol.* **46**:1433–1434.

110. **Lanz, R., P. Kuhnert, and P. Boerlin.** 2003. Antimicrobial resistance and resistance gene determinants in clinical *Escherichia coli* from different animal species in Switzerland. *Vet. Microbiol.* **91**:73–84.

111. **La Ragione, R. M., G. Casula, S. M. Cutting, and M. J. Woodward.** 2001. *Bacillus subtilis* spores competitively exclude *Escherichia coli* O78:K80 in poultry. *Vet. Microbiol.* **79**:133–142.

112. **La Ragione, R. M., A. Narbad, M. J. Gasson, and M. J. Woodward.** 2004. In vivo characterization of *Lactobacillus johnsonii* FI9785 for use as a defined competitive exclusion agent against bacterial pathogens in poultry. *Lett. Appl. Microbiol.* **38**:197–205.

113. **La Ragione, R. M., and M. J. Woodward.** 2002. Virulence factors of *Escherichia coli* serotypes associated with avian colisepticaemia. *Res. Vet. Sci.* **73**:27–35.

114. **Lee, C., B. E. Langlois, and K. A. Dawson.** 1993. Detection of tetracycline resistance determinants in pig isolates from three herds with different histories of antimicrobial agent exposure. *Appl. Environ. Microbiol.* **59**:1467–1472.

115. **Lehtolainen, T., A. Shwimmer, N. Y. Shpigel, T. Honkanen-Buzalski, and S. Pyorala.** 2003. In vitro antimicrobial susceptibility of *Escherichia coli* isolates from clinical bovine mastitis in Finland and Israel. *J. Dairy Sci.* **86**:3927–3932.

116. **Libal, M. C., and C. E. Gates.** 1982. Antimicrobial resistance in *Escherichia coli* strains isolated from pigs with diarrhea. *J. Am. Vet. Med. Assoc.* **180**:908–909.

117. **Linton, A. H., K. Howe, C. L. Hartley, H. M. Clements, M. H. Richmond, and A. D. Osborne.** 1977. Antibiotic resistance among *Escherichia coli* O-serotypes from the gut and carcases of commercially slaughtered broiler chickens: a potential public health hazard. *J. Appl. Bacteriol.* **42**:365–378.

118. **Linton, A. H., K. Howe, W. J. Sojka, and C. Wray.** 1979. A note on the range of Escherichia coli O-serotypes causing clinical bovine mastitis and their antibiotic resistance spectra. *J. Appl. Bacteriol.* **46**:585–590.

119. **Makovec, J. A., and P. L. Ruegg.** 2003. Antimicrobial resistance of bacteria isolated from dairy cow milk samples submitted for bacterial culture: 8,905 samples (1994–2001). *J. Am. Vet. Med. Assoc.* **222**:1582–1589.

120. **Margard, W. L., A. C. Peters, R. N. Pesut, and J. H. Litchfield.** 1971. Chlortetracycline resistance in enteric microorganisms in chickens and swine. *Dev. Ind. Microbiol.* **12**:376–392.

121. **Martel, J. L., M. Contrepois, H. C. Dubourguier, J. P. Girardeau, P. Gouet, C. Bordas, F. Hayers, A. Quilleriet-Eliez, J. Ramisse, and R. Sendral.** 1981. Frequence of K99 antigen and antibioresistance in *Escherichia coli* from calves in France. *Ann. Rech. Vet.* **12**:253–257. (In French.)

122. **Martins, M. F., N. M. Martinez-Rossi, A. Ferreira, M. Brocchi, T. Yano, A. F. Castro, and W. D. Silveira.** 2000. Pathogenic characteristics of *Escherichia coli* strains isolated from newborn piglets with diarrhea in Brazil. *Vet. Microbiol.* **76**:51–59.

123. **Mathew, A. G., W. G. Upchurch, and S. E. Chattin.** 1998. Incidence of antibiotic resistance in fecal *Escherichia coli* isolated from commercial swine farms. *J. Anim. Sci.* **76**: 429–434.

124. **Maynard, C., J. M. Fairbrother, S. Bekal, F. Sanschagrin, R. C. Levesque, R. Brousseau, L. Masson, S. Lariviere, and J. Harel.** 2003. Antimicrobial resistance genes in enterotoxigenic *Escherichia coli* O149:K91 isolates obtained over a 23-year period from pigs. *Antimicrob. Agents Chemother.* **47**: 3214–3221.

125. **McDermott, P. F., D. J. Eaves, L. J. V. Piddock, R. D. Walker, S. Zhao, S. Ayers, S. Bodeis, and D. G. White.** 2002. Characterization of multiple fluoroquinolone resistance among bovine pathogenic *Escherichia coli*, abstr. Z-44, p. 515. *Abstr. 102nd Gen. Meet. Am. Soc. Microbiol.* 2002. American Society for Microbiology, Washington, D.C.

126. **McGruder, E. D., and G. M. Moore.** 1999. Use of lipopolysaccharide (LPS) as a positive control for the evaluation of immunopotentiating drug candidates in experimental avian colibacillosis models. *Res. Vet. Sci.* **66**:33–37.

127. **Mellata, M., M. Dho-Moulin, C. M. Dozois, R. Curtiss III, P. K. Brown, P. Arne, A. Bree, C. Desautels, and J. M. Fairbrother.** 2003. Role of virulence factors in resistance of avian pathogenic *Escherichia coli* to serum and in pathogenicity. *Infect. Immun.* **71**:536–540.

128. **Mercer, H. D., D. Pocurull, S. Gaines, S. Wilson, and J. V. Bennett.** 1971. Characteristics of antimicrobial resistance of *Escherichia coli* from animals: relationship to veterinary and management uses of antimicrobial agents. *Appl. Microbiol.* **22**:700–705.

129. **Meunier, D., J. F. Acar, J. L. Martel, S. Kroemer, and M. Valle.** 2004. Seven years survey of susceptibility to marbofloxacin of bovine pathogenic strains from eight European countries. *Int. J. Antimicrob. Agents* **24**:268–278.

130. **Miniats, O. P., and C. K. Roe.** 1968. Escherichia coli infections in early weaned pigs. *Can. Vet. J.* **9**:210–217.

131. **Mitsuhashi, S., H. Hashimoto, and K. Suzuki.** 1967. Drug resistance of enteric bacteria. 13. Distribution of R factors in *Escherichia coli* strains isolated from livestock. *J. Bacteriol.* **94**:1166–1169.

132. **Moon, H. W., and T. O. Bunn.** 1993. Vaccines for preventing enterotoxigenic *Escherichia coli* infections in farm animals. *Vaccine* **11**:213–200.

133. **Nagy, B., and P. Z. Fekete.** 1999. Enterotoxigenic *Escherichia coli* (ETEC) in farm animals. *Vet. Res.* **30**: 259–284.

134. **Nataro, J. P., and J. B. Kaper.** 1998. Diarrheagenic *Escherichia coli*. *Clin. Microbiol. Rev.* **11**:142–201.

134a. **National Veterinary Institute.** *SVARM 2002: Swedish Veterinary Antimicrobial Resistance Monitoring*. National Veterinary Institute, Uppsala, Sweden.

135. **Nazer, A. H.** 1980. Transmissible drug resistance in *Escherichia coli* isolated from poultry and their carcasses in Iran. *Cornell Vet.* **70**:365–371.

136. **Normand, E. H., N. R. Gibson, S. W. Reid, S. Carmichael, and D. J. Taylor.** 2000. Antimicrobial-resistance trends in bacterial isolates from companion-animal community practice in the UK. *Prev. Vet. Med.* **46**:267–278.

137. **Oluoch, A. O., C. H. Kim, R. M. Weisiger, H. Y. Koo, A. M. Siegel, K. L. Campbell, T. J. Burke, B. C. McKiernan, and I. Kakoma.** 2001. Nonenteric *Escherichia coli* isolates from dogs: 674 cases (1990–1998). *J. Am. Vet. Med. Assoc.* **218**:381–384.

138. **Orden, J. A., J. A. Ruiz-Santa-Quiteria, S. Garcia, D. Cid, and R. de la Fuente.** 1999. In vitro activities of cephalosporins and quinolones against *Escherichia coli* strains isolated from diarrheic dairy calves. *Antimicrob. Agents Chemother.* **43**:510–513.

139. **Orden, J. A., J. A. Ruiz-Santa-Quiteria, S. Garcia, D. Cid, and R. de la Fuente.** 2000. In vitro susceptibility of *Escherichia coli* strains isolated from diarrhoeic dairy calves to 15 antimicrobial agents. *J. Vet. Med. B Infect. Dis. Vet. Public Health* **47**:329–335.

140. **Orskov, F., and I. Orskov.** 1990. The serology of capsular antigens. *Curr. Top. Microbiol. Immunol.* **150**:43–63.

141. **Orskov, I., and F. Orskov.** 1985. *Escherichia coli* in extraintestinal infections. *J. Hyg. Lond.* **95**:551–575.

142. **Osek, J.** 2000. Clonal analysis of *Escherichia coli* strains isolated from pigs with post-weaning diarrhea by pulsed-field gel electrophoresis. *FEMS Microbiol. Lett.* **186**:327–331.
143. **Osek, J.** 2003. Detection of the enteroaggregative *Escherichia coli* heat-stable enterotoxin 1 (EAST1) gene and its relationship with fimbrial and enterotoxin markers in *E. coli* isolates from pigs with diarrhoea. *Vet. Microbiol.* **91**:65–72.
144. **Osek, J., M. Truszczynski, K. Tarasiuk, and Z. Pejsak.** 1995. Evaluation of different vaccines to control of pig colibacillosis under large-scale farm conditions. *Comp. Immunol. Microbiol. Infect. Dis.* **18**:1–8.
145. **Piddock, L. J.** 1996. Does the use of antimicrobial agents in veterinary medicine and animal husbandry select antibiotic-resistant bacteria that infect man and compromise antimicrobial chemotherapy? *J. Antimicrob. Chemother.* **38**:1–3.
146. **Piddock, L. J.** 1998. Fluoroquinolone resistance: overuse of fluoroquinolones in human and veterinary medicine can breed resistance. *Br. Med. J.* **317**:1029–1030.
147. **Pyorala, S.** 2002. New strategies to prevent mastitis. *Reprod. Domest. Anim.* **37**:211–216.
148. **Pyorala, S. H., and E. O. Pyorala.** 1998. Efficacy of parenteral administration of three antimicrobial agents in treatment of clinical mastitis in lactating cows: 487 cases (1989–1995). *J. Am. Vet. Med. Assoc.* **212**:407–412.
149. **Rajala-Schultz, P. J., K. L. Smith, J. S. Hogan, and B. C. Love.** 2004. Antimicrobial susceptibility of mastitis pathogens from first lactation and older cows. *Vet. Microbiol.* **102**:33–42.
150. **Recchia, G. D., and R. M. Hall.** 1997. Origins of the mobile gene cassettes found in integrons. *Trends Microbiol.* **5**:389–394.
151. **Robins-Browne, R. M., and E. L. Hartland.** 2002. *Escherichia coli* as a cause of diarrhea. *J. Gastroenterol. Hepatol.* **17**:467–475.
152. **Rollins, L. D., D. W. Pocurull, H. D. Mercer, R. P. Natzke, and D. S. Postle.** 1974. Use of antibiotics in a dairy herd and their effect on resistance determinants in enteric and environmental *Escherichia coli. J. Dairy Sci.* **57**:944–950.
153. **Saenz, Y., M. Zarazaga, L. Brinas, F. Ruiz-Larrea, and C. Torres.** 2003. Mutations in *gyrA* and *parC* genes in nalidixic acid-resistant *Escherichia coli* strains from food products, humans and animals. *J. Antimicrob. Chemother.* **51**:1001–1005.
154. **Sallen, B., A. Rajoharison, S. Desvarenne, and C. Mabilat.** 1995. Molecular epidemiology of integron-associated antibiotic resistance genes in clinical isolates of *Enterobacteriaceae. Microb. Drug Resist.* **1**:195–202.
155. **Sanchez, S., M. A. McCrackin Stevenson, C. R. Hudson, M. Maier, T. Buffington, Q. Dam, and J. J. Maurer.** 2002. Characterization of multidrug-resistant *Escherichia coli* isolates associated with nosocomial infections in dogs. *J. Clin. Microbiol.* **40**:3586–3595.
156. **Sandholm, M., L. Kaartinen, and S. Pyorala.** 1990. Bovine mastitis—why does antibiotic therapy not always work? An overview. *J. Vet. Pharmacol. Ther.* **13**:248–260.
157. **Schwartz, B., D. M. Bell, and J. M. Hughes.** 1997. Preventing the emergence of antimicrobial resistance. A call for action by clinicians, public health officials, and patients. *JAMA* **278**:944–945.
158. **Sengelov, G., B. Halling-Sorensen, and F. M. Aarestrup.** 2003. Susceptibility of *Escherichia coli* and *Enterococcus faecium* isolated from pigs and broiler chickens to tetracycline degradation products and distribution of tetracycline resistance determinants in *E. coli* from food animals. *Vet. Microbiol.* **95**:91–101.
159. **Seriwatana, J., P. Echeverria, D. N. Taylor, L. Rasrinaul, J. E. Brown, J. S. Peiris, and C. L. Clayton.** 1988. Type II heat-labile enterotoxin-producing *Escherichia coli* isolated from animals and humans. *Infect. Immun.* **56**:1158–1161.
160. **Shiraki, Y., N. Shibata, Y. Doi, and Y. Arakawa.** 2004. *Escherichia coli* producing CTX-M-2 β-lactamase in cattle, Japan. *Emerg. Infect. Dis.* **10**:69–75.
161. **Shpigel, N. Y., D. Levin, M. Winkler, A. Saran, G. Ziv, and A. Bottner.** 1997. Efficacy of cefquinome for treatment of cows with mastitis experimentally induced using *Escherichia coli. J. Dairy Sci.* **80**:318–323.
162. **Singer, R. S., S. K. Patterson, A. E. Meier, J. K. Gibson, H. L. Lee, and C. W. Maddox.** 2004. Relationship between phenotypic and genotypic florfenicol resistance in *Escherichia coli. Antimicrob. Agents Chemother.* **48**:4047–4049.
163. **Smith, H. W.** 1958. Drug-resistant bacteria in domestic animals. *Proc. R. Soc. Med.* **51**:812–813.
164. **Smith, H. W.** 1966. The incidence of infective drug resistance in strains of Escherichia coli isolated from diseased human beings and domestic animals. *J. Hyg. Lond.* **64**: 465–474.
165. **Smith, H. W.** 1968. Antimicrobial drugs in animal feeds. *Nature* **218**:728–731.
166. **Smith, H. W.** 1971. The effect of the use of antibacterial drugs on the emergence of drug-resistant bacteria in animals. *Adv. Vet. Sci. Comp. Med.* **15**:67–100.
167. **Smith, H. W., and S. Halls.** 1966. Observations on infective drug resistance in Britain. *Br. Med. J.* **5482**:266–269.
168. **Smith, H. W., and M. A. Lovell.** 1981. *Escherichia coli* resistant to tetracyclines and to other antibiotics in the faeces of U.K. chickens and pigs in 1980. *J. Hyg. Lond.* **87**: 477–483.
169. **Sogaard, H.** 1982. In-vitro antibiotic susceptibility of *E. coli* isolated from acute and chronic bovine mastitis with reference to clinical efficacy. *Nord. Vetmed.* **34**:248–254.
170. **Sojka, W. J., and R. B. A. Carnaghan.** 1961. *Escherichia coli* infection in poultry. *Res. Vet. Sci.* **2**:340.
171. **Sunde, M., K. Fossum, A. Solberg, and H. Sorum.** 1998. Antibiotic resistance in *Escherichia coli* of the normal intestinal flora of swine. *Microb. Drug Resist.* **4**:289–299.
172. **Sundlof, S. F., J. B. Kaneene, and R. A. Miller.** 1995. National survey on veterinarian-initiated drug use in lactating dairy cows. *J. Am. Vet. Med. Assoc.* **207**:347–352.
173. **Swann, M. M.** 1969. Report of the Joint Committee on the Use of Antibiotics in Animal Husbandry and Veterinary Medicine. Health and Agriculture Ministers, London, United Kingdom.
174. **Teshager, T., L. Dominguez, M. A. Moreno, Y. Saenz, C. Torres, and S. Cardenosa.** 2000. Isolation of an SHV-12 β-lactamase-producing *Escherichia coli* strain from a dog with recurrent urinary tract infections. *Antimicrob. Agents Chemother.* **44**:3483–3484.
175. **Thiele, E. H., E. L. Dulaney, M. J. Carey, and D. Hendlin.** 1968. Detection of R factor-bearing microorganisms in laboratory animals. *J. Bacteriol.* **95**:1184.
176. **Tibbetts, R. J., D. G. White, N. W. Dyer, C. W. Giddings, and L. K. Nolan.** 2003. Characterization of *Escherichia coli* isolates incriminated in colisepticaemia in mink. *Vet. Res. Commun.* **27**:341–357.
177. **U.S. Department of Agriculture.** 2002. *Dairy 2002, Part I: Reference of Dairy Health and Management in the United States, 2002*, p. 1–92. Centers for Epidemiology and Animal Health, Animal and Plant Health Inspection Service, U.S. Department of Agriculture, Fort Collins, Colo.
178. **Vandemaele, F., M. Vereecken, J. Derijcke, and B. M. Goddeeris.** 2002. Incidence and antibiotic resistance of pathogenic *Escherichia coli* among poultry in Belgium. *Vet. Rec.* **151**:355–356.

179. **van den Bogaard, A. E., N. London, C. Driessen, and E. E. Stobberingh.** 2001. Antibiotic resistance of faecal *Escherichia coli* in poultry, poultry farmers and poultry slaughterers. *J. Antimicrob. Chemother.* **47:**763–771.

180. **van den Bogaard, A. E., and E. E. Stobberingh.** 2000. Epidemiology of resistance to antibiotics. Links between animals and humans. *Int. J. Antimicrob. Agents* **14:**327–335.

181. **Verdonck, F., E. Cox, and B. M. Goddeeris.** 2004. F4 fimbriae expressed by porcine enterotoxigenic *Escherichia coli*, an example of an eccentric fimbrial system? *J. Mol. Microbiol. Biotechnol.* **7:**155–169.

182. **Vulfson, L., K. Pedersen, M. Chriel, K. Frydendahl, T. H. Andersen, M. Madsen, and H. H. Dietz.** 2001. Serogroups and antimicrobial susceptibility among *Escherichia coli* isolated from farmed mink (Mustela vison Schreiber) in Denmark. *Vet. Microbiol.* **79:**143–153.

183. **Wallmann, J., K. Schroter, L. H. Wieler, and R. Kroker.** 2003. National antibiotic resistance monitoring in veterinary pathogens from sick food-producing animals: the German programme and results from the 2001 pilot study. *Int. J. Antimicrob. Agents* **22:**420–428.

184. **Walton, J. R.** 1966. Infectious drug resistance in *Escherichia coli* isolated from healthy farm animals. *Lancet* **ii:**1300–1302.

185. **Warren, A., K. Townsend, T. King, S. Moss, D. O'Boyle, R. Yates, and D. J. Trott.** 2001. Multi-drug resistant *Escherichia coli* with extended-spectrum beta-lactamase activity and fluoroquinolone resistance isolated from clinical infections in dogs. *Aust. Vet. J.* **79:**621–623.

186. **Wasteson, Y.** 2001. Zoonotic *Escherichia coli*. *Acta Vet. Scand. Suppl.* **95:**79–84.

187. **Watanabe, T.** 1963. Infective heredity of multiple drug resistance in bacteria. *Bacteriol. Rev.* **27:**87–115.

188. **Watts, J. L., S. A. Salmon, M. S. Sanchez, and R. J. Yancey, Jr.** 1997. In vitro activity of premafloxacin, a new extended-spectrum fluoroquinolone, against pathogens of veterinary importance. *Antimicrob. Agents Chemother.* **41:**1190–1192.

189. **Werckenthin, C., S. Seidl, J. Riedl, E. Kiossis, G. Wolf, R. Stolla, and O. R. Kaaden.** 2002. *Escherichia coli* isolates from young calves in Bavaria: in vitro susceptibilities to 14 antimicrobial agents. *J. Vet. Med. B* **49:**61–65.

190. **Wernicki, A., J. Krzyzanowski, and A. Puchalski.** 2002. Characterization of *Escherichia coli* strains associated with canine pyometra. *Pol. J. Vet. Sci.* **5:**51–56.

191. **White, D. G., C. Hudson, J. J. Maurer, S. Ayers, S. Zhao, M. D. Lee, L. Bolton, T. Foley, and J. Sherwood.** 2000. Characterization of chloramphenicol and florfenicol resistance in *Escherichia coli* associated with bovine diarrhea. *J. Clin. Microbiol.* **38:**4593–4598.

192. **White, D. G., L. J. Piddock, J. J. Maurer, S. Zhao, V. Ricci, and S. G. Thayer.** 2000. Characterization of fluoroquinolone resistance among veterinary isolates of avian *Escherichia coli*. *Antimicrob. Agents Chemother.* **44:**2897–2899.

193. **Wierup, M.** 1975. Antibiotic resistance and transferable antibiotic resistance of *Escherichia coli* isolated from Swedish calves 5 and 30 days old. *Nord. Vetmed.* **27:**77–84.

194. **Wierup, M.** 2001. The experience of reducing antibiotics used in animal production in the Nordic countries. *Int. J. Antimicrob. Agents* **18:**287–290.

195. **Williams, R. J., and D. L. Heymann.** 1998. Containment of antibiotic resistance. *Science* **279:**1153–1154.

196. **Wray, C., R. W. Hedges, K. P. Shannon, and D. E. Bradley.** 1986. Apramycin and gentamicin resistance in *Escherichia coli* and salmonellas isolated from farm animals. *J. Hyg. Lond.* **97:**445–456.

196a. **Wray, C., and M. J. Woodward.** 1997. *Escherichia coli* infections in farm animals, p. 49–84. *In* M. Sussman (ed.), Escherichia coli: *Mechanisms of Virulence*. Cambridge University Press, Cambridge, United Kingdom.

197. **Yang, H., S. Chen, D. G. White, S. Zhao, P. McDermott, R. Walker, and J. Meng.** 2004. Characterization of multiple-antimicrobial-resistant *Escherichia coli* isolates from diseased chickens and swine in China. *J. Clin. Microbiol.* **42:**3483–3489.

198. **Zhao, S., D. G. White, P. F. McDermott, S. Friedman, L. English, S. Ayers, J. Meng, J. J. Maurer, R. Holland, and R. D. Walker.** 2001. Identification and expression of cephamycinase bla(CMY) genes in *Escherichia coli* and *Salmonella* isolates from food animals and ground meat. *Antimicrob. Agents Chemother.* **45:**3647–3650.

Antimicrobial Resistance in Bacteria of Animal Origin
Edited by Frank M. Aarestrup

Chapter 11

Antimicrobial Resistance in Members of the Family *Pasteurellaceae*

Corinna Kehrenberg, Robert D. Walker, Ching Ching Wu, and Stefan Schwarz

THE FAMILY *PASTEURELLACEAE* AND ITS ROLE IN ANIMAL AND HUMAN INFECTIONS

The family *Pasteurellaceae* comprises a highly heterogeneous group of gram-negative bacteria. Evaluation by 16S rRNA sequencing, DNA-DNA hybridization, and analysis of the biochemical capacities identified a number of distinct genetic and phenotypic groups. As a consequence, the family *Pasteurellaceae* has undergone numerous reclassifications during the past years and currently contains 11 genera: *Pasteurella, Mannheimia, Actinobacillus, Haemophilus, Histophilus, Lonepinella, Phocoenobacter, Gallibacterium, Volucribacter, Nicoletella*, and *Avibacterium* (3, 4, 9, 29, 30, 84). Although many of these genera include pathogens of veterinary and human importance, this chapter focuses mainly on the genera *Pasteurella, Mannheimia, Actinobacillus, Haemophilus*, and *Histophilus*, for which sufficient data on antimicrobial susceptibility and the detection of resistance genes are currently available. Many isolates of these genera are commonly found on the mucous membranes of the respiratory and/or genital tracts of reptiles, birds, and numerous mammals, including a wide variety of food-producing animals. Some species, e.g., *Pasteurella multocida*, may be found in many different hosts, while others, such as *Actinobacillus pleuropneumoniae* and *Mannheimia haemolytica*, have a narrow host range, being found primarily in pigs and ruminants, respectively. Members of certain *Pasteurella, Mannheimia, Actinobacillus, Haemophilus*, and *Histophilus* species, such as *P. multocida, [Pasteurella] trehalosi, [Pasteurella] aerogenes, M. haemolytica, A. pleuropneumoniae, Actinobacillus suis, Actinobacillus equuli, Haemophilus parasuis*, and *Histophilus somni*, generally cause respiratory and/or septicemic diseases in the animal hosts they are commonly associated with. Some of these organisms, e.g., *P. multocida*, may also cause infections in humans who have contact with animals harboring these organisms as part of their normal oral flora.

P. multocida is the most relevant animal-pathogenic *Pasteurella* species. Various capsular types of *P. multocida* are known, some of which preferentially occur in connection with specific diseases in animals. For example, capsular type A is the causative agent of pneumonia in several animal species, including but not limited to cattle, sheep, and pigs; atrophic rhinitis in pigs; mastitis in sheep; snuffles in rabbits; and fowl cholera in poultry. *P. multocida* isolates of capsular types B and E are the causative agents of hemorrhagic septicemia of cattle and water buffaloes in Asia and Africa, respectively. Capsular type D is also an etiological agent of atrophic rhinitis and pneumonia in swine (116, 117). A recent report also showed that *P. multocida* capsular type F isolates may be involved in fatal peritonitis in calves (20). Bacteria assigned to the new species *[P.] trehalosi*, capsular types T3, T4, and T10, are encountered worldwide in sheep and goats, where they cause severe septicemia in young animals.

A. pleuropneumoniae causes a hemorrhagic pleuropneumonia in pigs of all ages (117), which causes huge economic losses in the swine industry worldwide. Currently, 2 biovars (the NAD-dependent biovar 1 and the NAD-independent biovar 2) and 15 serovars of *A. pleuropneumoniae* are distinguished. Serovars 1, 5, 9, 10, and 11 are considered to be more virulent than other serovars. Other animal-pathogenic *Actinobacillus* species include *A. suis*, which causes mastitis in sows and respiratory symptoms in growing pigs; *A. equuli*, which is involved in

Corinna Kehrenberg and Stefan Schwarz • Institut für Tierzucht, Bundesforschungsanstalt für Landwirtschaft, D-31535 Neustadt-Mariensee, Germany. **Robert D. Walker** • Office of Research, Center for Veterinary Medicine, U.S. Food and Drug Administration, Laurel, MD 20708. **Ching Ching Wu** • Animal Disease Diagnostic Laboratory, Department of Veterinary Pathobiology, Purdue University School of Veterinary Medicine, West Lafayette, IN 47907-2065.

several diseases in horses, and particularly with the usually fatal septicemia in neonatal foals; and *A. lignieresii*, which is associated with pyogranulomatous lesions in the upper alimentary tract of ruminants, known as "wooden tongue."

Several species of the genus *Haemophilus* are also animal pathogens, with *H. parasuis* being of major economic importance. *H. parasuis* is the etiological agent of Glässer's disease in pigs. More than 15 different serotypes have been identified, with serotypes 1, 5, 12, 13, and 14 thought to be the most virulent. Disease caused by this organism occurs most frequently in postweaning pigs and is characterized by high fevers, polyserositis, polysynovitis, respiratory distress, and meningitis. However, it may also occur in nursery-age animals and adult animals, primarily sows. *[Haemophilus] paragallinarum*—recently reclassified as *Avibacterium paragallinarum* (9)—is the etiological agent of infectious coryza, an upper respiratory disease of chickens that occurs worldwide. The organism may also cause disease in numerous game and companion birds.

[Haemophilus] somnus, [Haemophilus] ovis, and [Haemophilus] agni—recently reclassified as *Histophilus somni, Histophilus ovis*, and *Histophilus agni* (3)—are also pathogens of cattle, and sheep, respectively. *H. somni* is the etiological agent of thromboembolic meningoencephalitis in cattle. It has also been associated with various other diseases in sheep and diseases such as mastitis and abortions in dairy cattle and bronchopneumonia, necrotic laryngitis, myocarditis, arthritis, conjunctivitis, and myositis in lightweight feeder calves.

All the diseases in which the *Pasteurella, Mannheimia, Actinobacillus*, *Haemophilus*, or *Histophilus* isolates act as the primary pathogens commonly occur as peracute or acute forms and are accompanied by a high mortality rate, although subacute and chronic forms are also observed. As secondary pathogens, *P. multocida* and *M. haemolytica* play a major role in the final progression to severe bronchopneumonia and pleuropneumonia in cattle, sheep, and goats (57), as well as in enzootic pneumonia in calves (14), and *P. multocida* plays a role in progressive atrophic rhinitis of swine (93). *P. multocida* and *Pasteurella pneumotropica* play a role in pasteurellosis of small laboratory rodents and furbearing animals. Respiratory tract infections in which bacteria such as *P. multocida* and *M. haemolytica* isolates are involved are often multifactorial and polymicrobial diseases, with viruses and other bacteria such as *Mycoplasma* spp. representing the primary pathogens (14, 57, 93, 117). Under environmental and/or management conditions, such as transport, marketing, or change of feed, climate, or ventilation, which results in stress to the animals, especially in the presence of viruses and/or *Mycoplasma* spp. that may initiate damage to the host mucosal membranes, the bacterial pathogens can rapidly proliferate, resulting in high morbidity. Under conditions of low stress, the mortality rate may be low. As the amount of stress is increased, however, the mortality rate is also increased. Economic losses associated with acute pneumonic episodes are primarily due to increased costs in medications and retarded growth rates rather than mortality of the affected animals.

Pasteurella infections in humans are usually associated with bite wounds from animals that harbor these organisms as part of their oral flora. Dogs and cats are the most common source of these infections, although other animal species, such as hamsters and pigs, have also been associated with pasteurellosis in humans. Infection may also arise from an infected animal licking an open wound on a human. Isolates of *P. multocida* (15, 56), as well as *[P.] aerogenes* (46), *Pasteurella dagmatis* (43, 148), *Pasteurella canis* (58), *Pasteurella stomatis* (113), *P. multocida* subsp. *septica*, and *P. multocida* subsp. *gallicida* (134), have been isolated from infections of humans. Most cases of human pasteurellosis are limited to local wound infections, but sequelae such as meningitis, endocarditis, septic arthritis septicemia, and septic shock may also occur (134). The sequelae may require predisposing conditions such as immunosuppressive therapy or other ongoing infections in order to occur. *Pasteurella caballi* was isolated from an infected wound of a veterinary surgeon (8). *[P.] aerogenes*, which is considered to be a commensal in swine, was isolated from a case of stillbirth in a human and from vaginal swabs of the mother, who had been working on a swine farm (135). *M. haemolytica, A. pleuropneumoniae*, and animal pathogens of the genera *Haemophilus* and *Histophilus* rarely—if at all—play a role in human infections. However, other species within the families *Actinobacillus* and *Haemophilus*, such as *Actinobacillus actinomycetemcomitans* and *Haemophilus influenzae*, have been found to be associated with a wide range of infections in humans.

SUSCEPTIBILITY OF *PASTEURELLA, MANNHEIMIA, ACTINOBACILLUS, HAEMOPHILUS*, AND *HISTOPHILUS* TO ANTIMICROBIAL AGENTS

In vitro antimicrobial susceptibility testing is performed to predict how a bacterium may respond to an antimicrobial agent in vivo (clinical response) or to monitor changes in susceptibility in relation to time and geographic location. In both instances, results may be reported qualitatively, e.g., susceptible, intermediate, or resistant, or quantitatively, e.g., as the MIC. In antimicrobial susceptibility tests for surveillance purposes, the interpretive criteria are based on the bacterial population distributions relative to zone sizes and/or MICs. Interpretive criteria for clinical consideration require the generation of a bacterium's antibiogram in addition to knowledge of the pharmacokinetic parameters of the chosen drug in the target animal species and the pharmacodynamic indices associated with the in vivo bacterium-antimicrobial agent-host interactions. In either situation, to ensure intra- and interlaboratory reproducibility, it is essential that standardized testing methods be used.

The standardized testing methods should employ optimal growth conditions for the organism being tested. The in vitro antimicrobial susceptibility testing of *Pasteurella, Mannheimia, Actinobacillus, Haemophilus*, and *Histophilus* is no exception. Because these organisms are more fastidious in their growth requirements than the *Enterobacteriaceae* or staphylococci, they require different testing methods. Thus, while many studies have reported in vitro susceptibility data for isolates of these genera obtained from animal sources in various parts of the world, there has been a notable absence of standardization in testing methods. In most cases, it is difficult to compare the results because of the use of different methods and breakpoints. In the United States, the Clinical and Laboratory Standards Institute (CLSI) (formerly the National Committee for Clinical Laboratory Standards) has published two documents, M31-A2 (104) and M31-S1 (105), which provide the latest information on methods for in vitro susceptibility testing of *A. pleuropneumoniae* and *H. somni* and interpretive criteria for *P. multocida, M. haemolytica, A. pleuropneumoniae*, and *H. somni* for some veterinary-specific antimicrobial agents (e.g., ceftiofur, enrofloxacin, florfenicol, spectinomycin, tiamulin, and tilmicosin). However, specific testing methods for *P. multocida* and *M. haemolytica* have not yet been defined by the CLSI. Recognizing that *P. multocida* may be frequently encountered in clinical medicine, the CLSI has organized a working group to address the in vitro antimicrobial susceptibility testing needs of this organism and other bacteria that may be encountered in clinical medicine for which there is no defined testing method or interpretive criteria. The working group is charged with recommending the test media, quality control strain(s), testing conditions, and, where appropriate, interpretive criteria. These recommendations should be published in the spring of 2006. In general, recommendations for interpretive criteria for veterinary-specific antimicrobial agents will need to be generated by also taking into consideration host-specific pharmacokinetics and pharmacodynamics and addressed at future meetings of the CLSI Subcommittee on Veterinary Antimicrobial Susceptibility Testing.

Because of the lack of organism-specific testing methods and organism- and host-specific interpretive criteria and the fact that bacteria belonging to the genera *Pasteurella, Mannheimia, Actinobacillus, Haemophilus*, and *Histophilus* are not included in most national antimicrobial susceptibility testing monitoring and surveillance programs, there is a limited amount of data available on a national or international basis. For example, the National Antimicrobial Resistance Monitoring System (NARMS) in the United States, the Norwegian monitoring programs NORM and NORM-VET, and the Swedish Veterinary Antimicrobial Resistance Monitoring program do not test bacteria of any of the five genera. The Danish Integrated Antimicrobial Resistance Monitoring and Research Programme included *A. pleuropneumoniae* from pigs in the years 1997 and 1998 (35, 36). The Dutch program Monitoring of Antimicrobial Resistance and Antimicrobial Usage in Animals in The Netherlands from 2002 shows a year-by-year comparison of the percentages of resistant *P. multocida* and *M. haemolytica* isolates from cattle analyzed between 1996 and 2000 (98). However, this report also recognized that a large year-to-year variation in the percentages of resistant isolates exists for isolates of both bacterial species and most of the antimicrobial agents tested. Thus, it was concluded that real trends in antimicrobial resistance in bovine *P. multocida* and *M. haemolytica* isolates cannot be derived from these data. In Germany, the national resistance monitoring program GE*R*M-Vet was started in 2001. The pilot study from 2001 included *P. multocida* from respiratory tract infections in pigs (139), whereas the regular program starting in 2002 also included *P. multocida* and *M. haemolytica* from cattle (138). A complementary program in Germany, BfT-GermVet, was initiated in 2004 and includes *P. multocida* from dogs and cats. The GE*R*M-Vet program determines MIC data for a wide range of antimicrobial agents in accordance with the methods described in CLSI document M31-A2 (104). In the study period of 2002 and 2003, 132 bovine and 442 porcine *P. multocida* isolates were tested (Table 1). Less than 6% of the isolates were found to be resistant to newer antimicrobial agents such as ceftiofur, enrofloxacin, florfenicol, or tilmicosin (138). Similar results were found in a pilot national antimicrobial susceptibility monitoring program for veterinary pathogens for five major animal groups (dogs,

Table 1. In vitro susceptibility data for *P. multocida* isolates from different animal sources

Source	No. of isolates	Parameter	Value (μg/ml) for:							
			Ampicillin	Ceftiofur	Florfenicol	Gentamicin	Enrofloxacin	Tilmicosin	Tetracycline	Trimethoprim-sulfamethoxazole
Swine, United States	715[a]	MIC_{50}	0.25	≤0.06	0.25	2	≤0.03	4	1	≤0.5/9.5
		MIC_{90}	0.25	≤0.06	0.5	4	≤0.03	16	16	≤0.5/9.5
		Range	≤0.06–≥64	≤0.06–≥4	≤0.25–≥8	≤0.12–≥16	≤0.03–≥4	≤4–≥64	≤0.25–≥16	≤0.5/9.5–≥4/76
Swine, Germany	442[b]	MIC_{50}	≤0.12	≤0.004	≤2	1	0.015	4	0.5	0.12/2.4
		MIC_{90}	0.5	0.06	≤2	2	≤0.03	8	2	32/604
		Range	≤0.12–≥256	≤0.004–≥8	≤2–≥32	≤0.06–64	≤0.004–≥4	≤0.06–≥32	≤0.12–64	≤0.03/0.6–≥64/1,216
Cattle, Germany	132[b]	MIC_{50}	≤0.12	≤0.004	≤2	0.5	0.008	2	1	0.12/2.4
		MIC_{90}	1	0.12	≤2	2	0.03	8	8	4/76
		Range	≤0.12–≥256	≤0.004–≥8	≤2–≥32	≤0.06–≥128	≤0.004–2	≤0.06–≥32	≤0.12–128	≤0.03/0.6–≥64/1,216
Cattle, Germany	154[c]	MIC_{50}	0.12	≤0.03	0.25	2	ND[e]	ND	ND	0.06/1.2
		MIC_{90}	0.25	≤0.03	0.5	4	ND	ND	ND	0.12/2.4
		Range	≤0.03–≥32	≤0.03–0.12	≤0.12–2	≤0.03–8	ND	ND	ND	≤0.016/0.3–≥16/304
Dogs and cats, United States	112[d]	MIC_{50}	0.12	ND	ND	1	≤0.008[f]	ND	0.12	0.03/0.6
		MIC_{90}	0.25	ND	ND	2	0.015[f]	ND	0.5	0.12/2.4
		Range	≤0.03–0.5	ND	ND	≤0.12–4	≤0.008–0.5[f]	ND	≤0.03–2	≤0.008/0.15–≥0.25/4.8

[a]C. C. Wu, U.S. pilot monitoring data (unpublished).
[b]Reference 138.
[c]Reference 126.
[d]R. D. Walker, unpublished data.
[e]ND, not determined.
[f]Ciprofloxacin was tested instead of enrofloxacin.

horses, swine, cattle, and birds), funded by the American Veterinary Medical Association, the Association of American Veterinary Laboratory Diagnosticians, and Purdue University, which involves 27 states and uses CLSI broth microdilution methods to test against 17 antimicrobials (2001 to 2004). The data from 715 swine *P. multocida* isolates collected in the United States between 2001 and 2004 are included in Table 1. The MIC_{50} and the MIC_{90} (MICs at which 50% and 90%, respectively, of the strains are inhibited) for the U.S. isolates and the German isolates were the same or within one dilution of each other for five antimicrobial agents. While the annual data from the U.S. study are not shown in Table 1, the MIC distribution for the eight antibiotics reported either remained the same or tended to decrease, with the drugs having high MICs for fewer organisms (C. C. Wu, personal communication, 2005).

In North America, Watts and coworkers published a four-year survey of antimicrobial susceptibility of *P. multocida* and *[P.] haemolytica* involved in bovine respiratory disease (141). The isolates were collected between 1988 and 1992 at 9 to 13 laboratories in the United States and Canada. The study investigated their antimicrobial susceptibility by broth microdilution. Overall, resistance to ampicillin, tetracycline, erythromycin, and sulfonamides was frequently encountered among *P. multocida* and *[P.] haemolytica* isolates, whereas the MIC_{90} of ceftiofur was ≤0.06 μg/ml. Substantial variations in the year-to-year susceptibility of *P. multocida* and *[P.] haemolytica* to tilmicosin were observed (141). Data from the American Veterinary Medical Association pilot study indicated that 15 to 25% of the isolates were resistant to ampicillin, but the MIC_{90}s of ceftiofur (≤0.06 μg/ml), florfenicol (1 μg/ml), and tilmicosin (16 μg/ml) were all within the susceptible ranges (Wu, personal communication). A large-scale study of clinical isolates from porcine respiratory tract infections collected between 1994 and 1998 at various locations in the United States was conducted to determine the in vitro activity of tilmicosin. The overall MIC_{50} and MIC_{90} for the *P. multocida* isolates were 8 and 16 μg/ml, respectively (39). Studies of the in vitro susceptibility to florfenicol of bovine and porcine respiratory tract pathogens collected between 2000 and 2003 in Germany identified all the bovine *P. multocida* and *M. haemolytica* as well as all the porcine *P. multocida* and *A. pleuropneumoniae* isolates that were tested as susceptible, with MICs ranging between ≤0.12 and 2 μg/ml (70, 115). Another study in Germany, investigating the susceptibility of bovine isolates of *P. multocida* and *M. haemolytica* collected in 1999 to spectinomycin and comparator agents, showed that none of the 302 isolates tested were resistant to florfenicol, cefquinome, or ceftiofur, and only 6.5% of the *P. multocida* and 1.4% of the *M. haemolytica* isolates were classified as resistant to spectinomycin (126). In a study of the in vitro efficacy of cefquinome and other anti-infective drugs against bovine bacterial pathogens collected in Belgium, France, Germany, The Netherlands, and the United Kingdom, the MIC_{90}s of cefquinome and ceftiofur were 0.12 and ≤0.06 μg/ml, respectively, for both *P. multocida* and *[P.] haemolytica*. The MIC_{90}s of amoxicillin and enrofloxacin differed considerably between the *[P.] haemolytica* isolates (>2 and >4 μg/ml, respectively) and the *P. multocida* isolates (0.5 and 0.12 μg/ml, respectively). The MIC_{90}s for oxytetracycline and tylosin were >16 and >8 μg/ml, respectively, for *P. multocida* and *[P.] haemolytica* (11). While the *P. multocida* isolates from the different countries did not differ substantially, *[P.] haemolytica* isolates from The Netherlands were more resistant to enrofloxacin than the corresponding isolates from all other countries. Amoxicillin resistance was also seen at higher frequencies among the *[P.] haemolytica* isolates from The Netherlands and Belgium (11). These differences in the percentages of resistant isolates might reflect differences in the selective pressure due to preferences in the use of certain antimicrobial agents in the different countries or differences in testing methods and interpretive criteria.

In a recent study in the United States, using *Streptococcus pneumoniae* ATCC 49619 as the quality control organism and the broth microdilution in vitro susceptibility testing method recommended for *S. pneumoniae*, 112 canine and feline isolates were tested against eight antimicrobial agents that may be used to treat animal bite wounds in humans. The isolates were recovered from various wounds in dogs and cats between 1998 and 2002. A comparison of the results of this study with those of other studies is shown in Table 1.

Only a few reports have dealt with antimicrobial susceptibility testing of *Haemophilus* or *Histophilus* (1, 141, 143). Recent data from Denmark showed that virtually all porcine *H. parasuis* and bovine *H. somni* isolates were susceptible to the antimicrobial agents used for the control of the respective infections (1).

RESISTANCE GENES AND MECHANISMS IN *PASTEURELLA*, *MANNHEIMIA*, *ACTINOBACILLUS*, AND *HAEMOPHILUS*

Although antimicrobial agents are commonly used for the treatment of infections caused by bacteria of the family *Pasteurellaceae* and their resistance to several antimicrobial agents has been reported, little is known about the presence of genes and mutations conferring resistance to these antimicrobials (Table 2). The following sections provide an overview of the current knowledge of resistance genes and resistance-mediating mutations so far detected in bacteria of the genera *Pasteurella, Mannheimia, Actinobacillus,* and *Haemophilus.* Resistance genes have not yet been reported to be present in members of other genera within the family *Pasteurellaceae.*

Resistance to Tetracyclines

Seen from the molecular point of view, tetracycline resistance is a highly heterogeneous resistance property (28). In bacteria of the genera *Pasteurella, Mannheimia, Actinobacillus,* and *Haemophilus,* at least seven different tetracycline resistance genes (*tet* genes) representing two different resistance mechanisms have been detected.

Among the *tet* genes coding for proteins that mediate active efflux of tetracyclines from the bacterial cell, the genes *tet*(H), *tet*(B), *tet*(G), *tet*(K), and *tet*(L) have been identified in bacteria of these four genera. Several reports from the late 1970s and 1980s reported transferable tetracycline resistance among *P. multocida* and *[P.] haemolytica* isolates of animal origin (7, 53–55). However, the specific type of *tet* gene was not determined in any of these studies. In 1993 Hansen and coworkers identified a novel type of *tet* gene, designated *tet*(H) (52). The *tet*(H) gene was first detected on plasmid pVM111 that originated from a *P. multocida* isolate obtained from a turkey that had died of fowl cholera in the late 1970s in the United States (7). In a subsequent study Hansen et al. screened tetracycline-resistant *P. multocida* and *[P.] haemolytica* from infections of cattle and pigs in North America for the presence of the gene *tet*(H) and other *tet* genes (51). They found the *tet*(H) gene to be the predominant *tet* gene among the isolates screened. Since the *tet*(H) gene was located either in the chromosomal DNA or on plasmids, they speculated about the involvement of a transposable element in the spread of *tet*(H) (51). The corresponding transposon, Tn*5706*, was identified in 1998 on plasmid pPMT1 from a bovine *P. multocida* isolate (80). Tn*5706* is a small, nonconjugative composite transposon of 4378 bp and represents the first and so far only known resistance-mediating transposon identified among members of the genus *Pasteurella* (61). The *tetR-tet*(H) gene region in Tn*5706* is bracketed by inverted copies of the two closely related insertion sequences IS*1596* and IS*1597* (80). Truncated Tn*5706* elements in which these insertion sequences were deleted in part or completely have been found on small plasmids of 4.4 and 5.5 kb in isolates of *M. haemolytica, P. multocida*, and *[P.] aerogenes* (71, 73). All *tet*(H) genes sequenced so far code for membrane-associated efflux proteins of 400 amino acids, except that found on plasmid pPAT1. Due to a recombination between the terminal part of the *tet*(H) gene and the adjacent IS*1597* sequence (73), this gene codes for a protein of only 392 amino acids. Judging from the level of tetracycline resistance mediated by plasmid pPAT1, this terminal deletion, however, has no impact on the activity of the respective TetH efflux protein (73). Recent studies showed that the *tet*(H) gene is occasionally present in tetracycline-resistant *A. pleuropneumoniae* (10), but also in bacteria outside the family *Pasteurellaceae*, namely, in *Moraxella* spp. and *Acinetobacter radioresistens* (99), both obtained from salmon farms in Chile. The *A. radioresistens* isolate also harbored the insertion sequence IS*1599* (99), which is closely related to the Tn*5706*-associated insertion sequences IS*1596* and IS*1597*.

The gene *tet*(B) is located on the nonconjugative transposon Tn*10* (21, 87) and represents the most widely spread *tet* gene among *Enterobacteriaceae* (28). The *tet*(B) gene proved to be the dominant *tet* gene among porcine *[P.] aerogenes* isolates (74), whereas it has been detected in only a single bovine *[P.] haemolytica* isolate from France (26) and in two porcine *P. multocida* isolates from the United States and Germany (71). In all cases but one, the *tet*(B) gene was located in one or two copies on the chromosome. Hybridization studies using SfuI-digested whole cellular DNA of *tet*(B)-carrying *P. multocida* and *[P.] aerogenes* isolates suggested complete copies of Tn*10* in the majority of the isolates investigated (71, 74). In the only plasmid-borne case, the *tet*(B) gene proved to be part of a largely truncated Tn*10* element (74). Studies on tetracycline-resistant *A. pleuropneumoniae* from pigs (10, 108, 140) and *A. actinomycetemcomitans* from humans (119) also revealed the presence of the gene *tet*(B). Recently, the *tet*(B) gene, without the corresponding *tetR* repressor gene, however, was identified on the 5.1-kb plasmid pHS-Tet from *H. parasuis* (86). Tet(B)-mediated tetracycline resistance has also been found in other *Haemophilus* spp. from humans, including *H. parainfluenzae* (88), *H. influenzae*, and *H. ducreyi* (94).

The gene *tet*(G) was initially detected on a plasmid from *Vibrio anguillarum* (149). It has since been detected in *Pseudomonas* spp., isolated from leaves of tetracycline-treated apple trees (123), and found to be part of the multiresistance gene cluster present in *Salmonella enterica* serovar Typhimurium DT104 (12) and other *Salmonella* serovars. It has also been

Table 2. Antimicrobial resistance genes identified in *Pasteurella, Mannheimia, Actinobacillus*, and *Haemophilus*

Antimicrobial agent(s)	Resistance gene	Protein specified by the resistance gene	Detected in:			
			Pasteurella	*Mannheimia*	*Actinobacillus*	*Haemophilus*
Tetracycline	*tet*(H)	12-TMS[a] efflux protein	+	+	+	–
	tet(B)	12-TMS efflux protein	+	–	+	+
	tet(G)	12-TMS efflux protein	+	+	–	–
	tet(L)	14-TMS efflux protein	+	+	+	–
	tet(K)	14-TMS efflux protein	–	–	–	+
	tet(M)	Ribosome protective protein	+	–	+	+
	tet(O)	Ribosome protective protein	–	–	+	–
Penicillins	bla_{ROB-1}	β-Lactamase	+	+	+	+
	bla_{TEM-1}	β-Lactamase	+	–	–	+
	bla_{PSE-1}	β-Lactamase	+	–	–	–
Streptomycin	*strA*	Aminoglycoside-3″-phosphotransferase	+	+	+	+
	strB	Aminoglycoside-6-phosphotransferase	+	+	+	+
Streptomycin, spectinomycin	*aadA1*	Aminoglycoside-3″-adenyltransferase	+	–	–	–
	aadA14	Aminoglycoside-3″-adenyltransferase	+	–	–	–
Sulfonamides	*sul2*	Dihydropteroate synthase	+	+	+	+
Trimethoprim	*dfrA20*	Dihydrofolate reductase	+	–	–	–
Chloramphenicol	*catA1*	Type A chloramphenicol acetyltransferase	+	–	–	–
	catA2	Type A chloramphenicol acetyltransferase	–	–	–	+
	catA3	Type A chloramphenicol acetyltransferase	+	+	–	–
	catB2	Type B chloramphenicol acetyltransferase	+	–	–	–
Chloramphenicol, florfenicol	*floR*	12-TMS efflux protein	+	–	–	–
Macrolides	*erm*(A)	rRNA methylase	–	–	+	–
	erm(B)	rRNA methylase	–	–	+	+
	erm(C)	rRNA methylase	–	–	+	+
	erm(F)	rRNA methylase	–	–	+	+
	erm(Q)	rRNA methylase	–	–	+	–

[a]TMS, transmembrane segment.

found on the chromosome of six epidemiologically related *M. haemolytica* isolates from cattle (71) and on plasmid pJR1 from avian *P. multocida* (146). Surprisingly, the *tet*(G) structural gene in plasmid pJR1 was found in the absence of the corresponding *tetR* repressor gene, which is considered to be essential for the tetracycline-inducible expression of *tet*(G). Whether the lack of the repressor gene has an impact on the expression of *tet*(G)-mediated tetracycline resistance is unknown. It should be noted that plasmid pJR1 has not been transferred into susceptible recipient strains for phenotypic confirmation of the activity of the resistance genes found on this plasmid (146). The *tet*(L) gene, which is commonly found in gram-positive cocci and *Bacillus* spp., has also been identified on plasmids in porcine *A. pleuropneumoniae,* bovine *M. haemolytica,* and *Mannheimia glucosida* isolates (10, 69a) as well as in the chromosomal DNA of bovine *P. multocida* and *M. haemolytica* isolates (69a). The *tet*(K) gene, which is commonly found on small plasmids in human and animal staphylococci, was identified by PCR in *Haemophilus aphrophilus* (109). It is also noteworthy that a *tet*(D) tetracycline resistance gene (5) has been detected in isolates of the fish pathogen *Pasteurella piscicida.* In 1995 this organism was reclassified as *Photobacterium damselae* subsp. *piscicida* (48).

Two other tetracycline resistance genes, *tet*(M) and *tet*(O), both coding for ribosome protective proteins, have been identified in *P. multocida, H. ducreyi*, or *A. pleuropneumoniae.* The gene *tet*(M), which is associated with conjugative transposons such as Tn*916* (44), is the most widespread *tet* gene among gram-positive and gram-negative bacteria (28). It has been detected by hybridization in the chromosomal DNA of two bovine *P. multocida* isolates (26, 51), but also on a conjugative plasmid in *H. ducreyi* of human origin (94). The gene *tet*(O), previously identified in *Campylobacter* spp. and streptococci, was detected in the chromosomal DNA of a porcine *A. pleuropneumoniae* isolate (108).

Resistance to β-Lactams

Resistance to β-lactams among members of the *Pasteurellaceae* is often associated with small plasmids. These range in size between 4.1 and 4.4 kb in *P. multocida* (90, 103, 121), 4.2 and 5.2 kb in *[P.] haemolytica* (6, 23, 24, 33, 100, 122, 127), 2.5 and 6.8 kb in *A. pleuropneumoniae* (22, 25, 63, 67, 85), and 4.4 and 10.5 kb in *H. influenzae* and *H. ducreyi* (16, 92, 96, 97). Most of these β-lactam resistance plasmids have been identified phenotypically by transformation experiments. Three β-lactamase (*bla*) genes have been identified , bla_{ROB-1} (6, 66, 90, 91), bla_{TEM-1} (103), and bla_{PSE-1} (146). According to the existing classification schemes of β-lactamases, the enzymes ROB-1 and TEM-1 are assigned because of their structure to the Ambler class A and on the basis of their substrate profile to the Bush class 2b of β-lactamases (18). Members of this class can hydrolyze penicillins and narrow-spectrum cephalosporins but may be inactivated by β-lactamase inhibitors such as clavulanic acid. The PSE-1 β-lactamase belongs to the Ambler class A but to the Bush class 2c. This enzyme, also known as CARB-2 β-lactamase, can hydrolyze carbenicillin and is also inactivated by clavulanic acid. All these β-lactamases—ROB-1, TEM-1, and PSE-1—do not exhibit an extended spectrum of activity. They also do not mediate resistance to newer cephalosporins like ceftiofur or cefquinome.

Although initially identified in *H. influenzae* from a human infection (98), ROB-1 β-lactamases have been detected in porcine *A. pleuropneumoniae* isolates of various serotypes from North America (67) and in bovine and porcine *P. multocida, [P.] haemolytica*, and *[P.] aerogenes* isolates from France (90, 91, 112). Since bla_{ROB-1}-carrying plasmids from different bacterial sources were in the same size range, it appeared likely that they were also structurally related. Hybridization studies and restriction analysis supported the assumption of a close genetic relationship between the bla_{ROB-1}-encoding plasmids from *P. multocida, [P.] haemolytica*, and *H. influenzae* (91). Moreover, sequence comparisons of the five so far sequenced bla_{ROB-1} genes from *[P.] haemolytica, A. pleuropneumoniae,* and *H. influenzae* confirmed that all these genes coded for an identical β-lactamase protein of 305 amino acids. Mutations in the bla_{ROB-1} gene that resulted in resistance to extended-spectrum cephalosporins and β-lactamase inhibitors have been produced in vitro (47).

In contrast, only single reports described the detection of a TEM-1 β-lactamase in a *P. multocida* isolate of human origin (103) and a PSE-1 β-lactamase in an avian *P. multocida* isolate (146). The TEM-1 β-lactamase was confirmed by isoelectric focusing and sequence analysis of part of the bla_{TEM-1} gene, whereas the bla_{PSE-1} gene was completely sequenced. TEM-type β-lactamases have been identified in several *Haemophilus* spp. from humans, including *H. influenzae* and *H. ducreyi* (16, 92, 95, 96).

There is also evidence that mutations in the gene *ftsI* that result in amino acid substitutions at specific positions in penicillin-binding protein 3 (PBP3) of *H. influenzae* are responsible for resistance not only to β-lactam antibiotics but also to β-lactamase inhibitors (34, 95, 136).

Resistance to Aminoglycosides and Aminocyclitols

The first aminoglycoside resistance genes detected in *Pasteurella* and *Mannheimia* were those mediating streptomycin resistance. In 1978 Berman and Hirsh published a report on plasmids coding for streptomycin resistance along with sulfonamide resistance or sulfonamide and tetracycline resistance in *P. multocida* from turkeys (7). Streptomycin resistance is commonly associated with small, nonconjugative plasmids of less than 10 kb in *P. multocida* from turkeys (7, 53–55), pigs (32, 129, 147), and cattle (128, 129); *[P.] aerogenes* from pigs (75); *[P.] haemolytica* from cattle (23, 150); *Mannheimia varigena* from cattle (76); and *A. pleuropneumoniae* from pigs (22, 50, 63, 64, 83, 142). In one case, streptomycin resistance was mediated by a conjugative multiresistance plasmid of approximately 113 kb in an avian *P. multocida* isolate (55).

The *strA* gene is the predominant streptomycin resistance gene in bacteria of the genera *Pasteurella, Mannheimia*, and *Actinobacillus*. It codes for an aminoglycoside-3″-phosphotransferase of 269 amino acids and has been found together with the gene *strB*, which codes for an aminoglycoside-6-phosphotransferase of 278 amino acids. These genes are part of transposon Tn*5393* from *Erwinia amylovora* (27). In streptomycin-resistant *Pasteurella, Mannheimia*, and *Actinobacillus* isolates *strA* is usually complete, whereas various truncated *strB* genes have been identified (75, 76). Strains that carry a functionally active *strA* gene but a largely truncated *strB* gene have been shown to be highly resistant to streptomycin (75). Studies on the prevalence and distribution of the *strA-strB* genes showed that the *strA* gene—in combination with a complete or a truncated copy of *strB*—occurs on plasmids or in the chromosomal DNA of a wide range of commensal and pathogenic bacteria from humans, animals, and plants (131–133).

The *aadA1* gene, coding for an aminoglycoside-3″-adenyltransferase that mediates resistance to the aminoglycoside streptomycin and the aminocyclitol spectinomycin, has been detected on the 5.2-kb plasmid pJR2 from avian *P. multocida* (146). The *aadA1* gene is part of a gene cassette that is inserted into a relic of a class 1 integron in pJR2. The *intI1* gene, coding for the integrase in the 5′ conserved segment of this integron, is truncated, without affecting the promoter, however, and the *sul1* gene in the 3′ conserved fragment is missing completely. Attempts to identify the *aad* genes in bovine strains of *P. multocida* and *M. haemolytica* from Germany that are highly resistant to streptomycin and spectinomycin using PCR were unsuccessful (126). In all these isolates streptomycin resistance was based on the *strA* gene, whereas a spectinomycin resistance gene could not be identified.

Recently, a novel streptomycin-spectinomycin resistance gene, designated *aadA14*, was identified on a small 5.2-kb plasmid from bovine *P. multocida* from Belgium (69). The corresponding adenyltransferase protein of 261 amino acids exhibited only 51.4 to 56.0% identity to the known AadA proteins and hence proved to be only distantly related to AadA proteins previously found in other bacteria.

It is known that mutations in genes coding for specific ribosomal proteins can also confer streptomycin resistance. Comparative analysis of the chromosomal genes coding for the 124-amino-acid ribosomal protein S12 from a high-level streptomycin-resistant and a streptomycin-susceptible *H. influenzae* revealed two amino acid substitutions in the respective proteins (130).

Kanamycin resistance has been associated with the gene *aphA1*, also known as *aph(3′)-Ia*, which codes for an aminoglycoside-3′-phosphotransferase that mediates resistance to kanamycin and neomycin. This gene has been identified on transposon Tn*903* (107) but was later on detected together with the streptomycin resistance genes *strA-strB* and the sulfonamide resistance gene *sul2* on the broad-host-range plasmid pLS88 from *H. ducreyi* (40). A not further specified aminoglycoside-3′-phosphotransferase gene mediating kanamycin resistance was also found together with a $bla_{\text{ROB-1}}$ gene on the 6-kb plasmid pTMY2 from *A. pleuropneumoniae* (22).

Resistance to Sulfonamides

Sulfonamide resistance among *Pasteurella, Mannheimia*, and *Actinobacillus* isolates is commonly mediated by a type 2 dihydropteroate synthase (DHPS). The corresponding gene, *sul2*, is frequently found on small plasmids in *P. multocida* (32, 53, 145, 147), *[P.] haemolytica* (13, 23), *Mannheimia* spp. (75, 76), *A. pleuropneumoniae* (22, 62, 64, 65, 68, 142), *H. influenzae* (41), and *H. ducreyi* (40). The *sul2*-encoded DHPS proteins commonly consist of 271 amino acids. However, several variants ranging in size between 263 (40) and 289 amino acids (77) have also been reported. Sequence analysis showed that single-base-pair insertions downstream of codon 225 in the DHPS of the *H. ducreyi* plasmid pLS88 (40) resulted in a shortened carboxy terminus that differs from all so far known DHPS variants. A mutation in the translational stop codon of the DHPS from plasmids pYFC1 of *[P.] haemolytica* (23) and pTYM1 of *A. pleuropneumoniae* (22) led to an extension of 12 amino acids at the carboxy terminus. In plasmid pCCK154 from *P. multocida*, the loss of a single A at position 793 within the *sul2* gene caused a frameshift mutation that led to the substitution of 6 codons and extended the reading frame by 18 codons (77). Finally, a recombination in the 3′ end of the *sul2* reading frame changed the final three codons and extended the *sul2* reading frame by one codon in plasmid pVM111 from *P. multocida* (79). In addition to their location on small plasmids, *sul2* genes have also been detected on conjugative plasmids, such as pGS05 (118), or nonconjugative broad-host-range plasmids, such as RSF1010 (124) and pLS88 (40). Plasmids carrying *sul2* have also been identified in bacteria other than *Pasteurellaceae*, e.g., *E. coli* (124) and *P. damselae* subsp. *piscicida* (81).

Various studies revealed that the *sul2* gene is often linked to the *strA-strB* genes (23, 40, 75, 145). PCR assays were developed to confirm the linkage of *sul2* and *strA* in both orientations (75). In some cases, the *strA* gene followed by a truncated Δ*strB* gene was detected upstream of *sul2* (75, 145). However, in most of the *P. multocida, [P.] aerogenes*, and *Mannheimia* isolates studied, the genes were found in the orientation *sul2-strA*, whereas in one case a truncated Δ*strA* was found upstream of *sul2* (23, 40, 75). Detailed studies of the noncoding spacer between *sul2* and *strA* revealed different lengths (65, 75) and also showed that this region might represent a hot spot for recombination events. The *catA3* gene, coding for chloramphenicol resistance, was found to be inserted between *sul2* and *strA* via illegitimate recombination. Such *sul2-catA3-strA* clusters have been found on various plasmids as well as in the chromosomal DNA of *[P.] aerogenes, M. haemolytica, M. varigena*, and *Mannheimia* taxon 10 isolates (75, 76). In plasmid pVM111 from an avian *P. multocida* isolate (7, 52), a Tn*5706*-like *tetR-tet*(H) segment responsible for tetracycline resistance was also found to be inserted between *sul2* and *strA* via illegitimate recombination (79). The resulting *sul2-tetR-tet*(H)-*strA* cluster, however, has not yet been detected on plasmids other than pVM111 or in the chromosomal DNA of *Pasteurella, Mannheimia*, or *Actinobacillus* isolates.

In high-level sulfonamide-resistant *H. influenzae* which did not carry *sul1* or *sul2*, a 15-bp insertion into the chromosomal gene encoding DHPS, *folP*, was detected. This insertion was shown to increase the MIC of sulfamethoxazole from 32 to 1,024 μg/ml (41).

Resistance to Trimethoprim

High-level trimethoprim resistance is commonly due to trimethoprim-resistant dihydrofolate reductases (DHFRs); these genes (*dfr*, also referred to as *dhfr*) are frequently located on plasmids, transposons, or gene cassettes. However, mutations in the chromosomal DHFR genes can render the corresponding proteins resistant to trimethoprim, and overproduction of the susceptible DHFRs may increase the insensitivity of the bacteria to trimethoprim.

Studies on trimethoprim-resistant bovine *[P.] haemolytica* isolates from France revealed that trimethoprim resistance was not associated with plasmids and also was not transferable by conjugation. Hybridization experiments with gene probes specific for the genes *dhfr*I to *dhfr*V did not yield positive results (42). This observation led to the suggestion that either other trimethoprim resistance genes or other mechanisms are responsible for trimethoprim resistance in these isolates.

Recently, the 11-kb plasmid pCCK154 from bovine *P. multocida* was found to mediate high-level resistance to sulfonamides and trimethoprim (77). This plasmid was transferable into *E. coli*, where it was able to replicate and express both resistance properties. PCR analysis for the most frequently occurring *dfr* genes of gram-negative bacteria (45) did not give positive results. Sequence analysis identified the gene *sul2* for sulfonamide resistance and a novel gene, designated *dfrA20*, for trimethoprim resistance. The *dfrA20* gene codes for a trimethoprim-resistant DHFR of 169 amino acids that is only distantly related to the DHFRs of gram-negative bacteria, but upon cluster analysis appears to be related to those found in the gram-positive genera *Staphylococcus, Bacillus*, and *Listeria* (77).

Overproduction of a trimethoprim-sensitive DHFR, encoded by the gene *folH*, was considered to account for trimethoprim resistance in *H. influenzae* (37). Molecular analysis identified alterations in the promoter region, but also in the 5′ end and the central region, of the *folH* gene, which correspond to the trimethoprim-binding domains in the DHFR protein (38).

Resistance to Chloramphenicol and Florfenicol

Chloramphenicol resistance in gram-negative bacteria is commonly mediated by either chloramphenicol acetyltransferases or chloramphenicol exporters. The genes for both are often located on plasmids, transposons, or gene cassettes. Plasmids mediating chloramphenicol resistance have been identified in porcine *P. multocida* isolates (147), bovine *P. multocida* and *[P.] haemolytica* isolates (137), porcine *[P.] aerogenes* (75), bovine *Mannheimia* spp. (75, 76), and porcine *A. pleuropneumoniae* (50, 62, 68, 85). As previously seen with other resistance plasmids, those mediating chloramphenicol resistance were commonly less than 10 kb in size. Initial molecular studies on chloramphenicol resistance among *P. multocida* and *[P.] haemolytica* isolates included the detection of the three most frequently occurring *cat* genes among gram-negative bacteria, *catA1* to *catA3* (formerly known as *cat*I to *cat*III), by specific PCR assays (137). The *catA3* gene was detected on small plasmids of 5.1 kb whereas the *catA1* gene was located on plasmids of either 17.1 or 5.5 kb (137). More recently, *catA3* genes have been identified as parts of chromosomal or plasmid-borne resistance gene clusters in porcine *[P.] aerogenes* and bovine *Mannheimia* isolates (75, 76). The gene *catA1* was first identified on transposon Tn*9* (2) and the *catA3* gene on plasmid R387 from *Shigella flexneri* and *E. coli* (101). Similar or identical *catA1* and *catA3* genes have been detected in a wide variety of bacteria (125). Although the *catA2* gene is commonly found in *Haemophilus* spp. (102, 114), this gene has not yet been detected in chloramphenicol-resistant *Pasteurella, Mannheimia*, and *Actinobacillus*. However, the *catB2* gene, which codes for a different type of chloramphenicol acetyltransferase than the aforementioned *catA* genes (125), was found on plasmid pJR1 from avian *P. multocida* (146). The *catB2* gene is part of a gene cassette and thus needs the integron-associated promoter for its expression. In plasmid pJR1, the *catB2* cassette is located outside of an integron structure. Gene cassettes located at secondary sites outside of integrons may be expressed if a suitable promoter is available (106). However, such a promoter has not been identified in pJR1 (146).

A permeability barrier due to the downregulation of a 40-kDa outer membrane protein has also been reported to account for chloramphenicol resistance in *H. influenzae* (17).

So far, resistance to florfenicol, a structural analog of thiamphenicol, has rarely—if at all—been detected among *Pasteurellaceae*. A gene designated *pp-flo* that codes for a chloramphenicol/florfenicol exporter was identified in the fish pathogen *P. damselae* subsp. *piscicida* (formerly known as *Pasteurella piscicida*) (82). The gene *pp-flo* is closely related to the gene *floR*, which is part of the *S. enterica* serovar Typhimurium DT104 multiresistance gene cluster (12) and also has been found on plasmids or in the chromosome of various gram-negative bacteria (125). Monitoring studies to specifically determine the MICs of florfenicol among bovine and porcine respiratory tract pathogens showed that all *P. multocida, M. haemolytica*, and *A. pleuropneumoniae* isolates collected between 1994 and 2003 were susceptible to florfenicol (59, 60, 70, 115). Recently, the first florfenicol-resistant bovine *P. multocida* isolate from the United Kingdom was confirmed and shown to carry the gene *floR* on a 10.8-kb plasmid (78).

Resistance to Macrolides

Many gram-negative bacteria are believed to be innately resistant to macrolides due to permeability barriers or multidrug efflux pumps. Studies on the presence of macrolide resistance genes in bacteria of the genus *Actinobacillus* led to the identification of the rRNA methylase genes *erm*(A) and *erm*(C) in *A. pleuropneumoniae*. Mating experiments showed that these genes were transferred into *Moraxella catarrhalis* and/or *Enterococcus faecalis* (140). Similar studies with *A. actinomycetemcomitans* revealed the presence of the *erm*(A), *erm*(B), *erm*(C), *erm*(F), and/or *erm*(Q) genes. All of these genes except *erm*(A) could be transferred alone or in various combinations into either *E. faecalis* or *H. influenzae* (120). PCR-directed analysis of bovine *P. multocida* and *M. haemolytica* that exhibited erythromycin MICs of ≥16 μg/ml did not detect any of the three genes *erm*(A), *erm*(B), and *erm*(C) (C. Kehrenberg and S. Schwarz, unpublished data). Analysis of macrolide-resistant *H. influenzae* isolates from humans revealed occasional mutations in the genes coding for ribosomal proteins L4 and/or L22, in addition to mutations at various positions in the 23S rRNA (111). An unspecified efflux mechanism that accounted for reduced susceptibility (MICs of 0.25 to 4 μg/ml) was also detected in most clinical *H. influenzae* isolates (111).

Resistance to Quinolones and Fluoroquinolones

Very little is known about quinolone resistance in *Pasteurella, Mannheimia*, or *Actinobacillus*. A single report described the analysis of the quinolone resistance-determining region of the genes *gyrA* and *parC* in *P. multocida* isolates that exhibited different levels of resistance to nalidixic acid (19). A Ser83Ile alteration in GyrA was detected in an isolate for which the nalidixic acid MIC was 256 μg/ml, whereas Asp87Gly alterations were detected in isolates for which MICs were 4 and 12 μg/ml (19). None of these isolates exhibited resistance to fluoroquinolones.

In contrast, fluoroquinolone resistance has been detected occasionally in *H. influenzae*. Analysis of the quinolone resistance-determining regions in the target genes *gyrA, gyrB, parC*, or *parE* revealed a wide range of mutations in resistant clinical isolates and laboratory-selected mutants (31, 49, 89, 110).

DISSEMINATION, COSELECTION, AND PERSISTENCE OF RESISTANCE GENES

Molecular analysis of isolates of *Pasteurella, Mannheimia*, and *Actinobacillus* revealed that antimicrobial resistance genes were associated with plasmids in many cases (72). Most of the resistance plasmids identified to date are in the size range of <10 kb. Despite this relatively small size, many of them carry two or more resistance genes (Table 3 and Fig. 1). Up to now, only a few small resistance plasmids have been sequenced completely, including the plasmids pIG1 (145), pCCK381 (78), pCCK647 (69), and pJR1 and pJR2 (146) from *P. multocida*; pMS260 (65) and pTMY1 (22) from *A. pleuropneumoniae*; pYFC1 (23) and pAB2 (144) from *[P.] haemolytica*; pCCK3259 from *M. haemolytica* (69a); pMVSCS1 from *M. varigena* (76); pMHSCS1 from *Mannheimia* taxon 10 (initially identified as *M. haemolytica*) (75); pHS-Tet from *H. parasuis* (86); and pLS88 from *H. ducreyi* (40). In addition, the resistance gene regions of several other plasmids—listed in Table 3—have been sequenced. Sequence analysis of these resistance plasmids provided insight into (i) the genes involved in antimicrobial resistance of *Pasteurella, Mannheimia*, and *Actinobacillus* and their organization; (ii) the structural relationships between the resistance plasmids; and (iii) mechanisms resulting in the formation of multiresistance plasmids and plasmid-borne multiresistance gene clusters.

Some of the genes accounting for antimicrobial resistance in *Pasteurella, Mannheimia*, and *Actinobacillus*, such as the tetracycline resistance gene *tet*(H) and the β-lactamase gene bla_{ROB-1}, appear to be rather specific for these bacteria and have rarely—if at all—been detected outside of the family *Pasteurellaceae*. In contrast, other resistance genes such as the streptomycin resistance genes *strA-strB* have

Table 3. Resistance plasmids identified in *Pasteurella, Mannheimia, Actinobacillus*, and *Haemophilus*

Plasmid designation	Size (kb)	Resistance phenotype[a]	Resistance genotype	Bacterial source	Reference(s)
pIG1	5.4	Sm, Sul	*strA*, Δ*strB*, *sul2*	*P. multocida*	145
pPASS2	4.7	Sm, Sul	*strA*, Δ*strB*, *sul2*	*[P.] aerogenes*	75
pYFC1	4.2	Sul, Sm	*sul2*, *strA*, Δ*strB*	*[P.] haemolytica*	23
pPMSS1	4.2	Sul, Sm	*sul2*, *strA*, Δ*strB*	*P. multocida*	75
pPASS1	5.5	Sul, Sm	*sul2*, *strA*, Δ*strB*	*[P.] aerogenes*	75
pTMY1	4.2	Sul, Sm	*sul2*, *strA*, Δ*strB*	*A. pleuropneumoniae*	22
pMS260	8.1	Sul, Sm	*sul2*, *strA*, *strB*	*A. pleuropneumoniae*	65
pMVSCS1	5.6	Sul, Cm, Sm	*sul2*, *catA3*, *strA*, Δ*strB*	*M. varigena*	76
pMHSCS1	5.0	Sul, Cm, Sm	*sul2*, *catA3*, *strA*, Δ*strB*	*Mannheimia* taxon 10	75
pPASCS1	5.6	Sul, Cm, Sm	*sul2*, *catA3*, *strA*, Δ*strB*	*[P.] aerogenes*	75
pPASCS2	6.0	Sul, Cm, Sm	*sul2*, *catA3*, *strA*, Δ*strB*	*[P.] aerogenes*	75
pPASCS3	6.1	Sul, Cm, Sm	*sul2*, *catA3*, *strA*, Δ*strB*	*[P.] aerogenes*	75
pLS88	4.8	Sul, Sm, Km/Nm	*sul2*, *strA*, Δ*strB*, *aphA1*	*H. ducreyi*	40
pVM111	9.8	Sul, Tc, Sm	*sul2*, *tetR-tet*(H), *strA*, *strB*	*P. multocida*	52, 79
pPMT1	6.8	Tc	*tetR-tet*(H)	*P. multocida*	80
pPAT1	5.5	Tc	*tetR-tet*(H)	*[P.] aerogenes*	73
pMHT1	4.4	Tc	*tetR-tet*(H)	*M. haemolytica*	71
p9956H	5.7	Tc	*tetR-tet*(H)	*A. pleuropneumoniae*	10
p9555L	5.7	Tc	*tet*(L)	*A. pleuropneumoniae*	10
pCCK3259	5.3	Tc	*tet*(L)	*M. haemolytica*	69a
pPAT2	4.8	Tc	*tetR-tet*(B)	*[P.] aerogenes*	74
pHS-Tet	5.1	Tc	*tet*(B)	*H. parasuis*	86
pJR1	6.8	?[b]	*sul2*, *tet*(G), *catB2*	*P. multocida*	146
pJR2	5.3	?[b]	*aadA1*, bla_{PSE-1}	*P. multocida*	146
pCCK647	5.2	Sm, Sp	*aadA14*	*P. multocida*	69
pFAB-1	4.3	Pen	bla_{TEM-1}	*P. multocida*	103
pPH51	4.1	Pen	bla_{ROB-1}	*[P.] haemolytica*	91
pYFC2	4.2	Pen	bla_{ROB-1}	*[P.] haemolytica*	23
pR_{Rob}	4.4	Pen	bla_{ROB-1}	*H. influenzae*	66
Unknown	Unknown	Pen	bla_{ROB-1}	*A. pleuropneumoniae*	25
pAB2	4.3	Pen	bla_{ROB-1}	*[P.] haemolytica*	144
pCCK381	10.8	Cm, Ff	*floR*	*P. multocida*	78
pCCK154	11.0	Sul, Tmp	*sul2*, *dfrA20*	*P. multocida*	77

[a]Abbreviations for antimicrobial agent resistance: Cm, chloramphenicol; Ff, florfenicol; Km, kanamycin; Nm, neomycin; Pen, penicillins; Sm, streptomycin; Sp, spectinomycin; Tc, tetracycline.
[b]The resistance phenotype mediated by this plasmid has not been confirmed by transfer experiments.

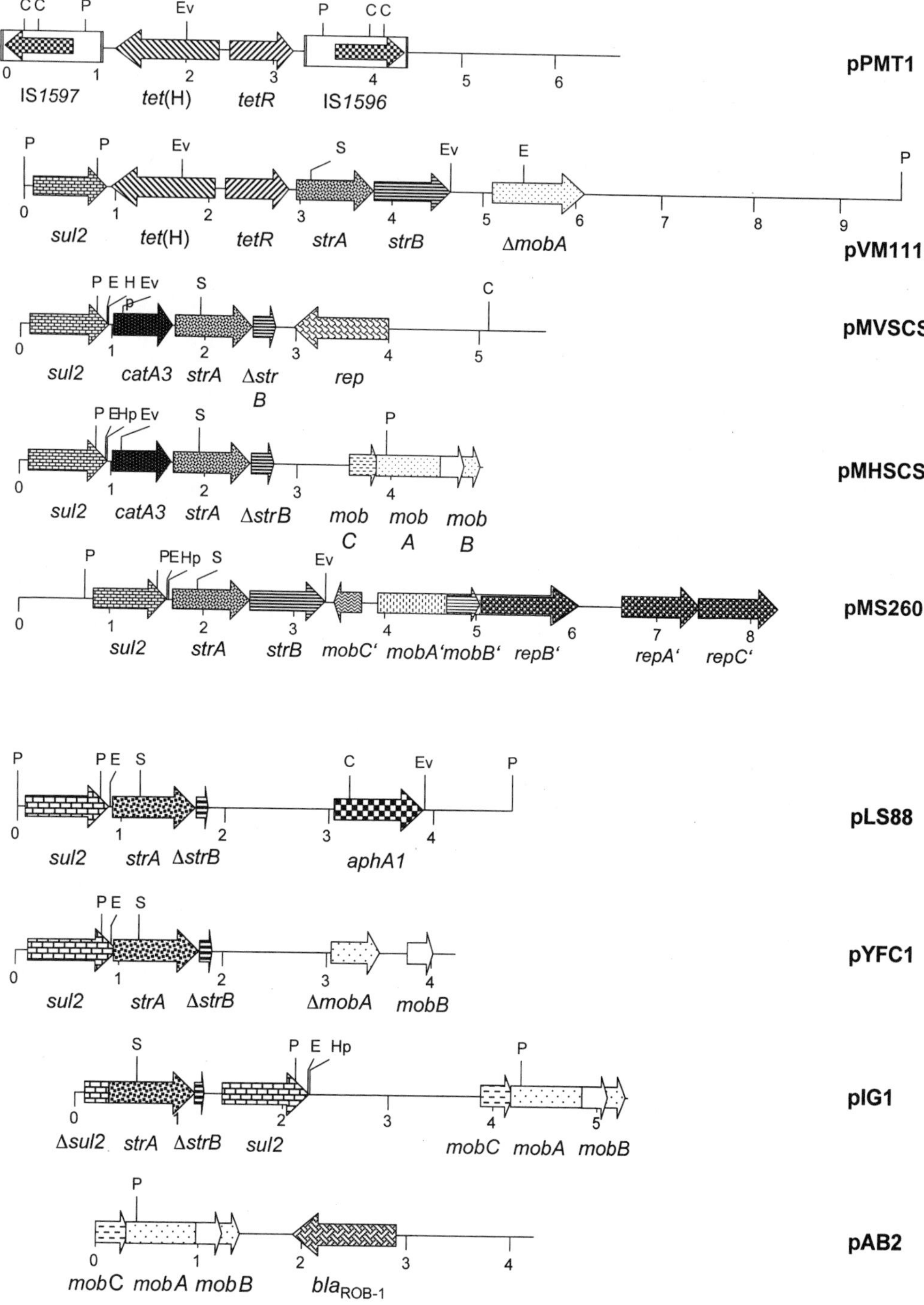

Figure 1. Structure and organization of selected resistance plasmids from members of the family *Pasteurellaceae* (Table 3). The genes are shown as arrows with the arrowhead indicating the direction of transcription. A distance scale in kilobases is given below each map. The following genes are involved in antimicrobial resistance: *tetR-tet*(H) (tetracycline resistance), *sul2* (sulfonamide resistance), *strA* and *strB* (streptomycin resistance), *catA3* (chloramphenicol resistance), *aphA1* (kanamycin and neomycin resistance), and $bla_{\text{ROB-1}}$ (β-lactam resistance). *rep, repA', repB'*, and *repC'* are involved in plasmid replication, and *mobA, mobB, mobC, mobA', mobB'*, and *mobC'* are involved in mobilization functions. The prefix Δ indicates a truncated, functionally inactive gene. The boxes in the map of pPMT1 indicate the insertion sequences IS*1596* and IS*1597*, with the arrows within these boxes marking the transposase genes. Restriction endonuclease cleavage sites are abbreviated as follows: C, ClaI; E, EcoRI; Ev, EcoRV; Hp, HpaI; P, PstI; S, SacI.

been detected in a wide range of gram-negative bacteria. The fact that these genes are associated with the transposon Tn*5393* (27), but also have been found on two mobilizable broad-host-range plasmids, pLS88 (40) and RSF1010 (124), might explain their widespread occurrence, which may be due to horizontal gene transfer. The location of resistance genes on mobile genetic elements allows the spread of the resistance genes into bacteria of other species and genera. This has been confirmed by the detection of plasmids, which were indistinguishable on the basis of their restriction maps, in different host bacteria. Examples are the *tet*(H)-carrying plasmids pMHT1, which was found in *P. multocida, M. haemolytica, M. varigena*, and *Mannheimia glucosida* (71), and pPAT1, present in *P. multocida* and *[P.] aerogenes* (73), as well as the *sul2-strA*-carrying plasmid pPMSS1, which was identified in *P. multocida, [P.] aerogenes*, and *M. haemolytica* (75). Plasmids from *H. influenzae, P. multocida*, and *[P.] haemolytica* carrying the β-lactamase gene $bla_{\text{ROB-1}}$ proved to be closely related on the basis of restriction fingerprints and hybridization patterns (67, 91). Several of these small plasmids carried *mob* genes, which allow mobilization in the presence of a conjugative element. Mobilization has also been confirmed for the 8.1-kb *sul2-strA*-carrying plasmid pMS260 from *A. pleuropneumoniae* (65). This plasmid, which closely resembles the broad-host-range plasmid RSF1010 (124), proved to be mobilizable into a wide variety of respiratory tract pathogens, including *P. multocida, Bordetella bronchiseptica*, and *Pseudomonas aeruginosa*, as well as other strains of *A. pleuropneumoniae* (64). Moreover, most of the small resistance plasmids found in *Pasteurella, Mannheimia*, and *Actinobacillus* are able to replicate and express their resistance properties in *E. coli*. On the other hand, most resistance plasmids of *Enterobacteriaceae* origin, harboring either *catA3, strA-strB, tet*(B), or *sul2*, usually cannot replicate in *Pasteurella, Mannheimia*, and *Actinobacillus* hosts. With the exception of the RSF1010-like plasmid pMS260 from *A. pleuropneumoniae* (65), analysis of the regions flanking the *sul2* and *strA-strB* genes in plasmids of *Pasteurella, Mannheimia*, or *Actinobacillus* did not reveal sequences similar to those of *Enterobacteriaceae* plasmids, but to those of plasmids known to occur in *Pasteurellaceae*. This observation suggests that recombination events between indigenous plasmids of *Pasteurellaceae* and resistance plasmids from other bacterial sources, which may be replication-deficient in *Pasteurellaceae*, have most likely occurred. As a result, the horizontally acquired resistance genes became inserted into new plasmidic replicons, which then have been stably maintained in *Pasteurellaceae*. Studies of the plasmid-borne *sul2-strA* gene cluster in *Pasteurella* and *Mannheimia* showed that the noncoding spacer region between the two resistance genes may represent the target site for further recombination events (75, 76). Thus, the *catA3* gene from plasmid R387 (101) was found to be integrated via illegitimate recombination into this spacer region (75, 76). Another example is plasmid pVM111, where recombination processes between the tetracycline resistance transposon Tn*5706* and the *sul2-strA* spacer region led to the integration of the entire *tetR-tet*(H) region between *sul2* and *strA* (79). However, the *tetR-tet*(H) region of Tn*5706* has also been detected in plasmids that do not carry additional resistance genes. Analysis of the sequences flanking the *tetR-tet*(H) area in these plasmids again suggested the involvement of recombination events in the truncation of the integrated transposon (79).

Based on the observation that many of the resistance plasmids so far detected in *Pasteurella, Mannheimia*, and *Actinobacillus* carry two or three resistance genes, coselection of these genes is likely. Once such a resistance plasmid is transferred to a new host, all resistance genes located on it are also transferred. As a consequence, a new host bacterium gains resistance to two or more antimicrobial agents or classes of antimicrobial agents, e.g., sulfonamides, streptomycin, and tetracyclines in the case of plasmid pVM111, by the acquisition of a single small plasmid. In these cases, selective pressure imposed by the use of one such antimicrobial agent, e.g., tetracyclines, is sufficient to favor the exchange of the multiresistance plasmid. The location of different resistance genes on the same plasmid also enables their persistence, in particular if the genes are organized in a cluster. A multiresistance gene cluster in which the genes *sul2, catA3*, and *strA* are organized as a transcriptional unit has been identified on several different plasmids, but also in the chromosomal DNA of *[P.] aerogenes* and several *Mannheimia* spp. (75, 76). It is highly unlikely that individual genes from such a cluster are lost. A study on the location of chloramphenicol resistance genes in *Pasteurella* and *Mannheimia* isolates from Germany showed that the dominant chloramphenicol resistance gene, *catA3*, was located in a *sul2-catA3-strA* cluster in all cases, except for a single bovine *M. glucosida* isolate (75). Although chloramphenicol has been prohibited for use in food-producing animals in the European Union and the United States for several years, amin glycosides including streptomycin, as well as sulfonamides, are still used. Streptomycin and/or sulfonamides might present the selective pressure that ensures the maintenance of the entire cluster.

Thus, clusters such as that containing the genes *sul2-catA3-strA* may play an important role in maintaining resistance genes without direct selective pressure.

Analysis of the resistance genes, their location, and their organization provides insight into (i) the gene pool to which bacteria of the genera *Pasteurella, Mannheimia*, and *Actinobacillus* have access; (ii) horizontal transfer processes that play a key role in the dissemination of the resistance genes between and beyond bacteria of the three aforementioned genera; and (iii) integration and recombination events that are of major importance for the development of novel resistance plasmids and the formation of multiresistance gene clusters in *Pasteurella, Mannheimia*, and *Actinobacillus* isolates.

CONCLUSION

Isolates of several genera within the family *Pasteurellaceae* cause a number of economically important diseases in cattle, swine, and other food-producing animals. Due to the multifactorial and polymicrobial nature of some of the infections in which *Pasteurella, Mannheimia*, and *Actinobacillus* isolates are involved, prevention is—except in confined production systems with high biosecurity—a cumbersome task that often yields unsatisfying results. Despite hygienic measures, improved management, and the use of vaccines, antimicrobial agents are indispensable tools for the control of infections in which bacteria of the family *Pasteurellaceae* are involved. Increasing numbers of resistant or multiresistant strains are reducing the efficacy of antimicrobial agents currently approved for use in animals. It is anticipated that in the near future, there will be no new classes of antimicrobial agents approved for use in veterinary medicine. Thus, veterinarians will have to rely on those antimicrobial agents currently available. To retain the efficacy of the antimicrobial drugs, prescription and administration of antimicrobial agents should be undertaken with discretion supported by an accurate diagnosis, a careful choice of the respective antimicrobial agent(s), and the most appropriate dosing regimen. Imprudent use of antimicrobials bears a high risk of selecting resistant bacteria. Many of the resistance genes known to be present in *Pasteurella, Mannheimia, Actinobacillus*, and *Haemophilus* are associated with plasmids or transposons and thus may be exchanged horizontally, not only between bacteria of the family *Pasteurellaceae* but also with other gram-negative bacteria. The examples given in this chapter illustrate that *Pasteurella, Mannheimia, Actinobacillus*, and *Haemophilus* have obviously acquired a number of resistance genes from other gram-negative or maybe even gram-positive bacteria. Knowledge of the location and colocation of the resistance genes on mobile genetic elements as well as the conditions for their coselection and persistence will be valuable for veterinarians and will assist them in selecting the most efficacious antimicrobial agents for the control of isolates of the family *Pasteurellaceae*.

REFERENCES

1. **Aarestrup, F. M., A. M. Seyfarth, and Ø. Angen.** 2004. Antimicrobial susceptibility of *Haemophilus parasuis* and *Histophilus somni* from pigs and cattle in Denmark. *Vet. Microbiol.* **101:**143–146.
2. **Alton, N. K., and D. Vapnek.** 1979. Nucleotide sequence analysis of the chloramphenicol resistance transposon Tn9. *Nature* **282:**864–869.
3. **Angen, Ø., P. Ahrens, P. Kuhnert, H. Christensen, and R. Mutters.** 2003. Proposal of *Histophilus somni* gen. nov., sp. nov. for the three species *incertae sedis* '*Haemophilus somnus*', '*Haemophilus agni*' and '*Histophilus ovis*.' *Int. J. Syst. Evol. Microbiol* **53:**1449–1456.
4. **Angen, Ø., R. Mutters, D. A. Caugant, J. E. Olsen, and M. Bisgaard.** 1999. Taxonomic relationships of [*Pasteurella*] *haemolytica* complex as evaluated by DNA-DNA hybridizations and 16S rRNA sequencing with proposal of *Mannheimia haemolytica* gen. nov., comb. nov., *Mannheima granulomatis* comb. nov., *Mannheimia glucosida* sp. nov., *Mannheimia ruminalis* sp. nov. and *Mannheimia varigena* sp. nov. *Int. J. Syst. Bacteriol.* **49:**67–86.
5. **Aoki, T., and A. Takahashi.** 1987. Class D tetracycline resistance determinants of R plasmids from the fish pathogens *Aeromonas hydrophila*, *Edwardsiella tarda*, and *Pasteurella piscicida*. *Antimicrob. Agents Chemother.* **31:**1278–1280.
6. **Azad, A. K., J. G. Coote, and R. Parton.** 1992. Distinct plasmid profiles of *Pasteurella haemolytica* serotypes and the characterization and amplification in *E. coli* of ampicillin-resistance plasmids encoding ROB1-β-lactamase. *J. Gen. Microbiol.* **138:**1185–1196.
7. **Berman, S. M., and D. C. Hirsh.** 1978. Partial characterization of R-plasmids from *Pasteurella multocida* isolated from turkeys. *Antimicrob. Agents Chemother.* **14:**348–352.
8. **Bisgaard, M., O. Heltberg, and W. Frederiksen.** 1991. Isolation of *Pasteurella caballi* from an infected wound of a veterinary surgeon. *APMIS* **99:**291–294.
9. **Blackall, P. J., H. Christensen, T. Beckenham, L. L. Blackall, and M. Bisgaard.** 2005. Reclassification of *Pasteurella gallinarum*, [*Haemophilus*] *paragallinarum*, *Pasteurella avium*, and *Pasteurella volantium* as *Avibacterium gallinarum* gen. nov., comb. nov., *Avibacterium paragallinarum* comb. nov., *Avibacterium avium* comb. nov. and *Avibacterium volantium* comb. nov. *Int. J. Syst. Evol. Microbiol.* **55:**353–362.
10. **Blanco, M., M. Fernandez, N. Garcia, C. B. Gutierrez, E. F. R. Ferri, and J. Navas.** 2003. Incidence, distribution and spread of tetracycline resistance determinants among Spanish isolates of the respiratory pathogen *Actinobacillus pleuropneumoniae*. *Abstr. 103rd Gen. Meet. Am. Soc. Microbiol.*, abstr. A-044, p. 9. American Society for Microbiology, Washington, D.C.
11. **Böttner, A., P. Schmid, and R. Humke.** 1995. *In vitro* efficacy of cefquinome (INN) and other anti-infective drugs against bovine bacterial isolates from Belgium, France, Germany, The

Netherlands, and the United Kingdom. *J. Vet. Med. B* **42:** 377–383.

12. **Briggs, C. E., and P. M. Fratamico.** 1999. Molecular characterization of an antibiotic resistance gene cluster of *Salmonella typhimurium* DT104. *Antimicrob. Agents Chemother.* **43:**846–849.
13. **Briggs, R. E., G. H. Frank, C. D. Purdy, E. S. Zehr, and R. W. Loan.** 1998. Rapid spread of a unique strain of *Pasteurella haemolytica* serotype 1 among transported calves. *Am. J. Vet. Res.* **59:**401–405.
14. **Brockmeier, S. L., P. G. Halbur, and E. L. Thacker.** 2002. Porcine respiratory disease complex, p. 231–258. *In* K. A. Brogden and J. M. Guthmiller (ed.), *Polymicrobial Diseases.* American Society for Microbiology, Washington, D.C.
15. **Brue, C., and O. Chosidow.** 1994. *Pasteurella multocida* wound infection and cellulitis. *Int. J. Dermatol.* **33:**471–473.
16. **Brunton, J. M. Meier, N. Erhman, D. Clare, and R. Almawy.** 1986. Origin of small β-lactamase-specifying plasmids in *Haemophilus* species and *Neisseria gonorrhoeae. J. Bacteriol.* **168:**374–379.
17. **Burns, J. L., P. M. Mendelman, J. Levy, T. L. Stull, and A. L. Smith.** 1985. A permeability barrier as a mechanism of chloramphenicol resistance in *Haemophilus influenzae. Antimicrob. Agents Chemother.* **27:**46–54.
18. **Bush, K., G. A. Jacoby, and A. A. Medeiros.** 1995. A functional classification scheme for β-lactamases and its correlation with molecular structure. *Antimicrob. Agents Chemother.* **39:**1211–1233.
19. **Cardenas, M., J. Barbe, M. Llagostera, E. Miro, F. Navarro, B. Mirelis, G. Prats, and I. Badiola.** 2001. Quinolone resistance-determining regions of *gyrA* and *parC* in *Pasteurella multocida* strains with different levels of nalidixic acid resistance. *Antimicrob. Agents Chemother.* **45:**990–991.
20. **Catry, B., K. Chiers, S. Schwarz, C. Kehrenberg, A. Decostere, and A. de Kruif.** 2005. A case of fatal peritonitis in calves caused by *Pasteurella multocida* capsular type F. *J. Clin. Microbiol.* **43:**1480–1483.
21. **Chalmers, S., R. Sewitz, K. Lipkow, and P. Crellin.** 2000. Complete nucleotide sequence of Tn*10*. *J. Bacteriol.* **182:**2970–2972.
22. **Chang, C.-F., T.-M. Yeh, C.-C. Chou, Y.-F. Chang, and T.-S. Chiang.** 2002. Antimicrobial susceptibility and plasmid analysis of *Actinobacillus pleuropneumoniae* isolated in Taiwan. *Vet. Microbiol.* **84:**169–177.
23. **Chang, Y. F., D. P. Ma, H. Q. Bai, R. Young, D. K. Struck, S. J. Shin, and D. H. Lein.** 1992. Characterization of plasmids with antimicrobial resistance genes in *Pasteurella haemolytica* A1. *DNA Sequence.* **3:**89–97.
24. **Chang, Y. F., H. W. Renshaw, and R. Young.** 1987. Pneumonic pasteurellosis: examination of typeable and untypeable *Pasteurella haemolytica* strains for leucotoxin production, plasmid content, and antimicrobial susceptibility. *Am. J. Vet. Res.* **48:**378–384.
25. **Chang, Y. F., J. Shi, S. J. Shin, and D. H. Lein.** 1992. Sequence analysis of the ROB-1 beta-lactamase gene from *Actinobacillus pleuropneumoniae. Vet. Microbiol.* **32:**319–325.
26. **Chaslus-Dancla, E., M.-C. Lesage-Descauses, S. Leroy-Sétrin, J.-L. Martel, and J.-P. Lafont.** 1995. Tetracycline resistance determinants, TetB and TetM, detected in *Pasteurella haemolytica* and *Pasteurella multocida* from bovine herds. *J. Antimicrob. Chemother.* **36:**815–819.
27. **Chiou, C.-S., and A. L. Jones.** 1993. Nucleotide sequence analysis of a transposon (Tn*5393*) carrying streptomycin resistance genes in *Erwinia amylovora* and other gram-negative bacteria. *J. Bacteriol.* **175:**732–740.
28. **Chopra, I., and M. C. Roberts.** 2001. Tetracycline antibiotics: mode of action, applications, molecular biology and epidemiology of bacterial resistance. *Microbiol. Mol. Biol. Rev.* **65:**232–260.
29. **Christensen, H., M. Bisgaard, B. Aalbaek, and J. E. Olsen.** 2004. Reclassification of Bisgaard taxon 33, with proposal of *Volucribacter psittacicida* gen. nov., sp. nov. and *Volucribacter amazonae* sp. nov. as new members of the *Pasteurellaceae. Int. J. Syst. Evol. Microbiol.* **54:**813–818.
30. **Christensen, H., M. Bisgaard, A. M. Bojesen, R. Mutters, and J. E. Olsen.** 2003. Genetic relationships among avian isolates classified as *Pasteurella haemolytica*, "*Actinobacillus salpingitidis*" or *Pasteurella anatis* with proposal of *Gallibacterium anatis* gen. nov., comb. nov. and description of additional genomospecies within *Gallibacterium* gen. nov. *Int. J. Syst. Evol. Microbiol.* **53:**275–287.
31. **Clark, C., K. Kosowska, B. Bozdogan, K. Credito, B. Dewasse, P. McGhee, M. R. Jacobs, and P. C. Appelbaum.** 2004. In vitro selection of resistance in *Haemophilus influenzae* by 4 quinolones and 5 β-lactams. *Diagn. Microbiol. Infect. Dis.* **49:**31–36.
32. **Cote, S., J. Harel, R. Higgins, and M. Jacques.** 1991. Resistance to antimicrobial agents and prevalence of R plasmids in *Pasteurella multocida* from swine. *Am. J. Vet. Res.* **52:** 1653–1657.
33. **Craig, F. F., J. G. Coote, R. Parton, J. H. Freer, and N. J. Gilmour.** 1989. A plasmid which can be transferred between *Escherichia coli* and *Pasteurella haemolytica* by electroporation and conjugation. *J. Gen. Microbiol.* **135:**2885–2890.
34. **Dabernat, H., C. Delmas, M. Seguy, R. Pelissier, G. Faucon, S. Bennamani, and C. Pasquier.** 2002. Diversity of β-lactam resistance conferring amino acid substitutions in penicillin-binding protein 3 of *Haemophilus influenzae. Antimicrob. Agents Chemother.* **46:**2208–2218.
35. **The Danish Integrated Antimicrobial Resistance Monitoring and Research Programme.** 1998. DANMAP 97—Consumption of antimicrobial agents and occurrence of antimicrobial resistance in bacteria from food animals, food and humans in Denmark. [Online.] http://www.dfvf.dk/Files/Filer/Zoonose-centret/Publikationer/Danmap/Danmap_1997.pdf.
36. **The Danish Integrated Antimicrobial Resistance Monitoring and Research Programme.** 1999. DANMAP 98—Consumption of antimicrobial agents and occurrence of antimicrobial resistance in bacteria from food animals, food and humans in Denmark. [Online.] http://www.dfvf.dk/Files/Filer/Zoonose-centret/Publikationer/Danmap/Danmap_1998.pdf.
37. **De Groot, R., J. Campos, S. L. Moseley, and A. L. Smith.** 1988. Molecular cloning and mechanism of trimethoprim resistance in *Haemophilus influenzae. Antimicrob. Agents Chemother.* **32:**477–484.
38. **De Groot, R., M. Sluijter, A. de Bruyn, J. Campos, W. H. Goessens, A. L. Smith, and P. W. Hermans.** 1996. Genetic characterization of trimethoprim resistance in *Haemophilus influenzae. Antimicrob. Agents Chemother.* **40:**2131–2136.
39. **DeRosa, D. C., M. F. Veenhuizen, D. J. Bade, and T. R. Shryock.** 2000. In vitro susceptibility of porcine respiratory pathogens to tilmicosin. *J. Vet. Diagn. Invest.* **12:**541–546.
40. **Dixon, L. G., W. L. Albritton, and P. J. Willson.** 1994. An analysis of the complete nucleotide sequence of the *Haemophilus ducreyi* broad-host-range plasmid pLS88. *Plasmid* **32:**228–232.
41. **Enne, V. I., A. King, D. M. Livermore, and L. M. Hall.** 2002. Sulfonamide resistance in *Haemophilus influenzae* mediated by acquisition of *sul2* or a short insertion in chromosomal *folP*. *Antimicrob. Agents Chemother.* **46:**1934–1939.
42. **Escande, F., G. Gerbaud, J.-L. Martel, and P. Courvalin.** 1991. Resistance to trimethoprim and 2,4-diamino-6,7-diisopropylpteridine (O/129) in *Pasteurella haemolytica. Vet. Microbiol.* **26:**107–114.

43. **Fajfar-Whetstone, C. J., L. Coleman, D. R. Biggs, and B. C. Fox.** 1995. *Pasteurella multocida* septicemia and subsequent *Pasteurella dagmatis* septicemia in a diabetic patient. *J. Clin. Microbiol.* **33:**202–204.

44. **Flannagan, S. E., L. A. Zitzow, Y. A. Su, and D. B. Clewell.** 1994. Nucleotide sequence of the 18-kb conjugative transposon Tn*916* from *Enterococcus faecalis*. *Plasmid* **32:**350–354.

45. **Frech, G., C. Kehrenberg, and S. Schwarz.** 2003. Resistance phenotypes and genotypes of multiresistant *Salmonella enterica* subsp. *enterica* serovar Typhimurium var. Copenhagen isolates from animal sources. *J. Antimicrob. Chemother.* **51:** 180–182.

46. **Freeman, A. F., X. T. Zheng, J. C. Lane, and S. T. Shulman.** 2004. *Pasteurella aerogenes* hamster bite peritonitis. *Pediatr. Infect. Dis. J.* **23:**368–370.

47. **Galan, J. C., M. I. Morosini, M. R. Baquero, M. Reig, and F. Baquero.** 2003. *Haemophilus influenzae* bla_{ROB-1} mutations in hypermutagenic Δ*ampC Escherichia coli* conferring resistance to cefotaxime and β-lactamase inhibitors and increased susceptibility to cefaclor. *Antimicrob. Agents Chemother.* **47:**2551–2557.

48. **Gauthier, G., B. Lafay, R. Ruimy, V. Breittmayer, J. L. Nicolas, M. Gauthier, and R. Christen.** 1995. Small subunit rRNA sequences and whole DNA relatedness concur for the reassignment of *Pasteurella piscicida* (Snieszko et al.) Janssen and Surgalla to the genus *Photobacterium* as *Photobacterium damsela* subsp. *piscicida* comb. nov. *Int. J. Syst. Bacteriol.* **45:** 139–144.

49. **Georgiu, M., R. Munoz, F. Roman, R. Canton, R. Gomez-Lus, J. Campos, and A. G. de la Campa.** 1996. Ciprofloxacin-resistant *Haemophilus influenzae* strains possess mutations in analogous positions of GyrA and ParC. *Antimicrob. Agents Chemother.* **40:**1741–1744.

50. **Gilbride, K. A., S. Rosendal, and J. L. Brunton.** 1989. Plasmid mediated antimicrobial resistance in Ontario isolates of *Actinobacillus (Haemophilus) pleuropneumoniae*. *Can. J. Vet. Res.* **53:**38–42.

51. **Hansen, L. M., P. C. Blanchard, and D. C. Hirsh.** 1996. Distribution of *tet*(H) among *Pasteurella* isolates from the United States and Canada. *Antimicrob. Agents Chemother.* **40:** 1558–1560.

52. **Hansen, L. M., L. M. McMurray, S. B. Levy, and D. C. Hirsh.** 1993. A new tetracycline resistance determinant, TetH, from *Pasteurella multocida* specifying active efflux of tetracycline. *Antimicrob. Agents Chemother.* **37:**2699–2705.

53. **Hirsh, D. C., D. L. Martin, and K. R. Rhoades.** 1981. Conjugal transfer of an R-plasmid in *Pasteurella multocida*. *Antimicrob. Agents Chemother.* **20:**415–417.

54. **Hirsh, D. C., D. L. Martin, and K. R. Rhoades.** 1985. Resistance plasmids of *Pasteurella multocida* isolated from turkeys. *Am. J. Vet. Res.* **46:**1490–1493.

55. **Hirsh, D. C., L. M. Hansen, L. C. Dorfman, K. P. Snipes, T. E. Carpenter, D. W. Hird, and R. H. McCapes.** 1989. Resistance to antimicrobial agents and prevalence of R plasmids in *Pasteurella multocida* from turkeys. *Antimicrob. Agents Chemother.* **33:**670–673.

56. **Ho, A. C., and C. J. Rapuano.** 1993. *Pasteurella multocida* keratitis and corneal laceration from a cat scratch. *Ophthalmic Surg.* **24:**346–348.

57. **Hodgins, D. C., J. A. Conlon, and P. E. Shewen.** 2002. Respiratory viruses and bacteria in cattle, p. 213–229. *In* K. A. Brogden and J. M. Guthmiller (ed.), *Polymicrobial Diseases*. American Society for Microbiology, Washington, D.C.

58. **Holst, E., J. Rollof, L. Larsson, and J. P. Nielsen.** 1992. Characterization and distribution of *Pasteurella* species recovered from infected humans. *J. Clin. Microbiol.* **30:**2984–2987.

59. **Hörmansdorfer, S., and J. Bauer.** 1996. Zur Resistenzsituation boviner Pasteurellen. *Berl. Münch. Tierärztl. Wochenschr.* **109:**168–171.

60. **Hörmansdorfer, S., and J. Bauer.** 1998. Zur Resistenz boviner und porciner Pasteurellen gegenüber Florfenicol und anderen Antibiotika. *Berl. Münch. Tierärztl. Wochenschr.* **111:**422–426.

61. **Hunt, M. L., B. Adler, and K. M. Townsend.** 2000. The molecular biology of *Pasteurella multocida*. *Vet. Microbiol.* **72:** 3–25.

62. **Ishii, H., T. Fukuyasu, S. Iyobe, and H. Hashimoto.** 1993. Characterization of newly isolated plasmids from *Actinobacillus pleuropneumoniae*. *Am. J. Vet. Res.* **54:**701–708.

63. **Ishii, H., F. Hayashi, S. Iyobe, and H. Hashimoto.** 1991. Characterization and classification of *Actinobacillus (Haemophilus) pleuropneumoniae* plasmids. *Am. J. Vet. Res.* **52:**1816–1820.

64. **Ishii, H., Y. Nakasone, S. Shigehara, K. Honma, Y. Araki, S. Iyobe, and H. Hashimoto.** 1990. Drug-susceptibility and isolation of a plasmid in *Haemophilus (Actinobacillus) pleuropneumoniae*. *Jpn. J. Vet. Sci.* **52:**1–9.

65. **Ito, H., H. Ishii, and M. Akiba.** 2004. Analysis of the complete nucleotide sequence of an *Actinobacillus pleuropneumoniae* streptomycin-sulfonamide resistance plasmid, pMS260. *Plasmid* **51:**41–47.

66. **Juteau, J.-M., and R. C. Levesque.** 1990. Sequence analysis and evolutionary perspectives of ROB1-β-lactamase. *Antimicrob. Agents Chemother.* **34:**1354–1359.

67. **Juteau, J.-M., M. Sirois, A. A. Medeiros, and R. C. Levesque.** 1991. Molecular distribution of ROB1-β-lactamase in *Actinobacillus pleuropneumoniae*. *Antimicrob. Agents Chemother.* **35:**1397–1402.

68. **Kawahara, K., H. Kawase, T. Nakai, K. Kume, and H. Danbara.** 1990. Drug resistance plasmids of *Actinobacillus pleuropneumoniae* serotype 2 strains isolated from swine. *Kitasato Arch. Exp. Med.* **63:**131–136.

69. **Kehrenberg, C., B. Catry, F. Haesebrouck, A. de Kruif, and S. Schwarz.** 2005. Novel spectinomycin/streptomycin resistance gene, *aadA14*, from *Pasteurella multocida*. *Antimicrob. Agents Chemother.* **49:**3046–3049.

69a. **Kehrenberg, C., B. Catry, F. Haesebrouck, A. de Kruif, and S. Schwarz.** 2005. *tet*(L)-mediated tetracycline resistance in bovine *Mannheimia* and *Pasteurella* isolates. *J. Antimicrob. Chemother.* **56:**403–406.

70. **Kehrenberg, C., J. Mumme, J. Wallmann, J. Verspohl, R. Tegeler, T. Kühn, and S. Schwarz.** 2004. Monitoring of florfenicol susceptibility among bovine and porcine respiratory tract pathogens collected in Germany during the years 2002 and 2003. *J. Antimicrob. Chemother.* **54:**572–574.

71. **Kehrenberg, C., S. A. Salmon, J. L. Watts, and S. Schwarz.** 2001. Tetracycline resistance genes in isolates of *Pasteurella multocida*, *Mannheimia haemolytica*, *Mannheimia glucosida*, and *Mannheimia varigena* from bovine and swine respiratory disease: intergeneric spread of plasmid pMHT1. *J. Antimicrob. Chemother.* **48:**631–640.

72. **Kehrenberg, C., G. Schulze-Tanzil, J.-L. Martel, E. Chaslus-Dancla, and S. Schwarz.** 2001. Antimicrobial resistance in *Pasteurella* and *Mannheimia*: epidemiology and genetic basis. *Vet. Res.* **32:**323–339.

73. **Kehrenberg, C., and S. Schwarz.** 2000. Identification of a truncated, but functionally active *tet*(H) tetracycline resistance gene in *Pasteurella aerogenes* and *Pasteurella multocida*. *FEMS Microbiol. Lett.* **188:**191–195.

74. **Kehrenberg, C., and S. Schwarz.** 2001. Molecular analysis of tetracycline resistance in *Pasteurella aerogenes*. *Antimicrob. Agents Chemother.* **45:**2885–2890.

75. **Kehrenberg, C., and S. Schwarz.** 2001. Occurrence and linkage of genes coding for resistance to sulfonamides, streptomycin and chloramphenicol in bacteria of the genera *Pasteurella* and *Mannheimia. FEMS Microbiol. Lett.* **205:**283–290.

76. **Kehrenberg, C., and S. Schwarz.** 2002. Nucleotide sequence and organisation of plasmid pMVSCS1 from *Mannheimia varigena*: identification of a multiresistance gene cluster. *J. Antimicrob. Chemother.* **49:**383–386.

77. **Kehrenberg, C., and S. Schwarz.** 2005. *dfrA20*, a novel trimethoprim resistance gene from *Pasteurella multocida. Antimicrob. Agents Chemother.* **49:**414–417.

78. **Kehrenberg, C., and S. Schwarz.** 2005. Plasmid-borne florfenicol resistance in *Pasteurella multocida. J. Antimicrob. Chemother.* **55:**773–775.

79. **Kehrenberg, C., N. T. T. Tham, and S. Schwarz.** 2003. New plasmid-borne antibiotic resistance gene cluster in *Pasteurella multocida. Antimicrob. Agents Chemother.* **47:**2978–2980.

80. **Kehrenberg, C., C. Werckenthin, and S. Schwarz.** 1998. Tn*5706*, a transposon-like element from *Pasteurella multocida* mediating tetracycline resistance. *Antimicrob. Agents Chemother.* **42:**2116–2118.

81. **Kim, E. H., and T. Aoki.** 1996. Sulfonamide resistance gene in a transferable R plasmid of *Pasteurella piscicida. Microbiol. Immunol.* **40:**397–399.

82. **Kim, E. H., and T. Aoki.** 1996b. Sequence analysis of the florfenicol resistance gene encoded in the transferable R-plasmid of a fish pathogen, *Pasteurella piscicida. Microbiol. Immunol.* **40:**665–669.

83. **Kiuchi, A., M. Hara, and K. Tabuchi.** 1992. Drug resistant plasmid of *Actinobacillus pleuropneumoniae* isolated from swine pleuropneumonia in Thailand. *Kansenshogaku Zasshi.* **66:**1243–1247.

84. **Kuhnert, P., B. Korczak, E. Falsen, R. Straub, A. Hoops, P. Boerlin, J. Frey, and R. Mutters.** 2004. *Nicoletella semolina* gen. nov., sp. nov., a new member of *Pasteurellaceae* isolated from horses with airway disease. *J. Clin. Microbiol.* **42:**5542–5548.

85. **Lalonde, G., J. F. Miller, L. S. Tompkins, and P. O'Hanley.** 1989. Transformation of *Actinobacillus pleuropneumoniae* and analysis of R factors by electroporation. *Am. J. Vet. Res.* **50:**1957–1960.

86. **Lancashire, J. F., T. D. Terry. P. J. Blackall, and M. P. Jennings.** 2005. Plasmid-encoded Tet B tetracycline resistance in *Haemophilus parasuis. Antimicrob. Agents Chemother.* **49:** 1927–1931.

87. **Lawley, T. D., V. D. Burland, and D. E. Taylor.** 2000. Analysis of the complete nucleotide sequence of the tetracycline resistance transposon Tn*10. Plasmid* **43:**235–239.

88. **Levy, S. B., A. Buu-Hoi, and B. Marshall.** 1984. Transposon Tn*10*-like tetracycline resistance determinants in *Haemophilus parainfluenzae. J. Bacteriol.* **160:**87–94.

89. **Li, X., N. Mariano, J. J. Rahal, C. M. Urban, and K. Drlica.** 2004. Quinolone-resistant *Haemophilus influenzae* in a long-term-care facility: nucleotide sequence characterization of alterations in the genes encoding DNA gyrase and DNA topoisomerase IV. *Antimicrob. Agents Chemother.* **48:** 3570–3572.

90. **Livrelli, V. O., A. Darfeuille-Richaud, C. Rich, B. H. Joly, and J.-L. Martel.** 1988. Genetic determinant of the ROB-1 β-lactamase in bovine and porcine *Pasteurella* strains. *Antimicrob. Agents Chemother.* **32:**1282–1284.

91. **Livrelli, V. O., J. Peduzzi, and B. Joly.** 1991. Sequence and molecular characterization of the ROB1-β-lactamase gene from *Pasteurella haemolytica. Antimicrob. Agents Chemother.* **35:**242–251.

92. **MacLean, I. W., L. Slaney, J.-M. Juteau, R. C. Levesque, W. L. Albritton, and A. R. Ronald.** 1992. Identification of a ROB-1 β-lactamase in *Haemophilus ducreyi. Antimicrob. Agents Chemother.* **36:**467–469.

93. **Magyar, T., and A. J. Lax.** 2002. Atrophic rhinitis, p. 169–197. *In* K. A. Brogden and J. M. Guthmiller (ed.), *Polymicrobial Diseases.* American Society for Microbiology, Washington, D.C.

94. **Marshall, B., M. Roberts, A. Smith, and S. B. Levy.** 1984. Homogeneity of transferable tetracycline resistance determinants in *Haemophilus* species. *J. Infect. Dis.* **149:**1028–1029.

95. **Matic, V., B. Bozdogan, M. R. Jacobs, K. Ubukata, and P. C. Appelbaum.** 2003. Contribution of β-lactamase and PBP amino acid substitutions to amoxicillin/clavulanate resistance in β-lactamase-positive, amoxicillin/clavulanate-resistant *Haemophilus influenzae. J. Antimicrob. Chemother.* **52:**1018–1021.

96. **McNicol, P. J., and A. R. Ronald.** 1984. The plasmids of *Haemophilus ducreyi. J. Antimicrob. Chemother.* **14:**561–573.

97. **Medeiros, A. A., R. C. Levesque, and G. A. Jacoby.** 1986. An animal source for the ROB1-β-lactamase of *Haemophilus influenzae* type b. *Antimicrob. Agents Chemother.* **29:**212–215.

98. **Mevius, D. J., and W. van Pelt (ed.).** 2003. *MARAN 2002: Monitoring of Antimicrobial Resistance and Antimicrobial Usage in Animals in the Netherlands in 2002.* [Online.] http://www.cidc-lelystad.nl/docs/MARAN-2002-web.pdf.

99. **Miranda, C. D., C. Kehrenberg, C. Ulep, S. Schwarz, and M. C. Roberts.** 2003. Diversity of tetracycline resistance genes from bacteria isolated from Chilean salmon farms. *Antimicrob. Agents Chemother.* **47:**883–888.

100. **Murphy, G. L., L. C. Robinson, and G. E. Burrows.** 1993. Restriction endonuclease analysis and ribotyping differentiate *Pasteurella haemolytica* serotype A1 isolates from cattle within a feedlot. *J. Clin. Microbiol.* **31:**2303–2308.

101. **Murray, I. A., J. Hawkins, J. W. Keyte, and W. V. Shaw.** 1988. Nucleotide sequence analysis and overexpression of the gene encoding a type III chloramphenicol acetyltransferase. *Biochem. J.* **252:**173–179.

102. **Murray, I. A., J. V. Martinez-Suarez, T. J. Close, and W. V. Shaw.** 1990. Nucleotide sequences of genes encoding the type II chloramphenicol acetyltransferases of *Escherichia coli* and *Haemophilus influenzae*, which are sensitive to inhibition by thiol-reactive reagents. *Biochem. J.* **272:**505–510.

103. **Naas, T., F. Benaoudia, L. Lebrun, and P. Nordmann.** 2001. Molecular identification of TEM-1 β-lactamase in a *Pasteurella multocida* isolate of human origin. *Eur. J. Clin. Microbiol. Infect. Dis.* **20:**210–213.

104. **National Committee for Clinical Laboratory Standards.** 2002. Performance standards for antimicrobial disk and dilution susceptibility tests for bacteria isolated from animals. Approved standard, 2nd ed. NCCLS document M31-A2. National Committee for Clinical Laboratory Standards, Wayne, Pa.

105. **National Committee for Clinical Laboratory Standards.** 2004. Performance standards for antimicrobial disk and dilution susceptibility tests for bacteria isolated from animals. Informational supplement (May 2004). NCCLS document M31-S1. National Committee for Clinical Laboratory Standards, Wayne, Pa.

106. **Ojo, K. K., C. Kehrenberg, H. A. Odelola, and S. Schwarz.** 2002. Identification of a complete *dfrA14* gene cassette integrated at a secondary site in a resistance plasmid of uropathogenic *Escherichia coli* from Nigeria. *Antimicrob. Agents Chemother.* **46:**2054–2055.

107. **Oka, A., H. Sugisaki, and M. Takanami.** 1981. Nucleotide sequence of the kanamycin resistance transposon Tn*903*. *J. Mol. Biol.* **147:**217–226.

108. **Ouellet, V., A. Forest, M. Nadeau, and M. Sirois.** 2004. Characterization of tetracycline resistance determinants in *Actinobacillus pleuropneumoniae*. *Abstr. 104th Gen. Meet. Am. Soc. Microbiol.*, abstr. A-113, p. 22. American Society for Microbiology, Washington, D.C.
109. **Pang, Y., T. Bosch, and M. C. Roberts.** 1994. Single polymerase chain reaction for the detection of the tetracycline resistance determinants TetK and TetL. *Mol. Cell. Probes* **8:** 417–422.
110. **Perez-Vazquez, M., F. Roman, B. Aracil, R. Canton, and J. Campos.** 2004. Laboratory detection of *Haemophilus influenzae* with decreased susceptibility to nalidixic acid, ciprofloxacin, levofloxacin, and moxifloxacin due to *gyrA* and *parC* mutations. *J. Clin. Microbiol.* **42:**1185–1191.
111. **Peric, M., B. Bozdogan, M. R. Jacobs, and P. C. Appelbaum.** 2003. Effects of an efflux mechanism and ribosomal mutations on macrolide susceptibility of *Haemophilus influenzae*. *Antimicrob. Agents Chemother.* **47:**1017–1022.
112. **Philippon, A., B. Joly, D. Reynaud, G. Paul, J.-L. Martel, D. Sirot, R. Cluzel, and P. Nevot.** 1986. Characterization of a beta-lactamase from *Pasteurella multocida*. *Ann. Inst. Pasteur Microbiol.* **137A:**153–158.
113. **Pouedras, P., P. Y. Donnio, Y. Le Tulzo, and J. L. Avril.** 1993. *Pasteurella stomatis* infection following a dog bite. *Eur. J. Clin. Microbiol. Infect. Dis.* **12:**65.
114. **Powell, M., and D. M. Livermore.** 1988. Mechanisms of chloramphenicol resistance in *Haemophilus influenzae* in the United Kingdom. *J. Med. Microbiol.* **27:**89–93.
115. **Priebe, S., and S. Schwarz.** 2003. In vitro activities of florfenicol against bovine and porcine respiratory tract pathogens. *Antimicrob. Agents Chemother.* **47:**2703–2705.
116. **Quinn, P. J., B. K. Markey, M. E. Carter, W. J. Donnelly, and F. C. Leonard.** 2002. *Veterinary Microbiology and Microbial Disease*. Blackwell Publishing, Ames, Iowa.
117. **Radostits, O. M., C. Gay, D. C. Blood, and K. W. Hinchcliff.** 2000. *A Textbook of the Diseases of Cattle, Sheep, Pigs, Goats, and Horses*, 9th ed., p. 829–867. The W. B. Saunders Co., Philadelphia, Pa.
118. **Radström, P., and G. Swedberg.** 1988. RSF1010 and a conjugative plasmid contain *sul*II, one of two known genes for plasmid-borne sulfonamide resistance dihydropteroate synthase. *Antimicrob. Agents Chemother.* **32:**1684–1692.
119. **Roe, D. E., P. H. Braham, A. Weinberg, and M. C. Roberts.** 1995. Characterization of tetracycline resistance in *Actinobacillus actinomycetemcomitans*. *Oral Microbiol. Immunol.* **10:**227–232.
120. **Roe, D. E., A. Weinberg, and M. C. Roberts.** 1996. Mobile rRNA methylase genes coding for erythromycin resistance in *Actinobacillus actinomycetemcomitans*. *J. Antimicrob. Chemother.* **37:**457–464.
121. **Rosenau, A., A. Labigne, F. Escande, P. Courcoux, and A. Philippon.** 1991. Plasmid-mediated ROB1-β-lactamase in *Pasteurella multocida* from human specimen. *Antimicrob. Agents Chemother.* **35:**2419–2422.
122. **Rossmanith, S. E. R., G. R. Wilt, and G. Wu.** 1991. Characterization and comparison of antimicrobial susceptibilities and outer membrane protein and plasmid DNA profiles of *Pasteurella haemolytica* and certain other members of the genus *Pasteurella*. *Am. J. Vet. Res.* **52:**2016–2022.
123. **Schnabel, E. L., and A. L. Jones.** 1999. Distribution of tetracycline resistance genes and transposons among phylloplane bacteria in Michigan apple orchards. *Appl. Environ. Microbiol.* **65:**4898–4907.
124. **Scholz, P., V. Haring, B. Wittmann-Liebold, K. Ashman, M. Bagdasarian, and E. Scherzinger.** 1989. Complete nucleotide sequence and gene organization of the broad-host-range plasmid RSF1010. *Gene* **75:**271–288.
125. **Schwarz, S., C. Kehrenberg, B. Doublet, and A. Cloeckaert.** 2004. Molecular basis of bacterial resistance to chloramphenicol and florfenicol. *FEMS Microbiol. Rev.* **28:**519–542.
126. **Schwarz, S., C. Kehrenberg, S. A. Salmon, and J. L. Watts.** 2004. *In vitro* activities of spectinomycin and comparator agents against *Pasteurella multocida* and *Mannheimia haemolytica* from respiratory tract infections of cattle. *J. Antimicrob. Chemother.* **53:**379–382.
127. **Schwarz, S., U. Spies, B. Reitz, H.-M. Seyfert, C. Lämmler, and H. Blobel.** 1989. Detection and interspecies-transformation of a β-lactamase-encoding plasmid from *Pasteurella haemolytica*. *Zentbl. Bakteriol. Mikrobiol. Hyg. A* **270:**462–469.
128. **Schwarz, S., U. Spies, F. Schäfer, and H. Blobel.** 1989. Isolation and interspecies-transfer of a plasmid from *Pasteurella multocida* encoding streptomycin resistance. *Med. Microbiol. Immunol.* **178:**121–125.
129. **Silver, R. P., B. Leming, C. F. Garon, and C. A. Hjerpe.** 1979. R-plasmids in *Pasteurella multocida*. *Plasmid* **2:**493–497.
130. **Stuy, J. H., and R. B. Walter.** 1992. Cloning, characterization, and DNA base sequence of the high-level-streptomycin resistance gene *strA1* of *Haemophilus influenzae* Rd. *J. Bacteriol.* **174:**5604–5608.
131. **Sundin, G. W.** 2000. Examination of base pair variants of the *strA-strB* streptomycin resistance genes from bacterial pathogens of humans, animals and plants. *J. Antimicrob. Chemother.* **46:**848–849.
132. **Sundin, G. W.** 2002. Distinct recent lineages of the *strA-strB* streptomycin-resistance genes in clinical and environmental bacteria. *Curr. Microbiol.* **45:**63–69.
133. **Sundin, G. W., and C. L. Bender.** 1996. Dissemination of the *strA-strB* streptomycin-resistance genes among commensal and pathogenic bacteria from humans, animals, and plants. *Mol. Ecol.* **5:**133–143.
134. **Talan, D. A., D. M. Citron, F. M. Abrahamian, G. J. Moran, and E. J. Goldstein for the Emergency Medicine Animal Bite Infection Study Group.** 1999. Bacteriologic analysis of infected dog and cat bites. *N. Engl. J. Med.* **340:**85–92.
135. **Thorsen, P. B., R. Moller, M. Apri, A. Bremmelgaard, and W. Frederiksen.** 1994. *Pasteurella aerogenes* isolated from stillbirth and mother. *Lancet* **343:**485–486.
136. **Ubukata, K., Y. Shibasaki, K. Yamamoto, N. Chiba, K. Hasegawa, Y. Takeuchi, K. Sunakawa, M. Inoue, and M. Konno.** 2001. Association of amino acid substitutions in penicillin-binding protein 3 with β-lactam resistance in β-lactamase-negative ampicillin-resistant *Haemophilus influenzae*. *Antimicrob. Agents Chemother.* **45:**1693–1699.
137. **Vassort-Bruneau, C., M.-C. Lesage-Decauses, J.-L. Martel, J.-P. Lafont, and E. Chaslus-Dancla.** 1996. CAT III chloramphenicol resistance in *Pasteurella haemolytica* and *Pasteurella multocida* isolated from calves. *J. Antimicrob. Chemother.* **38:**205–213.
138. **Wallmann, J., H. Kaspar, and R. Kroker.** 2005. Data on prevalence of antimicrobial susceptibility of veterinary pathogens from bovine and pigs: national antibiotic resistance monitoring 2002/2003 of the BVL. *Berl. Münch. Tierärztl. Wochenschr.* **117:**480–492.
139. **Wallmann, J., K. Schröter, L. H. Wieler, and R. Kroker.** 2003. National antibiotic resistance monitoring in veterinary pathogens from sick food-producing animals: the German programme and results from the 2001 pilot study. *Int. J. Antimicrob. Agents* **22:**420–428.
140. **Wasteson, Y., D. E. Roe, K. Falk, and M. C. Roberts.** 1996. Characterization of tetracycline and erythromycin resistance in *Actinobacillus pleuropneumoniae*. *Vet. Microbiol.* **48:**41–50.

141. **Watts, J. L., R. J. Yancey, Jr., S. A. Salmon, and C. A. Case.** 1994. A 4-year survey of antimicrobial susceptibility trends for isolates from cattle with bovine respiratory disease in North America. *J. Clin. Microbiol.* **32:**725–731.

142. **Willson, P. J., H. G. Deneer, A. Potter, and W. Albritton.** 1989. Characterization of a streptomycin-sulfonamide resistance plasmid from *Actinobacillus pleuropneumoniae. Antimicrob. Agents Chemother.* **33:**235–238.

143. **Wissing, A., J. Nicolet, and P. Boerlin.** 2001. Die aktuelle antimikrobielle Resistenzsituation in der schweizerischen Veterinärmedizin. *Schweiz. Arch. Tierheilkd.* **143:**503–510.

144. **Wood, A. R., F. A. Lainson, F. Wright, G. D. Baird, and W. Donachie.** 1995. A native plasmid of *Pasteurella haemolytica* serotype A1: DNA sequence analysis and investigation of its potential as a vector. *Res. Vet. Sci.* **58:**163–168.

145. **Wright, C. L., R. A. Strugnell, and A. L. M. Hodgson.** 1997. Characterization of a *Pasteurella multocida* plasmid and its use to express recombinant proteins in *P. multocida. Plasmid* **37:**65–79.

146. **Wu, J.-R., H. K. Shieh, J.-H. Shien, S.-R. Gong, and P.-C. Chang.** 2003. Molecular characterization of plasmids with antimicrobial resistant genes in avian isolates of *Pasteurella multocida. Avian Dis.* **47:**1384–1392.

147. **Yamamoto, J., T. Sakano, and M. Shimizu.** 1990. Drug resistance and R plasmids in *Pasteurella multocida* isolates from swine. *Microbiol. Immunol.* **34:**715–721.

148. **Zbinden, R., P. Sommerhalder, and U. von Wartburg.** 1988. Co-isolation of *Pasteurella dagmatis* and *Pasteurella multocida* from cat-bite wounds. *Eur. J. Clin. Microbiol. Infect. Dis.* **7:**203–204.

149. **Zhao, J., and T. Aoki.** 1992. Nucleotide sequence analysis of the class G tetracycline resistance determinant from *Vibrio anguillarum. Microbiol. Immunol.* **36:**1051–1060.

150. **Zimmerman, M. L., and D. C. Hirsh.** 1980. Demonstration of an R-plasmid in a strain of *Pasteurella haemolytica* isolated from feedlot cattle. *Am. J. Vet. Res.* **41:** 166–169.

Antimicrobial Resistance in Bacteria of Animal Origin
Edited by Frank M. Aarestrup

Chapter 12

Antimicrobial Resistance in Staphylococci and Streptococci of Animal Origin

FRANK M. AARESTRUP AND STEFAN SCHWARZ

Staphylococci and streptococci are among the most important gram-positive pathogens in both human and veterinary medicine. They cause a wide variety of infections, most of them with well-known epidemiology and pathogenesis. Antimicrobial agents are often essential in both the control of these bacteria and the treatment of the corresponding infections. A large number of species are described within the two groups, but only a limited number of species are of major importance (Table 1). In this chapter, summarized data on susceptibility patterns and prevalence and epidemiology of resistance are reviewed for the most clinically relevant staphylococcal and streptococcal pathogens in animals. An attempt is made to describe both the occurrence and trends in resistance. Problems in relation to human medicine are only dealt with when a zoonotic link is shown or suspected. In addition, the epidemiology of methicillin-resistant *Staphylococcus aureus* (MRSA) in animals is described.

STAPHYLOCOCCI

Staphylococci are a part of the natural skin flora of most mammals and birds. In addition, staphylococci normally colonize the skin or mucosal membranes of the respiratory, upper alimentary, and urogenital tracts and can easily spread between animals and humans through contact or vectors such as milking machines. To date, 48 different species and subspecies of staphylococci have been described, most of them with a preference for a specific host. The natural hosts of the different staphylococcal species are given in Table 2.

Not all staphylococci are equally important as pathogens. Thus, in veterinary medicine the most important species are *Staphylococcus aureus*, *Staphylococcus hyicus*, and *Staphylococcus intermedius*. *S. intermedius* was until 1976 (85) regarded as a canine variant of *S. aureus*. *S. aureus* and *S. intermedius* are both characterized by their ability to coagulate rabbit serum and are commonly termed coagulase-positive staphylococci. Both coagulase-positive and -negative strains of *S. hyicus* can be found. All other species of staphylococci are traditionally termed coagulase-negative staphylococci (CoNS) and were until the 1980s considered unimportant with regard to their role as causative agents of infections in both humans and animals (116). Since then, CoNS comprising a wide range of different species have been found to play a role in animal infections, mainly bovine mastitis.

S. aureus can cause a large number of different infections in most animal species but is mostly associated with bovine mastitis. *S. aureus* is also an important pathogen for humans, where this bacterium may cause a wide range of infections ranging from simple skin infections to osteomyelitis and septicemia. *S. hyicus* is most important as the causative agent of exudative epidermitis in pigs and *S. intermedius* as the cause of pyoderma in dogs. A number of other species causing infections in animals have also been found. These include *Staphylococcus schleiferi* subsp. *coagulans* from infections in dogs and *Staphylococcus felis* from infections in cats. Both species are also part of the natural skin flora of these animals, and like all other staphylococci, they are opportunistic pathogens. In the following sections, the focus is mainly on resistance in *S. aureus*, *S. hyicus*, and *S. intermedius*.

The different species differ in their intrinsic resistance (118, 119, 120) and probably also in their ability to acquire resistance. Thus, comparisons made without proper species identification are almost meaningless. Furthermore, susceptibility testing is not always performed in the same standardized way in the

Frank M. Aarestrup • Danish Institute for Food and Veterinary Research, Bülowsvej 27, DK-1790 Copenhagen V, Denmark. **Stefan Schwarz** • Institut für Tierzucht, Bundesforschungsanstalt für Landwirtschaft, D-31535 Neustadt-Mariensee, Germany.

Table 1. The most important pathogenic *Staphylococcus* and *Streptococcus* species in animals

Animal species	*Staphylococcus* spp.	*Streptococcus* spp.
Cattle	*S. aureus*, coagulase-negative staphylococci, *S. epidermidis*, *S. xylosus*, *S. chromogenes*, *S. sciuri*, *S. simulans*, *S. warneri*	*S. uberis*, *S. dysgalactiae*, *S. agalactiae*
Poultry	*S aureus*	
Pigs	*S. hyicus*	*S. suis*
Sheep and goats	*S. aureus*	
Horses	*S. aureus*	*S. zooepidemicus*, *S. equi*
Cats	*S. aureus*, *S. felis*, *S. intermedius*	
Dogs	*S. aureus*, *S. intermedius*, *S. schleiferi* subsp. *coagulans*	

different reports, which adds to the potential variation between studies.

Staphylococcus aureus

S. aureus is one of the most important human and veterinary pathogens, and the epidemiology, pathology, and antimicrobial resistance of this bacterium has been studied intensively in innumerable studies. Human and animal isolates of *S. aureus* have traditionally been seen as separate populations and classified into host-specific biovars (86). Bovine strains have mainly been characterized by their ability to produce beta-hemolysin, while human isolates have been characterized by the production of alpha-hemolysin. Most *S. aureus* isolates do, however, contain the genes for beta-hemolysin, and this seems to be an inducible phenotype (10). The zoonotic potential of bovine isolates of *S. aureus* has been discussed in several reports, but the most recent studies indicate that bovine and human isolates of *S. aureus* represent different populations even though some overlap might exist (104, 261), with the possible exception of MRSA (see below).

S. aureus was one of the first bacteria in which the development of antimicrobial resistance (penicillin resistance) was observed (15, 114, 154). The first observations on the inhibitory effect of *Penicillium* mold on bacteria seem to have been made by Sir John Burden-Sanderson in 1871 and Joseph Lister in 1872 (76, 135). In 1928 Alexander Fleming made similar observations (72), and when it later became possible to purify penicillin, the golden era of antibiotics took off. Since then, a large number of other antimicrobial agents have been discovered and intro-

Table 2. Species and subspecies of the genus *Staphylococcus* and their natural hosts[a]

Species	Subspecies	Natural host(s)[b]
S. arlettae		Mammals, birds
S. aureus	*anaerobius*	Sheep
S. aureus	*aureus*	Primates, humans, animals, birds
S. auricularis		Humans, primates
S. capitis	*capitis*	Humans
S. capitis	*urealyticus*	Humans, primates
S. caprae		Humans, goats
S. carnosus	*carnosus*	Unknown (meat and fish products)
S. carnosus	*utilis*	Unknown
S. chromogenes		Cattle, horses, goats
S. cohnii	*cohnii*	Humans
S. cohnii	*urealyticus*	Humans, primates
S. condimenti		Unknown (food products)
S. delphini		Dolphins
S. epidermidis		Humans (domestic animals)
S. equorum	*equorum*	Horses, cattle
S. equorum	*linens*	Unknown
S. felis		Cats
S. fleurettii		Unknown
S. gallinarum		Birds
S. haemolyticus		Humans, primates
S. hominis	*hominis*	Humans
S. hominis	*novobiosepticus*	Humans
S. hyicus		Pigs, cattle, goats, ungulates
S. intermedius		Canoidea (other mammals, birds)
S. kloosii		Mammals
S. lentus		Sheep, goats, cattle, dolphins
S. lugdunensis		Humans
S. lutrae		Otters
S. muscae		Domestic animals (flies)
S. nepalensis		Goats
S. pasteuri		Unknown
S. piscifermentans		Unknown
S. pulvereri		Humans, mammals
S. saccharolyticus		Humans
S. saprophyticus	*bovis*	Cattle
S. saprophyticus	*saprophyticus*	Humans, mammals
S. schleiferi	*coagulans*	Dogs, bears
S. schleiferi	*schleiferi*	Carnivora
S. sciuri	*carnaticus*	
S. sciuri	*rodentium*	Rodents
S. sciuri	*sciuri*	Mammals, birds
S. simulans		Humans, primates
S. succinus	*casei*	Unknown
S. succinus	*succinus*	Unknown
S. vitulinus		Cattle, ungulates, whales (meat products)
S. warneri		Humans, primates (domestic animals)
S. xylosus		Rodents, humans, mammals, birds

[a]Adapted from references 115–117, 120, 121, 165, 166, 170, 213, 232, and 262.
[b]Entries in parentheses are potential reservoirs.

duced for human and veterinary therapy, and in the course of the last 50 years antimicrobial agents have become the keystone in the therapy of bacterial infections in humans and animals (see chapter 2). Soon after the introduction of penicillin for treatment, resistance emerged rapidly among *S. aureus*, and at a hospital in England, Barber and Whitehead (16) found a 14% rate of resistance in 1946, a 38% rate in 1947, and a 59% rate in 1948. Today, a very high frequency of resistance to penicillin is recorded among *S. aureus* of human origin, and most studies report that more than 90% of isolates are resistant (263). Resistance to other antimicrobial agents varies between countries, regions, and hospitals. A recent study of resistance among 4,065 *S. aureus* isolates from 21 hospital laboratories in 19 countries found prevalences of resistance ranging from 0 to 63% for methicillin, 1 to 70% for erythromycin, and 1 to 73% for tetracycline (263). There was, however, a very strong association between methicillin resistance and resistance to the other antimicrobial agents. An association between usage of antimicrobial agents at hospitals and wards and the occurrence of resistance was also observed (249). The complex epidemiology of infections with *S. aureus* (especially MRSA) in human medicine, mainly at hospitals, has been reported in innumerable studies and will not be dealt with in this chapter (for recent reviews, see references 36, 64, and 66). The importance of MRSA in animals and the potential implications for human health are dealt with later.

Penicillin was introduced in veterinary medicine in the late 1940s, primarily in the treatment of or as part of eradication programs against *Streptococcus agalactiae*, which at that time was the primary etiologic agent in bovine mastitis (185). The eradication of *S. agalactiae* and increased usage of milking machines led to an increase in the absolute and relative importance of *S. aureus*, which since then has remained the most important agent causing bovine mastitis. The widespread usage of penicillin in the bovine environment led to an emergence and increase in the occurrence of penicillin-resistant *S. aureus* in the 1950s (4, 251), especially in countries with a liberal usage of antimicrobial agents. In countries with a restricted usage of antimicrobials, the occurrence of resistance has remained relatively low. Numerous reports on the occurrence of antimicrobial resistance among *S. aureus* from bovine mastitis have been made. However, the focus has been on penicillin resistance, which is widespread among *S. aureus* from bovine mastitis, whereas resistance to other antimicrobial agents is limited (123, 236, 244). Aarestrup and Jensen (4) reviewed the literature on penicillin resistance before 1998. They found the reported frequency of resistance to vary between 0 and 100%. In countries where data were available, an increase in the occurrence of resistance over time was observed. However, more recently resistance seems to have decreased in some countries where the frequency of resistance was very high in former times. This could perhaps be due to changes in therapeutic treatment, whereby other antimicrobial agents have replaced penicillin in these countries. The trends over time in occurrence of resistance are shown for Denmark and the United Kingdom in Fig. 1 and 2, which clearly indicate the different trends in these two countries. However, comparisons between studies over time and between countries have to be done with great care due to differences in sampling strategies and methods employed for susceptibility testing.

Recent data on the occurrence of resistance among *S. aureus* isolated from bovine mastitis in different countries are given in Table 3. Beside resistance to penicillin, which varies greatly, resistance is also observed to tetracycline, macrolides, chloramphenicol, and aminoglycosides. The frequency of resistance to these antimicrobials is, however, still low in most reports. Thus, with the exception of penicillin, most available antimicrobial agents can still be used in the treatment of bovine mastitis. Use of penicillin requires either prior susceptibility testing or thorough knowledge of the occurrence of resistance at the herd or local level. Also noteworthy is the fact that resistance to oxacillin or methicillin was detected at a low frequency in all countries, indicating that MRSA is present—although currently only in small numbers—among *S. aureus* from bovine mastitis.

There is only limited knowledge regarding the clonality of resistant isolates. In studies in Denmark it was shown that an increase in the occurrence of penicillin resistance among *S. aureus* causing infections in humans was caused by (i) the introduction and spread of penicillin-resistant clones, (ii) simultaneous disappearance of mainly susceptible types, and (iii) the emergence and spread of a 21-kb resistance plasmid among a phage group with a previous low frequency of resistance (175, 210).

In a minor study of 52 *S. aureus* isolates obtained between 1952 and 1956 and in 1992 from bovines with mastitis in Denmark, Aarestrup et al. (5) found that among the isolates from the 1950s penicillin resistance was exclusively seen in isolates of the same phage type and ribotype, whereas penicillin resistance was observed among several clones of the isolates from 1992. Thus, a single penicillin-resistant clone might have been introduced in the bovine environment in Denmark in the 1950s but since then become more widespread among several clones, probably due to horizontal transfer. A later study, which included more isolates, showed similar results (237). This study also revealed that the types of *S. aureus*

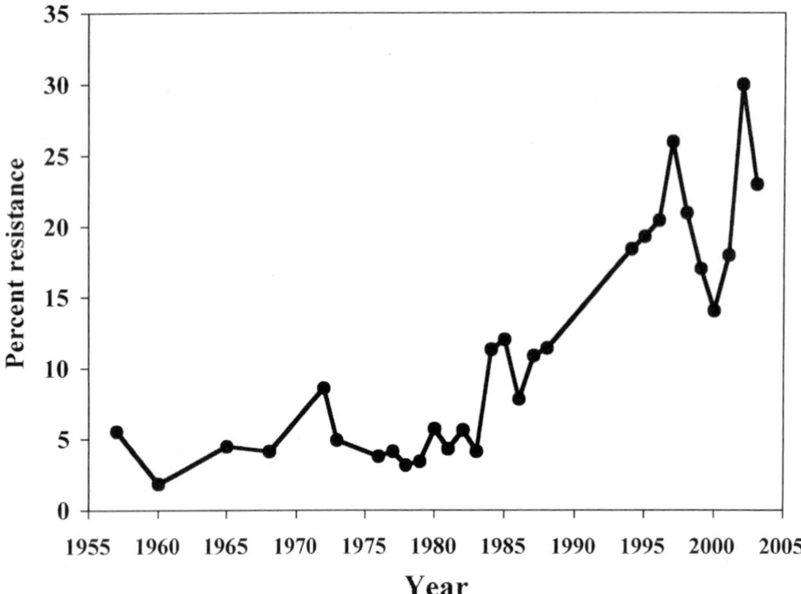

Figure 1. Trends in the occurrence of resistance to penicillin over time among *S. aureus* isolates from bovine mastitis in Denmark. Adapted from references 4 and 91a.

causing bovine mastitis in Denmark had remained relatively unchanged since the 1950s. Vintov et al. (236) examined the association between types of *S. aureus* and antimicrobial resistance in 815 isolates obtained from 10 countries. The isolates were in general susceptible to all antimicrobial agents tested except penicillin, where a variation in the frequency of resistance, from 2 to 71.4%, was found. Resistance to penicillin was associated with certain phage groups in countries with a high prevalence of penicillin resistance, whereas these phage types were rarely seen in countries with a low prevalence of penicillin resistance. This might indicate that the usage of penicillin has selected for penicillin-associated phage types in some countries as well as selected for a higher prevalence of resistance within types. In Norway, Waage et al. (238)

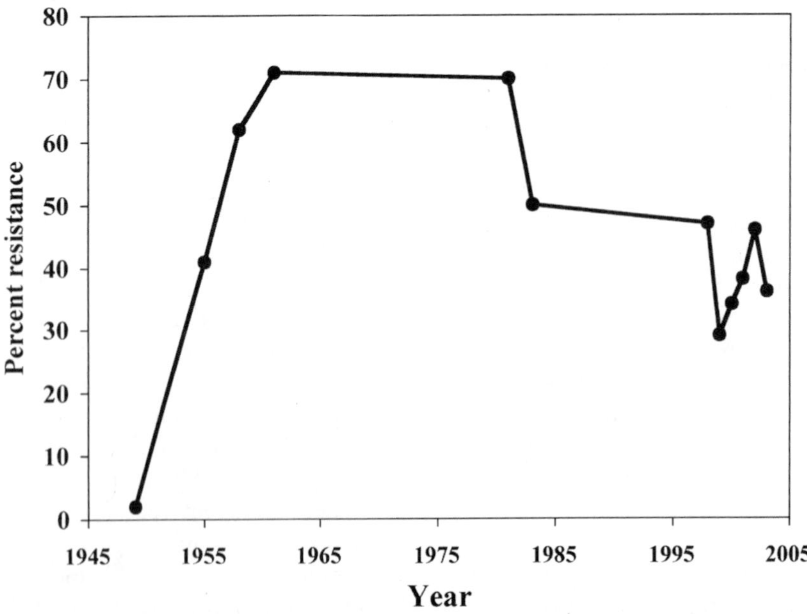

Figure 2. Trends in the occurrence of resistance to penicillin over time among *S. aureus* isolates from bovine mastitis in the United Kingdom. Adapted from references 4 and 219.

Table 3. Recent data on the occurrence of antimicrobial resistance among *S. aureus* from bovine mastitis in some selected countries[a]

Antimicrobial agent	% of isolates resistant												
	Argentina, 1996–1998 (n = 206)[b]	Brazil, 1999–2000 (n = 87)	Denmark, 2003 (n = 99)	England and Wales, 2003 (n = 378)	France, 2003 (n varies)	Italy, 2003 (n = 63)	Japan, 1997–1998 (n = 51)	Latvia, 2003 (n = 21)	The Netherlands, 2003 (n = 107)	Norway, 2003 (n = 117)	Spain, 2003 (n = 192)	Switzerland, 2003 (n = 60)	Germany, 2002–2003 (n = 227)
Chloramphenicol			0		1, 5	2	0	33		0	0		0
Macrolides	12	0	0	4	0	3	4	50	0	1	4	0	2
Neomycin				0				21		1		0	
Gentamicin	3	0	0		2	0	4	6		0		30	1
Oxacillin	0	0			1	0	0	3	0	1	0		0
Penicillin	40	87	23	36	1	40	27	100	24	5	40		23
Streptomycin			1		3	7	10		2	2	6	5	
Sulfonamides			0		8	0						0	
Tetracycline		0	2	3	2	17	4	58	3	0	2		4
Trimethoprim			1		9, 4			33			3	0	
Co-trimoxazole					0	0		33				-	
Vancomycin			0		0	0				0	0		0
Virginiamycin			1				0			0	0		0[c]

[a]Data are from references 13, 30, 78, 239, and 259.
[b]n = number of isolates.
[c]Quinupristin/dalfopristin was tested instead of virginiamycin.

found that 99 of 107 penicillin- and tetracycline-resistant *S. aureus* isolates obtained from bovine mastitis in 18 herds belonged to the same clone. Of the remaining eight isolates, seven had the same plasmid profile. The genetic location of the resistance genes was not determined, but it seems likely that the resistance to penicillin and tetracycline had spread mainly through the spread of a single clone in addition to the spread of a resistance plasmid.

In human medicine, most multiple-antimicrobial resistance in *S. aureus* is due to the spread of MRSA clones, whereas methicillin-susceptible *S. aureus* isolates in general show a limited frequency of resistance to other antimicrobial agents (73, 263). If MRSA isolates begin to emerge and spread in the bovine environment this will probably also lead to an increase of resistance to a large number of other antimicrobial agents, as has been observed in human medicine.

Staphylococcus hyicus

In pigs, *S. hyicus* is the causative agent of exudative epidermitis, a generalized infection of the skin characterized by greasy exudation, exfoliation, and vesicle formation. The infection is relatively rare but can be of considerable importance for individual pig breeders whose herds experience high mortality. Specific vaccines are currently not available, but autogenous vaccines are sometimes used. Antimicrobial agents are important, especially for the control of acute outbreaks. Nevertheless, relatively few data are available on the occurrence of antimicrobial resistance in *S. hyicus*. *S. hyicus* can also cause infections in other animal species (51, 91, 218), but such events are rare.

Some data on the occurrence of antimicrobial resistance among *S. hyicus* isolated from pigs from various countries are given in Table 4. The overall occurrence of resistance in *S. hyicus* is considerably higher than that observed among *S. aureus* from bovine mastitis (Table 3). The reason is probably the more widespread usage of different types and larger amounts of antimicrobial agents in pig production. However, it might also reflect differences in the ability of *S. hyicus* and *S. aureus* to acquire resistance. Whether such a difference between species exists is, however, not known.

The occurrence of antimicrobial resistance in *S. hyicus* has been monitored in Denmark since 1996 (3, 91a). As a result of this, it has been possible to follow trends in the occurrence of resistance over time. This has shown that the prevalence of resistance may vary considerably even within a few years. Thus, the occurrence of macrolide resistance increased from 33% in 1996 to 62% in 1997, followed by a decrease to 21% in 2003 (Fig. 3). For several years the macrolide tylosin was the most commonly used antimicrobial agent for growth promotion in pig production in Denmark (1). Its usage for growth promotion in Denmark was banned in 1999, but 10 to 20 tons are still used each year for therapy. The occurrence of resistance to macrolides among *S. hyicus* isolated from pigs in Denmark seems to have correlated relatively well with the usage of tylosin. This example shows that the prevalence of resistance might change rapidly if large changes in usage patterns occur, and it emphasizes that the choice of antimicrobial agents for treatment has to be based on recent data. Similarly, the occurrence of resistance to sulfonamides and trimethoprim has also decreased, probably due to the more limited usage of these antimicrobial compounds.

Comparison of the different studies in Table 4 is difficult because these data reflect different periods

Table 4. Occurrence of antimicrobial resistance in *S. hyicus* from different countries[a]

Antimicrobial agent	% of isolates resistant				
	Belgium, 1974–1976 (n = 46)[b]	Denmark, 2003 (n = 68)	Germany, 1989 (n = 32)	Japan, 1979–1984 (n = 124)[c]	United Kingdom, 1988 (n = 37)
Chloramphenicol		0	9	0	0
Florfenicol		0			
Fluoroquinolones		4			
Gentamicin		0		0	0
Macrolides	74	21	3	41	11
Penicillin	60	84	25	38	32
Streptomycin	72	44	43	23	51
Sulfonamides		2	100		
Tetracycline	60	35	66	54	41
Trimethoprim		24			

[a]Data are from references 46, 91a, 151, 189, and 220.
[b]n = number of isolates.
[c]Both healthy and diseased animals.

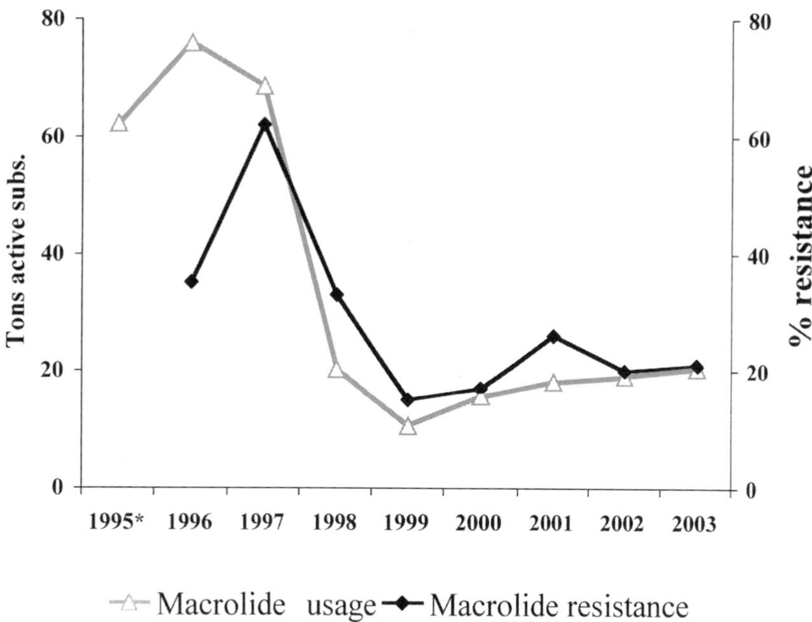

Figure 3. Trends in the occurrence of resistance to macrolides over time among *S. hyicus* isolates from exudative epidermitis in pigs in Denmark. Adapted from references 3 and 91a.

and sampling strategies. Nonetheless, resistance, especially to penicillin, streptomycin, and tetracycline, is very high in all studies, followed to some extent by resistance to macrolides. Isolates of *S. hyicus* can probably still be treated effectively with co-trimoxazole and cephalosporins such as ceftiofur. However, continuous monitoring of the occurrence of resistance at a regional level is necessary to guide therapy.

Staphylococcus intermedius

S. intermedius is probably part of the natural skin flora of all members of the Canoidea, and a certain host specificity seems to exist (2). In dogs, *S. intermedius* is a common cause of pyoderma and otitis, probably as a secondary invader following skin injuries. *S. intermedius* may, however, also be isolated from infections in other animals. Infections with *S. intermedius* are commonly treated with antimicrobial agents. Some data on the occurrence of antimicrobial resistance in *S. intermedius* from infections in dogs are given in Table 5. The overall occurrence of resistance in *S. intermedius* is considerably higher than that observed among *S. aureus* from bovine mastitis (Table 3). The reason is probably the more widespread usage of different types and larger amounts of antimicrobial agents for the treatment of pets such as dogs. However, it might also reflect differences in the ability of *S. intermedius* and *S. aureus* to acquire resistance. A frequent occurrence of resistance to penicillin, macrolides, and tetracycline has been observed in most studies (Table 5). The observed prevalences suggest that these antibiotics should not be used without prior susceptibility testing. Resistance to chloramphenicol, streptomycin, and co-trimoxazole has also been frequently reported. Most isolates seem to be susceptible to fluoroquinolones, florfenicol, and gentamicin. However, 24% of isolates from Spain were reported to be fluoroquinolone resistant (163), and some strains with resistance to gentamicin have also been observed. An increase in the prevalence of resistance over time has been reported (96, 132).

Other Species

CoNS from human wounds were first reported in 1884 (178). However, despite early reports on the importance of CoNS as hospital pathogens during the 1960s, the significance of CoNS as a major cause of infections in humans was unclear until the 1980s (116). The first report of CoNS in bovine mastitis is from 1916 (68). During the 1940s and 1950s the significance of CoNS in bovine mastitis was discussed, and it has even been suggested that these bacteria might protect the udder from more serious pathogens (26, 95). However, nowadays CoNS are regarded as significant mastitis pathogens that can cause substantial economical losses (44, 224). A large number of different CoNS species have been isolated from bovine milk, and even though a major part of them probably are contaminants, the most important species seem to be *S. chromogenes*, *S. simulans*, *S. epidermidis*,

Table 5. Occurrence of antimicrobial resistance in *S. intermedius* from infections in dogs in different countries[a]

Antimicrobial agent	% of isolates resistant[b]														
				France		Japan							United States		
	Denmark,[c] 1995 ($n = 50$)	England, 1980–1996 ($n = 2,296$)	Finland, 2002–2003 ($n = 95$)	1987–1988 ($n = 37$)	1992–1993 ($n = 50$)	1995–1996 ($n = 100$)	1982–1985 ($n = 12$)	1999 ($n = 47$)	Norway, 2002 ($n = 99$)	Spain, 1988–1992 ($n = 91$)	Sweden, 2002 ($n = 133$)	Switzerland, 1999–2000 ($n = 227$)	1982–1983 ($n = 109$)	1982–1984 ($n = 66$)	1986 ($n = 197$)
Chloramphenicol	16		6	16	18	18			2	0		30	18	6	11
Florfenicol							0	0							
Fluoroquinolones						1	0	0	0	24	2	4			
Gentamicin			0	3	0	2			0	0	0	3		0	0
Macrolides		9	25	19	24	22	17	4	18	35	20	37	24	12	26
Penicillin	60	79	77	5			0[d]	0[d]	86		78	76	52	38	83
Streptomycin			27						22			42	36		
Tetracycline	20	41	40	16	38	24	92	19	53	19	25	41	45	33	53
Co-trimoxazole	0	9	7	3	14	15			2	54	10	10	10		9

[a]Data are from references 41, 132, 141, 146a, 148a, 153, 158, 161, 163, 208, and 252.
[b]n = number of isolates.
[c]Both healthy and diseased dogs.
[d]Tested with ampicillin.

S. xylosus, and *S. haemolyticus* (6, 20, 99, 173, 225, 242). Some of these studies have reported high frequencies of *S. hyicus*. However, when only simple biochemical tests are used for species identification, it can be difficult to distinguish *S. chromogenes* from coagulase-negative *S. hyicus*, and hence *S. chromogenes* is likely to be misidentified as *S. hyicus*.

Recent reports on the occurrence of antimicrobial resistance among CoNS from bovine mastitis are given in Table 6. However, as mentioned above, due to the differences between species and lack of proper identification, comparisons have to be made with care. Nonetheless, the available data show that CoNS from bovine mastitis often are resistant to penicillin and to a lesser extent to macrolides and tetracycline, whereas resistances to other antimicrobials are low. Susceptibility testing, at least for penicillin, macrolides, and tetracyclines, should therefore always be performed prior to treatment.

CoNS might also be isolated from infections in other animal species, including poultry, dogs, cats, and pigs. There are only a few reports on antimicrobial resistance among CoNS from these reservoirs. Aarestrup et al. (11) found a frequent occurrence of resistance to macrolides (31%) and tetracycline (29%) among 35 CoNS isolates from infections in broilers, whereas most or all isolates were susceptible to chloramphenicol, penicillin, fluoroquinolones, and sulfonamides. DeBoer et al. (45) found three penicillin-resistant and one erythromycin-resistant CoNS isolates among 57 isolates from wild turkeys. Slaughter et al. (211) reported 219 of 222 CoNS isolates from gray tree frogs as penicillin resistant, 132 as resistant to oxacillin, and 3 as resistant to erythromycin. Lilenbaum et al. (128, 129, 130) reported a frequent occurrence of resistance to penicillin, tetracycline, gentamicin, and enrofloxacin among CoNS from dogs and cats.

Methicillin Resistance in *Staphylococcus* spp.

MRSA

During the past 20 years MRSA strains have become a major cause of hospital-acquired infections. The incidence of MRSA in hospitals varies by country. In general, these hospital-acquired MRSA strains (HA-MRSA) are resistant to many different classes of antibiotics (145, 223). In Europe, their prevalence varies from <1% in northern Europe to >40% in southern and western Europe (223, 263). In the United States, the proportion of nosocomial infections due to MRSA increased from 2.5% in 1975 to 54.5% in 1999 (214). In the last 2 decades an emergence of community-acquired MRSA (CA-MRSA) has been observed in individuals not specifically at risk for infection (36, 214). CA-MRSA strains seem in general to be more susceptible to other antimicrobial agents (12, 147) and more frequently associated with superficial skin and soft tissue infections than HA-MRSA, even though deaths have occurred in children with necrotizing CA-MRSA pneumonia (61, 214). Most *S. aureus* strains causing skin infection and necrotizing pneumonia harbor the Panton-Valentine leukocidin genes (61, 131). Clonally distributed CA-MRSA strains carrying the Panton-Valentine leukocidin genes have been described in Europe and the United States (61, 74, 240, 254). Reliable and accurate detection of methicillin resistance in *S. aureus* and CoNS in routine susceptibility testing has been a challenge ever since their emergence in the early 1960s, and several studies have shown the difficulties of reliable

Table 6. Recent data on the occurrence of antimicrobial resistance among CoNS from bovines with mastitis in selected countries[a]

Antimicrobial agent	% of isolates resistant				
	Argentina, 1998–2000 (n = 123)[b]	Denmark, 1995–1996 (n = 467)	Finland, 2001 (n = 335)	Germany, 2002–2003 (n = 162)	United States, 2001–2002 (n = 139)
Chloramphenicol		1		4	
Fluoroquinolones		0	0	1	
Gentamicin	0	0	0	1	
Macrolides	6		5	8	13
Penicillin	28	12	32	20	39
Streptomycin		6	7		
Sulfonamides		26			
Tetracycline		4	9	8	13
Co-trimoxazole			2		9

[a]Data are from references 9, 79, 164, 171, and 239.
[b]n = number of isolates.

phenotypic detection (35). Detection of the *mecA* gene and/or the resulting pencillin-binding protein 2a (PBB2a) has therefore been considered the gold standard (35).

MRSA is rarely isolated from animals, and most of the strains found are associated with exposure to infections in humans (48, 81, 136, 202, 229a, 243). MRSA has been described to occur in cattle (48, 125), chickens (125), and horses (90, 202, 243), as well as dogs and cats (62, 81, 136, 226, 229a).

The first isolation of MRSA from a veterinary specimen was reported from bovine mastitis in Belgium by Devriese et al. (50) in 1972. This strain was obtained from 20 different dairy herds and was probably one clone (48). Following this isolated incident, no immediate reports on the emergence of MRSA in dairy cattle were published. However, recently 12 MRSA isolates were found among 265 *S. aureus* isolates from bovine milk samples in South Korea (125). MRSA with the confirmed presence of the *mecA* gene was also reported in six bovine milk samples from two dairy herds in Hungary (105). A low frequency of methicillin resistance has also been reported in other countries (Table 3). In the later studies the genetic background for the resistance has not been investigated. These reports do, however, indicate that MRSA is emerging in the bovine environment, and monitoring should be implemented to determine its extent. MRSA in bovine milk might easily spread to humans, especially through the drinking of unpasteurized milk.

In dogs, MRSA isolates were probably first found in 1994 (34, 160) and have since then been reported in the United States (81, 136), United Kingdom (226), South Korea (157), Canada (155), and The Netherlands (229a). Recent data from the United Kingdom (24, 176) show that MRSA is widespread among small animals, and dogs should in some countries already be regarded as part of the epidemiology of MRSA. MRSA has been reported in three healthy cats in Brazil (128) and from abscesses in cats in Japan (156). MRSA in horses was first reported in South Korea, where 16 isolates were obtained from mares with metritis and a stallion with dermatitis (207). MRSA has also been reported in horses in the United States (90, 202). Seguin et al. (202) reported a nosocomial outbreak of MRSA involving 11 equine patients in a veterinary hospital. They found the same clone in humans handling the animals and suspected a human-to-animal spread of the strain. Weese et al. (243) reported colonization and clinical infections in horses at farms and a clinic and both human-to-horse and horse-to-human transmission of MRSA in Ontario, Canada. This study indicated that MRSA might spread between horses as well as between humans and horses.

Although human-to-animal transmission will play an important role in cases in companion and food animals, clonal distribution of MRSA in animals may also contribute to the dissemination of MRSA. The latter was described in horses in a veterinary teaching hospital in Michigan (202), in the report from Ontario (243), and in cattle and chickens in Korea (125). In both Michigan and Korea, the MRSA strains were multiple-drug resistant, which is indicative of their being related to HA-MRSA.

Methicillin resistance in other staphylococci

In human medicine, methicillin resistance is not only observed among *S. aureus*, but it is also prevalent among other staphylococcal species (55, 184). Methicillin-resistant staphylococci belonging to other species than *S. aureus* and containing the *mecA* gene have been isolated from animal sources in a number of studies. These include *S. intermedius*, *S. schleiferi* subsp. *schleiferi*, *S. schleiferi* subsp. *coagulans*, *S. epidermidis*, *S. haemolyticus*, *S. hominis*, and *S. xylosus* from dogs (81, 103, 229a); *S. haemolyticus* and CoNS from cows (79, 229a); *S. lentus* from cats (229a); *S. haemolyticus*, *S. lentus*, *S. sciuri*, *S. saprophyticus*, *S. xylosus*, and *S. epidermidis* from horses (227, 229a, 256, 257); and *S. sciuri*, *S. saprophyticus*, and *S. epidermidis* from chickens (108). A number of other reports on the occurrence of methicillin-resistant staphylococci from different animals have been published (29, 45, 75, 129, 130); however, the presence of *mecA* was not confirmed in these studies.

Mechanisms of Resistance in Staphylococci from Animals

The genetic background for resistance is described in chapter 6. The resistance genes found in staphylococci of animal origin are given in Table 7.

At least 38 different tetracycline resistance genes have been found to date. Four of these have been detected in staphylococci of animal origin. The *tet*(K) gene is considered indigenous to staphylococci and has been commonly found in a wide variety of staphylococcal species from animals (3, 11, 199, 228). The *tet*(L) gene was originally discovered in *Bacillus* spp. but has been found in *S. aureus*, *S. hyicus*, *S. lentus*, *S. sciuri*, and *S. xylosus* (3, 192, 199). The *tet*(M) gene is infrequently found in *S. aureus* (11) but seems to be the most common tetracycline resistance gene in *S. intermedius* (191, 199). The *tet*(O) gene has so far only rarely been found in staphylococci (199).

To date, seven different genes encoding macrolide resistance have been identified in staphylococci from animals, with *erm* genes coding for rRNA methylases

Table 7. Occurrence of antimicrobial resistance genes among staphylococci of animal origin

Antimicrobial agent	Resistance gene (resistance phenotype)	Reference(s)
Aminocyclitols	*spc* (spectinomycin)	110
Aminoglycosides	*aadD* (kanamycin, neomycin)	198
	aadE (streptomycin)	3, 25
	str (streptomycin)	190, 193, 194
	aadA-aphD (gentamicin, kanamycin, tobramycin)	124
	aphA-3 (kanamycin, neomycin)	25
Chloramphenicol	*catA*	33, 188, 193, 194, 195
Chloramphenicol, florfenicol	*cfr*	200
	fexA	109
Lincosamides	*lnu*(A)	54, 133, 134
	lsa(B)	110
Macrolides	*erm*(A)	3, 11, 100, 113, 149, 150, 247
	erm(B)	3, 25, 65, 245
	erm(C)	3, 65, 100, 196, 228, 248
	erm(F)	37
	erm(33)	201
	msr(A)	65, 134
	mph(C)	134
Mupirocin	*mupA*	246
Penicillin	*blaZ*	3, 233, 258
	mecA	81, 103, 108, 202, 229a
Streptogramin	*vga*(B)	11
	vat(A)	11
Streptothricins	*sat4*	25
Tetracycline	*tet*(K)	3, 11, 199, 228
	tet(L)	3, 192, 199
	tet(M)	11, 191, 199
	tet(O)	199
Quaternary ammonium compounds	*smr*	22
	qacJ	23

being the dominant genes. The most commonly reported macrolide resistance gene is the *erm*(C) gene. It has been found in a large number of species from various animal reservoirs (3, 65, 100, 196, 228, 248) and seems to be the most dominant macrolide resistance gene among staphylococci from animals. However, the *erm*(A) gene has also been commonly found in staphylococci of avian origin (11, 149, 150, 247) and has also been reported to be present in porcine and bovine staphylococci (3, 100, 113). The *erm*(B) gene seems to be the dominant gene among *S. intermedius* (25, 65) but has also been found in *S. hyicus* (3) and *S. lentus* (245). The gene *erm*(F) has only been identified in a few *S. intermedius* isolates from pigeons (37), and the *erm*(33) gene, which is believed to be a product of recombination between *erm*(C) and *erm*(A), has been detected in a single *S. sciuri* isolate of bovine origin (201). Finally, the *msr*(A) gene, which codes for a macrolide exporter, has been reported in a single isolate of porcine origin (65) but has recently also been detected in CoNS from bovine mastitis, alone or in combination with the gene *mph*(C), which codes for a macrolide phosphotransferase (134).

The *lnu*(A) gene (formerly also known as *linA*), which encodes a nucleotidyltransferase that mediates resistance to lincosamides, but not to macrolides, has been found in *S. aureus, S. chromogenes, S. xylosus, S. simulans*, and *S. warneri* from bovine mastitis (54, 133, 134). Recently, the gene *lsa*(B), which codes for an ABC transporter that mediates low-level lincosamide resistance, was identified on a multiresistance plasmid from bovine *S. sciuri* (110). Resistance to streptogramins has only rarely been reported among staphylococci. The streptogramin resistance genes *vga*(B) and *vat*(B) were reported to occur in two *S. xylosus* isolates of avian origin in Denmark (11).

Resistance to aminoglycosides and aminocyclitols is mainly due to enzymatic inactivation of the drugs (205; see also chapter 6). The different enzymes vary in their ability to degrade the different aminoglycosides, which in turn results in large variations in the resistance patterns. Six different genes encoding resistance to aminoglycosides or aminocyclitols have been found in staphylococci from animals. The *aadD* gene, encoding resistance to kanamycin and neomycin, has been found in porcine *S. epidermidis* isolates (198), whereas the *str* gene, encoding resistance to streptomycin, was identified in *S. hyicus* and *S. sciuri* (190, 193, 194). The Tn*4001*-associated *aadA-aphD* (180), encoding resistance to gentamicin, kanamycin, and tobramycin, was detected in *S. sciuri* and *S. warneri* from animals (124). In *S. intermedius* from pets, a Tn*5404*-like element carrying *aphA-3*, *sat4*, and *aadE*, encoding resistance to kanamycin and neomycin, to streptothricin, and to streptomycin, respectively, has been detected (25). The *aadE* gene has also been frequently detected in porcine *S. hyicus* (3). The gene *spc*, which codes for a spectinomycin adenyltransferase, is part of the *erm*(A)-carrying transposon Tn*554* and thus may occur preferentially in *erm*(A)-positive staphylococcal strains. It has recently also been detected on a multiresistance plasmid from *S. sciuri* (110).

In staphylococci, resistance to chloramphenicol is mainly due to plasmid-borne chloramphenicol acetyltransferases of type A. Three families of *catA* are currently known, of which two, $catA_{pC221}$ and $catA_{pC223}$, have been found in staphylococci of animal origin (33, 188, 194, 195). The *cat* genes do not encode resistance to florfenicol, a fluorinated chloramphenicol derivative that is licensed exclusively for veterinary use. Two different florfenicol resistance genes, both of which also mediate chloramphenicol resistance, have been found in bovine staphylococci: *cfr* in an *S. sciuri* isolate (200) and *fexA* in an *S. lentus* isolate (109).

The most common mechanism of resistance to β-lactams is the production of enzymes that degrade the drugs, namely β-lactamases. However, target modification is also seen. In staphylococci, four different closely related β-lactamases have been found, all mediating resistance to simple penicillins. The *blaZ* gene is located on the transposon Tn*552* (181). Studies on *S. aureus* from bovine mastitis (233, 258) and *S. hyicus* (3) from pigs also found the *blaZ* gene in all penicillin-resistant isolates. The *blaZ* gene can be located on both the chromosome and on plasmids. In bovine isolates the location seems to be mainly chromosomal (233). Sequencing and phylogenetic analyses of *blaZ* genes from *S. aureus* and CoNS from bovine mastitis in Denmark showed that the isolates could be separated into two large groups, roughly dividing strains carrying *blaZ* on the chromosome and those carrying the gene on plasmids. This suggests that the gene has followed two different evolutionary paths, one for plasmid-encoded and one for chromosomally encoded *blaZ* (J. Vintov et al., unpublished results). Resistance to β-lactamase-resistant penicillins, such as methicillin and oxacillin, is mediated by the chromosomally localized gene *mecA*, which encodes an accessory PBP, PBP2 (35).

There is only limited knowledge about the mechanism of resistance to sulfonamides, trimethoprim, and fluoroquinolones in staphylococci from animals. The general mechanisms of resistance are described in chapter 6. Resistance to mupirocin, an antistaphylococcal agent occasionally used for the treatment of canine pyoderma, is mediated by the gene *mupA*. This gene has so far been detected in only a single *S. aureus* strain of animal origin (246).

Disinfectants are widely used in food animal production. The use of disinfectants and mechanisms of resistance to them are described in chapter 8. The *smr* gene, encoding resistance to quaternary ammonium compounds, has been found in bovine *S. aureus* (22) and the *qacJ* gene in equine *S. aureus*, *S. simulans*, and *S. intermedius* (23).

STREPTOCOCCI

Bacteria belonging to the genus *Streptococcus* comprise a widespread group of important opportunistic and obligate pathogens, most of which have a high degree of host specificity. The genus includes some of the most important human pathogens, such as *Streptococcus pyogenes* and *Streptococcus pneumoniae*, as well as some very important veterinary pathogens, such as *Streptococcus agalactiae*, *Streptococcus equi*, *Streptococcus dysgalactiae*, and *Streptococcus uberis*. The name "streptococcus" was originally given to all gram-positive cocci forming small chains. Based on simple biochemical criteria, Sherman (206) divided the streptococci into four main groups: pyogenic, faecalis, viridans, and lactis. Lancefield (122) divided the pyogenic group into serogroups, of which there are at least 15 (A, B, C, D, E, F, G, H, K, L, M, N, O, R, and S). Serological methods have also been useful in the classification of the faecalis group (Lancefield group D) and lactis group (Lancefield group N). The faecalis group was later renamed as the genus *Enterococcus* (186), and the lactis group was renamed as the genus *Lactococcus* (187). Most pathogenic streptococci belong to the pyogenic group.

Antimicrobial agents play a very important role in the treatment of streptococcal infections. Traditionally, all streptococcal species have been regarded as highly susceptible to penicillins, which are the drugs of choice for the control of these bacteria. As with staphylococci, proper species identification and the use of quality-assured and standardized procedures for susceptibility testing is important to obtaining reliable results on the occurrence of antimicrobial resistance.

Streptococcus agalactiae

S. agalactiae is the only recognized species of group B streptococci (GBS). It is an important cause

Table 8. Occurrence of antimicrobial resistance in *S. dysgalactiae* from bovines with mastitis in different countries in 2003[a]

Antimicrobial agent	% of isolates resistant			
	England and Wales (n = 193)[b]	France (n varies)	The Netherlands (n = 94)	United States (n = 152)
Macrolides	5	17, 16, 24	13	7
Penicillin	0	0	0	1
Tetracycline	47	53, 12	77	41
Co-trimoxazole		4	0	

[a]Data are from references 13 and 179.
[b]n = number of isolates.

of neonatal septicemia and meningitis and other invasive diseases in humans. GBS are also an important cause of bovine mastitis. Before the 1950s, GBS were the leading cause of bovine mastitis in most countries. However, in the 1950s and 1960s, eradication programs were implemented in many countries, with such success that GBS now occur only occasionally in these countries. In other countries or regions, GBS are still the leading cause of bovine mastitis.

Human and bovine GBS have traditionally been regarded as separate populations, based mainly on the ability of bovine strains to utilize lactose (47). Genetic analyses have provided evidence that bovine and human isolates make up two generally separate populations but also that some exchange of strains between the two reservoirs probably takes place (21, 102, 139, 146). Human strains have been shown to cause bovine mastitis under experimental conditions (101).

Like most other streptococci, GBS are fully susceptible to β-lactam antimicrobials. This has been shown in numerous studies. A few reports on resistance or decreased susceptibility to penicillin in GBS have been published (18, 67, 140), but until these results are confirmed by genetic analysis, it must be assumed that this is simply a result of methodological failures. Studies on the susceptibility of GBS to antimicrobial agents revealed that the isolates are susceptible mainly to β-lactams, chloramphenicol, fluoroquinolones, and co-trimoxazole, whereas resistance of some strains to tetracyclines and macrolides has been recorded (59, 67, 84, 260).

Streptococcus dysgalactiae

The species *S. dysgalactiae* includes a variety of strains that are genetically very closely related but differ in serogroups, hemolysis, host association, and pathogenicity. The species includes two subspecies, *S. dysgalactiae* subsp. *dysgalactiae* and *S. dysgalactiae* subsp. *equisimilis* (70, 229, 234). The name *S. dysgalactiae* has traditionally been given to alpha-hemolytic group C streptococci from bovine mastitis (77). The bovine ecovar differs from all other ecovars by its appearance on blood agar as alpha-hemolytic. *S. dysgalactiae* subsp. *equisimilis* has been divided into four host-associated subgroups (47): human groups C and G and animal groups C and L. Members of the animal groups are frequently isolated from pigs with endocarditis (98). Moreover, alpha-hemolytic group C isolates identified as *S. dysgalactiae* have also been reported from infections in fish (152). *S. dysgalactiae* is commonly fully susceptible to β-lactams and chlorampenicol. Acquired resistance to tetracyclines and macrolides has been described (Table 8).

Streptococcus uberis

S. uberis is today one of the most important causes of bovine mastitis, being present in 15 to 35% of all cases (27). This species does not seem to cause infections in other animals. *S. uberis* was first described by Diernhofer (56) in 1932 and later separated into two species, *S. uberis* and *S. parauberis* (250). *S. parauberis* is only rarely isolated from cases of bovine mastitis (127). *S. uberis* mastitis occurs throughout the lactation period but is especially common in the dry period. Thus, antimicrobial therapy is in many cases important in the control of the infection.

In most reports on antimicrobial susceptibility of mastitis pathogens, identification that can separate *S. uberis* from enterococci has not been performed. In many other cases the separation is only based on morphology or insufficient tests. This can be a problem because enterococci are intrinsically resistant or show reduced susceptibility to several antimicrobial agents, including β-lactams. Furthermore, many studies have used their own procedures for susceptibility testing and not necessarily followed international standards such as those of the Clinical and Laboratory Standards Institute (148). Thus, reports from different laboratories have to be compared with great care.

Recent data on the occurrence of antimicrobial resistance in *S. uberis* from bovine mastitis for selected countries are given in Table 9. As with most other streptococci, *S. uberis* isolates are generally highly susceptible to β-lactam antibiotics and chloramphenicol but resistant to aminoglycosides. Acquired resistance to macrolides and tetracyclines is relatively common. Resistance to penicillin has been reported. Thus, Phuektes et al. (162) reported 12 (16%) of 74 isolates for which the species identity had been confirmed by PCR to be penicillin resistant. Similarly, Guérin-Faublee et al. (84) found that pencillin MICs were elevated (0.12 to 0.25 μg/ml) in 44% of 50 isolates. However, using the current Clinical and Laboratory Standards Institute breakpoints (148) for susceptibility to penicillin, these isolates have to be considered as intermediate resistant. Thus, unless genetic verification of acquired resistance to β-lactam antibiotics is provided, reports of such resistance should probably be regarded as results of either misidentification, methodological problems with the susceptibility testing, or use of breakpoints not appropriate for streptococci.

Streptococcus suis

S. suis is a very important cause of infections in the swine industry worldwide. The importance of the bacterium seems to be increasing, especially in countries with intensive agricultural production systems (92). In pigs, *S. suis* causes septicemia, meningitis, arthritis, endocarditis, bronchopneumonia, and abortion (92). *S. suis* also causes infections, mainly meningitis and septicemia, in humans (14, 217, 235). Human infections occur mainly in people working in close contact with pigs, such as farmers and slaughterhouse workers. Human infections are often lethal if not treated adequately. *S. suis* infections have also been reported to occur in cats, horses, ruminants, and other animals (49, 52, 53, 97, 112).

The upper respiratory tract, particularly the tonsils and nasal cavities, is considered the natural habitat of *S. suis* (92). *S. suis* is normally divided into different serotypes, of which 35 have been identified so far (82, 83, 94, 159). The prevalence of the different serotypes varies greatly (7, 93, 106, 137, 169, 230). In most countries, isolates of serotype 2 are most commonly observed, but serotypes 1/2, 3, 7, and 9 are also commonly reported.

S. suis can also be isolated from the tonsils of healthy pigs, and in the diagnostic laboratory it is often present as a contaminant of different organs, especially the lungs. Thus, in previous decades *S. suis* isolated from lung tissue was not necessarily regarded as the infectious agent and was therefore not included for further studies. In those older studies, isolates from the meninges and brain were typically included. In addition, it was mainly isolates of serotype 2 that were regarded as pathogenic. These aspects have to be remembered when comparing old and more recent studies.

Increases in antimicrobial resistance among *S. suis* over time have been found in some studies (8). Aarestrup et al. (8) compared isolates of serotypes 2 and 7 obtained in Denmark during the time periods 1968 to 1981 and 1992 to 1997 and found increases in resistance to macrolides and tetracyclines, which they attributed to the increased usage of tetracycline for therapy and tylosin for therapy and growth promotion. A comparison with isolates from Sweden revealed a very low frequency of resistance to macrolides. Since Sweden has not used tylosin for growth promotion since 1986, this finding supported the assumption that there is an association between macrolide resistance and tylosin usage.

Differences in the occurrence of antimicrobial resistance between different *S. suis* serotypes have been observed (7, 137). Thus, in Denmark, a much lower frequency of resistance to macrolides was found among isolates of serotype 2 than among other serotypes (7). The opposite was the case for resistance to tetracycline, where serotype 2 isolates were more frequently found to be resistant. In France, a much lower frequency of resistance to both

Table 9. Occurrence of antimicrobial resistance in *S. uberis* from bovines with mastitis in different countries in 2003[a]

Antimicrobial agent	% of isolates resistant					
	England and Wales (n = 775)[b]	Finland[c] (n = 89)	France (n varies)	Italy (n = 31)	The Netherlands (n = 83)	United States (n = 133)
Macrolides	8	0	17, 18, 29	23	19	41
Penicillin	0	0	1	3	0	0
Tetracycline	11	1	17, 8	39	41	70
Co-trimoxazole		0	0	74	1	

[a]Data are from references 13, 164, and 179.
[b]n = number of isolates.
[c]Data from 2001.

macrolides and tetracycline was observed among isolates of serotype 2 than among other serotypes (137). In Spain, isolates of serotype 9 were found to be more frequently associated with macrolide resistance than isolates of serotype 2 (231). In Denmark, a very high frequency of resistance to sulfonamides among serotype 7 isolates (>90%) was found (8, 221), which could indicate some association between serotype and resistance. There is currently no explanation for the observed differences in occurrence of resistance between the different serotypes. It might be related to the genotype and the ability of the different serotypes to acquire resistance. However, it might just as well be related to the exposure of the different serotypes to antimicrobial agents and thereby to selective pressure.

The association between type and antimicrobial resistance might not be restricted to serotypes. Rasmussen et al. (172) compared isolates of serotype 2 by ribotyping and susceptibility testing. They found an association between ribotype clusters, resistance to sulfonamides and tetracyclines, and clinical disease. All isolates belonging to one cluster were resistant to sulfonamides and were obtained mainly from meningitis cases in pigs. Isolates from meningitis cases in humans also belonged to this cluster. Isolates from a second cluster were mainly tetracycline resistant and obtained from cases of pneumonia or sepsis. In contrast, Tian et al. (221) compared isolates of serotype 7 and were not able to find any associations between ribotype, clinical disease, and antimicrobial resistance.

Most studies on susceptibility of *S. suis* do not make reference to serotypes, which may—as mentioned above—cause some problems in the comparison between countries and over time because of the differences in serotypes. The occurrence of antimicrobial resistance among *S. suis* in different countries is given in Table 10. In most reports *S. suis* isolates are fully susceptible to penicillins, although some studies have reported a low frequency of resistant isolates (Table 10). Some resistance to fluoroquinolones has also been observed. However, the normal distribution of the MICs of fluoroquinolones for *S. suis* is close to the breakpoint, and this probably indicates a general elevated level of insensitivity rather than acquired resistance. Monitoring of florfenicol susceptibility revealed a similar picture, with all *S. suis* isolates tested between 2000 and 2003 being susceptible, but the MICs at which 90% of the strains were inhibited were at the breakpoint for susceptibility (111, 168). Major variations in susceptibility to gentamicin have been reported. In some reports all isolates were susceptible, whereas in others a large proportion of the isolates were reported as resistant. Whether this reflects true acquired resistance or differences in the methodology and breakpoints used remains to be clarified. Acquired resistance to macrolides, tetracycline, and sulfonamides is widespread among *S. suis*. For this reason, penicillin currently seems to be the best choice for treatment of *S. suis* infections.

Mechanisms of Resistance in Streptococci

The genetic background for resistance in streptococci of animal origin has been determined in only a limited number of studies.

With regard to penicillin resistance, acquisition of genes encoding β-lactamases is by far the most common mechanism of resistance to β-lactam antibiotics (see chapter 6). Despite this, no β-lactamase-producing streptococci have so far been described. A much more sophisticated mechanism of resistance has evolved in *S. pneumoniae*. Thus, the entire target of penicillin, the PBP, has been restructured. Alterations in PBP1a, PBP2x, and PBP2b cause resistance in *S. pneumoniae* (17, 40, 87, 88). It has been suggested that penicillin resistance in *S. pneumoniae* arose following transformation and homologous recombination with PBP genes from a number of closely related species, including *Streptococcus mitis* (58). Horizontal transfer of PBP genes probably also plays a role in the spread of penicillin resistance both within *S. pneumoniae* and between streptococcal species (39, 57). Insertions in PBP2b have also been found (255). PBP modifications have also been suggested as the mechanism of penicillin resistance in *S. suis* (31). Recent sequencing studies of Danish and Polish penicillin-resistant and -susceptible isolates have also confirmed that resistant isolates contain base pair substitutions in the PBP genes at the same locations as in *S. pneumoniae* (A. Petersen and F. M. Aarestrup, unpublished results).

In *S. suis*, resistance to macrolides is encoded mainly by the *erm*(B) gene (100, 138, 221). Jensen et al. (100) found *erm*(B) in 69 of 77 *S. suis* isolates, Martel et al. (138) found *erm*(B) to be present in all of 71 macrolide-resistant isolates examined, whereas Tian et al. (221) found *erm*(B) in 39 of 42 isolates of serotype 7. Martel et al. (138) also examined their *S. suis* isolates for the presence of *mef*(A) or *mef*(E) and found all isolates to be negative. Sequence comparison has revealed 100% homology to the sequence of *erm*(B) obtained from *S. pneumoniae* and *S. pyogenes* (138). The *erm*(A), *erm*(B), *erm*(F), and/or *mre*(A) genes have been found in macrolide-resistant *S. agalactiae* isolates of bovine origin (60, 177). The *erm*(B), *erm*(F), and/or *erm*(Q) genes were detected in macrolide-resistant *S. dysgalactiae* and *S. uberis* isolates (177). In *S. agalactiae*, *S. pneumoniae*, and

Table 10. Recent data on the occurrence of antimicrobial resistance among *S. suis* isolated from swine in different countries[a]

Antimicrobial agent	% of isolates resistant																		
	Belgium, 1999–2000 ($n = 87$)[b]	Canada			Croatia, before 1995 ($n = 33$)[c]	Denmark		England and Wales, 2003 ($n = 34$)	France, 2003 (n differs)	Finland, 1984–1987 ($n = 35$)	Japan, 1987–1996 ($n = 689$)	The Nether-lands, 2003 ($n = 762$)	Norway, 1986 ($n = 21$)	Poland		Portugal, 2003 ($n = 14$)[d]	Spain		United States, before 1992 ($n = 48$)
		1986–1988 ($n = 59$)[c]	1988 ($n = 135$)	Before 1991 ($n = 80$)		1995–1996 ($n = 180$)	2003 ($n = 557$)							2002 ($n = 150$)	2003 ($n = 151$)		1992 ($n = 65$)	1999–2001 ($n = 151$)	
Fluoro-quinolones	1				9.1	2.2	0	0	2.9		0.3			8.6	9.9	64		2.0	
Macrolides	71	33.9	60.7	66.3	0	41.7	29.1	36	52.9	0		35	28.6	28.0		93, 71	63	90.7	58
Gentamicin		66.1	0.0	2.5					0.0						0.0	100		4.6	9
Penicillin		0	3.0	2.5	51.1	1.1	0.9	0		0	0.9	0		10.6	7.9	21	7	4.0	
Sulfonamides				47.5			0.9											96.0	44
Tetracycline	85	83.0	78.5	95.0	72.2	32.2	52.2	68	69.9	42.8	86.9	48	66.7	73.3	55.0	93, 79	61	95.4	63
Co-trimox-azole		39.0	11.5			1.7	51.5	3	15.5	31.4	0.0	8		30.0	16.6	100	61	0.0	

[a]Adapted from references 7, 13, 32, 89, 107, 138, 169, 183, 203, 209, 215, 231, and 241.
[b]n = number of isolates.
[c]Only serotype 2.
[d]Two values indicate data obtained with different substances.

S. pyogenes of human origin, the *erm*(B) gene seems to predominate, but *erm*(A) and *mef*(A) have also been frequently reported (19, 42, 45b, 69, 80, 142, 143, 167, 174, 222). These genes may also be found in the same isolates.

Both the *tet*(M) and *tet*(O) genes have been identified in tetracycline-resistant *S. suis*, whereas the genes *tet*(K), *tet*(L), *tet*(P), and *tet*(S) have not been not detected. Wasteson et al. (241) found *tet*(O) in 8 and *tet*(M) in 5 of 15 tetracycline-resistant isolates. Sachdé et al. (182) identified the *tet*(O) gene among 17 isolates from pigs, 3 isolates from cats, and single isolates of canine and human origin, while another 2 isolates from dogs were positive for *tet*(M). Tian et al. (221) found *tet*(M) in 11 and *tet*(O) in 6 of 25 tetracycline-resistant isolates of serotype 7. Eight isolates were negative for the *tet* genes examined. The *tet*(L), *tet*(M), and/or *tet*(O) genes have been found among tetracycline-resistant *S. agalactiae* isolates of bovine origin (28, 60, 197). Duarte et al. (60) found the *tet*(O) gene to be most common among bovine isolates, whereas *tet*(M) predominated among human isolates. Schwarz et al. (197) found the *tet*(M) gene to be most common among isolates from cattle, humans, and pigs, whereas *tet*(O) was only infrequently found. Brown and Roberts (28) found seven *S. agalactiae* isolates from bovine mastitis to hybridize with the *tet*(O) probe only, whereas three isolates did not hybridize with probes for *tet*(K), *tet*(L), *tet*(M), or *tet*(O). Brown and Roberts (28) examined 10 tetracycline-resistant *S. dysgalactiae* isolates and found 1 to hybridize with *tet*(O), 1 with *tet*(L), and 1 with *tet*(L) and *tet*(K), whereas no hybridization signal was found in the remaining 7 isolates. Soedarmanto et al. (212) identified the gene *tet*(M) in two canine and the gene *tet*(O) in three bovine group G streptococcal isolates, whereas *tet*(M) or *tet*(O) was found in four bovine, three porcine, and four avian group L streptococcal isolates. Brown and Roberts (28) found the *tet*(K) and *tet*(O) genes in one of two tetracycline-resistant *S. uberis* isolates examined.

Resistance to tetracycline and macrolides is often found in the same mobile unit, Tn*1545*, which is commonly found in streptococci and enterococci (38, 45a, 204; see also chapter 6). This mobile unit and similar transposons have a wide host range and are probably responsible for a large part of the tetracycline and macrolide resistance observed in streptococci.

The presence of other resistance genes and mechanisms has not been examined in streptococci of animal origin. Considering this and the large number of macrolide- and tetracycline-resistant isolates where no mechanism has been detected, it seems likely that new genes will be detected in the future.

CONCLUDING REMARKS

Staphylococci and streptococci constitute two important groups of pathogens of human, veterinary, and in some cases zoonotic relevance. Antimicrobial agents are most often used to control infections caused by these two groups of bacteria. The summary of the current knowledge on antimicrobial resistance of staphylococci and streptococci from animal sources, as presented in this chapter, still shows a rather incomplete picture in comparison to what is known about antimicrobial resistance in the corresponding organisms from human infections. The continuous monitoring of staphylococci and streptococci from animal infections is an essential prerequisite for early detection of new trends in the development of resistance to antimicrobials commonly used to control these infections. However, as mentioned several times in this chapter, standardized procedures need to be made available for unambiguous species identification and for in vitro susceptibility testing, and such procedures also need to be applied by researchers in this field to make the results of susceptibility testing more comparable. The ability of bacterial strains to acquire resistance varies among species, serotypes, phage types, and probably also clones. Thus, comparison of the prevalence of resistance between countries and over time must be based on proper and sufficient species and even subspecies identification. More knowledge about the ability of certain subtypes to acquire resistance, together with the development of means to control such clones, could perhaps provide new means of controlling the increase in resistance. In addition, molecular analysis of the genetic basis of resistance is essential to identify the gene flow between the different reservoirs and bacterial species and clones and to analyze which factors may contribute to increased or decreased resistance to specific antimicrobial agents. Moreover, knowledge of the colocation of resistance genes on multiresistance plasmids or transposons, as shown for the transposon Tn*1545*, will help us to understand why certain resistance genes emerge or persist even without direct selective pressure as imposed by the antimicrobial agents used. Certain resistance genes, such as *cfr* and *fexA*, have actually been found in only a few isolates of a certain staphylococcal species, whereas others, such as *tet*(K), *blaZ*, and *erm*(C), occur in a wide variety of staphylococcal species from various animal and human sources. A few other resistance genes, such as the tetracycline resistance gene *tet*(M) and the macrolide resistance gene *erm*(B), are even more widely disseminated among staphylococci, streptococci, and other gram-positive bacteria, including enterococci, lactococci, and listeriae (253). A point of additional interest is that *tet*(M) and *erm*(B) seem to be restricted to a few staphylococcal species. With more information becoming available on antimicrobial resistance of staphylococci and streptococci from animals, the more we see that these bacteria represent an integral part of the gene pool of gram-positive bacteria, in which not only the pathogenic species, but also those species which represent a part of the normal flora of the skin and the mucosal surfaces, play an important role as donors as well as recipients of antimicrobial resistance genes. Further studies on the exchange of resistance genes between staphylococci and streptococci isolated from animals and those isolated from humans are needed.

REFERENCES

1. **Aarestrup, F. M.** 2000. Occurrence, selection and spread of resistance to antimicrobial agents used for growth promotion for food animals in Denmark. *APMIS* **101:**1–48.
2. **Aarestrup, F. M.** 2001. Comparative ribotyping of *Staphylococcus intermedius* isolated from members of the Canoidea gives possible evidence for host-specificity and co-evolution of bacteria and hosts. *Int. J. Syst. Evol. Microbiol.* **51:**1343–1347.
3. **Aarestrup, F. M., and L. B. Jensen.** 2002. Trends in antimicrobial susceptibility in relation to antimicrobial usage and presence of resistance genes in *Staphylococcus hyicus* isolated from exudative epidermitis in pigs. *Vet. Microbiol.* **89:**83–94.
4. **Aarestrup, F. M., and N. E. Jensen.** 1998. Development of penicillin resistance among *Staphylococcus aureus* isolated from bovine mastitis in Denmark and other countries. *Microb. Drug Resist.* **4:**247–256.
5. **Aarestrup, F. M., H. C. Wegener, and V. T. Rosdahl.** 1995. A comparative study of *Staphylococcus aureus* strains isolated from bovine subclinical mastitis during 1952–1956 and 1992. *Acta Vet. Scand.* **36:**237–243.
6. **Aarestrup, F. M., H. C. Wegener, V. T. Rosdahl, and N. E. Jensen.** 1995. Staphylococcal and other bacterial species associated with intramammary infections in Danish dairy herds. *Acta Vet. Scand.* **36:**475–487.
7. **Aarestrup, F. M., S. E. Jorsal, and N. E. Jensen.** 1998. Serological characterization and antimicrobial susceptibility of *Streptococcus suis* isolates from diagnostic samples in Denmark during 1995 and 1996. *Vet. Microbiol.* **60:**59–66.
8. **Aarestrup, F. M., S. R. Rasmussen, K. Artursson, and N. E. Jensen.** 1998. Trends in resistance to antimicrobial agents of *Streptococcus suis* isolates from Denmark and Sweden. *Vet. Microbiol.* **63:**71–80.
9. **Aarestrup, F. M., F. Bager, N. E. Jensen, M. Madsen, A. Meyling, and H. C. Wegener.** 1998. Resistance to antimicrobial agents used for animal therapy in pathogenic-, zoonotic- and indicator bacteria isolated from different food animals in Denmark: a baseline study for the Danish Integrated Antimicrobial Resistance Monitoring Programme (DANMAP). *APMIS* **106:**745–770.
10. **Aarestrup, F. M., H. D. Larsen, N. H. Eriksen, C. S. Elsberg, and N. E. Jensen.** 1999. Frequency of alpha- and beta-haemolysin in *Staphylococcus aureus* of bovine and human origin. A comparison between pheno- and genotype and variation in phenotypic expression. *APMIS* **107:**425–430.
11. **Aarestrup, F. M., Y. Agersø, J. C. Ø. Christensen, M. Madsen, and L. B. Jensen.** 2000. Antimicrobial susceptibility and presence of resistance genes in staphylococci from poultry. *Vet. Microbiol.* **74:**353–364.
12. **Almer, L. S., V. D. Shortridge, A. M. Nilius, J. M. Beyer, N. B. Soni, M. H. Bui, G. G. Stone, and R. K. Flamm.** 2002. Antimicrobial susceptibility and molecular characterization of community-acquired methicillin-resistant Staphylococcus aureus. *Diagn. Microbiol. Infect. Dis.* **43:**225–232.
13. **Anonymous.** ARBAO-II: Antibiotic resistance in bacteria of animal origin—II. A concerted action funded by the European Commission. [Online.] http://www.dfvf.dk/Default.asp?ID=9753.
14. **Arends, J. P., and H. C. Zanen.** 1988. Meningitis caused by *Streptococcus suis* in humans. *Rev. Infect. Dis.* **10:**131–137.
15. **Barber, M.** 1947. Staphylococcal infection due to penicillin-resistant strains. *Br. Med. J.* **2:**863–865.
16. **Barber, M., and J. E. M. Whitehead.** 1949. Bacteriophage types in penicillin-resistant staphylococcal infection. *Br. Med. J.* **10:**565–569.
17. **Barcus, V. A., K. Ghanekar, M. Yeo, T. J. Coffey, and C. G. Dowson.** 1995. Genetics of high level penicillin resistance in clinical isolates of *Streptococcus pneumoniae*. *FEMS Microbiol. Lett.* **126:**299–303.
18. **Berghash, S. R., J. N. Davidson, J. C. Armstrong, and G. M. Dunny.** 1983. Effects of antibiotic treatment of nonlactating dairy cows on antibiotic resistance patterns of bovine mastitis pathogens. *Antimicrob. Agents Chemother.* **24:**771–776.
19. **Betriu, C., E. Culebras, I. Rodriguez-Avial, M. Gomez, B. A. Sanchez, and J. J. Picazo.** 2004. *In vitro* activities of tigecycline against erythromycin-resistant *Streptococcus pyogenes* and *Streptococcus agalactiae*: mechanisms of macrolide and tetracycline resistance. *Antimicrob. Agents Chemother.* **48:**323–325.
20. **Birgersson, A., P. Jonsson, and O. Holmberg.** 1992. Species identification and some characteristics of coagulase-negative staphylococci isolated from bovine udders. *Vet. Microbiol.* **31:**181–189.
21. **Bisharat, N., D. W. Crook, J. Leigh, R. M. Harding, P. N. Ward, T. J. Coffey, M. C. Maiden, T. Peto, and N. Jones.** 2004. Hyperinvasive neonatal group B streptococcus has arisen from a bovine ancestor. *J. Clin. Microbiol.* **42:**2161–2167.
22. **Bjorland, J., M. Sunde, and S. Waage.** 2001. Plasmid-borne *smr* gene causes resistance to quaternary ammonium compounds in bovine *Staphylococcus aureus*. *J. Clin. Microbiol.* **39:**3999–4004.
23. **Bjorland, J., T. Steinum, M. Sunde, S. Waage, and E. Heir.** 2003. Novel plasmid-borne gene *qacJ* mediates resistance to quaternary ammonium compounds in equine *Staphylococcus aureus*, *Staphylococcus simulans*, and *Staphylococcus intermedius*. *Antimicrob. Agents Chemother.* **47:**3046–3052.
24. **Boag, A., A. Loeffler, and D. H. Lloyd.** 2004. Methicillin-resistant *Staphylococcus aureus* isolates from companion animals. *Vet. Rec.* **154:**411.
25. **Boerlin, P., A. P. Burnens, J. Frey, P. Kuhnert, and J. Nicolet.** 2001. Molecular epidemiology and genetic linkage of macrolide and aminoglycoside resistance in *Staphylococcus intermedius* of canine origin. *Vet. Microbiol.* **79:**74–79.
26. **Bramley, A. J.** 1978. The effect of subclinical *Staphylococcus epidermidis* infection of the lactating bovine udder on its susceptibility to infection with *Streptococcus agalactiae* or *Escherichia coli*. *Br. Vet. J.* **134:**146–151.
27. **Bramley, A. J.** 1997. Environmental streptococci: summary and issues, p. 95–103. In *Proceedings of the Symposium on Udder Health Management for Environmental Streptococci*. Ontario Veterinary College, Guelph, Ontario, Canada.

28. **Brown, M. B., and M. C. Roberts.** 1991. Tetracycline resistance determinants in streptococcal species isolated from the bovine mammary gland. *Vet. Microbiol.* **29:**173–180.
29. **Burriel, A. R.** 1997. Resistance of coagulase-negative staphylococci isolated from sheep to various antimicrobial agents. *Res. Vet. Sci.* **63:**189–190.
30. **Cabral, K. G., C. Lammler, M. Zschock, H. Langoni, M. E. de Sa, C. Victoria, and A. V. Da Silva.** 2004. Pheno- and genotyping of *Staphylococcus aureus*, isolated from bovine milk samples from Sao Paulo State, Brazil. *Can. J. Microbiol.* **50:**901–909.
31. **Cain, D., F. Malouin, M. Dargis, J. Harel, and M. Gottschalk.** 1995. Alterations in penicillin-binding proteins in strains of *Streptococcus suis* possessing moderate and high levels of resistance to penicillin. *FEMS Microbiol. Lett.* **130:**121–127.
32. **Cantin, M., J. Harel, R. Higgins, and M. Gottschalk.** 1992. Antimicrobial resistance patterns and plasmid profiles of *Streptococcus suis* isolates. *J. Vet. Diagn. Investig.* **4:**170–174.
33. **Cardoso, M., and S. Schwarz.** 1992. Characterization of the chloramphenicol acetyltransferase variants encoded by the plasmids pSCS6 and pSCS7 from *Staphylococcus aureus*. *J. Gen. Microbiol.* **138:**275–281.
34. **Cefai, C., S. Ashurst, and C. Owens.** 1994. Human carriage of methicillin-resistant *Staphylococcus aureus* linked with pet dog. *Lancet* **344:**539–540.
35. **Chambers, H. F.** 1997. Methicillin resistance in staphylococci: molecular and biochemical basis and clinical implications. *Clin. Microbiol. Rev.* **10:**781–791.
36. **Chambers, H. F.** 2001. The changing epidemiology of *Staphylococcus aureus*? *Emerg. Infect. Dis.* **7:**178–182.
37. **Chung, W. O., C. Werckenthin, S. Schwarz, and M. C. Roberts.** 1999. Host range of the *erm*(F) rRNA methylase gene in bacteria of human and animal origin. *J. Antimicrob. Chemother.* **43:**5–14.
38. **Clewell, D. B., S. E. Flannagan, and D. D. Jaworski.** 1995. Unconstrained bacterial promiscuity: the Tn*916*-Tn*1545* family of conjugative transposons. *Trends Microbiol.* **3:**229–236.
39. **Coffey, T. J., C. G. Dowson, M. Daniels, and B. G. Spratt.** 1993. Horizontal spread of an altered penicillin-binding protein 2B gene between *Streptococcus pneumoniae* and *Streptococcus oralis*. *FEMS Microbiol. Lett.* **110:**335–339.
40. **Coffey, T. J., M. Daniels, L. K. McDougal, C. G. Dowson, F. C. Tenover, and B. G. Spratt.** 1995. Genetic analysis of clinical isolates of *Streptococcus pneumoniae* with high-level resistance to expanded-spectrum cephalosporins. *Antimicrob. Agents Chemother.* **39:**1306–1313.
41. **Cox, H. U., J. D. Hoskins, A. F. Roy, S. S. Newman, and D. G. Luther.** 1984. Antimicrobial susceptibility of coagulase-positive staphylococci isolated from Louisiana dogs. *Am. J. Vet. Res.* **45:**2039–2042.
42. **Culebras, E., I. Rodriguez-Avial, C. Betriu, M. Redondo, and J. J. Picazo.** 2002. Macrolide and tetracycline resistance and molecular relationships of clinical strains of *Streptococcus agalactiae*. *Antimicrob. Agents Chemother.* **46:**1574–1576.
43. Reference deleted.
44. **Davidson, T. J., I. R. Dohoo, A. W. Donald, H. Hariharan, and K. Collins.** 1992. A cohort study of coagulase-negative staphylococcal mastitis in selected dairy herds in Prince Edward island. *Can. J. Vet. Res.* **56:**275–280.
45. **DeBoer, L. R., D. M. Slaughter, R. D. Applegate, R. J. Sobieski, and S. S. Crupper.** 2001. Antimicrobial susceptibility of staphylococci isolated from the faeces of wild turkeys (*Meleagris gallopavo*). *Lett. Appl. Microbiol.* **33:**382–386.
45a. **de Leener, E., A. Martel, A. Decostere, and F. Haesebrouck.** 2004. Distribution of the *erm* (B) gene, tetracycline resistance genes, and Tn*1545*-like transposons in macrolide- and lincosamide-resistant enterococci from pigs and humans. *Microb. Drug Resist.* **10:**341–345.
45b. **de Mouy, D., J. D. Cavallo, R. Leclercq, R. Fabre; AFICORPI-BIO Network. Association de Formation Continue en Pathologie Infectieuse des Biologistes.** 2001. Antibiotic susceptibility and mechanisms of erythromycin resistance in clinical isolates of *Streptococcus agalactiae*: French multicenter study. *Antimicrob. Agents Chemother.* **45:**2400–2402.
46. **Devriese, L. A.** 1977. Antibiotic susceptibility of *Staphylococcus hyicus* isolated from exudative epidermitis cases in Belgium. *Vlaams Diergeeneskd. Tijdschr.* **46:**143–144.
47. **Devriese, L. A.** 1991. Streptococcal ecovars associated with different animal species: epidemiological significance of serogroups and biotypes. *J. Appl. Bacteriol.* **71:**478–483.
48. **Devriese, L. A., and J. Hommez.** 1975. Epidemiology of methicillin-resistant *Staphylococcus aureus* in dairy herds. *Res. Vet. Sci.* **19:**23–27.
49. **Devriese, L. A., and F. Haesebrouck.** 1992. *Streptococcus suis* infections in horses and cats. *Vet. Rec.* **130:**380.
50. **Devriese, L. A., L. R. Van Damme, and L. Fameree.** 1972. Methicillin (cloxacillin)-resistant *Staphylococcus aureus* strains isolated from bovine mastitis cases. *Zentbl. Veterinärmed. B* **19:**598–605.
51. **Devriese, L. A., D. Nzuambe, and C. Godard.** 1985. Identification and characteristics of staphylococci isolated from lesions and normal skin of horses. *Vet. Microbiol.* **10:**269–277.
52. **Devriese, L. A., B. Sustronck, T. Maenhout, and F. Haesebrouck.** 1990. *Streptococcus suis* meningitis in a horse. *Vet. Rec.* **127:**68.
53. **Devriese, L. A., M. Desmidt, S. Roels, J. Hoorens, and F. Haesebrouck.** 1993. *Streptococcus suis* infection in fallow deer. *Vet. Rec.* **132:**283.
54. **Devriese, L. A., M. Baele, M. Vaneechoutte, A. Martel, and F. Haesebrouck.** 2002. Identification and antimicrobial susceptibility of *Staphylococcus chromogenes* isolates from intramammary infections of dairy cows. *Vet. Microbiol.* **87:** 175–182.
55. **Diekema, D. J., M. A. Pfaller, F. J. Schmitz, J. Smayevsky, J. Bell, R. N. Jones, M. Beach, and the SENTRY Participants Group.** 2001. Survey of infections due to *Staphylococcus* species: frequency of occurrence and antimicrobial susceptibility of isolates collected in the United States, Canada, Latin America, Europe, and the Western Pacific region for the SENTRY Antimicrobial Surveillance Program, 1997–1999. *Clin. Infect. Dis.* **32:**114–132.
56. **Diernhofer, K.** 1932. Aesculinbouillon als Hilfmittel für die Differenzierung von Euter-und Milchstreptokokken bei Masseuntersuchungen. *Milchwirtsch. Forsch.* 368–374.
57. **Dowson, C. G., A. Hutchison, J. A. Brannigan, R. C. George, D. Hansman, J. Linares, A. Tomasz, J. M. Smith, and B. G. Spratt.** 1989. Horizontal transfer of penicillin-binding protein genes in penicillin-resistant clinical isolates of *Streptococcus pneumoniae*. *Proc. Natl. Acad. Sci. USA* **86:**8842–8846.
58. **Dowson, C. G., T. J. Coffey, C. Kell, and R. A. Whiley.** 1993. Evolution of penicillin resistance in *Streptococcus pneumoniae*; the role of *Streptococcus mitis* in the formation of a low affinity PBP2b in *S. pneumoniae*. *Mol. Microbiol.* **9:**635–643.
59. **Duarte, R. S., O. P. Miranda, B. C. Bellei, M. A. Brito, and L. M. Teixeira.** 2004. Phenotypic and molecular characteristics of *Streptococcus agalactiae* isolates recovered from milk of dairy cows in Brazil. *J. Clin. Microbiol.* **42:**4214–4222.
60. **Duarte, R. S., B. C. Bellei, O. P. Miranda, M. A. Brito, and L. M. Teixeira.** 2005. Distribution of antimicrobial resistance

and virulence-related genes among Brazilian group B streptococci recovered from bovine and human sources. *Antimicrob. Agents Chemother.* **49:**97–103.

61. **Dufour, P., Y. Gillet, M. Bes, G. Lina, F. Vandenesch, D. Floret, J. Etienne, and H. Richet.** 2002. Community-acquired methicillin-resistant *Staphylococcus aureus* infections in France: emergence of a single clone that produces Panton-Valentine leukocidin. *Clin. Infect. Dis.* **35:**819–824.
62. **Duquette, R. A., and T. J. Nuttall.** 2004. Methicillin-resistant *Staphylococcus aureus* in dogs and cats: an emerging problem? *J. Small Anim. Pract.* **45:**591–597.
63. Reference deleted.
64. **Eady, E. A., and J. H. Cove.** 2003. Staphylococcal resistance revisited: community-acquired methicillin resistant *Staphylococcus aureus*—an emerging problem for the management of skin and soft tissue infections. *Curr. Opin. Infect. Dis.* **16:** 103–124.
65. **Eady, E. A., J. I. Ross, J. L. Tipper, C. E. Walters, J. H. Cove, and W. C. Noble.** 1993. Distribution of genes encoding erythromycin ribosomal methylases and an erythromycin efflux pump in epidemiologically distinct groups of staphylococci. *J. Antimicrob. Chemother.* **31:**211–217.
66. **Enright, M. C.** 2003. The evolution of a resistant pathogen—the case of MRSA. *Curr. Opin. Pharmacol.* **3:**474–479.
67. **Erskine, R. J., R. D. Walker, C. A. Bolin, P. C. Bartlett, and D. G. White.** 2002. Trends in antibacterial susceptibility of mastitis pathogens during a seven-year period. *J. Dairy Sci.* **85:**1111–1118.
68. **Evans, A. C.** 1916. The bacteria of freshly drawn milk from normal udders. *J. Infect. Dis.* **18:**437–476.
69. **Farrell, D. J., and S. G. Jenkins.** 2004. Distribution across the USA of macrolide resistance and macrolide resistance mechanisms among *Streptococcus pneumoniae* isolates collected from patients with respiratory tract infections: PROTEKT US 2001–2002. *J. Antimicrob. Chemother.* **54:**17–22.
70. **Farrow, J. A. E., and M. D. Collins.** 1984. Taxonomic studies on streptococci of serological groups, C, G and L and possible related taxa. *Syst. Appl. Microbiol.* **5:**483–493.
71. Reference deleted.
72. **Fleming, A.** 1929. On the antibacterial action of cultures of a penicillum, with special reference to their use in the isolation of *B. influenzae*. *Br. J. Exp. Pathol.* **10:**226–236.
73. **Fluit, A. C., J. Verhoef, F. J. Schmitz; European SENTRY Participants.** 2001. Frequency of isolation and antimicrobial resistance of gram-negative and gram-positive bacteria from patients in intensive care units of 25 European university hospitals participating in the European arm of the SENTRY Antimicrobial Surveillance Program 1997–1998. *Eur. J. Clin. Microbiol. Infect. Dis.* **20:**617–625.
74. **Francis, J. S., M. C. Doherty, U. Lopatin, C. P. Johnston, G. Sinha, T. Ross, M. Cai, N. N. Hansel, T. Perl, J. R. Ticehurst, K. Carroll, D. L. Thomas, E. Nuermberger, and J. G. Bartlett.** 2005. Severe community-onset pneumonia in healthy adults caused by methicillin-resistant *Staphylococcus aureus* carrying the Panton-Valentine leukocidin genes. *Clin. Infect. Dis.* **40:**100–107.
75. **Frank, L. A., S. A. Kania, K. A. Hnilica, R. P. Wilkes, and D.A. Bemis.** 2003. Isolation of *Staphylococcus schleiferi* from dogs with pyoderma. *J. Am. Vet. Med. Assoc.* **222:**451–454.
76. **Fraser-Moodie, W.** 1971. Struggle against infection. *Proc. R. Soc. Med.* **64:**87–94.
77. **Garvie, E. I., J. A. E. Farrow, and A. J. Bramley.** 1983. *Streptococcus dysgalactiae* (Diernhofer) nom. rev. *Int. J. Syst. Bacteriol.* **33:**404–405.
78. **Gentilini, E., G. Denamiel, P. Llorente, S. Godaly, M. Rebuelto, and O. DeGregorio.** 2000. Antimicrobial susceptibility of *Staphylococcus aureus* isolated from bovine mastitis in Argentina. *J. Dairy Sci.* **83:**1224–1227.
79. **Gentilini, E., G. Denamiel, A. Betancor, M. Rebuelto, M. Rodriguez Fermepin, and R. A. De Torrest.** 2002. Antimicrobial susceptibility of coagulase-negative staphylococci isolated from bovine mastitis in Argentina. *J. Dairy Sci.* **85:** 1913–1917.
80. **Giovanetti, E., A. Brenciani, R. Lupidi, M. C. Roberts, and P. E. Varaldo.** 2003. Presence of the *tet*(O) gene in erythromycin- and tetracycline-resistant strains of *Streptococcus pyogenes* and linkage with either the *mef*(A) or the *erm*(A) gene. *Antimicrob. Agents Chemother.* **47:**2844–2849.
81. **Gortel, K., K. L. Campbell, I. Kakoma, T. Whittem, D. J. Schaeffer, and R. M. Weisiger.** 1999. Methicillin resistance among staphylococci isolated from dogs. *Am. J. Vet. Res.* **60:**1526–1530.
82. **Gottschalk, M., R. Higgins, M. Jacques, K. R. Mittal, and J. Henrichsen.** 1989. Description of 14 new capsular types of *Streptococcus suis*. *J. Clin. Microbiol.* **27:**2633–2635.
83. **Gottschalk, M., R. Higgins, M. Jacques, M. Beaudoin, and J. Henrichsen.** 1991. Characterization of six new capsular types (23 through 28) of *Streptococcus suis*. *J. Clin. Microbiol.* **29:**2590–2594.
84. **Guérin-Faublee, V., F. Tardy, C. Bouveron, and G. Carret.** 2002. Antimicrobial susceptibility of *Streptococcus* species isolated from clinical mastitis in dairy cows. *Int. J. Antimicrob. Agents* **19:**219–226.
85. **Hajek, V.** 1976. *Staphylococcus intermedius*, a new species isolated from animals. *Int. J. Syst. Bacteriol.* **26:**401–408.
86. **Hajek, V., and E. Marsalek.** 1971. The differentiation of pathogenic staphylococci and a suggestion for their taxonomic classification. *Zentbl. Bakteriol. Orig. A* **217:**176–182.
87. **Hakenbeck, R., M. Tarpay, and A. Tomasz.** 1980. Multiple changes of penicillin-binding proteins in penicillin-resistant clinical isolates of *Streptococcus pneumoniae*. *Antimicrob. Agents Chemother.* **17:**364–371.
88. **Hakenbeck, R., H. Ellerbrok, T. Briese, S. Handwerger, and A. Tomasz.** 1986. Penicillin-binding proteins of penicillin-susceptible and -resistant pneumococci: immunological relatedness of altered proteins and changes in peptides carrying the beta-lactam binding site. *Antimicrob. Agents Chemother.* **30:**553–558.
89. **Hariharan, H., J. Bryenton, J. St. Onge, N. McNair, and J. R. Long.** 1989. Antimicrobial drug susceptibility of *Streptococcus suis* type 2. *Ir. Vet. J.* **42:**113–114.
90. **Hartmann, F. A., S. S. Trostle, and A. A. Klohnen.** 1997. Isolation of methicillin-resistant *Staphylococcus aureus* from a postoperative wound infection in a horse. *J. Am. Vet. Med. Assoc.* **211:**590–592.
91. **Hazarika, R. A., P. N. Mahanta, G. N. Dutta, and L. A. Devriese.** 1991. Cutaneous infection associated with *Staphylococcus hyicus* in cattle. *Res. Vet. Sci.* **50:**374–375.

91a. **Heuer, O. E., and P. B. Larsen (ed.).** 2004. *DANMAP 2003—Use of Antimicrobial Agents and Occurrence of Antimicrobial Resistance in Bacteria from Food Animals, Foods and Humans in Denmark*. Danish Integrated Antimicrobial Resistance Monitoring and Research Programme, Copenhagen, Denmark.

92. **Higgins, R., and M. Gottschalk.** 1999. Streptococcal diseases, p. 563–578. *In* B. Straw, S. D'Allaire, W. L. Mengeling, and D. J. Taylor (ed.), *Diseases of Swine*. Iowa State University Press, Ames.
93. **Higgins, R., and M. Gottschalk.** 2001. Distribution of *Streptococcus suis* capsular types in 2000. *Can. Vet. J.* **42:**223.
94. **Higgins, R., M. Gottschalk, M. Boudreau, A. Lebrun, and J. Henrichsen.** 1995. Description of six new capsular types

(29–34) of *Streptococcus suis*. *J. Vet. Diagn. Investig.* **7:** 405–406.

95. **Hogan, J. S., K. L. Smith, D. A. Todhunter, and P. S. Schoenberger.** 1987. Rate of environmental mastitis in quarters infected with *Corynebacterium bovis* and *Staphylococcus* species. *J. Dairy Sci.* **71:**2520–2525.
96. **Holm, B. R., U. Petersson, A. Morner, K. Bergstrom, A. Franklin, and C. Greko.** 2002. Antimicrobial resistance in staphylococci from canine pyoderma: a prospective study of first-time and recurrent cases in Sweden. *Vet. Rec.* **151:** 600–605.
97. **Hommez, J., J. Wullepit, P. Cassimon, F. Castryck, K. Ceyssens, and L. A. Devriese.** 1988. *Streptococcus suis* and other streptococcal species as a cause of extramammary infection in ruminants. *Vet. Rec.* **123:**626–627.
98. **Hommez, J., L. A. Devriese, F. Castryck, and C. Miry.** 1991. β-hemolytic streptococci from pigs: bacteriological diagnosis. *J. Vet. Med. B* **38:**441–444.
99. **Honkanen-Buzalski, T., V. Myllys, and S. Pyörälä.** 1994. Bovine clinical mastitis due to coagulase-negative staphylococci and their susceptibility to antimicrobials. *J. Vet. Med. B* **41:**344–350.
100. **Jensen, L. B., N. Frimodt-Møller, and F. M. Aarestrup.** 1999. Presence of *erm* classes in Gram-positive bacteria of animal and human origin. *FEMS Microbiol. Lett.* **170:**151–158.
101. **Jensen, N. E.** 1982. Experimental bovine group-B streptococcal mastitis induced by strains of human and bovine origin. *Nord. Vetmed.* **34:**441–450.
102. **Jensen, N. E., and F. M. Aarestrup.** 1996. Epidemiological aspects of group B streptococci of bovine and human origin. *Epidemiol. Infect.* **117:**417–422.
103. **Kania, S. A., N. L. Williamson, L. A. Frank, R. P. Wilkes, R. D. Jones, and D. A. Bemis.** 2004. Methicillin resistance of staphylococci isolated from the skin of dogs with pyoderma. *Am. J. Vet. Res.* **65:**1265–1268.
104. **Kapur, V., W. M. Sisco, R. S. Greer, T. S. Whittam, and J. M. Musser.** 1995. Molecular population genetic analysis of *Staphylococcus aureus* recovered from cows. *J. Clin. Microbiol.* **33:**376–380.
105. **Kaszanyitzky, E. J., Z. Egyed, S. Janosi, J. Keseru, Z. Gal, I. Szabo, Z. Veres, and P. Somogyi.** 2004. Staphylococci isolated from animals and food with phenotypically reduced susceptibility to beta-lactamase-resistant beta-lactam antibiotics. *Acta Vet. Hung.* **52:**7–17.
106. **Kataoka, Y., C. Sugimoto, M. Nakazawa, T. Morozumi, and M. Kashiwazaki.** 1993. The epidemiological studies of *Streptococcus suis* infections in Japan from 1987 to 1991. *J. Vet. Med. Sci.* **55:**623–626.
107. **Kataoka, Y., T. Yoshida, and T. Sawada.** 2000. A 10-year survey of antimicrobial susceptibility of *Streptococcus suis* isolates from swine in Japan. *J. Vet. Med. Sci.* **62:**1053–1057.
108. **Kawano, J., A. Shimizu, Y. Saitoh, M. Yagi, T. Saito, and R. Okamoto.** 1996. Isolation of methicillin-resistant coagulase-negative staphylococci from chickens. *J. Clin. Microbiol.* **34:**2072–2077.
109. **Kehrenberg, C., and S. Schwarz.** 2004. *fexA*, a novel *Staphylococcus lentus* gene encoding resistance to florfenicol and chloramphenicol. *Antimicrob. Agents Chemother.* **48:** 615–618.
110. **Kehrenberg, C., K. K. Ojo, and S. Schwarz.** 2004. Nucleotide sequence and organisation of the multiresistance plasmid pSCFS1 from *Staphylococcus sciuri*. *J. Antimicrob. Chemother.* **54:**936–939.
111. **Kehrenberg, C., J. Mumme, J. Wallmann, J. Verspohl, R. Tegeler, T. Kühn, and S. Schwarz.** 2004. Monitoring of florfenicol susceptibility among bovine and porcine respiratory tract pathogens collected in Germany during the years 2002 and 2003. *J. Antimicrob. Chemother.* **54:**572–574.
112. **Keymer, I. F., S. E. Heath, and J. G. Wood.** 1983. *Streptococcus suis* type II infection in a raccoon dog (*Nyctereutes procyonoides*) family *Canidae*. *Vet. Rec.* **113:**624.
113. **Khan, S. A., M. S. Nawaz, A. A. Khan, R. S. Steele, and C. E. Cerniglia.** 2000. Characterization of erythromycin-resistant methylase genes from multiple antibiotic resistant *Staphylococcus* spp. isolated from milk samples of lactating cows. *Am. J. Vet. Res.* **61:**1128–1132.
114. **Kirby, W. M. M.** 1944. Extraction of a highly potent penicillin inactivator from penicillin resistant staphylococci. *Science* **99:**452–453.
115. **Kloos, W. E.** 1980. Natural populations of the genus *Staphylococcus*. *Annu. Rev. Microbiol.* **34:**559–592.
116. **Kloos, W. E., and T. L. Bannerman.** 1994. Update on clinical significance of coagulase-negative staphylococci. *Clin. Microbiol. Rev.* **7:**117–140.
117. **Kloos, W. E., and T. L. Bannerman.** 1999. *Staphylococcus* and *Micrococcus*, p. 264–282. *In* P. R. Murray et al. (ed.), *Manual of Clinical Microbiology, 7th ed.* ASM Press, Washington D.C.
118. **Kloos, W. E., and K. H. Schleifer.** 1976. Characterization of *Staphylococcus sciuri* sp. nov. and its subspecies. *Int. J. Syst. Bacteriol.* **26:**22–37.
119. **Kloos, W. E., D. N. Ballard, J. A. Webster, R. J. Hubner, A. Tomasz, I. Couto, G. L. Sloan, H. P. Dehart, F. Fiedler, K. Schubert, H. de Lencastre, I. S. Sanches, H. E. Heath, P. A. Leblanc, and A. Ljungh.** 1997. Ribotype delineation and description of *Staphylococcus sciuri* subspecies and their potential as reservoirs of methicillin resistance and staphylolytic enzyme genes. *Int. J. Syst. Bacteriol.* **47:**313–323.
120. **Kloos, W. E., C. G. George, J. S. Olgiate, L. Van Pelt, M. L. McKinnon, B. L. Zimmer, E. Muller, M. P. Weinstein, and S. Mirrett.** 1998. *Staphylococcus hominis* subsp. *novobiosepticus* subsp. nov., a novel trehalose- and *N*-acetyl-D-glucosamine-negative, novobiocin- and multiple-antibiotic-resistant subspecies isolated from human blood cultures. *Int. J. Syst. Bacteriol.* **48:**799–812.
121. **Lambert, L. H., T. Cox, K. Mitchell, R. A. Rossello-Mora, C. Del Cueto, D. E. Dodge, P. Orkand, and R. J. Cano.** 1998. *Staphylococcus succinus* sp. nov., isolated from Dominican amber. *Int. J. Syst. Bacteriol.* **48:**511–518.
122. **Lancefield, R. C.** 1933. A serological differentiation of human and other groups of hemolytic streptococci. *J. Exp. Med.* **57:**571–595.
123. **Lange, C. C., M. Cardoso, D. Senczek, and S. Schwarz.** 1999. Molecular subtyping of *Staphylococcus aureus* from cases of bovine mastitis in Brazil. *Vet. Microbiol.* **67:**127–141.
124. **Lange, C. C., C. Werckenthin, and S. Schwarz.** 2003. Molecular analysis of the plasmid-borne *aacA/aphD* resistance gene region of coagulase-negative staphylococci from chickens. *J. Antimicrob. Chemother.* **51:**1397–1401.
125. **Lee, J. H.** 2003. Methicillin (oxacillin)-resistant *Staphylococcus aureus* strains isolated from major food animals and their potential transmission to humans. *Appl. Environ. Microbiol.* **69:**6489–6494.
126. Reference deleted.
127. **Leigh, J. A.** 1999. *Streptococcus uberis*: a permanent barrier to the control of bovine mastitis? *Vet. J.* **157:**225–238.
128. **Lilenbaum, W., E. L. Nunes, and M. A. Azeredo.** 1998. Prevalence and antimicrobial susceptibility of staphylococci isolated from the skin surface of clinically normal cats. *Lett. Appl. Microbiol.* **27:**224–228.
129. **Lilenbaum, W., A. L. Esteves, and G. N. Souza.** 1999. Prevalence and antimicrobial susceptibility of staphylococci

isolated from saliva of clinically normal cats. *Lett. Appl. Microbiol.* **28:**448–452.

130. **Lilenbaum, W., M. Veras, E. Blum, and G. N. Souza.** 2000. Antimicrobial susceptibility of staphylococci isolated from otitis externa in dogs. *Lett. Appl. Microbiol.* **31:**42–45.

131. **Lina, G., Y. Piemont, F. Godail-Gamot, M. Bes, M. O. Peter, V. Gauduchon, F. Vandenesch, and J. Etienne.** 1999. Involvement of Panton-Valentine leukocidin-producing *Staphylococcus aureus* in primary skin infections and pneumonia. *Clin. Infect. Dis.* **29:**1128–1132.

132. **Lloyd, D. H., A. I. Lamport, and C. Feeney.** 1996. Sensitivity to antibiotics amongst cutaneous and mucosal isolates of canine pathogenic staphylococci in the UK, 1980–96. *Vet. Dermatol.* **7:**171–175.

133. **Loeza-Lara, P. D., M. Soto-Huipe, V. M. Baizabal-Aguirre, A. Ochoa-Zarzosa, J. J. Valdez-Alarcon, H. Cano-Camacho, and J. E. Lopez-Meza.** 2004. pBMSa1, a plasmid from a dairy cow isolate of *Staphylococcus aureus*, encodes a lincomycin resistance determinant and replicates by the rolling-circle mechanism. *Plasmid* **52:**48–56.

134. **Lüthje, P., G. Luhofer, M. Zschöck, P. Krabisch, and S. Schwarz.** 2004. Susceptibility of coagulase-negative staphylococci from cases of bovine subclinical mastitis to pirlimycin and other antimicrobial agents. *Int. J. Med. Microbiol.* **294:**222.

135. **MacFarlane, G.** 1984. *Alexander Fleming: the Man and the Myth.* Harvard University Press, Cambridge, Mass.

136. **Manian, F. A.** 2003. Asymptomatic nasal carriage of mupirocin-resistant, methicillin-resistant *Staphylococcus aureus* (MRSA) in a pet dog associated with MRSA infection in household contacts. *Clin. Infect. Dis.* **36:**e26–e28.

137. **Marie, J., H. Morvan, F. Berthelot-Herault, P. Sanders, I. Kempf, A. V. Gautier-Bouchardon, E. Jouy, and M. Kobisch.** 2002. Antimicrobial susceptibility of *Streptococcus suis* isolated from swine in France and from humans in different countries between 1996 and 2000. *J. Antimicrob. Chemother.* **50:**201–209.

138. **Martel, A., M. Baele, L. A. Devriese, H. Goossens, H. J. Wisselink, A. Decostere, and F. Haesebrouck.** 2001. Prevalence and mechanism of resistance against macrolides and lincosamides in *Streptococcus suis* isolates. *Vet. Microbiol.* **83:**287–297.

139. **Martinez, G., J. Harel, R. Higgins, S. Lacouture, D. Daignault, and M. Gottschalk.** 2000. Characterization of *Streptococcus agalactiae* isolates of bovine and human origin by randomly amplified polymorphic DNA analysis. *J. Clin. Microbiol.* **38:**71–78.

140. **Mdegela, R. H., L. J. Kusiluka, A. M. Kapaga, E. D. Karimuribo, F. M. Turuka, A. Bundala, F. Kivaria, B. Kabula, A. Manjurano, T. Loken, and D. M. Kambarage.** 2004. Prevalence and determinants of mastitis and milk-borne zoonoses in smallholder dairy farming sector in Kibaha and Morogoro districts in Eastern Tanzania. *J. Vet. Med. B* **51:**123–128.

141. **Medleau, L., R. E. Long, J. Brown, and W. H. Miller.** 1986. Frequency and antimicrobial susceptibility of *Staphylococcus* species isolated from canine pyodermas. *Am. J. Vet. Res.* **47:**229–231.

142. **Mendonca-Souza, C. R., M. da G. Carvalho, R. R. Barros, C. A. Dias, J. L. Sampaio, A. C. Castro, R. R. Facklam, and L. M. Teixeira.** 2004. Occurrence and characteristics of erythromycin-resistant *Streptococcus pneumoniae* strains isolated in three major Brazilian states. *Microb. Drug Resist.* **10:**313–320.

143. **Montanari, M. P., I. Cochetti, M. Mingoia, and P. E. Varaldo.** 2003. Phenotypic and molecular characterization of tetracycline- and erythromycin-resistant strains of *Streptococcus pneumoniae. Antimicrob. Agents Chemother.* **47:** 2236–2241.

144. Reference deleted.

145. **Munckhof, W. J., S. L. Kleinschmidt, and J. D. Turnidge.** 2004. Resistance development in community-acquired strains of methicillin-resistant *Staphylococcus aureus*: an in vitro study. *Int. J. Antimicrob. Agents* **24:**605–608.

146. **Musser, J. M., S. J. Mattingly, R. Quentin, A. Goudeau, and R. K. Selander.** 1989. Identification of a high-virulence clone of type III *Streptococcus agalactiae* (group B *Streptococcus*) causing invasive neonatal disease. *Proc. Natl. Acad. Sci. USA* **86:**4731–4735.

146a. **Myllyniemi, A.-L., V. Gindonis, S. Nykäsenoja, and J. Koppinen.** 2004. *FINRES-Vet 2002–2003, Finnish Veterinary Antimicrobial Resistance Monitoring and Consumption of Antimicrobial Agents.* National Veterinary and Food Research Institute, Helsinki, Finland.

147. **Naimi, T. S., K. H. LeDell, K. Como-Sabetti, S. M. Borchardt, D. J. Boxrud, J. Etienne, S. K. Johnson, F. Vandenesch, S. Fridkin, C. O'Boyle, R. N. Danila, and R. Lynfield.** 2003. Comparison of community- and health care-associated methicillin-resistant *Staphylococcus aureus* infection. *JAMA* **290:**2976–2984.

148. **National Committee for Clinical Laboratory Standards.** 2002. Performance standards for antimicrobial disk and dilution susceptibility tests for bacteria isolated from animals. Approved standard, 2nd ed. NCCLS document M31-A2. National Committee for Clinical Laboratory Standards, Wayne, Pa.

148a. **National Veterinary Institute.** 2003. *SVARM 2002: Swedish Veterinary Antimicrobial Resistance Monitoring.* National Veterinary Institute, Uppsala, Sweden.

149. **Nawaz, M. S., A. A. Khan, S. A. Khan, D. D. Paine, J. V. Pothuluri, and C. E. Cerniglia.** 1999. Biochemical and molecular characterization of erythromycin resistant avian *Staphylococcus* spp. isolated from chickens. *Poult. Sci.* **78:** 1191–1197.

150. **Nawaz, M. S., S. A. Khan, A. A. Khan, F. M. Khambaty, and C. E. Cerniglia.** 2000. Comparative molecular analysis of erythromycin-resistance determinants in staphylococcal isolates of poultry and human origin. *Mol. Cell. Probes* **14:** 311–319.

151. **Noble, W. C., and R. P. Allaker.** 1992. Staphylococci on the skin of pigs: isolates from two farms with different antibiotic policies. *Vet. Rec.* **130:**466–468.

152. **Nomoto, R., L. I. Munasinghe, D.-H. Jin, Y. Shimahara, H. Yasuda, A. Nakamura, N. Misawa, T. Itami, and T. Yoshida.** 2004. Lancefield group C *Streptococcus dysgalactiae* infection responsible for fish mortalities in Japan. *J. Fish Dis.* **27:**679–686.

153. **NORM and NORM-VET.** 2003. *NORM/NORM-VET 2002: Consumption of Antimicrobial Agents and Occurrence of Antimicrobial Resistance in Norway.* NORM, Tromsø, Norway, and NORM-VET, Oslo, Norway.

154. **North, E. A., and R. Christie.** 1946. Acquired resistance of staphylococci to the action of penicillin. *Med. J. Aust.* **1:**176–179.

155. **Oughton, M., H. Dick, B. M. Willey, A. McGeer, and D. E. Low.** 2001. Methicillin-resistant *Staphylococcus aureus* (MRSA) as a cause of infections in domestic animals: evidence for a new humanotic disease? *Can. Bacterial Surveill. Network Newsl.* **April:**1–2.

156. **Ozaki, K., T. Yamagami, K. Nomura, M. Haritani, Y. Tsutsumi, and I. Narama.** 2003. Abscess-forming inflammatory granulation tissue with Gram-positive cocci and prominent

eosinophil infiltration in cats: possible infection of methicillin-resistant *Staphylococcus. Vet. Pathol.* **40:** 283–287.

157. **Pak, S. I., H. R. Han, and A. Shimizu.** 1999. Characterization of methicillin-resistant *Staphylococcus aureus* isolated from dogs in Korea. *J. Vet. Med. Sci.* **61:**1013–1018.

158. **Pellerin, J. L., P. Bourdeau, H. Sebbag, and J. M. Person.** 1998. Epidemiosurveillance of antimicrobial compound resistance of *Staphylococcus intermedius* clinical isolates from canine pyodermas. *Comp. Immunol. Microbiol. Infect. Dis.* **21:**115–133.

159. **Perch, B., K. B. Pedersen, and J. Henrichsen.** 1983. Serology of capsulated streptococci pathogenic for pigs: six new serotypes of *Streptococcus suis. J. Clin. Microbiol.* **17:** 993–996.

160. **Petersen, A. D., R. D. Walker, M. M. Bowman, H. C. Schott II, and E. J. Rosser, Jr.** 2002. Frequency of isolation and antimicrobial susceptibility patterns of *Staphylococcus intermedius* and *Pseudomonas aeruginosa* isolates from canine skin and ear samples over a 6-year period (1992–1997). *J. Am. Anim. Hosp. Assoc.* **38:**407–413.

161. **Phillips, W. E., Jr., and B. J. Williams.** 1984. Antimicrobial susceptibility patterns of canine *Staphylococcus intermedius* isolates from veterinary clinical specimens. *Am. J. Vet. Res.* **45:**2376–2379.

162. **Phuektes, P., P. D. Mansell, R. S. Dyson, N. D. Hooper, J. S. Dick, and G. F. Brown.** 2001. Molecular epidemiology of *Streptococcus uberis* isolates from dairy cows with mastitis. *J. Clin. Microbiol.* **39:**1460–1466.

163. **Piriz, S., J. Valle, E. M. Mateos, R. de la Fuente, D. Cid, J. A. Ruiz-Santaquiteria, and S. Vadillo.** 1996. *In vitro* activity of fifteen antimicrobial agents against methicillin-resistant and methicillin-susceptible *Staphylococcus intermedius. J. Vet. Pharmacol. Ther.* **19:**118–123.

164. **Pitkälä, A., M. Haveri, S. Pyorala, V. Myllys, and T. Honkanen-Buzalski.** 2004. Bovine mastitis in Finland 2001—prevalence, distribution of bacteria, and antimicrobial resistance. *J. Dairy Sci.* **87:**2433–2441.

165. **Place, R. B., D. Hiestand, S. Burri, and M. Teuber.** 2002. *Staphylococcus succinus* subsp. *casei* subsp. nov., a dominant isolate from a surface ripened cheese. *Syst. Appl. Microbiol.* **25:**353–359.

166. **Place, R. B., D. Hiestand, H. R. Gallmann, and M. Teuber.** 2003. *Staphylococcus equorum* subsp. *linens*, subsp. nov., a starter culture component for surface ripened semi-hard cheeses. *Syst. Appl. Microbiol.* **26:**30–37.

167. **Poyart, C., L. Jardy, G. Quesne, P. Berche, and P. Trieu-Cuot.** 2003. Genetic basis of antibiotic resistance in *Streptococcus agalactiae* strains isolated in a French hospital. *Antimicrob. Agents Chemother.* **47:**794–797.

168. **Priebe, S., and S. Schwarz.** 2003. *In vitro* activities of florfenicol against bovine and porcine respiratory tract pathogens. *Antimicrob. Agents Chemother.* **47:**2703–2705.

169. **Prieto, C., J. Pena, P. Suarez, M. Imaz, and J. M. Castro.** 1993. Isolation and distribution of *Streptococcus suis* capsular types from diseased pigs in Spain. *Zentbl. Veterinärmed B* **40:**544–548.

170. **Probst, A. J., C. Hertel, L. Richter, L. Wassill, W. Ludwig, and W. P. Hammes.** 1998. *Staphylococcus condimenti* sp. nov., from soy sauce mash, and *Staphylococcus carnosus* (Schleifer and Fischer 1982) subsp. *utilis* subsp. nov. *Int. J. Syst. Bacteriol.* **48:**651–658.

171. **Rajala-Schultz, P. J., K. L. Smith, J. S. Hogan, and B. C. Love.** 2004. Antimicrobial susceptibility of mastitis pathogens from first lactation and older cows. *Vet. Microbiol.* **102:** 33–42.

172. **Rasmussen, S. R., F. M. Aarestrup, N. E. Jensen, and S. E. Jorsal.** 1999. Associations of *Streptococcus suis* serotype 2 ribotype profiles with clinical disease and antimicrobial resistance. *J. Clin. Microbiol.* **37:**404–408.

173. **Rather, P. N., A. P. Davis, and B. J. Wilkinson.** 1986. Slime production by bovine milk *Staphylococcus aureus* and identification of coagulase-negative staphylococcal isolates. *J. Clin. Microbiol.* **23:**858–862.

174. **Reinert, R. R., C. Franken, M. van der Linden, R. Lutticken, M. Cil, and A. Al-Lahham.** 2004. Molecular characterisation of macrolide resistance mechanisms of *Streptococcus pneumoniae* and *Streptococcus pyogenes* isolated in Germany, 2002–2003. *Int. J. Antimicrob. Agents* **24:**43–47.

175. **Renneberg, J., and V. T. Rosdahl.** 1992. Epidemiological studies of penicillin resistance in Danish *Staphylococcus aureus* strains in the period 1977–1990. *Scand. J. Infect. Dis.* **24:**401–409.

176. **Rich, M., and L. Roberts.** 2004. Methicillin-resistant *Staphylococcus aureus* isolates from companion animals. *Vet. Rec.* **154:**310.

177. **Roberts, M. C., and M. B. Brown.** 1994. Macrolide-lincosamide resistance determinants in streptococcal species isolated from the bovine mammary gland. *Vet. Microbiol.* **40:**253–261.

178. **Rosenbach, F. J.** 1884. *Mikroorganismen bei den Wundinfektionskrankheiten des Menschen.* J. F. Bergmann, Wiesbaden, Germany.

179. **Rossitto, P. V., L. Ruiz, Y. Kikuchi, K. Glenn, K. Luiz, J. L. Watts, and J. S. Cullor.** 2002. Antibiotic susceptibility patterns for environmental streptococci isolated from bovine mastitis in central California dairies. *J. Dairy Sci.* **85:**132–138.

180. **Rouch, D. A., M. E. Byrne, Y. C. Kong, and R. A. Skurray.** 1987. The *aacA-aphD* gentamicin and kanamycin resistance determinant of Tn*4001* from *Staphylococcus aureus*: expression and nucleotide sequence analysis. *J. Gen. Microbiol.* **133:**3039–3052.

181. **Rowland, S. J., and K. G. H. Dyke.** 1989. Characterization of the staphylococcal β-lactamase transposon Tn*552*. *EMBO J.* **8:**2761–2773.

182. **Sachdé, F., S. Schwarz, C. Werckenthin, and C. Lämmler.** 1997. Tetracycline and minocycline resistance in *Streptococcus suis. Med. Sci. Res.* **25:**11–13.

183. **Sandford, E. E., and A. M. E. Tilker.** 1989. *Streptococcus suis* antimicrobial susceptibility. *Can. Vet. J.* **30:**679–680.

184. **Santos Sanches, I., R. Mato, H. de Lencastre, and A. Tomasz; CEM/NET Collaborators and the International Collaborators.** 2000. Patterns of multidrug resistance among methicillin-resistant hospital isolates of coagulase-positive and coagulase-negative staphylococci collected in the international multicenter study RESIST in 1997 and 1998. *Microb. Drug Resist.* **6:**199–211.

185. **Schalm, O. W., E. J. Carroll, and N. C. Jain.** 1971. *Bovine Mastitis.* Lea and Febiger, Philadelphia, Pa.

186. **Schleifer, K. H., and R. Kilpper-Balz.** 1984. Transfer of *Streptococcus faecalis* and *Streptococcus faecium* to the genus *Enterococcus* nom. rev. as *Enterococcus faecalis* comb. nov. and *Enterococcus faecium* comb. nov. *Int. J. Syst. Bacteriol.* **34:**31–34.

187. **Schleifer, K. H., J. Kraus, C. Dvorak, R. Kilpper-Balz, M. D. Collins, and W. Fischer.** 1985. Transfer of *Streptococcus lactis* and related streptococci to the genus *Lactococcus* gen. nov. *Syst. Appl. Microbiol.* **6:**183–195.

188. **Schwarz, S.** 1994. Emerging chloramphenicol resistance in *Staphylococcus lentus* from mink following chloramphenicol treatment: characterisation of the resistance genes. *Vet. Microbiol.* **41:**51–61.

189. **Schwarz, S., and H. Blobel.** 1989 Plasmids and resistance to antimicrobial agents and heavy metals in *Staphylococcus hyicus* from pigs and cattle. *Zentbl. Veterinärmed. B* **36:** 669–673.
190. **Schwarz, S., and H. Blobel.** 1990. A new streptomycin-resistance plasmid from *Staphylococcus hyicus* and its structural relationship to other staphylococcal resistance plasmids. *J. Med. Microbiol.* **32:**201–205.
191. **Schwarz, S., and Z. Wang.** 1993. Tetracycline resistance in *Staphylococcus intermedius. Lett. Appl. Microbiol.* **17:**88–91.
192. **Schwarz, S., and W. C. Noble.** 1994. Tetracycline resistance genes in staphylococci from the skin of pigs. *J. Appl. Bacteriol.* **76:**320–326.
193. **Schwarz, S., and W.C. Noble.** 1994. Structure and putative origin of a plasmid from *Staphylococcus hyicus* that mediates chloramphenicol and streptomycin resistance. *Lett. Appl. Microbiol.* **18:**281–284.
194. **Schwarz, S., and S. Grölz-Krug.** 1991. A chloramphenicol-streptomycin-resistance plasmid from a clinical strain of *Staphylococcus sciuri* and its structural relationship to other staphylococcal plasmids. *FEMS Microbiol. Lett.* **66:**319–322.
195. **Schwarz, S., M. Cardoso, and H. Blobel.** 1989. Plasmid-mediated chloramphenicol resistance in *Staphylococcus hyicus. J. Gen. Microbiol.* **135:**3329–3336.
196. **Schwarz, S., H. C. Wegener, and H. Blobel.** 1990. Plasmid-encoded resistance to macrolides and lincosamides in *Staphylococcus hyicus. J. Appl. Bacteriol.* **69:**845–849.
197. **Schwarz, S., I. W. Wibawan, and C. Lammler.** 1994. Distribution of genes conferring combined resistance to tetracycline and minocycline among group B streptococcal isolates from humans and various animals. *Zentbl. Bakteriol.* **281:**526–533.
198. **Schwarz, S., P. D. Gregory, C. Werckenthin, S. Curnock, and K. G. H. Dyke.** 1996. A novel plasmid from *Staphylococcus epidermidis* specifying resistance to kanamycin, neomycin and tetracycline. *J. Med. Microbiol.* **45:**57–63.
199. **Schwarz, S., M. C. Roberts, C. Werckenthin, Y. Pang, and C. Lange.** 1998. Tetracycline resistance in *Staphylococcus* spp. from domestic animals. *Vet. Microbiol.* **63:**217–227.
200. **Schwarz, S., C. Werckenthin, and C. Kehrenberg.** 2000. Identification of a plasmid-borne chloramphenicol-florfenicol resistance gene in *Staphylococcus sciuri. Antimicrob. Agents Chemother.* **44:**2530–2533.
201. **Schwarz, S., C. Kehrenberg, and K. K. Ojo.** 2002. *Staphylococcus sciuri* gene *erm*(33), encoding inducible resistance to macrolides, lincosamides, and streptogramin B antibiotics, is a product of recombination between *erm*(C) and *erm*(A). *Antimicrob. Agents Chemother.* **46:**3621–3623.
202. **Seguin, J. C., R. D. Walker, J. P. Caron, W. E. Kloos, C. G. George, R. J. Hollis, R. N. Jones, and M. A. Pfaller.** 1999. Methicillin-resistant *Staphylococcus aureus* outbreak in a veterinary teaching hospital: potential human-to-animal transmission. *J. Clin. Microbiol.* **37:**1459–1463.
203. **Seol, B., Z. Kelneric, D. Hajsig, J. Madic, and T. Naglic.** 1996. Susceptibility to antimicrobial agents of *Streptococcus suis* capsular type 2 strains isolated from pigs. *Zentbl. Bakteriol.* **283:**328–331.
204. **Seral, C., F. J. Castillo, M. C. Rubio-Calvo, A. Fenoll, C. Garcia, and R. Gomez-Lus.** 2001. Distribution of resistance genes *tet*(M), *aph3'-III*, *catpC194* and the integrase gene of Tn*1545* in clinical *Streptococcus pneumoniae* harbouring *erm*(B) and *mef*(A) genes in Spain. *J. Antimicrob. Chemother.* **47:** 863–866.
205. **Shaw, K. J., P. N. Rather, R. S. Hare, and G. H. Miller.** 1993. Molecular genetics of aminoglycoside resistance genes and familial relationships of the aminoglycoside-modifying enzymes. *Microbiol. Rev.* **57:**138–163.
206. **Sherman, J. M.** 1937. The streptococci. *Bacteriol. Rev.* **1:** 3–97.
207. **Shimizu, A., J. Kawano, C. Yamamoto, O. Kakutani, T. Anzai, and M. Kamada.** 1997. Genetic analysis of equine methicillin-resistant *Staphylococcus aureus* by pulsed-field gel electrophoresis. *J. Vet. Med. Sci.* **59:**935–937.
208. **Shimizu, A., Y. Wakita, S. Nagase, M. Okabe, T. Koji, T. Hayashi, N. Nagase, A. Sasaki, J. Kawano, K. Yamashita, and M. Takagi.** 2001. Antimicrobial susceptibility of *Staphylococcus intermedius* isolated from healthy and diseased dogs. *J. Vet. Med. Sci.* **63:**357–360.
209. **Sihvonen, L., D. N. Kurl, and J. Henrichsen.** 1988. *Streptococcus suis* isolated from pigs in Finland. *Acta Vet. Scand.* **29:**9–13.
210. **Skov, R., T. J. Williams, L. Pallesen, V. T. Rosdahl, and F. Espersen.** 1995. Beta-lactamase production and genetic location in *Staphylococcus aureus*: introduction of a beta-lactamase plasmid in strains of phage group II. *J. Hosp. Infect.* **30:**111–124.
211. **Slaughter, D. M., T. G. Patton, G. Sievert, R. J. Sobieski, and S. S. Crupper.** 2001. Antibiotic resistance in coagulase-negative staphylococci isolated from Cope's gray treefrogs (*Hyla chrysoscelis*). *FEMS Microbiol. Lett.* **205:** 265–270.
212. **Soedarmanto, I., S. Schwarz, B. Liebisch, and C. Lämmler.** 1995. Tetracycline resistance determinants among streptococci of serological groups G and L. *Vet. Microbiol.* **45:** 331–337.
213. **Spergser, J., M. Wieser, M. Taubel, R. A. Rossello-Mora, R. Rosengarten, and H. J. Busse.** 2003. *Staphylococcus nepalensis* sp. nov., isolated from goats of the Himalayan region. *Int. J. Syst. Evol. Microbiol.* **53:**2007–2011.
214. **Stemper, M. E., S. K. Shukla, and K. D. Reed.** 2004. Emergence and spread of community-associated methicillin-resistant *Staphylococcus aureus* in rural Wisconsin, 1989 to 1999. *J. Clin. Microbiol.* **42:**5673–5680.
215. **Stuart, J. G., E. J. Zimmerer, and R. L. Maddux.** 1992. Conjugation of antibiotic resistance in *Streptococcus suis. Vet. Microbiol.* **30:**213–222.
216. Reference deleted.
217. **Tarradas, C., I. Luque, D. de Andres, Y. E. Abdel-Aziz Shahein, P. Pons, F. Gonzalez, C. Borge, and A. Perea.** 2001. Epidemiological relationship of human and swine *Streptococcus suis* isolates. *J. Vet. Med. B* **48:**347–355.
218. **Tate, C. R., W. C. Mitchell, and R. G. Miller.** 1993. *Staphylococcus hyicus* associated with turkey stifle joint osteomyelitis. *Avian Dis.* **37:**905–907.
219. **Teale, C. J., S. Cobb, P. K. Martin, and G. Watkins.** 2002. *VLA Antimicrobial Sensitivity Report—2002*. DEFRA, London, United Kingdom.
220. **Teranishi, H., A. Shimizu, J. Kawano, and S. Kimura.** 1987. Antibiotic resistance of *Staphylococcus hyicus* subsp. *hyicus* strains isolated from pigs, cattle and chickens. *Nippon Juigaku Zasshi* **49:**427–432.
221. **Tian, Y., F. M. Aarestrup, and C. P. Lu.** 2004. Characterization of *Streptococcus suis* serotype 7 isolates from diseased pigs in Denmark. *Vet. Microbiol.* **103:**55–62.
222. **Tiemei, Z., F. Xiangqun, and L. Youning.** 2004. Resistance phenotypes and genotypes of erythromycin-resistant *Streptococcus pneumoniae* isolates in Beijing and Shenyang, China. *Antimicrob. Agents Chemother.* **48:**4040–4041.
223. **Tiemersma, E. W., S. L. Bronzwaer, O. Lyytikainen, J. E. Degener, P. Schrijnemakers, N. Bruinsma, J. Monen, W. Witte, and H. Grundman.** 2004. Methicillin-resistant *Staphylococcus aureus* in Europe, 1999–2002. *Emerg. Infect. Dis.* **10:** 1627–1634.

224. **Timms, L. L., and L. H. Schultz.** 1987. Dynamics and significance of coagulase-negative staphylococcal intramammary infections. *J. Dairy Sci.* **70:**2648–2657.

225. **Todhunter, D. A., L. L. Cantwell, K. L. Smith, K. H. Hoblet, and J. S. Hogan.** 1993. Characteristics of coagulase-negative staphylococci isolated from bovine intramammary infections. *Vet. Microbiol.* **34:**373–380.

226. **Tomlin, J., M. J. Pead, D. H. Lloyd, S. Howell, F. Hartmann, H. A. Jackson, and P. Muir.** 1999. Methicillin-resistant *Staphylococcus aureus* infections in 11 dogs. *Vet. Rec.* **144:**60–64.

227. **Trostle, S. S., C. L. Peavey, D. S. King, and F. A. Hartmann.** 2001. Treatment of methicillin-resistant *Staphylococcus epidermidis* infection following repair of an ulnar fracture and humeroradial joint luxation in a horse. *J. Am. Vet. Med. Assoc.* **218:**554–559.

228. **Vancraeynest, D., K. Hermans, A. Martel, M. Vaneechoutte, L. A. Devriese, and F. Haesebrouck.** 2004. Antimicrobial resistance and resistance genes in *Staphylococcus aureus* strains from rabbits. *Vet. Microbiol.* **101:**245–251.

229. **Vandamme, P., B. Pot, E. Falsen, K. Kersters, and L. A. Devriese.** 1996. Taxonomic study of Lancefield streptococcal groups C, G, and L (*Streptococcus dysgalactiae*) and proposal of *S. dysgalactiae* subsp. *equisimilis* subsp. nov. *Int. J. Syst. Bacteriol.* **46:**774–781.

229a. **van Duijkeren, E., A. T. Box, M. E. Heck, W. J. Wannet, and A. C. Fluit.** 2004. Methicillin-resistant staphylococci isolated from animals. *Vet. Microbiol.* **103:**91–97.

230. **Vela, A. I., J. Goyache, C. Tarradas, I. Luque, A. Mateos, M. A. Moreno, C. Borge, J. A. Perea, L. Dominguez, and J. F. Fernandez-Garayzabal.** 2003. Analysis of genetic diversity of *Streptococcus suis* clinical isolates from pigs in Spain by pulsed-field gel electrophoresis. *J. Clin. Microbiol.* **41:**2498–2502.

231. **Vela, A. I., M. A. Moreno, J. A. Cebolla, S. Gonzalez, M. V. Latre, L. Dominguez, and J. F. Fernandez-Garayzabal.** 2005. Antimicrobial susceptibility of clinical strains of *Streptococcus suis* isolated from pigs in Spain. *Vet. Microbiol.* **105:**143–147.

232. **Vernozy-Rozand, C., C. Mazuy, H. Meugnier, M. Bes, Y. Lasne, F. Fiedler, J. Etienne, and J. Freney.** 2000. *Staphylococcus fleurettii* sp. nov., isolated from goat's milk cheeses. *Int. J. Syst. Evol. Microbiol.* **50:**1521–1527.

233. **Vesterholm-Nielsen, M., M. Ø. Larsen, J. E. Olsen, and F. M. Aarestrup.** 1999. Occurrence of the *blaZ* gene in penicillin resistant *Staphylococcus aureus* isolated from bovine mastitis in Denmark. *Acta Vet. Scand.* **40:**279–286.

234. **Vieira, V. V., L. M. Teixeira, V. Zahner, H. Momen, R. R. Facklam, A. G. Steigerwalt, D. J. Benner, and A. C. D. Castro.** 1998. Genetic relationship among the different phenotypes of *Streptococcus dysgalactiae* strains. *Int. J. Syst. Bacteriol.* **48:**1231–1243.

235. **Vilaichone, R. K., W. Vilaichone, P. Nunthapisud, and H. Wilde.** 2002. *Streptococcus suis* infection in Thailand. *J. Med. Assoc. Thail.* **85:**109–117.

236. **Vintov, J., F. M. Aarestrup, C. E. Zinn, and J. E. Olsen.** 2003. Association between phage types and antimicrobial resistance among bovine *Staphylococcus aureus* from 10 countries. *Vet. Microbiol.* **95:**133–147.

237. **Vintov, J., F. M. Aarestrup, C. E. Zinn, and J. E. Olsen.** 2003. Phage types and antimicrobial resistance among Danish bovine *Staphylococcus aureus* isolates since the 1950s. *Vet. Microbiol.* **97:**63–72.

238. **Waage, S., J. Bjorland, D. A. Caugant, H. Oppegaard, T. Tollersrud, T. Mørk, and F. M. Aarestrup.** 2002. Spread of *Staphylococcus aureus* resistant to penicillin and tetracycline within and between dairy herds. *Epidemiol. Infect.* **129:**193–202.

239. **Wallmann, J., H. Kaspar, and R. Kroker.** 2004. Data on the prevalence of antimicrobial susceptibility of veterinary pathogens from cattle and pigs: national antibiotic resistance monitoring 2002/2003 of the BVL. *Berl. Münch. Tierärztl. Wochenschr.* **117:**480–492.

240. **Wannet, W., M. Heck, G. Pluister, E. Spalburg, M. Van Santen, X. Huijsdans, E. Tiemersma, and A. J. de Neeling.** 2004. Panton-Valentine leukocidin positive MRSA in 2003: the Dutch situation. *Euro Surveill.* **9.**

241. **Wasteson, Y., S. Hoie, and M. C. Roberts.** 1994. Characterization of antibiotic resistance in *Streptococcus suis*. *Vet. Microbiol.* **41:**41–49.

242. **Watts, J. L., and W. E. Owens.** 1989. Prevalence of staphylococcal species in four dairy herds. *Res. Vet. Sci.* **46:**1–4.

243. **Weese, J. S., M. Archambault, B. M. Willey, H. Dick, P. Hearn, B. N. Kreiswirth, B. Said-Salim, A. McGeer, Y. Likhoshvay, J. F. Prescott, and D. E. Low.** 2005. Methicillin-resistant *Staphylococcus aureus* in horses and horse personnel, 2000–2002. *Emerg. Infect. Dis.* **11:**430–435.

244. **Werckenthin, C., M. Cardoso, J.-L. Martel, and S. Schwarz.** 2001. Antimicrobial resistance in staphylococci from animals with particular reference to bovine *Staphylococcus aureus*, porcine *Staphylococcus hyicus*, and canine *Staphylococcus intermedius*. *Vet. Res.* **32:**341–362.

245. **Werckenthin, C., S. Schwarz, and K. G. H. Dyke.** 1996. Macrolide-lincosamide-streptogramin B resistance in *Staphylococcus lentus* results from the integration of part of a transposon into a small plasmid. *Antimicrob. Agents Chemother.* **40:**2224–2225.

246. **Werckenthin, C., S. Schwarz, and M. C. Roberts.** 1996. Integration of pT181-like tetracycline resistance plasmids into large staphylococcal plasmids involves IS*257*. *Antimicrob. Agents Chemother.* **40:**2542–2544.

247. **Werckenthin, C., and S. Schwarz.** 2000. Molecular analysis of the translational attenuator of a constitutively expressed *erm*(A) gene from *Staphylococcus intermedius*. *J. Antimicrob. Chemother.* **46:**785–788.

248. **Werckenthin, C., S. Schwarz, and H. Westh.** 1999. Structural alterations in the translational attenuator of constitutively expressed *erm*C genes. *Antimicrob. Agents Chemother.* **43:**1681–1685.

249. **Westh, H., C. S. Zinn, V. T. Rosdahl, and the SARISA Study Group.** 2004. An international multicenter study of antimicrobial consumption and resistance in *Staphylococcus aureus* isolates from 15 hospitals in 14 countries. *Microb. Drug Resist.* **10:**169–176.

250. **Williams, A. M., and M. D. Collins.** 1990. Molecular taxonomic studies on *Streptococcus uberis* type I and II. Description of *Streptococcus parauberis* sp. nov. *J. Appl. Bacteriol.* **68:**485–490.

251. **Wilson, C. D.** 1961. The treatment of staphylococcal mastitis. *Vet. Rec.* **73:**1019–1024.

252. **Wissing, A., J. Nicolet, and P. Boerlin.** 2001. The current antimicrobial resistance situation in Swiss veterinary medicine. *Schweiz. Arch. Tierheilkd.* **143:**503–510.

253. **Witte, W.** 2004. Glycopeptide resistant *Staphylococcus*. *J. Vet. Med. B* **51:**370–373.

254. **Witte, W., C. Braulke, C. Cuny, B. Strommenger, G. Werner, D. Heuck, U. Jappe, C. Wendt, H. J. Linde, and D. Harmsen.** 2005. Emergence of methicillin-resistant *Staphylococcus aureus* with Panton-Valentine leukocidin genes in central Europe. *Eur. J. Clin. Microbiol. Infect. Dis.* **24:**1–5.

255. **Yamane, A., H. Nakano, Y. Asahi, K. Ubukata, and M. Konno.** 1996. Directly repeated insertion of 9-nucleotide

sequence detected in penicillin-binding protein 2B gene of penicillin-resistant *Streptococcus pneumoniae*. *Antimicrob. Agents Chemother.* **40:**1257–1259.

256. **Yasuda, R., J. Kawano, H. Onda, M. Takagi, A. Shimizu, and T. Anzai.** 2000. Methicillin-resistant coagulase-negative staphylococci isolated from healthy horses in Japan. *Am. J. Vet. Res.* **61:**1451–1455.
257. **Yasuda, R., J. Kawano, E. Matsuo, T. Masuda, A. Shimizu, T. Anzai, and S. Hashikura.** 2002. Distribution of *mecA*-harboring staphylococci in healthy mares. *J. Vet. Med. Sci.* **64:**821–827.
258. **Yazdankhah, S. P., H. Sørum, and H. Oppegaard.** 2000. Comparison of genes involved in penicillin resistance in staphylococci of bovine origin. *Microb. Drug Resist.* **6:** 29–36.
259. **Yoshimura, H., M. Ishimaru, and A. Kojima.** 2002. Minimum inhibitory concentrations of 20 antimicrobial agents against *Staphylococcus aureus* isolated from bovine intramammary infections in Japan. *J. Vet. Med. B* **49:** 457–460.
260. **Younan, M., Z. Ali, S. Bornstein, and W. Muller.** 2001. Application of the California mastitis test in intramammary *Streptococcus agalactiae* and *Staphylococcus aureus* infections of camels (*Camelus dromedarius*) in Kenya. *Prev. Vet. Med.* **51:**307–316.
261. **Zadoks, R., W. van Leeuwen, H. Barkema, O. Sampimon, H. Verbrugh, Y. H. Schukken, and A. van Belkum.** 2000. Application of pulsed-field gel electrophoresis and binary typing tools in veterinary clinical microbiology and molecular epidemiological analysis of bovine and human *Staphylococcus aureus* isolates. *J. Clin. Microbiol.* **38:**1931–1939.
262. **Zakrzewska-Czerwinska, J., A. Gaszewska-Mastalarz, B. Lis, A. Gamian, and M. Mordarski.** 1995. *Staphylococcus pulvereri* sp. nov., isolated from human and animal specimens. *Int. J. Syst. Bacteriol.* **45:**169–172.
263. **Zinn, C. S., H. Westh, V. T. Rosdahl, and the SARISA Study Group.** 2004. An international multicenter study of antimicrobial resistance and typing of hospital *Staphylococcus aureus* isolates from 21 laboratories in 19 countries and states. *Microb. Drug Resist.* **10:**160–168.

Antimicrobial Resistance in Bacteria of Animal Origin
Edited by Frank M. Aarestrup

Chapter 13

Antimicrobial Drug Resistance in Fish Pathogens

HENNING SØRUM

In addition to their use in land animal husbandry, antimicrobial drugs are used in fish farming, including food and pet fish production, to control bacterial and mycotic infections (117, 120). Infected fish are treated as groups or populations. The drug is administered through the feed. Diseased individual fish do not get optimal levels of the drug in the body tissues because of loss of appetite, while healthy fish are able to gain higher levels of administrated antimicrobial drugs. In addition, the environment surrounding the fish, i.e., water, sediments, wild fish, and other biological systems, is exposed to the antimicrobial drug in a direct manner because the drug is dissolved in the water or spread with particles transported in the water surrounding the fish during treatment (37, 48, 111). This situation is dramatically different from the case with land animals. Air is not a significant medium for spread to the environment of antimicrobial drugs used for treatment of infections in animals.

As in modern husbandry with terrestrial animals, a large number of individuals are concentrated in limited areas in fish farming. The high density of individuals makes the single individual vulnerable to contraction of infections and the population in general vulnerable with regard to spread of infectious diseases between the individuals. This is considered to be the result of several factors, of which physiological and social stress caused by intense production is important. Stressed individuals often have reduced immune system functionality (51, 64, 100).

Since the use of antibiotics in animal husbandry started in the 1950s, antibacterial drugs have been used in controlling bacterial diseases in fish. The first report on acquired antibacterial resistance in fish-pathogenic bacteria dealt with sulfathiazole and tetracycline resistance in *Aeromonas salmonicida* isolated from brook trout in the United States in 1959 (50). In the 1970s several reports of drug resistance in fish pathogens from Japanese fish farms linked antibiotic resistance to fish farming (8) (see Table 2). Cultured fish in both freshwater and marine water have been treated with antibacterials in Japan, including such species as ayu (*Plecoglossus altivelis*), carp (*Cyprinus carpio*), eel (*Anguilla japonica*), tilapia (*Tilapia nilotica*), channel catfish (*Ictalurus punctatus*), largemouth bass (*Micropterus salmoides*), mullets (*Muogil cephalus*), sea bream (*Evynnis japonicus*), the salmonids amago (*Oncorhynchus rhodurus* f. *macrostomus*) and yamame (*Oncorhynchus masou ishikawae*) (8, 12), and yellowtail (*Seriola quinqueradiata*) (70).

Farming of Atlantic salmon increased substantially in the 1980s and 1990s and is still expanding in regions with cold marine coastlines, like Norway, Scotland, Ireland, Iceland, Canada, the United States, Chile, and Tasmania (42). Before effective vaccines against *Vibrio* and *Aeromonas* infections were developed, large amounts of antibiotics were used in disease control in farms with Atlantic salmon (57, 58, 83, 87). Effective vaccines against piscirickettsiosis (which is caused by *Piscirickettsia salmonis*) still have not been developed, resulting in the use of large amounts of quinolones in controlling this disease in Chile (40).

ADMINISTRATION OF ANTIBACTERIAL DRUGS

To control infections before hatching, fish eggs may be dipped in solutions containing disinfectants to kill bacteria adhering to the egg surface (35). In fish hatcheries with yolk sac larvae and small fry, antibacterial drugs may be used in bath treatments added directly to the water. However, in larger fish and in all marine fish, infections are treated with antibacterial drugs added to the feed, except for a few cases of brood stock fish treated with intraperitoneal

Henning Sørum • Department of Food Hygiene and Infection Biology, Norwegian School of Veterinary Science, Oslo, Norway.

injections of antibiotics (35). The process of producing the medicated feed is normally performed by the same feed mills that also make the regular feed for the fish (56).

In marine water the high level of salts may reduce the effect of the antibiotics, so larger amounts of antibiotics have to be administered to secure a sufficient level of active drug molecules (85, 105).

PRESCRIPTIONS OF ANTIBIOTICS AND MONITORING OF CONSUMPTION

The routines of acquiring antibiotics for treatment of farmed fish vary between countries. Use of prescriptions made by fish health veterinarians after proper diagnostic routines before medication of farmed fish is mandatory in the European Union, Norway, and other countries (56). Norwegian prescriptions for antibiotics used in fish farming are stored in a national register available for control and research (83). Denmark, Norway, Sweden, and the United Kingdom are currently monitoring the consumption of antimicrobials in fish farming (4–7).

ANTIBIOTIC RESISTANCE IN *A. SALMONICIDA*

A. salmonicida causes disease in fish of temperate and colder areas. Subspecies *salmonicida* causes furunculosis in salmonid fish, while other subspecies, also referred to as atypical strains, cause septicemia and infections in skin, muscles, and various organs in both salmonids and several other marine fish species (31).

Furunculosis in salmonid hatcheries in the United States was treated primarily with sulfonamides in the 1950s, and an early report on acquired sulfonamide resistance in *Aeromonas salmonicida* from Leetown, W.Va., in 1955 showed resistance in 36 of 47 isolates from brook trout (*Salvelinus fontinalis*) and brown trout (*Salmo trutta*) (118). In this report, the devastating effect of acquired sulfonamide resistance in the treatment of furunculosis was demonstrated in clinical trials. A strain isolated from diseased brook trout in 1959 by Snieszko (in Leetown, W.Va.) was designated the type strain of the species (ATCC 14174 or NCMB 833). This strain was later shown to contain transferable resistance to both sulfonamides and tetracyclines (8, 116). For comparison, it was at the end of the 1950s in Japan that transferable drug resistance was documented for the first time in a human pathogen (*Shigella*) (135). Later it was shown that R plasmids were the responsible genetic factors behind the transfer of resistance in both *Shigella* (135) and *A. salmonicida* (8). Half of the drug-resistant *A. salmonicida* isolates from salmonids in Japan in the 1960s had R plasmids as drug resistance gene carriers. The drugs rendered ineffective were sulfonamides, tetracyclines, chloramphenicol, and streptomycin, of which streptomycin was not used in the control of fish diseases.

A French collection of 104 isolates of *A. salmonicida* was in 1971 reported to be completely (100%) resistant to sulfonamides, but only 11.5% of the isolates were resistant to the antibiotics tetracycline, streptomycin, and/or chloramphenicol (103). The combination of resistance against tetracycline and/or chloramphenicol was transferred to *Escherichia coli* K-12, *A. salmonicida*, and *Aeromonas hydrophila*, together with sulfonamide resistance. Sulfonamide resistance in this strain collection was not transferred as a single resistance feature.

At the beginning of the 1970s, a study of the occurrence of drug resistance in *A. salmonicida* isolated from the intestinal tract of diseased, pond-reared amago (*O. rhodurus macrostomus*) and yamame (*O. masou ishikawae*) was performed in Japan (10). A total of 24 fish ponds from the Nagano, Gifu, Shiga, and Tokyo districts were studied, and all ponds were supplied with fresh, flowing water from springs or mountain streams. The drugs used for treatment of diseased fish in the ponds involved in the study were chloramphenicol, sulfonamides, and to a minor extent tetracyclines. All 20 of the *A. salmonicida* isolates found on media with chloramphenicol contained transferable R plasmids conferring resistance to sulfonamides, streptomycin, and chloramphenicol. On nonselective media, 3 of 21 isolates of *A. salmonicida* contained transferable R plasmids with the same resistance profile. Of three drug-resistant *A. salmonicida* isolates from three ponds, two had transferable R plasmids with the same resistance profile. A large portion of the *Aeromonas hydrophila* strains isolated from the pond-reared fish in this study also contained a transferable R plasmid conferring resistance to the same agents: sulfonamides, streptomycin, and chloramphenicol (10).

The transferable R plasmids with resistance to sulfonamides, streptomycin, and chloramphenicol isolated from both *A. salmonicida* and *A. hydrophila* were found to be of same size and same incompatibility group (25). It was known that no exchange of salmonid fish between different areas had occurred because of restrictions of such activity applied to reduce transmission of various infectious diseases of fish. In spite of that, the same R plasmid was detected in all fish farms in the four different districts in Japan. This indicated that the plasmid occurred naturally in the environmental flora of the freshwater systems of these districts.

In the period from 1979 to 1981, *A. salmonicida* from fish farms in eight districts in Japan, including farms from three of the four districts studied by Aoki et al. in 1972 (10), was investigated for occurrence of antibiotic resistance (26). Of 129 isolates, only 5 were found to be susceptible to all antibiotic drugs tested. The other isolates were found to be resistant to up to six drugs, quinolones and nitrofurans in particular. Only 2 of the 124 resistant isolates of *A. salmonicida* were found to transfer drug resistance by R plasmids. These two isolates had an R plasmid with a molecular mass of 29 MDa and conferred resistance against sulfonamides, chloramphenicol, and streptomycin. One of the plasmids (pJA8102-1) from strain MZ8102, isolated in 1981, and a similar plasmid (pAr-32) from strain Ar-32, isolated in 1970 (9), were studied in more molecular detail (15). The two *A. salmonicida* strains (MZ8101 and MZ8102) with a transferable R plasmid of 29 MDa both contained a nonconjugative but mobilizable R plasmid of 7.6 MDa that conferred resistance against tetracycline (29) (Table 1).

In Atlantic salmon (*Salmo salar*) farms in a narrow fjord system on the western coast of Norway (Hordaland County) in 1989, it was found that infections caused by atypical *A. salmonicida* could not be controlled with the quinolone drug oxolinic acid because of chromosomal quinolone resistance. These strains were, in addition, found to carry transferable resistance to sulfonamides, trimethoprim, and tetracyclines (see Table 5). An R plasmid of 25 MDa was found to be identical to an R plasmid isolated from salmon with furunculosis caused by *A. salmonicida* subsp. *salmonicida* in farms in the same area in 1991 (123, 125). The R plasmid was found to transfer with higher frequency from atypical *A. salmonicida* than from *A. salmonicida* subsp. *salmonicida* and with higher frequency on agar surface compared to broth as transfer medium (see Table 5).

The 25-MDa plasmid (pRAS1) was found to be an IncU plasmid harboring a class 1 integron with a *dfr16* cassette and the sulfonamide resistance gene *sul1*. Directly downstream of the integron was a deleted Tn*1721* with the Tet A tetracycline resistance determinant (Fig. 1 and Table 1). Comparison of restriction digests and other features such as transfer frequencies of pRAS1 with published results from studies of other R plasmids led to the observation that pAr-32 (9, 25) and pJA8102-1 (15, 26) from *A. salmonicida*, isolated more than 10 years apart in the Shiga and Miyazaki prefectures in Japan, respectively, were similar. It was found that these three R plasmids had the same backbone structure, but that the drug resistance region differed; pRAS1 had an In*4* of Tn*1696* followed by a truncated Tn*1721*, and pAr-32 had a complex class 1 integron structure of In6, as seen in the plasmid Sa (125) (Fig. 1).

In Atlantic salmon farms in Scotland, *A. salmonicida* isolates from 229 outbreaks of furunculosis in 44 units at 34 locations over 2 years in 1988 to 1990 were investigated for occurrence of antibiotic resistance (66). Among 304 isolates, 55% were found to be resistant to tetracyclines, 37% resistant to oxolinic acid, 31% resistant to sulfonamides, and 10% resistant to the combination of sulfonamides and trimethoprim. Among 40 oxytetracycline-resistant isolates, 11 transferred an R plasmid that encoded resistance to oxytetracycline and/or sulfonamides, trimethoprim, and streptomycin to *E. coli* (67). In a study of 29 oxytetracycline-resistant *A. salmonicida* isolates from Scotland, 19 transferred their tetracycline resistance to *E. coli* (1). The Norwegian pRAS1 plasmids isolated from *A. salmonicida* were included in this study, and restriction digests showed obvious similarity to the Scottish R plasmids, which were of similar size even if the featured resistance patterns were not identical. In another study, R plasmids featuring oxytetracycline resistance from mesophilic, motile *Aeromonas* spp. isolated from freshwater in a fish hatchery and from hospital sewage in England were studied molecularly (108). Six of 91 isolates from the fish hatchery water and 11 of 72 isolates from the hospital sewage water were found to transfer oxytetracycline resistance. Seven of the 11 R plasmids from *Aeromonas* spp. from sewage were shown to belong to the IncU group. These plasmids, three R plasmids from *A. salmonicida* originating in Scottish fish farms (1), and both pRAS1 and pIE420 (133) were included in the study, and all were verified to be identical or similar in their major structure.

A collection of five plasmids isolated from human clinical infections and hospital sewage in the German Democratic Republic and Czechoslovakia in the period from 1976 to 1979 was found to belong to the IncU group (133) (Table 1). Comparison of the restriction digests of these plasmids and those of pRAS1 showed a similarity between pRAS1 and all these IncU plasmids, including the IncU prototype plasmid RA3 isolated from *A. hydrophila* in Japan (identical to pAr-32). This similarity was not fully recognized by the authors, probably because most of the restriction sites digested by the common restriction enzymes were located in the variable drug resistance region of the IncU plasmids, which made the interpretation of the digests unconventional.

In the Shannon River ecosystem in Ireland, antibiotic-resistant *A. salmonicida* from Atlantic salmon was isolated in a hatchery during a period of

Table 1. Global distribution of transferable[a] R plasmids in aeromonads

Plasmid	Incompatibility group[b]	Size	Drug resistance region[c]	Source	Location	Period	Reference(s)
RA3 (prototype)	U	29 MDa	*int1, aadA2, orf513, catAII, Sul1*	*A. hydrophila*, infected	Japan	1969	9
pAr-32	U	29 MDa	*int1, aadA2, orf513, catAII, sul1*	*A. salmonicida*, infected Biwamasu salmon	Japan	1970	19
pJA8102-1	U	30 MDa	*int1, aadA2, orf513* (2 copies), *catAII, sul1*	*A. salmonicida*, infected salmonid	Japan	1981	26
pUG1001	U	40 Mda	Sm, Su, Tc, Tp	*A. salmonicida*, infected Atlantic salmon	Ireland	1979–1983	63
pRAS1	U	25 MDa, 45 kb	*int1, dfr16, sul1* IS*6100*, Tn*1721′*, Tet A	*A. salmonicida*, infected Atlantic salmon	Western Norway	1989	125
pASOT	U	47 kb	*int1, aadA2/dfr2c*, Tn*1721*, Tet A, Su	*A. salmonicida*, infected Atlantic salmon	Scotland	1982–1993	5, 108, 125
pASOT2	U	47 kb	*int1, aadA2*, Su, Tet A	*A. salmonicida*, infected Atlantic salmon	Scotland	1988–1993	5, 125
pASOT3	U	39 kb	*int1, aadA2*, Su, Tet A	*A. salmonicida*, infected Atlantic salmon	Scotland	1986–1990	5, 125
pIE420	U	26 MDa, 45 kb	Tet A, Su, Tm	*E. coli*, human pyelonephritis	German Democratic Republic	1976–1979	108, 133
pFBAOT6	U		Tet A, Tn*1721*	*A. caviae*, hospital effluent	England	1997	108
pJA896	U	42 kb	Cm, Sm, Su	*A. hydrophila*, infected eel and carp	Japan	1970	2
pU12652-97	U	58 kb	Tet A	*A. salmonicida*, atypical, infected fish	Northeastern United States		41
pF1		50 kb	*int1, dfr2c*, TetA, Su	*A. salmonicida*, infected Atlantic salmon	Faroe Islands	1991	112
RA1	C	86 MDa	Tet D, Su	*A. hydrophila*, infected	Japan	1970?	9
pJA5017	C	125 kb	*sul2*, Tc	*A. hydrophila*, infected eel and carp	Japan	1969	2
pTW64	C	125 kb	Tc, Su	*A. hydrophila*, infected eel and carp	Taiwan	1977	2
R1491	C	100 MDa	Cm, Sm, Tc	*A. salmonicida*, infected salmonid	England		63
p950704-2/2		150 kb	*int1, dfr1, ant(3″) 1a*, Tet A, Su	*A. salmonicida*, infected rainbow trout	Denmark	1995	112
pES10		78 kb	*sul2*, Cm, Km, Sm, Tc	*A. hydrophila*, infected channel catfish	Southern United States	1974	2, 78
pRAS2		48 kb	Tet 31, *sul2, strA-strB*, Tn*5393c*	*A. salmonicida*, infected Atlantic salmon	Norway	1992	80
pJA8102-2		11.4 kb	Tet C	*A. salmonicida*, infected salmonid	Japan	1981	29
pRAS3		11.8 kb	Tet C (ay043298), complete sequence	*A. salmonicida*, infected Atlantic salmon	Norway	1980, 1991	79

[a]All plasmids in this table are conjugative except pJA8102-2 and pRAS3, which have to be mobilized.
[b]Plasmids in the same incompatibility group cannot be stably inherited, indicating similarity.
[c]Phenotypic resistance determinants: Cm, chloramphenicol; Km, kanamycin; Sm, streptomycin; Su, sulfonamides; Tc, tetracycline; Tp, trimethoprim.

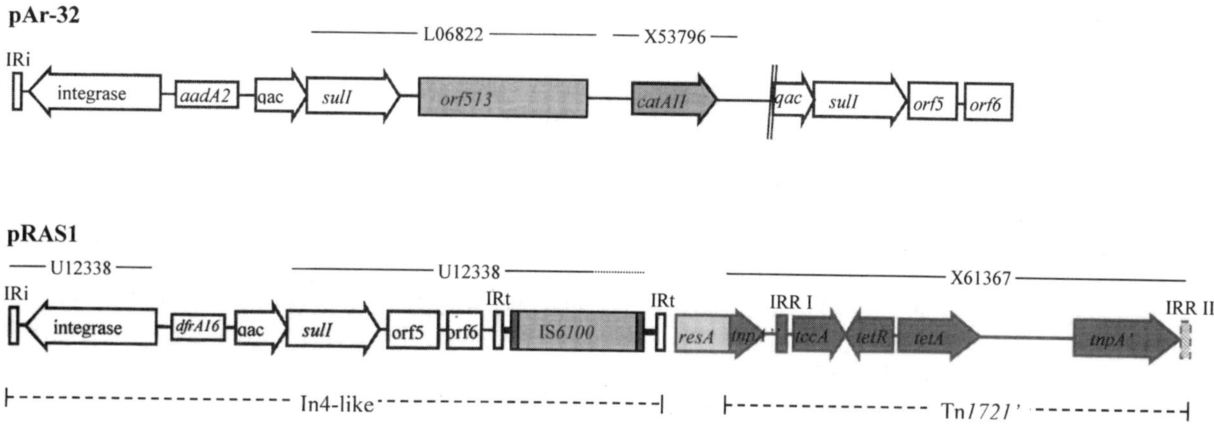

Figure 1. Comparison of the resistance-determining regions of pRAS1 and pAr-32. The areas of the plasmids that are the same as the sequences in Tn*1696* (EMBL accession number U12338), Tn*1721* (EMBL accession number X61367), pSa (EMBL accession number L06822), and *catA2* of *E. coli* (EMBL accession number X53796) are indicated by the lines at the top. The areas of pRAS1 with similarities to In*4* and Tn*1721* are indicated at the bottom. Reprinted from reference 125 with permission of the publisher.

8 years (1979 to 1986) (39). Forty-five isolates were studied, and only four were susceptible to all drugs included in the study. Resistance to sulfadiazine, spectinomycin, streptomycin, and trimethoprim was found in 24 strains, additional resistance to tetracycline was seen in 16 strains, and 1 strain was resistant to chloramphenicol as well. Chloramphenicol had been used in the control of furunculosis in the hatchery. All drug-resistant strains of *A. salmonicida* were found to harbor an IncU plasmid of 29 to 34 MDa. Restriction enzyme analysis using EcoRI showed a conserved pattern of seven DNA fragments from all plasmids. Transposition studies were performed, with combined transposition of trimethoprim, spectinomycin, and streptomycin as the result. These results indicated strongly that the IncU R plasmid that persisted in the hatchery resembled the Norwegian pRAS1, the German pIE420, and the similar plasmids isolated from the Scottish salmon farms. The transposition results might be explained by the occurrence of two drug resistance cassettes on the integron of the plasmid, probably the same *dfr1* and *ant(3")1a* cassette combination as was detected in *A. salmonicida* isolates from rainbow trout farms in Danish freshwater river systems (113).

After a period of 1 year with no disease in the hatchery in the Shannon River, an *A. salmonicida* isolate with the same R plasmid was isolated from a healthy carrier fish in the hatchery. This indicates that the sources of the strain with the IncU plasmid were the river water used in the hatchery and the feral fish. Alternatively, the R plasmid could have survived in bacteria on one of the mother fish. Subsequently, another year later, 49 isolates of *A. hydrophila* from the intake water to the hatchery were studied. In spite of a high level of multiple-drug-resistant isolates, only four isolates of *A. hydrophila* were found to transfer their drug resistance and the transconjugants were all found to contain an IncU R plasmid. A 60-MDa plasmid carrying resistance genes against chloramphenicol and tetracycline was also found in one strain of *A. hydrophila*, possibly explaining the source of chloramphenicol resistance in an isolate of *A. salmonicida* from the hatchery after use of chloramphenicol.

Transferable R plasmids from aeromonads isolated in Ireland (probably from the Shannon River study), England, France, and Japan (including pAr-32) were studied with regard to incompatibility (63). Both IncU and IncC plasmids were seen, in addition to a new Inc group. All the IncU plasmids were found to have a size of 30 to 40 MDa, while the other R plasmids were found to be larger. The authors suggested that the IncU plasmids belonged primarily to the aeromonads but that they might be transferred to other bacterial genera and acquire drug resistance factors that could be transferred back to aeromonads.

In a Danish study of 23 drug-resistant *A. salmonicida* isolates from 13 different freshwater rainbow trout farms, only 3 isolates transferred their R plasmid to *E. coli* (114). These three isolates transferred an R plasmid of 150 kb with resistance to oxytetracycline, sulfonamides, trimethoprim, and streptomycin. Also, three oxytetracycline- and sulfonamide-resistant isolates of *A. salmonicida* from Canada and one oxytetracycline-resistant isolate from the United States included as controls in the study transferred R plasmids of 140 to 160 kb. In the Danish study, drug-resistant isolates of *A. salmonicida* from Scotland (1) with transferable IncU R plasmids and an isolate with pRAS1 from Norway (125) were included as controls and the IncU plasmids were transferred. Five *A. salmonicida* isolates from the Faroe Islands resistant to oxytetracycline, sulfonamides, trimethoprim, and streptomycin were included in the study, and they transferred a 50-kb plasmid to *E. coli* encoding resistance to all the drugs that the donors were resistant against except streptomycin. Incompatibility typing was not performed; however, the R plasmids from the Faroe Islands were probably IncU plasmids, based on their size, the occurrence of integrons, and the drug resistance pattern.

Common to all the conjugable R plasmids, the majority of the strains containing plasmids of 150 kb, and all strains with reduced susceptibility to sulfonamides in the Danish study was that they contained class 1 integrons. The drug resistance cassette contents in *A. salmonicida* seemed to vary with the region from which they originated. Various trimethoprim resistance cassettes and the aminoglycoside resistance cassette *ant(3")1a* were found in the integrons. Three of four integrons from Canadian and U.S. strains of *A. salmonicida* did not contain any insert (114).

A. salmonicida strains from Norway, including 10 isolates of sulfonamide-resistant atypical strains representing the various groups of atypical *A. salmonicida* isolated in Norway (123), were screened for occurrence of class 1 integrons and sulfonamide resistance genes (78). In this study *A. salmonicida* isolates from Switzerland, Finland, France, Japan, Scotland, and the United States were also studied. It was shown that the class 1 integron was not widespread among sulfonamide-resistant atypical *A. salmonicida* strains isolated during a period of 25 years in Norway. Integrons were detected in the isolates of *A. salmonicida* from all the countries included. In isolates from France and Switzerland the *aadA1* cassette occurred in the integrons, while the *aadA2* cassette occurred in the Scottish integrons and in the pAr-32 from Japan. The *dfr16* cassette was isolated from both atypical and typical *A. salmonicida* isolates from Norway, while the *dfr2c* cassette was detected in trimethoprim-resistant Scottish isolates of *A. salmonicida*. In the French and Swiss isolates with tetracycline resistance the Tet E determinant was found, while in all other tetracycline-resistant isolates the Tet A determinant was present. In *A. hydrophila* isolates from farming of channel catfish in the southern United States, both Tet A and E determinants were found in combination in the same isolate (45).

In drug-resistant atypical *A. salmonicida* isolates from farmed and wild fish on the northeastern coasts of the United States and Canada, pRAS1-like R plasmids were detected. Seven of the nine isolates from the period 1992 to 2001 contained plasmids with the same genetic elements as pRAS1, including an integron with the *dfr16* cassette and a Tet A determinant in a Tn*1721* environment in the drug resistance region of the IncU plasmid, as was the case with pRAS1 isolated in salmon farms on the Norwegian coast (41). However, five of the seven pRAS1-like plasmids probably were identical to pRAS1, with an incomplete Tn*1721* with the Tet A determinant, while the other two strains had pRAS1-like plasmids that harbored a complete Tn*1721*.

A SMALL TETRACYCLINE RESISTANCE PLASMID

A nonconjugable R plasmid (pJA8102-2) of 11.4 kb (7.6 MDa) with a Tet C determinant responsible for tetracycline resistance was isolated from a Japanese *A. salmonicida* isolate (MZ8102) (29). This isolate originated from a diseased salmonid in a freshwater farm in 1981 (26). MZ8102 contained a conjugable R plasmid of 29 MDa (47 kb) (pJA81028-1) that was transferred to *E. coli* either alone or together with the small 11.4-kb pJA8102-2, which it mobilized. pJA8102-1 conferred resistance to chloramphenicol, sulfonamides, and streptomycin and was found to be closely related to the R plasmid pAr-32 isolated from *A. hydrophila* (15). The organization of the drug resistance region of pAr-32 and indirectly of pJA8102-1 was analyzed and compared to the drug resistance region of the R plasmid pRAS1 isolated from Norwegian *A. salmonicida* (125). These plasmids were identical except for differences in the compact drug resistance region.

The mobilizable pJA8102-2 was shown to contain a Tet C determinant similar to the Tet C in pSC101 originally isolated from a *Salmonella* isolate (29, 36) and later used in the construction of the plasmid vector pBR322. In both typical and atypical clinical isolates of *A. salmonicida* from Norway, a 12-kb mobilizable plasmid (pRAS3) containing the Tet C determinant has been found (79, 123). Comparison of complete DNA sequences of pRAS3 (11.8 kb) from both atypical and typical *A. salmonicida* isolates showed minor differences in the number of short repeats in the replication region and a limited number of single-base-pair differences in the Tet C determinant, indicating no recent or frequent transfer of pRAS3 between the two related *A. salmonicida* subspecies. It was found that the variant of pRAS3 from the typical strains, pRAS3.1, was the same as pJA8102-2 from Japan. A Scottish isolate of *A. salmonicida* with both the pRAS1-like IncU plasmid and a pRAS3-like plasmid was included in the study, and this isolate also contained a pRAS3.1 variant.

As with the Japanese pJA8102-2, pRAS3 was found to exist in the same isolate as pRAS1 in a few cases. In these instances pRAS3 could be transferred with the conjugable pRAS1 to *E. coli*, as was the case with pJA8102-2. This cotransfer of the coexisting pRAS1 and pRAS3 was the case with both pRAS3.1 in the typical *A. salmonicida* and pRAS3.2 in the atypical isolates (79).

Similarly, in a Danish study (114), another Scottish *A. salmonicida* isolate with a 13-kb plasmid with Tet C was found to mobilize this small plasmid by a coexisting integron-containing IncU R plasmid of 50 kb. In the Norwegian study (79), it was found that both pRAS3.1 in the typical *A. salmonicida* and pRAS3.2 in the atypical isolates in a few cases coexisted with and could be mobilized by pRAS1. In addition, it was found that pRAS3.1 coexisted with another conjugable, 49-kb R plasmid, pRAS2 (see next paragraph), in typical *A. salmonicida*. The coexistence of pRAS3 with pRAS1 or pRAS2 resulted in higher tetracycline MICs. The pRAS3 plasmid was shown to be highly related to a cryptic plasmid, pTF-FC2, seen in *Acidithiobacillus ferrooxidans* from mining environments in South Africa (79) except for the Tet C determinant, which seemed to be recombined from another source into the pTF-FC2 frame. The replication region of pTF-FC2 has some partial similarity to the replication region of the small R plasmid RSF1010.

In Norwegian isolates of *A. salmonicida*, both typical and atypical, a transferable R plasmid, pRAS2, of 27 MDa (49 kb) was found (80, 123). This plasmid contained the *sul2* gene, the *strA-strB* genes, and the novel Tet 31 determinant. The *strA-strB* genes resided in an active Tn*5393*-like transposon, as observed in plant-pathogenic bacteria (127). In animal- and human-pathogenic bacteria the *strA-strB* genes are often located on small RSF1010-like plasmids with only remnants of the Tn*5393* sequence and very close to the *sul2* gene. The organization of the *sul2* and *strA-strB* genes on pRAS2 indicated that this plasmid represented an ancestor of the common RSF1010-like plasmids in mammal pathogens (106).

OVERVIEW OF R PLASMIDS IN *A. SALMONICIDA*

The occurrence of a transferable R plasmid belonging to the IncU group in *A. salmonicida* isolates from various parts of the world in both freshwater systems and the marine environment is remarkable (Tables 1 and 2). This plasmid was identical except for the drug resistance region wherever it was sampled. Different drug resistance cassettes occurred in the integron. Directly downstream of the integron, genes of additional drug resistance factors located, for instance, in transposons might be present.

In Japan, it was found that *A. salmonicida* with the R plasmid (pJA8102-1) entered the various culture ponds of salmonids from the environment with no obvious epidemic spread of the salmonid pathogen between the different farms and districts. In Ireland, a similar scenario seemed to occur in the Shannon River. In the marine environment of the fjords of western Norway, pRAS1 was present. Since *A. salmonicida* may exist and produce disease in both freshwater and salt water, one could speculate that the plasmids were spread to the coastal waters by the rivers. However, in the sea farms of the Faroe Islands in the Atlantic Ocean, a parallel IncU plasmid was also seen in *A. salmonicida*. The Faroe Islands are small, with short rivers, and are surrounded by ocean water for hundreds of miles. There are reasons to believe that migrating anadrome Atlantic salmon may be responsible for the spread of drug-resistant isolates of *A. salmonicida* between the freshwater rivers of the Atlantic coasts and the marine environment of the Atlantic Ocean. A plausible explanation as to why the same R plasmid exists in Japanese isolates of *A. salmonicida* may be clearer if one considers the obvious global clonal appearance of the subspecies *salmonicida* of *A. salmonicida*. This subspecies was demonstrated to be very homogeneous in its genome and in its array of cryptic plasmids regardless of where the isolate originated (124). The IncU plasmid might be particularly successful in establishing itself in *A. salmonicida*.

However, the IncU plasmid is promiscuous and was found in *A. hydrophila* (see below), in atypical *A. salmonicida* on the coast of Norway and on the northern part of the east coast of North America, and in enterobacteria from humans in Eastern Europe. In 1985 Hedges et al. (63) suggested that the homogeneous IncU plasmids are characteristic of aeromonads but do occasionally transfer to and establish in other genera. The plasmids may acquire some of the genetic factors linked to drug resistance in the gene pools of these bacteria and subsequently ferry these back to aeromonads. However, one should not rule out the opposite possibility, namely, that these IncU plasmids may be ferrying antibiotic resistance factors from the ancient aquatic environments to our modern antibiotic-consuming microenvironments.

Table 2. Transferable[a] R plasmids in Japanese fish culturing

Plasmid	Incompatibility group[b]	Size	Resistance features[c]	Homology group[d]	Bacterial host	Fish host(s)	Yr	Reference
RA3	U	29 MDa	Cm, Sm, Su	1	*A. hydrophila*	Eel	1969	19
pAr-32	U	29 MDa	Cm, Sm, Su	1	*A. salmonicida*	Biwamasu salmon	1970	9
pJA8102-1	U	30 MDa	Cm, Sm, Su	1	*A. salmonicida*	Salmonid	1981	26
pJA8102-2		11.4 kb	Tc		*A. salmonicida*	Salmonid	1981	29
pJA896	U	42 kb	Cm, Sm, Su	1	*A. hydrophila*	Eel, carp	1970	2
RA1	C	86 MDa	Tc, Su	2	*A. hydrophila*	Eel	1969	19
pJA5017	C	125 kb	Tc, Su	2	*A. hydrophila*	Eel, carp	1969	2
pJA6018		120 kb	Tc, Su	2	*E. tarda*	Eel	1972	20
pJA6012		125 kb	Cm, Km, Sm, Su, Tc	2	*E. tarda*	Eel	1975	20
pAc8436		125 kb	Cm, Sm, Su, Tc	2	*E. tarda*	Eel	1984	27
p61K		120 kb	Tc, Su	3	*E. tarda*	Eel	1974	20
pAC8323		120 kb	Cm, Su, Tc	3	*E. tarda*	Eel	1983	27
pJAPE8232			Cm, Km, Su, Tc	2	*P. damselae* subsp. *piscicida*	Yellowtail	1982	70
pKP9033			Km, Su	2	*P. damselae* subsp. *piscicida*	Yellowtail	1990	70
pJA7324		185 kb	Cm, Sm, Su, Tc	4	*V. anguillarum*	Ayu	1973	91
pJA7600		185 kb	Cm, Sm, Su, Tc	4	*V. anguillarum*	Ayu	1976	91
			Cm	5	*V. anguillarum*	Ayu	1979	91
pPT8018	E	200 kb	Ap, Cm, Sm, Su	6	*V. anguillarum*	Ayu	1980	14
pJAPT8325		200 kb	Ap, Cm, Sm, Su, Tc	6	*V. anguillarum*	Ayu	1983	23
pPT86029				7	*V. anguillarum*	Ayu	1986	141
pAC8902			Cm, Km, Sm, Su, Tc, Tm	8	*V. anguillarum*	Ayu	1989	142
pSH90060			Cm, Km, Sm, Su, Tc, Tm	8	*V. anguillarum*	Ayu	1990	142

[a]All plasmids in this table are conjugative, except pJA8102-2, which has to be mobilized.
[b]Plasmids in the same incompatibility group cannot be stably inherited, indicating similarity.
[c]Phenotypic resistance determinants: Ap, ampicillin; Cm, chloramphenicol; Km, kanamycin; Sm, streptomycin; Su, sulfonamides; Tc, tetracycline; Tp, trimethoprim.
[d]Plasmids within each numbered group have nearly identical plasmid structures, including a common Inc group, except for the drug resistance region, which varies. Plasmids in groups 2 and 3 have similar drug resistance regions but different plasmid backbones.

The widespread occurrence of the small, nonconjugable R plasmid of 11.8 kb with the Tet C determinant and its seemingly close collaboration with the IncU plasmids in its spread among *A. salmonicida* (Table 1) indicate that the smaller R plasmids may be more common in the aquatic environments than believed so far.

A. salmonicida and its clonal appearance may lead us to believe that these bacteria contain fewer R plasmids in general compared to more heterogenous bacteria. Still, the existence of more R plasmids like pRAS2 and other less characterized R plasmids in *A. salmonicida* has been demonstrated in the studies published so far. It might also be that other subspecies of *A. salmonicida*, and maybe aeromonads in general, supply a larger variation of R plasmids than is currently recognized to the pathogenic *A. salmonicida* subspecies *salmonicida*.

DRUG RESISTANCE IN *A. SALMONICIDA* MEDIATED BY CHANGES IN CHROMOSOMAL GENES

The use of quinolones, oxolinic acid and later flumequine, in the control of bacterial infections in farmed fish from the 1980s resulted in detection of isolates of *A. salmonicida* with reduced susceptibility to quinolones (61, 65). Mutations in the gyrase A gene, *gyrA*, were found to be responsible for elevated quinolone MICs in clinical strains of *A. salmonicida* (99). A mutation changing the amino acid serine 83 to isoleucine in the gyrase A protein was found to be responsible for high-level resistance against quinolones. An additional mutation resulting in the change of alanine at position 67 to glycine raised the MIC of enrofloxacin fourfold in a strain with both mutations in *gyrA* compared to strains with a change only in serine 83. A study of 12 clinical *A. salmonicida* isolates from French marine fish farms in the period from 1998 to 2000 showed that all quinolone-resistant isolates carried a point mutation in *gyrA* that resulted in a change of aspartate at position 87 to asparagine (54) (Table 3). No mutations in the *parC* gene of the isolates were found.

In quinolone-resistant *E. coli* strains it was demonstrated that several amino acid substitutions in *gyrA*, concentrated in the region between amino acids 67 and 106, resulted in quinolone resistance; however, substitution in amino acid serine 83 is considered to be important (138).

Quinolone-resistant *A. salmonicida* isolates have been found to have changes in the outer membrane profile, with loss of a 38.5-kDa protein and occurrence of a 37-kDa protein probably linked to loss of porin function, resulting in low-level multiple-antibiotic resistance (32, 59).

In addition to amino acid substitutions in the gyrase A enzyme and porin changes in the outer membranes, it was recently indicated that an efflux mechanism might be involved in quinolone resistance in strains of *A. salmonicida* isolated from French marine fish farms (54).

Quinolones such as oxolinic acid and flumequine were used extensively in fish farming against infections caused by *A. salmonicida* from the end of the 1980s until effective vaccines containing oil adjuvants were introduced before the mid-1990s. In that period high quinolone MICs for *A. salmonicida* developed in all areas where furunculosis was endemic in salmon farming. Often, the result was repeated treatments of diseased fish in the summer months with only weeks between treatments. In Norway the first resistance to quinolones was discovered in 1989, about 1 year after the start of use of oxolinic acid in the control of furunculosis (65). That study included 138 clinical isolates of *A. salmonicida* subsp. *salmonicida* from 26 Atlantic salmon farms. It was found that 36% of the isolates were resistant to one or more of the drugs tested, including 30% that were resistant to quinolones. Resistance against tetracycline and trimethoprim occurred in 18 and 14% of isolates, respectively.

After 10 years of effective vaccination, there was minimal information on the occurrence of antimicrobial resistance in strains of *A. salmonicida* in general. Research has shown that *A. salmonicida* shares remarkably similar genetic tools worldwide when drug resistance develops (Table 1).

ANTIBIOTIC RESISTANCE IN *A. HYDROPHILA*: FARMED FISH

A. hydrophila may cause septicemia and mortality in farmed fish in temperate or warm freshwater all over the world. It is also an important pathogen in ornamental and pet fish. This bacterium is also a potential enteric pathogen in humans and other animals (http://www.bacterio.cict.fr/a/aeromonas.html). *A. hydrophila* comprises a group of motile aeromonads of which some have been given separate species names in the last decades, such as *Aeromonas bestiarum, A. media, A. punctata, A. sobria*, and *A. trota*. Some early studies included strains of motile aeromonads of several separate taxonomic species within the designation *A. hydrophila*. Transferable antibiotic resistance in the fish pathogen *A. hydrophila* was seen in isolates from farmed fish in Japan in the early 1960s (9). Tetracycline and sulfonamide

Table 3. Amino acid substitutions in the *gyrA* gene of fish-pathogenic bacteria causing quinolone resistance

Fish pathogen	Substituted amino acid[a]	Position[b]	New amino acid[c]	MIC[d]		Location	Reference
				Before	After		
A. salmonicida subsp. *salmonicida*	Serine (AGT)	83	Isoleucine (ATT)	0.02 (OXO), 0.04 (FLU)	2.56/3.20 (OXO), 1.60 (FLU)	Norway, marine Atlantic salmon farm	99
A. salmonicida subsp. *salmonicida*	Serine (AGT) Alanine (GCC)	83 67	Isoleucine (ATT) Glycine (GGC)	0.02 (OXO), 0.04 (FLU)	3.20 (OXO), 3.20 (FLU)	Norway, marine Atlantic salmon farm	99
A. salmonicida	Aspartate	87	Asparagine	<0.5 (OXO), <1 (FLU), <0.25 (CIP)	>2 (OXO), >4 (FLU), >0.125 (CIP)	France, marine farm	54
A. hydrophila, *A. caviae*, *A. sobria*	Serine	83	Isoleucine, arginine	<0.1 (OXO), <0.01 (FLU), <0.001 (CIP)	64/8/4 (OXO), 512/32/4 (FLU), 1/2/1 (CIP)	Arga River, Spain; Garonne River, France; water isolates	55
Y. ruckeri	Serine	83	Arginine	<0.125 (OXO), <0.5 (NAL)	>4 (OXO), >64 (NAL)	Spain, rainbow trout farm	53
F. psychrophilum	Threonine	83	Alanine, isoleucine	<0.8 (OXO), <3.1 (NAL)	~6.25 (OXO), 50–100 (NAL)	Japan, ayu and rainbow trout farms	68
F. psychrophilum	Aspartic acid	87	Tyrosine	<0.8 (OXO), <3.1 (NAL)	25 (OXO), 100 (NAL)	Japan, rainbow trout farm	68

[a]Amino acid before mutation with wild-type codon in parentheses.
[b]Numbering according to *gyrA* of *E. coli.*
[c]Amino acid after mutation with mutated codon in parentheses.
[d]MIC (μg/ml) of quinolones (OXO, oxolinic acid; FLU, flumequine; CIP, ciprofloxacin; NAL, nalidixic acid) before mutation for wild-type susceptible isolates and after mutation for wild-type resistant isolates.

resistance determinants were the most common. In 1970 *A. hydrophila* was isolated from many Japanese freshwater fish farms containing carp (5 farms), eel (26 farms), ayu (17 farms), and salmonids (26 farms), and it was shown that they harbored transferable R plasmids with resistance genes against sulfonamides, tetracyclines, chloramphenicol, and streptomycin (12). In a Japanese study of drug resistance in fish pathogens isolated from the intestines of diseased freshwater pond-reared salmonids and pond waters from various districts, it was found that isolates of *A. hydrophila* and *A. salmonicida* (Table 2) contained transferable R plasmids carrying resistance against a combination of tetracyclines, sulfonamides, trimethoprim, and streptomycin; a combination of tetracyclines and sulfonamides; and sulfonamides only (10). Drug-resistant isolates of the genus *Pseudomonas* and of the family *Enterobacteriaceae* did not transfer R plasmids in this study.

In a study of drug-resistant bacteria from the intestines of farmed eels (*A. japonica* and *Anguilla anguilla*) and from the water of the ponds of the farms in Japan, it was found that a relatively high proportion of the drug-resistant bacteria harbored R plasmids. The resistance features transferred with the plasmids were almost always the combination of tetracycline and sulfonamide resistance, especially from *A. hydrophila* isolates (28).

Representatives of R plasmids of *A. hydrophila* from the salmonid ponds in the various districts from 1969 to 1971 were studied in more detail later (2). All 10 R plasmids conferring combined resistance to tetracyclines and sulfonamides were found to belong to the IncA-C group. Six of these R plasmids originated from *A. hydrophila* isolated from salmonids in the ponds of the various districts of Japan, two of these plasmids came from *A. hydrophila* isolated in the United States, and two came from *A. hydrophila* isolated in Taiwan. All these R plasmids were found to be identical by restriction enzyme digest analysis, except for one of the plasmids from Taiwan, which had only a minor discrepancy in the restriction profile. The IncA-C group plasmids mediating tetracycline and sulfonamide resistance were found to have a size of about 125 kb. Plasmid RA1, which was isolated from *A. hydrophila* in Japan (9) and also mediates tetracycline and sulfonamide resistance, was compared to other R plasmids from aeromonads and found to belong to the IncC group and have a size of 86 MDa (i.e., about 130 kb) (63). Of the 13 R plasmids analyzed in this study, 2 other IncC plasmids harbored by *A. hydrophila* isolates from France (92), and 1 IncC plasmid of 100 MDa harbored by an *A. salmonicida* strain from the United Kingdom mediated resistance features different from those mediated by the Japanese plasmids. All these IncA-C or IncC plasmids are probably the same plasmid with variations in the genetic resistance factors of the drug resistance region. In a Danish study it was shown that transferable R plasmids of 150 kb harbored by *A. salmonicida* isolates from a Danish freshwater pond fish farm in 1995 mediated resistance to oxytetracycline, sulfonamides, trimethoprim, and streptomycin (114). In the same study three Canadian *A. salmonicida* isolates from 1986 and 1990 were found to harbor a 160-kb transferable R plasmid mediating resistance to oxytetracycline and sulfonamides. One strain of *A. salmonicida* from the United States isolated in 1989 was also found to contain a transferable R plasmid of 140 kb mediating only oxytetracycline resistance. Common to all these R plasmids with a size from 140 to 160 kb from *A. salmonicida* was the occurrence of an integron in each plasmid. The integron in the Danish R plasmids contained both a *dfr1* trimethoprim resistance cassette and an *ant(3")1a* aminoglycoside resistance cassette, the integron in one of the Canadian R plasmids contained only an *ant(3")1a* cassette, while the R plasmids from the two other Canadian *A. salmonicida* strains and the integron on the R plasmid from the U.S. strain of *A. salmonicida* did not contain any cassettes at all. The Danish R plasmids of 150 kb contained a tetracycline resistance determinant of class A, while the U.S. R plasmid contained a Tet C determinant. In conclusion, the resistance genes were probably in the same plasmid backbone in the IncC R plasmids of 130 to 160 kb of *A. hydrophila* and *A. salmonicida* from several regions around the world, as is the case with the IncU R plasmids already discussed (Table 1).

In the Japanese study of representatives of R plasmids of *A. hydrophila* from the salmonid ponds in the various districts from 1969 to 1971, two IncU R plasmids of 42 kb were also analyzed (2) (Table 2). They mediated resistance against chloramphenicol, sulfonamides, and streptomycin and were identical to pAr-32 (identical to RA3) isolated from *A. salmonicida*. The study also characterized a third R plasmid of about 70 kb found in two *A. hydrophila* isolates in 1974 in the United States (2). In addition, IncU R plasmids of 34 to 40 MDa from three French isolates and two Irish isolates of *A. hydrophila* have been studied together with pAr-32 and RA3 (63).

A study of motile aeromonads such as *A. hydrophila*, *Aeromonas veronii*, and *Aeromonas caviae* from a fish farm hatchery and hospital effluents in England showed that the aeromonads from the hospital effluents harbored IncU R plasmids but the motile aeromonads from the fish farm hatchery did not (108). The IncU plasmids of the motile aeromonads of the hospital effluent resembled the pRAS1-like plasmids from *A. salmonicida* from Norwegian and Scottish salmon farms, with a Tn*1721* environment for the Tet A determinant. One of these IncU R plasmids, pFBAOT6, was sequenced (109). An area of 30 kb of the 85-kb sequence of pFBAOT6 was very similar or identical to the the IncU backbone of pRAS1 (125). The genes located in this part of pFBAOT6 were related to functions like replication and conjugal transfer, demonstrating that this region of 30 kb was the IncU backbone common to all these plasmids while the other 50-kb part of the pFBAOT6 sequence constituted the variable drug resistance region of this IncU R plasmid. The variable region of pFBAOT6 contained an integron and a Tn*1721* environment similar to what was observed in pRAS1 but in addition contained various insertion elements and transposon structures (109). The R plasmids from motile aeromonads from the fish farm hatchery did not contain the Tet A determinant, and they were larger than the IncU plasmids and difficult to analyze by restriction fragment length polymorphism. The authors suggested that these R plasmids belonged to the IncC group.

In a Danish study (112) of 313 isolates of motile *Aeromonas* spp. (35.3% of which were *A. hydrophila*, 19% of which were *A. bestiarum*, and 15.3% of which were *A. veronii* biovar sobria) isolated from four freshwater fish farms (113), 69% of the isolates were resistant to oxytetracycline, 43% were resistant to sulfonamides and trimethoprim, and 20% were quinolone resistant. All the sulfonamides-trimethoprim-resistant aeromonads carried a class 1 integron. "Empty" integrons with no cassettes inserted were found in 23 isolates. The drug resistance cassettes most common were *dfr1* or *dfr2a*. These cassettes were without exception located directly downstream of the cassette promoter area. The aminoglycoside resistance cassette *ant(3")1a* occurred downstream of all the *dfr* cassettes (87 isolates). The chloramphenicol resistance cassette *catB2* was found in 31 isolates. The *catB2* cassette was always located as the most distant cassette from the cassette promoter. Only 30% of the 216 tetracycline-resistant isolates had either Tet A (19 isolates), Tet D (6 isolates), or Tet E (39 isolates). Among 17 strains that were able to transfer an R plasmid, the integron and the Tet determinant were transferred together on the R plasmid in 15 cases.

It can be said conclusively that both the IncU and IncC R plasmids are widespread within aeromonads and probably around the world (Table 1). The studies available so far indicate that both these plasmids originated when bacteria in the local environmental water sources adapted to the drugs used in fish farming locally and regionally. At first sight, variants of the two plasmids may look different, for instance, in the registration of their resistance features, but after more detailed molecular study of the DNA sequences of the plasmids their original similarity is revealed.

A. hydrophila isolates from channel catfish (*I. punctatus*) farmed in ponds in the southern United States have been typed for the determinants causing tetracycline resistance. It was shown that Tet E was the dominant genetic determinant, occurring in 69% of the tetracycline-resistant *A. hydrophila* isolates (45, 46). Tet A and D also occurred among the isolates. However, the tetracycline resistance determinants were in general not found to be transferable, indicating that the genes were located chromosomally or on R plasmids not easily transferred to *E. coli*.

In Japanese tetracycline-resistant *A. hydrophila* isolates (2), the Tet D determinant was responsible for the resistance (17). The Tet D determinant was located on the R plasmids belonging to the IncC group with plasmid sizes of about 130 kb. The 70-kb R plasmid of *A. hydrophila* from the United States also harbored the Tet D determinant.

A. hydrophila isolates from skin lesions of cultured tilapia (*Tilapia mossambica*) from Malaysia were screened for antibiotic resistance and plasmid contents (121). Of 21 isolates studied, all were resistant to ampicillin, 12 were resistant to streptomycin, 10 were resistant to tetracycline, and 9 were resistant to erythromycin. One isolate was resistant to 6 of the 10 drugs included in the study. One-third of the *A. hydrophila* isolates harbored plasmids in the size range of 3 to 64 kb. Only one strain was able to transfer plasmids (63 and 6.2 kb) to *E. coli*. No molecular genetic studies were performed.

Rainbow trout (*Oncorhynchus mykiss*) in northern Portugal with clinical lesions caused predominantly by *A. hydrophila* were investigated in 2001. The pathogenic isolates and isolates from the pond water were screened for resistance against β-lactams (110). Among the 51 strains, resistance to amoxicillin, carbenicillin, and ticarcillin was most common (between 76 and 88%). A few strains were also found to be resistant to imipenem. However, the level of resistance against β-lactam antibiotics among *A. hydrophila* isolates from rainbow trout was found to be lower than among isolates from human clinical infections.

ANTIBIOTIC RESISTANCE IN *A. HYDROPHILA*: PET FISH AND ORNAMENTAL FISH

Infection with *A. hydrophila* is an important cause of loss of fish in aquaria, and the use of antimicrobial drugs is common in the control of such infections. In a study of *A. hydrophila* isolated from the normal flora of commonly imported species of fish from Southeast Asia to two pet shops in the U.S. state of Georgia, it was found that about half of the isolates were resistant to one or more of the drugs tested and 25% of these isolates contained transferable R factors with resistance primarily to tetracyclines, sulfonamides, and ampicillin (115). One of the pet shops used tetracycline prophylaxis in the aquarium water. It was interesting that only the *A. hydrophila* isolates from the aquarium water of this shop carried transferable R factors; the drug-resistant *A. hydrophila* isolates from the other shop were not able to transfer their resistance in this study.

ANTIBIOTIC RESISTANCE IN *A. HYDROPHILA* ISOLATED FROM WILD FISH

The level of transferable R plasmids was low among isolates of *A. hydrophila* from eel living in rivers in Japan (28). Isolates of *A. hydrophila* from diseased wild fish in Lake Vrana on Cres Island in Croatia were not found to have acquired antibiotic resistance (131). The 26 isolates of *A. hydrophila* were isolated in the fall, winter, and spring, as this bacterium did not cause disease in fish of the lake in the summer months (131).

A screening in southern India of antibiotic resistance in *A. hydrophila* isolates from 536 fish and 278 prawns during a period of 2 years, with inclusion of 15 drugs in the study, revealed that only 3% of the strains were resistant to chloramphenicol (134). The fish and prawns studied were marketed from the commercial wild fisheries of coastal southern India.

OVERVIEW OF R PLASMIDS IN *A. HYDROPHILA*

A transferable R plasmid of the IncC group of 130 to 150 kb, depending on the organization of the drug resistance region, appears to be widespread among *A. hydrophila* globally (Table 1). This occurrence of the IncC R plasmid parallels the occurrence of the 45- to 50-kb IncU plasmid among *A. salmonicida*. The IncC R plasmid also occurs in *A. salmonicida* from Europe and North America. The IncU R plasmid has also been found among isolates of *A. hydrophila* in Japan, England, France, and Ireland (9, 63, 109). Future studies will probably verify that both the IncC and IncU plasmids are common to the aeromonads. In addition, other R plasmids, like the 60-kb plasmid harbored by isolates from the United States, occur in *A. hydrophila*.

DRUG RESISTANCE IN *A. HYDROPHILA*, *A. CAVIAE*, AND *A. SOBRIA* MEDIATED BY CHANGES IN CHROMOSOMAL GENES

Most of the *A. hydrophila*, *A. caviae*, and *A. sobria* isolates from the water in the rivers Arga in Spain and Garonne in France were found to have reduced susceptibility to quinolones (55) (Table 3). Fragments of the *gyrA*, *gyrB*, *parC*, and *parE* genes encompassing the quinolone resistance-determining regions were analyzed in 20 isolates. Amino acid substitutions caused by point mutations in *gyrA* and *parC* were found. However, the amino acid substitutions in *gyrA* seemed to have the greatest impact on increasing the quinolone MICs. The serine at position 83 was substituted with isoleucine and less frequently with arginine in all three species. In addition, the methionine at position 92 was replaced by leucine in isolates of *A. caviae*.

ANTIBIOTIC RESISTANCE OF FISH-PATHOGENIC SPECIES OF THE *ENTEROBACTERIACEAE*

Edwardsiella tarda

E. tarda has been a significant pathogen in Japanese eel farms. Modern eel farming is characterized by a high density of eels in freshwater ponds enclosed in greenhouses, with temperatures kept high partly by artificial heating. This enables effective production but also results in a high risk of bacterial infections, with the use antibiotics to control the diseases (24). Edwardsiellosis has also been recorded as an important disease in other freshwater cultured fish such as channel catfish (*I. punctatus*), Japanese flounder (*Paralichthys olivaceus*), largemouth bass (*M. salmoides*), and chinook salmon (*Oncorhynchus tshawytscha*) (139). Vaccine development has been difficult because of serological heterogenicity (69). *E. tarda* has also been described as a potential human pathogen and may cause disease in humans who handle fish and fish products (82).

Six strains of drug-resistant *E. tarda* isolated from farmed eels in Japan at the beginning of the 1970s were studied for occurrence of transferable R plasmids (21). Four strains harbored conjugative R plasmids. The conjugative R plasmids from three of the four strains mediated tetracycline and sulfonamide resistance, while the fourth plasmid had additional resistance genes against chloramphenicol, kanamycin, and streptomycin. The plasmids were stably hosted by *E. coli* and could be retransferred to *E. tarda*. Incompatibility grouping demonstrated that these plasmids belonged to the same group as the 120- to 150-kb R plasmids of *A. hydrophila*. A collection of 168 isolates of *E. tarda* from eels (*A. japonica*), channel catfish (*I. punctatus*), and the water of the culture ponds in the period from 1972 to 1979 in Japan were tested for their susceptibility against 10 antibacterial drugs (24). Thirty-two strains were susceptible to all the tested drugs. The strains were resistant to various combinations of eight different drugs. The most common combination of resistance features of the isolates was resistance against chloramphenicol, furazolidone, nalidixic acid, sulfonamides, and tetracycline. Transferable R plasmids were detected in 38 of the isolates. The transferred R plasmids conferred resistance combinations to sulfonamides, tetracycline, and chloramphenicol. One R plasmid was also carrying resistance to kanamycin and streptomycin. The drug resistance patterns mirrored the drugs used for controlling the bacterial infections in the fish. The eel isolates of *E. tarda* were more antibiotic resistant than the isolates from tilapia, consistent with a higher level of drug use in eel farming compared to the culturing of tilapia.

The genetic relationship between the various conjugative R plasmids of the eel-pathogenic isolates of *E. tarda* from Japan (Table 2) was studied and also compared to R plasmids of *E. tarda* from Taiwan (20). Restriction enzyme analysis of the 13 representative R plasmids combined with DNA-DNA hybridization in this study makes it possible to identify two separate groups of transferable R plasmids in *E. tarda*. One of these groups contained R plasmids that were identical to the IncC R plasmids of *A. hydrophila* (see above). The plasmids of this genetic group contain resistance genes against sulfonamides and tetracycline and sometimes chloramphenicol in addition. These two drug resistance profiles also occurred in plasmids in the other genetic group of R plasmids in *E. tarda*. The plasmids of this second group were of similar size, i.e., about 120 kb. They were identical except for a small variation in the drug resistance region. The results indicated that the two groups of R plasmids have sequences in the drug resistance region in common, and all information points to a class 1 integron as the common sequence between the two groups. The variations in drug resistance profile within and between the two plasmid groups of *E. tarda* were probably caused by the contents of different drug resistance cassettes. The transferable R plasmid from one of the two *E. tarda* isolates from Taiwan is identical to plasmids in the other Japanese group, while the other R plasmid from Taiwan does not belong to any of them.

One of the 13 R plasmids (pJA6012) from *E. tarda* (20) is similar to the plasmids in the first group but has an additional DNA fragment larger than one or two additional gene cassettes. It is possible that this DNA was inserted into the drug resistance region of the plasmid and is responsible for the additional kanamycin and streptomycin resistance this plasmid gives its host, unlike the other R plasmids of this group.

Another collection of isolates of *E. tarda* from 1983 and 1984 isolated from diseased eel in culture ponds in various districts of Japan was investigated for occurrence of drug resistance and R plasmids (27). A total of 152 of 186 isolates were found to be resistant to one or more of six drugs. Resistance against furazolidone and/or nalidixic acid that could not be transferred occurred in all 152 drug-resistant isolates. Transferable R plasmids were detected in 31 of the 152 resistant isolates. In 27 of the isolates with conjugative R plasmids, resistance against the combination of chloramphenicol, sulfonamides, and tetracycline was detected. Of the eight selected R plasmids studied, seven were found to be the same as the R plasmids of the second group that was identified from the previous study (20) of *E. tarda* from Japan and Taiwan. The last plasmid belonged to the first group of R plasmids. Common DNA sequences identified between the plasmids of the two groups were probably located in the drug resistance region and probably included a class 1 integron.

Edwardsiella ictaluri

E. ictaluri from diseased channel catfish (*I. punctatus*) in the southern United States was investigated for antibiotic resistance. None of the 10 strains were found to have acquired antibiotic resistance (107).

Citrobacter freundii

Isolates of *C. freundii* from various fish species in Spain and the United States, including rainbow trout, Atlantic salmon, channel catfish, and tilapia, were studied for the occurrence of drug resistance (132). Of 14 isolates, 13 were resistant to tetracycline alone or in combination with chloramphenicol and streptomycin, and 7 of these were able to transfer R plasmids conferring their resistance to *E. coli*. Genetic similarity between some of the transferable plasmids was found.

Yersinia ruckeri

Y. ruckeri is the primary cause of enteric redmouth disease of salmonid fish. Of 50 isolates of *Y. ruckeri* of various serotypes tested for susceptibility to 23 antibacterial drugs, 2 isolates were found to harbor a 36-MDa conjugative R plasmid encoding resistance to tetracyclines and sulfonamides (44).

On the Jutland peninsula in Denmark, four freshwater rainbow trout farms situated along a stream system were screened for occurrence of bacteria with drug resistance in fish, water, and sediment samples (113). The fish pathogen *Y. ruckeri* was included in the study, with 134 isolates from diseased fish. The *Y. ruckeri* isolates were found to be largely susceptible to all five antimicrobial agents included in the screening. However, the fish farming was found to increase the drug resistance in *Flavobacterium psychrophilum* (88 isolates included) and among 313 isolates of motile *Aeromonas* spp., in a comparison of bacteria at inlets and outlets of water to and from the farms, respectively.

In a French study of resistance to chloramphenicol and florfenicol among fish-pathogenic bacteria, no reduced susceptibility of *Y. ruckeri* to these drugs was revealed despite the wide use of florfenicol in fish farming in France (89).

Y. ruckeri isolates from diseased fish in one Spanish rainbow trout farm with enzootic enteric redmouth disease were collected in the period from 1994 to 2002 (53). Seven representative clinical isolates were selected for the studies. All isolates belonged to the same clone, as demonstrated by pulsed-field gel electrophoresis restriction patterns. For the isolates of *Y. ruckeri* from 2001 and 2002, the MICs of all the quinolones tested were significantly lower than those for the isolates from 1994 to 1998. Sequence analysis of the *gyrA* gene revealed a single amino acid substitution in position 83 from serine to arginine. The same mutation and similarly increased MICs of quinolones were discovered in *Y. ruckeri* isolates induced to quinolone resistance in the laboratory. The same single serine in position 83 of the GyrA enzyme was substituted, but to isoleucine, not arginine, in *A. salmonicida* subsp. *salmonicida* in Norway after use of oxolinic acid in the treatment of furunculosis (99) (Table 3).

ANTIBIOTIC RESISTANCE IN *PHOTOBACTERIUM DAMSELAE* SUBSP. *PISCICIDA*

P. damselae subsp. *piscicida* was given its standing position in the taxonomic system in 1995 after earlier being named *Pseudomonas piscicida* and then *Pasteurella piscicida* (52). Pasteurellosis or pseudotuberculosis, as are the clinical names of the disease, is a serious infection that has caused severe losses in the farming of marine yellowtail *(Seriola quinqueradiata)* in different areas of Japan since it was first observed in 1969 (11, 128). The disease was, however, first characterized in white perch *(Roccus americanus)* in the United States (119). It also affected cultured striped bass *(Morone saxatilis)* on the Gulf Coast of the United States (62, 119). In the Mediterranean marine farming of mainly gilthead sea bream *(Sparus aurata)* and sea bass *(Dicentrarchus labrax)*, pasteurellosis became a serious problem with the advent of epizootics in the farms at the beginning of the 1990s (86).

In a collection of 60 isolates of *P. damselae* subsp. *piscicida* isolated from cultured yellowtail in various districts of Japan in the period from 1975 to 1980, transferable resistance against chloramphenicol, kanamycin, sulfonamides, and tetracycline was found in 5 isolates (11). Nontransferable resistance to furazolidone was found in 21 isolates. All five isolates with transferable R plasmids were isolated in the same district. This was the first report of multiple-drug resistance in *P. damselae* subsp. *piscicida*, and the authors believed that the incidence could be explained by the abundant use of chemotherapeutics in yellowtail farming.

In the period from 1981 to 1983, another collection of 281 isolates of *P. damselae* subsp. *piscicida* was obtained from cultured yellowtail, mainly in the same districts in Japan (128). As many as 262 isolates were resistant to various combinations of seven drugs, and 168 isolates were able to transfer R plasmids to *E. coli*. The most common profile of drug resistance encoded by the R plasmids was one containing resistance features to chloramphenicol, kanamycin, sulfonamides, and tetracyclines.

An analysis of a random selection of 19 R plasmids from *P. damselae* subsp. *piscicida* isolates collected from 1980 to 1983 was performed (128). Patterns of restriction enzyme digests were compared and Southern blots were hybridized with labeled R plasmids to reveal similarities between the plasmids. It is interesting to note that all the plasmids were very similar, with only minor differences in the restriction profile. These differences can be related to the variations in resistance profiles of the R plasmids. Two plasmids lacked kanamycin resistance and in accordance with this had a DNA fragment that was shorter. One plasmid (pJAPW8201) without both the kanamycin and chloramphenicol resistance features lacked a large 6.2-kb fragment and a small fragment. This indicated that kanamycin resistance was encoded by a gene in a small resistance gene cassette located in an integron, while chloramphenicol resistance was caused by a larger gene, or a gene that was carried by a mobile transposon-like structure.

In genetic studies of the tetracycline resistance determinants of R plasmids from *A. hydrophila*, *E. tarda*, and *P. piscicida*, it was shown that it was the Tet D determinant that was responsible for tetracycline resistance in R plasmids from all three fish pathogens, including both groups of R plasmids in *E. tarda* and the IncC group R plasmid of *A. hydrophila* (17). It is also of particular interest (see figures in reference 17) that one of the R plasmids of *E. tarda* (pJA6012) is very similar to the R plasmids of *P. damselae* subsp. *piscicida*. The only difference is that pJA6012 carries an extra streptomycin resistance determinant. The pJA6012 plasmid represents one of the two groups of R plasmids detected in *E. tarda* causing infection in Japanese eels.

Continuous systematic collection of *P. damselae* subsp. *piscicida* isolates from diseased yellowtail in Japan and screening for drug resistance has also been performed for the periods 1984 to 1985 (307 isolates) (76), 1986 to 1988 (306 isolates) (77), and 1989 to 1991 (175 isolates) (70). The same resistance patterns of the isolates were found throughout Japan in all the years from 1975 to 1991, and the majority of the isolates were found to be multiresistant to a series of antibiotics (Table 2). Almost all drug-resistant isolates harbored the same type of transferable R plasmid, with variation only in the occurrence of the genes encoding the various resistance features in the drug resistance region of the plasmid. The resistance gene always residing on the R plasmid is the sulfonamide resistance gene.

The chloramphenicol resistance gene of the R plasmids of Japanese *P. damselae* subsp. *piscicida* was cloned and sequenced and found to encode a type I chloramphenicol acetyltransferase (CAT-I) with homology to the CAT-I gene from the chromosome of *Acinetobacter baumannii* (71).

The kanamycin and tetracycline resistance genes of the R plasmid of Japanese drug-resistant *P. damselae* subsp. *piscicida* isolates were found to be carried by a transposon-like structure with flanking copies of insertion sequence IS*26* (73). The tetracycline resistance determinant was verified to be Tet D, as shown earlier (17), and the kanamycin resistance was found to be encoded by the aminoglycoside phosphotransferase gene *aph-Ic*, being highly homologous to *aphA1* of Tn*903*. A similar IS*26*-based transposon structure with an identical kanamycin resistance gene is found in pBWH77 of *Klebsiella pneumoniae* (81).

The sulfonamide resistance gene of the R plasmid of Japanese drug-resistant *P. damselae* subsp. *piscicida* isolates was found to be the *sul2* gene (74).

A florfenicol resistance gene, *floR*, was present in the R plasmid of Japanese drug-resistant *P. damselae* subsp. *piscicida* isolates (72). This gene was located downstream of the *sul2* gene and has 47.4% identity with the chloramphenicol resistance gene *cmlA* of *Pseudomonas aeruginosa*. The *floR* gene of *P. damselae* subsp. *piscicida* was also later detected in the chromosomal drug resistance region of the genomic island of multidrug-resistant *Salmonella enterica* subsp. *enterica* serovar Typhimurium DT104 (30), and in bovine isolates of *E. coli* a florfenicol resistance gene with 98% homology is relatively widespread (136).

A recent molecular study of genes responsible for chloramphenicol resistance in Japanese drug-resistant *P. damselae* subsp. *piscicida* isolates resulted in detection of three transferable R plasmids of 100, 50, and 40 kb, all encoding chloramphenicol resistance in the isolates (93). A gene encoding a type II CAT (CAT-II) was cloned and sequenced from the 50-kb plasmid. The gene had 99.5% homology to the gene encoding the type II CAT of *Haemophilus influenzae*. There is no study available that reveals all the features and structures of the three different R plasmids of the Japanese *P. damselae* subsp. *piscicida* isolates from cultured yellowtail and that establishes how widespread the combined carriage of the three R plasmids is among *P. damselae* subsp. *piscicida*.

The ampicillin resistance gene of *P. damselae* subsp. *piscicida* isolated from diseased Japanese yellowtail in the Kyushu area was located on a 50-kb plasmid. It has been cloned and sequenced and found to be a novel ampicillin resistance gene in class A of β-lactamases (94).

P. damselae subsp. *piscicida* isolated from outbreaks of disease in the marine aquaculture of the Mediterranean countries also showed a high degree of genetic homology with Japanese and American strains (86). In the European strains, resistance to erythromycin, kanamycin, streptomycin, and sulfonamides was common. Plasmid profiling did not reveal a common R plasmid carrying the drug resistance genes in the *P. damselae* subsp. *piscicida* isolates. However, common DNA fragments of the plasmids were suggested to be carriers of drug resistance genes.

A recent study developed an auxotrophic strain of *P. damselae* subsp. *piscicida* with an interruption in the shikimate pathway as a promising candidate for a vaccine against disease caused by this pathogen of marine fish culture in temperate areas (130). Systematic use of effective vaccines seems to be the most effective way of reducing the use of antibiotic drugs in culture of fish.

ANTIBIOTIC RESISTANCE IN *VIBRIO ANGUILLARUM*

Vibrio bacteria have their primary habitats in marine ecosystems, and a few of them can cause disease in marine fish in general and particularly in farmed marine fish.

Infections with multiple-drug-resistant *V. anguillarum* occurred in farmed ayu *(P. altivelis)* in Japan in 1973 (22). Of 68 randomly selected *V. anguillarum* isolates from outbreaks of disease in 1973, 65 carried transferable R plasmids encoding resistance to chloramphenicol, sulfonamides, streptomycin, and tetracycline. Reduced susceptibility to furazolidone and nalidixic acid occurred widely, in more than half of the strains, but these features were not transferred to *E. coli*. It was assumed that use of antibacterial drugs in ayu farming exerted a selective pressure that resulted in the occurrence of transferable R plasmids in *V. anguillarum* isolates from diseased ayu.

A follow-up study including a collection of 259 *V. anguillarum* isolates from diseased ayu in farms of various districts of Japan from 1974 to 1977 revealed that 250 isolates were resistant to various combinations of six drugs (13). Transferable R plasmids were detected in 165 isolates (64%), and most R plasmids were found to carry resistance genes to chloramphenicol, sulfonamides, and tetracycline. The majority of the resistant isolates (59%) expressed resistance to five or six drugs. Nontransferable resistance to trimethoprim was discovered in the *V. anguillarum* isolates in 1976, only 1 year after trimethoprim had been introduced in the treatment of vibriosis in ayu farms.

Another follow-up study including 226 *V. anguillarum* isolates sampled from farmed ayu in the period from 1978 to 1980 showed that almost all strains had developed nontransferable resistance to furazolidone and nalidixic acid (14). A change was observed in the resistance patterns compared to the earlier studies. Only one isolate of *V. anguillarum* was found to be resistant to tetracycline, and this isolate could not transfer its tetracycline resistance to *E. coli*. Of the 112 isolates from 1978 and 1979, 22 carried a transferable R plasmid carrying resistance to only chloramphenicol. In 1980 isolates with a resistance pattern including resistance to ampicillin, streptomycin, sulfonamides, and trimethoprim increased rapidly in number. These strains harbored R plasmids with genes encoding resistance to various combinations of ampicillin, chloramphenicol, streptomycin, sulfonamides, and trimethoprim. A total of 75 of the 226 *V. anguillarum* isolates harbored a transferable R plasmid.

Another follow-up study on drug resistance in *V. anguillarum* from ayu with vibriosis investigated a collection of 139 isolates from various areas of Japan in the period from 1981 to 1983 (23). Two of the isolates were shown to be resistant to all 10 drugs used in the study. Transferable R plasmids were detected in 30 (22%) of the isolates, and they invariably encoded resistance to ampicillin, chloramphenicol, sulfonamides, and trimethoprim, with some variation in the occurrence of resistance genes to streptomycin and tetracycline. The transferable R plasmids were purified from *E. coli* transconjugants and analyzed by restriction fragment electrophoresis and Southern blot hybridization with one of the R plasmids as labeled probe. The R plasmids showed extensive homology, with minor variation in the drug resistance region.

The R plasmids of *V. anguillarum* isolated from ayu in Japan before 1980 belonged to two different groups, and both were different from the third group of R plasmids that appeared in 1980 (Table 2). This was evident from the pattern of resistance determinants encoded by the plasmids (23) and genetic analysis (91). The first group of R plasmids (approximately 185 kb, according to reported restriction patterns) was observed before 1978 and encoded resistance to chloramphenicol, sulfonamides, and tetracycline. The second group occurred in the period from 1978 to 1979 and carried only chloramphenicol resistance, and the third group of R plasmids (approximately 200 kb, according to reported restriction patterns) appeared in 1980, encoding resistance to ampicillin, chloramphenicol, sulfonamides, and trimethoprim and variable resistance to streptomycin and tetracycline. It was shown that the first and third groups of the Japanese R plasmids of *V. anguillarum* had drug resistance genetic structures in common with each other and with the IncU plasmid pJA8102-1 of *A. salmonicida* from Japan (91).

A collection of 114 isolates of *V. anguillarum* from Japanese ayu farms in various districts sampled in the period from 1989 to 1991 was analyzed for the occurrence of drug resistance (142). All except one isolate were resistant to various combinations of drugs. Transferable R plasmids with resistance to seven to nine drugs were detected in 21 isolates. Kanamycin was introduced as a resistance determinant in *V. anguillarum* in this period. The R plasmids were shown to be very similar in this period, but they were not found to be similar to the R plasmids seen earlier in *V. anguillarum* from ayu in Japan; i.e., they constituted a fourth group of R plasmids in this pathogen (Table 4).

The tetracycline resistance determinants of the R plasmids of *V. anguillarum* isolated from cultured

Table 4. Resistance determinants in representative R plasmids of *V. anguillarum* from Japanese ayu (*P. altivelis*) farms

Plasmid	Size (kb)	Resistance determinant(s)	Yr	Reference(s)
pJA7324	185	Tet B, CAT-VA	1973	91
pJA7601	185	Tet B, CAT-VA	1976	91
pJAPT8325	200	Tet G	1983	16, 23, 140
pPT86029		CAT-VA	1986	140–142
pAC8902		CAT-IV	1989	142
pSH90060		CAT-IV	1990	142

ayu in Japan were analyzed, and the first group of R plasmids, occurring from 1973 to 1977, were found to have the Tet B determinant. The second group, occurring from 1978 to 1979, did not carry any tetracycline resistance, and the third group of R plasmids, occurring in *V. anguillarum* from 1980 to 1983, hosted a novel tetracycline resistance determinant (16). This determinant was 60% homologous to Tet A and Tet C and 50% homologous to Tet B and was called Tet G (141). However, the Tet G determinant was not found in the fourth group of R plasmids, seen in *V. anguillarum* from ayu in the period from 1989 to 1991. Quite surprising and interesting is the fact that the Tet G determinant occurs in multidrug-resistant *S. enterica* serovar Typhimurium DT104 strains on the genomic island, called *Salmonella* genomic island 1, that contains an antibiotic resistance gene cluster with both Tet G and the *floR* gene (33). The *floR* gene was first detected in the fish pathogen *P. damselae* subsp. *piscicida*, also in Japan (72, 142).

The CAT enzyme encoded by the R plasmids of *V. anguillarum* isolated from ayu in 1989 to 1991 was found to be a novel type of CAT called CAT-IV (88). The CAT gene of the R plasmids occurring in *V. anguillarum* isolated from farmed ayu in Japan in 1973 was found to be 37 to 69% homologous with other CAT proteins of both gram-negative and -positive bacteria when comparing the predicted amino acid sequences (140).

V. anguillarum of serotypes not known to be pathogenic to farmed fish was sampled mainly from diseased fish in Galicia, Spain. Occurrence of drug resistance was analyzed in 46 isolates (101). Most of the isolates were resistant to streptomycin, approximately 25% of the isolates were resistant to the combination of sulfamethoxazole and trimethoprim, and only four isolates were resistant to tetracyclines.

A study of 520 *V. anguillarum* strains isolated from fish and the environment, mainly in Denmark but also from the rest of Europe, revealed minimal acquired resistance to antibacterial drugs (102). Most isolates were O1, O2, or non-O1-O10 serotypes, and among these there were two streptomycin-resistant, three tetracycline-resistant, five sulfonamide-resistant, and one trimethoprim-resistant isolate. The trimethoprim-resistant isolate *V. anguillarum* O2 was also cross-resistant to the diagnostic agent O/129, as was also shown in trimethoprim-resistant *V. anguillarum* from Japanese ayu farms (95). This cross-resistance between trimethoprim and the vibriostatic agent O/129 has been observed in other groups of bacteria with acquired trimethoprim resistance such as *P. damselae* subsp. *damselae* (102) and *Mannheimia (Pasteurella) haemolytica* (49). This phenomenon is of particular note in the diagnostic work with *Vibrio* isolates in fish health laboratories.

A total of 264 bacterial strains from Norway classified primarily as *V. anguillarum* were examined for drug resistance, among other features. The strains were isolated mostly from nine different species of diseased or healthy farmed fish after routine autopsy (96). Resistance against commonly used antibacterial compounds was not demonstrated among the *V. anguillarum* isolates.

ANTIBIOTIC RESISTANCE IN *VIBRIO SALMONICIDA*

Cold-water vibriosis caused by *V. salmonicida* was a devastating disease in Norwegian Atlantic salmon farming from the end of the 1970s to 1988, when an effective vaccine was developed (104). Before the vaccine was employed, medical feed with antimicrobial agents was the only measure used to control hundreds of outbreaks of cold-water vibriosis. Oxytetracycline, furazolidone, and sulfadiazine in combination with trimethoprim were the most important drugs in the treatment of salmon infected with *V. salmonicida* (57).

A collection of 463 isolates of *V. salmonicida* isolated in the period from 1980 to 1995, representing the majority of the outbreaks of cold-water vibriosis in Norway, was screened for resistance to antibacterial drugs. One-third of the isolates were resistant to tetracycline and one-third to trimethoprim, while 81% of the isolates were resistant to sulfonamides and 52% were resistant to furazolidone. The tetracycline resistance determinant found in all resistant isolates was Tet E (122, 126). The Tet E determinant has primarily been found in aquatic environments in both Europe and America (3, 45, 46, 78, 90).

ANTIBIOTIC RESISTANCE OF VARIOUS FISH-PATHOGENIC SPECIES OF MARINE *VIBRIO*

Six *Vibrio harveyi* strains were studied for occurrence of drug resistance (84). Four strains isolated from diseased penaeids and two reference strains isolated from seawater (ATCC 25919) and a diseased *Talorchestia* sp. (ATCC 14126) were used. All three strains isolated in Taiwan exhibited resistance against nitrofurantoin, novobiocin, and sulfonamide. The two reference strains and a strain from Indonesia were susceptible to these three antibiotics.

Among 32 isolates of *Vibrio vulnificus* isolated in 1996 from two disease outbreaks at a Danish eel farm that used brackish water, resistance to antibacterial drugs was not found (43).

A novel oxytetracycline resistance determinant, Tet 34, was cloned from chromosomal DNA of *Vibrio* sp. no. 6 isolated from intestinal contents of cultured yellowtail (*S. quinqueradiata*). This determinant needed extra Mg^{2+} to function (98).

So far there are no reports available on drug resistance in *Moritella viscosa*. *M. viscosa* is a psychrophilic *Vibrio*-like bacterium causing winter ulcer in farmed Atlantic salmon and cod on the northern coasts of the Atlantic Ocean (34).

ANTIBIOTIC RESISTANCE IN *F. PSYCHROPHILUM*

F. psychrophilum is an important fish pathogen of different species of fish in temperate to cold water. The bacterium often infects the skin of the fish and may cause considerable losses in fish farming. In a Danish study with a screening of samples in and around four freshwater fish farms situated along a stream in western Denmark during a 1-year period, 88 *F. psychrophilum* isolates were studied (113). A markedly decreased susceptibility of *F. psychrophilum* isolates to most antimicrobial agents presently available for use in Danish aquaculture was detected.

In Japan *F. psychrophilum* is the causative agent of bacterial cold-water disease and rainbow trout fry syndrome. It had been reported that isolates of *F. psychrophilum* were resistant to quinolones, and in a molecular study 27 isolates of the bacterium from Japan and the United States were investigated to detect potential amino acid substitutions in the *gyrA* gene as responsible for the quinolone resistance (68). Resistance to quinolones was detected in 14 of the isolates, and two amino acid substitutions in the deduced amino acid sequence of the gyrase A enzyme were found in all of them. The substitutions were at position 83, where threonine was replaced by an alanine or an isoleucine, and position 87, where aspartic acid was replaced by a tyrosine.

A substitution of the amino acid at position 83 in gyrase A seems to be important in the development of quinolone resistance among fish pathogens. Both *A. salmonicida* subsp. *salmonicida* from Norway (99) and *Y. ruckeri* from Spain (53) have a substitution of the amino acid at position 83 as the only mutation causing quinolone resistance in the isolates.

However, French isolates of *A. salmonicida* subsp. *salmonicida* have a substitution of the amino acid at position 87 as the only mutation detected in quinolone-resistant isolates (54) (Table 3).

ANTIBIOTIC RESISTANCE IN *PSEUDOMONAS FLUORESCENS*

Strains of *P. fluorescens* isolated from farmed channel catfish and yellowtail in Japan in 1973 contained R plasmids with genes encoding resistance to chloramphenicol, sulfonamides, and tetracyclines (12). Isolates of *P. fluorescens* from rainbow trout farms in Spain revealed resistance against a variety of drugs, with resistance to the combination of ticarcillin and clavulanic acid as the most common feature (60).

ANTIBIOTIC RESISTANCE IN *STREPTOCOCCUS* SPP.

Streptococci are uncommon as causes of infections in fish. However, a number of outbreaks of streptococci have been reported (47, 97). A *Streptococcus* sp. isolated from farmed yellowtail in Japan was found be resistant to macrolides, lincomycin, tetracyclines, and chloramphenicol (18). A group of these isolates could transfer their drug resistance to other streptococci.

ANTIBIOTIC RESISTANCE IN *RENIBACTERIUM SALMONINARUM*

Minimal information is available in the literature on antibiotic resistance in *R. salmoninarum*, the causative agent of bacterial kidney disease in salmonids.

CONJUGAL TRANSFER OF ANTIBIOTIC RESISTANCE BETWEEN BACTERIA RELATED TO AQUACULTURE

Several studies demonstrate transfer of R plasmids from fish pathogens to *E. coli* recipients. This is an important feature showing the potential mobility of antibiotic resistance genes between bacteria in general. However, it is not easy to compare the transfer frequencies reported in the various studies. Transfer frequencies vary between 1 and 10^{-12}. The transfer frequencies of the same R plasmid may vary a lot depending on the methods used for the conjugation. This phenomenon can be illustrated with the transfer capabilities of the IncU plasmid pRAS1. This plasmid may transfer almost 10^4 times faster on a solid surface compared to a liquid medium (Table 5) (38). The reason for this difference is the structure of the pili used for transfer of plasmid DNA. The short rigid pili encoded by the IncU plasmid make this plasmid transfer better on solid surfaces, while plasmids with long slender pili involved in the transfer prefer liquid media. Before transfer frequencies can be compared between studies, standardized transfer protocols should be accepted and used as part of the study.

IMPORTANCE OF RESISTANCE TO ANTIBACTERIAL DRUGS IN AQUACULTURE

A major challenge in human medicine is the increasing level of antibiotic resistance in bacterial pathogens. Scientists studying antibiotic resistance in aquaculture have reported results that may help us to understand how the pathogens in hospitals and other clinical arenas acquire and evolve the genetic structures important for their survival under the pressure of antibiotics used therapeutically. Human clinical pathogens probably have routes they frequently use for shipping resistance genes into hospitals or other similar environments. An example illustrating such a scenario may be the 51-kb R plasmid pTP10 from the multiresistant clinical isolate *Corynebacterium striatum* M82B. This R plasmid is composed of DNA fragments initially identified in soil bacteria and in pathogens of plants, animals, fish (*P. damselae* subsp. *piscicida*), and humans (129). R plasmids of fish pathogens and aquatic bacteria, such as the IncU plasmid, have been observed in bacteria of terrestrial, animal, and human bacterial floras and environments.

Transfer experiments in simulated natural microenvironments have shown that the IncU plasmid pRAS1 of *A. salmonicida* can transfer directly from the fish pathogen to human *E. coli* on a wooden cutting board in a kitchen where fresh salmon was prepared for the oven before vegetables were mixed into a salad. The transfer frequency (10^{-3}) was the same on the cutting board without laboratory media supplying necessary components for growth as it was in the laboratory on regular nutrition media (75).

Molecular genetic studies of antibiotic resistance in fish pathogens reveal that in general the degree of genetic recombination in the DNA segments carrying the resistance genes is considerably lower than what is documented in human clinical strains. This fact indicates that fish pathogens and other bacteria can utilize a natural pool of resistance genes in the environment when they need protection against a fish farmer who tries to control bacterial infections in his aquaculture. The sediments beneath the fish where feed and fecal material aggregate function like a potential incubator for the exchange of genes between fish pathogens and the environment.

In many ways, fish pathogens represent possible intermediate vectors for shipping antibiotic resistance genes between the environment and human beings (see chapter 20) for further recombination (Fig. 2). This situation makes it very exciting to study drug resistance in fish pathogens because it reveals keys to understanding how and why the antibiotic resistance of human pathogens represents a major threat to humankind.

Table 5. Conjugative transfer of pRAS1 measured by transfer frequencies[a]

Strain[b]	Transfer frequency[c] after indicated mating time in:									Frequency ratio of plate/broth mating
	Agar								Broth, 24 h	
	1 h	2 h	4 h	6 h	8 h	14 h	24 h	51 h		
2402/89	1.2×10^{-3}	4.0×10^{-3}	3.5×10^{-3}	0.13	0.18	0.25	0.48	0.59	1.1×10^{-3}	436
1995/91	1.6×10^{-6}	2.5×10^{-6}	3.3×10^{-5}	1.1×10^{-4}	4.1×10^{-4}	6.7×10^{-4}	6.5×10^{-3}	6.8×10^{-2}	8.7×10^{-5}	75

[a]Reprinted from reference 125 with permission of the publisher.
[b]Strain 2402/89 (freeze number 718) is an atypical *A. salmonicida* strain isolated in 1989, while strain 1995/91 is an *A. salmonicida* subsp. *salmonicida* strain isolated in 1991.
[c]Proportion of *E. coli* recipient cells receiving the plasmid after mating at 22°C after various periods either on a solid surface or in a liquid medium.

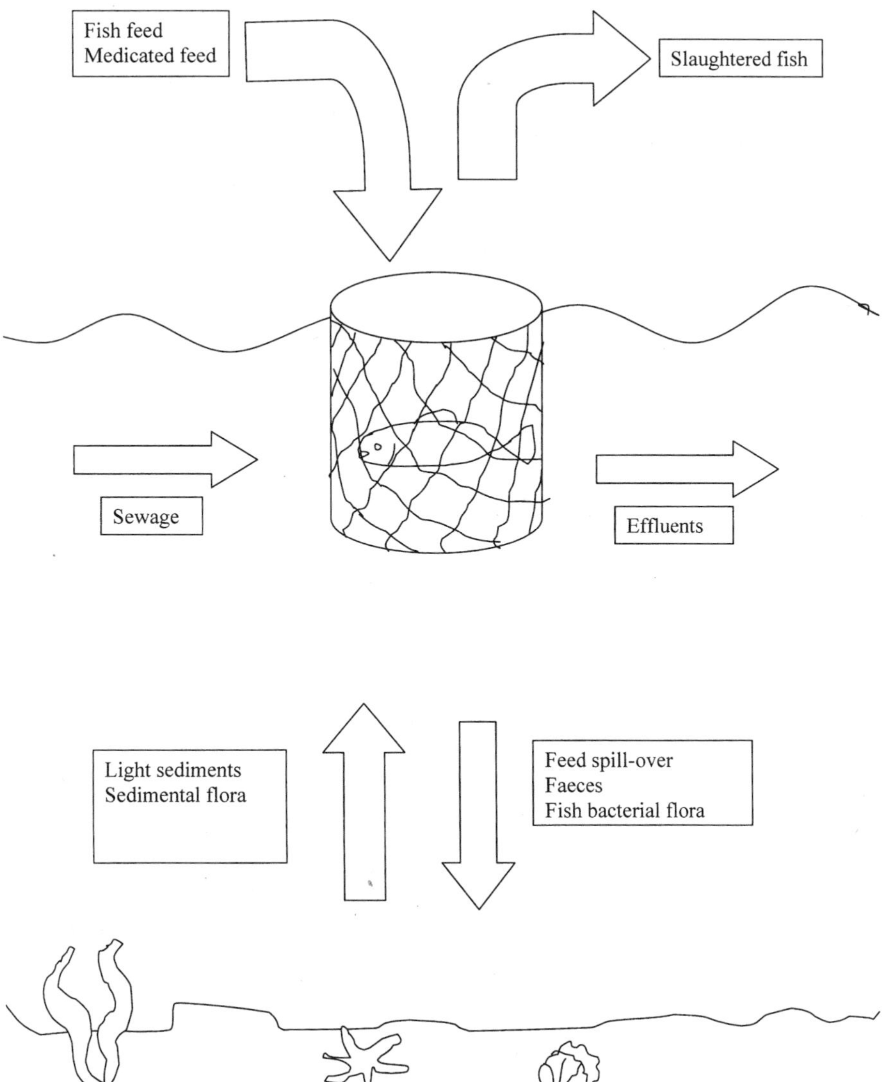

Figure 2. Schematic presentation of management and environmental factors in aquaculture that contribute to the spread of drug-resistant bacteria and their genetic factors.

CONCLUSION

Aquaculture produces about one-third (almost 40 million tonnes) of the fish consumed in the world. The use of antimicrobial agents has selected for resistance in several fish pathogens, making it increasingly difficult to control infections in fish with antimicrobial agents. Furthermore, fish pathogens and bacteria in the environments of the fish may also acquire resistance and act as reservoirs for bacteria pathogenic to humans and thereby constitute a human health problem. It is therefore crucial that the fish farming industry develop strategies of alternative infection control without the need for antibacterial drugs, for instance, by using vaccination and optimal management routines.

Acknowledgments. Trine L'Abée-Lund is acknowledged for reading the manuscript, and Kristina Sørum is acknowledged for assistance with Fig. 2.

REFERENCES

1. **Adams, C. A., B. Austin, P. G. Meaden, and D. McIntosh.** 1998. Molecular characterization of plasmid-mediated oxytetracycline resistance in *Aeromonas salmonicida*. *Appl. Environ. Microbiol.* **64:**4194–4201.
2. **Akashi, A., and T. Aoki.** 1986. Characterization of transferable R plasmids from *Aeromonas hydrophila*. *Bull. Jpn. Soc. Sci. Fish.* **52:**649–655.
3. **Andersen, S. R., and R. A. Sandaa.** 1994. Distribution of tetracycline resistance determinants among gram-negative bacteria isolated from polluted and unpolluted marine sediments. *Appl. Environ. Microbiol.* **60:**908–912.

4. **Anonymous.** 2003. *Sales of Antimicrobial Products Authorised for Use as Veterinary Medicines, Antiprotozoals, Growth Promoters, Antifungals and Coccidiostats, in the UK in 2002.* The Veterinary Medicines Directorate, Addlestone, United Kingdom. [Online.] http://www.vmd.gov.uk/general/publications/salesanti02.pdf.
5. **Anonymous.** 2004. *DANMAP 2003—Use of Antimicrobial Agents and Occurrence of Antimicrobial Resistance in Bacteria from Food Animals, Foods and Humans in Denmark.* Danish Integrated Antimicrobial Resistance Monitoring and Research Programme, Copenhagen, Denmark. [Online.] http://www.dfvf.dk/Files/Filer/Zoonosesenteret/Publikationer/Danmap/Danmap_2003.pdf.
6. **Anonymous.** 2004. *NORM/NORM-VET 2003: Usage of Antimicrobial Agents and Occurrence of Antimicrobial Resistance in Norway.* NORM, Tromsø, Norway, and NORM-VET, Oslo, Norway. [Online.] http://www.vetinst.no/Arkiv/Zoonosesenteret/NORM_NORM-VET_2003.pdf.
7. **Anonymous.** 2004. *SVARM 2003: Swedish Veterinary Antimicrobial Resistance Monitoring.* National Veterinary Institute, Uppsala, Sweden. [Online.] http://www.sva.se/pdf/svarm2003.pdf.
8. **Aoki, T.** 1988. Drug-resistant plasmids from fish pathogens. *Microbiol. Sci.* **5:**219–223.
9. **Aoki, T., S. Egusa, Y. Ogata, and T. Watanabe.** 1971. Detection of resistance factors in fish pathogen *Aeromonas liquefaciens. J. Gen. Microbiol.* **65:**343–349.
10. **Aoki, T., S. Egusa, C. Yada, and T. Watanabe.** 1972. Studies of drug resistance and R factors in bacteria from pond-cultured salmonids. I. Amago (*Oncorhynchus rhodurus macrostomus*) and yamame (*Oncorhynchus masou ishikawae*). *Jpn. J. Microbiol.* **16:**233–238.
11. **Aoki, T., and T. Kitao.** 1985. Detection of transferable R plasmids in strains of the fish-pathogenic bacterium, *Pasteurella piscicida. J. Fish Dis.* **8:**345–350.
12. **Aoki, T., T. Kitao, and T. Arai.** 1977. R plasmids in fish pathogens, p. 39–45. *In* S. Mitsuhashi (ed.), *Plasmids—Medical and Theoretical Aspects.* Avicenum—Czechoslovak Medical Press, Prague, Czechoslovakia.
13. **Aoki, T., T. Kitao, and K. Kawano.** 1981. Changes in drug resistance of *Vibrio anguillarum* in cultured ayu, *Plecoglossus altivelis* Temminck and Schlegel, in Japan. *J. Fish Dis.* **4:**223–230.
14. **Aoki, T., T. Kitao, S. Watanabe, and S. Takeshita.** 1984. Drug resistance and R plasmids in *Vibrio anguillarum* isolated in cultured ayu (*Plecoglossus altivelis*). *Microbiol. Immunol* **28:**1–9.
15. **Aoki, T., Y. Mitoma, and J. H. Crosa.** 1986. The characterization of a conjugative R-plasmid isolated from *Aeromonas salmonicida. Plasmid* **16:**213–218.
16. **Aoki, T., T. Satoh, and T. Kitao.** 1987. New tetracycline resistance determinant on R plasmids from *Vibrio anguillarum. Antimicrob. Agents Chemother.* **31:**1446–1449.
17. **Aoki, T., and A. Takahashi.** 1987. Class D tetracycline resistance determinants of R plasmids from the fish pathogens *Aeromonas hydrophila, Edwardsiella tarda,* and *Pasteurella piscicida. Antimicrob. Agents Chemother.* **31:**1278–1280.
18. **Aoki, T., K. Takami, and T. Kitao.** 1990. Drug resistance in a non-hemolytic *Streptococcus* sp. isolated from cultured yellowtail *Seriola quinqueradiata. Dis. Aquat. Org.* **8:**171–177.
19. **Aoki, T., S. Egusa, T. Kimura, and T. Watanabe.** 1971. Detection of R factors in naturally occurring *Aeromonas salmonicida* strains. *Appl. Microbiol.* **22:**716–717.
20. **Aoki, T., A. Akira, and T. Sakaguchi.** 1986. Phylogenetic relationships of transferable R plasmids from *Edwardsiella tarda. Bull. Jpn. Soc. Sci. Fish.* **52:**1173–1179.
21. **Aoki, T., T. Arai, and S. Egusa.** 1977. Detection of R plasmids in naturally occurring fish-pathogenic bacteria, *Edwardsiella tarda. Microbiol. Immunol.* **21:**77–83.
22. **Aoki, T., S. Egusa, and T. Arai.** 1974. Detection of R factors in naturally occurring *Vibrio anguillarum* strains. *Antimicrob. Agents Chemother.* **6:**534–538.
23. **Aoki, T., T. Kanazawa, and T. Kitao.** 1985. Epidemiological surveillance of drug resistant *Vibrio anguillarum* strains. *Fish Pathol.* **20:**199–208.
24. **Aoki, T., and T. Kitao.** 1981. Drug resistance and transferable R plasmids in *Edwardsiella tarda* from fish culture ponds. *Fish Pathol.* **15:**277–281.
25. **Aoki, T., T. Kitao, T. Ando, and T. Arai.** 1979. Incompatibility grouping of R plasmids detected in fish pathogenic bacteria, *Aeromonas salmonicida,* p. 219–222. *In* S. Mitsuhashi (ed.), *Microbial Drug Resistance.* University Park Press, Baltimore, Md.
26. **Aoki, T., T. Kitao, N. Iemura, Y. Mitoma, and T. Nomura.** 1983. The susceptibility of *Aeromonas salmonicida* strains isolated in cultured and wild salmonids to various chemotherapeutics. *Bull. Jpn. Soc. Sci. Fish.* **49:**17–22.
27. **Aoki, T., T. Sakaguchi, and T. Kitao.** 1987. Multiple drug-resistant plasmids from *Edwardsiella tarda* in eel culture ponds. *Nippon Suisan Gakkaishi* **53:**1821–1825.
28. **Aoki, T., and T. Watanabe.** 1973. Studies of drug-resistant bacteria isolated from eel-pond water and intestinal tracts of the eel (*Anguilla japonica* and *Anguilla anguilla*). *Bull. Jpn. Soc. Sci. Fish.* **39:**121–130.
29. **Aoki, T., and A. Takahashi.** 1986. Tetracycline-resistant gene of a non-transferable R plasmid from fish-pathogenic bacteria *Aeromonas salmonicida. Bull. Jpn. Soc. Sci. Fish.* **52:**1913–1917.
30. **Arcangioli, M. A., S. Leroy-Setrin, J. L. Martel, and E. Chaslus-Dancla.** 1999. A new chloramphenicol and florfenicol resistance gene flanked by two integron structures in *Salmonella typhimurium* DT104. *FEMS Microbiol. Lett.* **174:**327–332.
31. **Austin, B., and D. A. Austin.** 1993. *Bacterial Fish Pathogens: Disease in Farmed and Wild Fish,* p. 111–195. Ellis Horwood, Chichester, United Kingdom.
32. **Barnes, A. C., C. S. Lewin, T. S. Hastings, and S. G. Amyes.** 1990. Cross resistance between oxytetracycline and oxolinic acid in *Aeromonas salmonicida* associated with alterations in outer membrane proteins. *FEMS Microbiol. Lett.* **60:**337–339.
33. **Baucheron, S., S. Tyler, D. Boyd, M. R. Mulvey, E. Chaslus-Dancla, and A. Cloeckaert.** 2004. AcrAB-TolC directs efflux-mediated multidrug resistance in *Salmonella enterica* serovar Typhimurium DT104. *Antimicrob. Agents Chemother.* **48:**3729–3735.
34. **Benediktsdottir, E., L. Verdonck, C. Sproer, S. Helgason, and J. Swings.** 2000. Characterization of *Vibrio viscosus* and *Vibrio wodanis* isolated at different geographical locations: a proposal for reclassification of *Vibrio viscosus* as *Moritella viscosa* comb. nov. *Int. J. Syst. Evol. Microbiol.* **50**(Pt. 2): 479–488.
35. **Bergh, Ø., F. Nilsen, and O. B. Samuelsen.** 2001. Diseases, prophylaxis and treatment of the Atlantic halibut *Hippoglossus hippoglossus*: a review. *Dis. Aquat. Org.* **48:**57–74.
36. **Bernardi, A., and F. Bernardi.** 1984. Complete sequence of pSC101. *Nucleic Acids Res.* **12:**9415–9426.
37. **Björklund, H., J. Bondestam, and G. Bylund.** 1990. Residues of oxytetracycline in wild fish and sediments from fish farms. *Aquaculture* **86:**359–367.
38. **Bradley, D. E., T. Aoki, T. Kitao, T. Arai, and H. Tschäpe.** 1982. Specification of characteristics for the classification of plasmids in incompatibility group U. *Plasmid* **8:**89–93.

39. **Brazil, G., D. Curley, F. Gannon, and P. Smith.** 1986. *Persistence and Acquisition of Antibiotic Resistance Plasmids in* Aeromonas salmonicida. Cold Spring Harbor Laboratory, Cold Spring Harbor, N.Y.
40. **Cabello, F. C.** 2004. Antibiotics and aquaculture in Chile: implications for human and animal health. *Rev. Med. Chile* **132:**1001–1006. (In Spanish.)
41. **Casas, C., E. C. Anderson, K. K. Ojo, I. Keith, D. Whelan, D. Rainnie, and M. C. Roberts.** 2005. Characterization of pRAS1-like plasmids from atypical North American psychrophilic *Aeromonas salmonicida*. *FEMS Microbiol. Lett.* **242:**59–63.
42. **Chadwick, M., M. J. Waldock, R. J. Gowen, and D. Calamari.** 1993. Review of *The Atlantic Salmon: Natural History, Exploitation, and Future Management*, by W. M. Shearer; *Persistent Pollutants in Marine Ecosystems*, by Colin H. Walker and David L. Livingstone and *Aquaculture and the Environment*, by T. V. R. Pillay. *ICES J. Mar. Sci.* **50:** 325–327.
43. **Dalsgaard, I., L. Høi, R. J. Siebeling, and A. Dalsgaard.** 1999. Indole-positive *Vibrio vulnificus* isolated from disease outbreaks on a Danish eel farm. *Dis. Aquat. Org.* **35:**187–194.
44. **De Grandis, S. A., and R. M. Stevenson.** 1985. Antimicrobial susceptibility patterns and R plasmid-mediated resistance of the fish pathogen *Yersinia ruckeri*. *Antimicrob. Agents Chemother.* **27:**938–942.
45. **DePaola, A., P. A. Flynn, R. M. McPhearson, and S. B. Levy.** 1988. Phenotypic and genotypic characterization of tetracycline- and oxytetracycline-resistant *Aeromonas hydrophila* from cultured channel catfish (*Ictalurus punctatus*) and their environments. *Appl. Environ. Microbiol.* **54:** 1861–1863.
46. **DePaola, A., and M. C. Roberts.** 1995. Class D and E tetracycline resistance determinants in gram-negative bacteria from catfish ponds. *Mol. Cell. Probes* **9:**311–313.
47. **Duremdez, R., A. Al-Marzouk, J. A. Qasem, A. Al-Harbi, and H. Gharabally.** 2004. Isolation of *Streptococcus agalactiae* from cultured silver pomfret, *Pampus argenteus* (Euphrasen), in Kuwait. *J. Fish Dis.* **27:**307–310.
48. **Ervik, A., B. Thorsen, V. Eriksen, B. T. Lunestad, and O. B. Samuelsen.** 1994. Impact of administering antibacterial agents on wild fish and blue mussels *Mytilus edulis* in the vicinity of fish farms. *Dis. Aquat.Org.* **18:**45–51.
49. **Escande, F., G. Gerbaud, J. L. Martel, and P. Courvalin.** 1991. Resistance to trimethoprim and 2,4-diamino-6,7-diisopropylpteridine (O/129) in *Pasteurella haemolytica*. *Vet. Microbiol.* **26:**107–114.
50. **Ewing, J. H., R. Hugh, and J. Johnson.** 1961. *Studies on the* Aeromonas *Group*. Communicable Disease Center, U.S. Department of Health, Education and Welfare, Atlanta, Ga.
51. **Fleshner, M., and M. L. Laudenslager.** 2004. Psychoneuroimmunology: then and now. *Behav. Cogn. Neurosci. Rev.* **3:**114–130.
52. **Gauthier, G., B. Lafay, R. Ruimy, V. Breittmayer, J. L. Nicolas, M. Gauthier, and R. Christen.** 1995. Small-subunit rRNA sequences and whole DNA relatedness concur for the reassignment of *Pasteurella piscicida* (Snieszko et al.) Janssen and Surgalla to the genus *Photobacterium* as *Photobacterium damsela* subsp. *piscicida* comb. nov. *Int. J. Syst. Bacteriol.* **45:** 139–144.
53. **Gibello, A., M. C. Porrero, M. M. Blanco, A. I. Vela, P. Liebana, M. A. Moreno, J. F. Fernandez-Garayzabal, and L. Dominguez.** 2004. Analysis of the *gyrA* gene of clinical *Yersinia ruckeri* isolates with reduced susceptibility to quinolones. *Appl. Environ. Microbiol.* **70:**599–602.
54. **Giraud, E., G. Blanc, A. Bouju-Albert, F. X. Weill, and C. Donnay-Moreno.** 2004. Mechanisms of quinolone resistance and clonal relationship among *Aeromonas salmonicida* strains isolated from reared fish with furunculosis. *J. Med. Microbiol.* **53:**895–901.
55. **Goni-Urriza, M., C. Arpin, M. Capdepuy, V. Dubois, P. Caumette, and C. Quentin.** 2002. Type II topoisomerase quinolone resistance-determining regions of *Aeromonas caviae*, *A. hydrophila*, and *A. sobria* complexes and mutations associated with quinolone resistance. *Antimicrob. Agents Chemother.* **46:**350–359.
56. **Grave, K., A. Lillehaug, B. T. Lunestad, and T. E. Horsberg.** 1999. Prudent use of antibacterial drugs in Norwegian aquaculture? Surveillance by the use of prescription data. *Acta Vet. Scand.* **40:**185–195.
57. **Grave, K., M. Engelstad, N. E. Søli, and T. Håstein.** 1990. Utilization of antibacterial drugs in salmonid farming in Norway during 1980-1988. *Aquaculture* **86:**347–358.
58. **Grave, K., A. Markestad, and M. Bangen.** 1996. Comparison in prescribing patterns of antibacterial drugs in salmonid farming in Norway during the periods 1980–1988 and 1989–1994. *J. Vet. Pharmacol. Ther.* **19:**184–191.
59. **Griffiths, S. G., and W. H. Lynch.** 1989. Characterization of *Aeromonas salmonicida* mutants with low-level resistance to multiple antibiotics. *Antimicrob. Agents Chemother.* **33:** 19–26.
60. **Gutierrez, M. C., and M. L. Barros.** 1998. Antibiotic resistance of *Pseudomonas fluorescens* strains isolated from farmed rainbow trout (*Oncorhynchus mykiss*) in Spain. *Bull. Eur. Assoc. Fish Pathol.* **18:**168–171.
61. **Hastings, T. S., and A. McKay.** 1987. Resistance of *Aeromonas salmonicida* to oxolinic acid. *Aquaculture* **61:** 65–171.
62. **Hawke, J. P., S. M. Plakas, R. V. Minton, R. M. McPhearson, T. G. Snider, and M. Guarino.** 1987. Fish pasteurellosis of cultured striped bass, *Morone saxatilis*, in coastal Alabama. *Aquaculture* **65:**193–204.
63. **Hedges, R. W., P. Smith, and G. Brazil.** 1985. Resistance plasmids of aeromonads. *J. Gen. Microbiol.* **131:** 2091–2095.
64. **Hickman-Miller, H. D., and W. H. Hildebrand.** 2004. The immune response under stress: the role of HSP-derived peptides. *Trends Immunol.* **25:**427–433.
65. **Høie, S., B. Martinsen, S. Sohlberg, and T. E. Horsberg.** 1992. Sensitivity patterns of Norwegian clinical isolates of *Aeromonas salmonicida* subsp. *salmonicida* to oxolinic acid, flumequine, oxytetracycline, and sulphadiazine/trimethoprim. *Bull. Eur. Assoc. Fish Pathol.* **12:**142–144.
66. **Inglis, V., G. N. Frerichs, S. D. Millar, and R. H. Richards.** 1991. Antibiotic resistance of *Aeromonas salmonicida* isolated from Atlantic salmon, *Salmo salar* L., in Scotland. *J. Fish Dis.* **14:**353–358.
67. **Inglis, V., E. Yimer, E. J. Bacon, and S. Ferguson.** 1993. Plasmid-mediated antibiotic resistance in *Aeromonas salmonicida* isolated from Atlantic salmon, *Salmo salar* L., in Scotland. *J. Fish Dis.* **16:**593–599.
68. **Izumi, S., and F. Aranishi.** 2004. Relationship between *gyrA* mutations and quinolone resistance in *Flavobacterium psychrophilum* isolates. *Appl. Environ. Microbiol.* **70:**3968–3972.
69. **Kawai, K., Y. Liu, K. Ohnishi, and S. Oshima.** 2004. A conserved 37 kDa outer membrane protein of *Edwardsiella tarda* is an effective vaccine candidate. *Vaccine* **22:** 3411–3418.
70. **Kim, E., and T. Aoki.** 1993. Drug resistance and broad geographical distribution of identical R plasmids of *Pasteurella*

piscicida isolated from cultured yellowtail in Japan. *Microbiol. Immunol.* 37:103–109.

71. **Kim, E., and T. Aoki.** 1993. The structure of the chloramphenicol resistance gene on a transferable R plasmid from the fish pathogen, *Pasteurella piscicida. Microbiol. Immunol.* 37:705–712.
72. **Kim, E., and T. Aoki.** 1996. Sequence analysis of the florfenicol resistance gene encoded in the transferable R-plasmid of a fish pathogen, *Pasteurella piscicida. Microbiol. Immunol.* 40:665–669.
73. **Kim, E. H., and T. Aoki.** 1994. The transposon-like structure of IS*26*-tetracycline, and kanamycin resistance determinant derived from transferable R plasmid of fish pathogen, *Pasteurella piscicida. Microbiol. Immunol.* **38:**31–38.
74. **Kim, E. H., and T. Aoki.** 1996. Sulfonamide resistance gene in a transferable R plasmid of *Pasteurella piscicida. Microbiol. Immunol.* **40:**397–399.
75. **Kruse, H., and H. Sørum.** 1994. Transfer of multiple drug resistance plasmids between bacteria of diverse origins in natural microenvironments. *Appl. Environ. Microbiol.* **60:** 4015–4021.
76. **Kusuda, R., M. Itaoka, and K. Kawai.** 1988. Drug sensitivity of *Pasteurella piscicida* strains isolated from cultured yellowtail from 1984 to 1985. *Nippon Suisan Gakkaishi* **54:** 1521–1526.
77. **Kusuda, R., H. Sugiura, and K. Kawai.** 1990. Drug sensitivity of *Pasteurella piscicida* isolated from cultured yellowtail from 1986 to 1988. *Nippon Suisan Gakkaishi* **56:**239–242.
78. **L'Abée-Lund, T. M., and H. Sørum.** 2001. Class 1 integrons mediate antibiotic resistance in the fish pathogen *Aeromonas salmonicida* worldwide. *Microb. Drug Resist.* **7:**263–272.
79. **L'Abée-Lund, T. M., and H. Sørum.** 2002. A global non-conjugative Tet C plasmid, pRAS3, from *Aeromonas salmonicida. Plasmid* **47:**172–181.
80. **L'Abée-Lund, T. M., and H. Sørum.** 2001. Functional Tn*5393*-like transposon in the R plasmid pRAS2 from the fish pathogen *Aeromonas salmonicida* subspecies *salmonicida* isolated in Norway. *Appl. Environ. Microbiol.* **66:**5533–5535.
81. **Lee, K. Y., J. D. Hopkins, and M. Syvanen.** 1991. Evolved neomycin phosphotransferase from an isolate of *Klebsiella pneumoniae. Mol. Microbiol.* **5:**2039–2046.
82. **Lehane, L., and G. T. Rawlin.** 2000. Topically acquired bacterial zoonoses from fish: a review. *Med. J. Aust.* **173:** 256–259.
83. **Lillehaug, A., B. T. Lunestad, and K. Grave.** 2003. Epidemiology of bacterial diseases in Norwegian aquaculture—a description based on antibiotic prescription data for the ten-year period 1991 to 2000. *Dis. Aquat.Org.* **53:**115–125.
84. **Liu, P. C., K. K. Lee, and S. N. Chen.** 1997. Susceptibility of different isolates of *Vibrio harveyi* to antibiotics. *Microbios* **91:**175–180.
85. **Lunestad, B. T., and J. Goksøyr.** 1990. Reduction in the antibacterial effect of oxytetracycline in seawater by complex formation with magnesium and calcium. *Dis. Aquat. Org.* **9:** 67–72.
86. **Magarinos, B., J. L. Romalde, I. Bandin, B. Fouz, and A. E. Toranzo.** 1992. Phenotypic, antigenic, and molecular characterization of *Pasteurella piscicida* strains isolated from fish. *Appl. Environ. Microbiol.* **58:**3316–3322.
87. **Markestad, A., and K. Grave.** 1997. Reduction of antibacterial drug use in Norwegian fish farming due to vaccination. *Dev. Biol. Stand.* **90:**365–369.
88. **Masuyoshi, S., T. Okubo, M. Inoue, and S. Mitsuhashi.** 1988. Purification and some properties of a chloramphenicol acetyltransferase mediated by plasmids from *Vibrio anguillarum. J. Biochem.* (Tokyo) **104:**131–135.
89. **Michel, C., B. Kerouault, and C. Martin.** 2003. Chloramphenicol and florfenicol susceptibility of fish-pathogenic bacteria isolated in France: comparison of minimum inhibitory concentration, using recommended provisory standards for fish bacteria. *J. Appl. Microbiol.* **95:**1008–1015.
90. **Miranda, C. D., C. Kehrenberg, C. Ulep, S. Schwarz, and M. C. Roberts.** 2003. Diversity of tetracycline resistance genes in bacteria from Chilean salmon farms. *Antimicrob. Agents Chemother.* **47:**883–888.
91. **Mitoma, Y., T. Aoki, and J. H. Crosa.** 1984. Phylogenetic relationships among *Vibrio anguillarum* plasmids. *Plasmid* **12:** 143–148.
92. **Mizon, F. M., G. R. Gerbaud, H. Leclerc, and Y. A. Chabbert.** 1978. Occurrence of R plasmids belonging to incompatibility group *incC* in *Aeromonas hydrophila* strains isolated from sewage water. *Ann. Microbiol.* (Paris) **129B:**19–26. (In French with English abstract.)
93. **Morii, H., N. Hayashi, and K. Uramoto.** 2003. Cloning and nucleotide sequence analysis of the chloramphenicol resistance gene on conjugative R plasmids from the fish pathogen *Photobacterium damselae* subsp. *piscicida. Dis. Aquat. Org.* **53:**107–113.
94. **Morii, H., M. S. Bharadwaj, and N. Eto.** 2004. Cloning and nucleotide sequence analysis of the ampicillin resistance gene on a conjugative R plasmid from the fish pathogen *Photobacterium damselae* subsp. *piscicida. J. Aquat. Anim. Health* **16:**197–207.
95. **Muroga, K., N. Yoneyama, and Y. Jo.** 1979. Vibriostatic agent-nonsensitive *Vibrio anguillarum* isolated from ayu. *Fish Pathol.* **13:**159–162.
96. **Myhr, E., J. L. Larsen, A. Lillehaug, R. Gudding, M. Heum, and T. Håstein.** 1991. Characterization of *Vibrio anguillarum* and closely related species isolated from farmed fish in Norway. *Appl. Environ. Microbiol.* **57:**2750–2757.
97. **Nomoto, R. L., I. Munasinghe, D. H. Jin, Y. Shimahara, H. Yasuda, A. Nakamura, N. Misawa, T. Itami, and T. Yoshida.** 2004. Lancefield group C *Streptococcus dysgalactiae* infection responsible for fish mortalities in Japan. *J. Fish Dis.* **27:** 679–686.
98. **Nonaka, L., and S. Suzuki.** 2002. New Mg^{2+}-dependent oxytetracycline resistance determinant Tet 34 in *Vibrio* isolates from marine fish intestinal contents. *Antimicrob. Agents Chemother.* **46:**1550–1552.
99. **Oppegaard, H., and H. Sørum.** 1994. *gyrA* mutations in quinolone-resistant isolates of the fish pathogen *Aeromonas salmonicida. Antimicrob. Agents Chemother.* **38:**2460–2464.
100. **Padgett, D. A., and R. Glaser.** 2003. How stress influences the immune response. *Trends Immunol.* **24:**444–448.
101. **Pazos, F., Y. Santos, B. Magariños, I. Bandín, S. Núñez, and A. E. Toranzo.** 1993. Phenotypic characteristics and virulence of *Vibrio anguillarum*-related organisms. *Appl. Environ. Microbiol.* **59:**2969–2976.
102. **Pedersen, K., T. Tiainen, and J. L. Larsen.** 1995. Antibiotic resistance of *Vibrio anguillarum*, in relation to serovar and plasmid contents. *Acta Vet. Scand.* **36:**55–64.
103. **Popoff, M., and Y. Davaine.** 1971. Facteurs de résistance transférables chez *Aeromonas salmonicida. Ann. Inst. Pasteur* **121:**337–342.
104. **Press, C. M., and A. Lillehaug.** 1995. Vaccination in European salmonid aquaculture: a review of practices and prospects. *Br. Vet. J.* **151:**45–69.
105. **Pursell, L., O. B. Samuelsen, and P. Smith.** 1995. Reduction in the in-vitro activity of flumequine against *Aeromonas salmonicida* in the presence of the concentrations of Mg^{2+} and Ca^{2+} ions found in sea water. *Aquaculture* **135:**245–255.

106. **Rådström, P., G. Swedberg, and O. Sköld.** 1991. Genetic analyses of sulfonamide resistance and its dissemination in gram-negative bacteria illustrate new aspects of R plasmid evolution. *Antimicrob. Agents Chemother.* **35:**1840–1848.
107. **Reger, P. J., D. F. Mockler, and M. A. Miller.** 1993. Comparison of antimicrobial susceptibility, beta-lactamase production, plasmid analysis and serum bactericidal activity in *Edwardsiella tarda, E. ictaluri* and *E. hoshinae. J. Med. Microbiol.* **39:**273–281.
108. **Rhodes, G., G. Huys, J. Swings, P. McGann, M. Hiney, P. Smith, and R. W. Pickup.** 2000. Distribution of oxytetracycline resistance plasmids between aeromonads in hospital and aquaculture environments: implication of Tn*1721* in dissemination of the tetracycline resistance determinant Tet A. *Appl. Environ. Microbiol.* **66:**3883–3890.
109. **Rhodes, G., J. Parkhill, C. Bird, K. Ambrose, M. C. Jones, G. Huys, J. Swings, and R. W. Pickup.** 2004. Complete nucleotide sequence of the conjugative tetracycline resistance plasmid pFBAOT6, a member of a group of IncU plasmids with global ubiquity. *Appl. Environ. Microbiol.* **70:**7497–7510.
110. **Saavedra, M. J., S. Guedes-Novais, A. Alves, P. Rema, M. Tacao, A. Correia, and A. Martinez-Murcia.** 2004. Resistance to β-lactam antibiotics in *Aeromonas hydrophila* isolated from rainbow trout *(Oncorhynchus mykiss). Int. Microbiol.* 7:207–211.
111. **Samuelsen, O. B., B. T. Lunestad, B. Husevåg, T. Hølleland, and A. Ervik.** 1992. Residues of oxolinic acid in wild fauna following medication in fish farms. *Dis. Aquat. Org.* **12:** 111–119.
112. **Schmidt, A. S., M. S. Bruun, I. Dalsgaard, and J. L. Larsen.** 2001. Incidence, distribution, and spread of tetracycline resistance determinants and integron-associated antibiotic resistance genes among motile aeromonads from a fish farming environment. *Appl. Environ. Microbiol.* **67:**5675–5682.
113. **Schmidt, A. S., M. S. Bruun, I. Dalsgaard, K. Pedersen, and J. L. Larsen.** 2000. Occurrence of antimicrobial resistance in fish-pathogenic and environmental bacteria associated with four Danish rainbow trout farms. *Appl. Environ. Microbiol.* **66:**4908–4915.
114. **Schmidt, A. S., M. S. Bruun, J. L. Larsen, and I. Dalsgaard.** 2001. Characterization of class 1 integrons associated with R-plasmids in clinical Aeromonas salmonicida isolates from various geographical areas. *J. Antimicrob. Chemother.* **47:** 735–743.
115. **Shotts, E. B., V. L. Vanderwork, and L. M. Campbell.** 1976. Occurrence of R factors associated with *Aeromonas hydrophila* isolates from aquarium fish and waters. *J. Fish. Res. Board Can.* 33:736–740.
116. **Smith, I. W.** 1963. The classification of "*Bacterium salmonicida*". *J. Gen. Microbiol.* 33:263–274.
117. **Snieszko, S. F.** 1959. Antibiotics in fish diseases and fish nutrition. *Antibiot. Chemother.* **9:**541–545.
118. **Snieszko, S. F., and G. L. Bullock.** 1957. Treatment of sulfonamide-resistant furunculosis in trout and determination of drug sensitivity. *Fish. Bull.* **125:**555–564.
119. **Snieszko, S. F., G. L. Bullock, E. Hollis, and J. G. Boone.** 1964. *Pasteurella* sp. from an epizootic of white perch (*Roccus americanus*) in Chesapeake Bay tidewater areas. *J. Bacteriol.* 88:1814–1815.
120. **Snieszko, S. F., S. B. Friddle, and P. J. Griffin.** 1951. Successful treatment of ulcer disease in brook trout (*Salvelinus fontinalis*) with terramycin. *Science* **113:**717–718.
121. **Son, R., G. Rusul, A. M. Sahilah, A. Zainuri, A. R. Raha, and I. Salmah.** 1997. Antibiotic resistance and plasmid profile of *Aeromonas hydrophila* isolates from cultured fish, tilapia (*Tilapia mossambica*). *Lett. Appl. Microbiol.* **24:** 479–482.
122. **Sørum, H.** 2000. Farming of Atlantic salmon—an experience from Norway. *Acta Vet. Scand. Suppl.* **93:**129–134.
123. **Sørum, H., G. Holstad, T. Lunder, and T. Håstein.** 2000. Grouping by plasmid profiles of atypical *Aeromonas salmonicida* isolated from fish, with special reference to salmonid fish. *Dis. Aquat. Org.* **41:**159–171.
124. **Sørum, H., J. H. Kvello, and T. Håstein.** 1993. Occurrence and stability of plasmids in *Aeromonas salmonicida* ss *salmonicida*, isolated from salmonids with furunculosis. *Dis. Aquat. Org.* **16:**199–206.
125. **Sørum, H., T. M. L'Abée-Lund, A. Solberg, and A. Wold.** 2003. Integron-containing IncU R plasmids pRAS1 and pAr-32 from the fish pathogen *Aeromonas salmonicida. Antimicrob. Agents Chemother.* **47:**1285–1290.
126. **Sørum, H., M. C. Roberts, and J. H. Crosa.** 1992. Identification and cloning of a tetracycline resistance gene from the fish pathogen *Vibrio salmonicida. Antimicrob. Agents Chemother.* **36:**611–615.
127. **Sundin, G. W., and C. L. Bender.** 1995. Expression of the *strA-strB* streptomycin resistance genes in *Pseudomonas syringae* and *Xanthomonas campestris* and characterization of IS*6100* in *X. campestris. Appl. Environ. Microbiol.* **61:** 2891–2897.
128. **Takashima, N., T. Aoki, and T. Kitao.** 1985. Epidemiological surveillance of drug-resistant strains of *Pasteurella piscicida. Fish Pathol.* **20:**209–217.
129. **Tauch, A., S. Krieft, J. Kalinowski, and A. Puhler.** 2000. The 51,409-bp R-plasmid pTP10 from the multiresistant clinical isolate *Corynebacterium striatum* M82B is composed of DNA segments initially identified in soil bacteria and in plant, animal, and human pathogens. *Mol. Gen. Genet.* **263:**1–11.
130. **Thune, R. L., D. H. Fernandez, J. P. Hawke, and R. Miller.** 2003. Construction of a safe, stable, efficacious vaccine against *Photobacterium damselae* ssp. *piscicida. Dis. Aquat. Org.* 57:51–58.
131. **Topic, P. N., E. Teskeredzic, I. Strunjak-Perovic, and R. Coz-Rakovac.** 2000. *Aeromonas hydrophila* isolated from wild freshwater fish in Croatia. *Vet. Res. Commun.* **24:**371–377.
132. **Toranzo, A. E., J. M. Cutrin, B. S. Roberson, S. Nunez, J. M. Abell, F. M. Hetrick, and A. M. Baya.** 1994. Comparison of the taxonomy, serology, drug resistance transfer, and virulence of *Citrobacter freundii* strains from mammals and poikilothermic hosts. *Appl. Environ. Microbiol.* **60:**1789–1797.
133. **Tschäpe, H., E. Tietze, and C. Koch.** 1981. Characterization of conjugative R plasmids belonging to the new incompatibility group *IncU. J. Gen. Microbiol.* **127:**155–160.
134. **Vivekanandhan, G., K. Savithamani, A. A. Hatha, and P. Lakshmanaperumalsamy.** 2002. Antibiotic resistance of *Aeromonas hydrophila* isolated from marketed fish and prawn of South India. *Int. J. Food Microbiol.* **76:**165–168.
135. **Watanabe, T.** 1963. Infective heredity of multiple drug resistance in bacteria. *Bacteriol. Rev.* **27:**87–115.
136. **White, D. G., C. Hudson, J. J. Maurer, S. Ayers, S. Zhao, M. D. Lee, L. Bolton, T. Foley, and J. Sherwood.** 2000. Characterization of chloramphenicol and florfenicol resistance in *Escherichia coli* associated with bovine diarrhea. *J Clin. Microbiol.* **38:**4593–4598.
137. Reference deleted.
138. **Yoshida, H., M. Bogaki, M. Nakamura, and S. Nakamura.** 1990. Qulnolone resistance-determining region in the DNA gyrase *gyra* gene of *Escherichia coli. Antimicrob. Agents Chemother.* **34:**1271–1272.
139. **Yu, L., L. Yuan, H. Feng, and S. F. Li.** 2004. Determination of the bacterial pathogen *Edwardsiella tarda* in fish species

by capillary electrophoresis with blue light-emitting diode-induced fluorescence. *Electrophoresis* **25:**3139–3144.

140. **Zhao, J., and T. Aoki.** 1992. Cloning and nucleotide sequence analysis of a chloramphenicol acetyltransferase gene from *Vibrio anguillarum*. *Microbiol. Immunol.* **36:** 695–705.

141. **Zhao, J., and T. Aoki.** 1992. Nucleotide sequence analysis o the class G tetracycline resistance determinant from *Vibrio anguillarum*. *Microbiol. Immunol.* **36:**1051–1060.

142. **Zhao, J. A., E. Kim, T. Kobayashi, and T. Aoki.** 1992. Drug-resistance of *Vibrio anguillarum* isolated from ayu between 1989 and 1991. *Nippon Suisan Gakkaishi* **58:**1523–1527.

Antimicrobial Resistance in Bacteria of Animal Origin
Edited by Frank M. Aarestrup

Chapter 14

Mycoplasma

Frank M. Aarestrup and Isabelle Kempf

Mollicutes are the smallest free-living microorganisms. They are pleomorphic and approximately 0.2 to 0.3 μm in diameter. They do not have a cell wall and are thus not susceptible to β-lactam antibiotics, glycopeptides, and fosfomycin. They are also resistant to polymyxins, sulfonamides, trimethoprim, nalidixic acid, and rifampin (9). *Mollicutes* can probably be isolated from all mammalian and avian species (63, 75). They normally colonize mucous membranes as commensals or cause infections in the respiratory or urogenital tract, serous membranes, or mammary gland (63, 75). *Mollicutes* tend to show a high degree of host specificity. The main species that cause infections in animals belongs to the genera *Mycoplasma* and *Ureaplasma* (Table 1). Most *Mycoplasma* and *Ureaplasma* spp. are slowly growing, fastidious organisms with special growth requirements.

IMPORTANCE OF ANTIMICROBIAL TREATMENT

Infections with mycoplasmas normally lead to a good immune response (75), although some species possess sophisticated mechanisms (invasion of nonphagocytic host cells, surface antigenic variation) to escape the host immune system (70). However, vaccination is sometimes an effective way of reducing diseases with this group of organisms (63, 75). Furthermore, the International Office of Epizootics categorizes a number of *Mycoplasma* species as causes of group A or group B diseases, and eradication programs are initiated in many countries if these species are observed (55). However, for other species the use of antimicrobial agents is important in controlling infections. In veterinary medicine the most commonly used antimicrobial agents are fluoroquinolones, macrolides, tetracyclines, and tiamulin.

ANTIMICROBIAL SUSCEPTIBILITY TESTING

Susceptibility testing for *Mycoplasma* can, as for all other bacterial species, be performed by agar or broth dilution or disk diffusion. Because of their slow growth and fastidious medium requirements, susceptibility testing of mycoplasmas requires special media (Table 2). There have been only a limited number of attempts to determine the susceptibility of animal *Mycoplasma* by diffusion testing (2, 25), and MIC determinations are used in most studies. The MIC is the minimum concentration inhibiting the metabolism of a substrate, usually indicated by a color change of the broth medium, or preventing colony formation on agar media. For mycoplasmas fermenting glucose (*Mycoplasma hyopneumoniae, M. hyorhinis, M. gallisepticum*, and *M. synoviae*) or hydrolyzing arginine (*M. hyosynoviae*), the broth dilution method is usually based on the metabolism inhibition test and pH changes are visualized by use of phenol red. *M. bovis* neither ferments glucose nor hydrolyzes arginine, but metabolism of pyruvate (31), reduction of the colorless 2,3,5-triphenyltetrazolium to the red formazan and production of a film layer on top of the broth (77), or hydrolysis of Tween 80 (18) may be observed. Other authors record the growth or absence of growth of *M. bovis* or *M. agalactiae* according to medium turbidity measured by the opacimetric method (62) or centrifugation of plates and observation of wells with an inverted mirror (3, 52). Agar dilution methods are preferred when large numbers of strains are to be tested or for species that are difficult to grow in liquid medium, such as *M. meleagridis* (30).

Numerous studies on the determination of MICs of different antimicrobial agents for mycoplasmas have been published. However, there has been limited standardization of the procedures, making

Frank M. Aarestrup • Danish Institute for Food and Veterinary Research, Bülowsvej 27, DK-1790 Copenhagen V, Denmark.
Isabelle Kempf • Mycoplasmology Bacteriology Unit, French Agency for Food Safety (AFSSA), BP53, F-22440 Ploufragan, France.

Table 1. Pathogenic *Mycoplasma* and *Ureaplasma* species, animal hosts, diseases caused, and antimicrobial agents of importance in controlling infections[a]

Species	Animal host	Infection	Antimicrobial agents of importance in controlling infection	Vaccines available
Mycoplasma alkalescens	Cattle	Mastitis		
Mycoplasma agalactiae	Sheep, goats	Mastitis, arthritis, keratitis, pleuropneumonia, septicemia	Macrolides, tetracyclines	Yes
Mycoplasma bovigenitalium	Cattle	Mastitis		
Mycoplasma bovis	Cattle	Pneumonia, arthritis, mastitis	Macrolides, tilmicosin, linomycin, fluoroquinolones	
Mycoplasma bovoculi	Cattle	Keratoconjunctivitis	Oxytetracycline, polymyxin B	
Mycoplasma californicum	Cattle	Mastitis		
Mycoplasma canadense	Cattle	Mastitis		
Mycoplasma dispar	Cattle	Pneumonia		
Mycoplasma mycoides subsp. *mycoides* small colony	Cattle (sheep, goats)	Contagious bovine pleuropneumoniae	Treatment discouraged	Yes
Mycoplasma species bovine serogroup 7	Cattle	Mastitis, arthritis, pneumonia		
Mycoplasma capricolum subsp. *capricolum*	Goats, sheep	Mastitis, arthritis, keratitis, pleuropneumonia, septicemia	Macrolides, tetracyclines	
Mycoplasma conjunctivae	Goats, sheep	Keratoconjunctivitis	Tetracyclines	
Mycoplasma mycoides subsp. *capri*	Goats, sheep	Mastitis, arthritis, keratitis, pleuropneumonia, septicemia		
Mycoplasma mycoides subsp. *mycoides* large colony	Goats, sheep	Mastitis, arthritis, keratitis, pleuropneumonia, septicemia	Treatment discouraged	
Mycoplasma putrefaciens	Goats, sheep	Mastitis, arthritis, keratitis, pleuropneumonia, septicemia		
Mycoplasma capricolum subsp. *capripneumoniae*	Goats	Contagious caprine pleuropneumonia		
Mycoplasma ovipneumoniae	Sheep	Pneumonia		
Mycoplasma hyopneumoniae	Pigs	Enzootic pneumonia	Macrolides, tetracyclines	Yes
Mycoplasma hyorhinis	Pigs	Arthritis, polyserositis	Macrolides, tetracyclines	
Mycoplasma hyosynoviae	Pigs	Arthritis, polyarthritis	Macrolides, lincomycin, tiamulin, tetracyclines	
Mycoplasma gallisepticum	Chickens, turkeys	Chronic respiratory disease, infectious sinusitis	Tetracyclines, macrolides, tiamulin, fluoroquinolones	Yes
Mycoplasma synoviae	Chickens, turkeys	Infectious synovitis, respiratory infections	Tetracyclines, macrolides, tiamulin, fluoroquinolones	
Mycoplasma meleagridis	Turkeys	Airsacculitis, osteodystrophy, reduced hatchability	Fluoroquinolones	
Mycoplasma iowae	Turkeys	Reduced hatchability	Fluoroquinolones	
Ureaplasma diversum	Cattle	Granular vulvitis, infertility, calf pneumonia	Lincomycin-spectinomycin-tylosin, tetracyclines	

[a]From references 38, 49, 63, and 78.

Table 2. Recommendations for susceptibility testing of veterinary mycoplasmas[a]

Medium	The agar or broth giving the optimal growth for the specific species should be employed. Mycoplasma medium (24) and Frey's medium are most commonly used.
Inoculum	10^3 to 10^5 color-changing units
Incubation	Atmosphere suitable for the specific *Mycoplasma* species
Incubation time	In liquid medium, the time it takes for particular *Mycoplasma* species to cause color changes equivalent to controls; on agar, the time it takes for adequate growth of the specific species
Reading	Lowest drug concentration in which no color change occurs or lowest drug concentration causing >50% inhibition of colony growth
Interpretation	No international breakpoints are available. Isolates with clearly reduced susceptibility compared to the remaining population should be regarded as resistant.

[a]Based on reference 30.

comparison of the MICs between studies conducted in different laboratories difficult. Methods for testing human mycoplasmas, as recommended by the Mycoplasmal Chemotherapy Working Team of the International Research Program on Comparative Mycoplasmology, were recently published by Waites et al. (83). The general guidelines for storage, preparation of antimicrobial solutions, and dilutions also apply to susceptibility testing of mycoplasma. Recently, Hannan (30) published a review on the guidelines and recommendations for susceptibility testing of veterinary mycoplasmas. This guideline did not, however, include any recommendation on the media to use, since the different *Mycoplasma* species vary in their requirements. Thus, Friis' modified broth medium (22, 24) may be used for swine mycoplasmas (11, 25, 32, 54, 76, 86). For avian mycoplasmas, FM4 medium (23) was used by Kleven and Anderson (45) and Kempf et al. (44), Frey's medium (22) was used by Cerda et al. (14) and Wang et al. (84), and other media are also possible (14, 39, 40, 45, 74, 84). For MIC testing of mycoplasmas isolated from ruminants, Friis', Edward's, Hayflick's, and Eaton's media have been described (3, 30). A commercial medium (ME medium; Mycoplasma Experience, Ltd., Reigate, United Kingdom) is suitable for mycoplasmas from poultry, swine, or ruminants.

Both agar and broth dilutions have been used and seem to give reasonably comparable MICs for a number of *Mycoplasma* species (30, 76). The inoculum can greatly affect the MIC obtained (30, 39), which has also been observed for other bacteria. Thus, a careful standardization of inocula is required. Hannan (30) recommends 10^3 to 10^5 color-changing units/ml, which is also the concentration that has been most commonly used by other researchers. The different mycoplasma species vary in their ability to grow under different atmospheres. Thus, incubation should take place under the atmosphere where optimal growth normally is found with the given species. Incubation is normally good between 35 and 37°C. The incubation time also differs between species. Some mycoplasmas, such as *M. hyopneumoniae*, are very slow growing and may require incubation times up to 14 days. The MIC is normally read when the color of the control with no antimicrobial matches the preset pH control. However, when incubated further, the end point may shift considerably, especially in liquid medium (1). Thus, in some studies both the initial and the final reading are reported. On agar plates, reading is performed by comparing the growth on control plates without antimicrobial agents with that on plates containing dilutions of the antimicrobial agents. According to various authors, the MIC is the concentration that completely inhibits mycoplasmal growth (39), results in only a single colony or a layer of very small colonies (76), results in dwarf colonies not observed by the naked eye (46), or causes more than 50% inhibition of growth compared to the control plates (30, 32).

MBC TESTS

Few authors report MBC tests for mycoplasmas of veterinary interest. Kleven and Anderson (45) used subcultures onto agar to determine minimum lethal concentrations for *M. synoviae*. Among tested molecules, tylosin, lincomycin, and spectinomycin showed relatively better mycoplasmacidal activity than molecules of the tetracycline group. Ball et al. (4) and Ayling et al. (3) diluted antibiotics 1/200 and 1/20, respectively, to distinguish between mycoplasmastatic and mycoplasmacidal effects of different antimicrobials on *M. bovis*. Both groups reported mycoplasmacidal effects of fluoroquinolones. Hannan et al. (32) studied the killing curves of norfloxacin and one of its analogues against *M. hyopneumoniae* and concluded that both were mycoplasmacidal in vitro, whereas tiamulin was mycoplasmastatic.

In vitro susceptibility testing results should be used to predict the clinical effectiveness of a given antimicrobial agent in vivo. Thus, based on the MIC, the mycoplasma should be categorized as sensitive, intermediate resistant, or resistant. However, there are currently no international standards available, even though some researchers have attempted to establish breakpoints for different species and antimicrobial agents (31, 44, 76, 77). A synthesis of breakpoints suggested by various investigators is given by Hannan (30).

OCCURRENCE OF RESISTANCE

Pigs

Worldwide, there have been very few reports on the antimicrobial susceptibility of the different *Mycoplasma* species. In addition, several studies have reported only the MICs at which 50 or 90% of the strains were inhibited and not percent resistance.

Zimmermann and Ross (90) examined 43 isolates of *M. hyosynoviae* isolated between 1959 and 1971 in swineherds in Iowa and found a decrease in their susceptibility to tylosin among the isolates over time. Kobayashi et al. (46) determined the susceptibility of 27 Japanese *M. hyosynoviae* isolates from 1980 to 1984 and 25 from 1994 and 1995 to 13 antimicrobial agents. Two isolates from 1994 and 1995 were resistant to all 14- and 16-membered macrolides (tylosin, josamycin, kitasamycin, spiramycin, and lincomycin). For oxytetracycline, the MICs for most isolates from 1980 to 1984 were 0.1 to 0.78 μg/ml, while the oxytetracycline MICs for most isolates from 1994 and 1995 were 0.78 to 6.25 μg/ml. Otherwise, the isolates formed one population with susceptibilities to kanamycin, chloramphenicol, thiamphenicol, tiamulin, and enrofloxacin. Aarestrup and Friis (1) determined the susceptibility of 21 Danish *M. hyosynoviae* isolates from 1968 to 1971 and 21 from 1995 and 1996 to enrofloxacin, lincomycin, tetracycline, tiamulin, and tylosin. All isolates from 1968 to 1971 were highly susceptible to all antimicrobials tested, whereas 12 (57%) of the isolates from 1995 and 1996 showed reduced susceptibility to tylosin.

M. hyopneumoniae is intrinsically resistant to 14-membered macrolides such as erythromycin. Cooper et al. (15) examined 11 isolates from the United Kingdom and found all to be susceptible to danofloxacin and tylosin, whereas 5 (45%) of the isolates had reduced susceptibility to oxytetracycline. In The Netherlands all 10 isolates isolated from 1984 to 1989 were found to be susceptible to 16-membered macrolides, lincosamides, tetracyclines, tiamulin, and fluoroquinolones (76). More recently, Vicca et al. (81) studied the in vitro susceptibility of 21 *M. hyopneumoniae* field isolates and found acquired resistance to macrolides, lincosamides, and fluoroquinolones but not to tetracyclines, gentamicin, florfenicol, or tiamulin. Tanner et al. (73) examined 25 isolates from the United States and found all of them to be susceptible to tetracyclines, macrolides, lincosamides, and furaltadone. Several studies have been performed in Japan (35, 72, 87). These studies have shown susceptibility to macrolides, tiamulin, and lincosamides but also a decrease in the susceptibility to tetracyclines among more recent isolates.

M. hyorhinis from both The Netherlands and Japan has been found to be susceptible to tetracyclines and fluoroquinolones (47, 76). All 12 isolates from The Netherlands were susceptible to 16-membered macrolides and lincosamides, whereas 11 (10%) of 107 isolates from Japan were resistant.

Cattle

In Japan, Hirose et al. (33) determined MICs for 68 *M. bovirhinis*, 21 *M. alkalescens*, and 10 *M. bovis* isolates and found a frequent occurrence of resistance to tetracyclines and macrolides among all three species and resistance to enrofloxacin in *M. bovirhinis*. In The Netherlands, ter Laak et al. (77) examined 16 *M. bovis* and 19 *M. dispar* isolates and found that some of them had reduced susceptibility to tetracyclines. In Belgium, Thomas et al. (79) showed that many recent field isolates of *M. bovis* were resistant to macrolides and tetracyclines.

Poultry

M. gallisepticum is usually susceptible to erythromycin, spiramycin, lincomycin, tetracycline, tiamulin, and tylosin, but strains resistant to macrolides have been reported by different authors (41, 44, 54, 74, 85). The species is also susceptible to fluoroquinolones, but resistance may be observed in recent field isolates (63). Apparent natural resistance to apramycin has been observed (12, 74).

M. synoviae is intrinsically resistant to erythromycin (44, 45, 85) and flumequin (31). Most studied strains are susceptible to josamycin, spiramycin, lincomycin, tylosin, tilmicosin, tiamulin, danofloxacin, and enrofloxacin (31, 41, 44). According to Hannan et al. (31), Japanese isolates of *M. synoviae* were resistant to oxytetracycline, and Cerda et al. (14) reported a chlortetracycline-resistant isolate in Argentina. The fluoroquinolone concentrations inhibiting *M. synoviae* are higher than those inhibiting *M. gallisepticum* (12, 44).

GENETIC BACKGROUND FOR RESISTANCE

The genetic background for resistance has been studied only with mycoplasmas causing infections in humans. Thus, the following is based on studies with human-pathogenic species.

Macrolides

Macrolides bind to the 50S part of the ribosome and inhibit protein synthesis. Resistance to macrolides is most commonly caused by blockade of the entrance of the antibiotic into the cell, chemical inactivation of the antibiotic, lack of binding to the ribosomal target, or lack of inhibitory response upon binding to the target (see chapter 6). The most well-known mechanism for resistance among rapidly growing bacteria is lack of binding to the target due to target modification by dimethylation of an adenine residue in 23S rRNA (48; see also chapter 6), whereas in more slowly growing organisms with only a single or few ribosomal operon mutations in 23S rRNA genes at the same site are more commonly observed (37, 42, 80). Since mycoplasmas are slow growing and all species tested so far carry only one or two ribosomal operons (29), it would be expected that the mechanisms of resistance are mutations in the 23S rRNA gene.

Mycoplasmas present different phenotypes of intrinsic resistance to macrolides and lincosamides. However, a number of acquired mutations have also been observed both in in vitro-selected mutants and in clinical isolates (Table 3). In *M. pneumoniae*, which is naturally susceptible to all members of the macrolide-lincosamide-streptogramin-ketolide antibiotic group except lincomycin, it was found that provoked resistance to erythromycin obtained by long-term cultivation was caused by two different single-base-pair mutations in 23S rRNA genes (53, 56). These mutations were A to G at position 2058 and A to G at position 2059 (*Escherichia coli* numbering), where it also previously has been found that mutations cause resistance to macrolides and lincosamides (see chapter 6). The A2058G mutation has also been found in a clindamycin-resistant clinical isolate (56). Pereyre et al. (59) selected mutants of *M. pneumoniae* resistant to a number of different macrolides, lincosamides, and streptogramins. In josamycin- and quinupristin-dalfopristin-selected mutants they observed the A2062G mutations, whereas in erythromycin-, azithromycin-, and telithromycin-selected mutants they found C2611A mutations. At this later position a C2611U mutation was previously obtained in vitro (58). One mutant selected in the presence of clindamycin and three of five mutants selected in the presence of telithromycin harbored mutations giving rise to a single amino acid change at position 70 in ribosomal protein L4. Mutations at position 2062 have not been observed in other species, but both erythromycin and tylosin interact with this position (80).

M. hominis is naturally resistant to 14- and 15-membered macrolides such as erythromycin, but susceptible to 16-membered macrolides and lincosamides. Determination of the sequence of the peptidyltransferase loop of the region of the 23S rRNA genes associated with binding of macrolides showed

Table 3. Mutations in 23S rRNA genes conferring macrolide resistance in *Mycoplasma* spp.

Mutation in 23S rRNA gene	*Mycoplasma* species	Obtained	Resistance to: 14- and 15-membered macrolides	16-membered macrolides	Lincosamides	Reference(s)
G2057A		Intrinsic in *M. hominis*, *M. flocculare*, *M. fermentans*, *M. pulmonis*, and *M. hyopneumoniae*	+	–	–	26, 58
A2058G	*M. pneumoniae*	In vivo and in vitro	+	+	+	53, 56
A2059G	*M. pneumoniae*, *M. hominis*	In vivo and in vitro	+	+	+	53, 56
A2062G	*M. hominis*, *M. pneumoniae*	In vitro	+	+	–	26, 59
A2062T	*M. hominis*	In vitro	+	+	–	26
C2611A	*M. hominis*, *M. pneumoniae*	In vitro	+	–	–	58, 59

that this species, together with *M. flocculare*, *M. fermentans*, *M. pulmonis*, and *M. hyopneumoniae*, has a G to A transition at position 2057 (*E. coli* numbering) (26, 58), whereas *M. pneumoniae*, an erythromycin-susceptible mycoplasma, has a G. Alterations at this site in *E. coli* cause resistance to erythromycin and chloramphenicol but not clindamycin (20). Moreover, intracellular accumulation and ribosome binding of [^{14}C]erythomycin in *M. hominis* was reduced compared to *M. pneumoniae* (58). By selection of two mutant strains resistant to the 16-membered macrolide josamycin, it was found that two new mutations, A to G and A to T at position 2062 (*E. coli* numbering), also gave resistance to 16-membered macrolides, but not lincosamides (27). Pereyre et al. (58) examined two clinical isolates of *M. hominis* that were resistant to josamycin and lincosamides and found that they, in addition to the naturally occurring G2057A transition, also contained mutations at A2059G.

Positions 2057, 2058, 2059, and 2611 have been identified as hot spots for resistance mutations in the 23S rRNA gene (80), and it is not surprising that mycoplasma, with their limited number of operons, acquire macrolide resistance by mutations at these positions in the 23S rRNA gene.

Resistant mutants of bovine, porcine, and avian species have been obtained with tylosin, spiramycin, or erythromycin without elucidating the molecular support of such resistance (28, 31, 89). Field strains of *M. gallisepticum* or *M. meleagridis* with decreased susceptibility to tylosin were isolated by several authors (50, 51) after repeated exposure to this molecule, and resulted in therapeutic failures (54). Some strains of *M. hyorhinis* (46), *M. hyosynoviae* (1), *M. hyopneumoniae* (81), *M. gallisepticum* (12, 41, 44), and *M. bovis* (15) for which macrolide MICs are high have been reported.

Tetracyclines

Tetracyclines bind to the 30S part of ribosomes. Resistance to tetracyclines can occur by three mechanisms: active efflux, ribosomal protection, and enzymatic modification (see chapter 6). There are currently 35 different classes of tetracycline resistance genes (see chapter 6). A high frequency of tetracycline resistance has been reported in several *Mycoplasma* species. The only resistance mechanism observed so far has been the presence of *tet*(M)-like sequences in high-level-resistant *M. hominis* isolates and *Ureaplasma* spp. (67, 69). This gene is located on the conjugative transposon Tn*916*, which is widely distributed among urogenital bacteria of human origin (16, 68) and confers resistance to all tetracyclines. Strains of *M. bovis* (79), *M. hyopneumoniae* (81), *M. hyosynoviae* (32), *M. hyorhinis* (32), *M. gallisepticum* (12), and *M. synoviae* (32) for which antimicrobial MICs are increased have been reported, but the molecular mechanisms are unknown. However, *tet*(M) can be experimentally transferred to many species of animal mycoplasmas, including *M. gallisepticum* (13, 71), *M. arthritidis* (82), *M. pulmonis*, and *M. hyorhinis* (19).

Fluoroquinolones

Quinolones interfere with DNA replication by binding to DNA gyrase or topoisomerase IV (see Introduction). Resistance to quinolones is caused mainly by mutations in the genes encoding DNA gyrase (*gyrA* and *gyrB*) or topoisomerase IV (*parC* or *parE*) (Table 4) (see chapter 6). In gram-negative bacteria most mutations are found in *gyrA* and *gyrB*, whereas in gram-positive bacteria they are observed mainly in *parC* or *parE* (see chapter 6).

Bébéar et al. (5–8) found alterations in *gyrA*, *parC*, and *parE* in both fluoroquinolone-resistant clinical isolates of *M. hominis* and in in vitro-selected mutants. In *gyrA*, mutations were observed at position (*E. coli* numbering) 83 [TCA (Ser) → TTA (Leu) and TCA (Ser) → TGA (Trp)], position 84 [TCA (Ser) → TTA (Leu)], position 87 [GAA (Glu) → AAA (Lys)], and position 119 [GCA (Ala) → GTA (Val) and GCA (Ala) → GAA (Glu)] (5, 6, 8). In *parC*, mutations were observed at positions 69 [GAT (Asp) → TAT (Tyr)], 73 [CGT (Arg) → CAT (His), 80 (AGT (Ser) → ATT (Ile)], and 84 [GAA (Glu) → AAA (Lys)], and in *parE*, at position 420 [GAT (Asp) → AAT (Asn)] (6). In clinical *M. hominis* isolates, alterations were found at *gyrA* 83 [TCA (Ser) → TTA (Leu)], *gyrA* 87 [GAA (Glu) → AAA (Lys)], *parC* 81 [TCA (Ser) → CCA (Pro)], *parC* 84 [GAA (Glu) → AAA (Lys)], and *parE* 420 [GAT (Asp) → AAT (Asn)] (7).

Hirose et al. (33) reported a high frequency of resistance to enrofloxacin among *M. bovirhinis* isolated from cattle in Japan. Genetic examination of the *gyrA*, *gyrB*, *parC*, and *parE* genes revealed a TCA (Ser) → TTA (Leu) in position 80 of *parC* in resistant wild-type isolates and selected mutants compared to susceptible isolates (34).

Reinhardt et al. (66) selected fluoroquinolone-resistant *M. gallisepticum* mutants by passaging two strains in vitro in increasing concentrations of enrofloxacin. Sequencing of the quinolone resistance-determining region (QRDR) of the *gyrA*/*gyrB* and *parC*/*parE* genes revealed several mutations in the different targets. Ser83 → Arg and Ser80 → Trp in the GyrA and ParC QRDRs, respectively, seemed to

Table 4. Amino acid substitutions associated with fluoroquinolone resistance in *Mycoplasma* spp.

Gene	Amino acid substitution	*Mycoplasma* species	In vitro selection or clinical isolates	Likely involvement in quinolone resistance	Reference(s)
gyrA	Gly81 → Ala	*M. gallisepticum*	In vitro	ND[a]	66
	Ser83 → Leu	*M. hominis*	In vitro, clinical isolates	Yes	5, 6, 7, 8, 43
	Ser83 → Ile	*M. gallisepticum*	In vitro, clinical isolates	ND	64, 65, 66
	Ser83 → Asn	*M. gallisepticum*	In vitro	ND	65
	Ser83 → Arg	*M. gallisepticum*	In vitro	Yes	66
	Ser83 → Trp	*M. hominis*	In vitro	Yes	6, 43
	Ala84 → Pro	*M. gallisepticum*	In vitro	ND	66
	Ser84 → Leu	*M. hominis*	In vitro	Yes	6
	Glu87 → Gly	*M. gallisepticum*	In vitro	ND	66
	Glu87 → Lys	*M. hominis*	In vitro, clinical isolates	Yes	7, 8, 43, 66
		M. gallisepticum	In vitro	ND	
	Ala119 → Val	*M. hominis*	In vitro	Yes	8
	Ala119 → Glu	*M. hominis*	In vitro	Yes	8
gyrB	Asp426 → Asn	*M. gallisepticum*	In vitro	ND	66
	Asn464 → Asp	*M. gallisepticum*	In vitro	ND	66
	Glu465 → Lys	*M. gallisepticum*	In vitro	ND	66
	Glu465 → Gly	*M. gallisepticum*	In vitro	ND	66
parC	Ala64 → Ser	*M. gallisepticum*	In vitro	ND	66
	Asp69 → Tyr	*M. hominis*	In vitro	ND	6
	Arg73 → His	*M. hominis*	In vitro	ND	6
	Ser80 → Ile	*M. hominis*	In vitro	Yes	6, 8, 43
	Ser80 → Leu	*M. gallisepticum*	In vitro, clinical isolates	ND	33, 64, 66
		M. bovirhinis	In vitro and clinical isolates	Yes	
	Ser80 → Trp	*M. gallisepticum*	In vitro, clinical isolates	ND	64, 66
	Ser81 → Pro	*M. hominis*	Clinical isolates	Yes	7, 8, 66
		M. gallisepticum	In vitro	ND	Le Carrou et al., submitted
		M. synoviae	Experimental infection	Yes	
	Glu84 → Gly	*M. gallisepticum*	In vitro	ND	66
	Glu84 → Gln	*M. gallisepticum*	In vitro	ND	66
	Glu84 → Lys	*M. hominis*	In vitro, clinical isolates	Yes	6, 8, 43, 66
		M. gallisepticum	In vitro	ND	
parE	Asp420 → Asn	*M. hominis*	In vitro, clinical isolates	Yes	6, 7, 66
		M. gallisepticum	In vitro	ND	
	Asp420 → Lys	*M. gallisepticum*	In vitro	ND	65
	Ser463 → Leu	*M. gallisepticum*	In vitro	ND	66
	Cys467 → Phe	*M. gallisepticum*	In vitro	ND	66

[a]ND, not determined.

have greater influence on the resistance level. Mutations observed in two field isolates of *M. gallisepticum* were Ser83 → Ile in GyrA and Ser80 → Trp in ParC or Ser83 → Ile in GyrA and Ser80 → Leu in ParC (64). The persistence of *M. synoviae* in experimentally infected hens after two enrofloxacin treatments was studied (J. Le Carrou, A. K. Reinhardt, I. Kempf, and A. V. Gautier-Bouchardon, submitted for publication). A Ser81 → Pro substitution in the ParC QRDR of the DNA topoisomerase IV was associated with a slight increase in resistance in two *M. synoviae* clones isolated after the second treatment.

Mutations at positions 83, 87, and 119 in *gyrA* have been frequently found to be associated with quinolone resistance in several gram-negative bacterial species (61, 88; see also chapter 6), whereas changes at positions 81 and 84 seem to be infrequently found.

Substitutions at positions 80 and 84 in *parC* and at position 420 in *parE* seem to be frequent, especially in fluoroquinolone-resistant gram-positive bacteria (10, 21, 36, 57, 60; see also chapter 6), whereas the mutations at positions 69 and 73 of *parC* have not been observed in other species. The *parC* 81 substitution has also previously been described in *Neisseria gonorrhoeae* (17).

DISCUSSION

There are only a very limited number of reports on the antimicrobial susceptibility of the different *Mycoplasma* species pathogenic for animals, and there is an obvious need for standardization of methods and interpretation. However, based on the reports available, animal strains do not seem to have developed resistance to a major degree. Exceptions may be resistance to macrolides and lincosamides, where resistance in some countries is so high that routine use of these antimicrobial agents can no longer be recommended. In addition, strains with reduced susceptibility to tetracyclines seem to emerge. In contrast to *M. hominis*, these isolates are, with the possible exception of *M. bovirhinis*, not high-level resistant, and the mechanism of resistance is probably not due to the acquisition of *tet*(M). However, this has not been determined and is at present unknown. Fluoroquinolones can still be used against animal-pathogenic mycoplasmas, but the rapid emergence of resistance among human strains indicates that these strains may rapidly acquire resistance. Thus, at present, considering its very low MICs, tiamulin seems to be a valuable agent for the treatment of mycoplasmosis in poultry and pigs

REFERENCES

1. **Aarestrup, F. M., and N. F. Friis.** 1998. Antimicrobial susceptibility testing of *Mycoplasma hyosynoviae* isolated from pigs during 1968 to 1971 and during 1995 and 1996. *Vet. Microbiol.* **61:**33–39.
2. **Aarestrup, F. M., N. F. Friis, and J. Szancer.** 1998. Antimicrobial susceptibility of *Mycoplasma hyorhinis* in a liquid medium compared to a disc assay. *Acta Vet. Scand.* **39:**145–147.
3. **Ayling, R. D., S. E. Baker, M. L. Peek, A. J. Simon, and R. A. J. Nicholas.** 2000. Comparison of *in vitro* activity of danofloxacin, florfenicol, oxytetracycline, spectinomycin and tilmicosin against recent field isolates of *Mycoplasma bovis*. *Vet. Rec.* **146:**745–747.
4. **Ball, H. J., C. Reilly, and D. G. Bryson.** 1995. Antibiotic susceptibility of *Mycoplasma bovis* strains isolated in Northern Ireland. *Ir. Vet. J.* **48:**316–318.
5. **Bébéar, C. M., J. M. Bové, C. Bébéar, and J. Renaudin.** 1997. Characterization of *Mycoplasma hominis* mutations involved in resistance to fluoroquinolones. *Antimicrob. Agents Chemother.* **41:**269–273.
6. **Bébéar, C. M., H. Renaudin, A. Charron, J. M. Bové, C. Bébéar, and J. Renaudin.** 1998. Alterations in topoisomerase IV and DNA gyrase in quinolone-resistant mutants of *Mycoplasma hominis* obtained in vitro. *Antimicrob. Agents Chemother.* **42:**2304–2311.
7. **Bébéar, C. M., J. Renaudin, A. Charron, H. Renaudin, B. de Barbeyrac, T. Schaeverbeke, and C. Bébéar.** 1999. Mutations in the *gyrA*, *parC*, and *parE* genes associated with fluoroquinolone resistance in clinical isolates of *Mycoplasma hominis*. *Antimicrob. Agents Chemother.* **43:**954–956.
8. **Bébéar, C. M., O. Grau, A. Charron, H. Renaudin, D. Gruson, and C. Bébéar.** 2000. Cloning and nucleotide sequence of the DNA gyrase (*gyrA*) gene from *Mycoplasma hominis* and characterization of quinolone resistant mutants selected in vitro with trovafloxacin. *Antimicrob. Agents Chemother.* **44:**2719–2727.
9. **Bébéar, C. M., and C. Bébéar.** 2002. Antimycoplasmal agents, p. 545–566. *In* S. Razin and R. Herrmann (ed.), *Molecular Biology and Pathogenicity of Mycoplasmas*. Kluwer Academic/Plenum, New York, N.Y.
10. **Belland, R. J., S. G. Morrison, C. Ison, and W. M. Huang.** 1994. *Neisseria gonorrhoeae* acquires mutations in analogous regions of *gyrA* and *parC* in fluoroquinolone-resistant isolates. *Mol. Microbiol.* **14:**371–380.
11. **Bousquet, E., P. Pommier, S. Wessel-Robert, H. Morvan, H. Benoit-Valiergue, and A. Laval.** 1998. Efficacy of doxycycline in feed for the control of pneumonia caused by *Pasteurella multocida* and *Mycoplasma hyopneumoniae* in fattening pigs. *Vet. Rec.* **143:**269–272.
12. **Bradbury, J. M., C. A. Yavari, and C. J. Giles.** 1994. In vitro evaluation of various antimicrobials against *Mycoplasma gallisepticum* and *Mycoplasma synoviae* by the micro-broth method, and comparison with a commercially-prepared test system. *Avian Pathol.* **23:**105–115.
13. **Cao, J., P. A. Kapke, and F. C. Minion.** 1994. Transformation of *Mycoplasma gallisepticum* with Tn*916*, Tn*4001*, and integrative plasmid vectors. *J. Bacteriol.* **176:**4459–4462.
14. **Cerda, R. O., G. I. Giacoboni, J. A. Xavier, P. L. Sansalone, and M. F. Landoni.** 2002. *In vitro* antibiotic susceptibility of field isolates of *Mycoplasma synoviae* in Argentina. *Avian Dis.* **46:**215–218.
15. **Cooper, A. C., J. R. Fuller, M. K. Fuller, P. Whittlestone, and D. R. Wise.** 1993. *In vitro* activity of danofloxacin, tylosin and oxytetracycline against mycoplasmas of veterinary importance. *Res. Vet. Sci.* **54:**329–334.
16. **de Barbeyrac, B., M. Dupon, P. Rodriguez, H. Renaudin, and C. Bébéar.** 1996. A Tn1545-like transposon carries the tet(M) gene in tetracycline resistant strains of *Bacteroides ureolyticus* as well as *Ureaplasma urealyticum* but not *Neisseria gonorrhoeae*. *J. Antimicrob. Chemother.* **37:**223–232.
17. **Deguchi, T., M. Yasuda, M. Nakano, E. Kanematsu, S. Ozeki, Y. Nishino, T. Ezaki, S. Maeda, I. Saito, and Y. Kawada.** 1997. Rapid screening of point mutations of the *Neisseria gonorrhoeae parC* gene associated with resistance to quinolones. *J. Clin. Microbiol.* **35:**948–950.
18. **Devriese, L. A., and F. Haesebrouck.** 1991. Antibiotic susceptibility testing of *Mycoplasma bovis* using Tween 80 hydrolysis as an indicator of growth. *Zentbl. Veterinärmed. B* **38:**781–783.
19. **Dybvig, K., and J. Alderete.** 1988. Transformation of *Mycoplasma pulmonis* and *Mycoplasma hyorhinis*: transposition of Tn916 and formation of cointegrate structures. *Plasmid* **20:**33–41.
20. **Ettayebi, M., S. M. Prasad, and E. A. Morgan.** 1985. Chloramphenicol-erythromycin resistance mutations in a 23S rRNA gene of *Escherichia coli*. *J. Bacteriol.* **162:**551–557.
21. **Ferrero, L., B. Cameron, and J. Crouzet.** 1995. Analysis of *gyrA* and *grlA* mutations in stepwise-selected ciprofloxacin-resistant mutants of *Staphylococcus aureus*. *Antimicrob. Agents Chemother.* **39:**1554–1558.
22. **Freundt, E. A.** 1983. Culture media for classic mycoplasmes, p. 127–135. *In* J. G. Tully and S. Razin (ed.), *Methods in Mycoplasmology*. Academic Press, Inc., New York, N.Y.
23. **Frey, M. L., R. P. Hanson, and D. P. Anderson.** 1968. A medium for isolation of avian mycoplasmas. *Am. J. Vet. Res.* **29:**2163–2171.
24. **Friis, N. F.** 1975. Some recommendations concerning primary isolation of *Mycoplasma suipneumoniae* and *Mycoplasma flocculare*: a survey. *Nord. Vet. Med.* **27:**337–339.
25. **Friis, N. F., and J. Szancer.** 1994. Sensitivity of certain porcine and bovine mycoplasmas to antimicrobial agents in a liquid medium test compared to a disc assay. *Acta Vet. Scand.* **35:**389–394.
26. **Furneri, P. M., G. Rappazzo, M. P. Musumarra, G. Tempera, and L. S. Roccasalva.** 2000. Genetic basis of natural resistance

to erythromycin in *Mycoplasma hominis. J. Antimicrob. Chemother.* 45:547–548.

27. **Furneri, P. M., G. Rappazzo, M. P. Musumarra, P. Di Pietro, L. S. Catania, and L. S. Roccasalva.** 2001. Two new point mutations at A2062 associated with resistance to 16-membered macrolide antibiotics in mutant strains of *Mycoplasma hominis. Antimicrob. Agents Chemother.* 45:2958–2960.
28. **Gautier-Bouchardon, A. V., A. K. Reinhardt, M. Kobisch, and I. Kempf.** 2002. *In vitro* development of resistance to enrofloxacin, erythomycin, tylosin, tiamulin and oxytetracycline in *Mycoplasma gallisepticum*, *Mycoplasma synoviae* and *Mycoplasma iowae. Vet. Microbiol.* 88:47–58.
29. **Glasser, G., H. C. Hyman, and S. Razin.** 1992. Ribosomes, p. 169–177. *In* J. Maniloff, R. N. McElhaney, L. R. Finch, and J. B. Baseman (ed.), *Mycoplasmas: Molecular Biology and Pathogenesis.* American Society for Microbiology, Washington, D.C.
30. **Hannan, P. C. T.** 2000. Guidelines and recommendations for antimicrobial minimum inhibitory concentration (MIC) testing against veterinary mycoplasma species. International Research Programme on Comparative Mycoplasmology. *Vet. Res.* 31:373–395.
31. **Hannan, P. C. T., G. D. Windsor, A. de Jong, N. Schmeer, and M. Stegemann.** 1997. Comparative susceptibilities of various animal-pathogenic mycoplasmas to fluoroquinolones. *Antimicrob. Agents Chemother.* 41:2037–2040.
32. **Hannan, P. C. T., P. J. O'Hanlon, and N. H. Rogers.** 1989. *In vitro* evaluation of various quinolone antibacterial agents against veterinary mycoplasmas and porcine respiratory bacterial pathogens. *Res. Vet. Sci.* 46:202–211.
33. **Hirose, K., H. Kobayashi, N. Ito, Y. Kawasaki, M. Zako, K. Kotani, H. Ogawa, and H. Sato.** 2003. Isolation of Mycoplasmas from nasal swabs of calves affected with respiratory diseases and antimicrobial susceptibility of their isolates. *J. Vet. Med. B* 50:347–351.
34. **Hirose, K., Y. Kawasaki, K. Kotani, K. Abiko, and H. Sato.** 2004. Characterization of a point mutation in the *parC* gene of *Mycoplasma bovirhinis* associated with fluoroquinolone resistance. *J. Vet. Med. B* 51:169–175.
35. **Inamoto, T., H. Takahashi, K. Yamamoto, Y. Nakai, and K. Ogimoto.** 1994. Antibiotic susceptibility of *Mycoplasma hyopneumoniae* isolated from swine. *J. Vet. Med. Sci.* 56: 393–394.
36. **Ito, H., H. Yoshida, M. Bogaki-Shonai, T. Niga, H. Hattori, and S. Nakamura.** 1994. Quinolone resistance mutations in the DNA gyrase *gyrA* and *gyrB* genes of *Staphylococcus aureus. Antimicrob. Agents Chemother.* 38:2014–2023.
37. **Jensen, L. B., and F. M. Aarestrup.** 2001. Macrolide resistance in *Campylobacter coli* of animal origin in Denmark. *Antimicrob. Agents Chemother.* 45:371–372.
38. **Jordan, F. T. W.** 1990. Avian mycoplasmoses, p. 74–85. *In* F. T. W. Jordan (ed.), *Poultry Diseases*, 3rd ed. Bailliére Tindall, London, United Kingdom.
39. **Jordan, F. T. W., and D. Knight.** 1984. The minimum inhibitory concentration of kitasamycin, tylosin and tiamulin for *Mycoplasma gallisepticum* and their protective effect on infected chicks. *Avian Pathol.* 13:151–162.
40. **Jordan, F. T. W., S. Gilbert, D. L. Knight, and C. A. Yavari.** 1989. Effects of Baytril, tylosin and tiamulin on avian Mycoplasmas. *Avian Pathol.* 18:659–673.
41. **Jordan, F. T. W., and B. K. Horrocks.** 1996. The minimum inhibitory concentration of tilmicosin and tylosin for *Mycoplasma gallisepticum* and *Mycoplasma synoviae* and a comparison of their efficacy in the control of *Mycoplasma gallisepticum* infection in broiler chicks. *Avian Dis.* 40: 326–334.
42. **Karlsson, M., C. Fellstrom, M. U. Heldtander, K. E. Johansson, and A. Franklin.** 1999. Genetic basis of macrolide and lincosamide resistance in *Brachyspira (Serpulina) hyodysenteriae. FEMS Microbiol. Lett.* 172:255–260.
43. **Kenny, G. E., P. A. Young, F. D. Cartwright, K. E. Sjostrom, and W. M. Huang.** 1999. Sparfloxacin selects gyrase mutations in first-step *Mycoplasma hominis* mutants, whereas ofloxacin selects topoisomerase IV mutations. *Antimicrob. Agents Chemother.* 43:2493–2496.
44. **Kempf, I., C. Ollivier, R. L'Hospitalier, M. Guittet, and G. Bennejean.** 1989. Concentrations minimales inhibitrices de treize antibiotiques vis-à-vis de 21 souches de mycoplasmes de volailles. *Point Vet.* 20:935–940.
45. **Kleven, S. H., and D. P. Anderson.** 1971. In vitro activity of various antibiotics against *Mycoplasma synoviae. Avian Dis.* 15:551–557.
46. **Kobayashi, H., N. Sonmez, T. Morozumi, K. Mitani, N. Ito, H. Shiono, and K. Yamamoto.** 1996. *In vitro* susceptibility of *Mycoplasma hyosynoviae* and *M. hyorhinis* to antimicrobial agents. *J. Vet. Med. Sci.* 58:1107–1111.
47. **Kobayashi, H., T. Morozumi, G. Munthali, K. Mitani, N. Ito, and K. Yamamoto.** 1996. Macrolide susceptibility of *Mycoplasma hyorhinis* isolated from piglets. *Antimicrob. Agents Chemother.* 40:1030–1032.
48. **Leclercq, R., and P. Courvalin.** 1991. Bacterial resistance to macrolide, lincosamide, and streptogramin antibiotics by target modification. *Antimicrob. Agents Chemother.* 35: 1267–1272.
49. **Le Grand, D., M. A. Arcangioli, N. Giraud, F. Poumarat, and P. Bezille.** 2004. Pathologie infectieuse respiratoire chez les bovins: conduite à tenir lors de pneumopathies à mycoplasmes. *Point Vet.* 249:40–42.
50. **Levisohn, S.** 1981. Antibiotic sensitivity patterns in field isolates of *Mycoplasma gallisepticum* as a guide to chemotherapy. *Isr. J. Med. Sci.* 17:661–666.
51. **Levisohn, S., E. Berman, and Y. Weisman.** 1993. Effect of treatment of turkeys under field conditions with tylosin or enrofloxacin on frequency of isolation and sensitivity patterns of *Mycoplasma meleagridis. Public Health Res.* 20:183.
52. **Loria, G. R., C. Sammartino, R. A. Nicholas, and R. D. Ayling.** 2003. *In vitro* susceptibilities of field isolates of *Mycoplasma agalactiae* to oxytetracycline, tylosin, enrofloxacin, spiramycin and lincomycin-spectinomycin. *Res. Vet. Sci.* 75:3–7.
53. **Lucier, T. S., K. Heitzman, S. K. Liu, and P. C. Hu.** 1995. Transition mutations in the 23S rRNA of erythromycin-resistant isolates of *Mycoplasma pneumoniae. Antimicrob. Agents Chemother.* 39:2770–2773.
54. **Migaki, T. T., A. P. Avakian, H. J. Barnes, D. H. Ley, A. C. Tanner, and R. A. Magonigle.** 1993. Efficacy of danofloxacin and tylosin in the control of mycoplasmosis in chicks infected with tylosin-susceptible or tylosin-resistant field isolates of *Mycoplasma gallisepticum. Avian Dis.* 37: 508–514.
55. **Nicolet, J.** 1996. Animal mycoplasmoses: a general introduction. *Rev. Sci. Tech.* 15:1233–1240.
56. **Okazaki, N., M. Narita, S. Yamada, K. Izumikawa, M. Umetsu, T. Kenri, Y. Sasaki, Y. Arakawa, and T. Sasaki.** 2001. Characteristics of macrolide-resistant *Mycoplasma pneumoniae* strains isolated from patients and induced with erythromycin *in vitro. Microbiol. Immunol.* 45:617–620.
57. **Pan, X. S., J. Ambler, S. Mehtar, and L. M. Fisher.** 1996. Involvement of topoisomerase IV and DNA gyrase as ciprofloxacin targets in *Streptococcus pneumoniae. Antimicrob. Agents Chemother.* 40:2321–2326.
58. **Pereyre, S., P. Gonzalez, B. De Barbeyrac, A. Darnige, H. Renaudin, A. Charron, S. Raherison, C. Bébéar, and C. M. Bébéar.**

2002. Mutations in 23S rRNA account for intrinsic resistance to macrolides in *Mycoplasma hominis* and *Mycoplasma fermentans* and for acquired resistance to macrolides in *M. hominis*. *Antimicrob. Agents Chemother.* **46:**3142–3150.

59. **Pereyre, S., C. Guyot, H. Renaudin, A. Charron, C. Bébéar, and C. M. Bébéar.** 2004. *In vitro* selection and characterization of resistance to macrolides and related antibiotics in *Mycoplasma pneumoniae*. *Antimicrob. Agents Chemother.* **48:** 460–465.
60. **Perichon, B., J. Tankovic, and P. Courvalin.** 1997. Characterization of a mutation in the *parE* gene that confers fluoroquinolone resistance in *Streptococcus pneumoniae*. *Antimicrob. Agents Chemother.* **41:**1166–1167.
61. **Piddock, L. J.** 2002. Fluoroquinolone resistance in *Salmonella* serovars isolated from humans and food animals. *FEMS Microbiol. Rev.* **26:**3–16.
62. **Poumarat, F., and J. L. Martel.** 1989. Mise au point et évaluation d'une méthode opacimétrique pour la détermination de l'antibiosensibilité de *Mycoplasma bovis in vitro*. *Ann. Rech. Vet.* **20:**135–143.
63. **Radostits, O. M., C. C. Gay, D. C. Blood, and K. W. Hinchcliff.** 2000. *Veterinary Medicine: a Textbook of the Diseases of Cattle, Sheep, Pigs, Goats and Horses*, 9th ed. The W. B. Saunders Co., Philadelphia, Pa.
64. **Reinhardt, A. K.** 2002. Résistance aux fluoroquinolones liée à la cible chez *Mycoplasma gallisepticum*: sélection de mutants et analyse des mécanismes génétiques. Thèse d'Université. Université de Rennes, Rennes, France.
65. **Reinhardt, A. K., C. M. Bébéar, M. Kobisch, I. Kempf, and A. V. Gautier-Bouchardon.** 2002. Characterization of mutations in DNA gyrase and topoisomerase IV involved in quinolone resistance of *Mycoplasma gallisepticum* mutants obtained in vitro. *Antimicrob. Agents Chemother.* **46:**590–593.
66. **Reinhardt, A. K., I. Kempf, M. Kobisch, and A. V. Gautier-Bouchardon.** 2002. Fluoroquinolone resistance in *Mycoplasma gallisepticum*: DNA gyrase as primary target of enrofloxacin and impact of mutations in topoisomerases on resistance level. *J. Antimicrob. Chemother.* **50:**589–592.
67. **Roberts, M. C.** 1990. Characterization of the Tet M determinants in urogenital and respiratory bacteria. *Antimicrob. Agents Chemother.* **34:**476–478.
68. **Roberts, M. C.** 1992. Antibiotic resistance, p. 513–523. *In* J. Maniloff, R. N. McElhaney, L. R. Finch, and J. B. Baseman (ed.), *Mycoplasmas: Molecular Biology and Pathogenesis*. American Society for Microbiology, Washington, D.C.
69. **Roberts, M. C., L. A. Koutsky, K. K. Holmes, D. J. LeBlanc, and G. E. Kenny.** 1985. Tetracycline-resistant *Mycoplasma hominis* strains contain streptococcal *tetM* sequences. *Antimicrob. Agents Chemother.* **28:**141–143.
70. **Rosengarten, R., C. Citti, M. Glew, A. Lischewski, M. Droesse, P. Much, F. Winner, M. Brank, and J. Spergser.** 2000. Host-pathogen interactions in mycoplasma pathogenesis: virulence and survival strategies of minimalist prokaryotes. *Int. J. Med. Microbiol.* **290:**15–25.
71. **Ruffin, D. C., V. L. van Santen, Y. Zhang, L. L. Voelker, V. S. Panangala, and K. Dybvig.** 2000. Transposon mutagenesis of *Mycoplasma gallisepticum* by conjugation with *Enterococcus faecalis* and determination of insertion site by direct genomic sequencing. *Plasmid* **44:**191–195.
72. **Takahashi, K., C. Kuniyasu, Y. Yoshida, and E. Momotani.** 1978. Sensitivity *in vitro* to macrolide antibiotics and tetracyclines of *Mycoplasma hyopneumoniae* isolated from pneumonic porcine lungs. *Natl. Inst. Anim. Health Q.* (Tokyo) **18:** 41–42.
73. **Tanner, A. C., B. Z. Erickson, and R. F. Ross.** 1993. Adaptation of the Sensititre broth microdilution technique to antimicrobial susceptibility testing of *Mycoplasma hyopneumoniae*. *Vet. Microbiol.* **36:**301–306.
74. **Tanner, A. C., and C. C. Wu.** 1992. Adaptation of the Sensititre broth microdilution technique to antimicrobial susceptibility testing *of Mycoplasma gallisepticum*. *Avian Dis.* **36:**714–717.
75. **Taylor-Robinson, D.** 1995. *Mycoplasma* and *Ureaplasma*, p. 652–662. *In* P. R. Murray (ed.), *Manual of Clinical Microbiology*, 6th ed. ASM Press, Washington D.C.
76. **ter Laak, E. A., A. Pijpers, J. H. Noordergraaf, E. C. Schoevers, and J. H. Verheijden.** 1991. Comparison of methods for in vitro testing of susceptibility of porcine *Mycoplasma* species to antimicrobial agents. *Antimicrob. Agents Chemother.* **35:** 228–233.
77. **ter Laak, E. A., J. H. Noordergraaf, and M. H. Verschure.** 1993. Susceptibilities of *Mycoplasma bovis*, *Mycoplasma dispar*, and *Ureaplasma diversum* strains to antimicrobial agents in vitro. *Antimicrob. Agents Chemother.* **37:**317–321.
78. **Thiaucourt, F., and G. Bolske.** 1996. Contagious caprine pleuropneumonia and other pulmonary mycoplasmoses of sheep and goats. *Rev. Sci. Tech.* **15:**1397–1414.
79. **Thomas, A., C. Nicolas, I. Dizier, J. Mainil, and A. Linden.** 2003. Antibiotic susceptibilities of recent isolates of *Mycoplasma bovis* in Belgium. *Vet. Rec.* **153:**428–431.
80. **Vester, B., and S. Douthwaite.** 2001. Macrolide resistance conferred by base substitutions in 23S rRNA. *Antimicrob. Agents Chemother.* **45:**1–12.
81. **Vicca, J., T. Stakenborg, D. Maes, P. Butaye, J. Peeters, A. de Kruif, and F. Haesebrouck.** 2004. In vitro susceptibilities of *Mycoplasma hyopneumoniae* field isolates. *Antimicrob. Agents Chemother.* **48:**4470–4472.
82. **Voelker, L., and K. Dybvig.** 1996. Gene transfer in *Mycoplasma arthritidis:* transformation, conjugal transfer of Tn*916*, and evidence for a restriction system recognizing AGCT. *J. Bacteriol.* **178:**6078–6081.
83. **Waites, K. B., C. M. Bébéar, J. A. Robertson, D. F. Talkington, and G. E. Kenny.** 2001. *Cumitech 34, Laboratory Diagnosis of Mycoplasmal Infections*. Coordinating ed., F. S. Nolte. American Society for Microbiology, Washington D.C.
84. **Wang, C., M. Ewing, and S. Y. Aarabi.** 2001. *In vitro* susceptibility of avian mycoplasmas to enrofloxacin, sarafloxacin, tylosin, and oxytetracycline. *Avian Dis.* **45:**456–460.
85. **Whithear, K. G., D. D. Bowtell, E. Ghiocas, and K. L. Hughes.** 1983. Evaluation and use of a micro-broth dilution procedure for testing sensitivity of fermentative avian mycoplasmas to antibiotics. *Avian Dis.* **27:**937–949.
86. **Wu, C. C., T. R. Shryock, T. L. Lin, M. Faderan, and M. F. Veenhuizen.** 2000. Antimicrobial susceptibility of *Mycoplasma hyorhinis*. *Vet. Microbiol.* **76:**25–30.
87. **Yamamoto, K., K. Koshimizu, and M. Ogata.** 1986. In vitro susceptibility of *Mycoplasma hyopneumoniae* to antibiotics. *Jpn. J. Vet. Sci.* **48:**1–5.
88. **Yoshida, H., M. Bogaki, M. Nakamura, and S. Nakamura.** 1990. Quinolone resistance-determining region in the DNA gyrase *gyrA* gene of *Escherichia coli*. *Antimicrob. Agents Chemother.* **34:**1271–1272.
89. **Zanella, A., P., A. Martino, A. Pratelli, and M. Stonfer.** 1998. Development of antibiotic resistance in *Mycoplasma gallisepticum* in vitro. *Avian Pathol.* **27:**591–596.
90. **Zimmermann, B. J., and R. F. Ross.** 1975. Determination of sensitivity of *Mycoplasma hyosynoviae* to tylosin and selected antibacterial drugs by a microtiter technique. *Can. J. Comp. Med.* **39:**17–21.

Antimicrobial Resistance in Bacteria of Animal Origin
Edited by Frank M. Aarestrup

Chapter 15

Other Pathogens

FRANK M. AARESTRUP

A large number of different bacterial species can cause infections in animals and humans. The previous chapters described the occurrence of antimicrobial resistance in the most important groups. However, a number of other species are also isolated relatively frequently in diagnostic laboratories, and in some cases antimicrobial treatment is also of importance. International standards for susceptibility testing or breakpoints are in many cases not available for these species. Thus, susceptibility testing and interpretation of results are often based on the experience of the individual laboratory and knowledge of normal susceptibility patterns. Many laboratories will, however, use international standards developed for human or veterinary bacterial isolates of other species. This chapter describes the occurrence and mechanisms of resistance in some of these pathogens and some of the problems in susceptibility testing of these bacteria.

ACTINOBACULUM SUIS

Actinobaculum suis (172) (formerly *Corynebacterium suis*, *Eubacterium suis*, and *Actinomyces suis*) is an obligate anaerobic gram-positive bacterium that causes urinary tract infections, mainly cystitis and pyelonephritis, in sows (48, 236, 308). *A. suis* can be found in high prevalence in healthy boars, and it is in general considered a transmissible venereal disease (227, 264). In cases of infection, the disease is normally treated with penicillin, ampicillin, lincomycin, or tetracycline (70, 236, 316). There have been very few studies on the antimicrobial susceptibility of *A. suis*, probably due to the difficulties in cultivating this organism. There are no specific procedures for susceptibility testing, but the guidelines provided by the National Committee for Clinical Laboratory Standards for anaerobic bacteria can probably be used (209). *A. suis* seems to be susceptible to penicillin, ampicillin, ceftiofur, tetracyclines, macrolides, lincosamides, pleuromutilins, chloramphenicol, florfenicol, and spectinomycin but intrinsically resistant to the fluoroquinolones, aminoglycosides, and sulfamethoxazole-trimethoprim (co-trimoxazole or SXT) (32, 316).

ARCANOBACTERIUM PYOGENES

Arcanobacterium (*Actinomyces, Corynebacterium*) *pyogenes* (237) is a gram-positive pleomorphic coccus and a normal inhabitant of the mucous membranes of domestic animals, such as cattle, goats, sheep, and swine. *A. pyogenes* is also an opportunistic pathogen in these animals, where it causes a variety of purulent infections involving the skin, joints, and visceral organs (236). The bacterium has also been isolated from clinical cases in cats and dogs (34). Due to the formation of abscesses, infections with *A. pyogenes* normally respond poorly to antimicrobial therapy and drainage of abscesses is often necessary (236).

As with most gram-positive fastidious bacteria, susceptibility to antimicrobial agents can be tested by using conventional media supplemented with blood. In most studies MIC determinations have been performed, but disk diffusion shows good correlation with MIC determinations (125). *A. pyogenes* is intrinsically susceptible to β-lactams, fluoroquinolones, macrolides, lincosamides, aminoglycosides, tetracyclines, chloramphenicol, and vancomycin (124, 235, 260, 297, 334). Resistance to macrolides (12 to 28%), tetracyclines (45 to 86%), and streptomycin (52 to 86%) (124, 260, 297, 334) has been observed frequently. A few isolates resistant to chloramphenicol and fluoroquinolones (334) have also been reported, but otherwise *A. pyogenes* seems not

Frank M. Aarestrup • Danish Institute for Food and Veterinary Research, Bülowsvej 27, DK-1790 Copenhagen V, Denmark.

to have acquired resistance to other antimicrobial agents.

The genetic background for resistance has been examined in a limited number of studies. The *erm*(X) gene was found to mediate macrolide resistance in 9 out of 11 tylosin-resistant isolates (161) and the *erm*(B) gene in 10 out of 32 isolates (162). Later studies on isolates not containing *erm*(X) or *erm*(B) found mutations A2058T and C2611G in the 23S rRNA gene to mediate resistance to 14-membered macrolides and reduced susceptibility or resistance to 16-membered macrolides (163). The *tet*(W) gene, encoding tetracycline resistance, was found in all of 20 isolates examined (35). However, *tet*(33) was also detected in a single isolate during the total sequencing of a plasmid carrying *erm*(X) (161), but the occurrence of this determinant in *A. pyogenes* has not been determined.

BACILLUS SPP.

The genus *Bacillus* consists of gram-positive, aerobic or facultatively aerobic rods that produce endospora. The genus includes highly pathogenic species as well as species used as probiotics. The most important species belongs to the *Bacillus cereus* group, even though *Bacillus licheniformis* can cause bovine abortion (3). The *B. cereus* group consists of six closely related bacteria with highly diverse pathogenic potential (81, 175, 208). The group is taxonomically one single species (133), but because of their distinct pathogenic properties and human importance they have remained as individual species. *B. cereus* is a common cause of food poisoning in humans but may also cause infections in humans or bovine mastitis (81). *Bacillus thuringiensis* is mainly an insect pathogen, and toxins produced by this organism are widely used in organic farming as a pesticide (81). *Bacillus mycoides* and *Bacillus pseudomycoides* may also cause food poisoning and occasional infections in humans. The pathogenic importance of *Bacillus weihenstephanensis* is still unknown. The best-known member of the group is *Bacillus anthracis*, the causative agent of anthrax. Anthrax is one of the oldest known zoonotic diseases. It was described both in the Bible (Exodus 9), as the probable cause of the fifth Egyptian plague, and by the Romans (77, 276, 305). *B. anthracis* is highly pathogenic, especially for ungulates such as cattle, sheep, horses, pigs, and goats. In the 19th century, anthrax was an important cause of deaths in the food animal population in Europe (196, 276). The main symptom is sudden death following a peracute septicemia, but the disease may also take an acute form (236). Today anthrax is a relatively uncommon disease in animals, but some areas of endemicity with occasional outbreaks exist, mainly in countries with a subtropical or tropical climate (216, 217). The microorganism may, however, survive for several years in the soil (323) and can be found in almost any part of the world, leading to occasional sporadic cases. As an animal pathogen, the importance of the *B. cereus* group of microorganisms is limited. However, *B. anthracis* is regarded as a very potent biological weapon and its threat as a terrorist weapon in recent years has led to a multitude of research studies, publications, and reviews on this agent (45, 90, 196, 269, 317). The reader is referred to these reviews for a more comprehensive discussion of this organism.

Antimicrobial therapy can be crucial in the treatment of anthrax in humans (178, 313), and the bacterium is normally susceptible to most antimicrobials with activity against gram-positive organisms, including penicillins, macrolides, glycopeptides, tetracyclines, fluoroquinolones, and gentamicin (49, 63, 91, 103, 158, 197, 298), even though some penicillin-resistant strains have been observed (49, 63, 197, 298). A single high-level penicillin-resistant isolate was found to produce β-lactamase (197). Silent β-lactamases have been found on the chromosome of some strains (58, 187), but it is still not known whether increased expression of these β-lactamases will encode resistance in wild-type isolates. Traditionally, the recommended treatment has in most countries been penicillin for at least 7 to 10 days. However, recent studies indicate that *B. anthracis* may express a β-lactamase in vivo and that treatment with ampicillin may be associated with treatment failure (132).

B. anthracis has been found in vitro to develop resistance to fluoroquinolones, caused by amino acid substitutions in topoisomerase II (23). Resistant wild-type isolates have not been identified. Resistance to macrolides has been observed in several cases in bacterial species belonging to the genus *Bacillus*. The most commonly found mechanism is the *erm*(D) gene, encoding a ribosomal methylase, which has been found in *B. anthracis*, *B. licheniformis*, and *Bacillus halodurans* (123, 144, 167, 243). The genetic location of this gene has not been determined. A plasmid-borne *erm*(C) gene has been detected in *Bacillus subtilis* (198), as have chromosomally located *erm*(G) in *Bacillus sphaericus* (199), *erm*(B) in *B. cereus* group isolates from soil (153), and recently chromosomally located *erm*(34) in *Bacillus clausii* (40). Tetracycline-resistant *B. cereus*, *Bacillus stearothermophilus*, and *B. subtilis* have been shown to carry the *tet*(L) gene on a plasmid and/or the chromosome (25, 141, 251), and in *B. cereus* the *tet*(M) gene has been found on the transposon Tn*916* (4). Thus, given the right circumstances *B. anthracis* will probably develop resistance to the most commonly used agents for treatment. Antimicrobial agents used in food animal production are excreted in active forms in feces and urine, which subsequently are spread on fields (71, 256). Thus, veterinary use of antimicrobial agents may lead to selective pressure for resistance among several bacterial species in contact with food animals or their feces and urine. Recent studies have found a low frequency of antimicrobial resistance among isolates belonging to the *B. cereus* group isolated from soil treated with manure (152). Thus, it cannot be excluded that the veterinary use of antimicrobial agents will lead to the selection for resistance in *B. anthracis* and thereby compromise human health. It is, on the other hand, not likely that this will have any major importance.

BRUCELLA SPP.

Brucella spp. are obligate intracellular parasitic, slow-growing, gram-negative cocci and the causative agents of brucellosis. Today six different species are generally accepted: *Brucella abortus*, *Brucella canis*, *Brucella melitensis*, *Brucella neotomae*, *Brucella ovis* and *Brucella suis* (46, 143, 149, 157, 277). In addition, two new species from sea mammals have been proposed: *Brucella pinnipediae* and *Brucella cetaceae* (62, 94, 102). They are, however, closely related, and based on DNA-DNA homologies they should belong to the same species, *Brucella maris* (303, 304). Brucellosis is a zoonotic disease where animals serve as reservoirs (259), and it is also an important veterinary disease (236). Infections with *Brucella* spp. are mainly localized in the genital organs, with abortion in the female and infections such as orchitis or epididymitis in males (236, 259). Mastitis, mainly chronic, may also occur. The host range is extensive, but the different species show host preferences. *B. abortus* causes infections mainly in cattle, *B. melitensis* in goats and sheep, *B. suis* in pigs but possibly also commonly in cattle, *B. canis* in dogs, *B. ovis* in sheep, *B. neotomae* in rodents, and *B. maris* in marine animals. *B. abortus*, *B. canis*, *B. melitensis*, and *B. suis* have been isolated from infections in humans, whereas *B. ovis* and *B. neotomae* so far have not. *B. maris* has been identified in a single case (265). In humans, brucellosis may be confused with tuberculosis. *Brucella* spp. may cause a variety of infections in humans, with infections in almost any organ (259).

Antimicrobial treatment can be important in the control of the infection, especially in humans (266) and dogs (310). Brucellosis requires combination treatment for prolonged periods. Tetracyclines, aminoglycosides, rifampin, and SXT have been used successfully (200, 266, 310), whereas fluoroquinolones have had limited success (171).

Susceptibility testing is normally not performed or recommended for *Brucella* spp. because of the difficulties and dangers associated with handling these species. Furthermore, the importance of in vitro susceptibility has been questioned (16). Thus, there is only limited information available on the susceptibility of these species. When susceptibility testing is performed, it is necessary to use enriched media, such as Mueller-Hinton agar supplemented with blood or brucella agar or broth. Because of the slow growth of the bacteria, prolonged incubation is necessary and growth cannot normally be read for at least 48 h. Thus, susceptibility testing should be performed as MIC determinations on agar or in broth and not as diffusion tests.

Studies have been performed almost exclusively on *B. melitensis*, which in a number of studies has been found to be susceptible to antimicrobial agents that typically have activity against gram-negative bacteria, including aminoglycosides, tetracyclines, rifampin, ciprofloxacin, SXT, cefotaxime, and ceftriaxone (16, 29, 128, 170, 192, 203, 246). Acquired resistance to tetracyclines and streptomycin has not been observed, except by Memish et al. (192), who found 1 tetracycline- and 1 streptomycin-resistant isolate among 160 isolates tested. Resistance or reduced susceptibility to rifampin has been observed for a few isolates (25, 192).

There are conflicting reports as to the effect of macrolides against *Brucella* spp. Hall and Manion (128) found 27 isolates belonging to different *Brucella* spp. to be highly susceptible to erythromycin, whereas Mortensen et al. (203) found erythromycin to have limited activity against *Brucella*. Landinez et al. (170) examined 358 *B. melitensis* isolates from Spain and found all to be highly susceptible to azithromycin.

Resistance to SXT might be emerging in *Brucella*. Memish et al. (192) found 29% resistance among 160 isolates from 1983 to 1995 in Saudi Arabia, and Kinsara et al. (169) found 14 (38%) of 37 isolates obtained from 1995 to 1998 in Saudi Arabia to be susceptible. Also in Saudi Arabia, Almuneef et al. (11) found an increase from 22% resistance in 1996 to 66% in 2000. In Turkey, Baykam et al. (25) found 1 out of 42 isolates to be resistant to SXT. Hall and Manion (128) found two out of four *B. canis* isolates to be highly resistant to streptomycin.

The genetic background for antimicrobial resistance in *Brucella* spp. has not been studied, except for resistance to rifampin, which was found to be caused by mutations in the *rpoB* gene in resistant mutants in the laboratory (185).

BURKHOLDERIA MALLEI AND *BURKHOLDERIA PSEUDOMALLEI*

Burkholderia spp. are aerobic, gram-negative rods that can be found in water, in soil, and on plants and fruit worldwide (116). *B. mallei* is the causative agent of glanders in horses but can also cause serious infections in humans (14, 142, 236). *B. pseudomallei* causes melioidosis in both animals and humans (272, 319, 331). The two species should probably be considered to belong to one single species based on DNA-DNA homology (326) and multilocus sequence typing (119).

Glanders is a highly contagious disease in horses, mules, and donkeys caused by *B. mallei*. The disease is characterized by pneumonia and nodules or ulcers in the respiratory tract or skin (236). The disease has been known since ancient times and might have been the plague that afflicted the Greeks during the siege of Troy (139). The disease has been eradicated in most countries (73, 322) and is today of limited veterinary importance (216, 217). Melioidosis has a broad range of clinical manifestations ranging from asymptomatic infections to chronic infections and acute sepsis (272, 319). The infection is often associated with multiple abscesses in most organs (272, 319). Both bacteria are potential biological weapons (50). *B. mallei* is an obligate parasite, whereas *B. pseudomallei* can be found widely distributed in the environment.

In both horses and humans, infections with *Burkholderia* require long-term antimicrobial treatment. The bacteria are intrinsically resistant to many antimicrobial agents, including most β-lactams and aminoglycosides (68, 131, 151, 165, 226, 293). Recommended treatment is most often sulfonamides and trimethoprim, doxycycline, or the expanded-spectrum cephalosporin cefazidime (52, 53, 267, 320) and more recently meropenem (93, 262).

There have been only a limited number of studies on the antimicrobial susceptibility of *B. mallei* and *B. pseudomallei*. *B. pseudomallei* seems to be less susceptible than *B. mallei* (165, 293). Most isolates are fully susceptible to tetracyclines, carbapenam, cefazidime, and SXT (68, 131, 151, 165, 226, 293). However, isolates that are resistant to cefazidime and tetracycline have been observed (146, 151, 165, 293), indicating that additional resistance may also emerge in these bacteria. Development of resistance to doxycycline, cefazidime, and trimethoprim-sulfonamides has been observed in patients during treatment (68, 151), and it has been easy to select cefazidime-resistant mutants in vitro (68, 69, 211). It has been shown that both increased expression of the chromosomal class D β-lactamase and point mutations in the class A β-lactamase can confer resistance to cefazidime (118, 137, 211, 296). A carbapenem-hydrolyzing β-lactamase has been isolated from *Burkholderia cepacia*, indicating that metallo-β-lactamases may also emerge in *B. mallei* and *B. pseudomallei* (24).

CORYNEBACTERIUM SPP.

Corynebacterium spp. are irregularly shaped, aerobically growing, gram-positive rods with a high G+C content. There are a large number of species in the genus, but not all are important pathogens.

Corynebacterium pseudotuberculosis causes diseases in a number of food-producing animals, including arthritis and bursitis in lambs; caseous lymphadenitis in sheep, goats, and cattle; and contagious acne, abscessation, and ulcerative lymphadenitis in horses (5, 193, 221, 236, 332). The bacterium may also, through rarely, cause infections in humans (179, 195, 223). The species has been divided into two biotypes on the basis of the ability to reduce nitrate (30), a division that has been confirmed by biochemical and molecular characterization (64, 278). The nitrate-positive biovar seems to be specific for horses and cattle and the nitrate-negative biovar for sheep and goats. Antimicrobial therapy often has limited or no effect, but penicillin is most commonly used. *C. pseudotuberculosis* seems to be susceptible to β-lactams, tetracyclines, macrolides, chloramphenicol, lincosamides, vancomycin, and sulfonamides (2, 99, 164, 335). A few isolates resistant to fluoroquinolones and trimethoprim have been reported (99). Most studies have found that *C. pseudotuberculosis* shows reduced susceptibility or resistance to aminoglycosides (164, 335).

Corynebacterium renale causes pyelonephritis and cystitis in cattle and posthitis and vulvovaginitis in sheep and cattle (135, 219, 236, 238, 333). Infections in goats have also been found (10). Antimicrobial therapy is essential in the treatment of infections with *C. renale*, and penicillin remains the drug of choice. No reports on antimicrobial susceptibility testing of *C. renale* are available. *Corynebacterium pilosum* and *Corynebacterium cystitidis* have also been suggested as primary pathogens causing urinary tract infections in cattle (330), but it is still unknown whether they should be regarded as part of the normal flora.

Corynebacterium bovis is a frequent colonizer of the bovine teat. It has been debated whether infections with *C. bovis* should be considered true infections or whether these bacteria constitute part of the normal flora of the mammary teat and might even protect the mammary gland from infections with more-pathogenic bacteria (220). More-recent studies have indicated that infections with *C. bovis* are associated with production losses and should be eliminated if possible (78). Watts and Rossbach (312) determined the antimicrobial susceptibility of 46 *C. bovis* isolates on Mueller-Hinton II agar supplemented with 1% Tween 80 and found most of them to be susceptible to β-lactams, fluoroquinolones, tetracyclines, and macrolides.

No studies on the occurrence of antimicrobial resistance genes in *Corynebacterium* species causing infections in animals have been performed. However, a number of resistance genes have been identified in other *Corynebacterium* species (Table 1). Most of these genes, such as *tet*(M) and *erm*(B), have also been observed in other gram-positive bacterial species, but some of the genes, such as *strA*, *strB*, and integrons, have been mainly observed in gram-negative species. Thus, *Corynebacterium* seems to share genes with a large number of other species and genera, both gram positive and gram negative.

ERYSIPELOTHRIX RHUSIOPATHIAE

Erysipelothrix spp. are gram-positive, catalase- and oxidase-negative rods. The genus has two species, *Erysipelothrix rhusiopathiae* and *Erysipelothrix tonsillarum*, but only *E. rhusiopathiae* is pathogenic (283). *E. rhusiopathiae* is widely distributed in nature and causes infections in both humans and animals (33, 236, 239, 324). Infections in humans are normally cutaneous in fingers and hands (33, 42, 239). The infection normally occurs in people handling infected or contaminated material, e.g., veterinarians, slaughterhouse workers, butchers, and fish handlers (33, 42, 239). In animals, infections caused by *E. rhusiopathiae* are called erysipelas. The infection can take acute septicemic or chronic form (arthritis, lymphadenitis, endocarditis, and urticaria) (236, 324). The classic diamond-shaped, red, urticarial plaques in the skin are almost pathognomic. The disease is especially important in swine production, where the infection is commonly observed worldwide. Pigs become infected through contact with infected or carrier pigs or contaminated soil or environment (236). *E. rhusiopathiae* rarely causes infections in cattle and sheep, but more often in lambs, where the infection normally is manifested as polyarthritis with high mortality (236). In poultry, *E. rhusiopathiae* is also an important bacterial disease, especially in turkeys, where it can cause high mortality (202).

In animals, the most effective way of controlling the infection is vaccination (236). Medication with antimicrobial agents often fails or has a limited effect. If an antimicrobial is used, it is most often penicillin (236). In humans, antimicrobial treatment is also important and penicillin is also the drug of choice (33, 130, 275).

Susceptibility testing of *E. rhusiopathiae* has been performed as both agar and broth dilution using normal nonsupplemented medium (281, 282, 328) or medium for fastidious pathogens (159, 302). No specific international breakpoints for resistance in

Table 1. Occurrence of resistance genes in *Corynebacterium* spp.

Antimicrobial agent	Resistance gene	Species	Reference(s)
Chloramphenicol	*cmx* on Tn*5564*	*C. striatum*	288
	cmr on Tn*45*	*C. glutamicum*	261
Kanamycin	*aphA1*	*C. striatum*	287, 291
Lincosamide	*lmrB* (efflux)	*C. glutamicum*	166
Macrolide	*erm*(B)	*Corynebacterium* spp.	181
	erm(C)	*C. striatum*	241
	erm(X)	*C. jeikeium, C. diphtheriae, C. striatum*	138, 245, 287
	mef(A or E)	*C. jeikeium, Corynebacterium* spp.	181
Streptomycin	*addA9* as part of class I integron	*C. glutamicum*	292
	aadA2 as part of class I integron	*C. glutamicum*	210
	strA, strB	*C. striatum*	291
Sulfonamides	*sul1* as part of class I integron	*C. glutamicum*	292
Tetracycline	*tet*(M)	*C. striatum*	241
	tet(Z)	*C. glutamicum*	290
	tet(33)	*C. glutamicum*	292
	tetAB (efflux)	*C. striatum*	289

E. rhusiopathiae are given, but those provided for streptococci seem appropriate.

All isolates tested so far have shown high susceptibility to penicillin and other β-lactams (100, 159, 281, 282, 302, 328). *E. rhusiopathiae* is also highly susceptible to macrolides, lincosamides, virginiamycin, tiamulin, and fluoroquinolones and moderately susceptible to tetracyclines, florfenicol, and chloramphenicol (100, 159, 281, 282, 328). The bacterium is intrinsically resistant to kanamycin, sulfonamides, and vancomycin (100, 122, 282, 328).

In Japan, Takahashi et al. (281) found frequent resistance to erythromycin (6%), tetracycline (43%), and streptomycin (17%) among 258 *E. rhusiopathiae* strains isolated during 1980 to 1982 from chronic infections in pigs, while a later study reported 19% resistance to streptomycin and 100% susceptibility to erythromycin and tetracyclines among 63 *E. rhusiopathiae* strains isolated from tonsils of healthy pigs (282). In other studies from Japan, resistance has been observed to streptomycin (37%), tetracycline (53%), and erythromycin (2%) (328). The genetic background for resistance has only been determined in a single study, where the *tet*(M) gene was found in all of 114 tetracycline-resistant isolates from Japan (329).

FRANCISELLA TULARENSIS

Francisella tularensis is a strictly aerobic, pleomorphic gram-negative rod. *F. tularensis* is the causative agent of tularemia and an extremely infective bacterium with a broad host spectrum (85, 140). *F. tularensis* cases infections in a large number of different animal species (22, 36, 61, 126, 150, 201, 240, 306) but is mainly known for plaguelike disease in rodents, primarily wild mice, rats, and beavers, as well as hares (85, 140). Transmission occurs mainly with mites, ticks, and mosquitoes as vectors (85, 140). Humans are not normally part of the epidemiology but may become infected through contact with animals, inhalation of infected materials, digestion of contaminated food or water, or bites from bloodsucking insects (85, 140). In addition, *F. tularensis* may spread through inhalation or penetration of the skin. Because of its highly contagious nature and the severe infections it causes, the bacterium is one of the bacterial agents most likely to be used as biological weapons (72, 85). Historically, tularemia may have been one of the most important causes of major epidemics in humans that possibly changed the course of world history. For example, it has been suggested that tularemia was the cause of a major epidemic in Egypt in 1715 B.C., resulting in the internment of the Hebrews in labor camps and eventually leading to the Exodus (295).

Tularemia is normally restricted to the cooler regions of the Northern Hemisphere. At present, three subspecies of *F. tularensis* have been identified (85). *F. tularensis* subsp. *tularensis*, the most virulent type, is found mainly in North America. *F. tularensis* subsp. *holarctica* is more widespread in the Northern Hemisphere, and *F. tularensis* subsp. *mediasiatica* has been found only in Central Asia. *F. novicida* has been occacionally reported in North America.

Because of the severity of the infection, treatment with antimicrobial agents is essential for infected humans. Streptomycin, gentamicin, chloramphenicol, tetracyclines, and fluoroquinolones are available options for treating infections (26, 89, 247, 279). However, streptomycin seems to be especially efficient. Because of the growth requirements of the bacterium, susceptibility testing is normally performed as MIC determinations using modified Mueller-Hinton broth (21). *F. tularensis* is intrinsically resistant to all β-lactam antimicrobials, probably caused by the production of a β-lactamase (60, 145), but susceptible to aminoglycosides, tetracyclines, erythromycin, quinolones, chloramphenicol, and rifampin (21, 109, 145, 253, 279). Acquired resistance has not yet been found. However, it must be expected that the bacterium can acquire resistance genes from other species or mutate to resistance if exposed to antimicrobial agents. If *F. tularensis* establishes itself in the food animal reservoir or humans come into closer contact with infected rodents or pet animals exposed to antimicrobial agents, problems with treating tularemia might develop. Tularemia in cats and dogs and subsequent spread to humans has been detected (13, 20, 22, 126, 224, 240), and since antimicrobial agents are widely used for pet animals, development of resistance is likely to occur.

LEPTOSPIRA SPP.

The family *Leptospiraceae* belongs to the order *Spirochaetales* and consists of mobile, flexible, helical, gram-negative rods (177). *Leptospira* species are obligate aerobic bacteria with optimum growth at 28 to 30°C.

The classic taxonomy of *Leptospira* was based on serotyping, and more than 260 different serovars have been described (177). The pathogenic serovars were included in the species *Leptospira interrogans*, while the nonpathogenic serovars were included in the species *Leptospira biflexa* (318). Molecular studies have shown a high degree of genetic heterogeneity within the two classic species, which has led to proposals for new taxonomy (41). The serovars are, however, still widely used because of their usefulness in determining the pathogenicity of the isolates.

Pathogenic *Leptospira* species cause infections in both animals and humans (177, 236, 318). The bacteria can be transferred directly or indirectly from animals to humans and are a zoonosis (177, 318). Animals are often asymptomatic carriers, whereas humans are dead-end hosts. Some *L. interrogans* serovars have a host preference, such as Ballum in mice, Canicola in dogs, Icterohaemorrhagiae in rats, and Pomona in pigs, whereas others do not seem to prefer certain hosts (236, 318). Humans are infected by direct or indirect (via food or water) transfer of *Leptospira* from different animals. The infection occurs mainly in hot climates, which could indicate that environmental transmission is most common. Infections with *Leptospira* can result in meningitis, leptospiruria, icterus, and death (318).

In animals, *Leptospira* mainly causes subclinical and asymptomatic infections (236). However, in some cases it also causes acute, subacute, or chronic clinical infections in horses, sheep, cattle, goats, and pigs, with substantial deaths and production losses (236). The most common symptoms are abortion, stillbirths, infertility, loss of milk production, agalactiae, and failure to thrive (27, 37, 38, 59, 65, 75, 76, 79, 86, 88, 134, 176). In these cases, and in order to eradicate *Leptospira* for the protection of human health, the use of antimicrobial agents is important. Traditionally, the recommended antimicrobials for animals have been streptomycin, tetracyclines, tylosin, or penicillin (236). Dihydrostreptomycin has been found effective in stopping the shedding of *L. interrogans* serovar Hardjo from both naturally and experimentally infected cattle (111, 112), even though Ellis et al. (87) found that a single treatment with dihydrostreptomycin failed to eradicate genital and renal infection in experimentally infected heifers. Amoxillin, tetracycline, tilmicosin, dihydrostreptomycin plus penicillin, and ceftiofur have also been found effective in cattle (19, 263). Stalheim (274) found a single dose of dihydrostreptomycin as well as feed medication with chlortetracycline to remove *L. interrogans* serovar Pomona from the kidneys of experimentally infected pigs. Likewise, in swine experimentally infected with *L. interrogans* serovar Pomona, dihydrostreptomycin plus penicillin, oxytetracycline, tylosin, and erythromycin were found to be effective, whereas ceftiofur and ampicillin were ineffective (8).

Antimicrobial agents are important in the treatment of *Leptospira* infections in humans, where mainly penicillin or tetracyclines are preferred (82, 121, 129, 189, 248, 255, 280, 311), even though conflicting results have been observed, especially with penicillin (83, 114).

There have been a limited number of studies on the antimicrobial susceptibility of *Leptospira* species. This is probably due to the difficulty of cultivating this bacterium. *Leptospira* spp. are very slow-growing species, and clinical diagnosis often requires 10 to 14 days of incubation. Thus, initial therapy is often based on empirical treatment. Most studies have been performed on isolates from human patients. Most early studies on growth and susceptibility testing of *Leptospira* were performed using different media supplemented with serum (212, 299). In recent years the most widely used media for both isolation and susceptibility testing of *Leptospira* have been based on a commercially available oleic acid-albumin medium, Ellinghausen-McCullough-Johnson-Harris medium (84, 155).

Recently, Murray and Hospenthal (205) developed a microbroth method for susceptibility testing of *Leptospira* spp. This method is based on inoculating 100 µl of Ellinghausen-McCullough-Johnson-Harris medium containing approximately 2×10^6 organisms/ml in microtiter plates with known serial twofold dilutions of freeze-dried antimicrobials. After 3 days of incubation at 30°C, 20 µl of 10-times-concentrated alamarBlue (a growth indicator) is added to each well and the growth is read on day 5. This method seems to be reasonably easy to work with, and even though some variations between runs were detected (205, 206), this could form the basis for international standardization in the future.

There is currently no international standard for susceptibility testing of *Leptospira*, and it is virtually impossible to compare results between studies, both because of the lack of standardization but also because no control strains have been used and the MICs seem to vary greatly. Based on the available studies, *Leptospira* seems to be susceptible to most antimicrobial agents, including tetracyclines, β-lactams, fluoroquinolones, lincomycin, streptomycin, kanamycin, chloramphenicol, and quinupristin-dalfopristin, and highly susceptible to the macrolides erythromycin and tylosin (7, 43, 47, 96, 204, 206, 218, 234, 254, 258, 271, 273, 285, 325). However, some studies have reported high chloramphenicol MICs (28, 271, 273). *Leptospira* spp. are intrinsically resistant to metronidazole and vancomycin (107, 108). In addition, there might be some species- or serovar-specific differences in the susceptibility to β-lactams. Thus, both Murray and Hospenthal (206) and Oie et al. (218) found *L. biflexa* to be less susceptible to penicillin than the other serovars they tested. These findings are, however, based on so limited a number of isolates that this requires further testing.

Acquired resistance has only rarely been demonstrated. Petrov and Chernukha (225) were able to obtain streptomycin-resistant *L. interrogans* mutants in vitro at a frequency of 10^{-9} to 10^{-7}. Fukunaga and Mifuchi (106) studied the mechanism of streptomycin resistance in *L. biflexa* and found that the protein synthesis was insensitive to streptomycin in mutants, indicating that the mechanism of resistance is ribosomal.

LISTERIA MONOCYTOGENES

Members of the genus *Listeria* are short, regular, microaerophilic, oxidase-negative and catalase-positive, gram-positive rods with the ability to grow within a broad temperature interval. *Listeria* species are widely distributed in the environment and have been isolated from numerous reservoirs, including soil, plants, feedstuff, sewage, vegetables, silage, water, and a large number of food products (80, 97, 110, 222, 294, 314). The genus *Listeria* consists of six species, but only *Listeria monocytogenes* and *Listeria ivanovii* are isolated from clinical materials and only *L. monocytogenes* is of major importance as a causative agent of infections in animals and humans. *L. ivanovii* is an occasional cause of abortion in sheep and cattle (6, 51, 115, 257) but has also been isolated from other animals (168). *Listeria innocua* has also been reported from a case of ovine meningoencephalitis (307).

L. monocytogenes causes a number of different infections especially in ruminants, particularly sheep, but may also cause infections in horses and pigs (236). The most common clinical manifestations are encephalitis and abortion, but spinal myelitis, septicemia, uveitis, enteritis, and mastitis are also seen (154, 160, 180, 183, 236, 315, 321). The source of the infection is normally environmental and very often related to animal feed (98, 117, 300). Treatment with antimicrobial agents is essential for the resolution of infections. *L. monocytogenes* is also an important cause of infections in humans and an emerging food-borne disease that has caused numerous outbreaks during the past decades due to contaminated food (18, 67, 104, 182, 194). The annual number of cases may not be very high, but despite treatment with antibiotics the fatality rate might be as high as 30% (15, 136, 147, 186). In humans, ampicillin or penicillin, often in combination with gentamicin, remains the treatment of choice for infections with *L. monocytogenes* (156), but SXT is also an alternative (270). Ampicillin or tetracycline is recommended for treatment of infections in animals (236).

Susceptibility testing of *Listeria* spp. can be performed as for all other gram-positive bacterial species. Until 1988 acquired resistance in *L. monocytogenes* had not been reported (92, 228). The first tetracycline-resistant isolate was reported in this year, and in the same year a multiresistant isolate with a transferable plasmid conferring resistance to chloramphenicol, erythromycin, streptomycin, and tetracycline was found in France (230). Since then there have been several reports on the occurrence of resistance in *L. monocytogenes* isolated from various sources (55). However, these have been mainly sporadic clinical cases, and the frequency of resistance is still very low (19, 184, 188, 249, 301, 309).

A number of different resistance genes have been found in *Listeria* (Table 2), and it seems that this genus shares genes mainly with other gram-positive organisms such as enterococci, streptococci, and staphylococci (55). Resistance to quaternary ammonium compounds may also result from the expression of efflux pumps (1).

Table 2. Occurrence of resistance genes in *Listeria* spp.

Antimicrobial agent	Gene(s) or mechanism	Species	Reference(s)
Cadmium	*cadA* and *cadC*	*L. monocytogenes*	173, 174
Chloramphenicol	*cat221*	*L. monocytogenes*	127
Fluoroquinolones	Lde (efflux pump)	*L. monocytogenes*	120
Macrolides	*erm*(B)	*L. monocytogenes*	127
	erm(C)	*L. monocytogenes*	242
Streptomycin	*aad6*	*L. innocua, L. monocytogenes*	57, 127
Trimethoprim	*dfrD*	*L. monocytogenes*	54
Tetracycline	*tet*(K)	*L. innocua*	95
	tet(L)	*L. monocytogenes*	231
	tet(M)	*L. innocua, L. monocytogenes, L. welshimeri*	57, 95, 229, 231
	tet(S)	*L. innocua, L. monocytogenes, L. welshimeri*	56, 57, 127

RHODOCOCCUS EQUI

Rhodococcus equi is an aerobic, gram-positive rod that occasionally is found as an intracellular pathogen infecting foals and humans (191, 233). The bacterium is widely distributed in the environment and also commonly found in cervical lymph nodes in swine (44, 191, 233). In foals, *R. equi* most commonly causes chronic granulomatous pneumonia (191, 233). In humans, the bacterium mainly causes lung infections in immunocompromised patients (44, 191, 233). Infections in other species are rare, except in swine, where *R. equi* may cause submaxillary lymphadenitis (191, 233).

Antimicrobial agents are essential in the successful therapy of *R. equi* infections. Standard treatment for foals and humans is a combination of erythromycin and rifampin or each antimicrobial used alone (113, 191, 252), even through other drugs such as tetracyclines and SXT also have been used.

There is currently no international standard for susceptibility testing of *R. equi*, but testing of the bacterium can be performed with Mueller-Hinton II agar supplemented with blood. *R. equi* is susceptible to macrolides, chloramphenicol, aminoglycosides, tetracyclines, rifampin, glycopeptides, SXT, and oxazolidinones (2, 39, 148, 190, 213, 232, 268). The susceptibility to β-lactam antimicrobials seems to be more variable, with large MIC ranges that in several cases include the typically applied breakpoints (2, 39, 148, 190, 268). The same seems to be the case for susceptibility to fluoroquinolones (39, 148, 190, 244), florfenicol (39, 149), and streptogramins (268).

Acquired resistance has been reported in a number of studies (17, 105, 190, 284). The frequency of resistance still seems low, but some resistance to macrolides, tetracyclines, and especially rifampin has been observed.

The genetic background for resistance has been determined in only a few cases. Nordmann et al. (214) selected an imipenem-resistant isolate in vitro and found that resistance was mediated by an altered *pbp3* gene. This alteration caused reduced susceptibility to imipenem, cefoxitin, ceftriaxone, meropenem, moxalactam, and oxacillin, but no change in the MICs of amoxicillin, penicillin, or ticarcillion. Nordmann et al. (215) compared two β-lactam-susceptible and two -resistant isolates. They found three additional protein bands in the resistant isolates, but no β-lactamase production or differences in *pbp* patterns.

Resistance to rifampin has been found in a number of studies. Asoh et al. (17) examined the sequence of the *rpoB* gene in resistant and susceptible isolates and found Ser531Trp or His526Tyr mutations in two high-level rifampin-resistant (MICs of 64 and >128 μg/ml) isolates and a Ser509Pro mutation in one low-level-resistant (MIC of 16 μg/ml) isolate. Fines et al. (101) found His526Asp mutations in eight high-level-resistant (MIC of 128 μg/ml) isolates from two foals and His526Asn, Ser531Leu, and Asp516Val mutations in four low-level-resistant (MICs of 2 and 8 μg/ml) isolates. Mutations at positions 516, 526, and 531 are also the ones most commonly observed in *Mycobacterium tuberculosis* (207, 250, 327). Phosphorylation of the 21-OH group of rifampin has been observed in one strain of *Rhodococcus* (286). Subsequent cloning has identified a gene that may confer a 25-fold increase in the MIC of rifampin for *Rhodococcus* (12). This gene has not been reported in other studies.

Plasmid-borne resistance to arsenate, arsenite, cadmium, and chloramphenicol has also been reported in *Rhodococcus erythropolis* (66), but the genes encoding resistance have not been identified. A gene encoding resistance to chloramphenicol, probably through an efflux mechanism, has been identified in *Rhodococcus fascians* (74).

CONCLUDING REMARKS

Numerous bacterial species can cause infections in animals and humans or function as reservoirs for antimicrobial resistance genes. International standards for susceptibility testing are only available for a limited number of species, even though these few species comprise the vast majority of clinical isolations. The more rarely observed species cause problems for clinical laboratories due to the difficulties in cultivating these organisms or problems with interpretation of results due to lack of knowledge of the intrinsic susceptibility of these species or breakpoints for when the species should be considered resistant. Unless the individual laboratory has considerable experience with rarely isolated pathogens or includes control isolates with known susceptibilities, any interpretations and reporting have to be done with great care. For many of the species, a few researchers have performed studies and their methodology and results can be used as guidance for other researchers or microbiological diagnosticians. The first step in the development of interpretive criteria is a microbiological breakpoint based on MIC distributions (see chapter 3). The highest value of the normal distribution of the susceptible population is normally used as an initial breakpoint, if this value is within the achievable concentration of the antimicrobial agent at the infection site. If any clinical response data are available, then these are used as well. As antimicrobial susceptibility standards evolve, they will probably be expanded to include some of the atypical organisms mentioned in this chapter.

Some of the resistance genes found in rarely isolated pathogens are also well known from the more important pathogens. Thus, this emphasizes that all bacterial species to some extent share the same gene pool.

REFERENCES

1. **Aase, B., G. Sundheim, S. Langsrud, and L. M. Rorvik.** 2000. Occurrence of and a possible mechanism for resistance to a quaternary ammonium compound in *Listeria monocytogenes*. *Int. J. Food Microbiol.* **62:**57–63.
2. **Adamson, P. J., W. D. Wilson, D. C. Hirsh, J. D. Baggot, and L. D. Martin.** 1985. Susceptibility of equine bacterial isolates to antimicrobial agents. *Am. J. Vet. Res.* **46:**447–450.
3. **Agerholm, J. S., N. E. Jensen, V. Dantzer, H. E. Jensen, and F. M. Aarestrup.** 1999. Experimental infection of pregnant cows with *Bacillus licheniformis* bacteria. *Vet. Pathol.* **36:**191–201.
4. **Agersø, Y., L. B. Jensen, M. Givskov, and M. C. Roberts.** 2002. The identification of a tetracycline resistance gene *tet*(M), on a Tn*916*-like transposon, in the *Bacillus cereus* group. *FEMS Microbiol. Lett.* **214:**251–256.
5. **Aleman, M., S. J. Spier, W. D. Wilson, and M. Doherr.** 1996. *Corynebacterium pseudotuberculosis* infection in horses: 538 cases (1982–1993). *J. Am. Vet. Med. Assoc.* **209:**804–809.
6. **Alexander, A. V., R. L. Walker, B. J. Johnson, B. R. Charlton, and L. W. Woods.** 1992. Bovine abortions attributable to *Listeria ivanovii*: four cases (1988–1990). *J. Am. Vet. Med. Assoc.* **200:**711–714.
7. **Alston, J. M., and J. C. Broom.** 1944. The action of penicillin on *Leptospira* and on leptospiral infections in guinea-pigs. *Br. Med. J.* **ii:**718–719.
8. **Alt, D. P., and C. A. Bolin.** 1996. Preliminary evaluation of antimicrobial agents for treatment of *Leptospira interrogans* serovar *pomona* infection in hamsters and swine. *Am. J. Vet. Res.* **57:**59–62.
9. **Alt, D. P., R. L. Zuerner, and C. A. Bolin.** 2001. Evaluation of antibiotics for treatment of cattle infected with *Leptospira borgpetersenii* serovar *hardjo*. *J. Am. Vet. Med. Assoc.* **219:** 636–639.
10. **Altmaier, K. R., D. M. Sherman, S. H. Schelling, R. D. Fister, and C. R. Lamb.** 1994. Osteomyelitis and disseminated infection caused by *Corynebacterium renale* in a goat. *J. Am. Vet. Med. Assoc.* **204:**934–937.
11. **Almuneef, M., Z. A. Memish, M. Al Shaalan, E. Al Banyan, S. Al-Alola, and H. H. Balkhy.** 2003. *Brucella melitensis* bacteremia in children: review of 62 cases. *J. Chemother.* **15:** 76–80.
12. **Andersen, S. J., S. Quan, B. Gowan, and E. R. Dabbs.** 1997. Monooxygenase-like sequence of a *Rhodococcus equi* gene conferring increased resistance to rifampin by inactivating this antibiotic. *Antimicrob. Agents Chemother.* **41:**218–221.
13. **Anonymous.** 1982. Tularemia associated with domestic cats—Georgia, New Mexico. *Morb. Mortal. Wkly. Rep.* **31:**39–41.
14. **Anonymous.** 2000. Laboratory-acquired human glanders—Maryland, May 2000. *Morb. Mortal. Wkly. Rep.* **49:**532–535.
15. **Aouaj, Y., L. Spanjaard, N. van Leeuwen, and J. Dankert.** 2002. *Listeria monocytogenes* meningitis: serotype distribution and patient characteristics in The Netherlands, 1976–95. *Epidemiol. Infect.* **128:**405–409.
16. **Ariza, J., J. Bosch, F. Gudiol, J. Linares, P. F. Viladrich, and R. Martin.** 1986. Relevance of in vitro antimicrobial susceptibility of *Brucella melitensis* to relapse rate in human brucellosis. *Antimicrob. Agents Chemother.* **30:**958–960.
17. **Asoh, N., H. Watanabe, M. Fines-Guyon, K. Watanabe, K. Oishi, W. Kositsakulchai, T. Sanchai, K. Kunsuikmengrai, S. Kahintapong, B. Khantawa, P. Tharavichitkul, T. Sirisanthana, and T. Nagatake.** 2003. Emergence of rifampin-resistant *Rhodococcus equi* with several types of mutations in the *rpoB* gene among AIDS patients in northern Thailand. *J. Clin. Microbiol.* **41:**2337–2340.
18. **Aureli, P., G. C. Fiorucci, D. Caroli, G. Marchiaro, O. Novara, L. Leone, and S. Salmaso.** 2000. An outbreak of febrile gastroenteritis associated with corn contaminated by *Listeria monocytogenes*. *N. Engl. J. Med.* **342:**1236–1241.
19. **Aureli, P., A. M. Ferrini, V. Mannoni, S. Hodzic, C. Wedell-Weergaard, and B. Oliva.** 2003. Susceptibility of *Listeria monocytogenes* isolated from food in Italy to antibiotics. *Int. J. Food Microbiol.* **83:**325–330.
20. **Avashia, S. B., J. M. Petersen, C. M. Lindley, M. E. Schriefer, K. L. Gage, M. Cetron, T. A. DeMarcus, D. K. Kim, J. Buck, J. A. Montenieri, J. L. Lowell, M. F. Antolin, M. Y. Kosoy, L. G. Carter, M. C. Chu, K. A. Hendricks, D. T. Dennis, and J. L. Kool.** 2004. First reported prairie dog-to-human tularemia transmission, Texas, 2002. *Emerg. Infect. Dis.* **10:**483–486.
21. **Baker, C. N., D. G. Hollis, and C. Thornsberry.** 1985. Antimicrobial susceptibility testing of *Francisella tularensis* with a modified Mueller-Hinton broth. *J. Clin. Microbiol.* **22:** 212–215.
22. **Baldwin, C. J., R. J. Panciera, R. J. Morton, A. K. Cowell, and B. J. Waurzyniak.** 1991. Acute tularemia in three domestic cats. *J. Am. Vet. Med. Assoc.* **199:**1602–1605.
23. **Bast, D. J., A. Athamna, C. L. Duncan, J. C. de Azavedo, D. E. Low, G. Rahav, D. Farrell, and E. Rubinstein.** 2004. Type II topoisomerase mutations in *Bacillus anthracis* associated with high-level fluoroquinolone resistance. *J. Antimicrob. Chemother.* **54:**90–94.
24. **Baxter, I. A., and P. A. Lambert.** 1994. Isolation and partial purification of a carbapenem-hydrolysing metallo-beta-lactamase from *Pseudomonas cepacia*. *FEMS Microbiol. Lett.* **122:**251–256.
25. **Baykam, N., H. Esener, O. Ergonul, S. Eren, A. K. Celikbas, and B. Dokuzoguz.** 2004. *In vitro* antimicrobial susceptibility of *Brucella* species. *Int. J. Antimicrob. Agents* **23:**405–407.
26. **Bernard, W. V., C. Bolin, T. Riddle, M. Durando, B. J. Smith, and R. R. Tramontin.** 1993. Leptospiral abortion and leptospiruria in horses from the same farm. *J. Am. Vet. Med. Assoc.* **202:**1285–1286.
27. **Bernhard, K., H. Schrempf, and W. Goebel.** 1978. Bacteriocin and antibiotic resistance plasmids in *Bacillus cereus* and *Bacillus subtilis*. *J. Bacteriol.* **133:**897–903.
28. **Berson, R. C., and A. B. Harwell.** 1948. Streptomycin in the treatment of tularemia. *Am. J. Med. Sci.* **215:**243–249.
29. **Bessemans, A., P. Derom, I. Colle, and J. van Hoydonck.** 1954. Action *in vitro* précoce et tardive de divers antibiotiques sur les Leptospires. *Rev. Belg. Pathol. Med. Exp.* **23:** 351–358.
30. **Biberstein, E. L., H. D. Knight, and S. Jang.** 1971. Two biotypes of *Corynebacterium pseudotuberculosis*. *Vet. Rec.* **89:** 691–692.
31. Reference deleted.
32. **Biksi, I., A. Major, L. Fodor, O. Szenci, and F. Vetesi.** 2003. *In vitro* sensitivity of Hungarian *Actinobaculum suis* strains to selected antimicrobials. *Acta Vet. Hung.* **51:**53–59.
33. **Bille, J., J. Rocourt, and B. Swaminathan.** 1999. *Listeria, Erysipelothrix*, and *Kurthia*, p. 346–356. *In* P. R. Murray,

E. J. Baron, M. A. Pfaller, F. C. Tenover, and R. H. Yolken (ed.), *Manual of Clinical Microbiology*, 7th ed. ASM Press, Washington, D.C.

34. **Billington, S. J., K. W. Post, and B. H. Jost.** 2002. Isolation of *Arcanobacterium (Actinomyces) pyogenes* from cases of feline otitis externa and canine cystitis. *J. Vet. Diagn. Investig.* **14:**159–162.
35. **Billington, S. J., J. G. Songer, and B. H. Jost.** 2002. Widespread distribution of a Tet W determinant among tetracycline-resistant isolates of the animal pathogen *Arcanobacterium pyogenes. Antimicrob. Agents Chemother.* **46:**1281–1287.
36. **Bivin, W. S., and A. L. Hogge, Jr.** 1967. Quantitation of susceptibility of swine to infection with *Pasteurella tularensis. Am. J. Vet. Res.* **28:**1619–1621.
37. **Bolin, C. A., and J. A. Cassells.** 1990. Isolation of *Leptospira interrogans* serovar *bratislava* from stillborn and weak pigs in Iowa. *J. Am. Vet. Med. Assoc.* **196:**1601–1604.
38. **Bolin, C. A., J. A. Cassells, H. T. Hill, J. C. Frantz, and J. N. Nielsen.** 1991. Reproductive failure associated with *Leptospira interrogans* serovar *bratislava* infection of swine. *J. Vet. Diagn. Investig.* **3:**152–154.
39. **Bowersock, T. L., S. A. Salmon, E. S. Portis, J. F. Prescott, D. A. Robison, C. W. Ford, and J. L. Watts.** 2000. MICs of oxazolidinones for *Rhodococcus equi* strains isolated from humans and animals. *Antimicrob. Agents Chemother.* **44:**1367–1369.
40. **Bozdogan, B., S. Galopin, and R. Leclercq.** 2004. Characterization of a new *erm*-related macrolide resistance gene present in probiotic strains of *Bacillus clausii. Appl. Environ. Microbiol.* **70:**280–284.
41. **Brenner, D. J., A. F. Kaufmann, K. R. Sulzer, A. G. Steigerwalt, F. C. Rogers, and R. S. Weyant.** 1999. Further determination of DNA relatedness between serogroups and serovars in the family *Leptospiraceae* with a proposal for *Leptospira alexanderi* sp. nov. and four new *Leptospira* genomospecies. *Int. J. Syst. Bacteriol.* **49:**839–858.
42. **Brooke, C. J., and T. V. Riley.** 1999. *Erysipelothrix rhusiopathiae*: bacteriology, epidemiology and clinical manifestations of an occupational pathogen. *J. Med. Microbiol.* **48:** 789–799.
43. **Broughton, E. S., and L. E. Flack.** 1986. The susceptibility of a strain of *Leptospira interrogans* serogroup *icterohaemorrhagiae* to amoxycillin, erythromycin, lincomycin, tetracycline, oxytetracycline and minocycline. *Zentbl. Bakteriol. Mikrobiol. Hyg. A* **261:**425–431.
44. **Brown, J. M., M. M. McNeil, and E. P. Desmond.** 1999. *Norcadia, Rhodococcus, Gordona, Actinomadura, Streptomyces,* and other *Actinomycetes* of medical importance, p. 370–398. *In* P. R. Murray, E. J. Baron, M. A. Pfaller, F. C. Tenover, and R. H. Yolken (ed.), *Manual of Clinical Microbiology*, 7th ed. ASM Press, Washington, D.C.
45. **Bryskier, A.** 2002. *Bacillus anthracis* and antibacterial agents. *Clin. Microbiol. Infect.* **8:**467–478.
46. **Buddle, M. B.** 1956. Studies on *Brucella ovis* (n.sp.), a cause of genital disease of sheep in New Zealand and Australia. *J. Hyg. Lond.* **54:**351–364.
47. **Cameron, G. L.** 1977. The susceptibility of New Zealand isolates of *Leptospira* to three antibiotics. *N. Z. Med. J.* **86:** 93–94.
48. **Carr, J., and J. R. Walton.** 1993. Bacterial flora of the urinary tract of pigs associated with cystitis and pyelonephritis. *Vet. Rec.* **132:**575–577.
49. **Cavallo, J. D., F. Ramisse, M. Girardet, J. Vaissaire, M. Mock, and E. Hernandez.** 2002. Antibiotic susceptibilities of 96 isolates of *Bacillus anthracis* isolated in France between 1994 and 2000. *Antimicrob. Agents Chemother.* **46:**2307–2309.
50. **Centers for Disease Control and Prevention.** 2000. Biological and chemical terrorism: strategic plan for preparedness and response: recommendations of the CDC Strategic Planning Workgroup. *Morb. Mortal. Wkly. Rep.* **49:**6.
51. **Chand, P., and J. R. Sadana.** 1999. Outbreak of *Listeria ivanovii* abortion in sheep in India. *Vet. Rec.* **145:**83–84.
52. **Chaowagul, W., Y. Suputtamongkol, D. A. Dance, A. Rajchanuvong, J. Pattaraarechachai, and N. J. White.** 1993. Relapse in melioidosis: incidence and risk factors. *J. Infect. Dis.* **168:**1181–1185.
53. **Chaowagul, W., A. J. Simpson, Y. Suputtamongkol, M. D. Smith, B. J. Angus, and N. J. White.** 1999. A comparison of chloramphenicol, trimethoprim-sulfamethoxazole, and doxycycline with doxycycline alone as maintenance therapy for melioidosis. *Clin. Infect. Dis.* **29:**375–380.
54. **Charpentier, E., and P. Courvalin.** 1997. Emergence of the trimethoprim resistance gene *dfrD* in *Listeria monocytogenes* BM4293. *Antimicrob. Agents Chemother.* **41:**1134–1136.
55. **Charpentier, E., and P. Courvalin.** 1999. Antibiotic resistance in *Listeria* spp. *Antimicrob. Agents Chemother.* **43:**2103–2108.
56. **Charpentier, E., G. Gerbaud, and P. Courvalin.** 1993. Characterization of a new class of tetracycline-resistance gene *tet*(S) in *Listeria monocytogenes* BM4210. *Gene* **131:**27–34.
57. **Charpentier, E., G. Gerbaud, C. Jacquet, J. Rocourt, and P. Courvalin.** 1995. Incidence of antibiotic resistance in *Listeria* species. *J. Infect. Dis.* **172:**277–281.
58. **Chen, Y., J. Succi, F. C. Tenover, and T. M. Koehler.** 2003. β-Lactamase genes of the penicillin-susceptible *Bacillus anthracis* Sterne strain. *J. Bacteriol.* **185:**823–830.
59. **Clark, A. M.** 1994. *Leptospira hardjo* infection in sheep. *Vet. Rec.* **134:**283.
60. **Clarridge, J. E., III, T. J. Raich, A. Sjosted, G. Sandstrom, R. O. Darouiche, R. M. Shawar, P. R. Georghiou, C. Osting, and L. Vo.** 1996. Characterization of two unusual clinically significant *Francisella* strains. *J. Clin. Microbiol.* **34:**1995–2000.
61. **Claus, K. D., J. H. Newhall, and D. Mee.** 1959. Isolation of *Pasteurella tularensis* from foals. *J. Bacteriol.* **78:**294.
62. **Cloeckaert, A., J. M. Verger, M. Grayon, J. Y. Paquet, B. Garin-Bastuji, G. Foster, and J. Godfroid.** 2001. Classification of *Brucella* spp. isolated from marine mammals by DNA polymorphism at the *omp2* locus. *Microbes Infect.* **3:**729–738.
63. **Coker, P. R., K. L. Smith, and M. E. Hugh-Jones.** 2002. Antimicrobial susceptibilities of diverse *Bacillus anthracis* isolates. *Antimicrob. Agents Chemother.* **46:**3843–3845.
64. **Costa, L. R., S. J. Spier, and D. C. Hirsh.** 1998. Comparative molecular characterization of *Corynebacterium pseudotuberculosis* of different origin. *Vet. Microbiol.* **62:**135–143.
65. **Cousins, D. V., T. M. Ellis, J. Parkinson, and C. H. McGlashan.** 1989. Evidence for sheep as a maintenance host for *Leptospira interrogans* serovar *hardjo. Vet. Rec.* **124:** 123–124.
66. **Dabbs, E. R., and G. J. Sole.** 1988. Plasmid-borne resistance to arsenate, arsenite, cadmium, and chloramphenicol in a *Rhodococcus* species. *Mol. Gen. Genet.* **211:**148–154.
67. **Dalton, C. B., C. C. Austin, J. Sobel, P. S. Hayes, W. F. Bibb, L. M. Graves, B. Swaminathan, M. E. Proctor, and P. M. Griffin.** 1997. An outbreak of gastroenteritis and fever due to *Listeria monocytogenes* in milk. *N. Engl. J. Med.* **336:**100–105.
68. **Dance, D. A., V. Wuthiekanun, W. Chaowagul, and N. J. White.** 1989. The antimicrobial susceptibility of *Pseudomonas pseudomallei.* Emergence of resistance *in vitro* and during treatment. *J. Antimicrob. Chemother.* **24:**295–309.
69. **Dance, D. A., V. Wuthiekanun, W. Chaowagul, Y. Suputtamongkol, and N. J. White.** 1991. Development of resistance to ceftazidime and co-amoxiclav in *Pseudomonas pseudomallei. J. Antimicrob. Chemother.* **28:**321–324.

70. **Dee, S. A.** 1992. Porcine urogenital disease. *Vet. Clin. N. Am. Food Anim. Pract.* **8**:641–660.

71. **De Liguoro, M., V. Cibin, F. Capolongo, B. Halling-Sørensen, and C. Montesissa.** 2003. Use of oxytetracycline and tylosin in intensive calf farming: evaluation of transfer to manure and soil. *Chemosphere* **52**:203–212.

72. **Dennis, D. T., T. V. Inglesby, D. A. Henderson, J. G. Bartlett, M. S. Ascher, E. Eitzen, A. D. Fine, A. M. Friedlander, J. Hauer, M. Layton, S. R. Lillibridge, J. E. McDade, M. T. Osterholm, T. O'Toole, G. Parker, T. M. Perl, P. K. Russell, K. Tonat, and Working Group on Civilian Biodefense.** 2001. Tularemia as a biological weapon: medical and public health management. *JAMA* **285**:2763–2773.

73. **Derbyshire, J. B.** 2002. The eradication of glanders in Canada. *Can. Vet. J.* **43**:722–726.

74. **Desomer, J., D. Vereecke, M. Crespi, and M. Van Montagu.** 1992. The plasmid-encoded chloramphenicol-resistance protein of *Rhodococcus fascians* is homologous to the transmembrane tetracycline efflux proteins. *Mol. Microbiol.* **6**:2377–2385.

75. **Dhaliwal, G. S., R. D. Murray, H. Dobson, J. Montgomery, and W. A. Ellis.** 1996. Reduced conception rates in dairy cattle associated with serological evidence of *Leptospira interrogans* serovar *hardjo* infection. *Vet. Rec.* **139**:110–114.

76. **Dhaliwal, G. S., R. D. Murray, H. Dobson, J. Montgomery, and W. A. Ellis.** 1996. Effect of *Leptospira interrogans* serovar *hardjo* infection on milk yield in endemically infected dairy herds. *Vet. Rec.* **139**:319–320.

77. **Dirckx, J. H.** 1981. Virgil on anthrax. *Am. J. Dermatopathol.* **3**:191–195.

78. **Djabri, B., N. Bareille, F. Beaudeau, and H. Seegers.** 2002. Quarter milk somatic cell count in infected dairy cows: a meta-analysis. *Vet. Res.* **33**:335–357.

79. **Donahue, J. M., B. J. Smith, K. B. Poonacha, J. K. Donahoe, and C. L. Rigsby.** 1995. Prevalence and serovars of leptospira involved in equine abortions in central Kentucky during the 1991–1993 foaling seasons. *J. Vet. Diagn. Investig.* **7**:87–91.

80. **Donnelly, C. W.** 2001. *Listeria monocytogenes*: a continuing challenge. *Nutr. Rev.* **59**:183–194.

81. **Drobniewski, F. A.** 1993. *Bacillus cereus* and related species. *Clin. Microbiol. Rev.* **6**:324–338.

82. **Edwards, C. N., and P. N. Levett.** 2004. Prevention and treatment of leptospirosis. *Expert Rev. Anti-Infect. Ther.* **2**:293–298.

83. **Edwards, C. N., G. D. Nicholson, T. A. Hassell, C. O. Everard, and J. Callender.** 1988. Penicillin therapy in icteric leptospirosis. *Am. J. Trop. Med. Hyg.* **39**:388–390.

84. **Ellinghausen H. C., Jr., and W. G. McCullough.** 1965. Nutrition of *Leptospira* Pomona and growth of 13 other serotypes: fractionation of oleic albumin complex and a medium of bovine albumin and polysorbate 80. *Am. J. Vet. Res.* **26**:45–51.

85. **Ellis, J., P. C. Oyston, M. Green, and R. W. Titball.** 2002. Tularemia. *Clin. Microbiol. Rev.* **15**:631–646.

86. **Ellis, T. M., L. Hustas, G. M. Robertson, and C. Mayberry.** 1984. Kidney disease of sheep, associated with infection by leptospires of the Sejroe serogroup. *Aust. Vet. J.* **61**:304–306.

87. **Ellis, W. A., J. Montgomery, and J. A. Cassells.** 1985. Dihydrostreptomycin treatment of bovine carriers of *Leptospira interrogans* serovar *hardjo*. *Res. Vet. Sci.* **39**:292–295.

88. **Ellis, W. A., J. J. O'Brien, D. G. Bryson, and D. P. Mackie.** 1985. Bovine leptospirosis: some clinical features of serovar hardjo infection. *Vet. Rec.* **117**:101–104.

89. **Enderlin, G., L. Morales, R. F. Jacobs, and J. T. Cross.** 1994. Streptomycin and alternative agents for the treatment of tularemia: review of the literature. *Clin. Infect. Dis.* **19**:42–47.

90. **Erickson, M. C., and J. L. Kornacki.** 2003. *Bacillus anthracis*: current knowledge in relation to contamination of food. *J. Food Prot.* **66**:691–699.

91. **Esel, D., M. Doganay, and B. Sumerkan.** 2003. Antimicrobial susceptibilities of 40 isolates of *Bacillus anthracis* isolated in Turkey. *Int. J. Antimicrob. Agents* **22**:70–72.

92. **Espaze, E. P., and A. E. Reynaud.** 1988. Antibiotic susceptibilities of *Listeria*: *in vitro* studies. *Infection* **16**:160–164.

93. **European Agency for the Evaluation of Medical Products.** 2002. EMEA/CPMP guidance document on use of medical products for treatment and prophylaxis of biological agents that might be used as weapons of bioterrorism. [Online.] http://www.emea.eu.int/pdfs/human/bioterror/404801.pdf.

94. **Ewalt, D. R., J. B. Payeur, B. M. Martin, D. R. Cummins, and W. G. Miller.** 1994. Characteristics of a *Brucella* species from a bottlenose dolphin (*Tursiops truncatus*). *J. Vet. Diagn. Invest.* **6**:448–452.

95. **Facinelli, B., M. C. Roberts, E. Giovanetti, C. Casolari, U. Fabio, and P. E. Varaldo.** 1993. Genetic basis of tetracycline resistance in food-borne isolates of *Listeria innocua*. *Appl. Environ. Microbiol.* **59**:614–616.

96. **Faine, S., and W. J. Kaipainen.** 1955. Erythromycin in experimental leptospirosis. *J. Infect. Dis.* **97**:146–151.

97. **Farber, J. M., and P. I. Peterkin.** 1991. *Listeria monocytogenes*, a food-borne pathogen. *Microbiol. Rev.* **55**:476–511.

98. **Fenlon, D. R.** 1986. Rapid quantitative assessment of the distribution of *Listeria* in silage implicated in a suspected outbreak of listeriosis in calves. *Vet. Rec.* **118**:240–242.

99. **Fernandez, E. P., A. I. Vela, A. Las Heras, L. Dominguez, J. F. Fernandez-Garayzabal, and M. A. Moreno.** 2001. Antimicrobial susceptibility of corynebacteria isolated from ewe's mastitis. *Int. J. Antimicrob. Agents* **18**:571–574.

100. **Fidalgo, S. G., C. J. Longbottom, and T. V. Rjley.** 2002. Susceptibility of *Erysipelothrix rhusiopathiae* to antimicrobial agents and home disinfectants. *Pathology* **34**:462–465.

101. **Fines, M., S. Pronost, K. Maillard, S. Taouji, and R. Leclercq.** 2001. Characterization of mutations in the *rpoB* gene associated with rifampin resistance in *Rhodococcus equi* isolated from foals. *J. Clin. Microbiol.* **39**:2784–2787.

102. **Foster, G., A. P. MacMillan, J. Godfroid, F. Howie, H. M. Ross, A. Cloeckaert, R. J. Reid, S. Brew, and I. A. Patterson.** 2002. A review of *Brucella* sp. infection of sea mammals with particular emphasis on isolates from Scotland. *Vet. Microbiol.* **90**:563–580.

103. **Frean, J., K. P. Klugman, L. Arntzen, and S. Bukofzer.** 2003. Susceptibility of *Bacillus anthracis* to eleven antimicrobial agents including novel fluoroquinolones and a ketolide. *J. Antimicrob. Chemother.* **52**:297–299.

104. **Frye, D. M., R. Zweig, J. Sturgeon, M. Tormey, M. LeCavalier, I. Lee, L. Lawani, and L. Mascola.** 2002. An outbreak of febrile gastroenteritis associated with delicatessen meat contaminated with *Listeria monocytogenes*. *Clin. Infect. Dis.* **35**: 943–949.

105. **Fuhrmann, C., and C. Lämmler.** 1997. Characterization of *Rhodococcus equi* isolates from horse and man. *Berl. Munch. Tierarztl. Wochenschr.* **110**:54–59.

106. **Fukunaga, M., and I. Mifuchi.** 1988. Mechanism of streptomycin resistance in *Leptospira biflexa* strain Urawa. *Microbiol. Immunol.* **32**:641–644.

107. **Fuzi, M.** 1973. Vancomycin-resistance of leptospirae. *Zentbl. Bakteriol. Orig. A* **223**:368–371.

108. **Fuzi, M.** 1973. Metronidazole resistance, a genus-specific feature of leptospires. *Acta Microbiol. Acad. Sci. Hung.* **20**: 333–336.

109. **Garcia del Blanco, N., C. D. Gutierrez Martin, V. A. de la Puente Redondo, and E. F. Rodriguez Ferri.** 2004. *In vitro* susceptibility of field isolates of *Francisella tularensis* subsp. *holarctica* recovered in Spain to several antimicrobial agents. *Res. Vet. Sci.* **76**:195–198.

110. **Gellin, B. G., and C. V. Broome.** 1989. Listeriosis. *JAMA* **261**:1313–1320.

111. **Gerritsen, M. J., M. J. Koopmans, and T. Olyhoek.** 1993. Effect of streptomycin treatment on the shedding of and the serologic responses to *Leptospira interrogans* serovar *hardjo* subtype hardjobovis in experimentally infected cows. *Vet. Microbiol.* **38**:129–135.

112. **Gerritsen, M. J., M. J. Koopmans, T. C. Dekker, M. C. De Jong, A. Moerman, and T. Olyhoek.** 1994. Effective treatment with dihydrostreptomycin of naturally infected cows shedding *Leptospira interrogans* serovar *hardjo* subtype hardjobovis. *Am. J. Vet. Res.* **55**:339–343.

113. **Giguere, S., S. Jacks, G. D. Roberts, J. Hernandez, M. T. Long, and C. Ellis.** 2004. Retrospective comparison of azithromycin, clarithromycin, and erythromycin for the treatment of foals with *Rhodococcus equi* pneumonia. *J. Vet. Intern. Med.* **18**:568–573.

114. **Gilks, C. F., H. P. Lambert, E. S. Broughton, and C. C. Baker.** 1988. Failure of penicillin prophylaxis in laboratory acquired leptospirosis. *Postgrad. Med. J.* **64**:236–238.

115. **Gill, P. A., J. G. Boulton, G. C. Fraser, A. E. Stevenson, and L. A. Reddacliff.** 1997. Bovine abortion caused by *Listeria ivanovii. Aust. Vet.* J. **75**:214.

116. **Gilligan, P. H., and S. Whittier.** 1999. *Burkholderia, Stenotrophomonas, Ralstonia, Brevundimonas, Comamonas,* and *Acidovorax*, p. 526–538. *In* P. R. Murray, E. J. Baron, M. A. Pfaller, F. C. Tenover, and R. H. Yolken (ed.), *Manual of Clinical Microbiology*, 7th ed. ASM Press, Washington, D.C.

117. **Gitter, M., R. S. Stebbings, J. A. Morris, D. Hannam, and C. Harris.** 1986. Relationship between ovine listeriosis and silage feeding. *Vet. Rec.* **118**:207–208.

118. **Godfrey, A. J., S. Wong, D. A. Dance, W. Chaowagul, and L. E. Bryan.** 1991. *Pseudomonas pseudomallei* resistance to β-lactam antibiotics due to alterations in the chromosomally encoded β-lactamase. *Antimicrob. Agents Chemother.* **35**:1635–1640.

119. **Godoy, D., G. Randle, A. J. Simpson, D. M. Aanensen, T. L. Pitt, R. Kinoshita, and B. G. Spratt.** 2003. Multilocus sequence typing and evolutionary relationships among the causative agents of melioidosis and glanders, *Burkholderia pseudomallei* and *Burkholderia mallei. J. Clin. Microbiol.* **41**:2068–2079.

120. **Godreuil, S., M. Galimand, G. Gerbaud, C. Jacquet, and P. Courvalin.** 2003. Efflux pump Lde is associated with fluoroquinolone resistance in *Listeria monocytogenes. Antimicrob. Agents Chemother.* **47**:704–708.

121. **Gonsalez, C. R., J. Casseb, F. G. Monteiro, J. B. Paula-Neto, R. B. Fernandez, M. V. Silva, E. D. Camargo, J. M. Mairinque, and L. C. Tavares.** 1998. Use of doxycycline for leptospirosis after high-risk exposure in Sao Paulo, Brazil. *Rev. Inst. Med. Trop. Sao Paulo* **40**:59–61.

122. **Gorby, G. L., and J. E. Peacock, Jr.** 1988. *Erysipelothrix rhusiopathiae* endocarditis: microbiologic, epidemiologic, and clinical features of an occupational disease. *Rev. Infect. Dis.* **10**:317–325.

123. **Gryczan, T., M. Israeli-Reches, M. Del Bue, and D. Dubnau.** 1984. DNA sequence and regulation of *ermD*, a macrolide-lincosamide-streptogramin B resistance element from *Bacillus licheniformis. Mol. Gen. Genet.* **194**:349–356.

124. **Guerin-Faublee, V., J. P. Flandrois, E. Broye, F. Tupin, and Y. Richard.** 1993. *Actinomyces pyogenes*: susceptibility of 103 clinical animal isolates to 22 antimicrobial agents. *Vet. Res.* **24**:251–259.

125. **Guerin-Faublee, V., J. P. Flandrois, and Y. G. Richard.** 1993. Antimicrobial susceptibility testing of *Actinomyces pyogenes*: comparison of disk diffusion test and Api ATB Strep system with the agar dilution method. *Zentbl. Bakteriol.* **279**: 377–386.

126. **Gustafson, B. W., and L. J. DeBowes.** 1996. Tularemia in a dog. *J. Am. Anim. Hosp. Assoc.* **32**:339–341.

127. **Hadorn, K., H. Hachler, A. Schaffner, and F. H. Kayser.** 1993. Genetic characterization of plasmid-encoded multiple antibiotic resistance in a strain of *Listeria monocytogenes* causing endocarditis. *Eur. J. Clin. Microbiol. Infect. Dis.* **12**:928–937.

128. **Hall, W. H., and R. E. Manion.** 1970. In vitro susceptibility of *Brucella* to various antibiotics. *Appl. Microbiol.* **20**: 600–604.

129. **Hart, V. L.** 1944. A case of Weil's disease treated with penicillin. *Br. Med. J.* ii:720.

130. **Heilman, F. R., and W. E. Herrell.** 1944. Penicillin in the treatment of experimental infections due to *Erysipelothrix rhusiopathiae. Proc. Staff Meet. Mayo Clin.* **19**:340–345.

131. **Heine, H. S., M. J. England, D. M. Waag, and W. R. Byrne.** 2001. *In vitro* antibiotic susceptibilities of *Burkholderia mallei* (causative agent of glanders) determined by broth microdilution and E-test. *Antimicrob. Agents Chemother.* **45**: 2119–2121.

132. **Heine, H. S., J. Bassett, and L. Miller.** 2004. Does *Bacillus anthracis* (anthrax) express a beta-lactamase?, abstr. C1-301, p. 66. *Abstr. 44th Intersci. Conf. Antimicrob. Agents Chemother.* American Society for Microbiology, Washington, D.C.

133. **Helgason, E., O. A. Okstad, D. A. Caugant, H. A. Johansen, A. Fouet, M. Mock, I. Hegna, and AB Kolsto.** 2000. *Bacillus anthracis, Bacillus cereus,* and *Bacillus thuringiensis*—one species on the basis of genetic evidence. *Appl. Environ. Microbiol.* **66**:2627–2630.

134. **Higgins, R. J., J. F. Harbourne, T. W. Little, and A. E. Stevens.** 1980. Mastitis and abortion in dairy cattle associated with *Leptospira* of the serotype *hardjo. Vet. Rec.* **107**:307–310.

135. **Higgins, R. J., and C. R. Weaver.** 1981. *Corynebacterium renale* pyelonephritis and cystitis in a sheep. *Vet. Rec.* **109**:256.

136. **Hjaltested, E. K., S. Gudmundsdottir, K. Jonsdottir, K. G. Kristinsson, O. Steingrimsson, and M. Kristjansson.** 2002. Listeriosis in Iceland, 1978–2000: a description of cases and molecular epidemiology. *Scand. J. Infect. Dis.* **34**:735–741.

137. **Ho, P. L., T. K. Cheung, W. C. Yam, and K. Y. Yuen.** 2002. Characterization of a laboratory-generated variant of BPS β-lactamase from *Burkholderia pseudomallei* that hydrolyses ceftazidime. *J. Antimicrob. Chemother.* **50**:723–726.

138. **Hodgson, A. L., J. Krywult, and A. J. Radford.** 1990. Nucleotide sequence of the erythromycin resistance gene from the *Corynebacterium* plasmid pNG2. *Nucleic Acids Res.* **18**: 1891.

139. **Homer.** *Iliaden I*, 50–52. Translated into Danish by O. S. Due. Gyldendal, Copenhagen, Denmark. [1999 edition.]

140. **Hopla, C. E.** 1974. The ecology of tularemia. *Adv. Vet. Sci. Comp. Med.* **18**:25–53.

141. **Hoshino, T., T. Ikeda, N. Tomizuka, and K. Furukawa.** 1985. Nucleotide sequence of the tetracycline resistance gene of pTHT15, a thermophilic Bacillus plasmid: comparison with staphylococcal TcR controls. *Gene* **37**:131–138.

142. **Howe, C., and W. R. Miller.** 1947. Human glanders: report of six cases. *Ann. Intern. Med.* **26**:93–115.

143. **Huddleson, I. F.** 1929. The differentiation of the species of the genus *Brucella. Mich. Agric. Exp. Stn. Tech. Bull.* **100**:1–6.

144. **Hue, K. K., and D. H. Bechhofer.** 1992. Regulation of the macrolide-lincosamide-streptogramin B resistance gene *ermD. J. Bacteriol.* **174**:5860–5868.

145. **Ikaheimo, I., H. Syrjala, J. Karhukorpi, R. Schildt, and M. Koskela.** 2000. *In vitro* antibiotic susceptibility of *Francisella tularensis* isolated from humans and animals. *J. Antimicrob. Chemother.* **46:**287–290.
146. **Inglis, T. J., F. Rodrigues, P. Rigby, R. Norton, and B. J. Currie.** 2004. Comparison of the susceptibilities of *Burkholderia pseudomallei* to meropenem and ceftazidime by conventional and intracellular methods. *Antimicrob. Agents Chemother.* **48:**2999–3005.
147. **Iwarson, S., and S. Larsson.** 1979. Outcome of *Listeria monocytogenes* infection in compromised and non-compromised adults; a comparative study of seventy-two cases. *Infection* 7:54–56.
148. **Jacks, S. S., S. Giguere, and A. Nguyen.** 2003. *In vitro* susceptibilities of *Rhodococcus equi* and other common equine pathogens to azithromycin, clarithromycin, and 20 other antimicrobials. *Antimicrob. Agents Chemother.* **47:**1742–1745.
149. **Jahans, K. L., G. Foster, and E. S. Broughton.** 1997. The characterisation of *Brucella* strains isolated from marine mammals. *Vet. Microbiol.* **57:**373–382.
150. **Jellison, W., H. Jacobson, and S. Flora.** 1964. Tick-borne tularemia and tick paralysis in cattle and sheep. *Proc. Annu. Meet. U. S. Anim. Health Assoc.* **68:**60–64.
151. **Jenney, A. W., G. Lum, D. A. Fisher, and B. J. Currie.** 2001. Antibiotic susceptibility of *Burkholderia pseudomallei* from tropical northern Australia and implications for therapy of melioidosis. *Int. J. Antimicrob. Agents* **17:**109–113.
152. **Jensen, L. B., S. Baloda, M. Boye, and F. M. Aarestrup.** 2001. Antimicrobial resistance among *Pseudomonas* spp. and the *Bacillus cereus* group isolated from Danish agricultural soil. *Environ. Int.* **26:**581–587.
153. **Jensen, L. B., Y. Agersø, and G. Sengeløv.** 2002. Presence of *erm* genes among macrolide-resistant Gram-positive bacteria isolated from Danish farm soil. *Environ. Int.* **28:**487–491.
154. **Jensen, N. E., F. M. Aarestrup, J. Jensen, and H. C. Wegener.** 1996. *Listeria monocytogenes* in bovine mastitis. Possible implication for human health. *Int. J. Food Microbiol.* **32:**209–216.
155. **Johnson, R. C., and V. G. Harris.** 1967. Differentiation of pathogenic and saprophytic leptospires. I. Growth at low temperatures. *J. Bacteriol.* **94:**27–31.
156. **Jones, E. M., and A. P. MacGowan.** 1995. Antimicrobial chemotherapy of human infection due to *Listeria monocytogenes*. *Eur. J. Clin. Microbiol. Infect. Dis.* **14:**165–175.
157. **Jones, L. M., M. Zanardi, D. Leong, and J. B. Wilson.** 1968. Taxonomic position in the genus *Brucella* of the causative agent of canine abortion. *J. Bacteriol.* **95:**625–630.
158. **Jones, M. E., J. Goguen, I. A. Critchley, D. C. Draghi, J. A. Karlowsky, D. F. Sahm, R. Porschen, G. Patra, and V. G. DelVecchio.** 2003. Antibiotic susceptibility of isolates of *Bacillus anthracis*, a bacterial pathogen with the potential to be used in biowarfare. *Clin. Microbiol. Infect.* **9:**984–986.
159. **Jones, R. N., M. A. Pfaller, P. R. Rhomberg, and D. H. Walter.** 2002. Tiamulin activity against fastidious and nonfastidious veterinary and human bacterial isolates: initial development of in vitro susceptibility test methods. *J. Clin. Microbiol.* **40:**461–465.
160. **Jose-Cunilleras, E., and K. W. Hinchcliff.** 2001. *Listeria monocytogenes* septicaemia in foals. *Equine Vet. J.* **33:** 519–522.
161. **Jost, B. H., A. C. Field, H. T. Trinh, J. G. Songer, and S. J. Billington.** 2003. Tylosin resistance in *Arcanobacterium pyogenes* is encoded by an Erm X determinant. *Antimicrob. Agents Chemother.* **47:**3519–3524.
162. **Jost, B. H., H. T. Trinh, J. G. Songer, and S. J. Billington.** 2004. A second tylosin resistance determinant, Erm B, in *Arcanobacterium pyogenes*. *Antimicrob. Agents Chemother.* **48:**721–727.
163. **Jost, B. H., H. T. Trinh, J. G. Songer, and S. J. Billington.** 2004. Ribosomal mutations in *Arcanobacterium pyogenes* confer a unique spectrum of macrolide resistance. *Antimicrob. Agents Chemother.* **48:**1021–1023.
164. **Judson, R., and J. G. Songer.** 1991. *Corynebacterium pseudotuberculosis*: *in vitro* susceptibility to 39 antimicrobial agents. *Vet. Microbiol.* **27:**145–150.
165. **Kenny, D. J., P. Russell, D. Rogers, S. M. Eley, and R. W. Titball.** 1999. *In vitro* susceptibilities of *Burkholderia mallei* in comparison to those of other pathogenic *Burkholderia* spp. *Antimicrob. Agents Chemother.* **43:**2773–2775.
166. **Kim, H. J., Y. Kim, M. S. Lee, and H. S. Lee.** 2001. Gene *lmrB* of *Corynebacterium glutamicum* confers efflux-mediated resistance to lincomycin. *Mol. Cells* **12:**112–116.
167. **Kim, H. S., E. C. Choi, and B. K. Kim.** 1993. A macrolide-lincosamide-streptogramin B resistance determinant from *Bacillus anthracis* 590: cloning and expression of *ermJ*. *J. Gen. Microbiol.* **139:**601–607.
168. **Kimpe, A., A. Decostere, K. Hermans, M. Baele, and F. Haesebrouck.** 2004. Isolation of *Listeria ivanovii* from a septicaemic chinchilla (*Chinchilla lanigera*). *Vet. Rec.* **154:** 791–792.
169. **Kinsara, A., A. Al-Mowallad, and A. O. Osoba.** 1999. Increasing resistance of Brucellae to co-trimoxazole. *Antimicrob. Agents Chemother.* **43:**1531.
170. **Landinez, R., J. Linares, E. Loza, J. Martinez-Beltran, R. Martin, and F. Baquero.** 1992. In vitro activity of azithromycin and tetracycline against 358 clinical isolates of *Brucella melitensis*. *Eur. J. Clin. Microbiol. Infect. Dis.* **11:**265–267.
171. **Lang, R., and E. Rubinstein.** 1992. Quinolones for the treatment of brucellosis. *J. Antimicrob. Chemother.* **29:**357–360.
172. **Lawson, P. A., E. Falsen, E. Akervall, P. Vandamme, and M. D. Collins.** 1997. Characterization of some *Actinomyces*-like isolates from human clinical specimens: reclassification of *Actinomyces suis* (Soltys and Spratling) as *Actinobaculum suis* comb. nov. and description of *Actinobaculum schaalii* sp. nov. *Int. J. Syst. Bacteriol.* **47:**899–903.
173. **Lebrun, M., A. Audurier, and P. Cossart.** 1994. Plasmid-borne cadmium resistance genes in *Listeria monocytogenes* are similar to *cadA* and *cadC* of *Staphylococcus aureus* and are induced by cadmium. *J. Bacteriol.* **176:**3040–3048.
174. **Lebrun, M., A. Audurier, and P. Cossart.** 1994. Plasmid-borne cadmium resistance genes in *Listeria monocytogenes* are present on Tn*5422*, a novel transposon closely related to Tn*917*. *J. Bacteriol.* **176:**3049–3061.
175. **Lechner, S., R. Mayr, K. P. Francis, B. M. Pruss, T. Kaplan, E. Wiessner-Gunkel, G. S. Stewart, and S. Scherer.** 1998. *Bacillus weihenstephanensis* sp. nov. is a new psychrotolerant species of the *Bacillus cereus* group. *Int. J. Syst. Bacteriol.* **48:**1373–1382.
176. **Leon-Vizcaino, L., M. Hermoso de Mendoza, and F. Garrido.** 1987. Incidence of abortions caused by leptospirosis in sheep and goats in Spain. *Comp. Immunol. Microbiol. Infect. Dis.* **10:**149–153.
177. **Levett, P. N.** 2001. Leptospirosis. *Clin. Microbiol. Rev.* **14:** 296–326.
178. **Lohenry, K.** 2004. Anthrax exposure—stay alert, act swiftly. *JAAPA* **17:**29–33.
179. **Lopez, J. F., F. M. Wong, and J. Quesada.** 1966. *Corynebacterium pseudotuberculosis*. First case of human infection. *Am. J. Clin. Pathol.* **46:**562–567.
180. **Low, J. C., and C. P. Renton.** 1985. Septicaemia, encephalitis and abortions in a housed flock of sheep caused by *Listeria monocytogenes* type 1/2. *Vet. Rec.* **116:**147–150.

181. **Luna, V. A., P. Coates, E. A. Eady, J. H. Cove, T. T. Nguyen, and M. C. Roberts.** 1999. A variety of gram-positive bacteria carry mobile *mef* genes. *J. Antimicrob. Chemother.* **44:** 19–25.

182. **Lyytikainen, O., T. Autio, R. Maijala, P. Ruutu, T. Honkanen-Buzalski, M. Miettinen, M. Hatakka, J. Mikkola, V. J. Anttila, T. Johansson, L. Rantala, T. Aalto, H. Korkeala, and A. Siitonen.** 2000. An outbreak of *Listeria monocytogenes* serotype 3a infections from butter in Finland. *J. Infect. Dis.* **181:**1838–1841.

183. **Macleod, N. S., J. A. Watt, and J. C. Harris.** 1974. *Listeria monocytogenes* type 5 as a cause of abortion in sheep. *Vet. Rec.* **95:**365–367.

184. **Marco, F., M. Almela, J. Nolla-Salas, P. Coll, I. Gasser, M. D. Ferrer, M. de Simon, and The Collaborative Study Group of Listeriosis of Barcelona.** 2000. In vitro activities of 22 antimicrobial agents against *Listeria monocytogenes* strains isolated in Barcelona, Spain. *Diagn. Microbiol. Infect. Dis.* **38:**259–261.

185. **Marianelli, C., F. Ciuchini, M. Tarantino, P. Pasquali, and R. Adone.** 2004. Genetic bases of the rifampin resistance phenotype in *Brucella* spp. *J. Clin. Microbiol.* **42:**5439–5443.

186. **Mascola, L., F. Sorvillo, J. Neal, K. Iwakoshi, and R. Weaver.** 1989. Surveillance of listeriosis in Los Angeles County, 1985–1986. A first year's report. *Arch. Intern. Med.* **149:** 1569–1572.

187. **Materon, I. C., A. M. Queenan, T. M. Koehler, K. Bush, and T. Palzkill.** 2003. Biochemical characterization of β-lactamases Bla1 and Bla2 from *Bacillus anthracis*. *Antimicrob. Agents Chemother.* **47:**2040–2042.

188. **Mayrhofer, S., P. Paulsen, F. J. Smulders, and F. Hilbert.** 2004. Antimicrobial resistance profile of five major food-borne pathogens isolated from beef, pork and poultry. *Int. J. Food Microbiol.* **97:**23–29.

189. **McClain, J. B., W. R. Ballou, S. M. Harrison, and D. L. Steinweg.** 1984. Doxycycline therapy for leptospirosis. *Ann. Intern. Med.* **100:**696–698.

190. **McNeil, M. M., and J. M. Brown.** 1992. Distribution and antimicrobial susceptibility of *Rhodococcus equi* from clinical specimens. *Eur. J. Epidemiol.* **8:**437–443.

191. **Meijer, W. G., and J. F. Prescott.** 2004. *Rhodococcus equi*. *Vet. Res.* **35:**383–396.

192. **Memish, Z. A., M. W. Mah, S. Al Mahmoud, M. Al Shaalan, and M. Y. Khan.** 2000. *Brucella* bacteraemia: clinical and laboratory observations in 160 patients. *J. Infect.* **40:**59–63.

193. **Miers, K. C., and W. B. Ley.** 1980. *Corynebacterium pseudotuberculosis* infection in the horse: study of 117 clinical cases and consideration of etiopathogenesis. *J. Am. Vet. Med. Assoc.* **177:**250–253.

194. **Miettinen, M. K., A. Siitonen, P. Heiskanen, H. Haajanen, K. J. Bjorkroth, and H. J. Korkeala.** 1999. Molecular epidemiology of an outbreak of febrile gastroenteritis caused by *Listeria monocytogenes* in cold-smoked rainbow trout. *J. Clin. Microbiol.* **37:**2358–2360.

195. **Mills, A. E., R. D. Mitchell, and E. K. Lim.** 1997. *Corynebacterium pseudotuberculosis* is a cause of human necrotising granulomatous lymphadenitis. *Pathology* **29:**231–233.

196. **Mock, M., and A. Fouet.** 2001. Anthrax. *Annu. Rev. Microbiol.* **55:**647–671.

197. **Mohammed, M. J., C. K. Marston, T. Popovic, R. S. Weyant, and F. C. Tenover.** 2002. Antimicrobial susceptibility testing of *Bacillus anthracis*: comparison of results obtained by using the National Committee for Clinical Laboratory Standards broth microdilution reference and Etest agar gradient diffusion methods. *J. Clin. Microbiol.* **40:** 1902–1907.

198. **Monod, M., C. Denoya, and D. Dubnau.** 1986. Sequence and properties of pIM13, a macrolide-lincosamide-streptogramin B resistance plasmid from *Bacillus subtilis*. *J. Bacteriol.* **167:** 138–147.

199. **Monod, M., S. Mohan, and D. Dubnau.** 1987. Cloning and analysis of *ermG*, a new macrolide-lincosamide-streptogramin B resistance element from *Bacillus sphaericus*. *J. Bacteriol.* **169:**340–350.

200. **Montejo, J. M., I. Alberola, P. Glez-Zarate, A. Alvarez, J. Alonso, A. Canovas, and C. Aguirre.** 1993. Open, randomized therapeutic trial of six antimicrobial regimens in the treatment of human brucellosis. *Clin. Infect. Dis.* **16:**671–676.

201. **Morner, T., and K. Sandstedt.** 1983. A serological survey of antibodies against *Francisella tularensis* in some Swedish mammals. *Nord. Vetmed.* **35:**82–85.

202. **Morris, M. P., and O. J. Fletcher.** 1988. Diagnostic summary of 1986 turkey, broiler breeder, and layer necropsy cases at the University of Georgia. *Avian Dis.* **32:**391–403.

203. **Mortensen, J. E., D. G. Moore, J. E. Clarridge, and E. J. Young.** 1986. Antimicrobial susceptibility of clinical isolates of *Brucella*. *Diagn. Microbiol. Infect. Dis.* **5:**163–169.

204. **Murgia, R., and M. Cinco.** 2001. Sensitivity of *Borrelia* and *Leptospira* to quinupristin-dalfopristin (Synercid) *in vitro*. *New Microbiol.* **24:**193–196.

205. **Murray, C. K., and D. R. Hospenthal.** 2004. Broth microdilution susceptibility testing for *Leptospira* spp. *Antimicrob. Agents Chemother.* **48:**1548–1552.

206. **Murray, C. K., and D. R. Hospenthal.** 2004. Determination of susceptibilities of 26 *Leptospira* sp. serovars to 24 antimicrobial agents by a broth microdilution technique. *Antimicrob. Agents Chemother.* **48:**4002–4005.

207. **Musser, J. M.** 1995. Antimicrobial agent resistance in mycobacteria: molecular genetic insights. *Clin. Microbiol. Rev.* **8:**496–514.

208. **Nakamura, L. K.** 1998. *Bacillus pseudomycoides* sp. nov. *Int. J. Syst. Bacteriol.* **48:**1031–1035.

209. **National Committee for Clinical Laboratory Standards.** 2004. Methods for antimicrobial susceptibility testing of anaerobic bacteria. Approved standard, 6th ed. NCCLS document M11-A6. National Committee for Clinical Laboratory Standards, Wayne, Pa.

210. **Nesvera, J., J. Hochmannova, and M. Patek.** 1998. An integron of class 1 is present on the plasmid pCG4 from gram-positive bacterium *Corynebacterium glutamicum*. *FEMS Microbiol. Lett.* **169:**391–395.

211. **Niumsup, P., and V. Wuthiekanun.** 2002. Cloning of the class D β-lactamase gene from *Burkholderia pseudomallei* and studies on its expression in ceftazidime-susceptible and resistant strains. *J. Antimicrob. Chemother.* **50:**445–455.

212. **Noguchi, H.** 1918. Further studies on the cultural conditions of *Leptospira* (*Spirochaeta*) *icterohaemorrhagiae* (Inada and Ido). *J. Exp. Med.* **27:**575–592.

213. **Nordmann, P., and E. Ronco.** 1992. *In-vitro* antimicrobial susceptibility of *Rhodococcus equi*. *J. Antimicrob. Chemother.* **29:**383–393.

214. **Nordmann, P., M. H. Nicolas, and L. Gutmann.** 1993. Penicillin-binding proteins of *Rhodococcus equi*: potential role in resistance to imipenem. *Antimicrob. Agents Chemother.* **37:**1406–1409.

215. **Nordmann, P., M. Keller, F. Espinasse, and E. Ronco.** 1994. Correlation between antibiotic resistance, phage-like particle presence, and virulence in *Rhodococcus equi* human isolates. *J. Clin. Microbiol.* **32:**377–383.

216. **Office International des Épizooties.** 2003. *World Animal Health in 2002*. Office International des Épizooties, Paris, France.

217. **Office International des Épizooties.** 2004. *World Animal Health in 2003*. Office International des Épizooties, Paris, France.
218. **Oie, S., K. Hironaga, A. Koshiro, H. Konishi, and Z. Yoshii.** 1983. *In vitro* susceptibilities of five *Leptospira* strains to 16 antimicrobial agents. *Antimicrob. Agents Chemother.* **24:** 905–908.
219. **Otter, A., and C. Moynan.** 2000. *Corynebacterium renale* infection in calves. *Vet. Rec.* **146:**83–84.
220. **Pankey, J. W., S. C. Nickerson, R. L. Boddie, and J. S. Hogan.** 1985. Effects of *Corynebacterium bovis* infection on susceptibility to major mastitis pathogens. *J. Dairy Sci.* **68:** 2684–2693.
221. **Paton, M. W., S. B. Walker, I. R. Rose, an.d G. F. Watt.** 2003. Prevalence of caseous lymphadenitis and usage of caseous lymphadenitis vaccines in sheep flocks. *Aust. Vet. J.* **81:**91–95.
222. **Pearson, L. J., and E. H. Marth.** 1990. *Listeria monocytogenes*—threat to a safe food supply: a review. *J. Dairy Sci.* 73:912–928.
223. **Peel, M. M., G. G. Palmer, A. M. Stacpoole, and T. G. Kerr.** 1997. Human lymphadenitis due to *Corynebacterium pseudotuberculosis*: report of ten cases from Australia and review. *Clin. Infect. Dis.* **24:**185–191.
224. **Petersen, J. M., M. E. Schriefer, L. G. Carter, Y. Zhou, T. Sealy, D. Bawiec, B. Yockey, S. Urich, N. S. Zeidner, S. Avashia, J. L. Kool, J. Buck, C. Lindley, L. Celeda, J. A. Monteneiri, K. L. Gage, and M. C. Chu.** 2004. Laboratory analysis of tularemia in wild-trapped, commercially traded prairie dogs, Texas, 2002. *Emerg. Infect. Dis.* **10:**419–425.
225. **Petrov, E. M., and I. G. Chernukha.** 1975. Sensitivity of certain strains of pathogenic *Leptospira* to streptomycin, the nature of resistant variants and the frequency of their occurrence. *Antibiotiki* **20:**62–66. (In Russian.)
226. **Piliouras, P., G. C. Ulett, C. Ashhurst-Smith, R. G. Hirst, and R. E. Norton.** 2002. A comparison of antibiotic susceptibility testing methods for cotrimoxazole with *Burkholderia pseudomallei*. *Int. J. Antimicrob. Agents* **19:**427–429.
227. **Pleschakowa, V., W. Leibold, G. Amtsberg, D. Konine, and M. Wendt.** 2004. The prevalence of *Actinobaculum suis* in boars of breeding herds in the Omsk region (Russian Federation) by indirect immunofluorescence technique. *Dtsch. Tierarztl. Wochenschr.* **111:**67–69. (In German.)
228. **Poulsen, P. N., A. Carvajal, A. Lester, and J. Andreasen.** 1988. *In vitro* susceptibility of *Listeria monocytogenes* isolated from human blood and cerebrospinal fluid. A material from the years 1958–1985. *APMIS* **96:**223–228.
229. **Pourshaban, M., A. M. Ferrini, V. Mannoni, B. Oliva, and P. Aureli.** 2002. Transferable tetracycline resistance in *Listeria monocytogenes* from food in Italy. *J. Med. Microbiol.* **51:**564–566.
230. **Poyart-Salmeron, C., C. Carlier, P. Trieu-Cuot, A. L. Courtieu, and P. Courvalin.** 1990. Transferable plasmid-mediated antibiotic resistance in *Listeria monocytogenes*. *Lancet* **335:** 1422–1426.
231. **Poyart-Salmeron, C., P. Trieu-Cuot, C. Carlier, A. MacGowan, J. McLauchlin, and P. Courvalin.** 1992. Genetic basis of tetracycline resistance in clinical isolates of *Listeria monocytogenes*. *Antimicrob. Agents Chemother.* **36:**463–466.
232. **Prescott, J. F.** 1981. The susceptibility of isolates of *Corynebacterium equi* to antimicrobial drugs. *J. Vet. Pharmacol. Ther.* **4:** 27–31.
233. **Prescott, J. F.** 1991. *Rhodococcus equi*: an animal and human pathogen. *Clin. Microbiol. Rev.* **4:**20–34.
234. **Prescott, J. F., and V. M. Nicholson.** 1988. Antimicrobial drug susceptibility of *Leptospira interrogans* serovar *hardjo* isolated from cattle. *Can. J. Vet. Res.* **52:**286–287.
235. **Prescott, J. F., and K. M. Yielding.** 1990. *In vitro* susceptibility of selected veterinary bacterial pathogens to ciprofloxacin, enrofloxacin and norfloxacin. *Can. J. Vet. Res.* **54:**195–197.
236. **Radostits, O. M., C. C. Gay, D. C. Blood, and K. W. Hinchcliff.** 2000. *Veterinary Medicine: a Textbook of the Diseases of Cattle, Sheep, Pigs, Goats and Horses*, 9th ed. The W. B. Saunders Co., Philadelphia, Pa.
237. **Ramos, C. P., G. Foster, and M. D. Collins.** 1997. Phylogenetic analysis of the genus *Actinomyces* based on 16S rRNA gene sequences: description of *Arcanobacterium phocae* sp. nov., *Arcanobacterium bernardiae* comb. nov., and *Arcanobacterium pyogenes* comb. nov. *Int. J. Syst. Bacteriol.* **47:**46–53.
238. **Rebhun, W. C., S. G. Dill, J. A. Perdrizet, and C. E. Hatfield.** 1989. Pyelonephritis in cows: 15 cases (1982–1986). *J. Am. Vet. Med. Assoc.* **194:**953–955.
239. **Reboli, A. C., and W. E. Farrar.** 1989. *Erysipelothrix rhusiopathiae*: an occupational pathogen. *Clin. Microbiol. Rev.* **2:**354–359.
240. **Rhyan, J. C., T. Gahagan, and W. H. Fales.** 1990. Tularemia in a cat. *J. Vet. Diagn. Investig.* **2:**239–241.
241. **Roberts, M. C., R. B. Leonard, A. Briselden, F. D. Schoenknecht, and M.B. Coyle.** 1992. Characterization of antibiotic-resistant *Corynebacterium striatum* strains. *J. Antimicrob. Chemother.* **30:**463–474.
242. **Roberts, M. C., B. Facinelli, E. Giovanetti, and P. E. Varaldo.** 1996. Transferable erythromycin resistance in *Listeria* spp. isolated from food. *Appl. Environ. Microbiol.* **62:**269–270.
243. **Roberts, M. C., J. Sutcliffe, P. Courvalin, L. B. Jensen, J. Rood, and H. Seppala.** 1999. Nomenclature for macrolide and macrolide-lincosamide-streptogramin B resistance determinants. *Antimicrob. Agents Chemother.* **43:**2823–2830.
244. **Rolston, K. V., S. Frisbee-Hume, B. LeBlanc, H. Streeter, and D. H. Ho.** 2003. *In vitro* antimicrobial activity of moxifloxacin compared to other quinolones against recent clinical bacterial isolates from hospitalized and community-based cancer patients. *Diagn. Microbiol. Infect. Dis.* **47:**441–449.
245. **Rosato, A. E., B. S. Lee, and K. A. Nash.** 2001. Inducible macrolide resistance in *Corynebacterium jeikeium*. *Antimicrob. Agents Chemother.* **45:**1982–1989.
246. **Rubinstein, E., R. Lang, B. Shasha, B. Hagar, L. Diamanstein, G. Joseph, M. Anderson, and K. Harrison.** 1991. *In vitro* susceptibility of *Brucella melitensis* to antibiotics. *Antimicrob. Agents Chemother.* **35:**1925–1927.
247. **Russell, P., S. M. Eley, M. J. Fulop, D. L. Bell, and R. W. Titball.** 1998. The efficacy of ciprofloxacin and doxycycline against experimental tularaemia. *J. Antimicrob. Chemother.* **41:**461–465.
248. **Russell, R. W.** 1985. Treatment of leptospirosis with oxytetracycline. *Lancet* **ii:**1143–1145.
249. **Safdar, A., and D. Armstrong.** 2003. Antimicrobial activities against 84 *Listeria monocytogenes* isolates from patients with systemic listeriosis at a comprehensive cancer center (1955–1997). *J. Clin. Microbiol.* **41:**483–485.
250. **Sajduda, A., A. Brzostek, M. Poplawska, E. Augustynowicz-Kopec, Z. Zwolska, S. Niemann, J. Dziadek, and D. Hillemann.** 2004. Molecular characterization of rifampin- and isoniazid-resistant *Mycobacterium tuberculosis* strains isolated in Poland. *J. Clin. Microbiol.* **42:**2425–2431.
251. **Sakaguchi, R., H. Amano, and K. Shishido.** 1988. Nucleotide sequence homology of the tetracycline-resistance determinant naturally maintained in *Bacillus subtilis* Marburg 168 chromosome and the tetracycline-resistance gene of *B. subtilis* plasmid pNS1981. *Biochim. Biophys. Acta* **950:** 441–444.

252. **Sane, D. C., and D. T. Durack.** 1986. Infection with *Rhodococcus equi* in AIDS. *N. Engl. J. Med.* **314:**56–57.
253. **Scheel, O., T. Hoel, T. Sandvik, and B. P. Berdal.** 1993. Susceptibility pattern of Scandinavian *Francisella tularensis* isolates with regard to oral and parenteral antimicrobial agents. *APMIS* **101:**33–36.
254. **Schlipköter, H. W., and M. Beckers.** 1951. Die Wirkung von Chemotherapeutika und Antibiotika auf pathogene Leptospiren. *Z. Immunitaetsforsch. Exp. Ther.* **108:**301–317.
255. **Sehgal, S. C., A. P. Sugunan, M. V. Murhekar, S. Sharma, and P. Vijayachari.** 2000. Randomized controlled trial of doxycycline prophylaxis against leptospirosis in an endemic area. *Int. J. Antimicrob. Agents* **13:**249–255.
256. **Sengeløv, G., Y. Agersø, B. Halling-Sørensen, S. B. Baloda, J. S. Andersen, and L. B. Jensen.** 2003. Bacterial antibiotic resistance levels in Danish farmland as a result of treatment with pig manure slurry. *Environ. Int.* **28:**587–595.
257. **Sergeant, E. S., S. C. Love, and A. McInnes.** 1991. Abortions in sheep due to *Listeria ivanovii. Aust. Vet. J.* **68:**39.
258. **Shalit, I., A. Barnea, and A. Shahar.** 1989. Efficacy of ciprofloxacin against *Leptospira interrogans* serogroup *icterohaemorrhagiae. Antimicrob. Agents Chemother.* **33:**788–789.
259. **Shapiro, D. S., and J. D. Wong.** 1999. *Brucella*, p. 625–631. *In* P. R. Murray, E. J. Baron, M. A. Pfaller, F. C. Tenover, and R. H. Yolken (ed.), *Manual of Clinical Microbiology*, 7th ed. ASM Press, Washington, D.C.
260. **Sheldon, I. M., M. Bushnell, J. Montgomery, and A. N. Rycroft.** 2004. Minimum inhibitory concentrations of some antimicrobial drugs against bacteria causing uterine infections in cattle. *Vet. Rec.* **155:**383–387.
261. **Shen, T., P. Jia, S. Na, and D. Men.** 1993. Determination of nucleotide sequence of *Corynebacterium* plasmid pXZ10145. *Chin. J. Biotechnol.* **9:**171–178.
262. **Simpson, A. J., Y. Suputtamongkol, M. D. Smith, B. J. Angus, A. Rajanuwong, V. Wuthiekanun, P. A. Howe, A. L. Walsh, W. Chaowagul, and N. J. White.** 1999. Comparison of imipenem and ceftazidime as therapy for severe melioidosis. *Clin. Infect. Dis.* **29:**381–387.
263. **Smith, C. R., B. G. Corney, M. R. McGowan, C. S. McClintock, W. Ward, and P. J. Ketterer.** 1997. Amoxycillin as an alternative to dihydrostreptomycin sulphate for treating cattle infected with *Leptospira borgpetersenii* serovar *hardjo. Aust. Vet. J.* **75:**818–821.
264. **Sobestiansky, J., M. Wendt, R. Perestrelo, and A. Ambrogi.** 1993. Studies on the prevalence of *Eubacterium suis* in boars on farms in Brazil, Portugal and Argentina by indirect immunofluorescence technique. *Dtsch. Tierarztl. Wochenschr.* **100:**463–464.
265. **Sohn, A. H., W. S. Probert, C. A. Glaser, N. Gupta, A. W. Bollen, J. D. Wong, E. M. Grace, and W. C. McDonald.** 2003. Human neurobrucellosis with intracerebral granuloma caused by a marine mammal *Brucella* spp. *Emerg. Infect. Dis.* **9:**485–488.
266. **Solera, J., E. Martinez-Alfaro, and A. Espinosa.** 1997. Recognition and optimum treatment of brucellosis. *Drugs* **53:**245–256.
267. **Sookpranee, M., P. Boonma, W. Susaengrat, K. Bhuripanyo, and S. Punyagupta.** 1992. Multicenter prospective randomized trial comparing ceftazidime plus co-trimoxazole with chloramphenicol plus doxycycline and co-trimoxazole for treatment of severe melioidosis. *Antimicrob. Agents Chemother.* **36:**158–162.
268. **Soriano, F., R. Fernandez-Roblas, R. Calvo, and G. Garcia-Calvo.** 1998. *In vitro* susceptibilities of aerobic and facultative non-spore-forming gram-positive bacilli to HMR 3647 (RU 66647) and 14 other antimicrobials. *Antimicrob. Agents Chemother.* **42:**1028–1033.
269. **Spencer, R. C.** 2003. *Bacillus anthracis. J. Clin. Pathol.* **56:**182–187.
270. **Spitzer, P. G., S. M. Hammer, and A. W. Karchmer.** 1986. Treatment of *Listeria monocytogenes* infection with trimethoprim-sulfamethoxazole: case report and review of the literature. *Rev. Infect. Dis.* **8:**427–430.
271. **Spradbrow, P. B.** 1963. Sensitivity to drugs of Australian leptospiral serotypes. *Br. Pharm. Chemother.* **20:**230–236.
272. **Sprague, L. D., and H. Neubauer.** 2004. Melioidosis in animals: a review on epizootiology, diagnosis and clinical presentation. *J. Vet. Med. B* **51:**305–320.
273. **Stalheim, O. H.** 1966. Effects of antimicrobial agents on leptospiral growth, respiration, motility, and viability. *Am. J. Vet. Res.* **27:**797–802.
274. **Stalheim, O. H. V.** 1967. Chemotherapy of renal leptospirosis in swine. *Am. J. Vet. Res.* **28:**161.
275. **Stiles, G. W.** 1947. Chronic erysipeloid (swine erysipelas) in a man. The effect of treatment with penicillin. *JAMA* **134:**953–955.
276. **Sternbach, G.** 2003. The history of anthrax. *J. Emerg. Med.* **24:**463–467.
277. **Stoenner, H. G., and D. B. Lackman.** 1957. A new species of *Brucella* isolated from the desert wood rat, *Neotoma lepida* Thomas. *Am. J. Vet. Res.* **18:**947–951.
278. **Sutherland, S. S., R. A. Hart, and N. B. Buller.** 1996. Genetic differences between nitrate-negative and nitrate-positive *C. pseudotuberculosis* strains using restriction fragment length polymorphisms. *Vet. Microbiol.* **49:**1–9.
279. **Syrjala, H., R. Schildt, and S. Raisainen.** 1991. *In vitro* susceptibility of *Francisella tularensis* to fluoroquinolones and treatment of tularemia with norfloxacin and ciprofloxacin. *Eur. J. Clin. Microbiol. Infect. Dis.* **10:**68–70.
280. **Takafuji, E. T., J. W. Kirkpatrick, R. N. Miller, J. J. Karwacki, P. W. Kelley, M. R. Gray, K. M. McNeill, H. L. Timboe, R. E. Kane, and J. L. Sanchez.** 1984. An efficacy trial of doxycycline chemoprophylaxis against leptospirosis. *N. Engl. J. Med.* **310:**497–500.
281. **Takahashi, T., T. Sawada, K. Ohmae, N. Terakado, M. Muramatsu, K. Seto, T. Maruyama, and M. Kanzaki.** 1984. Antibiotic resistance of *Erysipelothrix rhusiopathiae* isolated from pigs with chronic swine erysipelas. *Antimicrob. Agents Chemother.* **25:**385–386.
282. **Takahashi, T., T. Sawada, M. Muramatsu, Y. Tamura, T. Fujisawa, Y. Benno, and T. Mitsuoka.** 1987. Serotype, antimicrobial susceptibility, and pathogenicity of *Erysipelothrix rhusiopathiae* isolates from tonsils of apparently healthy slaughter pigs. *J. Clin. Microbiol.* **25:**536–539.
283. **Takahashi, T., T. Fujisawa, Y. Tamura, S. Suzuki, M. Muramatsu, T. Sawada, Y. Benno, and T. Mitsuoka.** 1992. DNA relatedness among *Erysipelothrix rhusiopathiae* strains representing all twenty-three serovars and *Erysipelothrix tonsillarum. Int. J. Syst. Bacteriol.* **42:**469–473.
284. **Takai, S., K. Takeda, Y. Nakano, T. Karasawa, J. Furugoori, Y. Sasaki, S. Tsubaki, T. Higuchi, T. Anzai, R. Wada, and M. Kamada.** 1997. Emergence of rifampin-resistant *Rhodococcus equi* in an infected foal. *J. Clin. Microbiol.* **35:**1904–1908.
285. **Takashima, I., M. Ngoma, and N. Hashimoto.** 1993. Antimicrobial effects of a new carboxyquinolone drug, Q-35, on five serogroups of *Leptospira interrogans. Antimicrob. Agents Chemother.* **37:**901–902.
286. **Tanaka, Y., K. Yazawa, E. R. Dabbs, K. Nishikawa, H. Komaki, Y. Mikami, M. Miyaji, N. Morisaki, and S. Iwasaki.** 1996. Different rifampicin inactivation mechanisms in *Nocardia* and related taxa. *Microbiol. Immunol.* **40:**1–4.

287. **Tauch, A., F. Kassing, J. Kalinowski, and A. Puhler.** 1995. The *Corynebacterium xerosis* composite transposon Tn*5432* consists of two identical insertion sequences, designated IS*1249*, flanking the erythromycin resistance gene *ermCX*. *Plasmid* **34:**119–131.

288. **Tauch, A., Z. Zheng, A. Puhler, and J. Kalinowski.** 1998. *Corynebacterium striatum* chloramphenicol resistance transposon Tn*5564*: genetic organization and transposition in *Corynebacterium glutamicum*. *Plasmid* **40:**126–139.

289. **Tauch, A., S. Krieft, A. Puhler, and J. Kalinowski.** 1999. The *tetAB* genes of the *Corynebacterium striatum* R-plasmid pTP10 encode an ABC transporter and confer tetracycline, oxytetracycline and oxacillin resistance in *Corynebacterium glutamicum*. *FEMS Microbiol. Lett.* **173:**203–209.

290. **Tauch, A., A. Puhler, J. Kalinowski, and G. Thierbach.** 2000. TetZ, a new tetracycline resistance determinant discovered in gram-positive bacteria, shows high homology to gram-negative regulated efflux systems. *Plasmid* **44:**285–291.

291. **Tauch, A., S. Krieft, J. Kalinowski, and A. Puhler.** 2000. The 51,409-bp R-plasmid pTP10 from the multiresistant clinical isolate *Corynebacterium striatum* M82B is composed of DNA segments initially identified in soil bacteria and in plant, animal, and human pathogens. *Mol. Gen. Genet.* **263:**1–11.

292. **Tauch, A., S. Gotker, A. Puhler, J. Kalinowski, and G. Thierbach.** 2002. The 27.8-kb R-plasmid pTET3 from *Corynebacterium glutamicum* encodes the aminoglycoside adenyltransferase gene cassette *aadA9* and the regulated tetracycline efflux system Tet 33 flanked by active copies of the widespread insertion sequence IS*6100*. *Plasmid* **48:** 117–129.

293. **Thibault, F. M., E. Hernandez, D. R. Vidal, M. Girardet, and J. D. Cavallo.** 2004. Antibiotic susceptibility of 65 isolates of *Burkholderia pseudomallei* and *Burkholderia mallei* to 35 antimicrobial agents. *J. Antimicrob. Chemother.* **54:** 1134–1138.

294. **Tompkin, R. B.** 2002. Control of *Listeria monocytogenes* in the food-processing environment. *J. Food Prot.* **65:**709–725.

295. **Trevisanato, S. I.** 2004. Did an epidemic of tularemia in Ancient Egypt affect the course of world history? *Med. Hypotheses* **63:**905–910.

296. **Tribuddharat, C., R. A. Moore, P. Baker, and D. E. Woods.** 2003. *Burkholderia pseudomallei* class A β-lactamase mutations that confer selective resistance against ceftazidime or clavulanic acid inhibition. *Antimicrob. Agents Chemother.* **47:**2082–2087.

297. **Trinh, H. T., S. J. Billington, A. C. Field, J. G. Songer, and B. H. Jost.** 2002. Susceptibility of *Arcanobacterium pyogenes* from different sources to tetracycline, macrolide and lincosamide antimicrobial agents. *Vet. Microbiol.* **85:**353–359.

298. **Turnbull, P. C. B., N. M. Sirianni, C. I. LeBron, M. N. Samaan, F. N. Sutton, A. E. Reyes, and L. F. Peruski, Jr.** 2004. MICs of selected antibiotics for *Bacillus anthracis*, *Bacillus cereus*, *Bacillus thuringiensis*, and *Bacillus mycoides* from a range of clinical and environmental sources as determined by the Etest. *J. Clin. Microbiol.* **42:**3626–3634.

299. **Turner, L. H.** 1970. Leptospirosis. 3. Maintenance, isolation and demonstration of leptospires. *Trans. R. Soc. Trop. Med. Hyg.* **64:**623–646.

300. **Vazquez-Boland, J. A., L. Dominguez, M. Blanco, J. Rocourt, J. F. Fernandez-Garayzabal, C. B. Gutierrez, R. I. Tascon, and E. F. Rodriguez-Ferri.** 1992. Epidemiologic investigation of a silage-associated epizootic of ovine listeric encephalitis, using a new Listeria-selective enumeration medium and phage typing. *Am. J. Vet. Res.* **53:**368–371.

301. **Vela, A. I., J. F. Fernandez-Garayzabal, M. V. Latre, A. A. Rodriguez, L. Dominguez, and M. A. Moreno.** 2001. Antimicrobial susceptibility of *Listeria monocytogenes* isolated from meningoencephalitis in sheep. *Int. J. Antimicrob. Agents* **17:**215–220.

302. **Venditti, M., V. Gelfusa, A. Tarasi, C. Brandimarte, and P. Serra.** 1990. Antimicrobial susceptibilities of *Erysipelothrix rhusiopathiae*. *Antimicrob. Agents Chemother.* **34:**2038–2040.

303. **Verger, J. M., F. Grimont, P. A. D. Grimont, and M. Grayon.** 1985. *Brucella*, a monospecific genus as shown by deoxyribonucleic acid hybridisation. *Int. J. Syst. Bacteriol.* **35:** 292–295.

304. **Verger, J. M., M. Grayon, A. Cloeckaert, M. Lefevre, E. Ageron, and F. Grimont.** 2000. Classification of *Brucella* strains isolated from marine mammals using DNA-DNA hybridization and ribotyping. *Res. Microbiol.* **151:**797–799.

305. **Vergil, P. M. (Virgil).** *Om landbrug*. Translated into Danish by J. Frechland. [1818 edition.]

306. **Vyrostekova, V., G. Khanakah, E. Kocianova, D. Gurycova, and G. Stanek.** 2002. Prevalence of coinfection with *Francisella tularensis* in reservoir animals of *Borrelia burgdorferi* sensu lato. *Wien. Klin. Wochenschr.* **114:**482–488.

307. **Walker, J. K., J. H. Morgan, J. McLauchlin, K. A. Grant, and J. A. Shallcross.** 1994. *Listeria innocua* isolated from a case of ovine meningoencephalitis. *Vet. Microbiol.* **42:**245–253.

308. **Walker, R. L., and N. J. MacLachlan.** 1989. Isolation of *Eubacterium suis* from sows with cystitis. *J. Am. Vet. Med. Assoc.* **195:**1104–1107.

309. **Walsh, D., G. Duffy, J. J. Sheridan, I. S. Blair, and D. A. McDowell.** 2001. Antibiotic resistance among *Listeria*, including *Listeria monocytogenes*, in retail foods. *J. Appl. Microbiol.* **90:**517–522.

310. **Wanke, M. M.** 2004. Canine brucellosis. *Anim. Reprod. Sci.* **82–83:**195–207.

311. **Watt, G., L. P. Padre, M. L. Tuazon, C. Calubaquib, E. Santiago, C. P. Ranoa, and L. W. Laughlin.** 1988. Placebo-controlled trial of intravenous penicillin for severe and late leptospirosis. *Lancet* **i:**433–435.

312. **Watts, J. L., and S. Rossbach.** 2000. Susceptibilities of *Corynebacterium bovis* and *Corynebacterium amylocolatum* isolates from bovine mammary glands to 15 antimicrobial agents. *Antimicrob. Agents Chemother.* **44:**3476–3477.

313. **Wein, L. M., D. L. Craft, and E. H. Kaplan.** 2003. Emergency response to an anthrax attack. *Proc. Natl. Acad. Sci. USA* **100:**4346–4351.

314. **Weis, J., and H. P. Seeliger.** 1975. Incidence of *Listeria monocytogenes* in nature. *Appl. Microbiol.* **30:**29–32.

315. **Welsh, R. D.** 1983. Equine abortion caused by *Listeria monocytogenes* serotype 4. *J. Am. Vet. Med. Assoc.* **182:**291.

316. **Wendt, M., and J. Sobestiansky.** 1995. The therapy of urinary tract infections in sows. *Dtsch. Tierarztl. Wochenschr.* **102:**21–27. (In German.)

317. **Wenner, K. A., and J. R. Kenner.** 2004. Anthrax. *Dermatol. Clin.* **22:**247–256.

318. **Weyant, R. S., S. L. Bragg, and A. F. Kaufmann.** 1999. *Leptospira* and *Leptonema*, p. 739–745. *In* P. R. Murray, E. J. Baron, M. A. Pfaller, F. C. Tenover, and R. H. Yolken (ed.), *Manual of Clinical Microbiology*, 7th ed. ASM Press, Washington, D.C. (In German.)

319. **White, N. J.** 2003. Melioidosis. *Lancet* **361:**1715–1722.

320. **White, N. J., D. A. Dance, W. Chaowagul, Y. Wattanagoon, V. Wuthiekanun, and N. Pitakwatchara.** 1989. Halving of mortality of severe melioidosis by ceftazidime. *Lancet* **2:**697–701.

321. **Wiedmann, M., J. Czajka, N. Bsat, M. Bodis, M. C. Smith, T. J. Divers, and C. A. Batt.** 1994. Diagnosis and epidemiological association of *Listeria monocytogenes* strains in two outbreaks of listerial encephalitis in small ruminants. *J. Clin. Microbiol.* **32:**991–996.

322. **Wilkinson, L.** 1981. Glanders: medicine and veterinary medicine in common pursuit of a contagious disease. *Med. Hist.* **25:**363–384.
323. **Wilson, J. B., and K. E. Russell.** 1964. Isolation of *Bacillus anthracis* from soil stored 60 years. *J. Bacteriol.* **87:**237–238.
324. **Wood, R. L.** 1992. Erysipelas, p. 475–486. *In* A. D. Leman, B. E. Straw, W. L. Mengeling, S. D'Allaire, and E. D. J. Taylor (ed.), *Diseases of Swine*, 7th ed. Iowa State University Press, Ames.
325. **Wylie, J. A. H., and E. Vincent.** 1947. The sensitivity of organisms of the genus *Leptospira* to penicillin and streptomycin. *J. Pathol. Bacteriol.* **59:**247–254.
326. **Yabuuchi, E., Y. Kosako, H. Oyaizu, I. Yano, H. Hotta, Y. Hashimoto, T. Ezaki, and M. Arakawa.** 1992. Proposal of *Burkholderia* gen. nov. and transfer of seven species of the genus *Pseudomonas* homology group II to the new genus, with the type species *Burkholderia cepacia* (Palleroni and Holmes 1981) comb. nov. *Microbiol. Immunol.* **36:**1251–1275.
327. **Yam, W. C., C. M. Tam, C. C. Leung, H. L. Tong, K. H. Chan, E. T. Leung, K. C. Wong, W. W. Yew, W. H. Seto, K. Y. Yuen, and P. L. Ho.** 2004. Direct detection of rifampin-resistant *Mycobacterium tuberculosis* in respiratory specimens by PCR-DNA sequencing. *J. Clin. Microbiol.* **42:**4438–4443.
328. **Yamamoto, K., M. Kijima, H. Yoshimura, and T. Takahashi.** 2001. Antimicrobial susceptibilities of *Erysipelothrix rhusiopathiae* isolated from pigs with swine erysipelas in Japan, 1988–1998. *J. Vet. Med. B* **48:**115–126.
329. **Yamamoto, K., Y. Sasaki, Y. Ogikubo, N. Noguchi, M. Sasatsu, and T. Takahashi.** 2001. Identification of the tetracycline resistance gene, *tet*(M), in *Erysipelothrix rhusiopathiae*. *J. Vet. Med. B* **48:**293–301.
330. **Yanagawa, R.** 1986. Causative agents of bovine pyelonephritis: *Corynebacterium renale*, *C. pilosum* and *C. cystitidis*. *Prog. Vet. Microbiol. Immunol.* **2:**158–174.
331. **Yang, S.** 2000. Melioidosis research in China. *Acta Trop.* **77:**157–165.
332. **Yeruham, I., D. Elad, S. Friedman, and S. Perl.** 2003. *Corynebacterium pseudotuberculosis* infection in Israeli dairy cattle. *Epidemiol. Infect.* **131:**947–955.
333. **Yeruham, I., D. Elad, Y. Avidar, T. Goshen, and E. Asis.** 2004. Four-year survey of urinary tract infections in calves in Israel. *Vet. Rec.* **154:**204–206.
334. **Yoshimura, H., A. Kojima, and M. Ishimaru.** 2000. Antimicrobial susceptibility of *Arcanobacterium pyogenes* isolated from cattle and pigs. *J. Vet. Med. B* **47:**139–143.
335. **Zhao, H. K., H. Morimura, T. Hiramune, N. Kikuchi, R. Yanagawa, and S. Serikawa.** 1991. Antimicrobial susceptibility of *Corynebacterium pseudotuberculosis* isolated from lesions of caseous lymphadenitis in sheep in Hokkaido, Japan. *J. Vet. Med. Sci.* **53:**355–356.

Antimicrobial Resistance in Bacteria of Animal Origin
Edited by Frank M. Aarestrup

Chapter 16

Antimicrobial Resistance in *Campylobacter*

JØRGEN ENGBERG, MONIKA KEELAN, PETER GERNER-SMIDT, AND DIANE E. TAYLOR

Campylobacter, first identified as a human diarrheal pathogen in 1973, is the most frequently diagnosed bacterial cause of human gastroenteritis in the United States and throughout the world. As for other bacterial gastroenteric infections, most cases of *Campylobacter* infections do not require antimicrobial treatment, being clinically mild and self-limiting. However, some severe and prolonged cases of enteritis, septicemia, and other extraintestinal infections do require treatment. Macrolides are considered the drug of first choice for *C. jejuni* and *C. coli* enteritis, but fluoroquinolones are the drug of choice for empiric treatment of suspected bacterial gastroenteritis. Intravenous aminoglycosides should be included for the treatment of *Campylobacter* bacteremia in patients who appear very ill (18). In case of resistance, other antimicrobial agents may be used for treatment. Contaminated food is the usual source of human infections; therefore, the presence of antimicrobial-resistant strains in the food chain has raised concerns that the treatment of human infections will be compromised.

This chapter provides a review of prevalence and trends of resistance in *C. jejuni* and *C. coli* isolated from humans in different parts of the world and a more thorough description of the mechanisms of resistance, origin, spread, and clinical consequences of resistance.

PREVALENCE AND TRENDS OF RESISTANCE IN DIFFERENT PARTS OF THE WORLD

Macrolides

Table 1 shows data on macrolide resistance among *C. jejuni*, *C. coli*, and *C. jejuni* and *C. coli* combined, isolated from human sources around the world since 1997. There are notable differences between countries and species. Almost all studies report a higher frequency of erythromycin resistance in *C. coli* than in *C. jejuni*, with rates reported in proportions ranging from 0 to 20% in *C. jejuni* and 0 to 29% in *C. coli*. In a number of industrialized countries a higher proportion of *C. coli*, including macrolide-resistant *C. coli*, is reported among travel-related patients than among domestically acquired infections. Trends over time for macrolide resistance show stable low rates in most countries, which is comforting as erythromycin or, alternatively, one of the newer macrolides such as azithromycin is the drug of choice for treating enteritis caused by *C. jejuni* and *C. coli*.

Quinolones

In contrast to macrolide resistance, resistance to quinolones in *C. jejuni* and *C. coli* isolated from humans has emerged in numerous countries during the past 15 years (Fig. 1). The figure shows trends for quinolone resistance rates of *C. jejuni* and *C. coli* combined isolated from humans from 11 countries covering the period from 1989 to 2003. The use of fluoroquinolones (mainly enrofloxacin) in veterinary medicine is correlated with an increase in quinolone resistance in food animals; in retail food of animal origin, especially in poultry products; and most importantly in human *Campylobacter* infections. Before 1989 fluoroquinolones were mainly used in human medicine and resistance was rare, but with the introduction of fluoroquinolones in veterinary medicine, a rapid emergence of quinolone resistance in *Campylobacter* isolates from patients has been reported in a number of countries. The first study that

Jørgen Engberg and Peter Gerner-Smidt • Unit of Gastrointestinal Infections, Statens Serum Institut, Artillerivej 5, DK-2300 Copenhagen S, Denmark. **Monika Keelan** • Laboratory for Foodborne Zoonoses, Public Health Agency of Canada, and Department of Laboratory Medicine and Pathology, University of Alberta, Edmonton, Alberta T6G 2G3, Canada. **Diane E. Taylor** • Department of Medical Microbiology and Immunology, University of Alberta, Edmonton, Alberta T6G 2H7, Canada.

Table 1. Erythromycin or azithromycin resistance rates among *C. jejuni*, *C. coli*, and *C. jejuni* and *C. coli* combined isolated from humans worldwide since 1997

Country	Resistance rate (%) in:			Reference(s)
	C. jejuni	*C. coli*	*C. jejuni* and *C. coli*	
Argentina	3[a]	6[a]		52
Australia	3			151
Austria			<1–2	49–51
Belgium	4	6		190
Bosnia and Herzegovina	20	25	22	188
Canada	0–12			55, 62
Chile	6			52
Denmark	0–7[b]/0–7[c]	4–21		8, 45, 47
Egypt	0[a]	0[a]		137
Finland			0[b]/3[c]	139
France	3	11		107
Germany	0–4	0–29		101, 157, 193
Indonesia	0			181
Ireland			2	102
Italy	1	24		128
The Netherlands	4[b]/3[c]	6[b]/11[c]		7
New Zealand	3			64
Norway	0–2[b]/<1–3[c]			5, 11
Mexico	14			186
Spain	2–5[a]	35		145
Sweden	3		0[b]/5[c]	122, 143
Thailand	1[a]–2	17[a]–26		19, 77
United Kingdom	1–3	25	2	25, 110, 201
United States	1–5	4–9		30, 68, 113
Vietnam	0	0		77

[a]Isolates exclusively from children.
[b]Isolates acquired domestically.
[c]Isolates acquired abroad.

documented a link between veterinary use of fluoroquinolones and occurrence of resistant *Campylobacter* among both food animals and humans was from The Netherlands (44). The fluoroquinolone enrofloxacin was introduced for veterinary use in The Netherlands in 1987. No fluoroquinolone-resistant *Campylobacter* isolates were found in poultry products or in humans before 1987. The percentage of fluoroquinolone-resistant isolates in poultry products increased to 8.4% in 1987 and 14% in 1989 (44). In 1992 and 1993 the percentage of resistant isolates from broilers was 29% (79). This emergence of resistance among poultry products and broilers has been closely followed by the emergence and subsequent increase in resistance among isolates causing infections in humans. The rate of resistance was 8% from 1988 to 1989, 11% in 1989, and 29% in 1997 (44, 161). Veterinary use of quinolones has recently been reviewed by Wegener and Engberg (199) and is also described in more detail elsewhere in this book. Similar trends have been observed in other countries where fluoroquinolones are approved in veterinary medicine. In some countries the rise in resistance has been remarkably rapid and considerable, while in other countries the resistance rates have increased steadily. For instance, a recent report found that 86% of human *C. jejuni* isolates in Hong Kong were quinolone resistant (34).

Recent surveillance data from a number of countries show a significant difference in quinolone resistance rates between travel-related infections and domestically acquired infections, and document the importance of stratifying susceptibility data by travel status (Fig. 2). Travel-related infections from destinations with recognized high quinolone resistance in *Campylobacter* in poultry, as well as an established high risk of attracting quinolone-resistant human *Campylobacter* infections, are associated with a significantly higher prevalence of quinolone resistance compared to infections acquired domestically. The significantly lower prevalence of quinolone resistance among domestically acquired campylobacters likely reflects a more limited or lack of veterinary usage of fluoroquinolones in these countries. For instance, in Australia, where fluoroquinolones have not been licensed for use in food production animals,

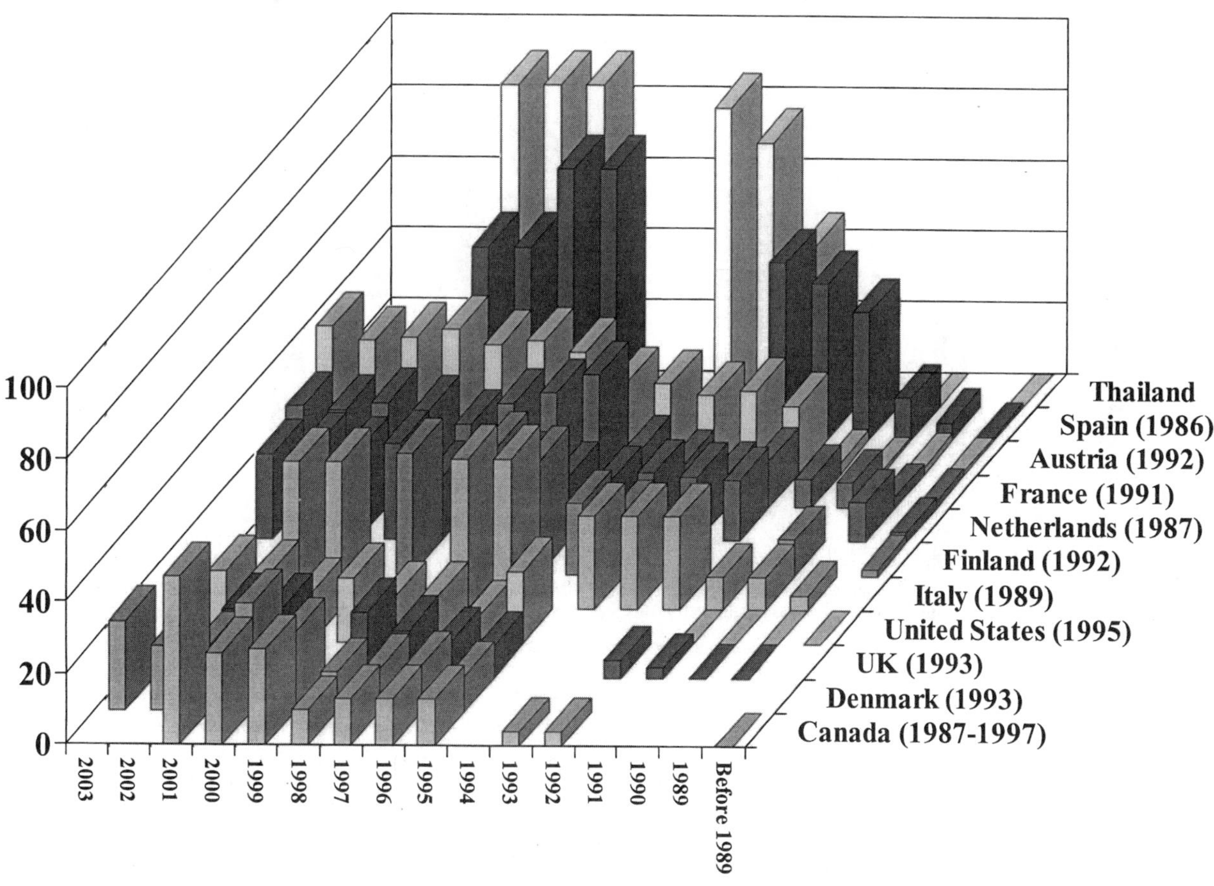

Figure 1. Trends for quinolone resistance rates (in percentages) among *C. coli* and *C. jejuni* combined from human sources around the world. The bars represent both nalidixic acid and fluoroquinolone resistance and are based on mean values of resistance from numerous reports. Updated and modified from reference 46. Additional data are from references 7, 9, 10, 19, 29, 30, 45, 47, 49–51, 107, 128, 139, and 201, and V. Prouzet-Mauléon (personal communication).

and only cooked chicken products may be imported, no fluoroquinolone resistance has been found in domestically acquired human infections (187). In contrast, while foreign travel is associated with quinolone-resistant infections in the United States, the majority of quinolone-resistant infections are domestically acquired in this country (68, 84).

Tetracyclines

Tetracyclines have been suggested as an alternative choice for the treatment of *C. jejuni* and *C. coli* enteritis (18, 106). However, as with other drug classes, major geographical differences in the susceptibility of *Campylobacter* have been reported. This reflects partly a domestic resistance problem and partly a lack of surveillance data stratified by travel status. For instance, recent rates of tetracycline and doxycycline resistance among domestically acquired and travel-related *C. jejuni* infections in Australia were 10 and 43%, respectively (151); in Denmark they were 13 and 43%, respectively (9); in Norway they were 10 and 63%, respectively (11); and in Sweden they were 1 to 5 and 45 to 51%, respectively (122, 143). In reports not stratified by travel status, examples of recent rates of resistance among *C. jejuni* or *C. jejuni*/*C. coli* were 21% in Austria (49), 15% in Bosnia and Herzegovina (188), 39 to 43% in Germany (101, 193), 17 to 21% in The Netherlands (10), 46% in Finland (70), 19% in France (107), 31% in Italy (128), 85 to 95% in Taiwan (94), 29% in the United Kingdom (201), and 43% in the United States (68). Two recent independent Canadian studies, by Gaudreau and Gilbert (55) and Gibreel and colleagues (61), reported a significant increase in the resistance of *C. jejuni* to tetracycline from 8 to 19% to 50 to 68% over the past 20 years. In Mexico, a study of 280 *C. jejuni* isolates from children (in an age group for whom tetracycline is not recommended) found that during the period from 1989 to

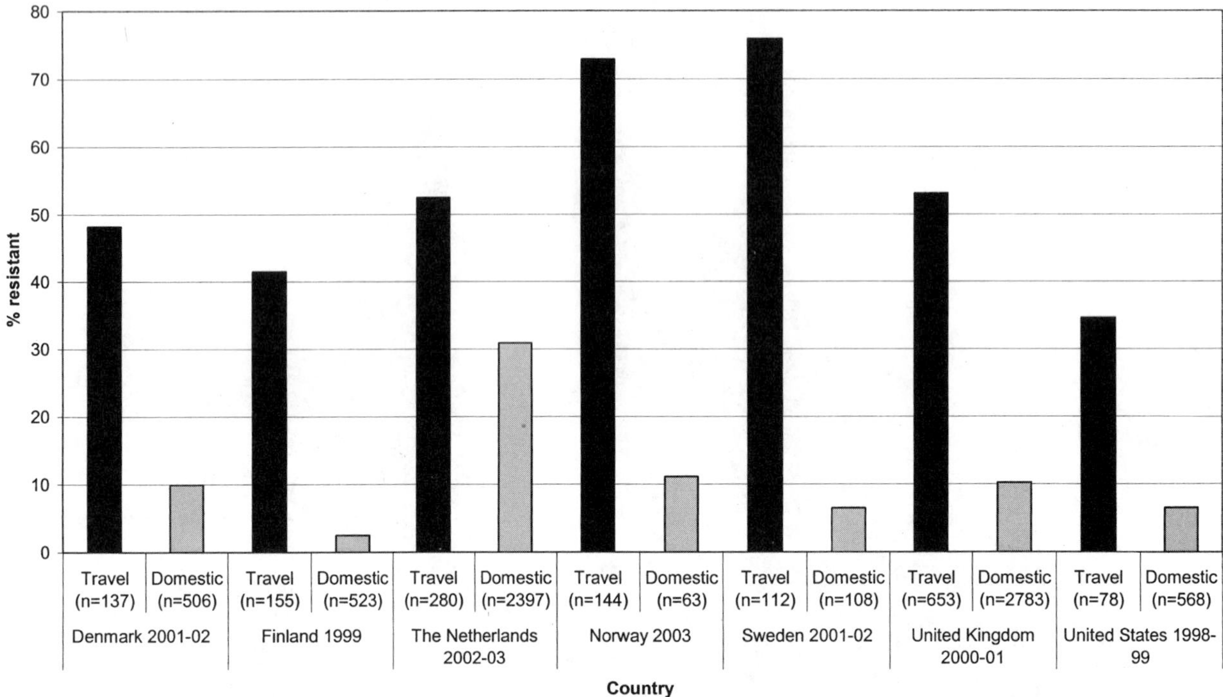

Figure 2. Quinolone resistance rates (in percentages) among *C. jejuni* (Denmark, The Netherlands, and Norway) and *C. jejuni* and *C. coli* combined (Finland, Sweden, the United Kingdom, and the United States) by history of travel. Data are from references 7, 11, 25, 47, 84, 139, and 143.

1999 resistance to tetracycline increased from 28 to 76% (186). No clear picture exists on the rates of resistance at the species level; some studies report higher levels among *C. coli* than among *C. jejuni* (128, 188), some report the opposite (101), while others report comparable proportions (68). Tetracyclines are ecologically disadvantageous drugs with a broad antibacterial spectrum, and their use is contraindicated in children. General clinical usage of tetracycline can therefore not be recommended, but tetracycline could be used in areas of low resistance to the agent, or better, after susceptibility testing of the clinical isolate in situations when other agents are contraindicated because of strain resistance or idiosyncratic responses in patients.

Aminoglycosides

Aminoglycosides exhibit rapid and significant bactericidal effects in vitro and should initially be included for the treatment of *Campylobacter* bacteremia in patients who appear very ill (18, 106). Resistance rates have been reported to be stable and low in most countries, making aminoglycosides a safe first-line drug for serious infections in most places (11, 43, 68, 101, 143). However, Sáenz et al. (145) found that <1% of *C. jejuni* but 9% of *C. coli* strains isolated from humans in Spain were gentamicin resistant. As a few strains are resistant to aminoglycosides, sensitivity testing is advised.

Multidrug Resistance

Multidrug resistance in *Campylobacter* species is on the increase, and an effective antimicrobial regimen to treat serious infections may be lacking in the future. Hakanen and colleagues (70) recently examined 376 *C. jejuni* isolates, of which 94% were travel related. Of 174 (46%) ciprofloxacin-resistant isolates, 68% were resistant to tetracycline and 3% were resistant to erythromycin, gentamicin, or clindamycin. One (0.6%) ciprofloxacin-resistant isolate was resistant to amoxicillin-clavulanic acid; imipenem was the only drug to which all isolates were susceptible. Multidrug resistance was significantly associated with ciprofloxacin resistance (33 versus 12%; $P < 0.01$). Eight (2%) strains were macrolide resistant, of which six were also ciprofloxacin resistant (70). Hoge et al. (74) found 100% coresistance between Thai isolates resistant to azithromycin and ciprofloxacin in 1994 and 1995. In addition, the level of tetracycline resistance in Thailand is so high that these agents now have no role in the treatment of *Campylobacter* or noncholera diarrhea. Li et al. (94) reported that concomitant resistance rates among nalidixic acid-resistant *C. jejuni* isolates from their patients (exclusively children) were as follows: gentamicin, 2%; erythromycin, 12%; clindamycin, 12%; tetracycline, 97%; and ciprofloxacin, 66%. All of the human erythromycin-resistant *C. jejuni* isolates and 90% of the *C. coli* isolates were also resistant to clindamycin.

MECHANISMS OF RESISTANCE

Completion of the genome sequence of *C. jejuni* NCTC 11168 reveals several homologies with genes known to encode multiple drug transporters. In contrast, the genome lacks other elements such as insertion sequences, prophages, and transposons that are often associated with genes encoding drug resistance in other human gram-negative pathogens (125). Antibiotic resistance observed in *Campylobacter* isolates from human and animal sources arises as a consequence of specific mutations in genes associated with protein synthesis or DNA replication, or through plasmid-mediated acquisition of foreign DNA. The latter is not surprising considering that antibiotic resistance genes are commonly located on plasmids originating from gram-positive and gram-negative organisms commonly residing in the human and animal intestine. In fact, plasmids may facilitate the acquisition of more than one resistance determinant (61, 197).

The bacterial ribosome is composed of a small 30S subunit with a single 16S rRNA strand and approximately 20 proteins; and a larger 50S subunit with a 23S rRNA strand, a 5S rRNA strand, and approximately 30 different proteins (111). High-resolution X-ray crystal structure models for prokaryotic ribosomal subunits have provided greater understanding of protein synthesis (14, 28, 35) and also insight into the sites where antibiotics may bind to the 30S ribosome (21, 27).

New perspectives on bacterial ribosome structure and how antibiotics interact with the ribosome are essential for the development of new therapeutics for the treatment of antibiotic-resistant bacteria. An overview of antibiotic resistance mechanisms present in *Campylobacter* spp. (Table 2) is discussed below.

Aminoglycosides

Aminoglycosides are bactericidal antimicrobials that bind irreversibly to ribosomes and inhibit protein synthesis (155). Kanamycin, streptomycin, and streptothricins primarily inhibit A-site binding of the ternary complex (Fig. 3A), resulting in translation errors. Spectinomycin blocks EF-G–GTP from binding

Table 2. Antibiotics and their resistance mechanisms in *Campylobacter* spp.

Antibiotic class	Gene	Protein	Mechanism
Aminoglycosides	*aphA-A3* *aphA-A1* *aphA-A7*	APH(3′)-III (aminoglycoside phosphotransferases)	Inactivation of antibiotic by phosphorylation
	aad4 *aadE*	AAD(3″)(9) AAD(6) (aminoglycoside adenyltransferases)	Inactivation of antibiotic by adenylation
	sat4	Streptothricin acetyltransferase	Inactivation of antibiotic by acetylation
β-lactams			Inactivation of antibiotic by:
		β-Lactamase	Breakdown of β-lactam ring
		Penicillin-binding protein	Decreased binding
		Porin	Decreased permeability
Chloramphenicol	*cat*	Chloramphenicol acetyltransferase	Inactivation of antibiotic by acetylation
Macrolides	*rrnB* operon of 23S rRNA domain V		Mutation inactivation of 2–3 copies of target gene: A2074C, A2074G, or A2075G[a]
Quinolones, including fluoroquinolones	*gyrA*	DNA gyrase (topoisomerase II)	Mutation inactivation of target gene: Thr-86, Asp-90, or Ala-70; Thr-86 and Asp-85 or Pro-104
	parC	Topoisomerase IV	Arg-139
Tetracycline	*tet*(O)	Tet(O)	Protection of ribosome target
Trimethoprim	*dfr1*, *dfr9*	Dihydrofolate reductase	Acquisition of resistant enzyme
Multidrug	*cmeR*	CmeR (transcriptional regulator of CmeABC)	Mutation inactivation of target gene: Gly-85-Ala

[a] A2058C, A2058G, or A2059G, respectively, by *E. coli* numbering.

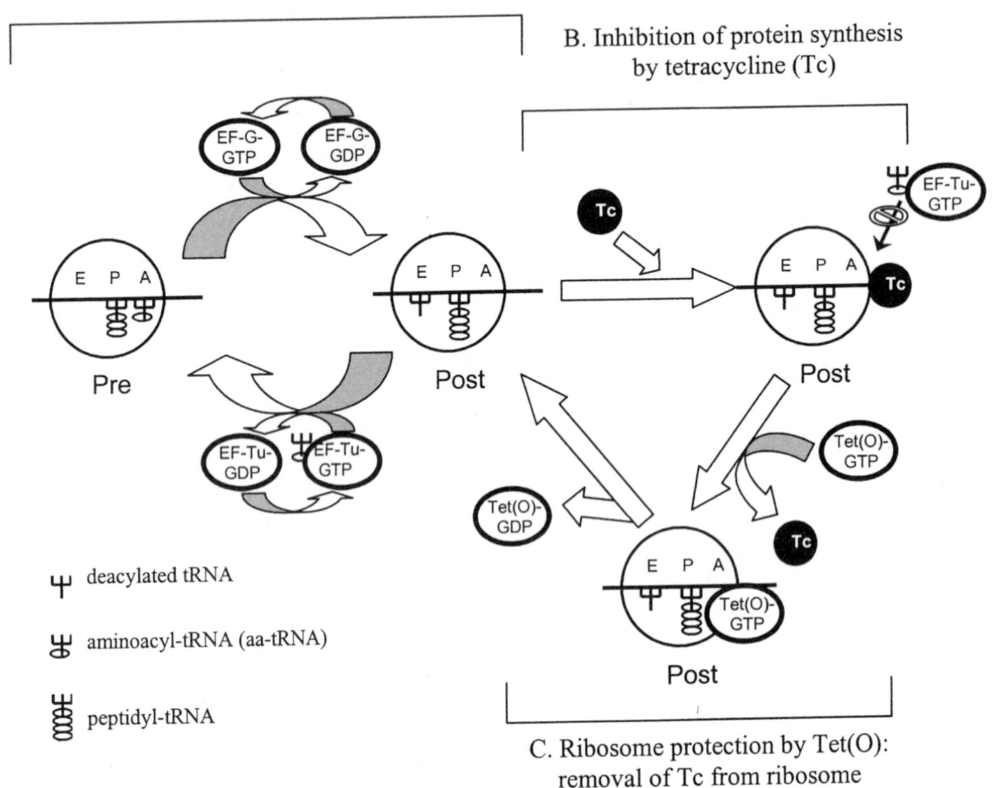

Figure 3. (A) Elongation cycle of protein synthesis; (B) inhibition by tetracycline (Tc); (C) model for Tet(O) action. (A) In the absence of antibiotics, the aa-tRNA–EF-Tu–GTP ternary complex catalyzes the binding of aa-tRNA to the open A site on the pretranslocation-state (Pre) ribosome. (B) Tc initially binds to the posttranslation-state (Post) ribosome and induces a conformational change (or steric clash) that blocks the aa-tRNA–EF-Tu–GTP ternary complex from occupying the A site, effectively inhibiting further protein synthesis. (C) If Tet(O) is present, it recognizes the Tc-blocked ribosome by virtue of its open A site, prolonged pausing, and possibly by a drug-induced conformational change. The interaction of Tet(O) with the ribosome induces rearrangements in the A site and triggers the release of Tc from the primary binding site prior to GTP hydrolysis. Tet(O) then hydrolyzes the bound GTP and likely leaves the ribosome with the GTPase-associated region in a configuration compatible with EF-Tu binding, thereby allowing protein synthesis to continue. Adapted from references 36 and 37.

to helix 34 of the 16S rRNA in the 30S ribosome subunit, inhibiting translocation of peptidyl-tRNAs from the ribosomal A site to the P site (17, 155). Resistance to aminoglycosides may arise through modification of the antibiotic or through mutations of ribosome proteins and rRNA.

Campylobacter resistance to aminoglycosides arises from modification of the antibiotic by aminoglycoside phosphotransferases (APH), aminoglycoside adenyltransferases (AAD), or acetyltransferases, which prohibit interaction and binding of the antibiotic to the ribosomes (88). These enzyme families are divided into subgroups according to their substrate modification site and characteristic substrate profile.

The most common enzyme found in *Campylobacter* spp. is APH(3′) type III, which phosphorylates kanamycin, butyrosine, lividomycin, and amikacin, but not tobramycin (173, 178). APH(3″) phosphorylates streptomycin but not spectinomycin (141). *C. jejuni* and *C. coli* kanamycin resistance is mediated by APH(3′) type III and type IV and APH(3″) (141, 173, 178).

Two AAD enzymes are also reported to occur in *C. jejuni* and *C. coli*. The presence of AAD(3′)(9), encoded by *aadA*, confers streptomycin and spectinomycin resistance, while the presence of AAD(6), encoded by *aadE*, confers streptomycin resistance only (131). These *aad* genes are chromosomally located and are common among class 1 integrons (26). Integrons contain an integrase gene that may link antibiotic resistance gene cassettes in tandem at a site-specific integration site. *Campylobacter* spp.

contain *aadA2*-encoding resistance determinants identical to gene cassettes in *Salmonella enterica* serovar Hadar and *E. coli*, suggesting that these organisms transmitted the gene cassettes to *Campylobacter* (121).

Streptothricin acetyltransferase, encoded by *sat4*, is present in human and animal streptothricin-resistant isolates of *C. coli* (78). An aminoglycoside 6′-*N*-acetyltransferase, AAC(6′)-Ib7, encoded by *aacA4*, confers resistance to purpurosamine ring-containing aminoglycosides such as tobramycin, kanamycin, and neomycin (138). A Thr-102-Ser point mutation confers additional resistance to gentamicin and amikacin. The *aacA4* gene does not confer resistance to streptomycin. Resistance to tobramycin (25 to 50 μg/ml) and gentamicin (10 to 50 μg/ml) is associated with the presence of the *aacA4* gene in *C. jejuni* isolated from water lines of a broiler chicken house, although none of the broilers were colonized with gentamicin-resistant *C. jejuni* strains (92).

Resistance to gentamicin is low in *C. jejuni* but higher in *C. coli* (145). The *aacA4* gene, which encodes aminoglycoside resistance, is found on class 1 and class 3 integrons in many bacteria. Class 1 integrons may play an important role in the spread of antimicrobial resistance in *Campylobacter* spp., since 21% of poultry *C. jejuni* isolates in one study possessed the integrase gene (92). Integron expression in *C. jejuni* may be controlled by translation of an upstream region similar to that observed in other bacteria (71).

Kanamycin resistance due to modification by APH(3″) is encoded by *aphA-3* and is most frequently found on plasmids 40 to 130 kb in size. The location of the *aphA-3* gene in six of eight kanamycin-resistant *C. jejuni* strains is downstream of an apparent insertion sequence, designated IS*607**, which is very similar to IS*607* characterized on the chromosome of some *Helicobacter pylori* strains (60). The IS*607** element was also observed in kanamycin-susceptible strains of *C. jejuni* on plasmids mediating tetracycline resistance (60). Kanamycin resistance in *C. jejuni* may also be mediated by *aphA-7*, found on small plasmids of 11.5 and 9.5 kb (179). An earlier study reports the chromosomal location of 3′-aminoglycoside phosphotransferase type I [APH(3′)-I], a kanamycin resistance marker nearly identical to the one in Tn*903* from *E. coli* (123). The *aphA-1* gene was adjacent to the insertion sequence IS*15*-delta, commonly found in gram-negative bacteria, and suggests that *aphA-1* may have originated in members of the family *Enterobacteriaceae* (123). Some plasmids in *C. jejuni* carry the *aphA-3* gene as a part of a resistance cluster that includes *aadE* and *sat*, which may have been acquired from a gram-positive organism (61).

Chromosomal mutations that alter the ribosome binding site do mediate aminoglycoside resistance in *E. coli* (155). Spontaneous streptomycin-resistant mutants are reported to occur when *C. coli* is plated out to streptomycin media, but these have not been thoroughly investigated and characterized beyond eliminating a mutation in the S12 protein (164, 184).

β-Lactams

Penicillins, cephalosporins, carbapenems, and monobactams are the four classes of β-lactam antibiotics, each containing a four-membered β-lactam ring. These bactericidal antibiotics irreversibly acylate and inactivate proteins associated with the synthesis and maintenance of the murein sacculus, including penicillin-binding proteins (PBPs), carboxypeptidases, and transpeptidases (156). Consequently, cell wall synthesis is discontinued, and murein hydrolases, responsible for nicking peptidoglycan to allow growth, are unchecked, which results in increasing osmotic pressure and ultimately lysis of the bacterial cell.

All campylobacters are resistant to cefoxitin, cefamandole, and cefoperazone, and most are resistant to cephalothin and cefazolin. Resistance to β-lactam antibiotics in *Campylobacter* spp. was first reported in 1981 and is likely to be of chromosomal origin (162). Resistance to β-lactams arises due to the presence of β-lactamase, low-affinity binding of antibiotic to PBPs, or failure of the antibiotic to penetrate to PBPs' targets. Hydrolysis of the β-lactam ring by β-lactamase renders the antibiotics inactive (40). The majority of *Campylobacter* spp. are intrinsically resistant to β-lactams due to their ability to produce β-lactamase or their limited ability to bind PBPs (160).

Campylobacter isolates are highly susceptible to imipenem, amoxicillin-clavulanic acid, and cefepime and, to a lesser degree, amoxicillin, ampicillin, and cefotaxime (160). The β-lactamase of *C. jejuni* is a penicillinase with a role in resistance to the overall neutrally charged amoxicillin, ampicillin, and ticarcillin but not to the negatively charged penicillin G or piperacillin (86). The negative charge on the latter two β-lactams may reduce the permeability across the *Campylobacter* outer membrane porins, as well as decrease the substrate specificity for the β-lactamases within the cell (124). The β-lactamase-positive strains are significantly less susceptible to amoxicillin, ampicillin, and ticarcillin than the β-lactamase-negative strains (87). All β-lactamase-positive strains become susceptible to amoxicillin and ampicillin upon the addition of the β-lactamase inhibitor clavulanic acid (56, 87).

Since imipenem binds well to PBPs and penetrates the outer membrane porins easily, it is an effective antibiotic against *Campylobacter* spp. (160). *Campylobacter* resistance to other β-lactams is proposed to arise primarily from a limited ability to bind the PBPs combined with a decreased ability to penetrate the outer membrane porins and the presence of β-lactamases (160). The mechanisms of β-lactam resistance have not been further characterized in *Campylobacter* species.

Chloramphenicol

Campylobacter resistance to chloramphenicol is rare, and rates of resistance have remained low (61, 89, 164). The only mechanism of chloramphenicol resistance identified in *Campylobacter* occurs through modification of chloramphenicol by chloramphenicol acetyltransferase, which prevents its binding to the ribosome (155). Chloramphenicol inhibits peptide chain elongation by reversibly binding to peptidyltransferase and competing with the aminoacyl-tRNA for the A site (Fig. 3A) of the ribosome (149, 155). Chloramphenicol acetyltransferase, encoded by *cat*, is constitutively produced by *C. coli* and shares 67% identity with *cat* in *Clostridium difficile* and *Clostridium perfringens* (196).

Macrolides

The macrolide erythromycin is the drug of choice for the treatment of *C. jejuni* infections. Erythromycin irreversibly binds to the ribosome and appears to cause dissociation of the peptidyl-rRNA (Fig. 3A), resulting in inhibition of protein synthesis (154). The ribosome binding site may include the 23S rRNA and proteins L2, L4, L15, L16, and L22 (154). Larger macrolides appear to block peptidyltransferase activity (154).

Mechanisms of resistance to erythromycin include target modification by mutation or methylation, antibiotic inactivation, or efflux (90). Erythromycin resistance in *C. jejuni* and *C. coli* occurs by modification of the ribosome site, through mutation in either the 23S rRNA or the proteins at the target binding site, and is not associated with rRNA methylation, modification of erythromycin, or efflux (81, 205). Neither are plasmids associated with erythromycin resistance in *C. jejuni* and *C. coli* (164). In *Helicobacter* spp. (closely related to *Campylobacter* spp.), alteration in one of two adenine residues at positions 2142 and 2143 (homologous to positions 2058 and 2059 in *E. coli* numbering) in the 23S rRNA genes at the erythromycin binding site is responsible for macrolide resistance (46, 169, 192, 194). Recently it has become clear that mutations in adenine residues in all three copies of the 23S rRNA gene (*rrnB* operon) are responsible for the majority of erythromycin resistance in *Campylobacter*, although in a few cases mutations in only two 23S rRNA genes are all that is necessary (57, 81, 183). The mutations are base substitutions at positions 2074 and 2075 (corresponding to positions 2058 and 2059 in the nomenclature for *E. coli* numbering) in the 23S rRNA genes of erythromycin-resistant *C. jejuni* and *C. coli* (81, 119, 183, 189). Mutations rarely occur at both 23S rRNA positions (A2074C and A2075G) in *C. jejuni* (189). In a recent study of *C. jejuni*, about 78% of the erythromycin-resistant isolates studied exhibited an A → G transition at 2059, whereas 13% of isolates had an A → C transversion at 2058 and a small percentage had an A → G transition at 2058 (using *E. coli* numbering) (57).

Quinolones

Quinolones are broad-spectrum bactericidal agents (63, 99, 140). Ciprofloxacin, a fluoroquinolone used to treat human infections since 1986, is the second treatment of choice for *Campylobacter* infections (3, 140). Fluoroquinolones are derived from the quinolone structure of nalidixic acid and contain a fluorine at the C-6 position. Other fluoroquinolones have equal (levafloxacin and ofloxacin) if not greater (trovafloxacin, clinafloxacin, and gatifloxacin) bactericidal activity in comparison with ciprofloxacin (15, 76). The newer fluoroquinolones, gatifloxacin and moxifloxacin, have the greatest anti-*Campylobacter* activity (85).

Quinolone resistance in *C. jejuni* and *C. coli* arises through chromosomal mutations, with nalidixic acid resistance often associated with cross-resistance to fluoroquinolones (65, 171). This differs from *C. fetus*, which is intrinsically resistant to nalidixic acid and susceptible to fluoroquinolones (171).

Quinolones stop cell growth by inhibiting DNA replication and transcription through alteration of DNA gyrase or topoisomerase IV, reduced permeability, or expression of efflux pumps (3). Quinolone resistance in *Campylobacter* is primarily mediated by single point mutations in *gyrA* in the presence of a constitutively expressed multidrug efflux pump, CmeABC (206). Ciprofloxacin accumulation studies suggest efflux likely plays a minor role in fluoroquinolone resistance (127). In *C. jejuni*, fluoroquinolones form a ternary complex with the DNA and type II topoisomerases DNA gyrase or topoisomerase IV, but do not directly bind either enzyme or the DNA (202). The quinolone-gyrase-DNA complex is more stable than the quinolone-topoisomerase IV-DNA complex (82).

DNA is cleaved following complex formation, and these double-stranded DNA breaks are proposed to be highly toxic to the cell (41).

Each topoisomerase structure is a tetramer of two subunits: $GyrA_2GyrB_2$ for gyrase and $ParC_2$-$ParE_2$ for topoisomerase IV (41). Mutations at Thr-86, Asp-90, and Ala-70 in the gene encoding DNA gyrase (*gyrA*) result in quinolone resistance in *C. jejuni* (195), although mutations at Thr-86 are the most common (69, 105). High-level resistance to nalidixic acid (64 to 128 μg/ml) and ciprofloxacin (16 to 64 mg/ml) is associated with mutations at Thr-86-Ile (16, 144, 195). Even higher resistance to ciprofloxacin (125 μg/ml) results when a mutation at Arg-139 in the *parC* gene encoding topoisomerase IV occurs together with a mutation at Thr-86 in *gyrA* (61). Other double mutations, such Thr-86 with Asp-85 or Pro-104, may also occur in ciprofloxacin-resistant *C. jejuni* (105, 129). A few silent mutations are reported in *gyrB* and may simply reflect natural polymorphisms in the gene (129). Mutations at Thr-86 in the *gyrA* gene of *C. coli* and *C. lari* (38, 129) or at Asp-90 in the *gyrA* gene of *C. coli* also result in ciprofloxacin resistance (13). An unusual resistance phenotype reported in *C. coli* is high-level resistance to ciprofloxacin and susceptibility to nalidixic acid with no mutations in DNA gyrase, suggesting that mutations may be present in topoisomerase IV (13).

C. fetus is intrinsically resistant to nalidixic acid, but sequence analysis reveals a conserved *gyrA* gene, suggesting mutations may be present in *gyrB*, *parC*, or *parE* (167). However, analysis of two ciprofloxacin-resistant *C. fetus* isolates found that resistance was associated with mutations at Asp-90 in *gyrA* (167).

Tetracycline

Tetracyclines are bacteriostatic broad-spectrum antibiotics. Atypical tetracyclines (anhydrotetracycline and 6-thiatetracycline) disrupt bacterial cell membranes (31), while typical tetracyclines (tetracycline, chlortetracycline, and minocycline) bind to the ribosome and inhibit protein synthesis (33). Tetracycline (Tc) is actively transported into the bacterial cell and binds to a high-affinity site at the 30S ribosome unit, as well as other low-affinity sites on both ribosome subunits (32, 147). Several pieces of experimental evidence support the high-affinity site as the primary Tc site (37).

Tc initially binds to the posttranslation-state ribosome (a ribosome with an open A site and occupied P and E sites) and induces a conformational change (or steric clash) that blocks the aminoacyl-tRNA complex from occupying the A site (Fig. 3B). At the primary binding site, Tc is bound with high affinity to the ribosomal A site by the irregular minor groove of helix 34 (h34) and the loop of helix 31 (h31) in the 16S rRNA of the 30S subunit (21, 132). As a result, Tc sterically interferes with aminoacyl-tRNA binding to the A site, preventing the addition of new amino acids to the growing polypeptide chain (159). This almost exclusive interaction of Tc with the sugar phosphate backbone of the RNA and lack of base-specific interactions may explain the broad specificity of this antibiotic (21, 132). Some of the secondary, lower-affinity Tc sites are associated with the switch helix (h27) of the 16S rRNA (100) and likely interfere with the transition between the open and closed states of the 30S ribosomal subunit. As a consequence, there is indirect interference with aminoacyl-tRNA binding to the ribosome (120). The impact of Tc binding to other sites is not as clearly associated with inhibition of protein synthesis (132).

The widespread use of Tc for over 50 years as a human therapeutic drug and as an animal growth promoter has increased the occurrence of tetracycline resistance (Tc^r) in microbial organisms (33). Tc^r occurs through efflux, modification of Tc, ribosomal protection, or mutation of 16S rRNA (33). In *Campylobacter*, resistance to Tc is mediated by the ribosomal protection protein Tet(O) (166) on a self-transmissible plasmid in *C. jejuni* and *C. coli* (162, 168). Although the Tc^r determinant may also be found on the chromosome, the mechanism for chromosomal insertion of the Tc^r determinant is unknown, but has not been associated with a transposon (164). The conjugative plasmid that carries *tet*(O) in *C. jejuni* transfers only within *Campylobacter* species (162, 177, 180). The sequence of *tet*(O), which encodes the ~72-kDa Tet(O) protein, reveals 76% similarity to Tet(M), found in gram-positive bacteria, and suggests a common ancestry (104). Many gram-positive organisms also carry the *tet*(O)-bearing plasmid (142). The *tet*(O) gene can be expressed in *E. coli*, specifying an MIC of 64 μg/ml (163), and appears to require an upstream element for full expression (198).

Ribosomal protection proteins (RPPs), including Tet(O), and their mechanisms of resistance have been extensively reviewed (36). RPPs share sequence similarity to the ribosomal elongation factors EF-G and EF-Tu, primarily in the N-terminal GTP binding region (146), and are members of the translation factor superfamily of GTPases (93). The ability of purified Tet(O) to hydrolyze GTP is stimulated 20-fold by the presence of 70S ribosomes and closely resembles the activity of EF-G (22, 23, 170). Mutations in the GTP binding domain of Tet(O) lead to a decrease in in vivo GTPase activity (37, 66). Although RPPs have lost their function as translocases, their ability to bind ribosomes and hydrolyze GTP suggests that they may be evolutionarily derived from EF-G and adapted to function in Tc[r] (37). A 16-Å-resolution reconstruction by cryoelectron microscopy demonstrates that Tet(O) and EF-G have a similar three-dimensional structure and overall shape, which allows them to bind at the interface of the ribosomal subunit on the A-site side (153). The majority of contacts between Tet(O) and the ribosome are mediated by the rRNA and one interaction with ribosomal protein S12 (153). Mutations in the S12 protein interfere with Tet(O) activity (172).

A model of Tet(O) interaction with the ribosome is shown in Fig. 3C. Tet(O) preferentially interacts with the posttranslation-state ribosome, which explains the selectivity for the Tc-inhibited ribosome over the active ribosome (36, 37). Only the GTP conformation of Tet(O) interacts with the ribosome (182). Tet(O) approaches the 70S ribosome from the open A-site side and binds in the intersubunit space, contacting the 50S subunit near the base of the L7/L12 stalk in the vicinity of both the α-sarcin/ricin loop (H95) (H = helix of 23S rRNA 50S subunit) and thiostrepton/L11 binding site (H43/H44) (153). On the 30S subunit, Tet(O) contacts ribosomal protein S12 and the 16S rRNA at h5, h18, and h34 of the decoding site (153). When the high-resolution X-ray structures depicting a Tc-ribosome complex (21) are combined with the cryoelectron microscopy maps of the 70S · Tet(O) complex, Tet(O) appears to approach, but does not overlap, the primary Tc binding site formed at h31 and h34 (153). This supports the concept of an allosteric mechanism for Tet(O)-mediated tetracycline release where Tet(O) does not bind at the primary Tc binding site. Instead, domain IV of Tet(O) is proposed to contact the base of h34 (h = helix of 16S rRNA 30S subunit) to induce a conformational change that disrupts the primary Tc binding site (153). Experimental evidence that Tet(O) induces conformational rearrangements within the ribosome obtained with an XTP-dependent mutant of Tet(O) is demonstrated by a stimulation in the GTPase activity of EF-Tu (36, 37). This suggests that the Tet(O)-induced conformation persists after Tet(O) has left the ribosome, which may prevent Tc rebinding and/or promote a productive A-site occupation by the ternary complex in the presence of Tc. The release of tetracycline from the ribosome allows aminoacyl-tRNA to bind to the A site and the continuation of protein synthesis.

Sequence analysis of *C. jejuni* isolates with very high-level Tc[r] (512 μg/ml) has identified seven specific nucleotide changes within the *tet*(O) gene that result in the substitution of seven amino acid residues on the Tet(O) protein (61). Characterization of the functionally important regions of Tet(O), the kinetics of the competition of Tc and Tet(O), as well as the possible role of rRNA mutations in the development of Tc[r] are the subject of future research studies.

Trimethoprim

Campylobacter is intrinsically resistant to trimethoprim, making this antibiotic useful in selective growth media (164). Trimethoprim selectively inhibits dihydrofolate reductase, an essential enzyme responsible for the regeneration of dihydrofolate to tetrahydrofolate, which is necessary for the biosynthesis of amino acids and nucleotides (40). Trimethoprim-resistant dihydrofolate reductase is encoded by the *dfr1* and *dfr9* genes, located in the context of remnants of an integron and a transposon, respectively (58). Although both genes are present in 10% of isolates, *dfr1* is present in most *Campylobacter* isolates (58, 80). The *dfr1* gene in one-third of *Campylobacter* isolates is identical to the gene present in *E. coli*, while a 90-bp direct repeat is present in the *dfr1* gene in 40% of isolates, and in another 5% of isolates this variant is present in two cassettes in tandem in an integron context (59). The higher G+C content of the *dfr* genes, the location of these genes on integron and transposon contexts, and the natural transformability of *C. jejuni* and *C. coli* suggest that these genes were likely acquired from a non-*Campylobacter* trimethoprim-resistant bacterium (58, 80, 197).

Multidrug Resistance

Multiple drug resistance (MDR) or multiple antibiotic resistance in bacteria is often associated with increased expression of an efflux system capable of transporting structurally unrelated antibiotics out of the bacterial cell. Genomic sequence analysis of *C. jejuni* NCTC 11168 reveals the presence of two putative resistance-nodulation-cell division (RND) and at least eight other non-RND efflux systems observed in other bacteria (125, 135). RND transporters are typically composed of approximately 1,000 amino acid residues predicted to form a 12-helical structure with two large-loop periplasmic or extracytoplasmic domains that are important in drug recognition (185). The periplasmic loops likely contain multiple binding sites for structurally unrelated compounds (20). Two RND systems, CmeABC and CmeDEF, are present in *Campylobacter* (136). CmeB, CmeF, and major outer membrane porin protein are known to transport many antibiotics, detergents, and dyes (135), but major outer membrane porin protein, encoded by *porA*, does not appear to play a role in the development of MDR in *Campylobacter* (136).

The sequence and structure of the CmeABC multidrug efflux system in *Campylobacter* is similar to a periplasmic fusion protein (CmeA), an inner membrane transporter (CmeB), and an outer membrane protein (CmeC) (96, 135). The genes are organized as an operon-encoding, energy-dependent, tripartite efflux system similar to MexAB/OprM observed in *Pseudomonas aeruginosa* (96, 114). A *tet*(R)-like transcriptional regulator, *cmeR*, located immediately upstream from *cmeA* shares similarities with the TetR/AcrR family of transcription suppressors of efflux systems (96, 135). In other RND efflux systems, a transcriptional regulator may modulate the expression of the efflux system by direct binding of the substrate as a means to monitor the substrate's intracellular level (67). Immunoblotting demonstrates that CmeABC is constitutively expressed in wild-type strains of *Campylobacter* (96). Overexpression of *cmeB* is observed with either mutation in *cmeR* or a knockout mutant of *cmeR* (98).

CmeABC is responsible for the active efflux of a variety of bile acids, antibiotics, heavy metals, and other antimicrobial agents (Table 3) and is essential for colonization of the chicken gut (96, 97). Inactivation of *cmeB* in *C. jejuni* NCTC 11168 and *C. jejuni* 81–176 by insertional mutagenesis results in increased susceptibility to β-lactams, fluoroquinolones, macrolides, chloramphenicol, tetracycline, ethidium bromide, acridine orange, and sodium dodecyl sulfate (135), as well as heavy metals and bile acids (96). Since tetracycline is also a substrate for CmeABC, acquired tetracyline resistance due to the presence of the *tet*(O) plasmid may be synergistically enhanced by this efflux pump activity. Resistance to ciprofloxacin and enrofloxacin is drastically decreased in *cmeB cmeC* mutants of fluoroquinolone-resistant isolates of *Campylobacter* (103). Decreased production of CmeB and CmeC following transposon insertion into the *cmeB* gene of *C. jejuni* 81–176 is most notably associated with a 100-fold decrease in resistance to rifampin and a 64- to 4,000-fold decrease in resistance to bile acids (96). The activity of CmeABC offers at least a partial explanation for the known intrinsic resistance of *Campylobacter* to rifampin, which allows it to be an effective selection agent in *Campylobacter* selection media. Since *Campylobacter* resides in the intestinal tract, the efflux of bile acids is a physiologically relevant function and suggests that CmeABC may play an important role in successful colonization of the intestine (97).

Accumulation of ciprofloxacin following interruption of CmeABC efflux indicates it is a substrate for CmeABC. In a recent study of 32 multiple-antibiotic-resistant *C. jejuni* strains, a mutation in *cmeR* (Gly-85–Ala) and overexpression of *cmeB* in nine isolates was associated with low-level accumulation of ciprofloxacin that could be restored to wild-type levels in the presence of carbonyl cyanide *m*-chlorophenyl hydrazone, a known efflux pump inhibitor (136).

Coresistance to fluoroquinolones and erythromycin represents a significant threat for the treatment of severe *Campylobacter* infections. Studies using the efflux pump inhibitor Phe–Arg–β-naphthylamide reveal that efflux plays a role in intrinsic and low-level acquired resistance to erythromycin in isolates of *C. coli* (126). Targeting the CmeABC efflux system may provide alternative antibacterial strategies to decrease the emergence of erythromycin-resistant strains of *Campylobacter* spp. (126) through the development of efflux pump inhibitors or antibacterials that bypass the efflux system (95, 133).

The second RND efflux system, CmeDEF, is present in *Campylobacter* (where CmeD is the outer membrane protein and CmeE is the integral membrane protein) and confers multiple-antibiotic resistance but does not transport ciprofloxacin (136). No

Table 3. Antimicrobial agents transported by CmeABC in *C. jejuni*

Bile acids	Antibiotics	Heavy metals	Other antimicrobials
Chenodeoxycholic acid	Aminoglycosides (e.g., gentamicin)	$CoCl_2$	Acridine orange
Cholic acid	β-Lactams (e.g., ampicillin, cefotaxime)	$CuCl_2$	Ethidium bromide
Deoxycholic acid	Chloramphenicol		Protamine
Taurocholic acid	Macrolides (e.g., erythromycin)		Sodium dodecyl sulfate
	Quinolones (e.g., ciprofloxacin, norfloxacin, nalidixic acid)		
	Rifampin		
	Tetracycline		

regulator has been identified for *cmeDEF*, and overexpression of *cmeF* occurs only when *cmeB* is also overexpressed (136). This is not surprising since most genes in *Campylobacter* are thought to be coregulated (125).

Intrinsic resistance of *Campylobacter* spp. to trimethoprim, cycloheximide, polymyxin B, and $ZnSO_4$ may be due to the activity of other efflux systems, since these antimicrobial agents do not appear to be substrates of CmeABC. *Campylobacter* isolates that overexpress an efflux pump(s) cannot easily be identified by analysis of antimicrobial susceptibility data, since more than one resistance mechanism may be present. Future studies are needed to discover agents capable of detecting the overexpression of efflux pumps (136).

EMERGENCE OF ANTIMICROBIAL RESISTANCE

Most of the antimicrobials used in veterinary medicine are tetracyclines and macrolides, which result in high and continuous selective pressure for the animal-colonizing bacteria, ultimately resulting in the acquisition of antimicrobial resistance genes (24). The possibility of zoonotic transfer of antimicrobial-resistant bacteria to humans presents a potential danger to human public health. In the absence of antimicrobial selective pressure, antimicrobial resistance in animal *Campylobacter* isolates may arise from human contamination of the farm environment where there is integron-mediated exchange of antibiotic resistance determinants from other bacteria (92). Accordingly, integrons may play an important role in the emergence of antimicrobial resistance in human and animal sources of bacteria. Surveillance programs are necessary to detect the emergence and prevalence of MDR in clinically important bacteria of human and animal origin. Estimating the prevalence of MDR may be difficult since several host and/or environmental conditions may alter the expression of MDR systems. Evaluation of the presence of MDR genes and their expression under different conditions will provide insight into novel strategies to control MDR-mediated resistance (24).

Investigation into the mechanisms of action of antimicrobials, as well as the transfer of resistance determinants, is necessary to gain effective control of antimicrobial resistance (24). In addition, insight into the mechanisms that efflux pumps use to accommodate a diverse range of compounds, as well as the conformational changes that occur to mediate substrate translocation outside the cell, will facilitate the identification of targets against these efflux pumps (20).

Spread of Resistance from Animals to Humans

It is generally agreed that use of antimicrobial agents is the most important factor in the selection of resistance in bacteria and that, in general, a close association exists between the rate of resistance development and the quantities of antimicrobial agents used (2). For *Campylobacter*, the resistance rates in isolates from humans are influenced by (i) the veterinary use of agents, (ii) recent or current antimicrobial treatment of the patients, and (iii) sampling strategy. These factors contribute to the complexity of the epidemiology and stress the need for caution in the interpretation and comparison of data from different centers.

The occurrence of macrolide and quinolone resistance is in general higher among *C. coli* compared to *C. jejuni* (1, 68, 107, 201). This is especially the case for macrolide resistance in *C. coli* from pigs. For instance, in a study by Sáenz et al. from Spain (145), rates of erythromycin and quinolone resistance in *C. coli* from pigs were 81% and 100%, respectively.

As described above, the macrolide resistance mechanism in *Campylobacter* is likely to be chromosomal mutations in the drug-sensitive target. Thus, resistance to macrolides in *Campylobacter* will spread with the bacteria and not be transferable to other bacteria. Development of resistance to macrolides in *Campylobacter* during therapy has not been documented in humans. The origin of resistant strains has been linked to the veterinary use of antibiotics of the macrolide-lincosamide group (1). This group of antibiotics has been used worldwide for treatment of food animals for several decades. The most commonly used antimicrobial agents have been lincomycin and tylosin for the control of dysentery and *Mycoplasma* infections in swine and spiramycin for the treatment of mastitis in cattle. In addition, for the past 20 years tylosin has been the most commonly used antimicrobial agent for growth promotion in swine production worldwide, whereas spiramycin has been commonly used for poultry. The use of macrolides for growth promotion was banned in all European Union countries in July 1999, but they are still used in a number of countries.

Most *Campylobacter* infections are sporadic, making the search for the source of infection difficult. The epidemiology of infections is not entirely elucidated, but the major sources have long been identified. Descriptive epidemiological studies have identified *Campylobacter* in the intestinal tracts of a wide variety of wild and domestic food animals and pets. Among food animals, *C. jejuni* predominates among cattle, broiler chickens, and turkeys, whereas *C. coli* is most common among pigs. As result of fecal contact during processing, the meat may be contaminated. The *Campylobacter* contamination rates at the retail level vary by food item and country, but in general beef and pork show low rates, whereas poultry, especially chicken, consistently shows high rates (8, 128, 200). In Denmark the rates of *Campylobacter*-positive retail chicken products were 33% for domestic and 50% for imported products and the corresponding quinolone resistance rates (QR) were 1% in *C. jejuni* in domestic and 8% in imported chicken products in 2003 (9); in Italy 81% of chicken products were *Campylobacter* positive, with 60% QR for *C. jejuni* and 79%QR for *C. coli* (128); in Ireland the figure was 29%, with 29% QR among *Campylobacter* spp. (102); in Spain it was 87%, with 99% QR for *C. jejuni* and 100% QR for *C. coli* (145); in Switzerland 22% of the products were positive, with 19% QR among domestic *Campylobacter* spp. and 53% QR among those from imported poultry (91); in the United Kingdom the figure was 44%, with 9% QR among domestic *Campylobacter* spp., versus 14% QR among those from imported chicken products (203); and in the United States the rate was 44% (exclusively U.S. production), with 29% QR for *C. jejuni* and 37% QR for *C. coli* (68).

Analytic epidemiological methods, e.g., case-control studies, have provided important information on the sources of human infections. At least 18 out of 23 case-control studies in the United States, Canada, New Zealand, Australia, and Western European countries have identified poultry (especially eating undercooked chicken) as a risk factor for sporadic *Campylobacter* infections. Additional, occasionally identified risk factors included contact with pet animals, drinking water, milk, barbecuing, swimming in water from natural sources, occupational exposure to animals, and traveling (53, 83, 108, 115, 134, 148, 176). Cross-contamination in the home and in the restaurant kitchen is probably a frequent route of transmission for *Campylobacter*, but also difficult to evaluate (83). In addition, poultry is a common food product frequently noted as a recent exposure among both cases and controls. Consequently, case-control studies of risk factors for sporadic *Campylobacter* infections have a relatively small population-attributable risk of exposures (115). Person-to-person transmission of *C. jejuni* and *C. coli* is rare and probably of no epidemiologic importance (44).

Other epidemiological data also support the assumption that poultry is an important source of human infections, e.g., the unintentional "intervention study" performed in Belgium during the dioxin crisis, where withdrawal of domestically produced poultry products from the market resulted in a 40% decrease in the *Campylobacter* infections (191).

In a number of countries, including Iceland, Norway, and Denmark, poultry consumption has increased steadily over the last 10 to 15 years and raw refrigerated products have become increasingly popular. In previous years a majority of the products were frozen. While frozen storage has been shown to reduce the number of viable campylobacters, *Campylobacter* survives well throughout the shelf life of fresh poultry products stored at refrigeration temperature in modified and normal atmospheres. Increased consumption of fresh poultry may have contributed to the rising incidence of *Campylobacter* infections in a number of countries. In Iceland the number of domestically acquired *Campylobacter* infections reached epidemic proportions in the years 1998 to 2000. Subsequently, a broad campaign was launched, directed at reducing *Campylobacter* in poultry during production, processing, and marketing and simultaneously focusing on consumer education. In order to reduce the distribution of *Campylobacter*-contaminated poultry, all positive flocks had to be frozen to reduce bacterial counts before going to retail. As a consequence, the incidence of domestically acquired *Campylobacter* infections dropped from 116 per 100,000 in 1999 to 33 per 100,000 in 2000, resulting in a 72% reduction in domestic infections. The combination of public education, enhanced on-farm biological security measures, carcass freezing, and other unidentified factors, such as variations in weather, contributed to the large reduction in poultry-borne campylobacteriosis. There was no immediate basis for assigning credit to any specific intervention (158). Based on the Icelandic experience, results from research projects in primary production, and results from a Danish risk assessment of campylobacteriosis associated with *Campylobacter* in chickens, comparable mitigation strategies have recently been adopted in Norway and Denmark (8, 12).

Veterinary use of fluoroquinolones is not the only selection pressure that acts upon *Campylobacter* to select for populations that are quinolone resistant. Resistance occurs naturally, but the selection and dissemination of resistance is an inevitable result of any antibiotic use. Fluoroquinolone use in humans can itself lead to emergence of quinolone-resistant *Campylobacter* in treated infections. At least four case-control studies have specifically addressed risk factors for quinolone-resistant *Campylobacter* infections in the United States, the United Kingdom, and Denmark (Table 4). Foreign travel was identified as a risk factor in all four studies. Three of the four studies evaluated current or recent treatment with antimicrobials.

Table 4. Studies evaluating the duration of illness in patients infected with quinolone-resistant *Campylobacter* strains versus quinolone-susceptible *Campylobacter* strains

Authors and reference	Resistant		Sensitive		*P*
	No. of patients	Duration of diarrhea (days)	No. of patients	Duration of diarrhea (days)	
Smith et al. (152)	69	10	115	7	0.03
Neimann et al. (116)[a]	5	14	31	9	0.13
The Campylobacter Sentinel Surveillance Scheme Collaborators (25)[b]		12.7,[d] 11.8[e]		13.5,[d] 11.2[e]	0.56,[d] 0.66[e]
Engberg et al. (47)[b]	86	13.2	381	10.3	0.001
Nelson et al. (117)[c]					
Model A	26	9	264	7	0.04
Model B	7	12	56	6	0.04
Model C	9	8	76	6	0.2

[a]Stratified by treatment, but not by antimicrobial agent used for treatment.
[b]Analysis not stratified by treatment.
[c]Model A: analysis of 290 persons who did not take antidiarrheal medications; model B: analysis of 63 persons who did not take antimicrobial agents or antidiarrheal medications; model C: analysis of 85 persons who took only fluoroquinolone antimicrobial agents.
[d]Domestically acquired infections.
[e]Travel-related infections.

An association between treatment with a fluoroquinolone before stool-specimen collection and having a quinolone-resistant *Campylobacter* infection was only observed in the study by Smith and colleagues (152), but their study also showed that treatment with a fluoroquinolone before stool culture accounted for a maximum of 15% of resistant isolates in Minnesota during 1996 and 1998. The studies suggest that quinolone use in humans is not the major selective force for quinolone resistance among *Campylobacter* spp. that cause human infection.

Available sero- and molecular typing methods are not suited for attribution analysis of *Campylobacter* infections, as can be done for *Salmonella*. The reason for this is the lack of host specificity of *Campylobacter* subtypes, the large diversity of *Campylobacter*, and the weak clonal structure of *Campylobacter*. However, valuable information has been gained by comparison of strains, including quinolone-resistant strains, from farm to fork. Recent Danish studies combining sero- and molecular typing of sporadic human infections suggest that almost one-third of apparently sporadic *Campylobacter* infections may be epidemiologically connected (54). In a comparison of human isolates to isolates from retail food samples and fecal samples from chickens, pigs, and cattle, 61% percent of the domestically acquired isolates from humans had a subtype that was also found in food (mainly chicken and turkey products) (118). The finding is in accordance with Finnish and Swedish studies (72, 75). Smith and colleagues (152) applied PCR-restriction fragment length polymorphism DNA typing, and documented fingerprints in quinolone-resistant *C. jejuni* from domestically (U.S.) produced poultry were identical to those in resistant *C. jejuni* from domestically acquired infections in humans.

In conclusion, there is ample evidence to indicate that contaminated fresh, raw, retail meat, especially poultry, is a major source of infection, even though other sources, such as raw milk, water, and pets, may contribute to human infections.

As a consequence, the CVM proposed to withdraw the approval of enrofloxacin (Baytril) in poultry in the United States in late 2000. The producer of Baytril requested a hearing before an administrative law judge. The verdict went largely against the manufacturer, the main conclusions being the following (39):

- Usage of enrofloxacin in poultry acts as a selection pressure, resulting in the emergence and dissemination of fluoroquinolone-resistant *Campylobacter*.
- There is evidence showing that fluoroquinolone-resistant *Campylobacter* in poultry can be transferred to humans and can contribute to fluoroquinolone-resistant *Campylobacter* infections in humans.
- Fluoroquinolone-resistant *Campylobacter* infections in humans have the potential to adversely affect human health.
- Enrofloxacin is not shown to be safe under the approved conditions of use.

Following the final decision, the approval of Baytril was withdrawn from the U.S. market in September 2005 (38a). In Canada, licensing of the veterinary use of fluoroquinolones was withdrawn in 1997.

CLINICAL IMPLICATIONS OF ANTIMICROBIAL RESISTANCE

Quinolone-resistant *Campylobacter* infections in humans have the potential to adversely affect human health. Table 5 shows case-comparison studies evaluating the duration of illness in patients infected with quinolone-resistant *Campylobacter* strains versus quinolone-sensitive *Campylobacter* strains (25, 47, 84, 152). The recent study by Nelson et al. (117) evaluated duration of illness across a variety of analytical models, including in a multivariable analysis-of-variance model, and identified a consistent correlation between quinolone resistance and prolonged duration of diarrhea. Although the results from these studies are not all statistically significant, the estimates point in the same direction and hence suggest that there is a longer duration of illness in patients infected with quinolone-resistant strains. Whether patients with resistant infections may suffer a longer duration of illness because the antibiotic provided to them simply does not work against resistant *Campylobacter* and/or due to increased inherent virulence associated with quinolone resistance remains to be fully determined.

Treatment failures, both clinical and bacteriological, with fluoroquinolones are common and may be due to selection of strains that were resistant at the time of ingestion or due to induction of fluoroquinolone resistance during treatment (4, 42, 47, 150, 174). It has been predicted that in 10 to

Table 5. Studies evaluating risk factors for quinolone-resistant *Campylobacter* infections[a]

Authors and reference	Potential risk factor	No. of patients with: Resistant isolates (%)	No. of patients with: Sensitive isolates (%)	Multivariate analysis: Matched odds ratio (95% confidence interval)	Multivariate analysis: *P*
Smith et al. (152)	Foreign travel:				
	To Mexico	47 (36)	30 (12)	26.0 (8.6–78. 6)	<0.001
	To Caribbean countries, South America, or Central America (not Mexico)	14 (11)	7 (3)	45.5 (9.7–214)	<0.001
	To Asia	23 (18)	8 (3)	40.7 (10.2–163.0)	<0.001
	To Spain	7 (5)	1 (<1)	48.6 (4.1–570.0)	0.002
	Use of a quinolone before the collection of stool specimens	26 (20)	7 (3)	7.5 (2.6–21.3)	<0.001
The Campylobacter Sentinel Surveillance Scheme Collaborators (25)	Travel-related infections:				
	Portugal	8 (2)	3 (2)	22.4 (4.4–115.0)	<0.001
	Cyprus	5 (1)	1 (<1)	11.7 (1.3–108.0)	0.03
	Spain	48 (14)	16 (11)	6.9 (3.5–13.4)	<0.001
	Consumption of chicken	92 (27)	82 (55)	5.0 (2.1–11.6)	<0.001
	Domestically acquired infections: Consumption of cold meats (precooked)	80 (27)	71 (4)	2.1 (1.4–3.1)	<0.001
Engberg et al. (47)	Foreign travel	30 (71)	12 (14)	16.8 (3.4–82.2)	0.001
	Consumption of fresh poultry other than chicken and turkey	14 (33)	58 (70)	19.1 (2.2–167.3)	0.008
	Swimming (pool, ocean, lake, or other places)	20 (48)	16 (19)	5.0 (1.14–22.0)	0.033
Kassenborg et al. (84)[b]	Consumption of chicken or turkey cooked at a commercial establishment	18 (55)	7 (21)	10.0 (1.3–78.0)	0.03

[a]Only risk factors associated with increased risk of infection are listed.
[b]Analysis of potential risk factors specifically on domestically acquired infections. Travel outside the United States was reported by 27 (42%) of 64 patients with fluoroquinolone-resistant *Campylobacter* and by 51 (9%) of 582 patients with fluoroquinolone-susceptible *Campylobacter* infection (odds ratio, 7.6; 95% confidence interval, 4.3–13.4).

20% of patients treated with a fluoroquinolone for *Campylobacter* enteritis, the *Campylobacter* strains will develop quinolone resistance (130, 204). However, in a study by Ellis-Pegler and colleagues (42), between 18 and 28% of the patients in their prospective trial developed fluoroquinolone resistance. Development of resistance has been registered in short-term treatments, but prolonged therapy, e.g., in immunosuppressed patients, is a risk factor and has been associated with both clinical and bacteriological failures (4, 109, 150, 174, 175). The public health impact of animal-related resistance in *Campylobacter* is described in more detail in chapter 19.

CONSEQUENCES OF RESISTANCE FOR THE CLINICAL DECISION-MAKING PROCESS

Infection with thermophilic *Campylobacter* spp. usually leads to an episode of acute gastroenteritis, which resolves within a few days to a few weeks. Fluid and electrolyte replacement constitutes the cornerstone of treatment of diarrheal diseases. Most cases of *Campylobacter* enteritis do not require antimicrobial treatment, as they are self-limiting. However, antimicrobial treatment is needed for systemic *Campylobacter* infections and for severe or long-lasting cases of *Campylobacter* enteritis. Erythromycin has been the agent of choice, but therapy with extended-spectrum macrolides, such as clarithromycin or azithromycin, should be equally effective (18, 48, 73, 165). It is seldom possible to establish the causative agent of an acute case of diarrhea in a patient before treatment is begun. The decision of which antimicrobial drug to use has to be taken on empirical basis in most cases in the clinical setting. Fluoroquinolones are the drug of choice in this situation. Increasing rates of quinolone resistance in *Campylobacter* and *Salmonella*, the predominant bacterial causes of community-acquired diarrhea, in most developed countries therefore constitute a major problem for public health. As presented in Fig. 2, the difference in resistance to quinolones between *Campylobacter* acquired abroad and domestically acquired infections in a number of countries is of such a magnitude that travel status should be considered when empiric antimicrobial therapy is deemed necessary. Therefore, the travel history should be considered not solely for surveillance purposes, but also in the clinical setting when considering therapeutic options. Antimicrobial resistance in *Campylobacter* spp. other than *C. jejuni* and *C. coli* and its clinical consequence have been reviewed elsewhere (112).

CONCLUSIONS AND FUTURE PERSPECTIVES

Campylobacter has become the leading cause of zoonotic enteric infections in developed and developing countries worldwide. Epidemiological and microbiological studies show that poultry is the most important source for quinolone-susceptible and quinolone-resistant *Campylobacter* infections in humans. Trends over time for macrolide resistance show stable low rates in most countries, and macrolides should remain the drug class of choice for *C. jejuni* and *C. coli* enteritis. However, macrolide resistance is emerging in some countries and needs to be monitored. Susceptibility to fluoroquinolones and tetracycline varies extensively by geographic origin of infection. In countries with widespread veterinary use of quinolones and among travelers returning from these destinations, fluoroquinolones are, at present, not safe drugs for the treatment of patients with *Campylobacter* enteritis.

The necessity for treating bacteremic episodes with agents other than a macrolide has not been established. For those patients who appear very ill, treatment with gentamicin, a carbapenem, cefotaxime, or chloramphenicol may be indicated, but susceptibility testing should be performed (18). For *Campylobacter*, as for any food-borne pathogen, the control of infections starts in agriculture and ends in the kitchen of the consumer.

Acknowledgments. Work in Edmonton on *Campylobacter* was supported by the Canadian Institutes of Health Research and the Natural Science and Engineering Research Council. D.E.T. is a Medical Scientist with the Alberta Heritage Foundation for Medical Research.

REFERENCES

1. **Aarestrup, F. M., E. M. Nielsen, M. Madsen, and J. Engberg.** 1997. Antimicrobial susceptibility patterns of thermophilic *Campylobacter* spp. from humans, pigs, cattle, and broilers in Denmark. *Antimicrob. Agents Chemother.* **41:**2244–2250.
2. **Aarestrup, F. M., and H. C. Wegener.** 1999. The effects of antibiotic usage in food animals on the development of antimicrobial resistance of importance for humans in *Campylobacter* and *Escherichia coli. Microbes Infect.* **8:**639–644.
3. **Acar, J. F., and F. W. Goldstein.** 1997. Trends in bacterial resistance to fluoroquinolones. *Clin. Infect. Dis.* **24**(Suppl. 1): S67–S73.
4. **Adler Mosca, H., J. Luthy Hottenstein, G. Martinetti Lucchini, A. Burnens, and M. Altwegg.** 1991. Development of resistance to quinolones in five patients with campylobacteriosis treated with norfloxacin or ciprofloxacin. *Eur. J. Clin. Microbiol. Infect. Dis.* **10:**953–957.
5. **Afset, J. E., and J. A. Maeland.** 2001. Erythromycin and ciprofloxacin resistant *Campylobacter jejuni. Tidsskr. Nor. Laegeforen.* **121:**2152–2154. (In Norwegian.)
6. Reference deleted.

7. **Anonymous.** 2003. *MARAN-2002: Monitoring of Antimicrobial Resistance and Antibiotic Usage in Animals in The Netherlands in 2002.* CIDC-Lelystad, Lelystad, The Netherlands.
8. **Anonymous.** 2004. Annual Report on Zoonoses in Denmark 2003, p. 1–31. Ministry of Food, Agriculture and Fisheries, Danish Zoonosis Centre, Søborg, Denmark.
9. **Anonymous.** 2004. *DANMAP 2003—Use of Antimicrobial Agents and Occurrence of Antimicrobial Resistance in Bacteria from Food Animals, Foods and Humans in Denmark.* Ministry of Food, Agriculture and Fisheries, Copenhagen, Denmark.
10. **Anonymous.** 2004. *MARAN 2003: Monitoring of Antimicrobial Resistance and Antibiotic Usage in Animals in The Netherlands in 2003.* CIDC-Lelystad, Lelystad, The Netherlands.
11. **Anonymous.** 2004. *NORM/NORM-VET 2003. Usage of Antimicrobial Agents and Occurrence of Antimicrobial Resistance in Norway.* Norwegian Zoonosis Centre, Oslo, Norway.
12. **Anonymous.** 2004. *Norwegian Action Plan against Campylobacter in Broilers.* Tromsø/Oslo, Norway.
13. **Bachoual, R., S. Ouabdesselam, F. Mory, C. Lascols, C. J. Soussy, and J. Tankovic.** 2001. Single or double mutational alterations of GyrA associated with fluoroquinolone resistance in *Campylobacter jejuni* and *Campylobacter coli. Microb. Drug Resist.* 7:257–261.
14. **Ban, N., P. Nissen, J. Hansen, M. Capel, P. B. Moore, and T. A. Steitz.** 1999. Placement of protein and RNA structures into a 5 Å-resolution map of the 50S ribosomal subunit. *Nature* **400**:841–847.
15. **Bauernfeind, A.** 1997. Comparison of the antibacterial activities of the quinolones Bay 12–8039, gatifloxacin (AM 1155), trovafloxacin, clinafloxacin, levofloxacin and ciprofloxacin. *J. Antimicrob. Chemother.* **40**:639–651.
16. **Beckmann, L., M. Muller, P. Luber, C. Schrader, E. Bartelt, and G. Klein.** 2004. Analysis of gyrA mutations in quinolone-resistant and -susceptible *Campylobacter jejuni* isolates from retail poultry and human clinical isolates by non-radioactive single-strand conformation polymorphism analysis and DNA sequencing. *J. Appl. Microbiol.* **96**:1040–1047.
17. **Bilgin, N., A. A. Richter, M. Ehrenberg, A. E. Dahlberg, and C. G. Kurland.** 1990. Ribosomal RNA and protein mutants resistant to spectinomycin. *EMBO J.* **9**:735–739.
18. **Blaser, M. J.** 2000. *Campylobacter jejuni* and related species, p. 2276–2285. *In* G. L. Mandell, J. E. Bennett, and R. Dolin (ed.), *Principles and Practice of Infectious Diseases.* Churchill Livingstone Inc., New York, N.Y.
19. **Bodhidatta, L., N. Vithayasai, B. Eimpokalarp, C. Pitarangsi, O. Serichantalergs, and D. W. Isenbarger.** 2002. Bacterial enteric pathogens in children with acute dysentery in Thailand: increasing importance of quinolone-resistant *Campylobacter. Southeast Asian J. Trop. Med. Public Health* **33**:752–757.
20. **Borges-Walmsley, M. I., K. S. McKeegan, and A. R. Walmsley.** 2003. Structure and function of efflux pumps that confer resistance to drugs. *Biochem. J.* **376**:313–338.
21. **Brodersen, D. E., W. M. Clemons, Jr., A. P. Carter, R. J. Morgan-Warren, B. T. Wimberly, and V. Ramakrishnan.** 2000. The structural basis for the action of the antibiotics tetracycline, pactamycin, and hygromycin B on the 30S ribosomal subunit. *Cell* **103**:1143–1154.
22. **Burdett, V.** 1991. Purification and characterization of Tet(M), a protein that renders ribosomes resistant to tetracycline. *J. Biol. Chem.* **266**:2872–2877.
23. **Burdett, V.** 1996. Tet(M)-promoted release of tetracycline from ribosomes is GTP dependent. *J. Bacteriol.* **178**:3246– 3251.
24. **Butaye, P., A. Cloeckaert, and S. Schwarz.** 2003. Mobile genes coding for efflux-mediated antimicrobial resistance in Gram-positive and Gram-negative bacteria. *Int. J. Antimicrob. Agents* **22**:205–210.
25. **The Campylobacter Sentinel Surveillance Scheme Collaborators.** 2002. Ciprofloxacin resistance in *Campylobacter jejuni*: case-case analysis as a tool for elucidating risks at home and abroad. *J. Antimicrob. Chemother.* **50**:561–568.
26. **Carattoli, A.** 2001. Importance of integrons in the diffusion of resistance. *Vet. Res.* **32**:243–259.
27. **Carter, A. P., W. M. Clemons, D. E. Brodersen, R. J. Morgan-Warren, B. T. Wimberly, and V. Ramakrishnan.** 2000. Functional insights from the structure of the 30S ribosomal subunit and its interactions with antibiotics. *Nature* **407**:340–348.
28. **Cate, J. H., M. M. Yusupov, G. Z. Yusupova, T. N. Earnest, and H. F. Noller.** 1999. X-ray crystal structures of 70S ribosome functional complexes. *Science* **285**:2095–2104.
29. **Centers for Disease Control and Prevention.** 2003. *National Antimicrobial Resistance Monitoring System for Enteric Bacteria (NARMS): 2001 Annual Report.* Centers for Disease Control and Prevention, U.S. Department of Health and Human Services, Atlanta, Ga.
30. **Centers for Disease Control and Prevention.** 2004. *National Antimicrobial Resistance Monitoring System for Enteric Bacteria (NARMS): 2002 Annual Report.* Centers for Disease Control and Prevention, U.S. Department of Health and Human Services, Atlanta, Ga.
31. **Chopra, I.** 1994. Tetracycline analogs whose primary target is not the bacterial ribosome. *Antimicrob. Agents Chemother.* **38**:637–640.
32. **Chopra, I., P. M. Hawkey, and M. Hinton.** 1992. Tetracyclines, molecular and clinical aspects. *J. Antimicrob. Chemother.* **29**:245–277.
33. **Chopra, I., and M. Roberts.** 2001. Tetracycline antibiotics: mode of action, applications, molecular biology, and epidemiology of bacterial resistance. *Microbiol. Mol. Biol. Rev.* **65**: 232–260.
34. **Chu, Y. W., M. Y. Chu, K. Y. Luey, Y. W. Ngan, K. L. Tsang, and K. M. Kam.** 2004. Genetic relatedness and quinolone resistance of *Campylobacter jejuni* strains isolated in 2002 in Hong Kong. *J. Clin. Microbiol.* **42**:3321–3323.
35. **Clemons, W. M., Jr., J. L. May, B. T. Wimberly, J. P. McCutcheon, M. S. Capel, and V. Ramakrishnan.** 1999. Structure of a bacterial 30S ribosomal subunit at 5.5 Å resolution. *Nature* **400**:833–840.
36. **Connell, S. R., D. M. Tracz, K. H. Nierhaus, and D. E. Taylor.** 2003. Ribosomal protection proteins and their mechanism of tetracycline resistance. *Antimicrob. Agents Chemother.* **47**:3675–3681.
37. **Connell, S. R., C. A. Trieber, G. P. Dinos, E. Einfeldt, D. E. Taylor, and K. H. Nierhaus.** 2003. Mechanism of Tet(O)-mediated tetracycline resistance. *EMBO J.* **22**:945–953.
38. **Cooper, R., H. Segal, A. J. Lastovica, and B. G. Elisha.** 2002. Genetic basis of quinolone resistance and epidemiology of resistant and susceptible isolates of porcine *Campylobacter coli* strains. *J. Appl. Microbiol.* **93**:241–249.
38a. **Crawford, L.** 2005. Final decision of the commissioner. Withdrawal of approval of the new animal drug application for enrofloxacin in poultry. U.S. Food and Drug Administration, Rockville, Md.
39. **Davidson, D. J.** 2004. Proposal to withdraw approval of the new animal drug application for enrofloxacin for poultry. Initial decision, p. 1–68. U.S. Food and Drug Administration, Rockville, Md.
40. **Dever, L. A., and T. S. Dermody.** 1991. Mechanisms of bacterial resistance to antibiotics. *Arch. Intern. Med.* **151**:886–895.

41. **Drlica, K., and X. Zhao.** 1997. DNA gyrase, topoisomerase IV, and the 4-quinolones. *Microbiol. Mol. Biol. Rev.* **61**: 377–392.
42. **Ellis-Pegler, R. B., L. K. Hyman, R. J. Ingram, and M. McCarthy.** 1995. A placebo controlled evaluation of lomefloxacin in the treatment of bacterial diarrhoea in the community. *J. Antimicrob. Chemother.* **36**:259–263.
43. **Emborg, H.-D., and O. E. Heuer (ed.).** 2003. *DANMAP 2002—Use of Antimicrobial Agents and Occurrence of Antimicrobial Resistance in Bacteria from Food Animals, Foods and Humans in Denmark*, p. 3–67. The Danish Zoonosis Centre, Copenhagen, Denmark.
44. **Endtz, H. P., G. J. Ruijs, B. van Klingeren, W. H. Jansen, T. van der Reyden, and R. P. Mouton.** 1991. Quinolone resistance in *Campylobacter* isolated from man and poultry following the introduction of fluoroquinolones in veterinary medicine. *J. Antimicrob. Chemother.* **27**:199–208.
45. **Engberg, J.** Unpublished data.
46. **Engberg, J., F. M. Aarestrup, D. E. Taylor, P. Gerner-Smidt, and I. Nachamkin.** 2001. Quinolone and macrolide resistance in *Campylobacter jejuni* and *C. coli*: resistance mechanisms and trends in human isolates. *Emerg. Infect. Dis.* **7**:24–34.
47. **Engberg, J., J. Neimann, E. M. Nielsen, F. M. Aarestrup, and V. Fussing.** 2004. Quinolone-resistant *Campylobacter* infections: risk factors and clinical consequences. *Emerg. Infect. Dis.* **10**:1056–1063.
48. **Engberg, J., K. Schønning, M. Voldstedlund, E. Dzajic, and N. Frimodt Moller.** 2004. Bactericidal activity of five antimicrobial agents against *Campylobacter jejuni* tested by time-kill studies. *Clin. Microbiol. Infect.* **10**:336.
49. **Feierl, G.** 2004. *Jahresbericht 2003 der Nationalen Referenzzentrale für* Campylobacter, *Mitteilungen der Sanitätsverwaltung*, p. 3–7. Institute of Hygiene, Graz, Austria.
50. **Feierl, G., C. Berghold, J. Posch, G. Gorkiewicz, E. Daghofer, and E. Marth.** 2003. Epidemiology, clinical features and therapy of campylobacteriosis in Styria, Austria. *Int. J. Med. Microbiol.* **293**(Suppl. 35):134.
51. **Feierl, G., U. Wagner, B. Sixl, A. Grisold, E. Daghofer, and E. Marth.** Epidemiology of campylobacteriosis and development of resistance in Styria, Austria. Presented at the 11th International Workshop on *Campylobacter*, *Helicobacter* and Related Organisms, Freiburg, Germany, 1 to 5 September 2001.
52. **Fernandez, H.** 2001. Emergence of antimicrobial resistance in *Campylobacter*: the consequences for incidence, clinical course, epidemiology and control, p. 67–72. *In The Increasing Incidence of Human Campylobacteriosis: Report and Proceedings of a WHO Consultation of Experts, Copenhagen, Denmark, 21–25 November 2000.* Department of Communicable Disease Surveillance and Response, World Health Organization, Geneva, Switzerland.
53. **Friedman, C. R., R. M. Hoekstra, M. Samuel, R. Marcus, J. Bender, B. Shiferaw, S. Reddy, S. D. Ahuja, D. L. Helfrick, F. Hardnett, M. Carter, B. Anderson, and R. V. Tauxe.** 2004. Risk factors for sporadic *Campylobacter* infection in the United States: a case-control study in FoodNet sites. *Clin. Infect. Dis.* **38**(Suppl. 3):S285–S296.
54. **Fussing, V., E. M. Nielsen, J. Engberg, and J. Neimann.** 2003. Intensive microbiologic and epidemiologic *Campylobacter* surveillance in two Danish counties. *Int. J. Med. Microbiol.* **293**(Suppl. 35):139.
55. **Gaudreau, C., and H. Gilbert.** 2003. Antimicrobial resistance of *Campylobacter jejuni* subsp. *jejuni* strains isolated from humans in 1998 to 2001 in Montreal, Canada. *Antimicrob. Agents Chemother.* **47**:2027–2029.
56. **Gaudreau, C. L., L. A. Lariviere, J. C. Lauzer, and F. F. Turgeon.** 1987. Effect of clavulanic acid on susceptibility of *Campylobacter jejuni* and *Campylobacter coli* to eight β-lactam antibiotics. *Antimicrob. Agents Chemother.* **31**:940–942.
57. **Gibreel, A., V. N. Kos, M. Keelan, C. A. Trieber, S. Levesque, S. Michaud, and D. E. Taylor.** 2004. Macrolide resistance in *Campylobacter jejuni* and *Campylobacter coli*: molecular mechanism and stability of the resistance phenotype. *Antimicrob. Agents Chemother.* **49**:2753–2759.
58. **Gibreel, A., and O. Skold.** 1998. High-level resistance to trimethoprim in clinical isolates of *Campylobacter jejuni* by acquisition of foreign genes (*dfr1* and *dfr9*) expressing drug-insensitive dihydrofolate reductases. *Antimicrob. Agents Chemother.* **42**:3059–3064.
59. **Gibreel, A., and O. Skold.** 2000. An integron cassette carrying *dfr1* with 90-bp repeat sequences located on the chromosome of trimethoprim-resistant isolates of *Campylobacter jejuni*. *Microb. Drug Resist.* **6**:91–98.
60. **Gibreel, A., O. Skold, and D. E. Taylor.** 2004. Characterization of plasmid-mediated *aphA-3* kanamycin resistance in *Campylobacter jejuni*. *Microb. Drug Resist.* **10**:98–105.
61. **Gibreel, A., D. M. Tracz, L. Nonaka, T. M. Ngo, S. R. Connell, and D. E. Taylor.** 2004. Incidence of antibiotic resistance in *Campylobacter jejuni* isolated in Alberta, Canada, from 1999 to 2002, with special reference to *tet*(O)-mediated tetracycline resistance. *Antimicrob. Agents Chemother.* **48**:3442–3450.
62. Reference deleted.
63. **Goldstein, E. J., D. M. Citron, C. V. Merriam, K. Tyrrell, and Y. Warren.** 1999. Activity of gatifloxacin compared to those of five other quinolones versus aerobic and anaerobic isolates from skin and soft tissue samples of human and animal bite wound infections. *Antimicrob. Agents Chemother.* **43**:1475–1479.
64. **Goodchild, C., B. Dove, D. Riley, and A. J. Morris.** 2001. Antimicrobial susceptibility of *Campylobacter* species. *N. Z. Med. J.* **114**:560–561.
65. **Gootz, T. D., and B. A. Martin.** 1991. Characterization of high-level quinolone resistance in *Campylobacter jejuni*. *Antimicrob. Agents Chemother.* **35**:840–845.
66. **Grewal, J., E. K. Manavathu, and D. E. Taylor.** 1993. Effect of mutational alteration of Asn-128 in the putative GTP-binding domain of tetracycline resistance determinant Tet(O) from *Campylobacter jejuni*. *Antimicrob. Agents Chemother.* **37**:2645–2649.
67. **Grkovic, S., M. H. Brown, and R. A. Skurray.** 2002. Regulation of bacterial drug export systems. *Microbiol. Mol. Biol. Rev.* **66**:671–701.
68. **Gupta, A., J. M. Nelson, T. J. Barrett, R. V. Tauxe, S. P. Rossiter, C. R. Friedman, K. W. Joyce, K. E. Smith, T. F. Jones, M. A. Hawkins, B. Shiferaw, J. L. Beebe, D. J. Vugia, T. Rabatsky-Ehr, J. A. Benson, T. P. Root, and F. J. Angulo.** 2004. Antimicrobial resistance among *Campylobacter* strains, United States, 1997–2001. *Emerg. Infect. Dis.* **10**:1102–1109.
69. **Hakanen, A., J. Jalava, P. Kotilainen, H. Jousimies-Somer, A. Siitonen, and P. Huovinen.** 2002. *gyrA* polymorphism in *Campylobacter jejuni*: detection of *gyrA* mutations in 162 *C. jejuni* isolates by single-strand conformation polymorphism and DNA sequencing. *Antimicrob. Agents Chemother.* **46**:2644–2647.
70. **Hakanen, A. J., M. Lehtopolku, A. Siitonen, P. Huovinen, and P. Kotilainen.** 2003. Multidrug resistance in *Campylobacter jejuni* strains collected from Finnish patients during 1995–2000. *J. Antimicrob.Chemother.* **52**:1035–1039.
71. **Hanau-Bercot, B., I. Podglajen, I. Casin, and E. Collatz.** 2002. An intrinsic control element for translational initiation in class 1 integrons. *Mol. Microbiol.* **44**:119–130.
72. **Hanninen, M. L., P. Perko-Makela, A. Pitkala, and H. Rautelin.** 2000. A three-year study of *Campylobacter jejuni* genotypes in humans with domestically acquired infections and in chicken

samples from the Helsinki area. *J. Clin. Microbiol.* 38:1998–2000.

73. **Hardy, D. J., D. M. Hensey, J. M. Beyer, C. Vojtko, E. J. McDonald, and P. B. Fernandes.** 1988. Comparative in vitro activities of new 14-, 15-, and 16-membered macrolides. *Antimicrob. Agents Chemother.* 32:1710–1719.
74. **Hoge, C. W., J. M. Gambel, A. Srijan, C. Pitarangsi, and P. Echeverria.** 1998. Trends in antibiotic resistance among diarrheal pathogens isolated in Thailand over 15 years. *Clin. Infect. Dis.* 26:341–345.
75. **Hook, H., M. B. Ekegren, H. Ericsson, I. Vagsholm, and M. L. Danielsson-Tham.** 2004. Genetic and epidemiological relationships among *Campylobacter* isolates from humans. *Scand. J. Infect. Dis.* 36:435–442.
76. **Hosaka, M., T. Yasue, H. Fukuda, H. Tomizawa, H. Aoyama, and K. Hirai.** 1992. In vitro and in vivo antibacterial activities of AM-1155, a new 6-fluoro-8-methoxy quinolone. *Antimicrob. Agents Chemother.* 36:2108–2117.
77. **Isenbarger, D. W., C. W. Hoge, A. Srijan, C. Pitarangsi, N. Vithayasai, L. Bodhidatta, K. W. Hickey, and P. D. Cam.** 2002. Comparative antibiotic resistance of diarrheal pathogens from Vietnam and Thailand, 1996–1999. *Emerg. Infect. Dis.* 8:175–180.
78. **Jacob, J., S. Evers, K. Bischoff, C. Carlier, and P. Courvalin.** 1994. Characterization of the sat4 gene encoding a streptothricin acetyltransferase in *Campylobacter coli* BE/G4. *FEMS Microbiol. Lett.* 120:13–17.
79. **Jacobs-Reitsma, W. F., P. M. Koenraad, N. M. Bolder, and R. W. Mulder.** 1994. In vitro susceptibility of *Campylobacter* and *Salmonella* isolates from broilers to quinolones, ampicillin, tetracycline, and erythromycin. *Vet. Q.* 16:206–208.
80. **Jansson, C., A. Franklin, and O. Skold.** 1992. Spread of a newly found trimethoprim resistance gene, *dhfrIX*, among porcine isolates and human pathogens. *Antimicrob. Agents Chemother.* 36:2704–2708.
81. **Jensen, L. B., and F. M. Aarestrup.** 2001. Macrolide resistance in *Campylobacter coli* of animal origin in Denmark. *Antimicrob. Agents Chemother.* 45:371–372.
82. **Kampranis, S. C., and A. Maxwell.** 1998. The DNA gyrase-quinolone complex. ATP hydrolysis and the mechanism of DNA cleavage. *J. Biol. Chem.* 273:22615–22626.
83. **Kapperud, G., G. Espeland, E. Wahl, A. Walde, H. Herikstad, S. Gustavsen, I. Tveit, O. Natas, L. Bevanger, and A. Digranes.** 2003. Factors associated with increased and decreased risk of *Campylobacter* infection: a prospective case-control study in Norway. *Am. J. Epidemiol.* 158:234–242.
84. **Kassenborg, H. D., K. E. Smith, D. J. Vugia, T. Rabatsky-Ehr, M. R. Bates, M. A. Carter, N. B. Dumas, M. P. Cassidy, N. Marano, R. V. Tauxe, and F. J. Angulo.** 2004. Fluoroquinolone-resistant *Campylobacter* infections: eating poultry outside of the home and foreign travel are risk factors. *Clin. Infect. Dis.* 38(Suppl. 3):S279–S284.
85. **Krausse, R., and U. Ullmann.** 2003. In vitro activities of new fluoroquinolones against *Campylobacter jejuni* and *Campylobacter coli* isolates obtained from humans in 1980 to 1982 and 1997 to 2001. *Antimicrob. Agents Chemother.* 47:2946–2950.
86. **Lachance, N., C. Gaudreau, F. Lamothe, and L. A. Lariviere.** 1991. Role of the β-lactamase of *Campylobacter jejuni* in resistance to β-lactam agents. *Antimicrob. Agents Chemother.* 35:813–818.
87. **Lachance, N., C. Gaudreau, F. Lamothe, and F. Turgeon.** 1993. Susceptibilities of β-lactamase-positive and -negative strains of *Campylobacter coli* β-lactam agents. *Antimicrob. Agents Chemother.* 37:1174–1176.
88. **Lambert, T., G. Gerbaud, P. Trieu-Cuot, and P. Courvalin.** 1985. Structural relationship between the genes encoding 3′-aminoglycoside phosphotransferases in *Campylobacter* and in gram-positive cocci. *Ann. Inst. Pasteur Microbiol.* **136B**:135–150.
89. **Lariviere, L. A., C. L. Gaudreau, and F. F. Turgeon.** 1986. Susceptibility of clinical isolates of *Campylobacter jejuni* to twenty-five antimicrobial agents. *J. Antimicrob. Chemother.* 18:681–685.
90. **Leclercq, R.** 2002. Mechanisms of resistance to macrolides and lincosamides: nature of the resistance elements and their clinical implications. *Clin. Infect. Dis.* 34:482–492.
91. **Ledergerber, U., G. Regula, R. Stephan, J. Danuser, B. Bissig, and K. D. Stark.** 2003. Risk factors for antibiotic resistance in *Campylobacter* spp. isolated from raw poultry meat in Switzerland. *BMC Public Health* 3:39.
92. **Lee, M. D., S. Sanchez, M. Zimmer, U. Idris, M. E. Berrang, and P. F. McDermott.** 2002. Class 1 integron-associated tobramycin-gentamicin resistance in *Campylobacter jejuni* isolated from the broiler chicken house environment. *Antimicrob. Agents Chemother.* 46:3660–3664.
93. **Leipe, D. D., Y. I. Wolf, E. V. Koonin, and L. Aravind.** 2002. Classification and evolution of P-loop GTPases and related ATPases. *J. Mol. Biol.* 317:41–72.
94. **Li, C. C., C. H. Chiu, J. L. Wu, Y. C. Huang, and T. Y. Lin.** 1998. Antimicrobial susceptibilities of *Campylobacter jejuni* and *coli* by using E-test in Taiwan. *Scand. J. Infect. Dis.* 30:39–42.
95. **Li, X. Z., and H. Nikaido.** 2004. Efflux-mediated drug resistance in bacteria. *Drugs* 64:159–204.
96. **Lin, J., L. O. Michel, and Q. Zhang.** 2002. CmeABC functions as a multidrug efflux system in *Campylobacter jejuni*. *Antimicrob. Agents Chemother.* 46:2124–2131.
97. **Lin, J., O. Sahin, L. O. Michel, and Q. Zhang.** 2003. Critical role of multidrug efflux pump CmeABC in bile resistance and in vivo colonization of *Campylobacter jejuni*. *Infect. Immun.* 71:4250–4259.
98. **Lin, J., O. Sahin, and Q. Zhang.** 2003. Regulatory mechanisms of the efflux pump CmeABC in *Campylobacter jejuni*. *Int. J. Med. Microbiol.* 293:49.
99. **Lode, H., and M. Allewelt.** 2002. Role of newer fluoroquinolones in lower respiratory tract infections. *J. Antimicrob. Chemother.* 50:151–154.
100. **Lodmell, J. S., and A. E. Dahlberg.** 1997. A conformational switch in *Escherichia coli* 16S ribosomal RNA during decoding of messenger RNA. *Science* 277:1262–1267.
101. **Luber, P., J. Wagner, H. Hahn, and E. Bartelt.** 2003. Antimicrobial resistance in *Campylobacter jejuni* and *Campylobacter coli* strains isolated in 1991 and 2001–2002 from poultry and humans in Berlin, Germany. *Antimicrob. Agents Chemother.* 47:3825–3830.
102. **Lucey, B., B. Cryan, F. O'Halloran, P. G. Wall, T. Buckley, and S. Fanning.** 2002. Trends in antimicrobial susceptibility among isolates of *Campylobacter* species in Ireland and the emergence of resistance to ciprofloxacin. *Vet. Rec.* 151:317–320.
103. **Luo, N., O. Sahin, J. Lin, L. O. Michel, and Q. Zhang.** 2003. In vivo selection of *Campylobacter* isolates with high levels of fluoroquinolone resistance associated with *gyrA* mutations and the function of the CmeABC efflux pump. *Antimicrob. Agents Chemother.* 47:390–394.
104. **Manavathu, E. K., K. Hiratsuka, and D. E. Taylor.** 1988. Nucleotide sequence analysis and expression of a tetracycline-resistance gene from *Campylobacter jejuni*. *Gene* 62:17–26.
105. **McIver, C. J., J. Hogan, P. A. White, and J. W. Tapsall.** 2004. Patterns of quinolone susceptibility in *Campylobacter*

jejuni associated with different gyrA mutations. *Pathology* 36:166–169.

106. **McNulty, C. A.** 1987. The treatment of *Campylobacter* infections in man. *J. Antimicrob. Chemother.* **19:**281–284.

107. **Mégraud, F., and V. Prouzet-Mauléon.** 2004. Évolution de la résistance des Campylobacters aux antibiotiques en France (1986–2002), p. 156–158. Institut de Veille Sanitaire, Saint-Maurice, France.

108. **Michaud, S., S. Ménard, and R. D. Arbeit.** 2004. Campylobacteriosis, Eastern Townships, Québec. *Emerg. Infect. Dis.* **10:**1844–1847.

109. **Molina, J., I. Casin, P. Hausfater, E. Giretti, Y. Welker, J. Decazes, V. Garrait, P. Lagrange, and J. Modai.** 1995. *Campylobacter* infections in HIV-infected patients: clinical and bacteriological features. *AIDS* **9:**881–885.

110. **Moore, J. E., M. Crowe, N. Heaney, and E. Crothers.** 2001. Antibiotic resistance in *Campylobacter* spp. isolated from human faeces (1980–2000) and foods (1997–2000) in Northern Ireland: an update. *J. Antimicrob. Chemother.* **48:** 455–457.

111. **Moore, P. B.** 2001. The ribosome at atomic resolution. *Biochemistry* **40:**3243–3250.

112. **Nachamkin, I., J. Engberg, and F. M. Aarestrup.** 2000. Diagnosis and antimicrobial susceptibility of *Campylobacter* species, p. 45–66. *In* I. Nachamkin and M. J. Blaser (ed.), *Campylobacter*, 2nd ed. ASM Press, Washington, D.C.

113. **Nachamkin, I., H. Ung, and M. Li.** 2002. Increasing fluoroquinolone resistance in *Campylobacter jejuni*, Pennsylvania, USA, 1982–2001. *Emerg. Infect. Dis.* **8:**1501–1503.

114. **Nakajima, A., Y. Sugimoto, H. Yoneyama, and T. Nakae.** 2000. Localization of the outer membrane subunit OprM of resistance-nodulation-cell division family multicomponent efflux pump in *Pseudomonas aeruginosa. J. Biol. Chem.* **275:** 30064–30068.

115. **Neimann, J., J. Engberg, K. Mølbak, and H. C. Wegener.** 2003. A case-control study of risk factors for sporadic *Campylobacter* infections in Denmark. *Epidemiol. Infect.* **130:**353–366.

116. **Neimann, J., K. Molbak, J. Engberg, F. M. Aarestrup, and H. C. Wegener.** Longer duration of illness among *Campylobacter* patients treated with fluoroquinolones. Presented at the 11th International Workshop on *Campylobacter*, *Helicobacter* and Related Organisms, Freiburg, Germany, 1 to 5 September 2001.

117. **Nelson, J. M., K. E. Smith, D. J. Vugia, T. Rabatsky-Ehr, S. D. Segler, H. D. Kassenborg, S. M. Zansky, K. Joyce, N. Marano, R. M. Hoekstra, and F. J. Angulo.** 2004. Prolonged diarrhea due to ciprofloxacin-resistant *Campylobacter* infection. *J. Infect. Dis.* **190:**1150–1157.

118. **Nielsen, E. M., V. Fussing, J. Engberg, N. L. Nielsen, and J. Neimann.** 2003. Subtypes of *Campylobacter* isolates from retail food compared with subtypes of human isolates from the same time period and geographical regions. *Int. J. Med. Microbiol.* **293**(Suppl. 35):135.

119. **Niwa, H., T. Chuma, K. Okamoto, and K. Itoh.** 2003. Simultaneous detection of mutations associated with resistance to macrolides and quinolones in *Campylobacter jejuni* and *C. coli* using a PCR-line probe assay. *Int. J. Antimicrob. Agents* **22:**374–379.

120. **Ogle, J. M., F. V. Murphy, M. J. Tarry, and V. Ramakrishnan.** 2002. Selection of tRNA by the ribosome requires a transition from an open to a closed form. *Cell* **111:**721–732.

121. **O'Halloran, F., B. Lucey, B. Cryan, T. Buckley, and S. Fanning.** 2004. Molecular characterization of class 1 integrons from Irish thermophilic *Campylobacter* spp. *J. Antimicrob. Chemother.* **53:**952–957.

122. **Osterlund, A., M. Hermann, and G. Kahlmeter.** 2003. Antibiotic resistance among *Campylobacter jejuni/coli* strains acquired in Sweden and abroad: a longitudinal study. *Scand. J. Infect. Dis.* **35:**478–481.

123. **Ouellette, M., G. Gerbaud, T. Lambert, and P. Courvalin.** 1987. Acquisition by a *Campylobacter*-like strain of *aphA-1*, a kanamycin resistance determinant from members of the family *Enterobacteriaceae. Antimicrob. Agents Chemother.* **31:**1021–1026.

124. **Page, W. J., G. Huyer, M. Huyer, and E. A. Worobec.** 1989. Characterization of the porins of *Campylobacter jejuni* and *Campylobacter coli* and implications for antibiotic susceptibility. *Antimicrob. Agents Chemother.* **33:**297–303.

125. **Parkhill, J., B. W. Wren, K. Mungall, J. M. Ketley, C. Churcher, D. Basham, T. Chillingworth, R. M. Davies, T. Feltwell, S. Holroyd, K. Jagels, A. V. Karlyshev, S. Moule, M. J. Pallen, C. W. Penn, M. A. Quail, M. A. Rajandream, K. M. Rutherford, A. H. M. vanVliet, S. Whitehead, and B. G Barrell.** 2000. The genome sequence of the food-borne pathogen *Campylobacter jejuni* reveals hypervariable sequences. *Nature* **403:**665–668.

126. **Payot, S., L. Avrain, C. Magras, K. Praud, A. Cloeckaert, and E. Chaslus-Dancla.** 2004. Relative contribution of target gene mutation and efflux to fluoroquinolone and erythromycin resistance, in French poultry and pig isolates of *Campylobacter coli. Int. J. Antimicrob. Agents* **23:**468–472.

127. **Payot, S., A. Cloeckaert, and E. Chaslus-Dancla.** 2002. Selection and characterization of fluoroquinolone-resistant mutants of *Campylobacter jejuni* using enrofloxacin. *Microb. Drug Resist.* **8:**335–343.

128. **Pezzotti, G., A. Serafin, I. Luzzi, R. Mioni, M. Milan, and R. Perin.** 2003. Occurrence and resistance to antibiotics of *Campylobacter jejuni* and *Campylobacter coli* in animals and meat in northeastern Italy. *Int. J. Food Microbiol.* **82:**281–287.

129. **Piddock, L. J., V. Ricci, L. Pumbwe, M. J. Everett, and D. J. Griggs.** 2003. Fluoroquinolone resistance in *Campylobacter* species from man and animals: detection of mutations in topoisomerase genes. *J. Antimicrob.Chemother.* **51:**19–26.

130. **Piddock, L. J. V.** 1997. Quinolone resistance and *Campylobacter*, p. 191–199. *In The Medical Impact of the Use of Antimicrobial Use in Food Animals. Report and Proceedings of a WHO Meeting, Berlin, Germany, 13–17 October 1997.* Division of Emerging and Other Communicable Diseases Surveillance and Control, World Health Organization, Geneva, Switzerland.

131. **Pinto-Alphandary, H., C. Mabilat, and P. Courvalin.** 1990. Emergence of aminoglycoside resistance genes *aadA* and *aadE* in the genus *Campylobacter. Antimicrob. Agents Chemother.* **34:**1294–1296.

132. **Pioletti, M., F. Schlunzen, J. Harms, R. Zarivach, M. Gluhmann, H. Avila, A. Bashan, H. Bartels, T. Auerbach, C. Jacobi, T. Hartsch, A. Yonath, and F. Franceschi.** 2001. Crystal structures of complexes of the small ribosomal subunit with tetracycline, edeine and IF3. *EMBO J.* **20:**1829–1839.

133. **Poole, K.** 2004. Efflux-mediated multiresistance in Gram-negative bacteria. *Clin. Microbiol. Infect.* **10:**12–26.

134. **Potter, R. C., J. B. Kaneene, and W. N. Hall.** 2003. Risk factors for sporadic *Campylobacter jejuni* infections in rural Michigan: a prospective case-control study. *Am. J. Public Health* **93:**2118–2123.

135. **Pumbwe, L., and L. J. Piddock.** 2002. Identification and molecular characterisation of CmeB, a *Campylobacter jejuni* multidrug efflux pump. *FEMS Microbiol. Lett.* **206:**185–189.

136. **Pumbwe, L., L. P. Randall, M. J. Woodward, and L. J. Piddock.** 2004. Expression of the efflux pump genes cmeB, cmeF and the porin gene porA in multiple-antibiotic-resistant *Campylobacter jejuni*. *J. Antimicrob. Chemother.* **54:**341–347.
137. **Putnam, S. D., R. W. Frenck, M. S. Riddle, A. El Gendy, N. N. Taha, B. T. Pittner, R. Abu-Elyazeed, T. F. Wierzba, M. R. Rao, S. J. Savarino, and J. D. Clemens.** 2003. Antimicrobial susceptibility trends in *Campylobacter jejuni* and *Campylobacter coli* isolated from a rural Egyptian pediatric population with diarrhea. *Diagn. Microbiol. Infect. Dis.* **47:**601–608.
138. **Rather, P. N., H. Munayyer, P. A. Mann, R. S. Hare, G. H. Miller, and K. J. Shaw.** 1992. Genetic analysis of bacterial acetyltransferases: identification of amino acids determining the specificities of the aminoglycoside 6′-*N*-acetyltransferase Ib and IIa proteins. *J. Bacteriol.* **174:**3196–3203.
139. **Rautelin, H., A. Vierikko, M. L. Hanninen, and M. Vaara.** 2003. Antimicrobial susceptibilities of *Campylobacter* strains isolated from Finnish subjects infected domestically or from those infected abroad. *Antimicrob. Agents Chemother.* **47:** 102–105.
140. **Rees, R. E., and R. F. Retts.** 1993. *Handbook of Antibiotics.* Little, Brown & Co., Boston, Mass.
141. **Rivera, M. J., J. Castillo, C. Martin, M. Navarro, and R. Gomez-Lus.** 1986. Aminoglycoside-phosphotransferases APH(3′)-IV and APH(3″) synthesized by a strain of *Campylobacter coli*. *J. Antimicrob. Chemother.* **18:**153–158.
142. **Roberts, M. C.** 1994. Epidemiology of tetracycline-resistance determinants. *Trends Microbiol.* **2:**353–357.
143. **Ronner, A. C., E. O. Engvall, L. Andersson, and B. Kaijser.** 2004. Species identification by genotyping and determination of antibiotic resistance in *Campylobacter jejuni* and *Campylobacter coli* from humans and chickens in Sweden. *Int. J. Food Microbiol.* **96:**173–179.
144. **Ruiz, J., P. Goni, F. Marco, F. Gallardo, B. Mirelis, T. Jimenez De Anta, and J. Vila.** 1998. Increased resistance to quinolones in *Campylobacter jejuni*: a genetic analysis of *gyrA* gene mutations in quinolone-resistant clinical isolates. *Microbiol. Immunol.* **42:**223–226.
145. **Sáenz, Y., M. Zarazaga, M. Lantero, M. J. Gastanares, F. Baquero, and C. Torres.** 2000. Antibiotic resistance in *Campylobacter* strains isolated from animals, foods, and humans in Spain in 1997–1998. *Antimicrob. Agents Chemother.* **44:**267–271.
146. **Sanchez-Pescador, R., J. T. Brown, M. Roberts, and M. S. Urdea.** 1988. Homology of the TetM with translational elongation factors: implications for potential modes of tetM-conferred tetracycline resistance. *Nucleic Acids Res.* **16:**1218.
147. **Schnappinger, D., and W. Hillen.** 1996. Tetracyclines: antibiotic action, uptake, and resistance mechanisms. *Arch. Microbiol.* **165:**359–369.
148. **Schönberg-Norio, D., J. Takkinen, M.-L. Hänninen, M.-L. Katila, S.-S. Kaukoranta, L. Mattila, and H. Rautelin.** 2004. Swimming and *Campylobacter* infections. *Emerg. Infect. Dis.* **10:**1474–1477.
149. **Schwarz, S., C. Kehrenberg, B. Doublet, and A. Cloeckaert.** 2004. Molecular basis of bacterial resistance to chloramphenicol and florfenicol. *FEMS Microbiol. Rev.* **28:**519–542.
150. **Segreti, J., T. D. Gootz, L. J. Goodman, G. W. Parkhurst, J. P. Quinn, B. A. Martin, and G. M. Trenholme.** 1992. High-level quinolone resistance in clinical isolates of *Campylobacter jejuni*. *J. Infect. Dis.* **165:**667–670.
151. **Sharma, H., L. Unicomb, W. Forbes, S. Djordjevic, M. Valcanis, C. Dalton, and J. Ferguson.** 2003. Antibiotic resistance in *Campylobacter jejuni* isolated from humans in the Hunter Region, New South Wales. *Commun. Dis. Intell.* **27**(Suppl.)**:**80–88.
152. **Smith, K. E., J. M. Besser, C. W. Hedberg, F. T. Leano, J. B. Bender, J. H. Wicklund, B. P. Johnson, K.A. Moore, and M. T. Osterholm.** 1999. Quinolone-resistant *Campylobacter jejuni* infections in Minnesota, 1992–1998. *N. Engl. J. Med.* **340:**1525–1532.
153. **Spahn, C. M., G. Blaha, R. K. Agrawal, P. Penczek, R. A. Grassucci, C. A. Trieber, S. R. Connell, D. E. Taylor, K. H. Nierhaus, and J. Frank.** 2001. Localization of the ribosomal protection protein Tet(O) on the ribosome and the mechanism of tetracycline resistance. *Mol. Cell* **7:** 1037–1045.
154. **Spahn, C. M., and C. D. Prescott.** 1996. Throwing a spanner in the works: antibiotics and the translation apparatus. *J. Mol. Med.* **74:**423–439.
155. **Spahn, C. M., M. A. Schafer, A. A. Krayevsky, and K. H. Nierhaus.** 1996. Conserved nucleotides of 23 S rRNA located at the ribosomal peptidyltransferase center. *J. Biol. Chem.* **271:**32857–32862.
156. **Spratt, B. G.** 1989. Resistance to β-lactam antibiotics mediated by alterations of penicillin-binding proteins., p. 77–100. *In* L. E. Bryan (ed.), *Microbial Resistance to Drugs*. Springer-Verlag KG, Berlin, Germany.
157. **Steinbruckner, B., F. Ruberg, M. Vetter-Knoll, and M. Kist,** Antimicrobial susceptibility of *Campylobacter jejuni* and *Campylobacter coli* isolated in Freiburg from 1992–2000. Presented at the 11th International Workshop on *Campylobacter, Helicobacter* and Related Organisms, Freiburg, Germany, 1 to 5 September 2001.
158. **Stern, N. J., K. L. Hiett, G. A. Alfredsson, K. G. Kristinsson, J. Reiersen, H. Hardardottir, H. Briem, E. Gunnarsson, F. Georgsson, R. Lowman, E. Berndtson, A. M. Lammerding, G. M. Paoli, and M. T. Musgrove.** 2003. *Campylobacter* spp. in Icelandic poultry operations and human disease. *Epidemiol. Infect.* **130:**23–32.
159. **Suarez, G., and D. Nathans.** 1965. Inhibition of aminoacyl tRNA binding to ribosomes by tetracycline. *Biochem. Biophys. Res. Commun.* **18:**743–750.
160. **Tajada, P., J. L. Gomez Graces, J. I. Alos, D. Balas, and R. Cogollos.** 1996. Antimicrobial susceptibilities of *Campylobacter jejuni* and *Campylobacter coli* to 12 β-lactam agents and combinations with β-lactamase inhibitors. *Antimicrob. Agents Chemother.* **40:**1924–1925.
161. **Talsma, E., W. G. Goettsch, H. L. Nieste, P. M. Schrijnemakers, and M. J. Sprenger.** 1999. Resistance in *Campylobacter* species: increased resistance to fluoroquinolones and seasonal variation. *Clin. Infect. Dis.* **29:**845–848.
162. **Taylor, D. E.** 1981. *Campylobacter jejuni*: characteristic features of the organism and identification of transmissible plasmids in tetracycline-resistant clinical isolates, p. 61–70. *In* S. B. Levy, R. C. Clowes, and E. L. Koenig (ed.), *Molecular Biology, Pathogenicity, and Ecology of Bacterial Plasmids*. Plenum Publishing Corporation, New York, N.Y.
163. **Taylor, D. E.** 1986. Plasmid-mediated tetracycline resistance in *Campylobacter jejuni*: expression in *Escherichia coli* and identification of homology with streptococcal class M determinant. *J. Bacteriol.* **165:**1037–1039.
164. **Taylor, D. E.** 1992. Antimicrobial resistance of *Campylobacter jejuni* and *Campylobacter coli* to tetracycline, chloramphenicol, and erythromycin, p. 74–86. *In* I. Nachamkin, M. J. Blaser, and L. S. Tompkins (ed.), Campylobacter jejuni: *Current Status and Future Trends*. American Society for Microbiology, Washington, D.C.
165. **Taylor, D. E., and N. Chang.** 1991. In vitro susceptibilities of *Campylobacter jejuni* and *Campylobacter coli* to azithromycin

and erythromycin. *Antimicrob. Agents Chemother.* 35:1917–1918.

166. **Taylor, D. E., and A. Chau.** 1996. Tetracycline resistance mediated by ribosomal protection. *Antimicrob. Agents Chemother.* 40:1–5.

167. **Taylor, D. E., and A. S. Chau.** 1997. Cloning and nucleotide sequence of the *gyrA* gene from *Campylobacter* fetus subsp. *fetus* ATCC 27374 and characterization of ciprofloxacin-resistant laboratory and clinical isolates. *Antimicrob. Agents Chemother.* 41:665–671.

168. **Taylor, D. E., R. S. Garner, and B. J. Allan.** 1983. Characterization of tetracycline resistance plasmids from *Campylobacter jejuni* and *Campylobacter coli. Antimicrob. Agents Chemother.* 24:930–935.

169. **Taylor, D. E., Z. Ge, D. Purych, T. Lo, and K. Hiratsuka.** 1997. Cloning and sequence analysis of two copies of a 23S rRNA gene from *Helicobacter pylori* and association of clarithromycin resistance with 23S rRNA mutations. *Antimicrob. Agents Chemother.* 41:2621–2628.

170. **Taylor, D. E., L. J. Jerome, J. Grewal, and N. Chang.** 1995. Tet(O), a protein that mediates ribosomal protection to tetracycline, binds, and hydrolyses GTP. *Can. J. Microbiol.* 41:965–970.

171. **Taylor, D. E., L. K. Ng, and H. Lior.** 1985. Susceptibility of *Campylobacter* species to nalidixic acid, enoxacin, and other DNA gyrase inhibitors. *Antimicrob. Agents Chemother.* 28: 708–710.

172. **Taylor, D. E., C. A. Trieber, G. Trescher, and M. Bekkering.** 1998. Host mutations (*miaA* and *rpsL*) reduce tetracycline resistance mediated by Tet(O) and Tet(M). *Antimicrob. Agents Chemother.* 42:59–64.

173. **Taylor, D. E., W. Yan, L. K. Ng, E. K. Manavathu, and P. Courvalin.** 1988. Genetic characterization of kanamycin resistance in *Campylobacter coli. Ann. Inst. Pasteur Microbiol.* 139:665–676.

174. **Tee, W., and A. Mijch.** 1998. *Campylobacter jejuni* bacteremia in human immunodeficiency virus (HIV)-infected and non-HIV-infected patients: comparison of clinical features and review. *Clin. Infect. Dis.* 26:91–96.

175. **Tee, W., A. Mijch, E. Wright, and A. Yung.** 1995. Emergence of multidrug resistance in *Campylobacter jejuni* isolates from three patients infected with human immunodeficiency virus. *Clin. Infect. Dis.* 21:634–638.

176. **Tenkate, T. D., and R. J. Stafford.** 2001. Risk factors for *Campylobacter* infection in infants and young children: a matched case-control study. *Epidemiol. Infect.* 127:399–404.

177. **Tenover, F. C., M. A. Bronsdon, K. P. Gordon, and J. J. Plorde.** 1983. Isolation of plasmids encoding tetracycline resistance from *Campylobacter jejuni* strains isolated from simians. *Antimicrob. Agents Chemother.* 23:320–322.

178. **Tenover, F. C., and P. M. Elvrum.** 1988. Detection of two different kanamycin resistance genes in naturally occurring isolates of *Campylobacter jejuni* and *Campylobacter coli. Antimicrob. Agents Chemother.* 32:1170–1173.

179. **Tenover, F. C., C. L. Fennell, L. Lee, and D. J. LeBlanc.** 1992. Characterization of two plasmids from *Campylobacter jejuni* isolates that carry the *aphA-7* kanamycin resistance determinant. *Antimicrob. Agents Chemother.* 36: 712–716.

180. **Tenover, F. C., S. Williams, K. P. Gordon, C. Nolan, and J. J. Plorde.** 1985. Survey of plasmids and resistance factors in *Campylobacter jejuni* and *Campylobacter coli. Antimicrob. Agents Chemother.* 27:37–41.

181. **Tjaniadi, P., M. Lesmana, D. Subekti, N. Machpud, S. Komalarini, W. Santoso, C. H. Simanjuntak, N. Punjabi, J. R. Cambell, K. Alexander, H. J. I. Beecham, A. L. Corwin, and B. A. Oyofo.** 2003. Antimicrobial resistance of bacterial pathogens associated with diarrheal patients in Indonesia. *Am. J. Trop. Med. Hyg.* 68:666–670.

182. **Trieber, C. A., N. Burkhardt, K. H. Nierhaus, and D. E. Taylor.** 1998. Ribosomal protection from tetracycline mediated by Tet(O): Tet(O) interaction with ribosomes is GTP-dependent. *Biol. Chem.* 379:847–855.

183. **Trieber, C. A., and D. E. Taylor.** 1999. Erythromycin resistance in *Campylobacter*, p. 3. *In* H. L. T. Mobley, I. Nachamkin, and D. McGee (ed.), *Proceedings of the 10th International Workshop on Campylobacter, Helicobacter and Related Organisms.* University of Maryland School of Medicine, Baltimore.

184. **Trieber, C. A., and D. E. Taylor.** 2000. Mechanisms of antibiotic resistance in *Campylobacter*, p. 455–464. *In* I. Nachamkin and M. J. Blaser (ed.), *Campylobacter*, 2nd ed. ASM Press, Washington, D.C.

185. **Tseng, T. T., K. S. Gratwick, J. Kollman, D. Park, D. H. Nies, A. Goffeau, and M. H. Saier, Jr.** 1999. The RND permease superfamily: an ancient, ubiquitous and diverse family that includes human disease and development proteins. *J. Mol. Microbiol. Biotechnol.* 1:107–125.

186. **Tuz-Dzib, F., M. L. Guerrero, L. E. Cervantes, L. K. Pickering, and G. M. Ruiz-Palacios.** 1999. Increased incidence of quinolone resistance among clinical isolates of *Campylobacter jejuni* in Mexico. *Abstr. 10th Int. Workshop Campylobacter, Helicobacter & Relat. Org.*

187. **Unicomb, L., J. Ferguson, T. V. Riley, and P. Collignon.** 2003. Fluoroquinolone resistance in *Campylobacter* absent from isolates, Australia. *Emerg. Infect. Dis.* 9:1482–1483.

188. **Uzunovic-Kamberovic, S.** 2003. Antibiotic susceptibility of *Campylobacter jejuni* and *Campylobacter coli* human isolates from Bosnia and Herzegovina. *J. Antimicrob. Chemother.* 51:1049–1051.

189. **Vacher, S., A. Menard, E. Bernard, and F. Megraud.** 2003. PCR-restriction fragment length polymorphism analysis for detection of point mutations associated with macrolide resistance in *Campylobacter* spp. *Antimicrob. Agents Chemother.* 47:1125–1128.

190. **Vandenberg, O., Y. Glupczynski, S. Ibekwem, K. Houf, A. Dediste, N. Douat, P. Retore, G. Zissis, and J. P. Butzler,** 2003. Trends in antimicrobial susceptibility among isolates of *Campylobacter* species isolated from humans in 1996 to 2002 in Belgium. *Int. J. Med. Microbiol.* 293(Suppl. 35):1–148.

191. **Vellinga, A., and F. Van Loock.** 2002. The dioxin crisis as experiment to determine poultry-related *Campylobacter* enteritis. *Emerg. Infect. Dis.* 8:19–22.

192. **Versalovic, J., D. Shortridge, K. Kibler, M. V. Griffy, J. Beyer, R. K. Flamm, S. K. Tanaka, D. Y. Graham, and M. F. Go.** 1996. Mutations in 23S rRNA are associated with clarithromycin resistance in *Helicobacter pylori. Antimicrob. Agents Chemother.* 40:477–480.

193. **Wagner, J., M. Jabbusch, M. Eisenblatter, H. Hahn, C. Wendt, and R. Ignatius.** 2003. Susceptibilities of *Campylobacter jejuni* isolates from Germany to ciprofloxacin, moxifloxacin, erythromycin, clindamycin, and tetracycline. *Antimicrob. Agents Chemother.* 47:2358-2361.

194. **Wang, G., and D. E. Taylor.** 1998. Site-specific mutations in the 23S rRNA gene of *Helicobacter pylori* confer two types of resistance to macrolide-lincosamide-streptogramin B antibiotics. *Antimicrob. Agents Chemother.* 42:1952–1958.

195. **Wang, Y., W. M. Huang, and D. E. Taylor.** 1993. Cloning and nucleotide sequence of the *Campylobacter jejuni gyrA*

gene and characterization of quinolone resistance mutations. *Antimicrob. Agents Chemother.* **37**:457–463.

196. **Wang, Y., and D. E. Taylor.** 1990. Chloramphenicol resistance in *Campylobacter coli*: nucleotide sequence, expression, and cloning vector construction. *Gene* **94**:23–28.
197. **Wang, Y., and D. E. Taylor.** 1990. Natural transformation in *Campylobacter* species. *J. Bacteriol.* **172**:949–955.
198. **Wang, Y., and D. E. Taylor.** 1991. A DNA sequence upstream of the *tet*(O) gene is required for full expression of tetracycline resistance. *Antimicrob. Agents Chemother.* **35**: 2020–2025.
199. **Wegener, H. C., and J. Engberg.** 2003. Veterinary use of quinolones and impact on human infections, p. 387–403. *In* D. C. Hooper and E. Rubinstein (ed.), *Quinolone Antimicrobial Agents*, 3rd ed. ASM Press, Washington, D.C.
200. **Whyte, P., K. McGill, D. Cowley, R. H. Madden, L. Moran, P. Scates, C. Carroll, A. O'Leary, S. Fanning, J. D. Collins, E. McNamara, J. E. Moore, and M. Cormican.** 2004. Occurrence of *Campylobacter* in retail foods in Ireland. *Int. J. Food Microbiol.* **95**:111–118.
201. **Wickins, H. V., R. Thwaites, and J. A. Frost.** 2001. Drug resistance in *Campylobacter jejuni* and *Campylobacter coli* in England & Wales 1993–2001. Presented at the 11th International Workshop on *Campylobacter, Helicobacter* and Related Organisms, Freiburg, Germany, 1 to 5 September 2001.
202. **Willmott, C. J., and A. Maxwell.** 1993. A single point mutation in the DNA gyrase A protein greatly reduces binding of fluoroquinolones to the gyrase-DNA complex. *Antimicrob. Agents Chemother.* **37**:126–127.
203. **Wilson, I. G.** 2003. Antibiotic resistance of *Campylobacter* in raw retail chickens and imported chicken portions. *Epidemiol. Infect.* **131**:1181–1186.
204. **Wistrom, J., and S. R. Norrby.** 1995. Fluoroquinolones and bacterial enteritis, when and for whom? *J. Antimicrob. Chemother.* **36**:23–39.
205. **Yan, W., and D. E. Taylor.** 1991. Characterization of erythromycin resistance in *Campylobacter jejuni* and *Campylobacter coli. Antimicrob. Agents Chemother.* **35**:1989–1996.
206. **Zhang, Q., J. Lin, and S. Pereira.** 2003. Fluoroquinolone-resistant *Campylobacter* in animal reservoirs: dynamics of development, resistance mechanisms and ecological fitness. *Anim. Health Res. Rev.* **4**:63–71.

Antimicrobial Resistance in Bacteria of Animal Origin
Edited by Frank M. Aarestrup
© 2006 ASM Press, Washington, D.C.

Chapter 17

Antimicrobial Resistance in Nontyphoidal Salmonellae

Patrick F. McDermott

The genus *Salmonella* was first identified as a distinct group of pathogens by Theobald Smith, stemming from his work on the etiologic agent of hog cholera. The genus is named after Daniel Salmon, at the time Smith's supervisor in the Veterinary Division at the U.S. Department of Agriculture, who first reported the discovery in 1886. However, it was Smith who carried out the work while at the Department of Agriculture (72) in an early application of Koch's postulates. Now *Salmonella enterica* is recognized as one of the most common bacterial causes of food-borne diarrheal illness worldwide. On a global scale, it has been estimated that annually there are about 1.3 billion cases of acute gastroenteritis due to nontyphoidal salmonellosis, resulting in 3 million deaths (169). *Salmonella* is widely distributed in nature, colonizing a range of animal hosts, including mammals, amphibians, reptiles, birds, and insects. In industrialized countries food animals are the main reservoir for human infections, the majority of which originate from contaminated meat products and eggs. Other food vehicles include milk, cheese, fish, shellfish, fresh fruits and juice, spices, chocolate, and vegetables (97).

Salmonella causes a number of different disease syndromes ranging from asymptomatic colonization to severe extraintestinal illness, such as meningitis or osteomyelitis (65). In infected humans the most common illness is a gastroenteritis that is indistinguishable from that caused by other enteric bacterial pathogens such as *Campylobacter* and *Escherichia coli*. Depending on host factors and inoculum size, symptoms typically follow 12 to 48 hours after ingestion of the organism with contaminated food or water and usually consist of nausea, vomiting, and diarrhea. The diarrhea can contain blood, lymphocytes, and mucus. Fever, cramping, and myalgia are common. Symptoms usually resolve within 3 to 7 days, wherein primary treatment consists of fluid and electrolyte replacement. In adults the organism continues to be shed in the feces at least 4 to 6 weeks after the cessation of symptoms (35). *Salmonella* can be shed in the feces for up to 20 weeks by children <5 years of age. In a small percentage of cases (1 to 3%), infected individuals become chronic carriers, shedding the bacterium for more than 1 year. The carriage rate may be higher in developing countries, where person-to-person transmission also likely plays a larger role in human illness.

The human burden of illness due to salmonellosis is difficult to estimate in many countries. While concerted efforts are under way to expand laboratory-based surveillance, improve data quality, and strengthen public health reporting capacities around the world (175), most countries lack systematic surveillance programs. In addition, only about 10% of food-borne cases are reported (235). Most are reported in the United States, the European Union, and parts of Southeast Asia, where laboratory-based surveillance systems are in place (240). While it can be difficult to compare data on incidence in different countries, the trends from these regions suggest that salmonellosis has declined in the past few years after several decades of steady increases (17, 46, 64, 88). In the United Kingdom it is estimated that over 93,000 food-borne cases occur annually, resulting in over 3,400 hospitalizations and 268 deaths within a population of almost 60 million (4). In the United States, with a population of around 293 million, it is estimated that over 1 million cases occur each year, with >95% being food borne (150). This represents national incidences of approximately 155 and 341 per 100,000 inhabitants, respectively. In Denmark the incidence of diagnosed cases has been reduced from 90 to 40 per 100,000 as a result of the national *Salmonella* control program (186). In the United States

Patrick F. McDermott • U.S. Food and Drug Administration, Center for Veterinary Medicine, Office of Research, Division of Animal and Food Microbiology, 8401 Muirkirk Road, Laurel, MD 20708.

the annual incidence represents about 26% of all infections caused by food-borne bacterial pathogens. Children, especially those <1 year of age, and adults ≥60 years old are most vulnerable to infection and tend to have more-severe disease. Among microbial causes of zoonotic, food-borne disease, *Salmonella* produces the highest overall mortality, with an annual estimate of 168,000 physician office visits, 15,000 hospitalizations, and 400 deaths (225), mostly (59%) among patients ≥60 years of age (129). The economic costs have been estimated at $2.3 billion to $3.6 billion annually (19, 106), due to loss of work, medical care, and mortality (106).

The proportion of *Salmonella* infections caused by antimicrobial-resistant strains has steadily increased around the world and now represents 20 to 40% of all isolates from human infections (45). In developing nations, where health care institutions are fewer and access to physicians more difficult, antimicrobials are made available to the public without prescription. In these areas antimicrobials are excessively and improperly used and resistance to more recently developed antimicrobial classes is more common. In addition, the greater proportion of cases due to nosocomial spread and person-to-person contact makes hospital and community drug use a more important driving factor in *Salmonella* resistance in developing nations. In developed countries, strategies to lessen antimicrobial selection pressure have focused on food animal production environments (12). The contribution of agricultural antimicrobial use to resistance in food-borne pathogens is a long-standing controversy (149). Antimicrobials have been used in livestock and poultry since the early 1950s to improve feed efficiency, prevent disease, and treat infections. The animal production industry relies heavily on these agents to protect animal health and believes that they are needed to provide affordable, high-quality products. While it is accepted that drug use selects for resistant pathogens in the animal environment, and that these resistant variants are transmitted to humans via the food supply, there is a great deal of debate on the magnitude of the public health impact. Holmberg et al. studied a multistate outbreak of food-borne salmonellosis due to resistant *Salmonella enterica* serovar Newport carrying a common ampicillin and tetracycline resistance plasmid (117). Epidemiologic data strongly associated hamburger meat originating from a single farm in South Dakota. Similarly, an outbreak study reported by Spika et al. (199) used antimicrobial resistance and plasmid profiling to trace chloramphenicol-resistant serovar Newport from the incriminated hamburger meat back through the abattoir and to the dairy farm from which the meat was derived. The cumulative evidence from multiple studies shows that antimicrobial-resistant *Salmonella* frequently comes from food animals and can cause serious human infections (13, 28, 86, 142, 154, 237).

While animal-derived food products are a well-established vehicle of transmission, less attention has been paid to the impact of fertilizing agricultural fields for crop production using untreated wastewater or manure, and the subsequent contamination of produce by resistant fecal pathogens. Wastewater is a known source of contamination in areas where it is used (6). As animal wastes are contaminated with significant levels of zoonotic agents (122), the practice may provide a pathway for resistant, food-borne pathogens, selected in the farm environment, to disseminate to uncooked food products. The importance of this has not been quantified, but it is expected to be much less important than transmission via animal products.

In addition to research aimed at understanding the ecology of *Salmonella*, substantial effort has been made to disclose the genetic means by which *Salmonella* has evolved to resist antimicrobials. Acquired resistance arises by two main avenues: by mutations in chromosomally encoded genetic elements (both structural and regulatory sequences) and by acquisition of exogenous mobile resistance genes in the form of plasmids, integrons, and transposons. Mutation is a relatively rare event (10^{-9} to 10^{-8} cells per generation) compared with gene transfer (10^{-5} to 10^{-4} cells per generation). While both mechanisms can lead to rapid and striking changes in the fitness of a bacterial population, horizontal gene transfer appears to be most important in the evolution of *Salmonella* resistance (39). Following transfer, plasmids can be maintained as extrachromosomal elements or incorporated wholly or partially into the chromosome, where they form "genomic islands," i.e., blocks of DNA with signatures of mobile genetic elements. All of these mechanisms play a role in the evolution of resistance in *Salmonella* and will be touched upon in succeeding sections.

ANTIMICROBIALS AND RESISTANCE

Due to the self-limiting nature of the illness, typical cases of acute *Salmonella* diarrhea are not usually treated with antimicrobials. However, in the immunocompromised, elderly, and newborns, as well as in cases of severe or systemic salmonellosis, antimicrobial therapy is warranted and can be lifesaving (185). In cases where susceptible strains are involved, it may be considered as a preemptive therapy to limit outbreaks among at-risk patients, such as those in long-term care facilities (174). Historically, the recommended antimicrobials for susceptible isolates included ampicillin, chloramphenicol, and trimethoprim-sulfamethoxazole. With increasing resistance to these agents in many regions, or in cases of severe disease, a fluoroquinolone or extended-spectrum cephalosporin may be needed (115). Presently, the use of fluoroquinolones in pediatric patients is not recommended due to the potential for arthropathy (36). In children, extended-spectrum cephalosporins such as ceftriaxone are currently considered front-line therapeutics (15). Because fluoroquinolones and extended-spectrum cephalosporins are central to the management of salmonellosis, emerging resistance to these two drug classes is a paramount concern.

There is evidence that antimicrobial resistance per se causes adverse health outcomes in patients with salmonellosis. These adverse effects are summarized by Barza (26) as excess cases of illness (the "attributable fraction" of infections that otherwise would not have occurred), worse outcomes from treatment failures, and increased severity of infection. Excess cases occur in patients taking an antimicrobial. Because antimicrobials disrupt the intestinal microflora and the colonization barrier they provide, prior or concurrent antimicrobial use is a risk factor for *Salmonella* infection (173), particularly by multidrug-resistant strains (96). Antimicrobial resistance in *Salmonella* has also been associated with increased hospitalization (116, 137). In studying *S. enterica* serovar Typhimurium infections, Helms et al. (112) examined the relationship between mortality and antimicrobial resistance in 2,047 Danish patients, 59 of whom died. Compared with the general population, individuals infected by susceptible strains were 2.3 times more likely to die 2 years after infection. In contrast, patients were 4.8 times more likely to die if infected by strains of serovar Typhimurium exhibiting the ACSSuT resistance phenotype (ampicillin, chloramphenicol, streptomycin, sulfonamides, and tetracycline) and 10.3 times more likely to die if infected with quinolone-resistant strains. In a study examining 1,323 patients with serovar Typhimurium infections, quinolone resistance was associated with a 3.15-fold higher risk of invasive disease or death within 90 days of infection (111). Varma et al. concluded from a study of 7,370 cases that bloodstream infections were more likely among patients infected with a resistant strain than among those infected with a susceptible strain (223). While the relationship between virulence and antimicrobial resistance is complex and unclear, the clinical evidence suggests that the greater health burden due to resistant serovar Typhimurium definitive phage type (DT) 104 is also due in part to increased virulence in these strains (146). The potential of antibiotic exposure to coselect for virulence traits is poorly understood (54, 101).

ANTIMICROBIAL RESISTANCE IN HUMAN CLINICAL SALMONELLAE

As with many bacterial pathogens, antimicrobial resistance in nontyphoidal *Salmonella* spp. is an international problem. The levels and extent of resistance vary in different places and are influenced by antimicrobial use practices in humans and animals, as well as geographical differences in the epidemiology of *Salmonella*. In developed countries drug resistance in *Salmonella* is driven largely by the use of antimicrobials in food-producing animals (13). In general, resistance profiles reflect the length of time an agent has been in use. Thus, irrespective of isolation source (humans, foods, or food animals), resistance is seen most frequently to older antimicrobials such as chloramphenicol, streptomycin, sulfamethoxazole, and tetracycline (45, 48, 64, 99, 162, 179, 195).

Strains displaying resistance to more than one of these agents have been noted at least since the 1960s (107). A study in Britain in 1965 found that 61% of 450 *Salmonella* strains were resistant to at least one antimicrobial and that many of the phenotypes were transferable (11). Resistance to these and other agents has spread over the past 4 decades (5, 34, 137, 211), with multiple-drug resistance (MDR, defined as resistance to ≥3 antimicrobials) becoming more common. A number of studies from many different regions illustrate recent trends in resistant *Salmonella*. In Great Britain antimicrobial resistance in serovar Typhimurium more than doubled between 1981 and 1989 (213). In Spain a 7-year study showed that ampicillin resistance increased from 8 to 44%, tetracycline resistance from 1 to 42%, chloramphenicol resistance from 1.7 to 26%, and nalidixic acid resistance from 0.1 to 11% (182). In the United States resistance to tetracycline in *Salmonella* species increased from 9% in 1980 to 24% in 1990, while ampicillin resistance rose from 10 to 14% (137). Among isolates submitted to the U.S. Centers for Disease Control and Prevention (CDC), the proportion of MDR isolates with the ACSSuT phenotype increased from less than 1% in 1979 and 1980 to 34% in 1996 (95), and declined to 21% in 2002 (Fig. 1). Similarly, in France MDR *Salmonella* appeared and spread rapidly among animals and humans by the late 1990s, with more than 70% of isolates showing resistance to ampicillin, sulfonamides, streptomycin, chloramphenicol, and tetracycline (34). In

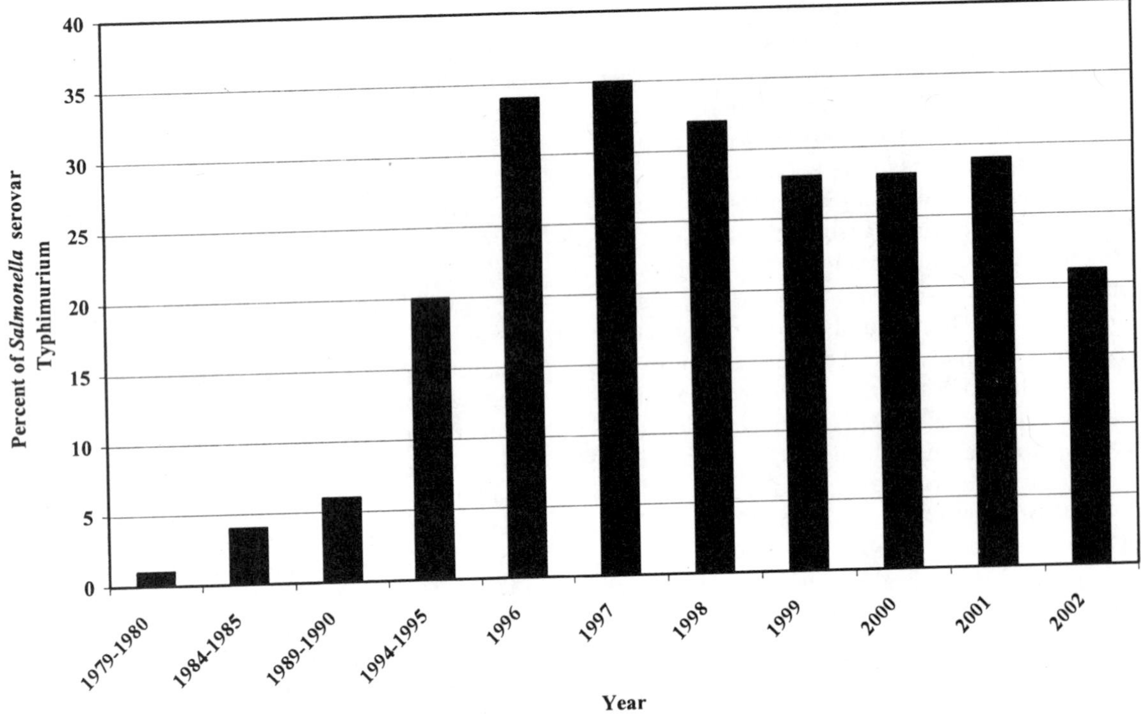

Figure 1. Proportion of *Salmonella* serovar Typhimurium isolates displaying DT104-like antimicrobial resistance in the United States. Adapted from references 45 and 95.

Canada, from 1997 to 2000, there was an increase in the proportion of *Salmonella* resistant to chloramphenicol (10 to 28%) and tetracycline (24 to 42%), with a high percentage (~20%) resistant to nitrofurantoin (55). Similarly, in Denmark resistance to ampicillin, chloramphenicol, sulfamethoxazole, and tetracycline increased two- to fourfold between 1997 and 2003, with higher levels among infections acquired abroad (64). These extensive resistance profiles among human isolates are mirrored in many nations. A report from Iran in the mid-1980s showed that 85.6% of the total *Salmonella* isolates displayed resistance to four to seven antimicrobials (85). The scientific literature is replete with similar findings from around the world (126, 127, 168, 186, 241).

In the United States, laboratory-based surveillance for antimicrobial susceptibility in human clinical isolates of nontyphoidal *Salmonella* began in 1996 and is conducted via the National Antimicrobial Resistance Monitoring System (NARMS) (45). NARMS data suggest that the level of resistance to many of the older compounds has stabilized or slightly declined. The prevalences of resistant isolates in 1996 and 2002, respectively, were as follows: for ampicillin, 21 and 13%; cephalothin, 3 and 5%; chloramphenicol, 11 and 9%; gentamicin, 5 and 1%; kanamycin, 5 and 4%; streptomycin, 21 and 13%; sulfamethoxazole, 23 and 13%; tetracycline, 24 and 15%; and trimethoprim-sulfamethoxazole, 4 and 1%. Extensive outbreaks caused by MDR *Salmonella* continue to occur. For the years 2000, 2001, and 2002, respectively, NARMS reported that 26, 28, and 21% of nontyphoidal *Salmonella* isolates were resistant to more than one drug, with 12, 12, and 9% resistant to five or more agents. Similarly, in 2000 the Enter-Net surveillance system reported data representing 10 European countries that showed that 40% of 27,059 clinical *Salmonella* isolates were resistant to at least one antimicrobial, with 18% resistant to four or more antimicrobials (210). Among these strains, 13% were resistant to chloramphenicol, 7% were resistant to trimethoprim, and 14% were resistant to nalidixic acid (210), the latter of which is a precursor to fluoroquinolone resistance (see below).

RESISTANCE IN *SALMONELLA* FROM FOOD ANIMALS AND HUMANS

The distribution of *Salmonella* strain types in humans, food animals, and retail meat products provides valuable information to understand the epidemiology of antimicrobial resistance. The association of certain serovars with animal hosts can be used to help estimate the contribution of antimicrobial use in each animal species with resistance in human isolates acquired via the food supply. Historically, serological strain typing based on surface antigen structure has been a mainstay of *Salmonella* epidemiology and a foundational tool for assessing food animals as a reservoir of resistant organisms. There are currently over 2,500 *Salmonella* serovars (178), some of which are highly adapted to specific animal hosts. For example, *Salmonella* serovar Typhi is found exclusively in humans, serovar Choleraesuis is host-adapted to swine, serovar Dublin is adapted to cattle, serovar Diarizonae is adapted to reptiles, and serovar Gallinarum is adapted to poultry. Serovars Choleraesuis and Dublin are important animal pathogens that rarely cause disease in humans. When zoonotic infections do occur, they are severe relative to illness caused by other serovars, often involving prolonged bacteremia. For example, a recent upsurge of serovar Choleraesuis infections in Taiwan was associated with an 18% mortality rate, as well as resistance to multiple antimicrobials (52). In contrast to the host-adapted serovars, others, such as serovar Typhimurium, have a broad host range and can be found in numerous wild and domesticated animal species.

Although many *Salmonella* serovars have been associated with a spectrum of human illnesses, a relatively small number of serovars are of public health importance. Most of the 2,500 *Salmonella* serovars have been implicated in human illness at some time. However, in many countries just two serovars, Enteritidis and Typhimurium, have accounted for the vast majority of disease for many years. An international study of 112,315 clinical isolates from 25 national institutions collected in the year 2000 showed that the most commonly identified serovars were Enteritidis (58%), Typhimurium (17%), and Newport (3%) (90). Following serovars Enteritidis and Typhimurium in prevalence is generally an assortment of various minor serovars that drift in regional prevalence from year to year, with occasional increases due to outbreaks. Surveillance data from Europe (210) show that in the year 2000, 79% of human infections were caused by serovars Enteritidis (54%) and Typhimurium (25%), followed by serovars Hadar (2.3%) and Virchow (1.7%). During the same time period in the United States 42% of human infections were due to serovars Enteritidis (23%) and Typhimurium (19%), followed by serovars Newport (9.3%) and Heidelberg (5.2%) (44). In other regions, such as the Caribbean (167), Mexico (243), and India (66), serovar Typhimurium is the most common, while serovar Enteritidis is relatively rare. By contrast, in Japan (17) and the United Kingdom (70) over half of infections were caused by serovar Enteritidis, with serovar Typhimurium causing a relatively minor number of cases. Different serovars may predominate in other areas (113). In 2000, for example, the most common serovars in Thailand were Weltevreden (16.1%), Anatum (10.1%), Enteritidis (7.5%), and Rissen (7.0%) (24). In Taiwan serovar Enteritidis is the most common, followed by serovars Schwarzengrund and Choleraesuis (49, 50).

The limited number of serovars causing human infections generally reflects their ability to persist in food animal reservoirs and be transmitted in the food chain. While targeted studies have been done in the past, extensive data on *Salmonella* serovars in food animal processing facilities have only recently become available. The U.S. Food Safety Inspection Service (FSIS) reported the *Salmonella* testing and serovar results for over 98,000 samples collected from broilers, cattle, pigs, ground chicken, ground turkey, and ground beef collected in the United States from January 1998 to December 2000 (191). In the following sections, the occurrence of resistance in these and other common serovars is given. It has not been possible to include all of the more than 2,500 serovars, and some that are important in individual countries may not have been included.

Serovar Typhimurium

Food-borne serovar Typhimurium infections are acquired mainly by ingesting organisms on beef and poultry that were contaminated by fecal material during processing. Other outbreaks have been linked to a variety of food products such as dairy, pork, lamb, seafood, and produce. Accordingly, Typhimurium is one of the most common serovars in food animals. Serovar Typhimurium represents 17.1% of total *Salmonella* isolations from beef carcasses, 16.6% from hog carcasses, 13.5% from chicken carcasses, 21.3% from raw ground chicken, and 12.3% from raw ground beef in the United States (191).

An important characteristic of outbreaks caused by MDR serovar Typhimurium is the emergence, widespread dissemination, and subsequent decline of various phage types over time (Fig. 2). In the United Kingdom, DT29 predominated in the late 1960s, followed by DT204 and DT193 in the 1970s and 1980s. Beginning in the 1990s, the increase in MDR *Salmonella* was driven largely by the global dissemination of serovar Typhimurium DT104 (95, 184, 209). This strain is typified by resistance to five antimicrobials: ampicillin, chloramphenicol or florfenicol, streptomycin, sulfonamides, and tetracycline (ACSSuT). This strain type first appeared in seagulls and cattle in the United Kingdom in 1984, where it was thought to have originated from gulls and exotic birds imported from Indonesia and Hong Kong (209). Since then, MDR DT104 has spread to many regions of the world (10, 22, 42, 84, 98, 171, 181, 190) and has been

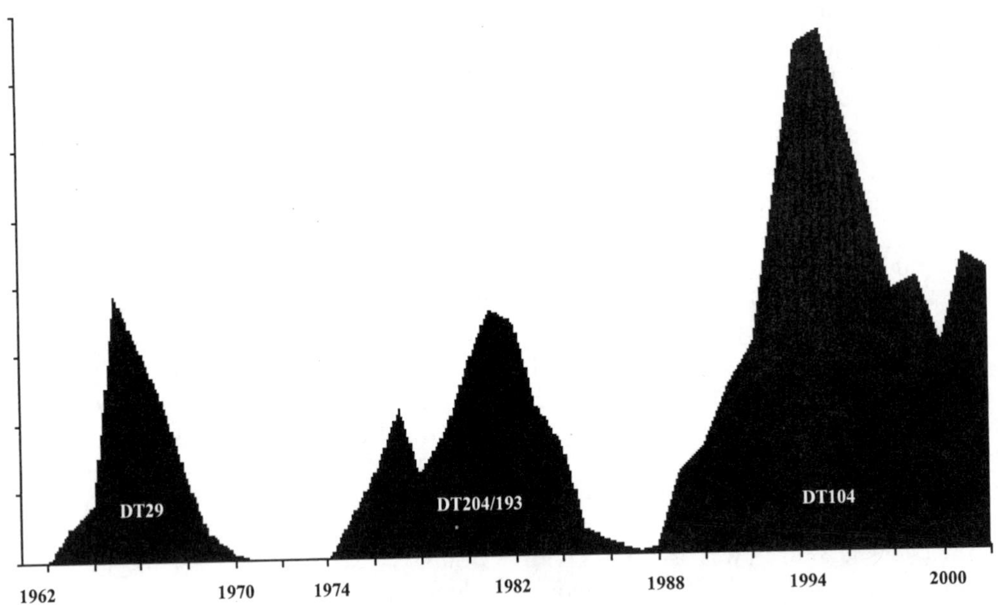

Figure 2. Changes in phage types of multidrug-resistant *Salmonella* serovar Typhimurium in England and Wales. Reprinted from reference 17a with permission from E. J. Threlfall.

isolated from many animal species, including poultry, cattle, pigs, sheep, and wild birds (121). In many countries DT104 has become the predominant Typhimurium strain type (42, 62, 197), whereas in other countries it remains rare (160b). In addition to the pentaresistance phenotype, DT104 has acquired other resistances, including trimethoprim, trimethoprim-sulfonamides, kanamycin, nalidixic acid, ciprofloxacin (214), and broad-spectrum cephalosporins (153). In recent years the importance of DT104 has decreased in the United Kingdom (Fig. 2) and elsewhere.

The genetic bases underlying multidrug resistance in serovar Typhimurium DT104 have been well characterized. The majority of isolates possess a discrete chromosomal gene cluster that encodes the entire ACSSuT resistance phenotype (33). The locus consists of the *floR* and *tet*(G) genes flanked by two class 1 integrons containing the *aadA2* and *pse-1* cassettes. The multidrug resistance region resides near the 3′ end of the 46-kb *Salmonella* genomic island 1 (SGI1). SGI1 has also been found in serovars Agona (30), Paratyphi B (152), Albany (74), Newport (75), and Typhimurium DT120 (30). It has been shown experimentally that the DT104 MDR cluster can be efficiently transduced by P22-like phages (196). Upstream of the first integron in the MDR locus is a gene encoding a putative resolvase enzyme, which demonstrates greater than 50% identity with the Tn*3* resolvase family (20). These findings support the potential for horizontal spread of the MDR gene cluster. Variations in the resistance region have also been identified, indicating recombination events independent of SGI1 transposition. In serovar Agona trimethoprim resistance has been linked to the insertion of *dfrA10* downstream of *pse-1* (73). In serovar Newport the resistance gene cluster has been found to contain *aac(3)-Id*, encoding gentamicin and sisomicin resistance, as well as a variant streptomycin and spectinomycin resistance gene, *aadA7* (75). This suggests that other *Salmonella* serovars can import SGI1 and adapt to any potential fitness costs associated with this type of acquired antimicrobial resistance.

Resistance associated with integrons has been studied extensively and is common in many MDR *Salmonella* serovars (187). While they are localized to the chromosome in DT104, they are often present on plasmids in conjunction with other resistance genes. Integrons have a specific structure consisting of two conserved segments flanking a central region in which antimicrobial resistance "gene cassettes" can be inserted in tandem (104a). The *sulI* gene, responsible for sulfonamide resistance, is located on the 3′ conserved segment. More than 70 distinct cassettes have been found in the central region of different integrons from diverse bacteria (194). Cassette-associated genes confer resistance to β-lactams, aminoglycosides, trimethoprim, chloramphenicol, and cephalosporins. There are four major integron classes, with class 1 being the most prevalent in *Salmonella* (80, 92, 100, 159, 187), both on the chromosome (61) and as passengers on plasmids (102, 220). In *Salmonella* integrons studies have uncovered one to four genes, most often encoding resistance to streptomycin and spectinomycin (*aadA*); gentamicin, kanamycin, and tobramycin (*aadB*); ampicillin (*bla*$_{PSE-1}$); and trimethoprim (*dfrV* and *dhfrXII*); as well as open reading frames of unknown function (63). Less common integron-associated phenotypes in *Salmonella* include streptothricin resistance (*sat-1*) (228, 244, 246), erythromycin resistance (*ere*A2) (91), chloramphenicol resistance (*catB*) (220), and extended-spectrum β-lactam resistance due to variants of *bla*$_{CTX-M}$ (71) and *bla*$_{OXA}$ (157). Salmonella isolates possessing multiple class 1 integrons have been identified, some with the same gene cassette (*aadA*) duplicated on different integrons within the same isolate (245). Since nearly all of these studies employed standard PCR parameters, it is not clear whether these elements are limited to a few contiguous cassettes in *Salmonella* or whether long-range PCR would reveal larger integron constructs. New gene cassettes and sequence variants are being reported regularly, highlighting the capacity of these DNA elements to mediate multiple resistances in *Salmonella* (39).

Serovar Enteritidis

Since the early 1980s chicken eggs have become recognized as the major source of serovar Enteritidis (172). The organism is present in between 1 in 12,000 and 1 in 30,000 eggs produced annually in the United States (79). Contamination of the egg can occur in the layer during ovigenesis before the shell is deposited (198) but is probably more commonly due to fecal contamination of the egg surface during passage through the cloaca. Regardless of the mode of transmission, the increasing incidence of serovar Enteritidis infection in chickens has paralleled the incidence of serovar Enteritidis infection in humans over the past 2 decades (201), making it one of the most common causes of salmonellosis in many regions (192).

In contrast to serovar Typhimurium, multiple-antimicrobial resistance in serovar Enteritidis is relatively rare, but it has been increasing in several geographical areas. A 9-year retrospective study in southern Italy found that only 2.3% of serovar Enteritidis strains were resistant to one or more antimicrobials (160). These findings were consistent with low levels reported in the United Kingdom (217), Japan (124), and Denmark. In Denmark in 2003, resistance in serovar Enteritidis was limited to nalidixic acid (14.3%) (64), which increased from 0.8% in 1995 and 8.5% in 2000. In Greece, by contrast, a 7-year study revealed a steady rise in the prevalence of resistant serovar Enteritidis between 1987 and 1991, with over 60% of strains from human and nonhuman sources showing resistance (206). In the United States serovar Enteritidis is responsible for 17% of documented human *Salmonella* infections, with 13% showing resistance to ≥1 antimicrobial and only 4% resistant to ≥2 antimicrobials (45). In Canada 27.3% of serovar Enteritidis isolates are resistant to one to four antimicrobials (55).

Serovar Heidelberg

Serovars Heidelberg and Hadar are mainly from poultry (191). Among broiler carcasses, Kentucky (25.9%) and Heidelberg (20.3%) were the two most common serovars, followed by Typhimurium (13.5%) and Hadar (7.5%) (191). These four serovars also were the most common in sampled ground chicken. Among FSIS ground turkey samples, serovar Heidelberg constituted 19.8% and serovar Hadar made up 18.6% of *Salmonella* isolates (191). Despite its prevalence in broiler carcasses, serovar Kentucky was not isolated from human clinical cases during this time period, suggesting that this serovar is not very virulent in humans. Serovar Heidelberg, on the other hand, ranked 4th (5.2%) among human cases, and Hadar ranked 16th (1% of human illness) (44). Epidemic outbreaks of serovar Heidelberg present a significant economic burden to health care systems in the United States and elsewhere (25).

Serovar Heidelberg has caused large outbreaks of food-borne illness in nursing homes, in hospitals, and within the community at large (53, 135, 142). Multiple-drug resistance in this serotype is notable. Resistance to at least ampicillin, amoxicillin-clavulanate, ceftiofur, and cephalothin was found in 8% of all serovar Heidelberg isolates submitted to the CDC in 2002 (45). These strains were also resistant to streptomycin (25%), tetracycline (25%), sulfamethoxazole (12%), chloramphenicol (12%), and trimethoprim-sulfamethoxazole (12%). This serovar derives mainly from poultry products, where ceftiofur is used in day-old chicks to control early chick mortality due to *E. coli* and *Staphylococcus aureus*. The occurrence of multiple-drug resistance in serovar Heidelberg is particularly concerning because of the propensity of this serovar to produce severe extraintestinal infections (230) such as septicemia (69) and myocarditis (37).

Serovar Hadar

In several studies from different geographical areas, serovar Hadar has been found associated with poultry (24, 123, 125, 180, 191). It is commonly found as a cause of infections in humans in many European countries (216), and isolates belonging to this serovar are often resistant to multiple antimicrobials (32, 60, 100, 239). Szych et al. (204) reported over 90% resistance to nalidixic acid among isolates from humans in Poland, as well as a frequent occurrence of resistance to ampicillin (58.5%), streptomycin

(100%), and tetracyclines (94.3%). A very high frequency of resistance to nalidixic acid (91.2%) and other antimicrobials has also been reported among serovar Hadar from human infections in Belgium (222). Threlfall et al. also reported a very high frequency of resistance to several antimicrobial agents (210, 216). For quinolones, the prevalence of resistance was 60% in 1996 and 70% in 1999 in England and Wales (216) and 57% among European isolates in 2000 (210).

Serovar Virchow

Serovar Virchow seems to be related mainly to chicken production. This serovar is a common cause of infections in humans in Europe (216), and isolates belonging to this serovar are very often multiply resistant (100, 204, 216, 239). Serovar Virchow is distinguished by its resistance to quinolone antimicrobials. In Poland, Szych et al. (204) reported 45% resistance to nalidixic acid among isolates from humans, as well as a frequent occurrence of resistance to ampicillin (13.3%), streptomycin (95.5%), and tetracyclines (85.8%). A very high, and seemingly increasing, occurrence of resistance to nalidixic acid (46.2% in 2000 and 80.9% in 2002) has been reported among serovar Virchow from human infections in Belgium (239). Similarly, Threlfall et al. reported a very high and increasing proportion of serovar Virchow isolates resistant to nalidixic acid, rising from 11% in 1996 to 39% in 1999 (216) to 53% in 2000 (210). This is particularly concerning because of the potential of this serovar to cause bloodstream infections (212).

Serovar Weltevreden

In the 1980s serovar Weltevreden emerged to supplant Enteritidis and Typhimurium as the dominant serovar associated with food-borne, nontyphoidal salmonellosis in Malaysia and Thailand (29, 242), and it is common in other countries of Southeast Asia. Enter-Net surveillance showed that 11 of 29 cases were in patients returning to Europe from travel to this region (87). Boonmar et al. (29) and Thong et al. (208) reported low levels of antimicrobial resistance in serovar Weltevreden. This was confirmed in an extensive study of 503 isolates from 10 countries, in which only 48 (9.5%) were resistant to one or more of the antimicrobial agents (2). Observed resistances included streptomycin (4.4%), sulfamethoxazole (4.2%), tetracycline (4.0%), ampicillin (1.8%), chloramphenicol (1.6%), nalidixic acid (1.6%), trimethoprim (1.4%), neomycin (0.6%), and florphenicol (0.4%). All isolates were susceptible to amoxicillin-clavulanate, colistin, gentamicin, ceftiofur, and ciprofloxacin. Resistance was also present in a low proportion of serovar Weltevreden isolates from retail foods imported to the United States from Southeast Asia, where resistance was limited to sulfamethoxazole in 1 of 24 isolates (244).

While the low prevalence of resistance in serovar Weltevreden may reflect a low past exposure to antimicrobials, it also raises the possibility that some serovars (including Enteritidis) may be less disposed to acquire resistance. Serovar Typhi, which is also generally susceptible to antimicrobials, also appears to be a poor host for plasmids. This has been attributed to a rearrangement and destabilization of plasmids received in conjugation from other *Enterobacteriaceae* (151). Whether similar systems exist in non-Typhi salmonellae is not known.

Serovar Newport

Outbreak investigations and targeted studies have identified dairy cattle as the main reservoir of serovar Newport in the United States (103). According to the FSIS, serovar Newport was detected in 10% of cattle carcasses and 6.2% of ground beef samples (191). While serovar Typhimurium DT104 has been the most prevalent MDR *Salmonella* for many years, a recent emergence of MDR serovar Newport strains in the United States and Canada, known as Newport MDR-AmpC (77), represents a new challenge. An outbreak of serovar Newport MDR-AmpC reported by the CDC identified raw or undercooked ground beef as the vehicle of transmission (16). Serovar Newport MDR-AmpC is a particular concern because of its resistance to at least nine antimicrobials, including extended-spectrum cephalosporins (16). In addition to the DT104-like resistance to ampicillin, chloramphenicol, streptomycin, sulfamethoxazole, and tetracycline, Newport-MDRAmpC isolates also are resistant to amoxicillin-clavulanic acid, cephalothin, cefoxitin, and ceftiofur and exhibit decreased susceptibility to ceftriaxone (MIC of ≥16 μg/ml). Some strains also show resistance to gentamicin, kanamycin, and trimethoprim-sulfamethoxazole. The prevalence of Newport MDR-AmpC among serovar Newport isolates from humans in the United States increased from 0% during 1996 and 1997 to 26% in 2001 (103), declining slightly to 22% in 2002 (45). This trend was mirrored in cattle isolates, rising from 0% of slaughter isolates in 1997 to 8.3% in 1998 and 27.3% in 1999, with comparable upward trends in diagnostic isolates sent to the National Veterinary Services Laboratories. Whether or not this represents a long-term epidemiological shift remains to be seen. The management practices that promote its spread are unknown. In cattle, it has been suggested that the use of tetracycline-containing milk replacer, along with other antimicrobials commonly used to treat diseases in dairy cattle, may contribute to the dissemination of Newport MDR-AmpC (118, 183).

The spread of Newport MDR-AmpC signifies a notable and troubling feature of recent surveillance trends, namely, the rise in high-number drug-resistant (HNDR) *Salmonella*, i.e., isolates resistant to ≥8 antimicrobials. The HNDR phenotype is frequently associated with the plasmid-mediated AmpC β-lactamase, bla_{CMY-2} (8, 86, 188, 232). NARMS data show that HNDR *Salmonella* increased from 0.3% of all *Salmonella* isolates in 1996 to 3% in 2002. Novel HNDR phenotypes, first widespread in serovars Typhimurium and Newport, are emerging in other serovars. This development can be explained largely by the accumulation of linked genes on large (>100 kb), transmissible MDR plasmids in *Salmonella* (86, 166, 246), *E. coli* (234), and other *Enterobacteriaceae*. These plasmids often transmit resistance to all antimicrobials except carbapenems, extended-spectrum cephalosporins, and fluoroquinolones. From an epidemiological standpoint, this is a departure from historical trends in resistance development. Whereas in the past, resistance in human pathogens typically emerged incrementally from low levels to high and from single resistances to multiple, the situation today is such that a single genetic (conjugation) event can confer resistance in *Salmonella* to as many as 12 antimicrobials (86). In addition to the obvious and serious implications for treatment, this situation can thwart attempts to mitigate resistance in both humans and animals through restricted-use practices. Since MDR plasmids can be maintained in a population by selection pressure from a single antimicrobial, or by the presence of plasmid addiction systems, populations carrying these plasmids may be very difficult to eradicate (202). Moreover, with additional, chromosomally encoded resistance mechanisms in strains harboring these plasmids, it is possible to have isolates resistant to all antimicrobial classes. The confluence of plasmid-mediated, extended-spectrum β-lactum resistance with quinolone resistance represents a serious challenge to therapy. Thus, resistance to these two important antimicrobial classes will be considered separately.

RESISTANCE TO QUINOLONES AND EXTENDED-SPECTRUM CEPHALOSPORINS

Quinolone Resistance

Fluoroquinolones are the first-line agents used in the treatment of invasive salmonellosis. Resistance to the quinolone nalidixic acid (MIC of ≥32 μg/ml) is used as a sentinel phenotype for incipient fluoroquinolone resistance. Both classes exert their antimicrobial effects by binding to DNA gyrase; thus, nalidixic acid-resistant strains display decreased susceptibility to ciprofloxacin (MIC of 0.125 to 2 μg/ml). There is disagreement on the appropriate resistance breakpoint for fluoroquinolones (and β-lactams). The Clinical and Laboratory Standards Institute (CLSI; formerly the National Committee for Clinical Laboratory Standards [NCCLS]) suggests a breakpoint for the fluoroquinolone ciprofloxacin at ≥4 μg/ml, while the breakpoint for resistance to the veterinary compound enrofloxacin is ≥2 μg/ml. Even though the CLSI does not provide specific breakpoints for bacteria associated with gastrointestinal infections in humans, this breakpoint has been widely used by medical clinicians, veterinarians, and microbiologists. However, in a recent supplement the CLSI notes that fluoroquinolone-susceptible strains of *Salmonella* that are resistant to nalidixic acid may be associated with clinical failure (56). Clinical reports have shown that isolates with a single mutation in *gyrA* are, to some extent, refractory to the bactericidal effect of fluoroquinolones (3). In several countries a resistance breakpoint of ≥1 μg/ml for fluoroquinolones is now recommended, both for evaluating laboratory susceptibility test results and when tabulating surveillance data for this group of antimicrobials in both human and veterinary medicine in order to detect the mutation responsible for resistance to quinolones (160a; EUCAST [www.escmid.org]; www.srga.org/eucastwt/MICTAB/index.html). Thus, when comparing reports on fluoroquinolone resistance from various countries, it is essential to take into account the breakpoints used in different regions.

As noted above, quinolone resistance in specific serovars of *S. enterica* has been reported from various regions around the globe. An extensive retrospective study in Spain examined susceptibility to nalidixic acid in 10,504 *Salmonella* isolates from patients with acute enteric disease between 1981 and 2003. In this time period the prevalence of resistant isolates increased from <0.5% to 38.5%, mainly in serovar Enteritidis (145). In the United States, the prevalence of nalidixic acid resistance increased from 0.4% in 1996 to 2% in 2002 (45), mainly among serovars Enteritidis, Typhimurium, Paratyphi, and Virchow. In Belgium, resistance to nalidixic acid is very high in serovar Virchow, increasing from 46.2% of isolates in 2000 to 80.9% in 2002 (239). At the same time resistance to ciprofloxacin was detected in three serovar Typhimurium isolates. In Saudi Arabia, the prevalence of resistance to nalidixic acid increased from 0.1% in 1999 to 5.5% in 2002, while ciprofloxacin resistance increased significantly, from 0.1 to 0.9% of isolates (170). In this study, 29 quinolone-resistant isolates from 2002 displayed nalidixic acid MICs of >256 μg/ml and ciprofloxacin MICs of 8 to 16 μg/ml. In serovar Typhimurium DT104, nalidixic acid resistance has also appeared. An outbreak of quinolone-resistant DT104 in Denmark, originating in swine, resulted in 11 hospitalizations and the death of 2 patients due to therapeutic failure (155).

Resistance of nontyphoidal *Salmonella* to fluoroquinolones also has become more common (43, 48, 51, 119, 170, 219). Recent data from Europe show ciprofloxacin resistance among 7.7% of human clinical isolates (88). This phenotype first appeared in limited regions of Europe in the 1990s among human and animal isolates of serovar Typhimurium (var. Copenhagen) DT204 (110) that were highly resistant (ciprofloxacin MIC of 32 μg/ml). Since then fluoroquinolone-resistant *Salmonella* has been reported in other countries (141, 158, 219). One troubling example comes from Taiwan's laboratory-based surveillance system, which began in 1997. This program tracked the rapid emergence of fluoroquinolone resistance in serovar Choleraesuis (51, 120) and its spread from pigs to humans (120). In early 2000 no isolates were resistant to ciprofloxacin. By the third quarter of 2001, 60% of serovar Choleraesuis isolates were resistant (51). This trend is of particular concern since serovar Choleraesuis, along with serovars Heidelberg, Virchow, and Dublin, is among the more invasive serovars, causing severe bacteremic infections in humans, and has historically been susceptible to most antimicrobials (200).

Intercontinental spread of fluoroquinolone resistance has been noted. While resistance to ciprofloxacin (MIC of ≥4 μg/ml) has not been reported among autochthonous isolates in the United States, an outbreak of fluoroquinolone-resistant serovar Schwarzengrund occurred in 1997 (165). This outbreak spread nosocomially in long-term-care facilities and was linked to a patient previously hospitalized in the Philippines. Travel has been associated with quinolone resistance in cases of salmonellosis from Denmark, where national control programs have been effective in limiting indigenous cases (64). Among travelers returning to Finland from Thailand, quinolone resistance increased from 3.9% to 23.5% from 1995 to 1999 (104). The emergence of quinolone resistance in *Salmonella* is an unwelcome development and underscores the need for vigorous control measures to limit the impact on public health and patient care.

The mechanisms of quinolone cell killing and the genetic bases of fluoroquinolone resistance have been studied extensively and are reviewed in the scientific literature (76, 109). Quinolones function by inhibiting the bacterial topoisomerases DNA gyrase (encoded by *gyrA*/*gyrB*) and topoisomerase IV (encoded by *parC*/*parE*), thereby disrupting transcription and replication. Mutations in these genes cluster within a specific topoisomerase subdomain termed the quinolone resistance-determining region (QRDR). These mutations function to decrease quinolone affinity for the enzyme-DNA complex (147) and allow DNA replication to continue in the presence of fluoroquinolone concentrations that are inhibitory to wild-type cell growth.

Most amino acid changes occur at Ser83 (to Phe or Tyr) and Asp87 (to Asn, Tyr, or Gly) in *gyrA* (141) and at Ser80 (to Arg) and Thr57 (to Ser) in *parC* (78). A single QRDR mutation, usually at Ser83, confers resistance to nalidixic acid and decreases susceptibility to fluoroquinolones (ciprofloxacin MICs of 0.125 to 2 μg/ml from a wild-type baseline of 0.015 to 0.03 μg/ml). Higher MICs (≥4 μg/ml) are most often associated with double *gyrA* mutations (Ser83 plus Asp87) (78, 105, 141) alone or in conjunction with *parC* (141), with less frequent changes in *gyrB* (93, 110) and *parE* (78). While these generalizations are consistent with what has been reported in other bacterial species, a recent examination of 182 *Salmonella* isolates by Eaves et al. (78) showed that the pattern and location of amino acid substitutions outside of *gyrA* and their influence on fluoroquinolone susceptibility varies by serovar.

Not all quinolone resistance is explained by topoisomerase mutations. Resistance in both clinical isolates and those selected in vitro also involves reduced drug access to the intracellular targets by decreased cell wall permeability and expression of energy-dependent drug efflux systems (94, 176). While resistance due to topoisomerase mutations characteristically results in decreased susceptibility or resistance to other members of the quinolone class, resistance due to permeability and efflux changes often generates multidrug resistance (177). In *E. coli* the AcrAB::TolC efflux pump plays a central role in MDR fluoroquinolone-resistant phenotypes (163, 164). Based on this finding, Giraud et al. (94) showed that de-repression of the AcrAB efflux pump likewise contributes to *Salmonella* fluoroquinolone resistance and may be more important than secondary mutations in topoisomerase genes. Indeed, based on an association of increased ciprofloxacin (but not nalidixic acid) susceptibility among *Salmonella* isolates with a Thr57-Ser mutation in *parC*, it has been hypothesized that some secondary mutations in *parC* may be compensatory mutations (78). Overexpression of AcrAB appears to occur before QRDR mutations and is necessary for high-level resistance (94). As in *E. coli* (163), deletion of the *Salmonella* AcrAB::TolC efflux pump reduced ciprofloxacin MICs to near wild-type levels in cells carrying topoisomerase mutations. Thus, fluoroquinolone resistance in *Salmonella* is explained, to a large extent, by a combination of target gene mutations and efflux. In *E. coli*, *acrAB-tolC* expression is part of the Mar regulon (7), which controls resistance to multiple antimicrobials and organic solvents. The *mar* locus is induced by exposure to a variety of compounds with aromatic rings, such as bile salts and tetracycline antimicrobials. Normally repressed by MarR, expression of the *mar* operon produces the transcriptional activator MarA, which in turn triggers AcrAB::TolC synthesis. The influence of *mar* in *Salmonella* was first described in a fluoroquinolone-resistant clinical isolate of serovar Typhimurium (133), and later in other serovars (9, 218). In addition to *acrAB-tolC*, *mar* regulates decreased drug uptake via downregulation of OmpF synthesis (57). While the role of efflux and mutations is obviously important, it is not clear whether decreased permeability alone is sufficient to confer clinical resistance in *Salmonella*. A number of cell wall proteins are differentially expressed in antimicrobial-resistant strains, but their functions are not known (58).

Extended-Spectrum β-Lactam Resistance

While fluoroquinolone resistance has become relatively common, resistance to extended-spectrum β-lactam agents is less prevalent: these agents may be the only efficacious therapies in some regions (48). Since the late 1980s, however, a growing number of reports have described human *Salmonella* isolates with decreased susceptibility to ceftriaxone (MIC of 16 to 32 μg/ml) or resistance to this drug (MIC of ≥64 μg/ml) (77, 229, 232). These strains produce either an extended-spectrum β-lactamase (ESBL) or a plasmid-mediated AmpC β-lactamase (153, 233). ESBLs are class A β-lactamases that hydrolyze oxyimino-cephalosporins and monobactams, but not cephamycins, and are inhibited by clavulanic acid. Most are point mutation derivatives of SHV or TEM enzymes, which are widely distributed in members of the *Enterobacteriaceae* (38). In addition—and perhaps subsequent—to gaining variants of SHV and TEM, *Salmonella* strains have acquired other plasmid-mediated class A β-lactamases such as CTX-M, KPC, PER, and OXA (153).

It is difficult to assess the prevalence of ESBL-producing *Salmonella* due to the limited number of surveillance studies. These strains first became important, and appear to be most prevalent, in developing countries, where they initially emerged and spread in the hospital setting. Some of the early cases of ESBL-producing salmonellae were in isolates from pediatric patients in Tunisia (27). Such strains are now widespread in North Africa and may be endemic in other parts of Africa, as well as India and the western Pacific region (31). In South Africa a recent survey of 160 isolates from 13 hospitals over 5 months showed that 15.6% of isolates produced SHV or TEM ESBLs and 2% produced CMY-2 (134). A survey in Europe of ESBL-producing *Salmonella* blood isolates showed that 28% carried TEM, OXA, or the combination (221).

While sporadic in most regions, ESBL-producing *Salmonella* appeared suddenly in Argentine pediatric units in 1989. Within a few years resistance spread in serovars Typhimurium, Agona, and Infantis throughout the country. A survey of five Buenos Aires hospitals from 1991 to 1994 showed strikingly high levels of coresistance to extended-spectrum cephalosporins (59%) and aminoglycosides (66%) in *Salmonella* (193). These strains were found to carry the CTX-M type of plasmid-mediated ESBLs. Over 40 types of CTX-M enzymes have been described, which are characterized by the preferential hydrolysis of cefotaxime and ceftriaxone. The CTX-M2 subtype is most prevalent in Argentina, while other variants are found in isolates from other countries (81, 156, 205). The variety of ESBL variants among *Salmonella* suggests multiple independent environmental sources for these β-lactamases. The level of genetic identity between the *Salmonella* variants and other enterics suggests that *Salmonella* acquired class A β-lactamases from hospital strains of *E. coli*, *Enterobacter cloacae*, or other nosocomial enterobacteria. Other evidence suggests food animals as reservoirs of these resistances (40). Regardless of the relative contributions of hospital and agricultural antimicrobial selection, resistance due to ESBLs spreads both clonally (19) and horizontally (136) in *Salmonella* and has been associated with strains causing enteritis and systemic infections.

More recently, a second mechanism of β-lactam resistance has appeared, due to plasmid-mediated AmpC β-lactamases. AmpC β-lactamases are mainly cephalosporinases but have some hydrolytic activity against all β-lactam antimicrobials. They impart resistance to all the β-lactam drugs except for the methoxyimino-cephalosporins and carbapenems (207), and they are not inhibited by clavulanic acid. These resistance determinants are derived from the chromosomally encoded enzymes of organisms such as *E. cloacae*, *Citrobacter freundii*, and others. Long thought to be only chromosomal genes, *ampC*-like genes appear to have been picked up by plasmids fairly recently and now spread, often undetected, among various *Enterobacteriaceae*, including *Salmonella*. The majority of *Salmonella* AmpC β-lactamases belong to the CMY gene family, whose sequence similarity suggests an origin in *C. freundii.* Two other plasmid-borne *ampC* genes have been identified in *Salmonella.* The DHA gene (derived from *Morganella morganii*) has been found in various serovars in Saudi Arabia (224), the United Kingdom (138), and Korea (132), and the ACC-1 gene (from *Hafnia alvei*) has been found in Tunisian strains of serovars Livingstone (189) and Mbandaka (143).

The emergence of the AmpC β-lactamase $bla_{CMY\text{-}2}$ has been monitored carefully in North America, where it emerged first in serovar Typhimurium (77, 232) and later as part of the multiple-antibiotic resistance genotype in livestock (86) and food-borne (16) isolates of serovar Newport MDR-AmpC. A number of CMY-2-producing *Salmonella* serovars have been detected in Europe, Africa, Australia, and Taiwan. CMY-producing salmonellae have spread from North America to Europe via the international food trade. The first report of CMY-2 *Salmonella* in the United Kingdom showed the strain to be identical to a Canadian turkey isolate (140). In Denmark in 2003 the first case of CMY-2-producing serovar Heidelberg in food animals occurred in a live boar imported from Canada (1). This finding highlights the role of live animals, which are sold worldwide for breeding purposes, in the international spread of resistant *Salmonella.* While no conclusive link was made, an outbreak of serovar Newport MDR-AmpC in northern France associated with consumption of horse meat included some meats imported from North America (83). CMY-2 is also present in *E. coli*, including isolates from raw beef, and can acquire the gene by conjugation with *Salmonella* (247). It has been speculated that the evolution of this genotype may be related to the veterinary use of ceftiofur (229), an agent in use since 1988 for treating bovine respiratory disease and other food animal infections.

The movement of the *ampC* gene onto plasmids and transmission to *Salmonella* (and other organisms) is of major concern, because it threatens the efficacy of ceftriaxone therapy, is difficult to detect, and often spreads on plasmids that carry numerous resistance determinants. Case reports from endemic regions suggest that β-lactam-resistant, multidrug-resistant *Salmonella* strains are becoming pervasive. A recent report showed that *Salmonella* isolates may acquire the capacity to produce both ESBLs and AmpC-like enzymes. An isolate of serovar Typhimurium recovered from the stool of a 14-month-old child after traveling through the Middle East was found to produce the SHV-9, CMY-7, and OXA-30 β-lactamases (106), in addition to other resistances. A case report from Honduras (139) described a child infected with a serovar Infantis strain exhibiting resistance to ampicillin, amoxicillin-clavulanic acid, ceftiofur, cefuroxime, ceftazidime, cefotaxime, ceftriaxone, cefoperazone, cefoxitin, cefpodoxime, aztreonam, amikacin, chloramphenicol, colistin sulfate, gentamicin, and sulfamethoxazole-trimethoprim. It was susceptible to imipenem and several older agents such as nalidixic acid, neomycin, tetracycline, furazolidone, and streptomycin. This isolate carried four β-lactamase genes ($bla_{TEM\text{-}1b}$, $bla_{SHV\text{-}5}$, $bla_{CTX\text{-}M\text{-}15}$, and $bla_{CMY\text{-}2}$) conferring resistance to all β-lactams except imipenem. While MDR strains carrying ESBLs and AmpC-like enzymes are a serious public health threat, none of these enzymes confers imipenem resistance. Resistance to agents in this class, however, has been discovered recently in ESBL-producing, MDR isolates. A strain of serovar Wien isolated in 2001 in Tunis was resistant to all β-lactams including imipenem, plus tetracycline, chloramphenicol, sulfonamides, gentamicin, kanamycin, and tobramycin (21). Resistance was linked to the loss of the porin OmpF and the presence of CMY-4. A second strain in the study, susceptible to imipenem, was resistant to netilmicin, amikacin, and trimethoprim-sulfamethoxazole. This strain was found to carry four different β-lactamase genes, including three ESBLs (TEM-1, SHV-2a, and CTX-M3), and the cephamycinase CMY-4 (21).

ANTIMICROBIAL-RESISTANT SALMONELLAE IN RETAIL MEATS

In conducting antimicrobial resistance surveillance and monitoring for food-borne pathogens, the World Health Organization (WHO) recommends a tripartite approach that includes isolates from human clinical cases, food animals, and retail meats (236). There is also a need to harmonize methods, sampling schemes, and reporting formats to facilitate international comparability of results (89). To date only Denmark, with the Danish Integrated Antimicrobial Resistance Monitoring and Research Programme (DANMAP) (64), has fully integrated representative monitoring of all three environments. In the United States (NARMS [45]) and Canada (Canadian Integrated Program for Antimicrobial Resistance Surveillance [55]), monitoring currently entails isolates from carcasses at slaughter in lieu of animals on farms. Other countries have established, or are in the early stages of integrating, standardized monitoring programs for various national purposes (82, 128, 161, 226).

In most areas to date, available reports of *Salmonella* resistance in animal-derived foods consist mainly of point-prevalence studies of domestic or imported foods or limited temporal surveillance data. A survey in Spain tested 112 isolates from 691 frozen and fresh chicken meat products (114). Almost half (46%) were susceptible to all antimicrobials tested. The most common resistances were to chloramphenicol (45%), ampicillin (35%), and tetracycline (34%). Resistance to multiple antimicrobials was observed in 44% of isolates, including resistance to imipenem. Serovar Typhimurium isolates tended to be more resistant than other serovars tested. A study from southern Italy (144) reported the distribution of serovars and drug resistances of 206 *Salmonella* isolates obtained between 1998 and 2000 from 172 samples of raw meats, 22 food animal fecal samples, and 12 animal feed samples. Among non-Typhimurium isolates tested, 46 of 122 (38%) strains were resistant to ≥3 antimicrobials. Typhimurium was the predominant serovar recovered, with 35 of 67 (52%) isolates displaying multidrug resistance. The characteristic DT104 antimicrobial resistance phenotype of ACSSuT was identified in 17 (8.2%) of these isolates. In Northern Ireland a survey of retail chicken products found resistance limited to sulfonamide (52%), streptomycin (26%), tetracycline (22%), and ampicillin (17%), with low rates of multidrug resistance (231).

In a 1998 U.S. pilot survey (229), *Salmonella* was recovered from 41 of 200 (21%) ground meat samples (51 chicken, 50 beef, 50 turkey, and 49 pork) purchased in the greater Washington, D.C., area. *Salmonella* was isolated more frequently from poultry (33% of chicken and 24% of turkey samples) than red meats (18% of pork and 6% of beef samples), and 84% (38 of 45) of isolates were resistant to at least one antimicrobial. The most common resistances were to older agents: tetracycline (80%), streptomycin (73%), sulfamethoxazole (69%), and ampicillin (27%). Sixteen percent of isolates displayed resistance to amoxicillin-clavulanic acid, cephalothin, ceftiofur, and ceftriaxone. Ceftriaxone-resistant *Salmonella* was isolated from ground turkey, chicken, and beef. After this initial study, the U.S. Food and Drug Administration conducted a larger pilot project (41) in Iowa over 15 months (March 2001 to June 2002), sampling randomly from 300 retail outlets across the state. One hundred thirty-one *Salmonella* strains were recovered from 126 of 981 (13%) meat samples, all but 5 of which were from ground turkey and chicken breast samples. Antimicrobial resistance was common, with 12% of isolates showing resistance to 3 antimicrobials, 5% to 7 antimicrobials, and 1% to 12 antimicrobials. Resistance to nalidixic acid ($n = 5$) and ceftiofur ($n = 2$) was seen only in isolates from ground turkey.

Following the WHO recommendations, the U.S. NARMS program expanded in 2002 to include ongoing surveillance of retail meats for antimicrobial-resistant, food-borne pathogens (http://www.fda.gov/cvm/index/narms/narms_pg.html). Data from the first 2 years of sampling showed an overall 6% *Salmonella* contamination rate for both 2002 and 2003, coming mainly from chicken breast (9.7% and 9.3%, respectively) and ground turkey (11.5% and 13.3%, respectively) products. Comparing ground turkey isolates for 2003 and 2002, respectively, resistance was common for streptomycin (45.6 versus 37.8% of isolates), tetracycline (39.5 versus 55.4%), and sulfamethoxazole (33.3 versus 20.3%). Resistance to ceftiofur decreased from 8.1% of isolates in 2002 to 2.6% in 2003, and nalidixic acid resistance decreased from 8.1 to 4.4%. For chicken breast isolates, resistance was most frequent to ampicillin (34.9% of isolates in 2003 versus 16.7% in 2002), cephalothin (30.1% versus 13.3%), and tetracycline (28.9 versus 33.3%), with increases in the number of isolates resistant to ceftiofur (26.5 versus 10%), amoxicillin-clavulanic acid (26.5 versus 10%), and cefoxitin (26.5 versus 10%) in this commodity. All isolates from both years were susceptible to amikacin, ceftriaxone, ciprofloxacin, and trimethoprim-sulfamethoxazole.

Chen et al. (47) compared antimicrobial susceptibilities of 133 isolates of *Salmonella* from retail meats acquired in the United States and China. Resistance was more common in the U.S. isolates, with 82% resistant to at least one agent, compared with 64% among Chinese isolates. Both strain sets were resistant most frequently to tetracycline (68 and 43%, respectively) streptomycin (61 and 27%), sulfamethoxazole (42 and 16%), and ampicillin (29 and 39%). Nineteen percent of U.S. retail meat isolates in this study were resistant or showed intermediate susceptibility to ceftriaxone and harbored the $bla_{\text{CMY-2}}$ gene on a mobile plasmid (47). In contrast, all of the *Salmonella* isolates from China were susceptible to ceftriaxone and none had $bla_{\text{CMY-2}}$. It was suggested that the reason for this is that ceftiofur, the only cephalosporin approved for therapeutic use in food animals, has been used in the United States since 1988, whereas it was approved for use in the People's Republic of China in 2002. In contradistinction, nalidixic acid resistance was common among China isolates (32%) and absent among U.S. isolates, likely reflecting the longer use of quinolones in China.

A study in Austria (148) conducted over 3 years examined 922 samples of pork ($n = 220$), beef ($n = 134$), chicken ($n = 288$), turkey ($n = 266$), and minced meat ($n = 14$) collected randomly from supermarkets, butchers, street markets, and abattoirs across the country. *Salmonella* was present in 16.4%

of chicken samples but was rare or absent from the other meat types. In contrast to other reports, the most common resistance among the Austrian isolates was to nalidixic acid (42% of isolates). This was followed by resistance to tetracycline (33%), streptomycin (27%), ampicillin (17%), and chloramphenicol (17%). Ciprofloxacin resistance was detected in five strains (9.6%). The limited data currently available indicate that ciprofloxacin resistance among meat isolates of *Salmonella* is not common (130). Given the absence of other known selection pressures, these findings strongly suggest that the use of fluoroquinolones in poultry production is driving the observed quinolone resistance.

Denmark's DANMAP program, begun in 1995, tests isolates from food animals, foods, and humans (64). The Danish food production model stipulates that meat and eggs from any flock infected with *Salmonella* will be heat treated and not marketed as fresh product. This control program all but ensures that domestically raised meats will be free of *Salmonella*. Thus, of the 146 *Salmonella* isolates recovered from broiler and beef samples in 2003, only 4 were derived from animals raised in Denmark (64). DANMAP is a success story in national food safety monitoring and can be considered a model program for countries where it can be implemented (227).

GLOBAL ASPECTS OF ANTIMICROBIAL-RESISTANT SALMONELLAE

Salmonella clones have shown a remarkable ability to spread worldwide. During the last decades the international spread of a number of MDR *Salmonella* clones has been observed. The striking example of global dissemination illustrated by MDR DT104 is a case in point. This strain has contributed to the prevalence of resistance reported in many regions (68) and may be present in almost all countries (23, 67, 215). The mode of transmission is not definitively known but is most likely related to trade of breeding animals, human travel, and international sales of food products.

Food is an important vehicle for the national and international transmission of antimicrobial-resistant bacteria and antimicrobial resistance genes from food animals to humans, and international outbreaks have been reported (59, 108, 131, 215). Crook et al. (59) reported a European outbreak of MDR serovar Typhimurium DT204b involving 392 people in England and Wales, Germany, Iceland, Scotland, and The Netherlands. The source was probably imported lettuce originating from a common source. In Denmark a much higher frequency of antimicrobial resistance and multiple-drug resistance has been observed in salmonellae from imported food products compared to isolates from domestic products (M. N. Skov et al., submitted for publication). Furthermore, it was estimated for 2003 that, while 75% of all human cases with serovar Typhimurium could be attributed to Danish products and only 25% to imported food, 60% of all infections with MDR serovar Typhimurium were related to imported food products (18). Therefore, more infections with MDR serovar Typhimurium occur in humans in Denmark as a consequence of imported foods than domestically raised products. The global trade in food products is expected to increase in the future. Thus, endeavors to improve food safety have to take into account the importance of resistant *Salmonella* in imported food products. As food is distributed worldwide, attempts to control the spread of antimicrobial resistance must be approached internationally, in order to reduce or eliminate contamination by antimicrobial-resistant *Salmonella* at the primary production site. Recently, the WHO has launched the Global Salm Surv program (238) in an attempt to determine the global importance and occurrence of different *Salmonella* serovars and their antimicrobial susceptibility. This is an important first step in controlling *Salmonella* and antimicrobial resistance in the modern globalized economy.

CONCLUDING REMARKS

Given the importance of *Salmonella* as a pathogen, its ability to acquire antimicrobial resistance, and its capacity for intercontinental transmission, national and regional surveillance systems are needed to measure and monitor drug resistance in these organisms. Given the steady loss of antimicrobial efficacy over the past decades, this information is becoming an indispensable component of patient care and is needed to revise the canon of preferred antimicrobial therapeutics. In addition, special emphasis on the resistance mechanisms involved and a refinement of genetic methods to understand the biology of resistant *Salmonella* will help counteract the emergence and spread of resistant strains.

REFERENCES

1. **Aarestrup, F. M., H. Hasman, I. Olsen, and G. Sorensen.** 2004. International spread of bla_{CMY-2}-mediated cephalosporin resistance in a multiresistant *Salmonella enterica* serovar Heidelberg isolate stemming from the importation of a boar by Denmark from Canada. *Antimicrob. Agents Chemother.* 48: 1916–1917.
2. **Aarestrup, F. M., M. Lertworapreecha, M. C. Evans, A. Bangtrakulnonth, T. Chalermchaikit, R. S. Hendriksen, and**

H. C. Wegener. 2003. Antimicrobial susceptibility and occurrence of resistance genes among *Salmonella enterica* serovar Weltevreden from different countries. *J. Antimicrob. Chemother.* **52:**715–718.

3. **Aarestrup, F. M., C. Wiuff, K. Molbak, and E. J. Threlfall.** 2003. Is it time to change fluoroquinolone breakpoints for *Salmonella* spp.? *Antimicrob. Agents Chemother.* **47:**827–829.
4. **Adak, G. K., S. M. Long, and S. J. O'Brien**. 2002. Trends in indigenous foodborne disease and deaths, England and Wales: 1992 to 2000. *Gut* **51:**832–841.
5. **Agarwal, K. C., R. K. Garg, B. R. Panhotra, A. D. Verma, A. Ayyagari, and J. Mahanta**. 1980. Drug resistance in Salmonellae isolated at Chandigarh (India) during 1972–1978. *Antonie Leeuwenhoek* **46:**383–390.
6. **Ait Melloul, A., L. Hassani, and L. Rafouk**. 2001. *Salmonella* contamination of vegetables irrigated with untreated wastewater. *World J. Microbiol. Biotechnol.* **17:**207–209.
7. **Alekshun, M. N., and S. B. Levy**. 1999. The *mar* regulon: multiple resistance to antibiotics and other toxic chemicals. *Trends Microbiol.* **7:**410–413.
8. **Allen, K. J., and C. Poppe**. 2002. Occurrence and characterization of resistance to extended-spectrum cephalosporins mediated by β-lactamase CMY-2 in *Salmonella* isolated from food-producing animals in Canada. *Can. J. Vet. Res.* **66:** 137–144.
9. **Allen, K. J., and C. Poppe**. 2002. Phenotypic and genotypic characterization of food animal isolates of *Salmonella* with reduced sensitivity to ciprofloxacin. *Microb. Drug Resist.* **8:** 375–383.
10. **Alvseike, O., T. Leegaard, P. Aavitsland, and J. Lassen**. 2002. Trend of multiple drug resistant *Salmonella* Typhimurium in Norway. *Eur. Surveill.* **7:**5–7.
11. **Anderson, E. S., and M. J. Lewis**. 1965. Drug resistance and its transfer in *Salmonella typhimurium*. *Nature* **206:**579–583.
12. **Angulo, F. J., K. R. Johnson, R. V. Tauxe, and M. L. Cohen**. 2000. Origins and consequences of antimicrobial-resistant nontyphoidal *Salmonella*: implications for the use of fluoroquinolones in food animals. *Microb. Drug Resist.* **6:**77–83.
13. **Angulo, F. J., V. N. Nargund, and T. C. Chiller**. 2004. Evidence of an association between use of anti-microbial agents in food animals and anti-microbial resistance among bacteria isolated from humans and the human health consequences of such resistance. *J. Vet. Med. B* **51:**374–379.
14. Reference deleted.
15. **Anonymous**. 2000. *Salmonella* infections, p. 501–506. *In* L. K. Pickering (ed.), *Red Book: Report of the Committee on Infectious Diseases*. American Academy of Pediatrics, Committee on Infectious Diseases, Elk Grove Village, Ill.
16. **Anonymous**. 2002. Outbreak of multidrug-resistant *Salmonella* Newport—United States, January-April 2002. *JAMA* **288:**951–953.
17. **Anonymous**. 2003. Salmonellosis in Japan as of June 2003. *Infect. Agents Surveill. Rep.* **24:**179–180.

17a. **Anonymous.** 2003. *Annual Report 2002*. Division of Gastrointestinal Infections, Central Public Health Laboratory, Health Protection Agency, London, United Kingdom. [Online.] http://www.hpa.org.uk/srmd/div_dgi/dgi_annual_report_02.pdf.

18. **Anonymous**. 2004. *Annual Report on Zoonoses in Denmark 2003*. Ministry of Agriculture, Food and Fisheries, Copenhagen, Denmark.
19. **Antunes, P., J. Machado, J. C. Sousa, and L. Peixe**. 2004. Dissemination amongst humans and food products of animal origin of a *Salmonella typhimurium* clone expressing an integron-borne OXA-30 β-lactamase. *J. Antimicrob. Chemother.* **54:** 429–434.
20. **Arcangioli, M. A., S. Leroy-Setrin, J. L. Martel, and E. Chaslus-Dancla**. 1999. A new chloramphenicol and florfenicol resistance gene flanked by two integron structures in *Salmonella typhimurium* DT104. *FEMS Microbiol. Lett.* **174:**327–332.
21. **Armand-Lefevre, L., V. Leflon-Guibout, J. Bredin, F. Barguellil, A. Amor, J. M. Pages, and M. H. Nicolas-Chanoine**. 2003. Imipenem resistance in *Salmonella enterica* serovar Wien related to porin loss and CMY-4 β-lactamase production. *Antimicrob. Agents Chemother.* **47:**1165–1168.
22. **Baggesen, D. L., and F. M. Aarestrup**. 1998. Characterisation of recently emerged multiple antibiotic-resistant *Salmonella enterica* serovar Typhimurium DT104 and other multiresistant phage types from Danish pig herds. *Vet. Rec.* **143:** 95–97.
23. **Baggesen, D. L., D. Sandvang, and F. M. Aarestrup**. 2000. Characterization of *Salmonella enterica* serovar Typhimurium DT104 isolated from Denmark and comparison with isolates from Europe and the United States. *J. Clin. Microbiol.* **38:** 1581–1586.
24. **Bangtrakulnonth, A., S. Pornreongwong, C. Pulsrikarn, P. Sawanpanyalert, R. S. Hendriksen, D. M. Lo Fo Wong, and F. M. Aarestrup**. 2004. *Salmonella* serovars from humans and other sources in Thailand, 1993–2002. *Emerg. Infect. Dis.* **10:**131–136.
25. **Barnass, S., M. O'Mahony, P. N. Sockett, J. Garner, J. Franklin, and S. Tabaqchali**. 1989. The tangible cost implications of a hospital outbreak of multiply-resistant Salmonella. *Epidemiol. Infect.* **103:**227–234.
26. **Barza, M.** 2002. Potential mechanisms of increased disease in humans from antimicrobial resistance in food animals. *Clin. Infect. Dis.* **34**(Suppl. 3):S123–S125.
27. **Ben Hassen, A., G. Fournier, A. Kechrid, C. Fendri, S. Ben Redjeb, and A. Philippon**. 1990. Enzymatic resistance to cefotaxime in 56 strains of Klebsiella spp., Escherichia coli and Salmonella spp. at a Tunisian hospital (1984–1988). *Pathol. Biol.* (Paris) **38:**464–469. (In French.)
28. **Bezanson, G. S., R. Khakhria, and E. Bollegraaf**. 1983. Nosocomial outbreak caused by antibiotic-resistant strain of *Salmonella typhimurium* acquired from dairy cattle. *Can. Med. Assoc. J.* **128:**426–427.
29. **Boonmar, S., A. Bangtrakulnonth, S. Pornrunangwong, N. Marnrim, K. Kaneko, and M. Ogawa**. 1998. Predominant serovars of *Salmonella* in humans and foods from Thailand. *J. Vet. Med. Sci.* **60:**877–880.
30. **Boyd, D., G. A. Peters, A. Cloeckaert, K. S. Boumedine, E. Chaslus-Dancla, H. Imberechts, and M. R. Mulvey**. 2001. Complete nucleotide sequence of a 43-kilobase genomic island associated with the multidrug resistance region of *Salmonella enterica* serovar Typhimurium DT104 and its identification in phage type DT120 and serovar Agona. *J. Bacteriol.* **183:** 5725–5732.
31. **Bradford, P. A.** 2001. Extended-spectrum β-lactamases in the 21st century: characterization, epidemiology, and detection of this important resistance threat. *Clin. Microbiol. Rev.* **14:** 933–951.
32. **Breuil, J., A. Brisabois, I. Casin, L. Armand-Lefevre, S. Fremy, and E. Collatz**. 2000. Antibiotic resistance in salmonellae isolated from humans and animals in France: comparative data from 1994 and 1997. *J. Antimicrob. Chemother.* **46:**965–971.
33. **Briggs, C. E., and P. M. Fratamico**. 1999. Molecular characterization of an antibiotic resistance gene cluster of *Salmonella typhimurium* DT104. *Antimicrob. Agents Chemother.* **43:**846–849.
34. **Brisabois, A., I. Cazin, J. Breuil, and E. Collatz**. 1997. Surveillance of antibiotic resistance in *Salmonella*. *Eur. Surveill.* **2:** 19–20.

35. **Buchwald, D. S., and M. J. Blaser.** 1984. A review of human salmonellosis: II. Duration of excretion following infection with nontyphi Salmonella. *Rev. Infect. Dis.* **6:**345–356.
36. **Burkhardt, J. E., J. N. Walterspiel, and U. B. Schaad.** 1997. Quinolone arthropathy in animals versus children. *Clin. Infect. Dis.* **25:**1196–1204.
37. **Burt, C. R., J. C. Proudfoot, M. Roberts, and R. H. Horowitz.** 1990. Fatal myocarditis secondary to Salmonella septicemia in a young adult. *J. Emerg. Med.* **8:**295–297.
38. **Bush, K., G. A. Jacoby, and A. A. Medeiros.** 1995. A functional classification scheme for β-lactamases and its correlation with molecular structure. *Antimicrob. Agents Chemother.* **39:** 1211–1233.
39. **Carattoli, A., L. Villa, C. Pezzella, E. Bordi, and P. Visca.** 2001. Expanding drug resistance through integron acquisition by IncFI plasmids of *Salmonella enterica* Typhimurium. *Emerg. Infect. Dis.* **7:**444–447.
40. **Cardinale, E., P. Colbachini, J. D. Perrier-Gros-Claude, A. Gassama, and A. Aidara-Kane.** 2001. Dual emergence in food and humans of a novel multiresistant serotype of *Salmonella* in Senegal: *Salmonella enterica* subsp. *enterica* serotype 35:c:1,2. *J. Clin. Microbiol.* **39:**2373–2374.
41. **Carter, P. J., L. L. English, B. Cook, T. Proescholdt, and D. G. White.** 2002. Prevalence and antimicrobial susceptibility profiles of *Salmonella* and *Campylobacter* isolated from retail meats, abstr. P-84. *Abstr. 102nd Gen. Meet. Am. Soc. Microbiol.* American Society for Microbiology, Washington, D.C.
42. **Casin, I., J. Breuil, A. Brisabois, F. Moury, F. Grimont, and E. Collatz.** 1999. Multidrug-resistant human and animal *Salmonella typhimurium* isolates in France belong predominantly to a DT104 clone with the chromosome- and integron-encoded β-lactamase PSE-1. *J. Infect. Dis.* **179:**1173–1182.
43. **Casin, I., J. Breuil, J. P. Darchis, C. Guelpa, and E. Collatz.** 2003. Fluoroquinolone resistance linked to GyrA, GyrB, and ParC mutations in *Salmonella enterica* Typhimurium isolates in humans. *Emerg. Infect. Dis.* **9:**1455–1457.
44. **Centers for Disease Control and Prevention.** 2001. Salmonella *Surveillance: Annual Summary, 2000.* Centers for Disease Control and Prevention, U.S. Department of Health and Human Services, Atlanta, Ga.
45. **Centers for Disease Control and Prevention.** 2004. *National Antimicrobial Resistance Monitoring System for Enteric Bacteria (NARMS): 2002 Annual Report.* Centers for Disease Control and Prevention, U.S. Department of Health and Human Services, Atlanta, Ga.
46. **Centers for Disease Control and Prevention.** 2004. Preliminary FoodNet data on the incidence of infection with pathogens transmitted commonly through food—selected sites, United States, 2003. *Morb. Mortal. Wkly. Rep.* **53:**338–343.
47. **Chen, S., S. Zhao, D. G. White, C. M. Schroeder, R. Lu, H. Yang, P. F. McDermott, S. Ayers, and J. Meng.** 2004. Characterization of multiple-antimicrobial-resistant *Salmonella* serovars isolated from retail meats. *Appl. Environ. Microbiol.* **70:**1–7.
48. **Chiappini, E., L. Galli, P. Pecile, A. Vierucci, and M. de Martino.** 2002. Results of a 5-year prospective surveillance study of antibiotic resistance among *Salmonella enterica* isolates and ceftriaxone therapy among children hospitalized for acute diarrhea. *Clin. Ther.* **24:**1585–1594.
49. **Chiu, C. H., T. Y. Lin, and J. T. Ou.** 1999. Predictors for extraintestinal infection of non-typhoidal *Salmonella* in patients without AIDS. *Int. J. Clin. Pract.* **53:**161–164.
50. **Chiu, C. H., T. Y. Lin, and J. T. Ou.** 1999. Prevalence of the virulence plasmids of nontyphoid *Salmonella* in the serovars isolated from humans and their association with bacteremia. *Microbiol. Immunol.* **43:**899–903.
51. **Chiu, C. H., T. L. Wu, L. H. Su, C. Chu, J. H. Chia, A. J. Kuo, M. S. Chien, and T. Y. Lin.** 2002. The emergence in Taiwan of fluoroquinolone resistance in *Salmonella enterica* serotype Choleraesuis. *N. Engl. J. Med.* **346:**413–419.
52. **Chiu, S., C. H. Chiu, and T. Y. Lin.** 2004. *Salmonella enterica* serotype Choleraesuis infection in a medical center in northern Taiwan. *J. Microbiol. Immunol. Infect.* **37:**99–102.
53. **Choi, M., T. T. Yoshikawa, J. Bridge, A. Schlaifer, D. Osterweil, D. Reid, and D. C. Norman.** 1990. Salmonella outbreak in a nursing home. *J. Am. Geriatr. Soc.* **38:**531–534.
54. **Chu, C., C. H. Chiu, W. Y. Wu, C. H. Chu, T. P. Liu, and J. T. Ou.** 2001. Large drug resistance virulence plasmids of clinical isolates of *Salmonella enterica* serovar Choleraesuis. *Antimicrob. Agents Chemother.* **45:**2299–2303.
55. **CIPARS.** 2004. Canadian Integrated Program for Antimicrobial Resistance Surveillance (CIPARS), Annual Report, 2002. [Online.] http://www.phac-aspc.gc.ca/cipars-picra/pdf/cipars-picra-2002_e.pdf.
56. **Clinical and Laboratory Standards Institute.** 2004. Performance standards for antimicrobial susceptibility testing. CLSI document M100-S14, 14th informational supplement. Clinical and Laboratory Standards Institute, Wayne, Pa.
57. **Cohen, S. P., L. M. McMurry, and S. B. Levy.** 1988. *marA* locus causes decreased expression of OmpF porin in multiple-antibiotic-resistant (Mar) mutants of *Escherichia coli. J. Bacteriol.* **170:**5416–5422.
58. **Coldham, N. G., and M. J. Woodward.** 2004. Characterization of the *Salmonella typhimurium* proteome by semi-automated two dimensional HPLC-mass spectrometry: detection of proteins implicated in multiple antibiotic resistance. *J. Proteome Res.* **3:**595–603.
59. **Crook, P. D., J. F. Aguilera, E. J. Threlfall, S. J. O'Brien, G. Sigmundsdottir, D. Wilson, I. S. Fisher, A. Ammon, H. Briem, J. M. Cowden, M. E. Locking, H. Tschape, W. van Pelt, L. R. Ward, and M. A. Widdowson.** 2003. A European outbreak of *Salmonella enterica* serotype Typhimurium definitive phage type 204b in 2000. *Clin. Microbiol. Infect.* **9:**839–845.
60. **Cruchaga, S., A. Echeita, A. Aladuena, J. Garcia-Pena, N. Frias, and M. A. Usera.** 2001. Antimicrobial resistance in salmonellae from humans, food and animals in Spain in 1998. *J. Antimicrob. Chemother.* **47:**315–321.
61. **Daly, M., J. Buckley, E. Power, and S. Fanning.** 2004. Evidence for a chromosomally located third integron in *Salmonella enterica* serovar Typhimurium DT104b. *Antimicrob. Agents Chemother.* **48:**1350–1352.
62. **Daly, M., J. Buckley, E. Power, C. O'Hare, M. Cormican, B. Cryan, P. G. Wall, and S. Fanning.** 2000. Molecular characterization of Irish *Salmonella enterica* serotype Typhimurium: detection of class I integrons and assessment of genetic relationships by DNA amplification fingerprinting. *Appl. Environ. Microbiol.* **66:**614–619.
63. **Daly, M., and S. Fanning.** 2004. Integron analysis and genetic mapping of antimicrobial resistance genes in *Salmonella enterica* serotype Typhimurium. p. 15–32. *In* J. F. T. Spencer and A. L. Ragout de Spencer (ed.), *Public Health Microbiology: Methods and Protocols.* Humana Press, Inc., Totowa, N.J.
64. **DANMAP.** 2004. DANMAP 2003—Use of antimicrobial agents and occurrence of antimicrobial resistance in bacteria from food animals, foods and humans in Denmark. [Online.] http://www.dfvf.dk/Files/Filer/Zoonosecentret/Publikationer/Danmap/Danmap_2003.pdf.
65. **Darwin, K. H., and V. L. Miller.** 1999. Molecular basis of the interaction of *Salmonella* with the intestinal mucosa. *Clin. Microbiol. Rev.* **12:**405–428.
66. **Das, S., S. Gupta, and Mukesh.** 2002. Serotypic and antibiotic susceptibility pattern of *Salmonella* species isolated from cases

of gastroenteritis at Infectious Diseases Hospital (IDH), Delhi from 1997–2000. *J. Commun. Dis.* **34:**237–244.

67. **Davis, M. A., D. D. Hancock, and T. E. Besser.** 2002. Multiresistant clones of *Salmonella enterica*: the importance of dissemination. *J. Lab. Clin. Med.* **140:**135–141.
68. **Davis, M. A., D. D. Hancock, T. E. Besser, D. H. Rice, J. M. Gay, C. Gay, L. Gearhart, and R. Digiacomo.** 1999. Changes in antimicrobial resistance among *Salmonella enterica* serovar Typhimurium isolates from humans and cattle in the Northwestern United States, 1982–1997. *Emerg. Infect. Dis.* **5:**802–806.
69. **Demczuk, W., R. Ahmed, D. Woodward, C. Clark, and F. Rodgers.** 2000. *Laboratory Surveillance for Enteric Pathogens in Canada, 2000 Annual Summary.* The Canadian Science Centre for Human and Animal Health, Winnipeg, Manitoba, Canada.
70. **Department for Environment, Food and Rural Affairs.** 2004. Salmonella *in Livestock Production in Great Britain in 2003*, p. 17. Veterinary Laboratories Agency, Addlestone, Surrey, United Kingdom.
71. **Di Conza, J., J. A. Ayala, P. Power, M. Mollerach, and G. Gutkind.** 2002. Novel class 1 integron (InS21) carrying $bla_{CTX-M-2}$ in *Salmonella enterica* serovar Infantis. *Antimicrob. Agents Chemother.* **46:**2257–2261.
72. **Dolman, C. E., and R. J. Wolfe.** 2003. *Suppressing the Diseases of Animals and Man: Theobald Smith, Microbiologist.* Harvard University Press, Boston, Mass.
73. **Doublet, B., P. Butaye, H. Imberechts, D. Boyd, M. R. Mulvey, E. Chaslus-Dancla, and A. Cloeckaert.** 2004. *Salmonella* genomic island 1 multidrug resistance gene clusters in *Salmonella enterica* serovar Agona isolated in Belgium in 1992 to 2002. *Antimicrob. Agents Chemother.* **48:**2510–2517.
74. **Doublet, B., R. Lailler, D. Meunier, A. Brisabois, D. Boyd, M. R. Mulvey, E. Chaslus-Dancla, and A. Cloeckaert.** 2003. Variant *Salmonella* genomic island 1 antibiotic resistance gene cluster in *Salmonella enterica* serovar Albany. *Emerg. Infect. Dis.* **9:**585–591.
75. **Doublet, B., F. X. Weill, L. Fabre, E. Chaslus-Dancla, and A. Cloeckaert.** 2004. Variant *Salmonella* genomic island 1 antibiotic resistance gene cluster containing a novel *3′-N*-aminoglycoside acetyltransferase gene cassette, *aac*(3)-*Id*, in *Salmonella enterica* serovar Newport. *Antimicrob. Agents Chemother.* **48:**3806–3812.
76. **Drlica, K., and M. Malik.** 2003. Fluoroquinolones: action and resistance. *Curr. Top. Med. Chem.* **3:**249–282.
77. **Dunne, E. F., P. D. Fey, P. Kludt, R. Reporter, F. Mostashari, P. Shillam, J. Wicklund, C. Miller, B. Holland, K. Stamey, T. J. Barrett, J. K. Rasheed, F. C. Tenover, E. M. Ribot, and F. J. Angulo.** 2000. Emergence of domestically acquired ceftriaxone-resistant *Salmonella* infections associated with AmpC beta-lactamase. *JAMA* **284:**3151–3156.
78. **Eaves, D. J., L. Randall, D. T. Gray, A. Buckley, M. J. Woodward, A. P. White, and L. J. Piddock.** 2004. Prevalence of mutations within the quinolone resistance-determining region of *gyrA*, *gyrB*, *parC*, and *parE* and association with antibiotic resistance in quinolone-resistant *Salmonella enterica*. *Antimicrob. Agents Chemother.* **48:**4012–4015.
79. **Ebel, E., and W. Schlosser.** 2000. Estimating the annual fraction of eggs contaminated with *Salmonella enteritidis* in the United States. *Int. J. Food Microbiol.* **61:**51–62.
80. **Ebner, P., K. Garner, and A. Mathew.** 2004. Class 1 integrons in various *Salmonella enterica* serovars isolated from animals and identification of genomic island SGI1 in *Salmonella enterica* var. Meleagridis. *J. Antimicrob. Chemother.* **53:**1004–1009.
81. **Edelstein, M., M. Pimkin, T. Dmitrachenko, V. Semenov, N. Kozlova, D. Gladin, A. Baraniak, and L. Stratchounski.** 2004. Multiple outbreaks of nosocomial salmonellosis in Russia and Belarus caused by a single clone of *Salmonella enterica* serovar Typhimurium producing an extended-spectrum β-lactamase. *Antimicrob. Agents Chemother.* **48:**2808–2815.
82. **Esaki, H., A. Morioka, K. Ishihara, A. Kojima, S. Shiroki, Y. Tamura, and T. Takahashi.** 2004. Antimicrobial susceptibility of *Salmonella* isolated from cattle, swine and poultry (2001–2002): report from the Japanese Veterinary Antimicrobial Resistance Monitoring Program. *J. Antimicrob. Chemother.* **53:**266–270.
83. **Espié, E., and F. X. Weill.** 2003. Outbreak of multidrug resistant *Salmonella* Newport due to the consumption of horsemeat in France. *Eur. Surveill.* **7:**2.
84. **Faldynova, M., M. Pravcova, F. Sisak, H. Havlickova, I. Kolackova, A. Cizek, R. Karpiskova, and I. Rychlik.** 2003. Evolution of antibiotic resistance in *Salmonella enterica* serovar Typhimurium strains isolated in the Czech Republic between 1984 and 2002. *Antimicrob. Agents Chemother.* **47:**2002–2005.
85. **Farhoudi-Moghaddam, A. A., M. Katouli, A. Jafari, M. A. Bahavar, M. Parsi, and F. Malekzadeh.** 1990. Antimicrobial drug resistance and resistance factor transfer among clinical isolates of salmonellae in Iran. *Scand. J. Infect. Dis.* **22:**197–203.
86. **Fey, P. D., T. J. Safranek, M. E. Rupp, E. F. Dunne, E. Ribot, P. C. Iwen, P. A. Bradford, F. J. Angulo, and S. H. Hinrichs.** 2000. Ceftriaxone-resistant salmonella infection acquired by a child from cattle. *N. Engl. J. Med.* **342:**1242–1249.
87. **Fisher, I.** 2004. Enter-net Quarterly *Salmonella* Report: Jul.–Sept. 2004. [Online.] http://www.hpa.org.uk/hpa/inter/enter-net_reports.htm. Health Protection Agency, London, United Kingdom.
88. **Fisher, I. S.** 2004. International trends in salmonella serotypes 1998–2003—a surveillance report from the Enter-net international surveillance network. *Eur. Surveill.* **9:**9–10.
89. **Franklin, A., J. Acar, F. Anthony, R. Gupta, T. Nicholls, Y. Tamura, S. Thompson, E. J. Threlfall, D. Vose, M. van Vuuren, D. G. White, H. C. Wegener, and M. L. Costarrica.** 2001. Antimicrobial resistance: harmonisation of national antimicrobial resistance monitoring and surveillance programmes in animals and in animal-derived food. *Rev. Sci. Tech.* **20:**859–870.
90. **Galanis, E., F. L., D. M. Wong, M. Patrick, and H. C. Wegener.** 2004. Characterizing the worldwide distribution of *Salmonella* serotypes: the role of WHO Global Salm-Surv, abstr. 78, p. 177. *Abstr. Int. Conf. Emerg. Infect. Dis.*, Atlanta, Ga.
91. **Gassama-Sow, A., A. Aidara-Kane, N. Raked, F. Denis, and M. C. Ploy.** 2004. Integrons in Salmonella Keurmassar, Senegal. *Emerg. Infect. Dis.* **10:**1339–1341.
92. **Gebreyes, W. A., P. R. Davies, P. K. Turkson, W. E. Morrow, J. A. Funk, C. Altier, and S. Thakur.** 2004. Characterization of antimicrobial-resistant phenotypes and genotypes among *Salmonella enterica* recovered from pigs on farms, from transport trucks, and from pigs after slaughter. *J. Food Prot.* **67:**698–705.
93. **Gensberg, K., Y. F. Jin, and L. J. Piddock.** 1995. A novel *gyrB* mutation in a fluoroquinolone-resistant clinical isolate of *Salmonella typhimurium*. *FEMS Microbiol. Lett.* **132:**57–60.
94. **Giraud, E., A. Cloeckaert, D. Kerboeuf, and E. Chaslus-Dancla.** 2000. Evidence for active efflux as the primary mechanism of resistance to ciprofloxacin in *Salmonella enterica* serovar Typhimurium. *Antimicrob. Agents Chemother.* **44:**1223–1228.
95. **Glynn, M. K., C. Bopp, W. Dewitt, P. Dabney, M. Mokhtar, and F. J. Angulo.** 1998. Emergence of multidrug-resistant *Salmonella enterica* serotype Typhimurium DT104 infections in the United States. *N. Engl. J. Med.* **338:**1333–1338.
96. **Glynn, M. K., V. Reddy, L. Hutwagner, T. Rabatsky-Ehr, B. Shiferaw, D. J. Vugia, S. Segler, J. Bender, T. J. Barrett, and F. J. Angulo.** 2004. Prior antimicrobial agent use increases the

risk of sporadic infections with multidrug-resistant *Salmonella enterica* serotype Typhimurium: a FoodNet case-control study, 1996–1997. *Clin. Infect. Dis.* **38**(Suppl. 3):S227–S236.

97. **Gomez, T. M., Y. Motarjemi, S. Miyagawa, F. K. Kaferstein, and K. Stohr.** 1997. Foodborne salmonellosis. *World Health Stat. Q.* **50**:81–89.

98. **Gorman, R., and C. C. Adley.** 2004. Characterization of *Salmonella enterica* serotype Typhimurium isolates from human, food, and animal sources in the Republic of Ireland. *J. Clin. Microbiol.* **42**:2314–2316.

99. **Grant, R. B., and L. Di Mambro.** 1977. Antimicrobial resistance and resistance plasmids in *Salmonella* from Ontario, Canada. *Can. J. Microbiol.* **23**:1266–1273.

100. **Guerra, B., S. Soto, S. Cal, and M. C. Mendoza.** 2000. Antimicrobial resistance and spread of class 1 integrons among *Salmonella* serotypes. *Antimicrob. Agents Chemother.* **44**:2166–2169.

101. **Guerra, B., S. Soto, R. Helmuth, and M. C. Mendoza.** 2002. Characterization of a self-transferable plasmid from *Salmonella enterica* serotype Typhimurium clinical isolates carrying two integron-borne gene cassettes together with virulence and drug resistance genes. *Antimicrob. Agents Chemother.* **46**:2977–2981.

102. **Guerra, B., S. M. Soto, J. M. Argüelles, and M. C. Mendoza.** 2001. Multidrug resistance is mediated by large plasmids carrying a class 1 integron in the emergent *Salmonella enterica* serotype [4,5,12:i:–]. *Antimicrob. Agents Chemother.* **45**:1305–1308.

103. **Gupta, A., J. Fontana, C. Crowe, B. Bolstorff, A. Stout, S. Van Duyne, M. P. Hoekstra, J. M. Whichard, T. J. Barrett, and F. J. Angulo.** 2003. Emergence of multidrug-resistant *Salmonella enterica* serotype Newport infections resistant to expanded-spectrum cephalosporins in the United States. *J. Infect. Dis.* **188**:1707–1716.

104. **Hakanen, A., P. Kotilainen, P. Huovinen, H. Helenius, and A. Siitonen.** 2001. Reduced fluoroquinolone susceptibility in *Salmonella enterica* serotypes in travelers returning from Southeast Asia. *Emerg. Infect. Dis.* **7**:996–1003.

104a. **Hall, R.M.** 1997. Mobile gene cassettes and integrons: moving antibiotic resistance genes in gram-negative bacteria. *Ciba Found. Symp.* **207**:192–202.

105. **Hansen, H., and P. Heisig.** 2003. Topoisomerase IV mutations in quinolone-resistant salmonellae selected in vitro. *Microb. Drug Resist.* **9**:25–32.

106. **Hanson, N. D., E. S. Moland, A. Hossain, S. A. Neville, I. B. Gosbell, and K. S. Thomson.** 2002. Unusual *Salmonella enterica* serotype Typhimurium isolate producing CMY-7, SHV-9 and OXA-30 β-lactamases. *J. Antimicrob. Chemother.* **49**:1011–1014.

107. **Harada, K., M. Kameda, M. Suzuki, and S. Mitsuhashi.** 1963. Drug resistance of enteric bacterial II. Tranduction of transmissible drug-resistance (R) factors with phage epsilon. *J. Bacteriol.* **86**:1332–1338.

108. **Hastings, L., A. Burnens, B. de Jong, L. Ward, I. Fisher, J. Stuart, C. Bartlett, and B. Rowe.** 1996. Salm-Net facilitates collaborative investigation of an outbreak of *Salmonella tosamanga* infection in Europe. *Commun. Dis. Rep. CDR Rev.* **6**:R100–R102.

109. **Hawkey, P. M.** 2003. Mechanisms of quinolone action and microbial response. *J. Antimicrob. Chemother.* **51**(Suppl. 1):29–35.

110. **Heisig, P.** 1993. High-level fluoroquinolone resistance in a *Salmonella typhimurium* isolate due to alterations in both *gyrA* and *gyrB* genes. *J. Antimicrob. Chemother.* **32**:367–377.

111. **Helms, M., J. Simonsen, and K. Molbak.** 2004. Quinolone resistance is associated with increased risk of invasive illness or death during infection with *Salmonella* serotype Typhimurium. *J. Infect. Dis.* **190**:1652–1654.

112. **Helms, M., P. Vastrup, P. Gerner-Smidt, and K. Molbak.** 2002. Excess mortality associated with antimicrobial drug-resistant *Salmonella typhimurium. Emerg. Infect. Dis.* **8**:490–495.

113. **Herikstad, H., Y. Motarjemi, and R. V. Tauxe.** 2002. Salmonella surveillance: a global survey of public health serotyping. *Epidemiol. Infect.* **129**:1–8.

114. **Hernandez, T., C. Rodriguez-Alvarez, M. P. Arevalo, A. Torres, A. Sierra, and A. Arias.** 2002. Antimicrobial-resistant *Salmonella enterica* serovars isolated from chickens in Spain. *J. Chemother.* **14**:346–350.

115. **Hohmann, E. L.** 2001. Nontyphoidal salmonellosis. *Clin. Infect. Dis.* **32**:263–269.

116. **Holmberg, S. D., S. L. Solomon, and P. A. Blake.** 1987. Health and economic impacts of antimicrobial resistance. *Rev. Infect. Dis.* **9**:1065–1078.

117. **Holmberg, S. D., J. G. Wells, and M. L. Cohen.** 1984. Animal-to-man transmission of antimicrobial-resistant *Salmonella*: investigations of U.S. outbreaks, 1971–1983. *Science* **225**:833–835.

118. **Hornish, R. E., and S. F. Kotarski.** 2002. Cephalosporins in veterinary medicine—ceftiofur use in food animals. *Curr. Top. Med. Chem.* **2**:717–731.

119. **Howard, A. J., T. D. Joseph, L. L. Bloodworth, J. A. Frost, H. Chart, and B. Rowe.** 1990. The emergence of ciprofloxacin resistance in *Salmonella typhimurium. J. Antimicrob. Chemother.* **26**:296–298.

120. **Hsueh, P. R., L. J. Teng, S. P. Tseng, C. F. Chang, J. H. Wan, J. J. Yan, C. M. Lee, Y. C. Chuang, W. K. Huang, D. Yang, J. M. Shyr, K. W. Yu, L. S. Wang, J. J. Lu, W. C. Ko, J. J. Wu, F. Y. Chang, Y. C. Yang, Y. J. Lau, Y. C. Liu, C. Y. Liu, S. W. Ho, and K. T. Luh.** 2004. Ciprofloxacin-resistant *Salmonella enterica* Typhimurium and Choleraesuis from pigs to humans, Taiwan. *Emerg. Infect. Dis.* **10**:60–68.

121. **Hudson, C. R., C. Quist, M. D. Lee, K. Keyes, S. V. Dodson, C. Morales, S. Sanchez, D. G. White, and J. J. Maurer.** 2000. Genetic relatedness of *Salmonella* isolates from nondomestic birds in Southeastern United States. *J. Clin. Microbiol.* **38**: 1860–1865.

122. **Hutchison, M. L., L. D. Walters, S. M. Avery, B. A. Synge, and A. Moore.** 2004. Levels of zoonotic agents in British livestock manures. *Lett. Appl. Microbiol.* **39**:207–214.

123. **Irwin, R. J., C. Poppe, S. Messier, G. G. Finley, and J. Oggel.** 1994. A national survey to estimate the prevalence of *Salmonella* species among Canadian registered commercial turkey flocks. *Can. J. Vet. Res.* **58**:263–267.

124. **Izumiya, H., N. Nojiri, Y. Hashiwata, K. Tamura, J. Terajima, and H. Watanabe.** 2003. *Salmonella enterica* serovar Enteritidis, Japan. *Emerg. Infect. Dis.* **9**:1650–1651.

125. **Jorgensen, F., R. Bailey, S. Williams, P. Henderson, D. R. Wareing, F. J. Bolton, J. A. Frost, L. Ward, and T. J. Humphrey.** 2002. Prevalence and numbers of *Salmonella* and *Campylobacter* spp. on raw, whole chickens in relation to sampling methods. *Int. J. Food Microbiol.* **76**:151–164.

126. **Kam, K. M.** 1996. Serotype epidemiology and patterns of antibiotic susceptibilities of salmonellae isolated in Hong Kong 1983–93. *Chin. Med. J. (Engl. Ed.)* **109**:276–281.

127. **Kariuki, S., G. Revathi, N. Kariuki, J. Muyodi, J. Mwituria, A. Munyalo, D. Kagendo, L. Murungi, and C. A. Hart.** 2005. Increasing prevalence of multidrug-resistant non-typhoidal salmonellae, Kenya, 1994–2003. *Int. J. Antimicrob. Agents* **25**:38–43.

128. **Kaszanyitzky, E. J., A. Tarpai, S. Janosi, M. Papp, J. Skare, and G. Semjen.** 2002. Development of an antibiotic resistance monitoring system in Hungary. *Acta Vet. Hung.* **50**:189–197.

129. **Kennedy, M., R. Villar, D. J. Vugia, T. Rabatsky-Ehr, M. M. Farley, M. Pass, K. Smith, P. Smith, P. R. Cieslak, B. Imhoff, and P. M. Griffin.** 2004. Hospitalizations and deaths due to Salmonella infections, FoodNet, 1996–1999. *Clin. Infect. Dis.* 38(Suppl. 3):S142–S148.
130. **Kiessling, C. R., J. H. Cutting, M. Loftis, W. M. Kiessling, A. R. Datta, and J. N. Sofos.** 2002. Antimicrobial resistance of food-related Salmonella isolates, 1999–2000. *J. Food Prot.* **65:**603–608.
131. **Killalea, D., L. R. Ward, D. Roberts, J. de Louvois, F. Sufi, J. M. Stuart, P. G. Wall, M. Susman, M. Schwieger, P. J. Sanderson, I. S. Fisher, P. S. Mead, O. N. Gill, C. L. Bartlett, and B. Rowe.** 1996. International epidemiological and microbiological study of outbreak of Salmonella agona infection from a ready to eat savoury snack—I: England and Wales and the United States. *Br. Med. J.* **313:**1105–1107.
132. **Kim, J. Y., Y. J. Park, S. O. Lee, W. Song, S. H. Jeong, Y. A. Yoo, and K. Y. Lee.** 2004. Case report: bacteremia due to *Salmonella enterica* serotype Montevideo producing plasmid-mediated AmpC beta-lactamase (DHA-1). *Ann. Clin. Lab Sci.* **34:**214–217.
133. **Koutsolioutsou, A., E. A. Martins, D. G. White, S. B. Levy, and B. Demple.** 2001. A *soxRS*-constitutive mutation contributing to antibiotic resistance in a clinical isolate of *Salmonella enterica* (serovar Typhimurium). *Antimicrob. Agents Chemother.* **45:**38–43.
134. **Kruger, T., D. Szabo, K. H. Keddy, K. Deeley, J. W. Marsh, A. M. Hujer, R. A. Bonomo, and D. L. Paterson.** 2004. Infections with nontyphoidal *Salmonella* species producing TEM-63 or a novel TEM enzyme, TEM-131, in South Africa. *Antimicrob. Agents Chemother.* **48:**4263–4270.
135. **Layton, M. C., S. G. Calliste, T. M. Gomez, C. Patton, and S. Brooks.** 1997. A mixed foodborne outbreak with *Salmonella heidelberg* and *Campylobacter jejuni* in a nursing home. *Infect. Control Hosp. Epidemiol.* **18:**115–121.
136. **Lee, K., D. Yong, J. H. Yum, H. H. Kim, and Y. Chong.** 2003. Diversity of TEM-52 extended-spectrum beta-lactamase-producing non-typhoidal *Salmonella* isolates in Korea. *J. Antimicrob. Chemother.* **52:**493–496.
137. **Lee, L. A., N. D. Puhr, E. K. Maloney, N. H. Bean, and R. V. Tauxe.** 1994. Increase in antimicrobial-resistant Salmonella infections in the United States, 1989–1990. *J. Infect. Dis.* **170:**128–134.
138. **Liebana, E., M. Batchelor, F. A. Clifton-Hadley, R. H. Davies, K. L. Hopkins, and E. J. Threlfall.** 2004. First report of *Salmonella* isolates with the DHA-1 AmpC β-lactamase in the United Kingdom. *Antimicrob. Agents Chemother.* **48:**4492.
139. **Liebana, E., M. Batchelor, C. Torres, L. Brinas, L. A. Lagos, B. Abdalhamid, N. D. Hanson, and J. Martinez-Urtaza.** 2004. Pediatric infection due to multiresistant *Salmonella enterica* serotype Infantis in Honduras. *J. Clin. Microbiol.* **42:**4885–4888.
140. **Liebana, E., M. Gibbs, C. Clouting, L. Barker, F. A. Clifton-Hadley, E. Pleydell, B. Abdalhamid, N. D. Hanson, L. Martin, C. Poppe, and R. H. Davies.** 2004. Characterization of β-lactamases responsible for resistance to extended-spectrum cephalosporins in *Escherichia coli* and *Salmonella enterica* strains from food-producing animals in the United Kingdom. *Microb. Drug Resist.* **10:**1–9.
141. **Ling, J. M., E. W. Chan, A. W. Lam, and A. F. Cheng.** 2003. Mutations in topoisomerase genes of fluoroquinolone-resistant salmonellae in Hong Kong. *Antimicrob. Agents Chemother.* **47:**3567–3573.
142. **Lyons, R. W., C. L. Samples, H. N. DeSilva, K. A. Ross, E. M. Julian, and P. J. Checko.** 1980. An epidemic of resistant *Salmonella* in a nursery. Animal-to-human spread. *JAMA* **243:**546–547.
143. **Makanera, A., G. Arlet, V. Gautier, and M. Manai.** 2003. Molecular epidemiology and characterization of plasmid-encoded β-lactamases produced by Tunisian clinical isolates of *Salmonella enterica* serotype Mbandaka resistant to broad-spectrum cephalosporins. *J. Clin. Microbiol.* **41:**2940–2945.
144. **Mammina, C., L. Cannova, S. Massa, E. Goffredo, and A. Nastasi.** 2002. Drug resistances in salmonella isolates from animal foods, Italy 1998–2000. *Epidemiol. Infect.* **129:**155–161.
145. **Marimon, J. M., M. Gomariz, C. Zigorraga, G. Cilla, and E. Perez-Trallero.** 2004. Increasing prevalence of quinolone resistance in human nontyphoid *Salmonella enterica* isolates obtained in Spain from 1981 to 2003. *Antimicrob. Agents Chemother.* **48:**3789–3793.
146. **Martin, L. J., M. Fyfe, K. Dore, J. A. Buxton, F. Pollari, B. Henry, D. Middleton, R. Ahmed, F. Jamieson, B. Ciebin, S. A. McEwen, and J. B. Wilson.** 2004. Increased burden of illness associated with antimicrobial-resistant *Salmonella enterica* serotype Typhimurium infections. *J. Infect. Dis.* **189:**377–384.
147. **Maxwell, A., and S. E. Critchlow.** 1998. Mode of action, p. 119–166. *In* J. Kuhlman, A. Dalhoff, and H. J. Zeiler (ed.), *Quinolone Antibacterials*. Springer-Verlag, Berlin, Germany.
148. **Mayrhofer, S., P. Paulsen, F. J. Smulders, and F. Hilbert.** 2004. Antimicrobial resistance profile of five major food-borne pathogens isolated from beef, pork and poultry. *Int. J. Food Microbiol.* **97:**23–29.
149. **McDermott, P. F., S. Zhao, D. D. Wagner, S. Simjee, R. D. Walker, and D. G. White.** 2002. The food safety perspective of antibiotic resistance. *Anim. Biotechnol.* **13:**71–84.
150. **Mead, P. S., L. Slutsker, V. Dietz, L. F. McCaig, J. S. Bresee, C. Shapiro, P. M. Griffin, and R. V. Tauxe.** 1999. Food-related illness and death in the United States. *Emerg. Infect. Dis.* **5:**607–625.
151. **Mendoza-Medellin, A., E. Curiel-Quesada, and R. Camacho-Carranza.** 2004. *Escherichia coli* R-factors unstable in *Salmonella typhi* are deleted before being segregated in this host. *Plasmid* **51:**75–86.
152. **Meunier, D., D. Boyd, M. R. Mulvey, S. Baucheron, C. Mammina, A. Nastasi, E. Chaslus-Dancla, and A. Cloeckaert.** 2002. *Salmonella enterica* serotype Typhimurium DT 104 antibiotic resistance genomic island I in serotype paratyphi B. *Emerg. Infect. Dis.* **8:**430–433.
153. **Miriagou, V., P. T. Tassios, N. J. Legakis, and L. S. Tzouvelekis.** 2004. Expanded-spectrum cephalosporin resistance in non-typhoid *Salmonella. Int. J. Antimicrob. Agents* **23:**547–555.
154. **Molbak, K.** 2004. Spread of resistant bacteria and resistance genes from animals to humans—the public health consequences. *J. Vet. Med. B Infect. Dis. Vet. Public Health* **51:**364–369.
155. **Molbak, K., D. L. Baggesen, F. M. Aarestrup, J. M. Ebbesen, J. Engberg, K. Frydendahl, P. Gerner-Smidt, A. M. Petersen, and H. C. Wegener.** 1999. An outbreak of multidrug-resistant, quinolone-resistant *Salmonella enterica* serotype typhimurium DT104. *N. Engl. J. Med.* **341:**1420–1425.
156. **Moubareck, C., F. Doucet-Populaire, M. Hamze, Z. Daoud, and F. X. Weill.** 2005. First extended-spectrum-β-lactamase (CTX-M-15)-producing *Salmonella enterica* serotype Typhimurium isolate identified in Lebanon. *Antimicrob. Agents Chemother.* **49:**864–865.
157. **Mulvey, M. R., D. A. Boyd, L. Baker, O. Mykytczuk, E. M. Reis, M. D. Asensi, D. P. Rodrigues, and L. K. Ng.** 2004. Characterization of a *Salmonella enterica* serovar Agona strain harbouring a class 1 integron containing novel OXA-type beta-lactamase (bla_{OXA-53}) and 6′-*N*-aminoglycoside

acetyltransferase genes [aac(6')-I30]. *J. Antimicrob. Chemother.* 54:354–359.

158. **Nakaya, H., A. Yasuhara, K. Yoshimura, Y. Oshihoi, H. Izumiya, and H. Watanabe.** 2003. Life-threatening infantile diarrhea from fluoroquinolone-resistant *Salmonella enterica* Typhimurium with mutations in both *gyrA* and *parC*. *Emerg. Infect. Dis.* **9**:255–257.
159. **Nastasi, A., and C. Mammina.** 2001. Presence of class I integrons in multidrug-resistant, low-prevalence *Salmonella* serotypes, Italy. *Emerg. Infect. Dis.* **7**:455–458.
160. **Nastasi, A., C. Mammina, and L. Cannova.** 2000. Antimicrobial resistance in *Salmonella enteritidis*, southern Italy, 1990–1998. *Emerg. Infect. Dis.* **6**:401–403.

160a. **National Committee for Clinical Laboratory Standards.** 2003. *Performance Standards for Antimicrobial Susceptibility Testing; Thirteenth Informational Supplement.* NCCLS document M100-S13. National Committee for Clinical Laboratory Standards, Wayne, Pa.

160b. **National Veterinary Institute.** 2001. *SVARM 2000: Swedish Veterinary Antimicrobial Resistance Monitoring.* National Veterinary Institute, Uppsala, Sweden.

161. **Nel, H., M. van Vuuren, and G. E. Swan.** 2004. Towards the establishment and standardization of a veterinary antimicrobial resistance surveillance and monitoring programme in South Africa. *Onderstepoort J. Vet. Res.* **71**:239–246.
162. **Neu, H. C., C. E. Cherubin, E. D. Longo, B. Flouton, and J. Winter.** 1975. Antimicrobial resistance and R-factor transfer among isolates of Salmonella in the northeastern United States: a comparison of human and animal isolates. *J. Infect. Dis.* **132**:617–622.
163. **Oethinger, M., W. V. Kern, A. S. Jellen-Ritter, L. M. McMurry, and S. B. Levy.** 2000. Ineffectiveness of topoisomerase mutations in mediating clinically significant fluoroquinolone resistance in *Escherichia coli* in the absence of the AcrAB efflux pump. *Antimicrob. Agents Chemother.* **44**:10–13.
164. **Okusu, H., D. Ma, and H. Nikaido.** 1996. AcrAB efflux pump plays a major role in the antibiotic resistance phenotype of *Escherichia coli* multiple-antibiotic-resistance (Mar) mutants. *J. Bacteriol.* **178**:306–308.
165. **Olsen, S. J., E. E. DeBess, T. E. McGivern, N. Marano, T. Eby, S. Mauvais, V. K. Balan, G. Zirnstein, P. R. Cieslak, and F. J. Angulo.** 2001. A nosocomial outbreak of fluoroquinolone-resistant salmonella infection. *N. Engl. J. Med.* **344**:1572–1579.
166. **Orman, B. E., S. A. Pineiro, S. Arduino, M. Galas, R. Melano, M. I. Caffer, D. O. Sordelli, and D. Centron.** 2002. Evolution of multiresistance in nontyphoid *Salmonella* serovars from 1984 to 1998 in Argentina. *Antimicrob. Agents Chemother.* **46**:3963–3970.
167. **Orrett, F. A., and S. M. Shurland.** 2001. Susceptibility patterns and serotypes of non-typhoidal *Salmonella* in Trinidad. *Saudi Med. J.* **22**:852–855.
168. **Oundo, J. O., S. Kariuki, J. K. Maghenda, and B. S. Lowe.** 2000. Antibiotic susceptibility and genotypes of non-typhi *Salmonella* isolates from children in Kilifi on the Kenya coast. *Trans. R. Soc. Trop. Med. Hyg.* **94**:212–215.
169. **Pang, T., Z. A. Bhutta, B. B. Finlay, and M. Altwegg.** 1995. Typhoid fever and other salmonellosis: a continuing challenge. *Trends Microbiol.* **3**:253–255.
170. **Panhotra, B. R., A. K. Saxena, and A. M. Al-Ghamdi.** 2004. Emerging nalidixic acid and ciprofloxacin resistance in nontyphoidal *Salmonella* isolated from patients having acute diarrhoeal disease. *Ann. Saudi Med.* **24**:270–272.
171. **Paszti, J., V. G. Laszlo, I. Gado, H. Milch, K. Krisztalovics, M. Kiraly, J. Orban, and V. Koppany.** 2001. The spread and antibiotic resistance of *Salmonella enterica* serotype Typhimurium DT104 in Hungary. *Acta Microbiol. Immunol. Hung.* **48**:95–105.
172. **Patrick, M. E., P. M. Adcock, T. M. Gomez, S. F. Altekruse, B. H. Holland, R. V. Tauxe, and D. L. Swerdlow.** 2004. *Salmonella* Enteritidis infections, United States, 1985–1999. *Emerg. Infect. Dis.* **10**:1–7.
173. **Pavia, A. T., L. D. Shipman, J. G. Wells, N. D. Puhr, J. D. Smith, T. W. McKinley, and R. V. Tauxe.** 1990. Epidemiologic evidence that prior antimicrobial exposure decreases resistance to infection by antimicrobial-sensitive Salmonella. *J. Infect. Dis.* **161**:255–260.
174. **Pegues, D. A., M. E. Ohl, and S. I. Miller.** 2002. *Salmonella*, including *Salmonella typhi*, p. 669–697. *In* M. J. Blaser, P. D. Smith, J. I. Ravdin, H. B. Greenberg, and R. L. Guerrant (ed.), *Infections of the Gastrointestinal Tract.* Lippincott Williams & Wilkins, Philadelphia, Pa.
175. **Petersen, A., F. M. Aarestrup, F. J. Angulo, S. Wong, K. Stohr, and H. C. Wegener.** 2002. WHO Global Salm-Surv External Quality Assurance System (EQAS): an important step toward improving the quality of *Salmonella* serotyping and antimicrobial susceptibility testing worldwide. *Microb. Drug Resist.* **8**:345–353.
176. **Piddock, L. J., D. G. White, K. Gensberg, L. Pumbwe, and D. J. Griggs.** 2000. Evidence for an efflux pump mediating multiple antibiotic resistance in *Salmonella enterica* serovar Typhimurium. *Antimicrob. Agents Chemother.* **44**:3118–3121.
177. **Poole, K.** 2004. Efflux-mediated multiresistance in Gram-negative bacteria. *Clin. Microbiol. Infect.* **10**:12–26.
178. **Popoff, M. Y., J. Bockemuhl, and L. L. Gheesling.** 2004. Supplement 2002 (no. 46) to the Kauffmann-White scheme. *Res. Microbiol.* **155**:568–570.
179. **Poppe, C., M. Ayroud, G. Ollis, M. Chirino-Trejo, N. Smart, S. Quessy, and P. Michel.** 2001. Trends in antimicrobial resistance of *Salmonella* isolated from animals, foods of animal origin, and the environment of animal production in Canada, 1994–1997. *Microb. Drug Resist.* **7**:197–212.
180. **Poppe, C., R. J. Irwin, S. Messier, G. G. Finley, and J. Oggel.** 1991. The prevalence of *Salmonella enteritidis* and other *Salmonella* sp. among Canadian registered commercial chicken broiler flocks. *Epidemiol. Infect.* **107**:201–211.
181. **Poppe, C., K. Ziebell, L. Martin, and K. Allen.** 2002. Diversity in antimicrobial resistance and other characteristics among *Salmonella typhimurium* DT104 isolates. *Microb. Drug Resist.* **8**:107–122.
182. **Prats, G., B. Mirelis, T. Llovet, C. Munoz, E. Miro, and F. Navarro.** 2000. Antibiotic resistance trends in enteropathogenic bacteria isolated in 1985–1987 and 1995–1998 in Barcelona. *Antimicrob. Agents Chemother.* **44**:1140–1145.
183. **Quigley, J. D., J. J. Drewry, L. M. Murray, and S. J. Ivey.** 1997. Body weight gain, feed efficiency, and fecal scores of dairy calves in response to galactosyl-lactose or antibiotics in milk replacers. *J. Dairy Sci.* **80**:1751–1754.
184. **Rabatsky-Ehr, T., J. Whichard, S. Rossiter, B. Holland, K. Stamey, M. L. Headrick, T. J. Barrett, and F. J. Angulo.** 2004. Multidrug-resistant strains of *Salmonella enterica* Typhimurium, United States, 1997–1998. *Emerg. Infect. Dis.* **10**:795–801.
185. **Rabsch, W., H. Tschape, and A. J. Baumler.** 2001. Non-typhoidal salmonellosis: emerging problems. *Microbes Infect.* **3**:237–247.
186. **Rahman, M., H. Islam, D. Ahmed, and R. B. Sack.** 2001. Emergence of multidrug-resistant Salmonella Gloucester and Salmonella typhimurium in Bangladesh. *J. Health Popul. Nutr.* **19**:191–198.
187. **Randall, L. P., S. W. Cooles, M. K. Osborn, L. J. Piddock, and M. J. Woodward.** 2004. Antibiotic resistance genes,

integrons and multiple antibiotic resistance in thirty-five serotypes of *Salmonella enterica* isolated from humans and animals in the UK. *J. Antimicrob. Chemother.* 53:208–216.

188. **Rankin, S. C., H. Aceto, J. Cassidy, J. Holt, S. Young, B. Love, D. Tewari, D. S. Munro, and C. E. Benson.** 2002. Molecular characterization of cephalosporin-resistant *Salmonella enterica* serotype Newport isolates from animals in Pennsylvania. *J. Clin. Microbiol.* 40:4679–4684.
189. **Rhimi-Mahjoubi, F., M. Bernier, G. Arlet, Z. B. Jemaa, P. Jouve, A. Hammami, and A. Philippon.** 2002. Identification of plasmid-encoded cephalosporinase ACC-1 among various enterobacteria (*Klebsiella pneumoniae, Proteus mirabilis, Salmonella*) isolated from a Tunisian hospital (Sfax 997–2000). *Pathol. Biol.* (Paris) 50:7–11. (In French.)
190. **Ribot, E. M., R. K. Wierzba, F. J. Angulo, and T. J. Barrett.** 2002. *Salmonella enterica* serotype Typhimurium DT104 isolated from humans, United States, 1985, 1990, and 1995. *Emerg. Infect. Dis.* 8:387–391.
191. **Rigney, C. P., B. P. Salamone, N. Anandaraman, B. E. Rose, R. L. Umholtz, K. E. Ferris, D. R. Parham, and W. James.** 2004. *Salmonella* serotypes in selected classes of food animal carcasses and raw ground products, January 1998 through December 2000. *J. Am. Vet. Med. Assoc.* 224:524–530.
192. **Rodrigue, D. C., R. V. Tauxe, and B. Rowe.** 1990. International increase in *Salmonella* Enteritidis: a new pandemic? *Epidemiol. Infect.* 105:21–27.
193. **Rossi, M. S., M. Tokumoto, E. Couto, A. Di Bella, M. Alstchuler, N. Gomez, F. Dujovney, L. Galanternik, M. Woloj, N. Hardie, J. Stelling, M. Schlipak, and T. O'Brien.** 1995. Survey of the levels of antimicrobial resistance in Argentina: WHONET program—1991 to 1994. *Int. J. Antimicrob. Agents* 6:103–110.
194. **Rowe-Magnus, D. A., and D. Mazel.** 2001. Integrons: natural tools for bacterial genome evolution. *Curr. Opin. Microbiol.* 4:565–569.
195. **Ryder, R. W., P. A. Blake, A. C. Murlin, G. P. Carter, R. A. Pollard, M. H. Merson, S. D. Allen, and D. J. Brenner.** 1980. Increase in antibiotic resistance among isolates of Salmonella in the United States, 1967–1975. *J. Infect. Dis.* 142:485–491.
196. **Schmieger, H., and P. Schicklmaier.** 1999. Transduction of multiple drug resistance of *Salmonella enterica* serovar *typhimurium* DT104. *FEMS Microbiol. Lett.* 170:251–256.
197. **Schroeter, A., B. Hoog, and R. Helmuth.** 2004. Resistance of *Salmonella* isolates in Germany. *J. Vet. Med. B Infect. Dis. Vet. Public Health* 51:389–392.
198. **Snoeyenbos, G. H., C. F. Smyser, and H. Van Roekel.** 1969. Salmonella infections of the ovary and peritoneum of chickens. *Avian Dis.* 13:668–670.
199. **Spika, J. S., S. H. Waterman, G. W. Hoo, M. E. St. Louis, R. E. Pacer, S. M. James, M. L. Bissett, L. W. Mayer, J. Y. Chiu, B. Hall, et al.** 1987. Chloramphenicol-resistant *Salmonella newport* traced through hamburger to dairy farms. A major persisting source of human salmonellosis in California. *N. Engl. J. Med.* 316:565–570.
200. **Stephen, J. M., M. A. Toleman, T. R. Walsh, and R. N. Jones.** 2003. *Salmonella* bloodstream infections: report from the SENTRY Antimicrobial Surveillance Program (1997–2001). *Int. J. Antimicrob. Agents* 22:395–405.
201. **St. Louis, M. E., D. L. Morse, M. E. Potter, T. M. DeMelfi, J. J. Guzewich, R. V. Tauxe, and P. A. Blake.** 1988. The emergence of grade A eggs as a major source of *Salmonella* Enteritidis infections. New implications for the control of salmonellosis. *JAMA* 259:2103–2107.
202. **Summers, A. O.** 2002. Generally overlooked fundamentals of bacterial genetics and ecology. *Clin. Infect. Dis.* 34(Suppl. 3):S85–S92.
203. Reference deleted.
204. **Szych, J., A. Cieslik, J. Paciorek, and S. Kaluzewski.** 2001. Antibiotic resistance in *Salmonella enterica* subsp. *enterica* strains isolated in Poland from 1998 to 1999. *Int. J. Antimicrob. Agents* 18:37–42.
205. **Tassios, P. T., M. Gazouli, E. Tzelepi, H. Milch, N. Kozlova, S. Sidorenko, N. J. Legakis, and L. S. Tzouvelekis.** 1999. Spread of a *Salmonella typhimurium* clone resistant to expanded-spectrum cephalosporins in three European countries. *J. Clin. Microbiol.* 37:3774–3777.
206. **Tassios, P. T., A. Markogiannakis, A. C. Vatopoulos, E. Katsanikou, E. N. Velonakis, J. Kourea-Kremastinou, and N. J. Legakis.** 1997. Molecular epidemiology of antibiotic resistance of *Salmonella enteritidis* during a 7-year period in Greece. *J. Clin. Microbiol.* 35:1316–1321.
207. **Thomson, K. S., and M. E. Smith.** 2000. Version 2000: the new β-lactamases of Gram-negative bacteria at the dawn of the new millennium. *Microbes. Infect.* 2:1225–1235.
208. **Thong, K. L., Y. L. Goh, S. Radu, S. Noorzaleha, R. Yasin, Y. T. Koh, V. K. Lim, G. Rusul, and S. D. Puthucheary.** 2002. Genetic diversity of clinical and environmental strains of *Salmonella enterica* serotype Weltevreden isolated in Malaysia. *J. Clin. Microbiol.* 40:2498–2503.
209. **Threlfall, E. J.** 2000. Epidemic *Salmonella typhimurium* DT 104—a truly international multiresistant clone. *J. Antimicrob. Chemother.* 46:7–10.
210. **Threlfall, E. J., I. S. Fisher, C. Berghold, P. Gerner-Smidt, H. Tschape, M. Cormican, I. Luzzi, F. Schnieder, W. Wannet, J. Machado, and G. Edwards.** 2003. Antimicrobial drug resistance in isolates of *Salmonella enterica* from cases of salmonellosis in humans in Europe in 2000: results of international multi-centre surveillance. *Eur. Surveill.* 8:41–45.
211. **Threlfall, E. J., J. A. Frost, L. R. Ward, and B. Rowe.** 1994. Epidemic in cattle and humans of *Salmonella typhimurium* DT 104 with chromosomally integrated multiple drug resistance. *Vet. Rec.* 134:577.
212. **Threlfall, E. J., M. L. Hall, and B. Rowe.** 1992. Salmonella bacteraemia in England and Wales, 1981–1990. *J. Clin. Pathol.* 45:34–36.
213. **Threlfall, E. J., B. Rowe, and L. R. Ward.** 1993. A comparison of multiple drug resistance in salmonellas from humans and food animals in England and Wales, 1981 and 1990. *Epidemiol. Infect.* 111:189–197.
214. **Threlfall, E. J., L. R. Ward, J. A. Frost, and G. A. Willshaw.** 2000. The emergence and spread of antibiotic resistance in food-borne bacteria. *Int. J. Food Microbiol.* 62:1–5.
215. **Threlfall, E. J., L. R. Ward, M. D. Hampton, A. M. Ridley, B. Rowe, D. Roberts, R. J. Gilbert, P. Van Someren, P. G. Wall, and P. Grimont.** 1998. Molecular fingerprinting defines a strain of Salmonella enterica serotype Anatum responsible for an international outbreak associated with formula-dried milk. *Epidemiol. Infect.* 121:289–293.
216. **Threlfall, E. J., L. R. Ward, J. A. Skinner, and A. Graham.** 2000. Antimicrobial drug resistance in non-typhoidal salmonellas from humans in England and Wales in 1999: decrease in multiple resistance in Salmonella enterica serotypes Typhimurium, Virchow, and Hadar. *Microb. Drug Resist.* 6: 319–325.
217. **Threlfall, E. J., L. R. Ward, J. A. Skinner, and B. Rowe.** 1997. Increase in multiple antibiotic resistance in nontyphoidal salmonellas from humans in England and Wales: a comparison of data for 1994 and 1996. *Microb. Drug Resist.* 3:263–266.
218. **Tibbetts, R. J., T. L. Lin, and C. C. Wu.** 2003. Phenotypic evidence for inducible multiple antimicrobial resistance in *Salmonella choleraesuis*. *FEMS Microbiol. Lett.* 218:333–338.
219. **Tjaniadi, P., M. Lesmana, D. Subekti, N. Machpud, S. Komalarini, W. Santoso, C. H. Simanjuntak, N. Punjabi, J. R.**

Campbell, W. K. Alexander, H. J. Beecham III, A. L. Corwin, and B. A. Oyofo. 2003. Antimicrobial resistance of bacterial pathogens associated with diarrheal patients in Indonesia. *Am. J. Trop. Med. Hyg.* **68:**666–670.

220. **Tosini, F., P. Visca, I. Luzzi, A. M. Dionisi, C. Pezzella, A. Petrucca, and A. Carattoli.** 1998. Class 1 integron-borne multiple-antibiotic resistance carried by IncFI and IncL/M plasmids in *Salmonella enterica* serotype Typhimurium. *Antimicrob. Agents Chemother.* **42:**3053–3058.

221. **Tzouvelekis, L. S., V. Lukova, P. T. Tassios, A. C. Fluit, R. N. Jones, and N. J. Legakis.** 2003. Resistance to β-lactams among blood isolates of *Salmonella* spp. in European hospitals: results from the SENTRY Antimicrobial Surveillance Program 1997–98. *Clin. Microbiol. Infect.* **9:**149–152.

222. **Van Looveren, M., M. L. Chasseur-Libotte, C. Godard, C. Lammens, M. Wijdooghe, L. Peeters, and H. Goossens.** 2001. Antimicrobial susceptibility of nontyphoidal Salmonella isolated from humans in Belgium. *Acta Clin. Belg.* **56:**180–186.

223. **Varma, J. K., K. Molbak, T. J. Barrett, J. L. Beebe, T. F. Jones, T. Rabatsky-Ehr, K. E. Smith, D. J. Vugia, H. G. Chang, and F. J. Angulo.** 2005. Antimicrobial-resistant nontyphoidal *Salmonella* is associated with excess bloodstream infections and hospitalizations. *J. Infect. Dis.* **191:**554–561.

224. **Verdet, C., G. Arlet, G. Barnaud, P. H. Lagrange, and A. Philippon.** 2000. A novel integron in *Salmonella enterica* serovar Enteritidis, carrying the bla_{DHA-1} gene and its regulator gene *ampR*, originated from *Morganella morganii*. *Antimicrob. Agents Chemother.* **44:**222–225.

225. **Voetsch, A. C., T. J. Van Gilder, F. J. Angulo, M. M. Farley, S. Shallow, R. Marcus, P. R. Cieslak, V. C. Deneen, and R. V. Tauxe.** 2004. FoodNet estimate of the burden of illness caused by nontyphoidal *Salmonella* infections in the United States. *Clin. Infect. Dis.* **38**(Suppl. 3)**:**S127–S134.

226. **Wang, M., L. Ran, Z. Wang, and Z. Li.** 2004. Study on national active monitoring for food borne pathogens and antimicrobial resistance in China 2001. *Wei Sheng Yan Jiu* **33:** 49–54. (In Chinese.)

227. **Wegener, H. C., T. Hald, W. D. Lo Fo, M. Madsen, H. Korsgaard, F. Bager, P. Gerner-Smidt, and K. Molbak.** 2003. *Salmonella* control programs in Denmark. *Emerg. Infect. Dis.* **9:**774–780.

228. **White, D. G., A. Datta, P. McDermott, S. Friedman, S. Qaiyumi, S. Ayers, L. English, S. McDermott, D. D. Wagner, and S. Zhao.** 2003. Antimicrobial susceptibility and genetic relatedness of *Salmonella* serovars isolated from animal-derived dog treats in the USA. *J. Antimicrob. Chemother.* **52:**860–863.

229. **White, D. G., S. Zhao, R. Sudler, S. Ayers, S. Friedman, S. Chen, P. F. McDermott, S. McDermott, D. D. Wagner, and J. Meng.** 2001. The isolation of antibiotic-resistant salmonella from retail ground meats. *N. Engl. J. Med.* **345:**1147–1154.

230. **Wilmshurst, P., and H. Sutcliffe.** 1995. Splenic abscess due to *Salmonella* heidelberg. *Clin. Infect. Dis.* **21:**1065.

231. **Wilson, I. G.** 2004. Antimicrobial resistance of Salmonella in raw retail chickens, imported chicken portions, and human clinical specimens. *J. Food Prot.* **67:**1220–1225.

232. **Winokur, P. L., A. Brueggemann, D. L. DeSalvo, L. Hoffmann, M. D. Apley, E. K. Uhlenhopp, M. A. Pfaller, and G. V. Doern.** 2000. Animal and human multidrug-resistant, cephalosporin-resistant *Salmonella* isolates expressing a plasmid-mediated CMY-2 AmpC β-lactamase. *Antimicrob. Agents Chemother.* **44:**2777–2783.

233. **Winokur, P. L., R. Canton, J. M. Casellas, and N. Legakis.** 2001. Variations in the prevalence of strains expressing an extended-spectrum β-lactamase phenotype and characterization of isolates from Europe, the Americas, and the Western Pacific region. *Clin. Infect. Dis.* **32**(Suppl. 2)**:**S94–S103.

234. **Winokur, P. L., D. L. Vonstein, L. J. Hoffman, E. K. Uhlenhopp, and G. V. Doern.** 2001. Evidence for transfer of CMY-2 AmpC β-lactamase plasmids between *Escherichia coli* and *Salmonella* isolates from food animals and humans. *Antimicrob. Agents Chemother.* **45:**2716–2722.

235. **World Health Organization.** 1992. *Surveillance Programme for Control of Foodborne Infections and Intoxication in Europe.* Fifth Report 1985–1989. Robert von Istertag Institue, FAO/WHO Collaborating Centre, Berlin, Germany.

236. **World Health Organization.** 2001. *WHO Global Principles for the Containment of Antimicrobial Resistance in Animals Intended for Food.* Report of a WHO Consultation with the Participation of the Food and Agriculture Organization of the United Nations and the Office International des Epizooties, Geneva, Switzerland 5–9 June 2000. World Health Organization, Geneva, Switzerland.

237. **World Health Organization.** 2002. *Monitoring Antimicrobial Usage in Food Animals for the Protection of Human Health.* Report of a WHO Consultation, Oslo, Norway 10–13 September 2001. World Health Organization, Geneva, Switzerland.

238. **World Health Organization.** 2004. Global Salm Surv (GSS). [Online.] http://www.who.int/salmsurv/en/.

239. **Wybot, I., C. Wildemauwe, C. Godard, S. Bertrand, and J. M. Collard.** 2004. Antimicrobial drug resistance in nontyphoid human *Salmonella* in Belgium: trends for the period 2000–2002. *Acta Clin. Belg.* **59:**152–160.

240. **Yang, S.** 1998. FoodNet and Enter-net: emerging surveillance programs for foodborne diseases. *Emerg. Infect. Dis.* **4:**457–458.

241. **Yang, Y. J., C. C. Liu, S. M. Wang, J. J. Wu, A. H. Huang, and C. P. Cheng.** 1998. High rates of antimicrobial resistance among clinical isolates of nontyphoidal *Salmonella* in Taiwan. *Eur. J. Clin. Microbiol. Infect. Dis.* **17:**880–883.

242. **Yasin, R. M., M. M. Jegathesan, and C. C. Tiew.** 1996. Salmonella serotypes isolated in Malaysia over the ten-year period 1983–1992. *Asia Pac. J. Public Health* **9:**1–5.

243. **Zaidi, M. B., P. F. McDermott, C. Perez, S. Hubert, C. Canche, D. Melka, M. Leon, S. Zhao, L. Tollefson, and M. Headrick.** 2004. Increasing trends in multidrug resistance in *Salmonella Typhimurium* from Mexico, p. 121, abstr. C2-1717. *Abstr. 44th Intersci. Conf. Antimicrob. Agents Chemother.* American Society for Microbiology, Washington, D.C.

244. **Zhao, S., A. R. Datta, S. Ayers, S. Friedman, R. D. Walker, and D. G. White.** 2003. Antimicrobial-resistant *Salmonella* serovars isolated from imported foods. *Int. J. Food Microbiol.* **84:**87–92.

245. **Zhao, S., A. R. Datta, S. Ayers, S. Friedman, R. D. Walker, and D. G. White.** 2004. Characterization of *Salmonella* Typhimurium from diagnostic samples and food animal carcasses, abstr. C2-1994. *Abstr. 44th Intersci. Conf. Antimicrob. Agents Chemother.* American Society for Microbiology, Washington, D.C.

246. **Zhao, S., S. Qaiyumi, S. Friedman, R. Singh, S. L. Foley, D. G. White, P. F. McDermott, T. Donkar, C. Bolin, S. Munro, E. J. Baron, and R. D. Walker.** 2003. Characterization of *Salmonella enterica* serotype Newport isolated from humans and food animals. *J. Clin. Microbiol.* **41:**5366–5371.

247. **Zhao, S., D. G. White, P. F. McDermott, S. Friedman, L. English, S. Ayers, J. Meng, J. J. Maurer, R. Holland, and R. D. Walker.** 2001. Identification and expression of cephamycinase bla_{CMY} genes in *Escherichia coli* and *Salmonella* isolates from food animals and ground meat. *Antimicrob. Agents Chemother.* **45:**3647–3650.

Antimicrobial Resistance in Bacteria of Animal Origin
Edited by Frank M. Aarestrup

Chapter 18

Enterococcus

SHABBIR SIMJEE, LARS B. JENSEN, SUSAN M. DONABEDIAN, AND MARCUS J. ZERVOS

Enterococcus is an extremely versatile bacterial genus. Enterococci form part of the normal human and animal gut flora, and some strains are used for the manufacturing of foods or as probiotics. Enterococcal strains have been implicated in serious diseases in animals and humans and over the last 2 decades have emerged as one of the leading causes of nosocomial bloodstream infections in humans (see reference 115 and http://www.cdc.gov/ncidod/hip/Surveill/nnis.htm). This has been further compounded by the fact that enterococci are able to acquire antimicrobial resistance and have increasingly become resistant to a number of antibiotics. This ability to acquire antimicrobial resistance has made enterococci the obvious choice as indicator organisms for antimicrobial resistance in gram-positive bacteria, and prevalence of resistance has been monitored in surveillance programs (see reference 13 and http://www.cdc.gov/ncidod/hip/Surveill/nnis.htm). Although not classic food-borne pathogens, they have been associated with food-borne outbreaks due to their presence in foods and their capacity to carry and disseminate antibiotic resistance genes. In this chapter we will focus on the presence of virulence and antimicrobial resistance genes in enterococci of animal origin and the possible spread of resistance between the animal and human reservoir, probably through the food chain. Pathogenicity of enterococci will be described, with a focus on the problems enterococci cause for humans.

CLASSIFICATION AND IDENTIFICATION

Although classically considered as a major division of the genus *Streptococcus*, in 1984 *Enterococcus* became recognized as a separate genus (50, 141). Enterococci are catalase-negative, gram-positive cocci that occur singly, in pairs, or in short chains. They are facultative anaerobes, exhibiting versatility in that they are tolerant to extremes of temperatures, salinity, and pH; thus they grow in 6.5% NaCl broth at pH 9.6 and at temperatures ranging from 10 to 45°C, with optimum growth at 35°C (141). Enterococci hydrolyze esculin in the presence of 40% bile salts. Most enterococci hydrolyze L-pyrrolidonyl-β-naphthylamide, and all strains hydrolyze leucine-β-naphthylamide by producing leucine aminopeptidase. Some species, such as *Enterococcus gallinarum* and *E. casseliflavus*, are motile.

Current criteria for inclusion into the *Enterococcus* genus are a combination of DNA-DNA reassociation values, 16S rRNA gene sequencing, whole-cell protein analysis, and conventional phenotypic tests (50, 107, 141).

At least 23 distinct *Enterococcus* species are recognized (Table 1) (see reference 50 and http://www.ncbi.nlm.nih.gov/Taxonomy/Browser/wwtar.cgi), and new species continue to be identified (34). The defined species have been separated into five groups on the basis of acid formation in mannitol and sorbose broths and hydrolysis of arginine (Table 1) (50).

Three new species of *Enterococcus* were recently identified from human clinical sources by analysis of whole-cell protein profiles and DNA-DNA reassociation experiments, in conjunction with conventional physiological tests. These new enterococcal species, provisionally designated *Enterococcus* sp. nov. CDC PNS-E1, *Enterococcus* sp. nov. CDC PNS-E2, and *Enterococcus* sp. nov. CDC PNS-E3, resemble physiological groups I, II, and IV, respectively; two were isolated from human blood and one from human brain tissue.

The species most broadly distributed in nature are *E. faecalis* and *E. faecium*. Identification of the

Shabbir Simjee • Center for Veterinary Medicine, U.S. Food and Drug Administration, Laurel, MD 20708. Lars B. Jensen • Danish Institute for Food and Veterinary Research, Bülowsvej 27, DK-1790 Copenhagen V, Denmark. Susan M. Donabedian • Division of Infectious Diseases, William Beaumont Hospital, Royal Oak, MI 40873. Marcus J. Zervos • Division of Infectious Diseases, William Beaumont Hospital, Royal Oak, MI 40873, and Wayne State University School of Medicine, Detroit, MI 48202.

Table 1. Phenotypic characteristics used for identification of *Enterococcus* species

Species	Phenotypic characteristic[a]											
	MAN	SOR	ARG	ARA	SBL	RAF	TEL	MOT	PIG	SUC	PYU	MGP
Group I												
E. avium	+	+	–	+	+	–	–	–	–	+	+	V
E. malodoratus	+	+	–	–	+	+	–	–	–	+	+	V
E. raffinosus	+	+	–	+	+	+	–	–	–	+	+	V
E. pseudoavium	+	+	–	–	+	–	–	–	–	+	+	+
E. saccharolyticus	+	+	–	–	+	+	–	–	–	+	–	+
E. pallens	+	+	–	–	+	+	–	–	+	+	–	+
E. gilvus	+	+	–	–	+	+	–	–	+	+	+	–
Group II												
E. faecalis	+	–	+	–	+	–	+	–	–	V	+	–
E. faecium	+	–	+	+	V	V	–	–	–	V	–	–
E. casseliflavus	+	–	+	+	V	+	V	V	+	+	V	+
E. mundtii	+	–	+	+	V	+	–	–	+	+	–	–
E. gallinarum	+	–	+	+	–	+	–	V	–	+	–	+
Group III												
E. durans	–	–	+	V	–	V	V	–	–	V	V	V
E. villorum	–	–	+	V	–	V	V	–	–	V	V	V
E. ratti	–	–	+	V	–	V	V	–	–	V	V	V
E. hirae	–	–	+	V	–	V	V	–	–	V	V	V
E. dispar	–	–	+	V	–	V	V	–	–	V	V	V
E. faecalis	–	–	+	V	–	V	V	–	–	V	V	V
E. faecium	–	–	+	V	–	V	V	–	–	V	V	V
Group IV												
E. asini	–	–	–	–	–	–	–	–	–	+	–	–
E. sulfureus	–	–	–	–	–	+	–	–	+	+	–	+
E. cecorum	–	–	–	–	+	+	–	–	–	+	+	–
Group V												
E. casseliflavus	+	–	–	+	V	+	V	+	+	+	V	+
E. gallinarum	+	–	–	+	–	+	–	+	–	+	–	+
E. faecalis	+	–	–	–	+	–	+	–	–	+	+	–
E. columbae	+	–	–	+	+	+	–	–	–	+	+	–

[a]MAN, mannitol; SOR, sorbose; ARG, arginine; ARA, arabinose; SBL, sorbitol; RAF, raffinose; TEL, 0.04% tellurite; MOT, motility; PIG, pigment; SUC, sucrose; PYU, pyruvate; MGP, methyl-α-D-glucopyranoside; +, >90% positive; –, <10% positive; V, variable.

different *Enterococcus* species can be done by conventional physiological tests, by commercial systems, or by molecular methods (73). Correct species identification is important due to varying intrinsic resistance among the different species; misidentification may lead to improper antimicrobial treatment, inaccurate data on the prevalence of antimicrobial resistance in epidemiologic surveillance, and incorrect choice of starter strains or labeling of the product to which the starter is added.

RESERVOIRS

Enterococci have the capacity to grow and survive in very harsh environments and thus occupy a variety of ecological niches. They can be found in soil, water, food, plants, insects, birds, and mammals, including humans. The major natural habitat of these organisms appears to be the gastrointestinal tract of animals and humans, where they make up a significant portion of the normal aerobic gut flora (107). With the increase in antimicrobial-resistant enterococci worldwide and their implication in serious human diseases, there has been growing interest in identifying reservoirs of these organisms and of the antimicrobial resistance genes that they carry.

The Animal Reservoir

Enterococci are a natural part of the intestinal flora in most mammals and birds. Insects and reptiles have been found to harbor these organisms. Some *Enterococcus* species are host specific, while others are more broadly distributed. Several species, although identifiable in a number of hosts, appear to have some host-specific properties (4). Examples of host-specific enterococci are *E. columbae*, specific for pigeons, and *E. asini*, found so far only in donkeys.

The most often encountered enterococcal species in the intestines of farm animals are *E. faecalis*, *E. faecium*, *E. hirae*, and *E. durans*. In chickens, *E. faecalis*, found early in life, is later replaced by *E. faecium*, then by *E. cecorum*. Other species occasionally isolated from chickens are *E. casseliflavus*, *E. gallinarum*, and *E. mundtii*.

The Food Reservoir

Enterococci are present in high numbers in food of animal origin (88). As contaminants from the intestinal tract, they have been found in raw meat in concentrations of 10^2 to 10^4 CFU g^{-1}.

In fermented food products, enterococci survive easily due to their ability to survive harsh environments, and they have been found in the range of 10^2 to 10^5 CFU g^{-1} in salami (88). Enterococci can also be isolated from vegetables (59). Enterococci have important implications in dairy products. They are used as starters for cheeses, especially in Europe (61), are used in the production of mozzarella cheese (61), and can be found in ripening cheese in the range of 10^5 to 10^7 CFU g^{-1} (88). Enterococci can also be used as starter adjuncts as producers of enterocin, which inhibits the presence of *Listeria monocytogenes* and *Staphylococcus aureus* (59, 91).

Enterococci have been implicated in spoilage of meat. If present in high numbers, they can survive heat processing (52). They have been identified in spoilage of pasteurized canned ham and today cannot be avoided in processed food. The most abundant enterococci in food are *E. faecium* and *E. faecalis* (52), but *E. durans* has also been isolated from cheese (59).

The Human Reservoir

Enterococci make up approximately 1% of the normal intestinal flora of humans (140), being the predominant gram-positive cocci in stool, with concentrations ranging from 10^5 to 10^7 CFU/g of feces (81). *E. faecalis* is normally found in the stool of 90 to 100% of animals and humans, while *E. faecium* is found in 25%. Small numbers of enterococci also occur in oropharyngeal secretions, the urogenital tract, and on the skin, especially in the perineal area (107, 141). The prevalence of the different species varies according to the host and is also influenced by age, diet, underlying diseases, and prior antimicrobial therapy (58, 141). The species most commonly isolated from human clinical specimens is *E. faecalis*, followed by *E. faecium*. Infections caused by *E. casseliflavus* and *E. raffinosus* have also been reported (141). Rarely, other species, including *E. avium*, *E. cecorum*, *E. dispar*, *E. durans*, *E. gilvus*, *E. gallinarum*, *E. hirae*, *E. mundtii*, and *E. pallens*, have also been isolated from human sources (141).

ENTEROCOCCAL INFECTIONS

Virulence Determinants in Enterococci

Several potential virulence factors have been identified in enterococci (Table 2) (47, 152), but none has been established as having a major or consistent contribution to virulence in humans. The best described are cytolysin (38, 58, 82), aggregation substance (38, 56, 89), pheromones (49, 81), lipoteichoic acid (22, 48), the metalloendopeptidase gelatinase (99, 139), hyaluronidase (125), and AS-48, a bacteriocin with activity against gram-positive and gram-negative bacteria (57). Cytolysin has lytic activity against gram-positive bacteria and selected eukaryotic cells; in combination with aggregation substance, it was shown to increase mortality in a rabbit model of endocarditis (38,81). Aggregation substance facilitates binding of donor to recipient cells in the pheromone mating response, thus allowing exchange of plasmids carrying virulence traits or antibiotic resistance genes (81) (see "Mobile DNA Elements in Enterococci" below).

Other putative virulence factors include the adhesin called enterococcal surface protein (Esp) and surface carbohydrates (4, 24, 54, 81, 161). Most virulence factors have been described in *E. faecalis*, and many reside on conjugative plasmids that can spread between strains in a natural environment, such as the

Table 2. Function of the enterococcal virulence factors

Virulence factor	Role of virulence factor
GelE	Toxin; extracellular metalloendopeptidase, hydrolyzes gelatin, collagen, hemoglobin, and other bioactive compounds
CylA	Activation of cytolysin
CylB	Transport of cytolysin
CylM	Posttranslational modification of cytolysin
Esp	Cell wall-associated protein involved in immune evasion, may be associated with *cyl* genes on a pathogenicity island
EfaAfm	Cell wall adhesins expressed in serum
Cpd and Cob	Sex pheromones, chemotactic for human leukocytes; facilitate conjugation

gastrointestinal tract (81). Virulence traits are less well characterized in *E. faecium*, but EfaAfm has been indicated as a possible virulence factor (134) and an open reading frame, hyl_{Efm}, has been identified in *E. faecium* (119).

Virulence factors such as hemolysin, aggregation substance, Esp, and gelatinase can also be present in food isolates (47, 54, 102), and *esp* has been identified in *E. faecalis* isolates from production animals (66). In general, the incidence of these virulence traits is lower among *E. faecium* strains than among *E. faecalis* strains, and *E. faecium* harbors fewer virulence traits than *E. faecalis* (47, 54). In a comparative study, *E. faecalis* strains causing human infection had more virulence determinants than did food strains, which in turn had more than did starter strains (47). It was also demonstrated that starter strains, added intentionally to certain cheeses and other fermented milk products, can acquire known virulence genes by conjugation, a natural gene transfer process (47). Recently, pathogenicity islands (PAIs) have been detected both in *E. faecium* and *E. faecalis* (93, 126). A study of *esp*-positive *E. faecalis* of porcine origin indicated the presence of a PAI very similar to the PAI in a virulent *E. faecalis* of human origin (N. Shankar, unpublished data).

Infection in Animals

Enterococci can cause a number of infections in animals, including bovine mastitis. Most cases are related to poor hygiene, and an improvement could reduce the number of cases. The most prevalent enterococci in these cases are *E. faecalis*, followed by *E. faecium*. Other enterococci, like *E. durans*, *E. avium*, *E. hirae*, and *E. pseudoavium*, have also been detected (11).

In poultry, infections occur primarily in the animals' first weeks (32). Enterococci have also been isolated from focal necrosis of the brain, septicemia, and endocarditis in poultry. Enterococci can cause diarrhea. In production animals, cases caused by *E. durans* have been reported in calves (122) and piglets, as have cases caused by *E. villorum* (147).

Infection in Humans

With the exception of *E. faecium* and *E. faecalis*, enterococci are rarely reported to be pathogens in humans (52). In fact, until 2 decades ago, when they started emerging as important nosocomial pathogens, enterococci were considered rather innocuous. They were previously regarded as endogenous pathogens acquired from the patient's own flora, until person-to-person transmission was first demonstrated in 1987 (153). Spread of enterococci among patients and even from one institution to another has been documented (153).

Enterococci have been associated with high mortality rates (12 to 68%) in patients with bacteremia (26, 29, 63, 65, 83, 90, 101, 107, 121, 127, 153, 163), but these studies have nonetheless failed to establish unequivocally the pathogenicity of the causative organism in this setting. In one large study of bloodstream infections, enterococci were the only gram-positive pathogens independently associated with a high risk of death (154). Due to the facts that most of the patients are severely debilitated and that enterococci are often part of a polymicrobic bacteremia, it has been difficult to determine the independent contribution of enterococci to morbidity and mortality in these patients.

Enterococci are able to adhere to left-sided heart valves and renal epithelial cells, properties which likely enable them to cause endocarditis and urinary tract infections (107). Although they are natural inhabitants of the gastrointestinal tract, they are not known to cause gastroenteritis in humans except for possibly a strain of *E. hirae* isolated from a patient with diarrhea. This strain was able to cause diarrhea in suckling rats (107). In intra-abdominal and wound infections, it has been suggested that enterococci act synergistically with other bacteria, but their exact role in those settings still remains to be defined (107).

Food-Borne Outbreaks

E. faecalis and *E. faecium* are suspected but unconfirmed causative agents of food-borne illness in its classic sense. They were first associated with food-borne illness in 1926, when two outbreaks of gastroenteritis from cheese were reported (138). Enterococci were implicated due to their presence in large numbers in the incriminated foods and the absence of other pathogens such as *S. aureus* or *Salmonella* spp. (120). On the other hand, it is felt that enterococci can cause food intoxication through the production of biogenic amines, but both these observations are still awaiting confirmation (59). Efforts to prove that enterococci cause food-borne illness, including animal experiments and studies using human volunteers, have yielded contradictory results (120, 138). Food intoxication caused by ingestion of biogenic amines is associated with a number of symptoms, including headache, vomiting, increased blood pressure, and even allergic reactions (59). The ability to produce biogenic amines in cheese and fermented sausages has been reported for bacteria of the genus *Enterococcus* (27, 59).

ANTIMICROBIAL RESISTANCE IN ENTEROCOCCI

The emergence of antimicrobial resistance represents the greatest threat to the treatment of human enterococcal infections. Enterococci are intrinsically resistant to a number of antimicrobial agents normally used to treat infections cause by gram-positive organisms. In addition, they have a remarkable ability to acquire new mechanisms of resistance and to transfer resistance determinants, by way of conjugation, among themselves and between themselves and other organisms. In this section, we focus on the antimicrobial resistance selected for in animals that can be transferred to humans, causing treatment failures. Several studies have indicated transfer of antimicrobial resistance between the animal and human reservoir. Reduced use of antimicrobials in animal production has affected the prevalence of antimicrobial resistance among enterococci of human origin.

Resistance in Food Animals

Antimicrobial agents are used in animals for therapy; for prophylaxis of infection during times of stress, such as early weaning; for metaphylaxis (treatment of clinically healthy animals belonging to the same flock or pen as sick animals); and for growth promotion (4). The latter use has been seriously questioned in recent years (4). Often, members of the same classes of antimicrobials are used for treatment or growth promotion in food animals and for treatment of human infections. Unfortunately, the use of antimicrobial agents in food animals has created a large reservoir of antimicrobial-resistant enterococci and resistance genes, the dissemination of which to humans may pose a significant threat to human health.

Aminoglycoside resistance

Several aminoglycosides are used for treatment of animals. Among these are gentamicin, kanamycin, and streptomycin. Gentamicin is commonly used in swine and widely used in chickens and turkeys. High-level gentamicin-resistant enterococci have been isolated from broilers and pigs in Europe (4, 149, 150). Gentamicin resistance has also been detected in enterococci of animal origin in the United States (73, 144), and one study from the United States found that when gentamicin resistance genes were present in resistant enterococci isolated from animals, they were also present in the enterococci isolated from food products of the same animal species (32). Gentamicin-resistant enterococci have also been isolated from bovine mastitis (75). Gentamicin resistance is predominantly encoded by the *aac(6)′-aph(2″)* gene (Table 3).

Table 3. Antimicrobial resistance genes in enterococci of animal origin

Antimicrobial agent	Genetic background for resistance	Reference(s)
Aminoglycosides	*aadE*	155
	aac(6′)-aph(2″)	2, 42, 144
	aphA-3	2, 155
Chloramphenicol	*catA*	2, 4, 158
Glycopeptide	*vanA*	2, 78, 148, 151
	vanB	42
	vanC1, *vanC2*	98, 117
Macrolides	*erm*(A)	77
	erm(B)	77, 103, 157
	mrs(C)	156
Oxazolidinone (linezolid)		159
Oligosaccharides	*emtA*	106
Penicillin	*pbp5*	5
Streptogramin B	*vgb*	79
Streptogramin A	*vat*(D) [*sat*(G)]	79, 135
	vat(E)	79, 135
Streptothricin	*sat4*	157
Tetracycline	*tet*(K)	25
	tet(L)	2
	tet(M)	2
	tet(O)	2
	tet(S)	5

Kanamycin-resistant enterococci have been isolated from pigs and poultry in Europe (5) and in the United States (123). Kanamycin-resistant enterococci have been isolated from bovine mastitis (74). Resistance mediated by the *aph(3′)* gene has been found in both *E. faecium* and *E. faecalis* (2).

Streptomycin-resistant enterococci have been isolated from pigs and poultry in Europe (2) and in the United States, as well as in cattle (74). Resistance was found in *E. faecium* and *E. faecalis*, but the genetic background for the resistance was not determined.

Aminoglycoside-resistant enterococci (resistant to gentamicin, kanamycin, and streptomycin) have been isolated from sewage and seawater in the United States (118).

Macrolide resistance

High levels of macrolide-resistant enterococci have been detected among enterococci of animal origin in Europe (10, 55). Prior to 1999 the macrolide tylosin was used in large amounts for growth promotion in Europe; tylosin and erythromycin are still used for treatment of animal infections. After the ban on use of the growth promoter tylosin in Europe in 1999, a substantial reduction in the prevalence of macrolide-resistant enterococci was observed in

Denmark (see Fig. 1 in chapter 23) and in The Netherlands. Resistance to macrolides in most enterococci is encoded by the *erm*(B) gene (Table 3).

Oligosaccharide resistance

The oligosaccharide avilamycin has been used for growth promotion, mainly in poultry, for many years in Europe. A high prevalence of avilamycin resistance in enterococci has been detected in several countries (31, 43), and an association between use of avilamycin and occurrence of resistance has been detected (43). Resistance is mostly encountered in *E. faecium* but has also been detected in *E. faecalis* (9). After a voluntary withdrawal of usage of avilamycin in Denmark, the prevalence of avilamycin resistance was reduced (see Fig. 1 in chapter 23) (10). Cross-resistance to the oligosaccharide evernimicin has been detected. The *emtA* gene was identified (9) in some of the avilamycin-resistant enterococci of animal origin. This gene also encodes high-level resistance to evernimicin. Point mutations in the L16 ribosomal protein have been associated with reduced susceptibility to both avilamycin and evernimicin (8).

Streptogramin resistance

Virginiamycin (a streptogramin) was used in Europe until 1999. High levels of streptogramin-resistant *E. faecium* (SREF) were detected in production animals in several European countries (5, 79), and SREF has been found in food (128, 130, 132). A study of different ecological sources in Germany discovered rates of resistance to streptogramins of up to 100% among *E. faecium* isolates from sewage, poultry manure, and pig manure, whereas rates of resistance among broiler chickens, pork meat, human stool samples, and hospitalized patients were 46%, 10%, 14%, and 7.4%, respectively (158). Virginiamycin was banned in Europe, pending further studies on the possible relationship of its use in food animals and cross-resistance to streptogramins used clinically to treat infections in humans. Reduced prevalence of SREF has been detected since the ban on virginiamycin as a growth promoter in Europe.

Virginiamycin has been used for over 2 decades in poultry and swine feed in the United States. Data suggest that SREF is more common in farms that use virginiamycin (70). Concerns exist that the agricultural use of virginiamycin has generated SREF, and SREF is common in isolates recovered from food animals (158). Resistance to streptogramins is encoded by a combination of resistance genes. Since streptogramins consist of a combination of a streptogramin A and a streptogramin B, resistance to both is required. Among the enterococci, *E. faecalis* is intrinsically resistant to streptogramins of type A, but like all other enterococci, it must acquire genes to become resistant to streptogramins of type B. This is generally encoded, together with macrolide and lincosamide resistance, by the *erm*(B) gene. Streptogramin A resistance is encoded in enterococci by either *vat*(D) or *vat*(E) (Table 3). Genetic links between genes encoding streptogramins of types A and B have been detected in several enterococcal isolates (79).

Tetracycline resistance

Tetracycline resistance has in Europe been detected among *E. faecium* from broilers, cattle, and pigs and among *E. faecalis* from pigs and broilers (2, 30). In the United States high levels of tetracycline-resistant enterococci have been isolated from poultry (68).

In enterococci, tetracycline resistance is most commonly encoded by *tet*(M), which is widely distributed among gram-positive bacteria. *tet*(M) is normally positioned in Tn*916* or derivatives of this transposon. Other resistance genes and mechanisms, such as *tet*(K), *tet*(L), *tet*(O), and *tet*(S), have been detected in enterococci (4), but frequencies vary in enterococci from different reservoirs.

Vancomycin resistance

In Europe, the prevalence of vancomycin-resistant enterococci (VRE) in production animals was linked to the use of avoparcin (a glycopeptide related to vancomycin) as a growth promoter in food animals (18). In Europe, VRE was found throughout the community, the food supply and urban and rural sewage systems. After the ban on usage of avoparcin in 1995 in Europe, a reduced prevalence of VRE in animals was found in several European countries. In Denmark, the prevalence of VRE in production animals has been reduced since the ban of avoparcin (see Fig. 1 in chapter 23). In contrast, in the United States, where avoparcin was never approved for use in animals, VRE are rarely found in production animals or in the environment.

Six types of glycopeptide resistance have been identified, with three of them being most common. The VanA acquired phenotype is associated with inducible high-level resistance to both vancomycin and teicoplanin. The VanB acquired phenotype is associated with moderate to high levels of inducible resistance to vancomycin only. VanA and VanB are found most often in *E. faecium*, but also in *E. faecalis* and occasional isolates of other species. In contrast, the intrinsic VanC phenotype, which is usually associated with low-level, noninducible resistance to vancomycin (141), is found in *E. gallinarum* and *E. casseliflavus*.

The *vanA* gene cluster, encoded by Tn*1546*, encodes almost exclusively for vancomycin resistance in enterococci of animal origin.

Resistance in Pets

Antimicrobial resistance in pet animals may play a very central role in the spread of resistance to humans. Antimicrobials used for the treatment of pets include antimicrobials prescribed for human use (64), and pets are in very close contact with humans. The transfer of resistance from pets might be underestimated. Antimicrobial-resistant enterococci have been isolated from pet animals (69, 129). These include VRE isolated from pets in Europe and in the United States (129), where VRE have not been isolated from production animals. Resistance to macrolides, tetracyclines, and aminoglycosides has also been demonstrated.

Resistance in Food Products of Animal Origin

Antimicrobial resistance to aminoglycosides, penicillin, chloramphenicol, macrolides, and vancomycin has been identified in food derived from animal products (59). In a study from Scandinavia a high prevalence of resistant enterococci was noted in isolates from pork and poultry (116). Studies from the United States found high levels of SREF (130, 132) and gentamicin-resistant enterococci (44) in retail poultry. Tetracycline resistance is probably the most common resistance phenotype in enterococci from food. However, enterococci with resistance to more than one antimicrobial have been isolated from beef products like minced meat, tenderloin beef, and raw meat sausages (137) and from cheese (71). The focus on antimicrobial resistance in food of animal origin has been on the prevalence of VRE, which have been found in beef, chicken, pork, and other meat products (30, 137, 160).

Foods other than meat have also been found to harbor resistant enterococci. A study carried out in Argentina found high-level resistance to streptomycin and gentamicin in *E. faecium* and resistance to streptomycin alone in *E. faecalis* from farm lettuce (124). In study of 24 enterococcal strains isolated from traditional Italian cheeses, 1 *E. faecium* strain showed the *vanA* vancomycin resistance genotype while 4 strains showed beta-hemolysis on human blood (12).

Antimicrobial Resistance in Humans

Beta-lactam resistance

Clinical isolates of enterococci, in particular *E. faecium*, have become increasingly resistant to ampicillin. In some hospitals over 90% of the *E. faecium* isolates are resistant to ampicillin (MIC of ≥32 μg/ml) (84). High-level resistance to penicillins is due predominantly either to the overproduction of a penicillin-binding protein with low affinity for penicillins or to mutations that make the low-affinity penicillin-binding protein even less susceptible to inhibition by penicillins (84). Beta-lactam resistance in *E. faecium* has recently been linked to hospital-specific clones belonging to the CC17 complex (R. Willems, *Antimicrob. Agents Chemother.*, in press).

Some rare *E. faecalis* strains produce beta-lactamase; importantly, these strains may appear to be susceptible to penicillins in vitro when standard MIC testing is done since they produce the enzyme in small amounts. These strains caused outbreaks in the 1980s but have not been seen in significant numbers in the last 15 years (100).

Aminoglycoside resistance

Enterococci with high-level resistance to streptomycin and/or kanamycin are commonly detected, but high-level resistance to gentamicin has become a clinical problem only since the 1980s (107). Clinical failures and relapses after therapy in patients with endocarditis due to *E. faecalis* and *E. faecium* with high-level resistance to all aminoglycosides are increasingly being encountered. Some isolates with high-level gentamicin resistance remain susceptible in vitro to streptomycin, which can be used in combination with a cell wall-active agent for therapy of endocarditis.

Oxazolidinone and streptogramin resistance

Resistance to the most recently introduced anti-gram-positive agents, oxazolidinones and streptogramins, has already emerged among enterococci (37, 46, 62, 105, 128, 130, 132). Although rare, SREF has been documented in humans (135). Of concern, emergence of resistance during therapy was observed and resulted in clinical failure (108). At the Centers for Disease Control and Prevention, a multistate surveillance study found a 1 to 2% rate of SREF isolated from human stool samples.

Vancomycin resistance

In the late 1980s, VRE were described, first in Europe and then in the United States (94). Strains of VRE are often multidrug resistant. Ampicillin and vancomycin resistance are associated with *E. faecium* far more commonly than with other species (141). In the United States VRE is largely confined to hospitals, where it is likely thriving under selective pressure from widespread vancomycin use (23). The percentage of nosocomial infections caused by VRE increased more than 20-fold between 1989 and 1993, from 0.3 to 7.9%, and the trend has continued since then, with rates now approaching 20% of all enterococcal isolates (107, 112). In a comparison of National Nosocomial Infections Surveillance pathogens from 1994 through 1998 and January through May 1999, there was a 47% increase in VRE (13). In 1997 data obtained from more than 100 clinical laboratories showed that 52% of *E. faecium* and 1.9% of *E. faecalis* isolates were resistant to vancomycin (28, 40, 92, 96, 97, 104, 107, 109, 110, 113, 146). The risk factors and epidemiology of vancomycin-resistant *E. faecalis* were recently analyzed (113). Transfer of VanA-mediated vancomycin resistance from VRE to methicillin-resistant *S. aureus* has been detected in hospital settings recently (35, 51, 142), raising serious concerns.

There is clear evidence that with an increase in the consumption of antimicrobial agents by humans and animals there is a resultant increase in antimicrobial resistance (33, 44). Some studies have indicated that reduction in the use of antimicrobials and the presence of antimicrobial-resistant isolates in animals have influenced the prevalence of resistance in humans. In studies in Germany (85) and The Netherlands a reduced prevalence of VRE was detected in nonhospitalized humans, and a study in Belgium (72) showed reduced prevalence of the *vanA* gene, the most abundant resistance gene in VRE of animal origin, after the ban on using avoparcin as a growth promoter.

Other antimicrobials

In the case of the recently approved antibiotic daptomycin, spontaneous acquisition of resistance in vitro is rare, and it is hoped that this will extrapolate into the clinical setting (33).

MOBILE DNA ELEMENTS IN ENTEROCOCCI

Enterococci have an ability to become resistant to antimicrobials. Most of this resistance is due to acquisition of mobile DNA elements like plasmids, transposons, or combinations of these by horizontal gene transfer. Several experiments have shown high transfer rates of antimicrobial resistance between enterococci both in vitro (67) and in vivo (95, 111). In *E. faecalis*, specialized sex pheromone-based conjugational plasmids have been detected (39). These conjugational systems are based on production of aggregation substance, which enables the enterococci to be in close contact and transfer plasmids very efficiently. The system is largely confined to enterococci, with the only similar system detected in *Bacillus* spp., and is predominantly found in *E. faecalis*. Recent studies have detected *E. faecium* isolates containing sex pheromone-responsive plasmids. Several of the sex pheromone plasmids have been sequenced, such as pAD1 (D. Clewell, personal communication), pCF10 (G. Dunny, personal communication), and pAM373 (41). Recently, with the total sequencing of *E. faecalis* V583, three additional plasmids (pTEF1, pTEF2, and pTEF3) have been sequenced (114). The plasmid pRE25 was isolated from food and its sequence determined (143). Data on total plasmid sequences make comparison of plasmids from different reservoirs possible.

Transposons are widely detected among enterococci, in particular Tn*916*, carrying the tetracycline resistance determinant *tet*(M), and Tn*917*, conferring macrolide resistance [*erm*(B)]. For vancomycin the *vanA* transposon Tn*1546* is detected in enterococci of both animal and human origin while Tn*1547* (*vanB*) is predominantly found in enterococci of human origin.

TRANSFER OF ENTEROCOCCI AND ANTIMICROBIAL RESISTANCE GENES BETWEEN NONHUMAN RESERVOIRS AND HUMANS

After the introduction of avoparcin as a growth promoter for livestock in Europe in 1974, animals presumably started developing VRE. In the late 1980s VRE emerged in humans. Epidemiologic studies examining glycopeptide use in animal husbandry have provided evidence that *vanA*-mediated VRE are now ubiquitous in European communities, the organism readily colonizing intestinal tracts of animals for which avoparcin was used as a feed supplement (1, 20, 86, 87, 112). Subsequent enteric colonization of humans has been documented (19, 112). Genetic characterization of the VanA element has identified identical elements in isolates of human and animal origin (78, 160), and one study indicated transfer of VRE from animals to humans (76).

In the United States the use of virginiamycin in animal food and the emergence of SREF mirror the avoparcin-VRE situation in Europe. Virginiamycin is used worldwide and has been approved in the United States for use in chickens, turkeys, swine, and cattle, mainly for growth promotion. Molecular analysis of gentamicin-resistant enterococcal strains from humans, food, and farm animals provided evidence of the spread of such isolates from animals to humans over a broad geographical area through the food supply (44).

SUMMARY AND CONCLUSIONS

Although part of the normal intestinal flora and once felt to be innocuous, enterococci have proven to have much more complex interactions with the human host, having emerged in recent years as important nosocomial pathogens. Strains with resistance to multiple antimicrobials are on the rise, posing significant therapeutic and epidemiological challenges. Virulence factors have also been described for these organisms, which traditionally are regarded as having low pathogenicity.

The role of enterococci in disease raises valid concerns regarding their safety for use in foods or as probiotics. If *Enterococcus* strains are selected for use as starter or probiotic cultures, ideally such strains should harbor no virulence determinants and should be susceptible to clinically relevant antibiotics.

In 1994, as the imminent crisis of emergent antimicrobial resistance became more and more recognized, the World Health Organization recommended immediate and drastic reductions in the use of antibiotics in animals, plants, and fish, as well as in human medicine (21, 162). Even if they occur, such reductions are unlikely to be sufficient in curtailing the emergence of resistant bacteria. In order to achieve this goal, a more comprehensive, multidisciplinary effort is needed, including a better understanding of the epidemiology and pathogenicity of these microorganisms, judicious use of antimicrobials, effective infection control measures in hospitals, and reduction of resistance in reservoirs such as the environment and animal husbandry.

REFERENCES

1. **Aarestrup, F. M.** 1995. Occurrence of glycopeptide resistance among Enterococcus faecium isolates from conventional and ecological poultry farms. *Microb. Drug Resist.* **1:**255–257.
2. **Aarestrup, F. M., Y. Agerso, P. Gerner-Smidt, M. Madsen, and L. B. Jensen.** 2000. Comparison of antimicrobial resistance phenotypes and resistance genes in Enterococcus faecalis and Enterococcus faecium from humans in the community, broilers, and pigs in Denmark. *Diagn. Microbiol. Infect. Dis.* **37:**127–137.
3. Reference deleted.
4. **Aarestrup, F. M., P. Butaye, and W. Whitte.** 2002. Nonhuman reservoirs of enterococci, p. 55–99. *In* M. S. Gilmore, D. B. Clewell, P. Courvalin, G. M. Dunny, B. E. Murray, and L. B. Rice (ed.), *The Enterococci: Pathogenesis, Molecular Biology, and Antibiotic Resistance.* ASM Press, Washington, D.C.
5. **Aarestrup, F. M., H. Hasman, L. B. Jensen, M. Moreno, I. A. Herrero, L. Dominguez, M. Finn, and A. Franklin.** 2002. Antimicrobial resistance among enterococci from pigs in three European countries. *Appl. Environ. Microbiol.* **68:**4127–4129.
6. Reference deleted.
7. Reference deleted.
8. **Aarestrup, F. M., and L. B. Jensen.** 2000. Presence of variations in ribosomal protein L16 corresponding to susceptibility of enterococci to oligosaccharides (avilamycin and evernimicin). *Antimicrob. Agents Chemother.* **44:**3425–3427.
9. **Aarestrup, F. M., and P. M. McNicholas.** 2002. Incidence of high-level evernimicin resistance in *Enterococcus faecium* among food animals and humans. *Antimicrob. Agents Chemother.* **46:**3088–3090.
10. **Aarestrup, F. M., A. M. Seyfarth, H. D. Emborg, K. Pedersen, R. S. Hendriksen, and F. Bager.** 2001. Effect of abolishment of the use of antimicrobial agents for growth promotion on occurrence of antimicrobial resistance in fecal enterococci from food animals in Denmark. *Antimicrob. Agents Chemother.* **45:**2054–2059.
11. **Aarestrup, F. M., H. C. Wegener, V. T. Rosdahl, and N. E. Jensen.** 1995. Staphylococcal and other bacterial species associated with intramammary infections in Danish dairy herds. *Acta Vet. Scand.* **36:**475–487.
12. **Andrighetto, C., E. Knijff, A. Lombardi, S. Torriani, M. Vancanneyt, K. Kersters, J. Swings, and F. Dellaglio.** 2001. Phenotypic and genetic diversity of enterococci isolated from Italian cheeses. *J. Dairy Res.* **68:**303–316.
13. **Anonymous.** 1999. National Nosocomial Infections Surveillance (NNIS) System report, data summary from January 1990–May 1999, issued June 1999. *Am. J. Infect. Control* **27:**520–532.
14. Reference deleted.
15. Reference deleted.
16. Reference deleted.
17. Reference deleted.
18. **Bager, F., M. Madsen, J. Christensen, and F. M. Aarestrup.** 1997. Avoparcin used as a growth promoter is associated with the occurrence of vancomycin-resistant Enterococcus faecium on Danish poultry and pig farms. *Prev. Vet. Med.* **31:**95–112.
19. **Bates, J.** 1997. Epidemiology of vancomycin-resistant enterococci in the community and the relevance of farm animals to human infection. *J. Hosp. Infect.* **37:**89–101.
20. **Bates, J., J. Z. Jordens, and D. T. Griffiths.** 1994. Farm animals as a putative reservoir for vancomycin-resistant enterococcal infection in man. *J. Antimicrob. Chemother.* **34:**507–514.
21. **Bengmark, S.** 2000. Colonic food: pre- and probiotics. *Am. J. Gastroenterol.* **95:**S5–S7.
22. **Bhakdi, S., T. Klonisch, P. Nuber, and W. Fischer.** 1991. Stimulation of monokine production by lipoteichoic acids. *Infect. Immun.* **59:**4614–4620.
23. **Bonten, M. J., S. Slaughter, A. W. Ambergen, M. K. Hayden, J. van Voorhis, C. Nathan, and R. A. Weinstein.** 1998. The role of "colonization pressure" in the spread of vancomycin-resistant enterococci: an important infection control variable. *Arch. Intern. Med.* **158:**1127–1132.
24. **Bonten, M. J., R. Willems, and R. A. Weinstein.** 2001. Vancomycin-resistant enterococci: why are they here, and where do they come from? *Lancet Infect. Dis.* **1:**314–325.
25. **Borgen, K., M. Sorum, Y. Wasteson, H. Kruse, and H. Oppegaard.** 2002. Genetic linkage between erm(B) and vanA in Enterococcus hirae of poultry origin. *Microb. Drug Resist.* **8:**363–368.
26. **Boulanger, J. M., E. L. Ford-Jones, and A. G. Matlow.** 1991. Enterococcal bacteremia in a pediatric institution: a four-year review. *Rev. Infect. Dis.* **13:**847–856.
27. **Bover-Cid, S., M. Hugas, M. Izquierdo-Pulido, and M. C. Vidal-Carou.** 2001. Amino acid-decarboxylase activity of bacteria isolated from fermented pork sausages. *Int. J. Food Microbiol.* **66:**185–189.
28. **Boyce, J. M., S. M. Opal, J. W. Chow, M. J. Zervos, G. Potter-Bynoe, C. B. Sherman, R. L. Romulo, S. Fortna, and A. A. Medeiros.** 1994. Outbreak of multidrug-resistant *Enterococcus*

faecium with transferable *vanB* class vancomycin resistance. *J. Clin. Microbiol.* **32:**1148–1153.

29. **Bryan, C. S., K. L. Reynolds, and J. J. Brown.** 1985. Mortality associated with enterococcal bacteremia. *Surg. Gynecol. Obstet.* **160:**557–561.
30. **Busani, L., M. Del Grosso, C. Paladini, C. Graziani, A. Pantosti, F. Biavasco, and A. Caprioli.** 2004. Antimicrobial susceptibility of vancomycin-susceptible and -resistant enterococci isolated in Italy from raw meat products, farm animals, and human infections. *Int. J. Food Microbiol.* **97:** 17–22.
31. **Butaye, P., L. A. Devriese, and F. Haesebrouck.** 2003. Antimicrobial growth promoters used in animal feed: effects of less well known antibiotics on gram-positive bacteria. *Clin. Microbiol. Rev.* **16:**175–188.
32. **Cardona, C. J., A. A. Bickford, B. R. Charlton, and G. L. Cooper.** 1993. Enterococcus durans infection in young chickens associated with bacteremia and encephalomalacia. *Avian Dis.* **37:**234–239.
33. **Carpenter, C. F., and H. F. Chambers.** 2004. Daptomycin: another novel agent for treating infections due to drug-resistant gram-positive pathogens. *Clin. Infect. Dis.* **38:**994–1000.
34. **Carvalho, M. G., A. G. Steigerwalt, R. E. Morey, P. L. Shewmaker, L. M. Teixeira, and R. R. Facklam.** 2004. Characterization of three new enterococcal species, *Enterococcus* sp. nov. CDC PNS-E1, *Enterococcus* sp. nov. CDC PNS-E2, and *Enterococcus* sp. nov. CDC PNS-E3, isolated from human clinical specimens. *J. Clin. Microbiol.* **42:**1192–1198.
35. **Chang, S., D. M. Sievert, J. C. Hageman, M. L. Boulton, F. C. Tenover, F. P. Downes, S. Shah, J. T. Rudrik, G. R. Pupp, W. J. Brown, D. Cardo, and S. K. Fridkin.** 2003. Infection with vancomycin-resistant Staphylococcus aureus containing the vanA resistance gene. *N. Engl. J. Med.* **348:**1342–1347.
36. **Cheon, D. S., and C. Chae.** 1996. Outbreak of diarrhea associated with Enterococcus durans in piglets. *J. Vet. Diagn. Invest.* **8:**123–124.
37. **Chow, J. W., S. M. Donahedian, and M. J. Zervos.** 1997. Emergence of increased resistance to quinupristin/dalfopristin during therapy for Enterococcus faecium bacteremia. *Clin. Infect. Dis.* **24:**90–91.
38. **Chow, J. W., L. A. Thal, M. B. Perri, J. A. Vazquez, S. M. Donabedian, D. B. Clewell, and M. J. Zervos.** 1993. Plasmid-associated hemolysin and aggregation substance production contribute to virulence in experimental enterococcal endocarditis. *Antimicrob. Agents Chemother.* **37:**2474–2477.
39. **Clewell, D. B.** 1990. Movable genetic elements and antibiotic resistance in enterococci. *Eur. J. Clin. Microbiol. Infect. Dis.* **9:**90–102.
40. **D'Agata, E. M., W. K. Green, G. Schulman, H. Li, Y. W. Tang, and W. Schaffner.** 2001. Vancomycin-resistant enterococci among chronic hemodialysis patients: a prospective study of acquisition. *Clin. Infect. Dis.* **32:**23–29.
41. **De Boever, E. H., D. B. Clewell, and C. M. Fraser.** 2000. Enterococcus faecalis conjugative plasmid pAM373: complete nucleotide sequence and genetic analyses of sex pheromone response. *Mol. Microbiol.* **37:**1327–1341.
42. **del Campo, R., P. Ruiz-Garbajosa, M. P. Sanchez-Moreno, F. Baquero, C. Torres, R. Canton, and T. M. Coque.** 2003. Antimicrobial resistance in recent fecal enterococci from healthy volunteers and food handlers in Spain: genes and phenotypes. *Microb. Drug Resist.* **9:**47–60.
43. **Delsol, A. A., L. Randall, S. Cooles, M. J. Woodward, J. Sunderland, and J. M. Roe.** 2005. Effect of the growth promoter avilamycin on emergence and persistence of antimicrobial resistance in enteric bacteria in the pig. *J. Appl. Microbiol.* **98:** 564–571.
44. **Donabedian, S. M., L. A. Thal, E. Hershberger, M. B. Perri, J. W. Chow, P. Bartlett, R. Jones, K. Joyce, S. Rossiter, K. Gay, J. Johnson, C. Mackinson, E. Debess, J. Madden, F. Angulo, and M. J. Zervos.** 2003. Molecular characterization of gentamicin-resistant enterococci in the United States: evidence of spread from animals to humans through food. *J. Clin. Microbiol.* **41:**1109–1113.
45. Reference deleted.
46. **Dowzicky, M., G. H. Talbot, C. Feger, P. Prokocimer, J. Etienne, and R. Leclercq.** 2000. Characterization of isolates associated with emerging resistance to quinupristin/dalfopristin (Synercid) during a worldwide clinical program. *Diagn. Microbiol. Infect. Dis.* **37:**57–62.
47. **Eaton, T. J., and M. J. Gasson.** 2001. Molecular screening of *Enterococcus* virulence determinants and potential for genetic exchange between food and medical isolates. *Appl. Environ. Microbiol.* **67:**1628–1635.
48. **Ehrenfeld, E. E., R. E. Kessler, and D. B. Clewell.** 1986. Identification of pheromone-induced surface proteins in *Streptococcus faecalis* and evidence of a role for lipoteichoic acid in formation of mating aggregates. *J. Bacteriol.* **168:**6–12.
49. **Ember, J. A., and T. E. Hugli.** 1989. Characterization of the human neutrophil response to sex pheromones from Streptococcus faecalis. *Am. J. Pathol.* **134:**797–805.
50. **Facklam, R. R., Carvalho, M. D. G. S. and L. M. Teixeira.** 2002. History, taxonomy, biochemical characteristics, and antibiotic susceptibility testing of enterococci, p. 1–54. *In* M. S. Gilmore, D. B. Clewell, P. Courvalin, G. M. Dunny, B. E. Murray, and L. B. Rice (ed.), *The Enterococci: Pathogenesis, Molecular Biology, and Antibiotic Resistance*. ASM Press, Washington, D.C.
51. **Flannagan, S. E., J. W. Chow, S. M. Donabedian, W. J. Brown, M. B. Perri, M. J. Zervos, Y. Ozawa, and D. B. Clewell.** 2003. Plasmid content of a vancomycin-resistant *Enterococcus faecalis* isolate from a patient also colonized by *Staphylococcus aureus* with a VanA phenotype. *Antimicrob. Agents Chemother.* **47:**3954–3959.
52. **Franz, C. M., W. H. Holzapfel, and M. E. Stiles.** 1999. Enterococci at the crossroads of food safety? *Int. J. Food Microbiol.* **47:**1–24.
53. Reference deleted.
54. **Franz, C. M., A. B. Muscholl-Silberhorn, N. M. Yousif, M. Vancanneyt, J. Swings, and W. H. Holzapfel.** 2001. Incidence of virulence factors and antibiotic resistance among enterococci isolated from food. *Appl. Environ. Microbiol.* **67:**4385–4389.
55. **Frei, A., D. Goldenberger, and M. Teuber.** 2001. Antimicrobial susceptibility of intestinal bacteria from Swiss poultry flocks before the ban of antimicrobial growth promoters. *Syst. Appl. Microbiol.* **24:**116–121.
56. **Galli, D., and R. Wirth.** 1991. Comparative analysis of *Enterococcus faecalis* sex pheromone plasmids identifies a single homologous DNA region which codes for aggregation substance. *J. Bacteriol.* **173:**3029–3033.
57. **Galvez, A., M. Maqueda, M. Martinez-Bueno, and E. Valdivia.** 1991. Permeation of bacterial cells, permeation of cytoplasmic and artificial membrane vesicles, and channel formation on lipid bilayers by peptide antibiotic AS-48. *J. Bacteriol.* **173:** 886–892.
58. **Gilmore, M. S., and J. J. Ferretti.** 2003. Microbiology. The thin line between gut commensal and pathogen. *Science* **299:**1999–2002.
59. **Giraffa, G.** 2002. Enterococci from foods. *FEMS Microbiol. Rev.* **26:**163–171.
60. Reference deleted.
61. **Giraffa, G.** 2003. Functionality of enterococci in dairy products. *Int. J. Food Microbiol.* **88:**215–222.

62. **Gonzales, R. D., P. C. Schreckenberger, M. B. Graham, S. Kelkar, K. DenBesten, and J. P. Quinn.** 2001. Infections due to vancomycin-resistant Enterococcus faecium resistant to linezolid. *Lancet* **357:**1179.
63. **Graninger, W., and R. Ragette.** 1992. Nosocomial bacteremia due to Enterococcus faecalis without endocarditis. *Clin. Infect. Dis.* **15:**49–57.
64. **Guardabassi, L., and A. Dalsgaard.** 2004. Occurrence, structure, and mobility of Tn1546-like elements in environmental isolates of vancomycin-resistant enterococci. *Appl. Environ. Microbiol.* **70:**984–990.
65. **Gullberg, R. M., S. R. Homann, and J. P. Phair.** 1989. Enterococcal bacteremia: analysis of 75 episodes. *Rev. Infect. Dis.* **11:**74–85.
66. **Hammerum, A. M., and L. B. Jensen.** 2002. Prevalence of *esp*, encoding the enterococcal surface protein, in *Enterococcus faecalis* and *Enterococcus faecium* isolates from hospital patients, poultry, and pigs in Denmark. *J. Clin. Microbiol.* **40:**4396.
67. **Hammerum, A. M., C. H. Lester, J. Neimann, L. J. Porsbo, K. E. Olsen, L. B. Jensen, H. D. Emborg, H. C. Wegener, and N. Frimodt-Moller.** 2004. A vancomycin-resistant Enterococcus faecium isolate from a Danish healthy volunteer, detected 7 years after the ban of avoparcin, is possibly related to pig isolates. *J. Antimicrob. Chemother.* **53:**547–549.
68. **Hayes, J. R., L. L. English, L. E. Carr, D. D. Wagner, and S. W. Joseph.** 2004. Multiple-antibiotic resistance of *Enterococcus* spp. isolated from commercial poultry production environments. *Appl. Environ. Microbiol.* **70:**6005–6011.
69. **Herrero, I. A., J. F. Fernandez-Garayzabal, M. A. Moreno, and L. Dominguez.** 2004. Dogs should be included in surveillance programs for vancomycin-resistant enterococci. *J. Clin. Microbiol.* **42:**1384–1385.
70. **Hershberger, E., S. Donabedian, K. Konstantinou, and M. J. Zervos.** 2004. Quinupristin-dalfopristin resistance in gram-positive bacteria: mechanism of resistance and epidemiology. *Clin. Infect. Dis.* **38:**92–98.
71. **Huys, G., K. D'Haene, J. M. Collard, and J. Swings.** 2004. Prevalence and molecular characterization of tetracycline resistance in *Enterococcus* isolates from food. *Appl. Environ. Microbiol.* **70:**1555–1562.
72. **Ieven, M., E. Vercauteren, C. Lammens, D. Ursi, and H. Goossens.** 2001. Significant decrease of GRE colonization rate in hospitalized patients after avoparcin ban in animals, abstr. LB-8. *Abstr. 41st Intersci. Conf. Antimicrob. Agents Chemother.* American Society for Microbiology, Washington, D.C.
73. **Jackson, C. R., P. J. Fedorka-Cray, and J. B. Barrett.** 2004. Use of a genus- and species-specific multiplex PCR for identification of enterococci. *J. Clin. Microbiol.* **42:**3558–3565.
74. **Jayarao, B. M., J. J. Dore, Jr., and S. P. Oliver.** 1992. Restriction fragment length polymorphism analysis of 16S ribosomal DNA of *Streptococcus* and *Enterococcus* species of bovine origin. *J. Clin. Microbiol.* **30:**2235–2240.
75. **Jayarao, B. M., and S. P. Oliver.** 1992. Aminoglycoside-resistant Streptococcus and Enterococcus species isolated from bovine mammary secretions. *J. Dairy Sci.* **75:**991–997.
76. **Jensen, L. B.** 1998. Differences in the occurrence of two base pair variants of Tn*1546* from vancomycin-resistant enterococci from humans, pigs, and poultry. *Antimicrob. Agents Chemother.* **42:**2463–2464.
77. **Jensen, L. B., Y. Agerso, and G. Sengelov.** 2002. Presence of erm genes among macrolide-resistant Gram-positive bacteria isolated from Danish farm soil. *Environ. Int.* **28:**487–491.
78. **Jensen, L. B., P. Ahrens, L. Dons, R. N. Jones, A. M. Hammerum, and F. M. Aarestrup.** 1998. Molecular analysis of Tn*1546* in *Enterococcus faecium* isolated from animals and humans. *J. Clin. Microbiol.* **36:**437–442.
79. **Jensen, L. B., A. M. Hammerum, F. Bager, and F. M. Aarestrup.** 2002. Streptogramin resistance among Enterococcus faecium isolated from production animals in Denmark in 1997. *Microb. Drug Resist.* **8:**369–374.
80. Reference deleted.
81. **Jett, B. D., M. M. Huycke, and M. S. Gilmore.** 1994. Virulence of enterococci. *Clin. Microbiol. Rev.* **7:**462–478.
82. **Jett, B. D., H. G. Jensen, R. E. Nordquist, and M. S. Gilmore.** 1992. Contribution of the pAD1-encoded cytolysin to the severity of experimental *Enterococcus faecalis* endophthalmitis. *Infect. Immun.* **60:**2445–2452.
83. **Jones, W. G., P. S. Barie, R. W. Yurt, and C. W. Goodwin.** 1986. Enterococcal burn sepsis. A highly lethal complication in severely burned patients. *Arch. Surg.* **121:**649–653.
84. **Kak, V., and J. W. Chow.** 2002. Acquired antibiotic resistance in enterococci, p. 355–383. *In* M. S. Gilmore, D. B. Clewell, P. Courvalin, G. M. Dunny, B. E. Murray, and L. B. Rice (ed.), *The Enterococci: Pathogenesis, Molecular Biology, and Antibiotic Resistance.* ASM Press, Washington, D.C.
85. **Klare, I., D. Badstubner, C. Konstabel, G. Bohme, H. Claus, and W. Witte.** 1999. Decreased incidence of VanA-type vancomycin-resistant enterococci isolated from poultry meat and from fecal samples of humans in the community after discontinuation of avoparcin usage in animal husbandry. *Microb. Drug Resist.* **5:**45–52.
86. **Klare, I., H. Heier, H. Claus, R. Reissbrodt, and W. Witte.** 1995. vanA-mediated high-level glycopeptide resistance in Enterococcus faecium from animal husbandry. *FEMS Microbiol. Lett.* **125:**165–171.
87. **Klare, I., H. Heier, H. Claus, and W. Witte.** 1993. Environmental strains of Enterococcus faecium with inducible high-level resistance to glycopeptides. *FEMS Microbiol. Lett.* **106:**23–29.
88. **Klein, G.** 2003. Taxonomy, ecology and antibiotic resistance of enterococci from food and the gastro-intestinal tract. *Int. J. Food Microbiol.* **88:**123–131.
89. **Kreft, B., R. Marre, U. Schramm, and R. Wirth.** 1992. Aggregation substance of *Enterococcus faecalis* mediates adhesion to cultured renal tubular cells. *Infect. Immun.* **60:**25–30.
90. **Landry, S. L., D. L. Kaiser, and R. P. Wenzel.** 1989. Hospital stay and mortality attributed to nosocomial enterococcal bacteremia: a controlled study. *Am. J. Infect. Control* **17:**323–329.
91. **Laukova, A., S. Czikkova, S. Laczkova, and P. Turek.** 1999. Use of enterocin CCM 4231 to control Listeria monocytogenes in experimentally contaminated dry fermented Hornad salami. *Int. J. Food Microbiol.* **52:**115–119.
92. **Lautenbach, E., W. B. Bilker, and P. J. Brennan.** 1999. Enterococcal bacteremia: risk factors for vancomycin resistance and predictors of mortality. *Infect. Control Hosp. Epidemiol.* **20:**318–323.
93. **Leavis, H., J. Top, N. Shankar, K. Borgen, M. Bonten, J. van Embden, and R. J. Willems.** 2004. A novel putative enterococcal pathogenicity island linked to the *esp* virulence gene of *Enterococcus faecium* and associated with epidemicity. *J. Bacteriol.* **186:**672–682.
94. **Leclercq, R., E. Derlot, J. Duval, and P. Courvalin.** 1988. Plasmid-mediated resistance to vancomycin and teicoplanin in Enterococcus faecium. *N. Engl. J. Med.* **319:**157–161.
95. **Lester, C. H., N. Frimodt-Moller, and A. M. Hammerum.** 2004. Conjugal transfer of aminoglycoside and macrolide resistance between Enterococcus faecium isolates in the intestine of streptomycin-treated mice. *FEMS Microbiol. Lett.* **235:**385–391.

96. **Linden, P. K., A. W. Pasculle, R. Manez, D. J. Kramer, J. J. Fung, A. D. Pinna, and S. Kusne.** 1996. Differences in outcomes for patients with bacteremia due to vancomycin-resistant Enterococcus faecium or vancomycin-susceptible E. faecium. *Clin. Infect. Dis.* **22:**663–670.

97. **Loeb, M., S. Salama, M. Armstrong-Evans, G. Capretta, and J. Olde.** 1999. A case-control study to detect modifiable risk factors for colonization with vancomycin-resistant enterococci. *Infect. Control Hosp. Epidemiol.* **20:**760–763.

98. **Mac, K., H. Wichmann-Schauer, J. Peters, and L. Ellerbroek.** 2003. Species identification and detection of vancomycin resistance genes in enterococci of animal origin by multiplex PCR. *Int. J. Food Microbiol.* **88:**305–309.

99. **Makinen, P. L., D. B. Clewell, F. An, and K. K. Makinen.** 1989. Purification and substrate specificity of a strongly hydrophobic extracellular metalloendopeptidase ("gelatinase") from Streptococcus faecalis (strain 0G1-10). *J. Biol. Chem.* **264:**3325–3334.

100. **Malani, P. N., C. A. Kauffman, and M. J. Zervos.** 2002. Enterococcal disease, epidemiology, and treatment, p. 385–408. *In* M. S. Gilmore, D. B. Clewell, P. Courvalin, G. M. Dunny, B. E. Murray, and L. B. Rice (ed.), *The Enterococci: Pathogenesis, Molecular Biology, and Antibiotic Resistance.* ASM Press, Washington, D.C.

101. **Malone, D. A., R. A. Wagner, J. P. Myers, and C. Watanakunakorn.** 1986. Enterococcal bacteremia in two large community teaching hospitals. *Am. J. Med.* **81:**601–606.

102. **Mannu, L., A. Paba, E. Daga, R. Comunian, S. Zanetti, I. Dupre, and L. A. Sechi.** 2003. Comparison of the incidence of virulence determinants and antibiotic resistance between Enterococcus faecium strains of dairy, animal and clinical origin. *Int. J. Food Microbiol.* **88:**291–304.

103. **Martel, A., L. A. Devriese, A. Decostere, and F. Haesebrouck.** 2003. Presence of macrolide resistance genes in streptococci and enterococci isolated from pigs and pork carcasses. *Int. J. Food Microbiol.* **84:**27–32.

104. **Mayhall, C. G.** 1999. The epidemiology and control of VRE: still struggling to come of age. *Infect. Control Hosp. Epidemiol.* **20:**650–652.

105. **McDonald, L. C., S. Rossiter, C. Mackinson, Y. Y. Wang, S. Johnson, M. Sullivan, R. Sokolow, E. Debess, L. Gilbert, J. A. Benson, B. Hill, and F. J. Angulo.** 2001. Quinupristin-dalfopristin-resistant Enterococcus faecium on chicken and in human stool specimens. *N. Engl. J. Med.* **345:**1155–1160.

106. **McNicholas, P. M., D. J. Najarian, P. A. Mann, D. Hesk, R. S. Hare, K. J. Shaw, and T. A. Black.** 2000. Evernimicin binds exclusively to the 50S ribosomal subunit and inhibits translation in cell-free systems derived from both gram-positive and gram-negative bacteria. *Antimicrob. Agents Chemother.* **44:**1121–1126.

107. **Moellering, R. C.** 2000. *Enterococcus* species, *Streptococcus bovis*, and *Leuconostoc* species, p. 2147–2152. *In* D. Mandell, J. E. Bennett, and R. Dolin (ed.), *Principles and Practice of Infectious Diseases.* Churchill Livingstone, Philadelphia, Pa.

108. **Moellering, R. C., P. K. Linden, J. Reinhardt, E. A. Blumberg, F. Bompart, and G. H. Talbot.** 1999. The efficacy and safety of quinupristin/dalfopristin for the treatment of infections caused by vancomycin-resistant Enterococcus faecium. Synercid Emergency-Use Study Group. *J. Antimicrob. Chemother.* **44:**251–261.

109. **Montecalvo, M. A., H. Horowitz, C. Gedris, C. Carbonaro, F. C. Tenover, A. Issah, P. Cook, and G. P. Wormser.** 1994. Outbreak of vancomycin-, ampicillin-, and aminoglycoside-resistant *Enterococcus faecium* bacteremia in an adult oncology unit. *Antimicrob. Agents Chemother.* **38:**1363–1367.

110. **Montecalvo, M. A., D. K. Shay, P. Patel, L. Tacsa, S. A. Maloney, W. R. Jarvis, and G. P. Wormser.** 1996. Bloodstream infections with vancomycin-resistant enterococci. *Arch. Intern. Med.* **156:**1458–1462.

111. **Moubareck, C., N. Bourgeois, P. Courvalin, and F. Doucet-Populaire.** 2003. Multiple antibiotic resistance gene transfer from animal to human enterococci in the digestive tract of gnotobiotic mice. *Antimicrob. Agents Chemother.* **47:**2993–2996.

112. **Mundy, L. M., D. F. Sahm, and M. Gilmore.** 2000. Relationships between enterococcal virulence and antimicrobial resistance. *Clin. Microbiol. Rev.* **13:**513–522.

113. **Oprea, S. F., N. Zaidi, S. M. Donabedian, M. Balasubramaniam, E. Hershberger, and M. J. Zervos.** 2004. Molecular and clinical epidemiology of vancomycin-resistant Enterococcus faecalis. *J. Antimicrob. Chemother.* **53:**626–630.

114. **Paulsen, I. T., L. Banerjei, G. S. Myers, K. E. Nelson, R. Seshadri, T. D. Read, D. E. Fouts, J. A. Eisen, S. R. Gill, J. F. Heidelberg, H. Tettelin, R. J. Dodson, L. Umayam, L. Brinkac, M. Beanan, S. Daugherty, R. T. DeBoy, S. Durkin, J. Kolonay, R. Madupu, W. Nelson, J. Vamathevan, B. Tran, J. Upton, T. Hansen, J. Shetty, H. Khouri, T. Utterback, D. Radune, K. A. Ketchum, B. A. Dougherty, and C. M. Fraser.** 2003. Role of mobile DNA in the evolution of vancomycin-resistant Enterococcus faecalis. *Science* **299:**2071–2074.

115. **Pfaller, M. A., R. N. Jones, S. A. Marshall, M. B. Edmond, and R. P. Wenzel.** 1997. Nosocomial streptococcal blood stream infections in the SCOPE Program: species occurrence and antimicrobial resistance. The SCOPE Hospital Study Group. *Diagn. Microbiol. Infect. Dis.* **29:**259–263.

116. **Quednau, M., S. Ahrne, A. C. Petersson, and G. Molin.** 1998. Antibiotic-resistant strains of Enterococcus isolated from Swedish and Danish retailed chicken and pork. *J. Appl. Microbiol.* **84:**1163–1170.

117. **Rice, E. W., L. A. Boczek, C. H. Johnson, and J. W. Messer.** 2003. Detection of intrinsic vancomycin resistant enterococci in animal and human feces. *Diagn. Microbiol. Infect. Dis.* **46:**155–158.

118. **Rice, E. W., J. W. Messer, C. H. Johnson, and D. J. Reasoner.** 1995. Occurrence of high-level aminoglycoside resistance in environmental isolates of enterococci. *Appl. Environ. Microbiol.* **61:**374–376.

119. **Rice, L. B., L. Carias, S. Rudin, C. Vael, H. Goossens, C. Konstabel, I. Klare, S. R. Nallapareddy, W. Huang, and B. E. Murray.** 2003. A potential virulence gene, hylEfm, predominates in Enterococcus faecium of clinical origin. *J. Infect. Dis.* **187:**508–512.

120. **Riemann, H., and F. L. Bryan.** 1979. *Foodborne Infections and Intoxications.* Academic Press, Inc., New York, N. Y.

121. **Rimailho, A., E. Lampl, B. Riou, C. Richard, E. Rottman, and P. Auzepy.** 1988. Enterococcal bacteremia in a medical intensive care unit. *Crit. Care Med.* **16:**126–129.

122. **Rogers, D. G., D. H. Zeman, and E. D. Erickson.** 1992. Diarrhea associated with Enterococcus durans in calves. *J. Vet. Diagn. Invest.* **4:**471–472.

123. **Rollins, L. D., L. N. Lee, and D. J. LeBlanc.** 1985. Evidence for a disseminated erythromycin resistance determinant mediated by Tn*917*-like sequences among group D streptococci isolated from pigs, chickens, and humans. *Antimicrob. Agents Chemother.* **27:**439–444.

124. **Ronconi, M. C., L. A. Merino, and G. Fernandez.** 2002. Detection of Enterococcus with high-level aminoglycoside and glycopeptide resistance in Lactuca sativa (lettuce). *Enferm. Infecc. Microbiol. Clin.* **20:**380–383.

125. **Rosan, B., and N. B. Williams.** 1964. Hyaluronidase production by oral enterococci. *Arch. Oral Biol.* **11:**291–298.

126. **Shankar, N., P. Coburn, C. Pillar, W. Haas, and M. Gilmore.** 2004. Enterococcal cytolysin: activities and association with other virulence traits in a pathogenicity island. *Int. J. Med. Microbiol.* **293:**609–618.
127. **Shlaes, D. M., J. Levy, and E. Wolinsky.** 1981. Enterococcal bacteremia without endocarditis. *Arch. Intern. Med.* **141:**578–581.
128. **Simjee, S., P. F. McDermott, D. D. Wagner, and D. G. White.** 2001. Variation within the *vat*(E) allele of *Enterococcus faecium* isolates from retail poultry samples. *Antimicrob. Agents Chemother.* **45:**2931–2932.
129. **Simjee, S., D. G. White, P. F. McDermott, D. D. Wagner, M. J. Zervos, S. M. Donabedian, L. L. English, J. R. Hayes, and R. D. Walker.** 2002. Characterization of Tn1546 in vancomycin-resistant Enterococcus faecium isolated from canine urinary tract infections: evidence of gene exchange between human and animal enterococci. *J. Clin. Microbiol.* **40:**4659–4665.
130. **Simjee, S., D. G. White, J. Meng, D. D. Wagner, S. Qaiyumi, S. Zhao, J. R. Hayes, and P. F. McDermott.** 2002. Prevalence of streptogramin resistance genes among Enterococcus isolates recovered from retail meats in the Greater Washington DC area. *J. Antimicrob. Chemother.* **50:**877–882.
131. Reference deleted.
132. **Simjee, S., D. G. White, D. D. Wagner, J. Meng, S. Qaiyumi, S. Zhao, and P. F. McDermott.** 2002. Identification of *vat*(E) in *Enterococcus faecalis* isolates from retail poultry and its transferability to *Enterococcus faecium*. *Antimicrob. Agents Chemother.* **46:**3823–3828.
133. Reference deleted.
134. **Singh, K. V., T. M. Coque, G. M. Weinstock, and B. E. Murray.** 1998. In vivo testing of an Enterococcus faecalis efaA mutant and use of efaA homologs for species identification. *FEMS Immunol. Med. Microbiol.* **21:**323–331.
135. **Soltani, M., D. Beighton, J. Philpott-Howard, and N. Woodford.** 2000. Mechanisms of resistance to quinupristin-dalfopristin among isolates of *Enterococcus faecium* from animals, raw meat, and hospital patients in Western Europe. *Antimicrob. Agents Chemother.* **44:**433–436.
136. Reference deleted.
137. **Son, R., F. Nimita, G. Rusul, E. Nasreldin, L. Samuel, and M. Nishibuchi.** 1999. Isolation and molecular characterization of vancomycin-resistant Enterococcus faecium in Malaysia. *Lett. Appl. Microbiol.* **29:**118–122.
138. **Stiles, M. E.** 1989. Less recognized or presumptive foodborne pathogenic bacteria, p. 674–735. *In* M. P. Doyle (ed.), *Foodborne Bacterial Pathogens*. Marcel Dekker, Inc., New York, N.Y.
139. **Su, Y. A., M. C. Sulavik, P. He, K. K. Makinen, P. L. Makinen, S. Fiedler, R. Wirth, and D. B. Clewell.** 1991. Nucleotide sequence of the gelatinase gene (*gelE*) from *Enterococcus faecalis* subsp. *liquefaciens*. *Infect. Immun.* **59:**415–420.
140. **Tannock, G. W., and G. Cook.** 2002. Enterococci as members of the intestinal microflora of humans, p. 101–132. *In* M. S. Gilmore, D. B. Clewell, P. Courvalin, G. M. Dunny, B. E. Murray, and L. B. Rice (ed.), *The Enterococci: Pathogenesis, Molecular Biology, and Antibiotic Resistance*. ASM Press, Washington, D.C.
141. **Teixeira, L. M., and R. R. Facklam.** 2003. *Enterococcus*, p. 422–429. *In* P. R. Murray, E. J. Baron, J. H. Jorgensen, M. A. Pfaller, and H. Y. Yolker (ed.), *Manual of Clinical Microbiology*. ASM Press, Washington, D.C.
142. **Tenover, F. C., L. M. Weigel, P. C. Appelbaum, L. K. McDougal, J. Chaitram, S. McAllister, N. Clark, G. Killgore, C. M. O'Hara, L. Jevitt, J. B. Patel, and B. Bozdogan.** 2004. Vancomycin-resistant *Staphylococcus aureus* isolate from a patient in Pennsylvania. *Antimicrob. Agents Chemother.* **48:**275–280.
143. **Teuber, M., F. Schwarz, and V. Perreten.** 2003. Molecular structure and evolution of the conjugative multiresistance plasmid pRE25 of Enterococcus faecalis isolated from a raw-fermented sausage. *Int. J. Food Microbiol.* **88:**325–329.
144. **Thal, L. A., J. W. Chow, R. Mahayni, H. Bonilla, M. B. Perri, S. A. Donabedian, J. Silverman, S. Taber, and M. J. Zervos.** 1995. Characterization of antimicrobial resistance in enterococci of animal origin. *Antimicrob. Agents Chemother.* **39:**2112–2115.
145. Reference deleted.
146. **Tornieporth, N. G., R. B. Roberts, J. John, A. Hafner, and L. W. Riley.** 1996. Risk factors associated with vancomycin-resistant Enterococcus faecium infection or colonization in 145 matched case patients and control patients. *Clin. Infect. Dis.* **23:**767–772.
147. **Vancanneyt, M., C. Snauwaert, I. Cleenwerck, M. Baele, P. Descheemaeker, H. Goossens, B. Pot, P. Vandamme, J. Swings, F. Haesebrouck, and L. A. Devriese.** 2001. Enterococcus villorum sp. nov., an enteroadherent bacterium associated with diarrhoea in piglets. *Int. J. Syst. Evol. Microbiol.* **51:**393–400.
148. **van den Bogaard, A. E., N. Bruinsma, and E. E. Stobberingh.** 2000. The effect of banning avoparcin on VRE carriage in The Netherlands. *J. Antimicrob. Chemother.* **46:**146–148.
149. **van den Bogaard, A. E., L. B. Jensen, and E. E. Stobberingh.** 1997. Vancomycin-resistant enterococci in turkeys and farmers. *N. Engl. J. Med.* **337:**1558–1559.
150. **van den Bogaard, A. E., N. London, and E. E. Stobberingh.** 2000. Antimicrobial resistance in pig faecal samples from the Netherlands (five abattoirs) and Sweden. *J. Antimicrob. Chemother.* **45:**663–671.
151. **van den Bogaard, A. E., R. Willems, N. London, J. Top, and E. E. Stobberingh.** 2002. Antibiotic resistance of faecal enterococci in poultry, poultry farmers and poultry slaughterers. *J. Antimicrob. Chemother.* **49:**497–505.
152. **Vankerckhoven, V., T. Van Autgaerden, C. Vael, C. Lammens, S. Chapelle, R. Rossi, D. Jabes, and H. Goossens.** 2004. Development of a multiplex PCR for the detection of *asa1*, *gelE*, *cylA*, *esp*, and *hyl* genes in enterococci and survey for virulence determinants among European hospital isolates of *Enterococcus faecium*. *J. Clin. Microbiol.* **42:**4473–4479.
153. **Vergis, E. N., M. K. Hayden, J. W. Chow, D. R. Snydman, M. J. Zervos, P. K. Linden, M. M. Wagener, B. Schmitt, and R. R. Muder.** 2001. Determinants of vancomycin resistance and mortality rates in enterococcal bacteremia. a prospective multicenter study. *Ann. Intern. Med.* **135:**484–492.
154. **Weinstein, M. P., J. R. Murphy, L. B. Reller, and K. A. Lichtenstein.** 1983. The clinical significance of positive blood cultures: a comprehensive analysis of 500 episodes of bacteremia and fungemia in adults. II. Clinical observations, with special reference to factors influencing prognosis. *Rev. Infect. Dis.* **5:**54–70.
155. **Werner, G., B. Hildebrandt, and W. Witte.** 2001. Aminoglycoside-streptothricin resistance gene cluster *aadE-sat4-aphA-3* disseminated among multiresistant isolates of *Enterococcus faecium*. *Antimicrob. Agents Chemother.* **45:**3267–3269.
156. **Werner, G., B. Hildebrandt, and W. Witte.** 2001. The newly described *msrC* gene is not equally distributed among all isolates of *Enterococcus faecium*. *Antimicrob. Agents Chemother.* **45:**3672–3673.
157. **Werner, G., B. Hildebrandt, and W. Witte.** 2003. Linkage of erm(B) and aadE-sat4-aphA-3 in multiple-resistant Enterococcus faecium isolates of different ecological origins. *Microb. Drug Resist.* 9(Supp. 1):S9–S16.

158. **Werner, G., I. Klare, H. Heier, K. H. Hinz, G. Bohme, M. Wendt, and W. Witte.** 2000. Quinupristin/dalfopristin-resistant enterococci of the satA (vatD) and satG (vatE) genotypes from different ecological origins in Germany. *Microb. Drug Resist.* **6:**37–47.
159. **Werner, G., B. Strommenger, I. Klare, and W. Witte.** 2004. Molecular detection of linezolid resistance in *Enterococcus faecium* and *Enterococcus faecalis* by use of 5′ nuclease real-time PCR compared to a modified classical approach. *J. Clin. Microbiol.* **42:**5327–5331.
160. **Woodford, N., A. M. Adebiyi, M. F. Palepou, and B. D. Cookson.** 1998. Diversity of VanA glycopeptide resistance elements in enterococci from humans and nonhuman sources. *Antimicrob. Agents Chemother.* **42:**502–508.
161. **Woodford, N., M. Soltani, and K. J. Hardy.** 2001. Frequency of esp in Enterococcus faecium isolates. *Lancet* **358:**584.
162. **World Health Organization.** 1994. WHO Scientific Working Group on monitoring and management of bacterial resistance to antimicrobial agents. World Health Organization, Geneva, Switzerland.
163. **Zervos, M. J., C. A. Kauffman, P. M. Therasse, A. G. Bergman, T. S. Mikesell, and D. R. Schaberg.** 1987. Nosocomial infection by gentamicin-resistant Streptococcus faecalis. An epidemiologic study. *Ann. Intern. Med.* **106:**687–691.

Antimicrobial Resistance in Bacteria of Animal Origin
Edited by Frank M. Aarestrup

Chapter 19

The Clinical Importance of Animal-Related Resistance

KÅRE MØLBAK

The clinical importance and public health significance of antimicrobial drug-resistant bacteria transferred from food-producing animals via the food chain to humans has been debated for many years. One of the early occasions was in 1968, in a description of a rise in *Salmonella enterica* serovar Typhimurium DT29 infection in calves in Britain during the period from 1964 to 1966 (4). The increase was observed following the adoption of intensive farming methods. Attempts to treat and control the disease among the animals with a range of antibiotics proved to be ineffective but resulted in the acquisition of transferable multiple-drug resistance in type DT29, which, in turn, resulted in human infections. Anderson (5) underlined that transferable drug resistance transmitted to humans from *Enterobacteriaceae* of animal origin may ultimately reach human pathogens. He also stressed the need for a reassessment of the methods of using antibiotics to conserve their long-term efficacy. As is often recognized, current scientific controversies are in fact not new, and dated papers continue to be relevant to public health today. The aim of this chapter is to review the clinical and public health consequences of antimicrobial drug resistance in bacteria transferred from food animals to humans.

MECHANISMS THROUGH WHICH ANIMAL-RELATED DRUG RESISTANCE MAY CAUSE EXCESS MORBIDITY AND MORTALITY IN HUMANS

To address the clinical importance of animal-related drug resistance, we must review how resistant bacteria may be a cause of increased morbidity and mortality (Table 1) (4, 6, 10). One important mechanism is increased transmission as a result of the unrelated use of antimicrobial agents to which a pathogen is resistant. This mechanism has recently been reviewed in detail (6, 7) and will also be discussed in the present chapter. Another potential factor is horizontal transmission of resistance genes from one bacterial species or subtype to another, which will be discussed in other sections of this book. Reduced efficacy of early empirical treatment and limited treatment choices may be the consequences if and when resistance to clinically important antimicrobial drugs is acquired. Finally, because a number of studies have indicated increased risk of invasive infections and hospitalization associated with antimicrobial drug-resistant, food-borne pathogens, it is likely that resistance in some "drug-bug combinations" may be associated with increased virulence. The underlying mechanisms could be coselection of virulence traits (e.g., by integration of virulence and resistance plasmids [16]), upregulation of virulence, or improved fitness of the bacteria. The present chapter will cover reduced efficacy of treatment and increased virulence from a public health perspective, i.e., by summarizing observational studies that address the clinical and public health consequences of animal-related resistance.

INCREASED TRANSMISSION

The use of antimicrobial drugs causes a transient decrease in resistance to infection after exposure to a food-borne pathogen. This notion has been corroborated by several epidemiological studies identifying unrelated antimicrobial use as a risk factor for infection with antimicrobial drug-resistant bacteria of animal origin. Thus, case-control studies of risk factors for food-borne bacterial infections have identified preinfection antimicrobial therapy as a risk factor for *Campylobacter* (42) and zoonotic *Salmonella* infections (Table 2) (12, 28, 41). In Denmark this has not been the case for *S. enterica* serovar Enteritidis, in

Kåre Mølbak • Department of Epidemiology, Statens Serum Institut, Artillerivej 5, DK-2300 Copenhagen S, Denmark.

Table 1. Mechanisms by which human health may be affected by the emergence of animal-related antimicrobial drug resistance in food-borne bacteria

Mechanism	Effect on human health
Increased transmission	Resistant, food-borne bacteria have a selective advantage in patients treated with antimicrobial drugs for other reasons. Resistant strains may easily gain a foothold in settings where antimicrobials are used, such as hospitals.
Horizontal transmission of resistance	Genes encoding antimicrobial drug resistance are often located on mobile genetic elements such as plasmids, transposons, and integrons. These may be transferred to other bacteria.
Reduced efficacy of early empirical treatment	Antimicrobial drug treatment is not advocated for most cases of gastroenteritis. However, in patients with severe underlying illness or with suspected extraintestinal spread, treatment should be initiated prior to microbiological diagnosis. In these cases, resistance to clinically important drugs will increase the risk of treatment failure.
Limited choice of treatment after diagnosis	Drug resistance to clinically important classes of antimicrobial drugs will limit the choices of drugs and lead to increasing costs of treatment
Increased virulence	There is evidence that resistant bacteria cause more-invasive infections and increased mortality, perhaps due to coselection of virulence traits and improved fitness of drug-resistant bacterial pathogens

which levels of resistance are much lower than for *Salmonella* serovar Typhimurium (33).

The fact that preinfection antimicrobial therapy is pointed out as a general risk factor in epidemiological studies may be due to several reasons. A decreased susceptibility may be separated into a so-called competitive effect and a selective effect that offers a specific advantage for a certain resistant pathogen (7). In other words, due to the selective effect, drug-resistant gastrointestinal pathogens such as *Salmonella* and *Campylobacter* may preferentially cause illness in persons taking antimicrobial drugs for unrelated medical conditions (Table 2).

The competitive effect is independent of resistance. Persons receiving antimicrobial treatment may already be enfeebled by other underlying diseases and consequently be more susceptible to infections. Furthermore, antimicrobial treatment will affect the composition of the normal intestinal flora, and thereby the conditions for the establishment of an infection. The latter is one of the reasons why, in antimicrobial therapy, it is generally recommended to use narrow-spectrum antimicrobial agents acting on a few bacterial species rather than broad-spectrum antimicrobial agents affecting a larger proportion of the normal flora.

The selective effect is a more direct consequence of exposure to drug-resistant, food-borne bacteria such as *Salmonella* and *Campylobacter*. Antimicrobial therapy carried out during asymptomatic colonization with antimicrobial-resistant bacteria may cause the colonization to progress to clinical disease. Rosenthal (39) was one of the first to report on a convalescent who, after a mild *Salmonella* serovar Typhimurium infection, commenced with ampicillin treatment and subsequently developed a severe infection caused by the ampicillin-resistant serovar Typhimurium strain.

Holmberg et al. (26) reported on a *Salmonella* outbreak in the United States in which 18 persons fell ill, presumably after having eaten hamburgers contaminated with an ampicillin-, carbenicillin-, and tetracycline-resistant strain of *S. enterica* serovar Newport. Between 24 and 48 h before the onset of diarrhea, 12 of the 18 persons had been taking penicillin derivatives for reasons other than diarrhea. The investigation of this outbreak demonstrated that there may be a direct connection between antimicrobial treatment and the risk of disease caused by resistant *Salmonella* bacteria. The contaminated hamburgers probably originated from beef cattle in South Dakota that had received subtherapeutic doses of chlorotetracycline as a growth promoter.

In 1985 a large outbreak of *Salmonella* serovar Typhimurium involved more than 16,000 patients with culture-confirmed infection (40). The causal vehicle was contaminated milk that had not been properly pasteurized. The strain causing the outbreak showed a characteristic resistance profile (resistant to ampicillin, tetracycline, carbenicillin, and streptomycin; sensitive

Table 2. Summary of selected epidemiological studies demonstrating that recent antimicrobial use is a risk factor for infection with drug-resistant salmonellae

Setting	Resistant pathogens	No. of cases with recent antimicrobial use among patients with drug- or multidrug-resistant strains/total no. of cases	Risk of infection associated with drug use [OR (95% CI)]	Reference
Outbreak in a pediatric ward	Multidrug-resistant *Salmonella enterica* serovar Indiana	28/36	3.2 (1.1–9.9)[a]	3
Case-control study of sporadic cases	Multidrug-resistant *Salmonella* serovar Typhimurium (ACSSuT, AKSSuT, ACKSSuT)[c]	13/61	5.7 (1.8–17.4)[a]	17
Case-case comparison of sporadic cases, 2000–2002	Multidrug-resistant *Salmonella* serovar Typhimurium (ACSSuT)[c]	7/27	5.1 (1.5–17.8)[b]	21
Outbreak investigation	Multidrug-resistant *Salmonella* serovar Newport associated with beef	12/18	Not calculated	26
Case-case comparison of sporadic cases, 1989–1990	Several different serotypes	49/126	5.1 (3.2–8.0)[b]	29
Case-case comparison of sporadic cases, 1984–1985	Several different serotypes	13/117	5.7 (1.8–17.4)[b]	30
Outbreak in nursing home	Fluoroquinolone-resistant *Salmonella enterica* serovar Schwarzengrund	4/5	22.0 (1.1–1177)[a]	37
Case-case comparison of sporadic cases, 1979–1980	Several different serotypes	13/59	3.7 (1.7–8.0)[b]	38
Case and case-family members in an outbreak investigation	Outbreak of multidrug-resistant *Salmonella* enterica Typhimurium associated with contaminated milk	16/54	6.4 (2.2–18.8)[a]	40
Outbreak investigation	Outbreak of multidrug-resistant *Salmonella* serovar Newport associated with contaminated ground beef	11/45	14.1 (2.8–134.3)[a]	43

[a]Compared with controls.
[b]Compared with patients who had infection with susceptible strains.
[c]Resistant to: A, ampicillin; C, chloramphenicol; K, kanamycin; S, streptomycin; Su, sulfonamides; T, tetracycline.

to chloramphenicol, gentamicin, kanamycin, trimethoprim, cephalothin, and nalidixic acid). Subsequent analyses revealed that patients who were undergoing antimicrobial therapy using one of the antimicrobials to which the bacteria were resistant had drunk significantly less milk than persons who had not been taking antimicrobials. This suggested that the infectious dose is lower for patients receiving antimicrobial therapy than for those who do not receive treatment. The study further attempted to estimate the attributable fraction of persons experiencing illness due to antimicrobial resistance in the concerned strain. The authors concluded that 16% of the disease cases could be attributed to the antimicrobial drug resistance of the strain. Theoretically, a proportion of these patients might thus not have developed disease had the milk been contaminated by a fully sensitive *Salmonella* strain (40). Cohen and Tauxe (10) have estimated the attributable fraction in relation to antimicrobial treatment in four outbreaks by resistant *Salmonella*. If the strain had been sensitive (or if the patients had not received antimicrobial treatment), between 16 and 64% of the cases would have been asymptomatic. The attributable fraction (and its counterpart in veterinary medicine) is further discussed by Barza and Travers (6, 7).

A recent American case-control study (17) identified preinfection antimicrobial treatment as the only risk factor for multidrug-resistant *Salmonella* serovar Typhimurium DT104 infection. Compared with both control subjects and patients infected with pansensitive strains of serovar Typhimurium, patients with multidrug-resistant serovar Typhimurium infection were significantly more likely to have received an antimicrobial agent, particularly an agent to which the *Salmonella* isolate was resistant, during the 4 weeks preceding illness onset. Helms et al. (21) corroborated this observation. However, antimicrobial drug treatment was only a risk factor for infection with serovar Typhimurium with a DT104-like resistance pattern (i.e., resistant to ampicillin, chloramphenicol, streptomycin, sulfonamide, and tetracycline) but not for other drug-resistant serovar Typhimurium isolates.

The interaction between drug resistance in food-borne bacteria and the unrelated use of antimicrobial drugs in humans has at least two consequences. First, it contributes to increased transmission of resistant bacteria among individuals receiving treatment for other reasons, including an increased risk of outbreaks in hospital settings and other places where antimicrobial drugs are used. Thus, if the prevalence of drug resistance among food-borne gastrointestinal pathogens increases, the total burden of illness will also increase. Also, persons who have underlying illness or are treated for other disorders may face more severe clinical consequences of the infection. This interaction may in some situations explain why infections with antimicrobial drug-resistant bacteria may appear more virulent than those caused by drug-sensitive bacteria.

REDUCED CLINICAL EFFICACY AND INCREASED MORBIDITY AND MORTALITY

Treatment of Infections with Zoonotic Gastrointestinal Bacteria

Treatment of infections with most food-borne bacteria, such as *Salmonella* infections other than typhoid fever, as well as infections with *Campylobacter*, *Escherichia coli* O157, other Shiga toxin-producing *E. coli* strains, and *Yersinia enterocolitica*, is supportive. Antibiotic therapy is not indicated in uncomplicated cases of gastrointestinal illness in patients without underlying illness. However, therapy is needed and may be lifesaving in selected patients with underlying illness and in patients with a prolonged febrile course, where invasive illness is suspected. If the bacteria have acquired resistance to clinically important drugs, early empirical therapy may be less efficacious. Furthermore, after the results from bacterial culture and susceptibility testing are made available, the clinician's choice of drugs is limited. Currently, there is an increasing number of reported multidrug-resistant, food-borne *Salmonella* infections, with few options left for antimicrobial treatment (1, 9, 18, 34).

In fact, antimicrobial drugs are quite commonly prescribed in the management of food-borne infections. In the United States, for instance, up to 40% of patients with *Salmonella* infections are given antimicrobial treatment (10), and in a recent study in Denmark 36% of patients with *Salmonella* serovar Typhimurium infection were treated with antibiotics (21). With the increasing prevalence of resistance along with the high treatment rates, it is likely that there will be still more cases with a mismatch between prescribed treatment and resistance pattern. It is biologically plausible that patients in such situations will be worse off with treatment than without.

Resistance to clinically important antimicrobial drugs such as fluoroquinolones, expanded-spectrum cephalosporins (e.g., ceftriaxone and cefotaxime), and macrolides warrants special consideration. A fluoroquinolone (e.g., ciprofloxacin) is the drug of first choice in early empirical treatment of severe gastroenteritis in adults, whereas expanded-spectrum cephalosporins frequently are the chosen antimicrobial agents in the treatment of pediatric patients with invasive *Salmonella* infections (25). Macrolides are commonly prescribed for the treatment of severe *Campylobacter* infections.

Therapeutic failures due to reduced sensitivity of *Salmonella* to fluoroquinolones have been reported since the early 1990s. Several reports have described reduced efficacy of fluoroquinolones in treating infections with *Salmonella* isolates resistant to nalidixic acid but ciprofloxacin MICs of <4 mg/liter, i.e., strains that would have been considered susceptible to ciprofloxacin by the current standards of the National Committee for Clinical Laboratory Standards (2, 11). End points have included failure to clear the pathogen, prolonged fever, and death.

In 1999 we described an outbreak in Denmark in which 25 patients acquired multidrug-resistant *Salmonella* serovar Typhimurium DT104 infection. Beyond being resistant to the antimicrobials ampicillin, chloramphenicol, streptomycin, sulfonamide, and tetracycline, the strain was resistant to nalidixic acid. The investigation described treatment failures due to reduced efficacy of fluoroquinolones (32).

More recently, there has been an increasing number of reports on expanded-spectrum beta-lactamase resistance in non-Typhi *Salmonella* and other *Enterobacteriaceae* (1, 4, 9, 13, 50, 51). Fey et al. (15) described a case of ceftriaxone-resistant *Salmonella* serovar Typhimurium infection in a child living on a farm. Cephalosporins were widely used in the cattle, and in the investigation of the outbreak identical strains were identified in the cattle reservoir. In the United States, between 1998 and 2001, a fivefold increase in the prevalence of *Salmonella* resistant to expanded-spectrum cephalosporins was primarily due to the emergence of the so-called serovar Newport MDR-AmpC strains (18).

Early Epidemiological Studies

Several epidemiological studies have attempted to measure the clinical and public health consequences of antimicrobial drug resistance in food-borne bacteria. The outcomes have been rate of admission to hospital, duration of illness, risk of spread to the bloodstream, risk of acute or late-onset complications, and, finally, increase in mortality.

The clinical consequences of antimicrobial drug resistance were illustrated for the first time in American studies in the 1980s. Holmberg et al. (27) examined 52 nontyphoid *Salmonella* outbreaks investigated by the Centers for Disease Control and Prevention during the period from 1971 to 1983. Of the 52 outbreaks, 17 were caused by antimicrobial-resistant isolates, resulting in a total of 312 cases. Thirteen patients (4.2%) died, whereas the corresponding mortality rate was 0.2% for patients with infections caused by sensitive isolates (27). This study was recently repeated for outbreaks investigated from 1984 to 2002 (47). Among 32 outbreaks in this period, 22% of 13,286 persons in 10 outbreaks caused by resistant *Salmonella* isolates were hospitalized, compared with 8% of 2,194 persons in 22 outbreaks caused by pan-susceptible isolates ($P < 0.01$). A greater proportion of persons died in outbreaks caused by resistant strains than pan-susceptible strains. However, the overall mortality was low, and the difference was not statistically significant.

Lee et al. (29) carried out a prospective study during the period from 1989 to 1990 and found that patients infected with resistant nontyphoid *Salmonella* were more frequently hospitalized than patients with infections caused by sensitive bacteria, were more frequently <1 year old, were more frequently African-American, and had more frequently received antimicrobial therapy prior to the diagnosis. In a subgroup of 84 patients with *Salmonella* resistant to ampicillin, 12 (14%) had taken ampicillin or amoxicillin, compared with 29 (6%) of 521 infected with ampicillin-susceptible strains (odds ratio [OR], 2.8; 95% confidence interval [CI], 1.3 to 6.0). Three variables—hospitalization due to salmonellosis, underlying disease, and exposure to antimicrobials—were analyzed in a multivariate logistic regression model. Hospitalization and exposure to antimicrobials were found to be independently associated with having a resistant infection, whereas underlying disease could not be associated with having infection with a resistant isolate. As regards complications, no differences could be demonstrated between diseases due to resistant and sensitive strains (29).

The Emergence of Multidrug-Resistant *Salmonella* Serovar Typhimurium DT104

The debate about the clinical consequences of drug resistance in bacteria of animal origin resurfaced after the emergence of multidrug-resistant *Salmonella* serovar Typhimurium DT104, which is often resistant to five antimicrobial drugs: ampicillin, chloramphenicol, streptomycin, sulfonamides, and tetracycline (R-type ACSSuT) (19).

Salmonella spp. are highly clonal bacteria, and "successful clones" of drug-resistant *Salmonella* may spread in the food animal reservoir, with or even without the selective pressure of antimicrobial drugs (44). It is difficult to predict when this will happen, but it is clearly related to both transmission dynamics and bacterial factors, e.g., the strain having a broad reservoir and being easily adaptable and fit. To understand the transmission of these strains, it is also important to understand the organization of modern food production, with separate systems for central rearing, breeding, rearing, and production. If a "clonal lineage" with adequate fitness enters at the narrow top of this production pyramid, it may spread throughout the food chain. Trade of live animals amplifies this spread and is a major risk factor for introduction of *Salmonella* in a herd. Serovar Typhimurium DT104 is one recent example of a multidrug-resistant *Salmonella* clone that has spread internationally (19, 44, 46). Multidrug-resistant serovar Newport, which is now very common in North America, is another example (18).

One of the first papers to describe the emergence of DT104 was a case-control study by Wall et al. (49). The prime objective of this study was to determine the risk factors for infection. Wall et al. found that illness was independently associated with the consumption of several food items and contact with animals, ill farm animals in particular. In addition, they reported a hospitalization rate of 41% and a risk of death of 3.0%. This case-fatality rate—in line with that reported by Holmberg et al. (27)—suggested that DT104 could be slightly more virulent than most other *Salmonella* serovar Typhimurium strains. The increased morbidity and mortality could not easily be explained by therapeutic failures, as the drugs in the ACSSuT complex are rarely used for the management of food-borne infections in adults. Instead, the excess morbidity and mortality could be related to (i) resistance on top of R-type ACSSuT (which DT104 readily develops), (ii) increased virulence of DT104 (which raised the hypothesis that virulence factors could be coselected by the use of antimicrobial drugs), or (iii) host factors in patients infected with DT104.

The possibility of increased virulence of multidrug-resistant *Salmonella* serovar Typhimurium DT104 was subsequently addressed in a study in England and Wales from 1994 to 1996. Of 10,149 mutlidrug-resistant DT104 isolates, 1.3% were from blood, compared with 1.0% of 7,277 serovar Typhimurium isolates of other phage types and 1.3% of 59,821 *Salmonella* serovar Enteritidis isolates. In other words, the frequency of multidrug-resistant DT104 from blood culture of human beings was not significantly greater than that of other subtypes of serovar Typhimurium. The main limitation of this study was that the reference group (other serovar Typhimurium isolates) contained many other multidrug-resistant strains of serovar Typhimurium that were very common in England and Wales at the time. Pansusceptible strains of serovar Typhimurium would have been a better reference. In addition, possibly confounding factors (e.g., age) were not taken into account (45).

Hence, the question whether a DT104-like resistance pattern is associated with excess morbidity and mortality has not been resolved. A recent series of studies from the United States, Canada, and Denmark has shed more light on this issue and has examined the effect of DT104-like resistance as well as resistance to clinically important antimicrobial drugs (20, 23, 24, 31, 48).

Recent Epidemiological Studies

The series of new studies addressing the clinical and public health consequences of drug resistance in *Salmonella* and *Campylobacter* spp. was prompted partly by the emergence of DT104 and other animal-related, drug-resistant bacteria. Furthermore, the studies from the 1980s were based mainly on surveillance data or clinical case reports with limited possibilities for sophisticated data analysis. The problem is that surveillance data often include inadequate information on outcome, whereas outcome-based registries have inadequate data on infections. Additionally, there are a number of confounding factors, such as variation by subtype and contributions from comorbidity. In studies of mortality, it is furthermore crucial to subtract background mortality data to gain a more detailed understanding of the mortality due to *Salmonella* and other food-borne agents.

In Denmark a series of registry-based studies was initiated to determine mortality associated with gastrointestinal infections, adjusting for comorbidity and underlying mortality. From 1995 to 1999, 2,047 patients with *Salmonella* serovar Typhimurium infection were registered. To determine the survival of these patients, the registry of gastrointestinal pathogens was linked to the Danish Civil Registry System. Furthermore, to determine the survival of nonexposed individuals, 10 persons per case from the Civil Registry System were randomly selected and matched by age, sex, and county. Data on comorbidity were obtained from the national patient registry. A total of 59 deaths among the 2,047 patients were identified. Overall, patients with serovar Typhimurium infection had a mortality rate 3.0 times higher than the Danish population in general. After adjustment for comorbidity, this figure declined to 2.3. Looking at the resistance pattern, patients infected with pansusceptible strains had a 2.3-fold higher relative mortality compared with the general population, whereas patients with R-type ACSSuT had a mortality rate 4.8 times higher. Those patients who were infected with a quinolone-resistant (nalidixic acid, or Nx) strain had a 10.3-fold higher relative mortality, and 40 patients who had R-type ACSSuTNx had a mortality rate 13.1 times higher than the general Danish population. All the estimates were adjusted for comorbidity (Table 3). Excess mortality due to resistance in serovar Typhimurium was mainly related to resistance to quinolones (23).

Table 3. Survival after infection with *Salmonella* serovar Typhimurium according to antimicrobial drug resistance

Resistance pattern	No. of patients	Relative mortality compared with the general population (95% CI)[a]
Pansusceptible	953	2.3 (1.5–3.5)
ACSSuT[b]	283	4.8 (2.2–10.2)
Nx[c]	83	10.3 (2.8–37.8)
ACSSuTNx	40	13.1 (3.3–51.9)

[a]All estimates are hazard ratios, calculated by conditional proportional hazard regression analysis, compared with an age- and gender-matched sample of the general Danish population and adjusted for underlying illness. Data collected in Denmark from 1995 to 1999. Data from reference 20.
[b]Resistant to at least ampicillin, chloramphenicol, streptomycin, sulfonamide, and tetracycline.
[c]Resistant to at least nalidixic acid (i.e., a first-generation quinolone; these strains have reduced susceptibility to fluoroquinolones such as ciprofloxacin).

In a more recent Danish study, the excess risk of death or invasive illness due to quinolone resistance in *Salmonella* serovar Typhimurium was determined. Of 1,323 patients infected with serovar Typhimurium, 46 (3.5%) were hospitalized due an invasive illness within 90 days of infection and 16 (1.2%) died within 90 days of infection. After adjustment for age, sex, and comorbidity, infection with quinolone-resistant serovar Typhimurium was associated with a significant, 3.15-fold-higher risk of invasive illness or death within 90 days of infection, compared with that observed for infection with pansusceptible strains (20).

In Canada, increased risk of hospitalization was found in patients with multidrug-resistant *Salmonella* serovar Typhimurium (31). Hospitalization was more likely to occur among case subjects whose infections were resistant to at least ampicillin, chloramphenicol and/or kanamycin, streptomycin, sulfamethoxazole, and tetracycline (R-type AK/CSSuT) (OR, 2.3; $P = 0.003$) compared with case subjects with AK/CSSuT-susceptible infections, and among case subjects with non-DT104 R-type AKSSuT infections (OR, 3.6; $P = 0.005$) compared with case subjects with non-DT104 AKSSuT-susceptible infections. In contrast, hospitalization rates did not differ between case subjects with DT104 infections and case subjects with non-DT104 infections, or between case subjects with DT104 R-type ACSSuT infections and case subjects with DT104 ACSSuT-susceptible infections.

Recent data from the United States corroborate that resistance in *Salmonella* is associated with increased morbidity. Varma et al. (48) used data from the National Antimicrobial Resistance Monitoring System (NARMS), which performs susceptibility testing on nontyphoid *Salmonella* isolates. Data on resistance were linked with outcome data collected partly through the Foodborne Diseases Active Surveillance Network (FoodNet). Isolates defined as resistant to a clinically important agent were resistant to one or more of the following agents: ampicillin, ceftriaxone, ciprofloxacin, gentamicin, and/or trimethoprim-sulfa methoxazole.

In the period from 1996 to 2001, NARMS received 7,370 serotyped, nontyphoid *Salmonella* isolates from blood or stool. Bloodstream infection occurred more frequently among patients infected with an isolate resistant to ≥1 clinically important agent (adjusted OR, 1.6; 95% CI, 1.2 to 2.1) compared with patients with pansusceptible infection. During 1996 to 2001, FoodNet staff ascertained outcomes for 1,415 patients who had isolates tested in NARMS. Hospitalization with bloodstream infection occurred more frequently among patients infected with an isolate resistant to ≥1 clinically important agent (adjusted OR, 3.1; 95% CI, 1.4 to 6.6) compared with patients with pansusceptible infection. The risk of hospital admission was particularly high for patients infected with strains with R-type ACSSuT (OR, 4.6; 95% CI, 1.3 to 16.7) (48).

Fluoroquinolone and Macrolide Resistance in *Campylobacter*

The hazards of fluoroquinolone resistance have also been demonstrated for *Campylobacter* spp. Table 4 in chapter 16 summarizes information from five studies evaluating the duration of illness in patients infected with fluoroquinolone-resistant versus fluoroquinolone-sensitive *Campylobacter* isolates (8, 14, 35, 36, 42). Although the results of these studies are not all statistically significant, the estimates point in the same direction. Taken together, they suggest that there is a longer duration of illness in patients infected with resistant strains. Additionally, it has been determined that there is an excess risk of death or invasive illness following infection with fluoroquinolone- or macrolide-resistant *Campylobacter* compared with susceptible strains (22). In 3,471 patients with *Campylobacter* infections, a total of 22 (0.63%) had an adverse event, defined as invasive illness or death within 90 days of the date of sample receipt.

Patients with quinolone-resistant *Campylobacter* infections had an increased risk of an adverse event within 30 days compared with quinolone- and erythromycin-susceptible *Campylobacter* infections (adjusted OR, 6.17; 95% CI, 1.62 to 23.47). Compared with quinolone- and erythromycin-susceptible *Campylobacter* infection, infection with erythromycin-resistant strains was associated with a more than five-fold higher risk of an adverse event within 90 days of receipt of sample (adjusted OR, 5.51; 95% CI, 1.19 to 25.50).

CONCLUSION

The food chain contains an abundance of antimicrobial drug-resistant pathogens, including *Salmonella* and *Campylobacter*. There is growing evidence that this has significant public health consequences. One consequence is increased transmission, supported by the unrelated use of antimicrobials in humans. Other consequences are related to reduced efficacy of early empirical treatment, limited treatment choices after microbiological diagnosis has been confirmed, and finally, a possible coselection or upregulation of virulence traits in resistant agents. This contributes to the excess mortality and morbidity observed in outbreaks and in sporadic cases of drug-resistant *Salmonella* and *Campylobacter*. Mitigation of antimicrobial resistance in food-borne bacteria such as *Salmonella* and *Campylobacter* will likely benefit human health.

REFERENCES

1. **Aarestrup, F. M., H. Hasman, I. Olsen, and G. Sørensen.** 2004. International spread of bla_{CMY-2}-mediated cephalosporin resistance in a multiresistant *Salmonella enterica* serovar Heidelberg isolate stemming from the importation of a boar by Denmark from Canada. *Antimicrob. Agents Chemother.* **48:**1916–1917.
2. **Aarestrup, F. M., C. Wiuff, K. Mølbak, and E. J. Threlfall.** 2003. Is it time to change fluoroquinolone breakpoints for *Salmonella* spp.? *Antimicrob. Agents Chemother.* **47:**827–829.
3. **Adler, J. L., R. L. Anderson, J. R. Boring III, and A. J. Nahmias.** 1970. A protracted hospital-associated outbreak of salmonellosis due to a multiple-antibiotic-resistant strain of *Salmonella indiana*. *J. Pediatr.* **77:**970–975.
4. **Anderson, A. D., J. M. Nelson, S. Rossiter, and F. J. Angulo.** 2003. Public health consequences of use of antimicrobial agents in food animals in the United States. *Microb. Drug Resist.* **9:**373–379.
5. **Anderson, E. S.** 1968. Drug resistance in *Salmonella typhimurium* and its implications. *Br. Med. J.* **3:**333–339.
6. **Barza, M.** 2002. Potential mechanisms of increased disease in humans from antimicrobial resistance in food animals. *Clin. Infect. Dis.* **34** (Suppl. 3):S123–S125.
7. **Barza, M., and K. Travers.** 2002. Excess infections due to antimicrobial resistance: the "attributable fraction." *Clin. Infect. Dis.* **34**(Suppl. 3):S126–S130.
8. ***Campylobacter* Sentinel Surveillance Scheme Collaborators.** 2002. Ciprofloxacin resistance in *Campylobacter jejuni*: case-case analysis as a tool for elucidating risks at home and abroad. *J. Antimicrob. Chemother.* **50:**561–568.
9. **Carattoli, A., F. Tosini, W. P. Giles, M. E. Rupp, S. H. Hinrichs, F. J. Angulo, T. J. Barrett, and P. D. Fey.** 2002. Characterization of plasmids carrying CMY-2 from expanded-spectrum cephalosporin-resistant *Salmonella* strains isolated in the United States between 1996 and 1998. *Antimicrob. Agents Chemother.* **46:**1269–1272.
10. **Cohen, M. L., and R. V. Tauxe.** 1986. Drug-resistant *Salmonella* in the United States: an epidemiologic perspective. *Science* **234:**964–969.
11. **Crump, J. A., T. J. Barrett, J. T. Nelson, and F. J. Angulo.** 2003. Reevaluating fluoroquinolone breakpoints for *Salmonella enterica* serotype Typhi and for non-Typhi salmonellae. *Clin. Infect. Dis.* **37:**75–81.
12. **Delarocque-Astagneau, E., C. Bouillant, V. Vaillant, P. Bouvet, P. A. Grimont, and J. C. Desenclos.** 2000. Risk factors for the occurrence of sporadic *Salmonella enterica* serotype Typhimurium infections in children in France: a national case-control study. *Clin. Infect. Dis.* **31:**488–492.
13. **Dunne, E. F., P. D. Fey, P. Kludt, R. Reporter, F. Mostashari, P. Shillam, J. Wicklund, C. Miller, B. Holland, K. Stamey, T. J. Barrett, J. K. Rasheed, F. C. Tenover, E. M. Ribot, and F. J. Angulo.** 2000. Emergence of domestically acquired ceftriaxone-resistant *Salmonella* infections associated with AmpC beta-lactamase. *JAMA* **284:**3151–3156.
14. **Engberg, J., J. Neimann, E. M. Nielsen, F. M. Aarestrup, and V. Fussing.** 2004. Quinolone-resistant *Campylobacter* infections: risk factors and clinical consequences. *Emerg. Infect. Dis.* **10:**1056–1063.
15. **Fey, P. D., T. J. Safranek, M. E. Rupp, E. F. Dunne, E. Ribot, P. C. Iwen, P. A. Bradford, F. J. Angulo, and S. H. Hinrichs.** 2000. Ceftriaxone-resistant salmonella infection acquired by a child from cattle. *N. Engl. J. Med.* **342:**1242–1249.
16. **Fluit, A. C.** 2005. Towards more virulent and antibiotic-resistant *Salmonella*. *FEMS Immunol. Med. Microbiol.* **43:** 1–11.
17. **Glynn, M. K., V. Reddy, L. Hutwagner, T. Rabatsky-Ehr, B. Shiferaw, D. J. Vugia, S. Segler, J. Bender, T. J. Barrett, and F. J. Angulo.** 2004. Prior antimicrobial agent use increases the risk of sporadic infections with multidrug-resistant *Salmonella enterica* serotype Typhimurium: a FoodNet case-control study, 1996–1997. *Clin. Infect. Dis.* **38** (Suppl. 3):S227–S236.
18. **Gupta, A., J. Fontana, C. Crowe, B. Bolstorff, A. Stout, S. Van Duyne, M. P. Hoekstra, J. M. Whichard, T. J. Barrett, and F. J. Angulo.** 2003. Emergence of multidrug-resistant *Salmonella enterica* serotype Newport infections resistant to expanded-spectrum cephalosporins in the United States. *J. Infect. Dis.* **188:**1707–1716.
19. **Helms, M., S. Ethelberg, K. Mølbak, and the DT104 Study Group.** 2005. International *Salmonella* Typhimurium DT104 infections, 1992–2001. *Emerg. Infect. Dis.* **11:**859–867. [Online.] http://www.cdc.gov/ncidod/EID/vol11no6/04-1017.htm.
20. **Helms, M., J. Simonsen, and K. Mølbak.** 2004. Quinolone resistance is associated with increased risk of invasive illness or death during infection with *Salmonella* serotype Typhimurium. *J. Infect. Dis.* **190:**1652–1654.
21. **Helms, M., J. Simonsen, J. Neimann, L. J. Porsbo, H. D. Emborg, and K. Mølbak.** *Salmonella* Typhimurium in Denmark: clinical consequences and the impact of antimicrobial drug resistance, a case comparison study. Submitted for publication.
22. **Helms, M., J. Simonsen, K. E. P. Olsen, and K. Mølbak.** 2005. Adverse health events associated with antimicrobial drug resistance in *Campylobacter* species: a registry-based cohort study. *J. Infect. Dis.* **191:**1050–1055.
23. **Helms, M., P. Vastrup, P. Gerner-Smidt, and K. Mølbak.** 2002. Excess mortality associated with antimicrobial drug-resistant *Salmonella* Typhimurium. *Emerg. Infect. Dis.* **8:**490–495.
24. **Helms, M., P. Vastrup, P. Gerner-Smidt, and K. Mølbak.** 2003. Short and long term mortality associated with foodborne bacterial gastrointestinal infections: registry based study. *Br. Med. J.* **326:**357.
25. **Hohmann, E. L.** 2001. Nontyphoidal salmonellosis. *Clin. Infect. Dis.* **32:**263–269.
26. **Holmberg, S. D., M. T. Osterholm, K. A. Senger, and M. L. Cohen.** 1984. Drug-resistant *Salmonella* from animals fed antimicrobials. *N. Engl. J. Med.* **311:**617–622.
27. **Holmberg, S. D., J. G. Wells, and M. L. Cohen.** 1984. Animal-to-man transmission of antimicrobial-resistant *Salmonella*:

investigations of U.S. outbreaks, 1971–1983. *Science* **225:** 833–835.

28. **Kass, P. H., T. B. Farver, J. J. Beaumont, C. Genigeorgis, and F. Stevens.** 1992. Disease determinants of sporadic salmonellosis in four northern California counties. A case-control study of older children and adults. *Ann. Epidemiol.* **2:**683–696.
29. **Lee, L. A., N. D. Puhr, E. K. Maloney, N. H. Bean, and R. V. Tauxe.** 1994. Increase in antimicrobial-resistant *Salmonella* infections in the United States, 1989–1990. *J. Infect. Dis.* **170:** 128–134.
30. **MacDonald, K. L., M. L. Cohen, N. T. Hargrett-Bean, J. G. Wells, N. D. Puhr, S. F. Collin, and P. A. Blake.** 1987. Changes in antimicrobial resistance of *Salmonella* isolated from humans in the United States. *JAMA* **258:**1496–1499.
31. **Martin, L. J., M. Fyfe, K. Dore, J. A. Buxton, F. Pollari, B. Henry, D. Middleton, R. Ahmed, F. Jamieson, B. Ciebin, S. A. McEwen, and J. B. Wilson.** 2004. Increased burden of illness associated with antimicrobial-resistant *Salmonella enterica* serotype Typhimurium infections. *J. Infect. Dis.* **189:** 377–384.
32. **Mølbak, K., D. L. Baggesen, F. M. Aarestrup, J. M. Ebbesen, J. Engberg, K. Frydendahl, P. Gerner-Smidt, A. M. Petersen, and H. C. Wegener.** 1999. An outbreak of multidrug-resistant, quinolone-resistant *Salmonella enterica* serotype Typhimurium DT104. *N. Engl. J. Med.* **341:**1420–1425.
33. **Mølbak, K., and J. Neimann.** 2002. Risk factors for sporadic infection with *Salmonella* Enteritidis, Denmark, 1997–1999. *Am. J. Epidemiol.* **156:**654–661.
34. **Nakaya, H., A. Yasuhara, K. Yoshimura, Y. Oshihoi, H. Izumiya, and H. Watanabe.** 2003. Life-threatening infantile diarrhea from fluoroquinolone-resistant *Salmonella enterica* Typhimurium with mutations in both *gyrA* and *par*C. *Emerg. Infect. Dis.* **9:**255–257.
35. **Neimann, J., K. Mølbak, J. Engberg, F. M. Aarestrup, and H. C. Wegener.** 2001. Longer duration of illness among *Campylobacter* patients treated with fluoroquinolones. Presented at the 11th International Workshop on *Campylobacter*, *Helicobacter* and related organisms, Freiburg, Germany, 1 to 5 September 2001.
36. **Nelson, J. M., K. E. Smith, D. J. Vugia, T. Rabatsky-Ehr, S. D. Segler, H. D. Kassenborg, S. M. Zansky, K. Joyce, N. Marano, R. M. Hoekstra, and F. J. Angulo.** 2004. Prolonged diarrhea due to ciprofloxacin-resistant *Campylobacter* infection. *J. Infect. Dis.* **190:**1150–1157.
37. **Olsen, S. J., E. E. DeBess, T. E. McGivern, N. Marano, T. Eby, S. Mauvais, V. K. Balan, G. Zirnstein, P. R. Cieslak, and F. J. Angulo.** 2001. A nosocomial outbreak of fluoroquinolone-resistant *Salmonella* infection. *N. Engl. J. Med.* **344:**1572–1579.
38. **Riley, L. W., M. L. Cohen, J. E. Seals, M. J. Blaser, K. A. Birkness, N. T. Hargrett, S. M. Martin, and R. A. Feldman.** 1984. Importance of host factors in human salmonellosis caused by multiresistant strains of *Salmonella*. *J. Infect. Dis.* **149:**878–883.
39. **Rosenthal, S. L.** 1969. Exacerbation of salmonella enteritis due to ampicillin. *N. Engl. J. Med.* **280:**147–148.
40. **Ryan, C. A., M. K. Nickels, N. T. Hargrett-Bean, M. E. Potter, T. Endo, L. Mayer, C. W. Langkop, C. Gibson, R. C. McDonald, R. T. Kenney, N. D. Puhr, P. J. McDonnell, R. J. Martin, M. L. Cohen, and P. A. Blake.** 1987. Massive outbreak of antimicrobial-resistant salmonellosis traced to pasteurized milk. *JAMA* **258:**3269–3274.
41. **Schmid, H., A. P. Burnens, A. Baumgartner, and J. Oberreich.** 1996. Risk factors for sporadic salmonellosis in Switzerland. *Eur. J. Clin. Microbiol. Infect. Dis.* **15:**725–732.
42. **Smith, K. E., J. M. Besser, C. W. Hedberg, F. T. Leano, J. B. Bender, J. H. Wicklund, B. P. Johnson, K. A. Moore, and M. T. Osterholm.** 1999. Quinolone-resistant *Campylobacter jejuni* infections in Minnesota, 1992–1998. *N. Engl. J. Med.* **340:**1525–1532.
43. **Spika, J. S., S. H. Waterman, G. W. Hoo, M. E. St. Louis, R. E. Pacer, S. M. James, M. L. Bissett, L. W. Mayer, J. Y. Chiu, B. Hall, et al.** 1987. Chloramphenicol-resistant *Salmonella newport* traced through hamburger to dairy farms. A major persisting source of human salmonellosis in California. *N. Engl. J. Med.* **316:**565–570.
44. **Tauxe, R. V.** 1999. *Salmonella* Enteritidis and *Salmonella* Typhimurium DT104: successful subtypes in the modern world, p. 37–52. *In* W. M. Scheld, W. A. Craig, and J. M. Hughes (ed.), *Emerging Infections 3*. ASM Press, Washington, D.C.
45. **Threlfall, E. J., L. R. Ward, and B. Rowe.** 1998. Multiresistant *Salmonella typhimurium* DT 104 and salmonella bacteraemia. *Lancet* **352:**287–288.
46. **Threlfall, E. J.** 2000. Epidemic *Salmonella* Typhimurium DT 104—a truly international multiresistant clone. *J. Antimicrob. Chemother.* **46:**7–10.
47. **Varma, J. K., K. D. Greene, J. Ovitt, F. Medalla, and F. J. Angulo.** 2005. Hospitalization and antimicrobial resistance in *Salmonella* outbreaks, 1984–2002. *Emerg. Infect. Dis.* **11:**943–946.
48. **Varma, J. K., K. Mølbak, T. J. Barrett, J. L. Beebe, T. F. Jones, T. Rabatsky-Ehr, K. E. Smith, D. J. Vugia, H. G. Chang, and F. J. Angulo.** 2005. Antimicrobial-resistant nontyphoidal *Salmonella* is associated with excess bloodstream infections and hospitalizations. *J. Infect. Dis.* **191:**554–561.
49. **Wall, P. G., D. Morgan, K. Lamden, M. Ryan, M. Griffin, E. J. Threlfall, L. R. Ward, and B. Rowe.** 1994. A case control study of infection with an epidemic strain of multiresistant *Salmonella* Typhimurium DT104 in England and Wales. *Commun. Dis. Rep. CDR Rev.* **4:**R130–R135.
50. **Winokur, P. L., R. Canton, J. M. Casellas, and N. Legakis.** 2001. Variations in the prevalence of strains expressing an extended-spectrum β-lactamase phenotype and characterization of isolates from Europe, the Americas, and the Western Pacific region. *Clin. Infect. Dis.* 32 (Suppl. 2):S94–S103.
51. **Winokur, P. L., D. L. Vonstein, L. J. Hoffman, E. K. Uhlenhopp, and G. V. Doern.** 2001. Evidence for transfer of CMY-2 AmpC β-lactamase plasmids between *Escherichia coli* and *Salmonella* isolates from food animals and humans. *Antimicrob. Agents Chemother.* **45:**2716–2722.

Antimicrobial Resistance in Bacteria of Animal Origin
Edited by Frank M. Aarestrup

Chapter 20

The Origin, Evolution, and Local and Global Dissemination of Antimicrobial Resistance

FRANK M. AARESTRUP

The global emergence of antimicrobial-resistant bacteria has had serious consequences for human and animal health. The speediness with which antimicrobial resistance has emerged, evolved, and spread worldwide has been without comparison and clearly shows the great adaptive ability of bacteria. The origin of acquired antimicrobial resistance is in general believed to be adoption of resistance genes from antimicrobial-producing organisms and/or nucleotide changes in housekeeping genes. A large number of different mechanisms encoding resistance have been identified in bacteria (see chapter 6). These genes have transferred to susceptible bacteria and become localized on different mobile elements, from where they have spread to other bacteria. Bacteria have evolved many different mechanisms that facilitate gene transfer. Most of these mechanisms have also been involved in the dissemination of antimicrobial resistance genes, and most studies have in fact been done using transfer of antimicrobial resistance as a model. Identical bacterial clones and identical resistance genes often carried on mobile DNA elements like transposons and plasmids have been detected in a large number of reservoirs all around the world. It is unlikely that this is caused by independent evolutionary events; it must be caused by horizontal spread both between bacterial species and around the world.

In addition to the many genetic mechanisms that facilitate gene transfer, the modern globalized world has provided efficient ways for bacteria and resistance genes to rapidly disseminate worldwide through trade of food products, live animals, and travel. Further globalization will only increase trade and international contacts in the future. Besides the many benefits thereof, this can also create serious health problems. Therefore, how we handle the control of antimicrobial resistance in human pathogens, including those of animal origin, will have important public health consequences for the future.

This chapter provides a brief overview of the putative origins of some of the most important antimicrobial resistance determinants and some of the genetic mechanisms whereby they have spread among different bacterial clones and genera. In addition, some of the modes whereby resistance genes and resistant bacteria may have disseminated worldwide are described.

ORIGIN OF ANTIMICROBIAL RESISTANCE

Bacteria may acquire resistance by mutations in their DNA, changing the target; by hyperproduction of genes that are already present; or by acquisition of heterologous resistance genes. The different mechanisms of resistance are reviewed in chapter 6. The most important mechanism of acquired resistance in most bacterial pathogens is horizontal acquisition of resistance genes. The actual origin of antimicrobial resistance genes is unknown, but environmental microbes, including the natural producers of antimicrobial substances, are believed to be important primary sources. It has been speculated that microbes surrounding antibiotic-producing organisms acquired the resistance gene from the producers and thereby acquired the ability to survive and thrive in an otherwise hostile environment. This theory is supported by the substantial genetic and biochemical similarities between resistance determinants from antibiotic-producing organisms and some of the most important and widespread resistance genes found in both gram-negative and gram-positive bacteria (Table 1). Various housekeeping genes are also a likely origin for several

Frank M. Aarestrup • Danish Institute for Food and Veterinary Research, Bülowsvej 27, DK-1790 Copenhagen V, Denmark.

Table 1. Origin of antimicrobial resistance genes

Antimicrobial agent	Resistance determinant(s)	Putative origin
Aminoglycosides	Acetyltransferases, phosphotransferases, nucleotidyltransferases	Aminoglycoside-producing organisms
Chloramphenicol	Acetyltransferases	Housekeeping genes
Streptogramins	Acetyltransferases	
Glycopeptides	VanHAX cluster	VanHAX-like cluster from the glycopeptide-producing organisms
Macrolides	rRNA methylation	*erm* genes from the macrolide-producing organisms
Penicillins	β-lactamases, modified penicillin-binding proteins	Penicillin-binding proteins of bacteria
Tetracyclines	Ribosomal protection proteins	Ribosomal protection proteins from the tetracycline-producing organisms

resistance determinants. This is especially the case for the different efflux genes, where these transmembrane transport proteins also can play a role in protecting bacteria from antimicrobials. Our knowledge is still incomplete, since most DNA sequences are from various clinical and pathogenic isolates, with comparatively few from environmental species. In the following examples, the likely origin of some of the most important mechanisms of resistance is given.

β-Lactams

The β-lactamases are believed to have evolved from enzymes involved in cell wall biosynthesis. Because these proteins interact with penicillins, they are referred to collectively as the penicillin-binding proteins (PBPs) (112, 131). PBPs and β-lactamases are related enzymes: the former are the targets for β-lactam antibiotics and the latter are enzymes responsible for resistance to these antibiotics. The two families of enzymes share sequence homology, structural topologies, and mechanistic features. Many bacterial species, including *Escherichia coli*, contain chromosally encoded β-lactamases. These genes are normally expressed at a low level, which is not sufficient to give clinical resistance, and their normal function is unknown. Mutations in the regulatory gene(s) and promoter upregulation can, however, increase enzyme activity and render cells clinically resistant. The primary means of acquired β-lactam resistance is by importing transferable genes encoding β-lactamases (121). The rapid and widespread development of resistance to these drugs is an instructive example of evolution occurring on a timescale of a few years, as well as the dramatic effect that single and multiple mutations can have on the structure and function of β-lactamases (135, 149). Ampicillin was introduced into clinical use more than 40 years ago, and the first plasmid-borne β-lactamase was detected in an *E. coli* strain in 1965 (55), mediated by the TEM-1 gene. When resistance rapidly spread, a new combination treatment including an inhibitor of the enzyme was developed. However, a single mutation in TEM-1 altered the enzyme to escape the action of the inhibitor while retaining activity toward the β-lactams. Subsequently, the cephalosporins were developed, but upon the introduction of every new β-lactam the TEM genes mutated in new directions, leading to 128 different TEM β-lactamases in various bacterial strains at present (see chapter 6). Some of these enzymes have activity against almost all β-lactam antibiotics. Other important genes are the CTX-M, CMY, SHV, and OXA genes, which are believed to have their origin in the chromosome of bacterial genera such as *Citrobacter*, *Kluyvera*, etc. (28, 87, 150, 162, 220). These genes have, apparently just recently, escaped the chromosome and spread rapidly on plasmids among pathogenic bacteria such as *Salmonella* and *E. coli* (75, 87, 150, 175, 221).

Another important mechanism of resistance is acquisition of new PBPs with reduced affinity for β-lactam antibiotics (chapter 6). This is the mechanism of resistance that has emerged in *Streptococcus pneumoniae* and methicillin-resistant staphylococci (see chapter 12). The origin of the *mecA* gene in staphylococci is not known, but it may be a gene homolog naturally present in *Staphylococcus sciuri* (219).

Aminoglycosides

The main mechanism of resistance to aminoglycosides is enzymatic inactivation (chapter 6). Aminoglycoside-inactivating enzymes are encoded by a large group of genes, most of which are unrelated at the DNA level (177). Thus, these genes most likely have a variety of different microbial origins. Some appear to have originated in aminoglycoside-producing bacteria, such as *Streptomyces*, *Micromonospora*, and *Bacillus* (29, 56, 111, 177, 195). Other aminoglycoside-modifying enzymes have probably also originated from genes involved in normal cellular metabolism (151, 177).

Macrolides

Target modification by rRNA methylases, encoded by *erm* genes, is the most common mechanism of resistance to macrolide antibiotics (161; see also chapter 6). Comparison of the DNA and deduced amino acid sequence of the *erm* genes from macrolide-producing organisms and macrolide-resistant bacteria strongly suggests that the origin of macrolide resistance is macrolide-synthesizing organisms (22). The sequence diversity is, however, so extensive that innumerable evolutionary steps must have occurred to generate the variety of genes found in bacteria today (99). Furthermore, comparison of the sequences and the species in which they are found could indicate that the *erm* genes were transferred into different bacterial species a long time ago and subsequently have evolved independently in these different bacterial species (99).

Tetracyclines

Resistance to tetracyclines is mediated either by genes encoding ribosomal protection proteins (RPPs) or efflux pumps (chapter 6). The RPPs found in pathogenic and saprophytic bacteria show a high degree of sequence similarity to genes found in tetracycline-producing strains (9). Furthermore, mycobacteria have been found to contain sequences similar to those encoding RPPs in the producing organisms (144). Thus, it seems plausible that the genes encoding RPPs have transferred from the tetracycline-producing strains to other bacteria and evolved to the genes we observe today. Efflux of tetracyclines can be mediated by several chromosomal transporters, some of which are specific to the class (*tet*) and others (*acr*) that efflux multiple classes of antimicrobials. Thus, efflux-mediated tetracycline resistance most likely evolved from various transporter proteins (178).

Glycopeptides

Acquired resistance to glycopeptides has been detected mainly in enterococci and is mediated mainly through modification of the target site, where the terminal dipeptide D-alanine–D-alanine in the peptido-glycal precursor is replaced by D-alanine–D-lactate or D-alanine–D-serine (chapter 6). In isolates from animals, the most common resistance gene is *vanA*, located on the transposon Tn*1546* (chapter 18). Genes encoding homologs to three determinants essential for glycopeptide resistance (*vanHAX*) have been found in the glycopeptide-producing organisms *Streptomyces toyocaensis* and *Amycolatopsis orientalis* (128, 129). Furthermore, the three genes have the same orientation and sequence overlap in both the producing organisms and in enterococci with acquired resistance. Hybridization experiments have shown that homologs to *vanHAX* are also present in other glycopeptide-producing organisms, including the avoparcin-producing organism *Amycolatopsis coloradensis* (129). This could indicate that the enterococci acquired the resistance genes en bloc from the producing organisms. It seems unlikely that a genetic structure such as the *vanHAX* cluster evolved independently. This cluster mediates resistance through a sophisticated mechanism that involves degradation of already established structures in the cell wall by VanX, reduction of pyruvate to D-lactate by VanH, and generation of a new linkage with reduced affinity to glycopeptides by VanA (23).

Evolution of Resistance Genes

DNA from antibiotic-producing organisms, including their resistance genes, has been found in antibiotic preparations intended for animal or human use. Thus, nucleotide sequences related to the *erm* genes encoding macrolide resistance, ribosomal protection genes encoding tetracycline resistance, phosphotransferase encoding streptomycin resistance, and the *vanHAX* cluster encoding glycopeptide resistance have been found in antibiotic preparations (124, 207), presumably as remnant genetic material from the antimicrobial-producing organism. Thus, the antibiotic could have provided both the resistance genes and the selective environment favoring their devolvement to recipient bacteria. This would imply that the evolution from the original gene to the resistance genes we see in pathogenic bacteria today has taken place within the antibiotic era, i.e., in just around 50 years. In environmental bacteria, evolutionary selection and dissemination of resistance determinants has been operating for hundreds of millions of years, resulting in many of the resistance genes we see today. The intensive and global use of antibiotic drug preparations containing associated resistance genes represents a type of Trojan horse scenario, which may have played a vital role in accelerating the evolution and spread of important resistance phenotypes in the past few decades.

Even though major similarities exist between resistance genes in their putative organisms of origin and those identified in clinical pathogens, there are also striking differences in the DNA sequences, CG content, and codon usage. Changes in the genes might have occurred to optimize the usage of available tRNA, lowering the burden of acquired coding sequences. Quite naturally, the question arises as to how the gene evolved from the putative origin in the producing organism to the resistance gene we know today. In theory, gene evolution is a process where single point mutations occur with a certain frequency. This mutation establishes itself in the population when it constitutes an advantage for the bacterium in comparison to the ancestor. Furthermore, the new mutation should give the bacterium a sufficient advantage for this new gene to survive an evolutionary bottleneck (103, 116). This implies that the evolutionary process from the gene in the producing organism to the final resistance gene should be a long process of sequential mutations, each giving the bacterium an advantage over the prior mutant. This would mean 480 base pair changes (in a gene 1,048 bp in length) from the *vanA* homolog in *A. orientalis* to the *vanA* gene located on Tn*1546*. It can be argued that this simplest model is possible given the enormous number of bacterial species found in the intestinal tract of animals and in the environment, the long time frame of evolution, and the short generation time of bacteria. As mentioned, it is unlikely that this gene was transferred directly from one of the antibiotic-producing organisms into enterococci. Given the molecular complexity of the *van* gene locus, it seems more likely that intermediate bacterial hosts moderated its evolution. Some variants of the *vanA* gene have been detected in several different bacterial genera, including *Oerskovia turbata* (152), *Bacillus circulans* (119), *Paenibacillus popilliae* (145), and *Paenibacillus apiarius* and *Paenibacillus thiaminolyticus* (82), which may play a role as intermediate hosts. Furthermore, the genes may have adapted in one or several of the organisms, which we so far have been unable to cultivate (86). Nonetheless, the evolution from a producing organism, even through intermediate hosts, to the genes found in enterococci requires an enormous number of bacterial generations occurring within favorable environments. It has also been suggested that new variants arise in bacterial subpopulations with a very high rate of mutations (e.g., *mutS* mutants). In this way, evolution might be hastened by simultaneous point mutations taking place within relatively few generations, thus avoiding the need for successive single mutations to gain independent ascendancy.

Besides mutation, recombination of related genes also appears to play an important role in the evolution of resistance genes. Recombination has been indicated both for *erm* genes (171) and tetracycline resistance genes (141, 188), either creating a mosaic structure of the genes or even giving rise to new genes (171). Recombination would also help to speed up the evolutionary process. In addition, some genes might have a higher evolutionary potential than others. Tertiary and secondary structures of both DNA and protein sequences play an important role in determining how freely genes can change their sequences and still attain functionality (10, 176). Much more knowledge about the adaptive and evolutionary processes is needed for us to truly understand gene evolution.

MOLECULAR MECHANISMS OF DISSEMINATION

Horizontal exchange of DNA plays a profound role in the evolution of prokaryotes. Acquisition of genes from other organisms provides an efficient way to acquire new traits and adapt to new or changing environments. Most evidence for horizontal gene transfer is based on comparison of DNA nucleotide sequence data. Analyses of total genome sequences of different bacterial species have indicated that large parts of bacterial genomes have resulted from horizontal gene transfer (31, 133, 146). For example, comparison of three *E. coli* isolates found only 39% of their proteins to be common for all three strains (208). Such comparative analyses have even indicated interkingdom transfer between eukaryotes and prokaryotes (62, 147, 185). This possibility has also been verified in vitro (223), showing that gene transfer is not restricted to closely related organisms.

While it is debatable whether the evolution of the resistance determinants we see among pathogenic bacteria today from their potential origins in antibiotic-producing organisms has occurred over a long time span or is a more recent event, there can be no doubt that the rapid dissemination of resistance genes among different commensal and pathogenic bacteria is a very recent evolutionary event. This dissemination has occurred within the antibiotic era as a consequence of horizontal transfer mediated by a diverse array of mobile DNA elements, such as plasmids, transposons, genomic islands, and integrons, as well as natural transformation (Table 2) (142). These mechanisms provide almost endless avenues for resistance genes to disseminate into any given clone or bacterial species (Fig. 1). Some mobile elements might not transfer effectively between all species. However, identical resistance genes have been found in many genetic contexts, indicating that they can become members of different DNA vectors and bypass host restrictions imposed on a given mobile element. The increase in sequence data within the last decade has given us new insights into the

Table 2. Transfer mechanisms in gram-positive and gram-negative bacteria

Bacteria	Mechanism	Example	Antimicrobial resistance	Reference(s)
Gram-positive	Sex pheromone conjugative plasmids	pCF10	Tetracycline [*tet*(M)]	44
	Nonpheromone conjugative plasmids	pGO1	Gentamicin [*aac(6′)-aph(2″)*], quaternary ammonium compounds (*smr*), streptomycin (*aadD*), and trimethoprim (*dfrA*)	137
	Nonconjugative plasmids	pC221	Chloramphenicol (*cat*)	153
	Conjugative transposons	Tn*916* family	Tetracycline [*tet*(M)]	47, 158
	Transformation	*pbp2*	Penicillin resistance in *S. pneumoniae*	65
Gram-negative	Conjugative plasmids	R751	Trimethoprim and quaternary ammonium compounds	102
	Nonconjugative plasmids	RSF1010	Streptomycin (*strA-strB*) and sulfonamides (*sul1*)	167
	Genomic islands	SG11	Ampicillin (*pse-1*), chloramphenicol (*floR*), streptomycin (*aadA*), sulfonamides (*sul1*), and tetracycline [*tet*(G)]	35
	Transposons	Tn*21*	Streptomycin (*aadA1*)	118

multiple mechanisms bacteria have developed to share advantageous DNA sequences, and we have probably just begun to see the number of possibilities. Transfer of different DNA elements has mainly been conducted in vitro. However, the situation in vivo might be quite different, where the multitude of heterogeneous bacterial communities might facilitate the spread of resistance genes (60). In the following sections, a few of the most important mobile DNA elements are discussed.

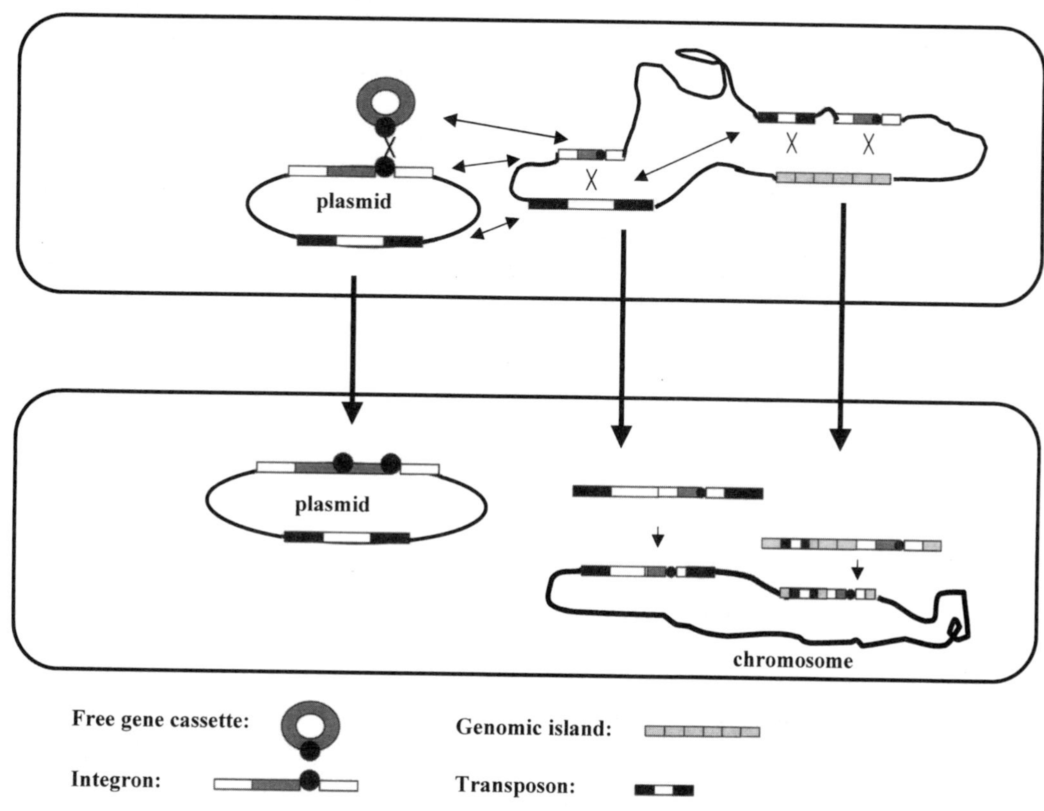

Figure 1. Mechanisms of gene transfer within and between bacteria. Picture by Yvonne Agersø.

Plasmids

A large number of different plasmids have been found in bacteria, and they have probably been the most important single mediator of the dissemination of resistance. A plasmid is defined as extrachromosomal DNA that replicates in an autonomous, self-controlled way (104). They normally range in size from 300 bp to 2,400 kb.

Lederberg first introduced the term "plasmid" in 1952 (115). The importance of plasmids in the emergence and spread of antimicrobial resistance became increasingly clear in the following decades. Today, many plasmids with many different structures and capabilities have been identified (for recent reviews, see references 59, 79, 107–109, and 186). Early classification of plasmids divided them into different incompatibility (Inc) groups (53), where plasmids of the same Inc group were unable to exist together in a cell. Total sequencing of plasmids has revealed a large degree of instability and crossover between different plasmids. Several plasmids show a mosaic structure of DNA sequences from different plasmids, transposons, and phage DNA (36, 166). Insertion sequences play an important role in the evolution of plasmids as mediators of crossover recombination. The backbone of the plasmid is its replicon (i.e., those genes required for plasmid maintenance), and today plasmids are increasingly classified according to the sequence of their replicons (72). Nonetheless, plasmids are still often divided into conjugative, nonconjugative, mobilizable, and cryptic plasmids. Some plasmid replicons can only be maintained in a single or a few closely related bacterial hosts, while others have a broad host range. Thus, conjugative and mobilizable plasmids are again divided into broad-spectrum and narrow-spectrum plasmids. A few examples are given below, but for more thorough reviews see references 59, 72, 79, 107–109, and 186.

The best-described plasmid conjugation system is probably the F plasmid of *E. coli*. This plasmid encodes genes for the F pilus, which establishes physical contact between donor and recipient, forming a conjugation junction where plasmid DNA is transferred (165, 180). Conjugation is initiated when the F pilus interacts with a suitable recipient, which results in retraction and aggregation formation (114).

Among gram-positive bacteria, enterococci contain sex pheromone-responsive conjugative plasmids (79). These plasmids encode responses to small peptides (pheromones) that are produced by the recipients. These pheromones activate the donors to produce aggregation substances, which lead to clumping between donors and recipients and highly efficient plasmid transfer, with rates as high as 10^{-1} transconjugants per donor (48, 66). A typical example is pCF10 from *Enterococcus faecalis* (44). Similar systems have been detected in the *Bacillus cereus* group (12). The importance of pheromone-responding plasmids in the dissemination of antimicrobial resistance is still unclear. However, the *vanA* gene cluster, encoding glycopeptide resistance, has been found on pheromone-responsive plasmids (90). It has been speculated that pheromone-responsive plasmids were responsible for the spread of glycopeptide resistance from enterococci to *Staphylococcus aureus* (42, 70).

Conjugative plasmids have been described in a large number of gram-positive and gram-negative bacterial species. The precise mechanism of transfer in gram-positive species has not been determined, but broad-host-range plasmids are important in the dissemination of antimicrobial resistance, even though they transfer at a much lower frequency than sex pheromone plasmids. This type of plasmid has been best characterized in staphylococci (139, 182). The prototype of these plasmids is pGO1, which mediates resistance to gentamicin, quaternary ammonium compounds, streptomycin, and trimethoprim (137). In gram-negative bacteria, plasmids belonging to the IncP incompatibility group seem to be prevalent. The prototype IncP-1 β resistance plasmid R751 carries resistance to trimethoprim and quaternary ammonium compounds mediated by *dhfrIIc* and *qacE*, respectively (102, 198). Conjugative plasmids have evolved to contain an astonishing number of resistance determinants. In *Salmonella*, for example, up to nine resistance phenotypes have been transmitted in a single in vitro conjugation with susceptible recipients (70). This development highlights an important and confounding phenomenon, namely, that multiple antimicrobial resistance plasmids may be maintained and disseminated by selection pressure from a single antimicrobial agent. The consequence of this is that attempts to mitigate resistance by antimicrobial use restrictions may not have the desired outcome unless all agents are restricted. This was found to be the case in Denmark, where macrolide use continued to select for glycopeptide resistance since the resistance genes were present on the same plasmid (2). Once both drugs were no longer used, both glycopeptide and macrolide resistance abated (4; see also chapter 6).

In gram-positive organisms, nonconjugative plasmids have mainly been described in *S. aureus*. These are small plasmids that can be mobilized by larger conjugative plasmids. They normally contain only one or a few resistance genes. A typical example is pC221, which mediates resistance to chloramphenicol. Small mobilizable plasmids can be found in a wide range of gram-negative species and are important in the dissemination of antimicrobial resistance.

Recently, a classification based on replicons has been proposed (72). In gram-negative bacteria, a typical example is the plasmid RSF1010, which has been given considerable attention because of its wide host range (167).

Transposons

Conjugative transposons are mobile DNA sequences that can transfer from one bacterium to another without a plasmid intermediate (79). They are present in a wide range of gram-positive and gram-negative bacterial species. The first identified conjugative transposon was Tn*916* from *E. faecalis* (74), which together with the closely related Tn*1545* forms the basis for a family of conjugative transposons with a wide host range (47, 158). The different transposons are often cointegrates of transposons and DNA sequences from different bacteria and plasmids. One example is Tn*5385*, which is approximately 65 kb and consists of both enterococcal and staphylococcal DNA and four different transposons (159). This conjugative transposon carries resistance to gentamicin [*aac(6′)-aph(2″)*], penicillins (β-lactamase production), macrolides [*erm*(B)], mercury, streptomycin (*aadE*), and tetracycline [(*tet*(M)].

One of the most widely distributed transposons in gram-negative bacteria is the nonconjugative Tn*21* subgroup belonging to the Tn*3* family (78, 118). Tn*21* carry a class I integron with an *aadA1* gene cassette and mercury resistance. Mobilizable transposons are also commonly found in *Bacteroides* spp. (163).

Bacteriophages

Bacteriophage-mediated transduction has been speculated to play an important role, especially in the transfer of β-lactamases in staphylococci (125), mainly through a mistaken incorporation of resistance plasmids into the bacteriophage head. The importance of this in the spread of antimicrobial resistance has not been verified. Bacteriophages do, however, play an important role in the spread of virulence factors such as TSST in *S. aureus* (140).

Transformation

Transformation is believed to have played a vital role in the overall evolution of bacterial genomes. The importance of transformation in the dissemination of resistance is difficult to estimate. However, it is believed that resistance to penicillin has emerged in *Streptococcus pneumoniae* as a result of transformation (65). Natural transformation was first observed in *S. pneumoniae* (77) but has since been identified in more than 40 different bacterial species (123). Natural transformation is considered to be an important factor in the evolution of *Campylobacter* and probably also contributes to the evolution of antimicrobial resistance in this bacterial group (59a, 160, 190, 206).

Conjugative Self-Transmissible Elements (Genomic Islands and Integrated and Conjugative Elements)

Conjugative self-transmissible elements have been detected in several gram-negative bacterial species. Such elements are also often referred to as genomic islands. The first element was R391 (51), which mediates resistance to kanamycin and mercury. This element consists of a mosaic of phage, plasmid, and transposon elements (32). Recently, another chromosomally located self-transferable element called SXT, mediating resistance to chloramphenicol, streptomycin, sulfonamides, and tetracycline, has been found in *Vibrio cholerae* in Asia (205). This element has spread rapidly and is today common in clinical isolates (93). This element is almost 100 kb in size and is also a mosaic of phage, plasmids, and transposons (27). Genomic islands, of which a large number contain genes involved in metabolic pathways, have today been detected in many different bacterial species, mainly though total genome analyses (38, 61). The *mecA* gene, encoding resistance to β-lactam antibiotics in *S. aureus*, is located on a genetic element called staphylococcal cassette chromosome (SCC), which is transferable between different staphylococci (95–97, 106). Different SCCmecs have been identified, and their dissemination has been responsible for the emergence of methicillin resistance in new clones and thereby contributed to the spread of methicillin-resistant *S. aureus* and methicillin-resistant, coagulase-negative staphylococci (88, 97, 189).

An example from animals is *Salmonella* genomic island 1 (SGI1) from *Salmonella enterica* serovar Typhimurium DT104. Most *S.* Typhimurium DT104 isolates are resistant to ampicillin, chloramphenicol, florfenicol, quaternary ammonium compounds, spectinomycin, streptomycin, sulfonamides, and tetracyclines, with the genes encoding resistance located on a 14-kb fragment in the chromosome (49). The *floR* and *tet*(G) genes are located between two class I integrons containing *pse-1* and *aadA1*, respectively. It has been shown that this resistance gene cluster is part of a large, 43-kb element designated SGI1 (35). SGI1 has not been found to be transferable in vitro, but has been detected in a number of other *Salmonella* serovars, including Agona, Albany, Meleagridis, Newport, and Paratyphi B (35, 63, 64, 67, 136), which indicates that this segment may transfer horizontally. So far, eight different variants of SGI1 have been found, some of them with additional resistance genes, showing the ongoing and continuous evolution of this element.

Integrons

Integrons are not known to be self-transmissible, but they are often located on conjugative elements such as plasmids and transposons. Integrons are natural genetic engineering systems that capture and incorporate open reading frames and convert them into functional genes (52, 71, 85, 130). They thereby facilitate the spread of genes between bacterial clones and species. At present, four different types of integrons have been found.

Class 1 integrons are the most common and widely distributed (40). The widespread occurrence of class 1 integrons might also be due in part to the fact that many researchers have looked intensively for them, and their importance might therefore be overreported. Class 1 integrons consist of an integrase gene at the 5′ conserved sequence followed by a primary recombination site just downstream. The integrase catalyzes recombination between the recombination site and a secondary target (*attC* site or 59-bp element) that is associated with a single open reading frame. The recombination leads to the insertion of the open reading frame downstream of a resident promoter within the integron. The most commonly detected open reading frames are those encoding antimicrobial resistance, and more than 70 different resistance genes covering most classes of antimicrobials have been found as gene cassettes. The integron can incorporate several gene cassettes, and as many as seven different genes have been found within one single integron (201). Located in the 3′ conserved sequence are the *sul1* and *qacE*Δ*1* genes, encoding resistance to sulfonamides and quaternary ammonium compounds, respectively. Class 1 integrons were originally thought to be restricted to gram-negative bacteria. However, class 1 integrons have also been detected in gram-positive bacteria (46, 138), and it seems that these structures have facilitated the emergence in gram-positive bacteria of resistance genes originally thought restricted to gram-negative species.

Class 2 integrons are included in the Tn7 family of transposons (85, 154). Tn7 transposons contain three integrated gene cassettes (*dhfrI-sat-aadA1*), a defective integrase, and genes that promote transposition (154).

A class 3 integron has been found in a number of different gram-negative species in Japan (21, 179). It contains the bla_{IMP} gene, encoding broad-spectrum β-lactam resistance. Resistance to imipenem is still rare, and even though only a few attempts have been made to look for class 3 integrons, the prevalence of this integron type is probably still low.

The likely ancestors of the previously mentioned integrons are the chromosomal superintegrons that were originally described in *V. cholerae* (132) but have also been found in *Pseudomonas* (202). The opposite might, however, also be the case. The *V. cholerae* superintegron is 126 kb and contains 214 open reading frames in 179 gene cassettes (91), of which most of the functions are unknown. The superintegrons differ from antimicrobial resistance integrons in that the latter are associated with mobile DNA elements while the genes in superintegrons are stationary. In addition, the recombination sites (attC) of superintegrons are highly homogeneous compared to those of antimicrobial resistance integrons. It has also been shown that the range of attC sites recombined by superintegrons is narrower than the range of attC sites recombined by class 1 integrons (30).

MODES OF DISSEMINATION

Multiple-resistant bacterial clones have in several cases spread worldwide. In animal populations, examples have primarily included the international dissemination of different *Salmonella* clones. One of the most striking examples has been the worldwide spread of multiple-resistant serovar Typhimurium DT104. Multiresistant DT104 was first reported in large numbers in cattle in the United Kingdom in 1989 (199). During the late 1990s DT104 was reported in an increasing number of countries worldwide, and today it can probably be found in almost all countries (25, 58, 199). This multiple-resistant *Salmonella* type has contributed to the prevalence of resistance reported in many countries (57). The mode of transmission is not definitively known but is probably related to trade of breeding animals, traveling, and international sale of food products. Most information regarding international spread has been based on the detection of international outbreaks of resistant *Salmonella* due to international trade of food products, of which several have been reported (54, 89, 110, 192, 200). Besides *Salmonella*, a large number of other resistant bacteria have also emerged worldwide in the food animal population, from where they constitute a reservoir of resistance genes that may transfer to and cause problems for humans. A recent example is the worldwide emergence of bla_{CMY-2}, which was first identified in a *Klebsiella pneumoniae* isolate causing infection in a patient in Greece in 1990 (26), emerged in *Salmonella* in Algiers in 1994 (113), and has since spread to America, Asia, and Europe, where it is found on similar plasmids in both *E. coli* and *Salmonella* from different animal and human reservoirs (8, 69, 156, 211, 212, 222). Other extended-spectrum β-lactamases, such as CTX-M enzymes, have also emerged and spread worldwide within the last few decades (34, 37).

From gram-positive bacteria, *vanA*-mediated glycopeptide resistance in enterococci seems to have emerged in the food animal population in all countries where avoparcin is or has been used for growth promotion (1).

Antimicrobial-resistant bacteria and resistance genes may disseminate via many different routes (Fig. 2). Traditionally, the focus has been on the local or national spread of new problems. Different countries have implemented national policies to regulate and control the emergence and spread of various pathogenic bacterial species. However, in the future more emphasis should be put on the international routes of dissemination. Some of the routes are only speculative and have not yet been shown to play a major role, whereas the importance of other routes is well established. Some examples hereof are outlined below.

Animals to Humans

The importance of meat and eggs in the direct transmission of pathogenic zoonotic bacteria, including antimicrobial-resistant organisms, from animals to humans is well documented in numerous studies (see chapters 16 to 19). This direct transmission is quantitatively the most important mode of transmission of antimicrobial-resistant bacteria and resistance genes from the farm to the consumer. The importance of meat and eggs in the transmission of resistance genes is less well documented. However, it must be assumed that if organisms such as *Campylobacter*, *Salmonella*, and *E. coli* can survive and transfer from farm animals to the human gut, then this will also be the case for other bacterial species and the resistance genes they contain. Antimicrobial resistance genes are not only present in the pathogenic bacteria, but they are also prevalent in the normal commensal flora that makes up the major part of the gastrointestinal flora. These bacteria may function as a reservoir of resistance genes that can transfer to pathogenic bacteria (164).

Antimicrobial-resistant bacteria may also transfer from animals to humans though direct contact. This is the case for companion animals, where it has been shown, for example, that humans may become colonized with *Staphylococcus intermedius* from dogs (81). Bacteria may be transferred from food animals to farmers or other humans in contact with the animals. Thus, transmission of vancomycin- and streptogramin-resistant enterococci between farmers

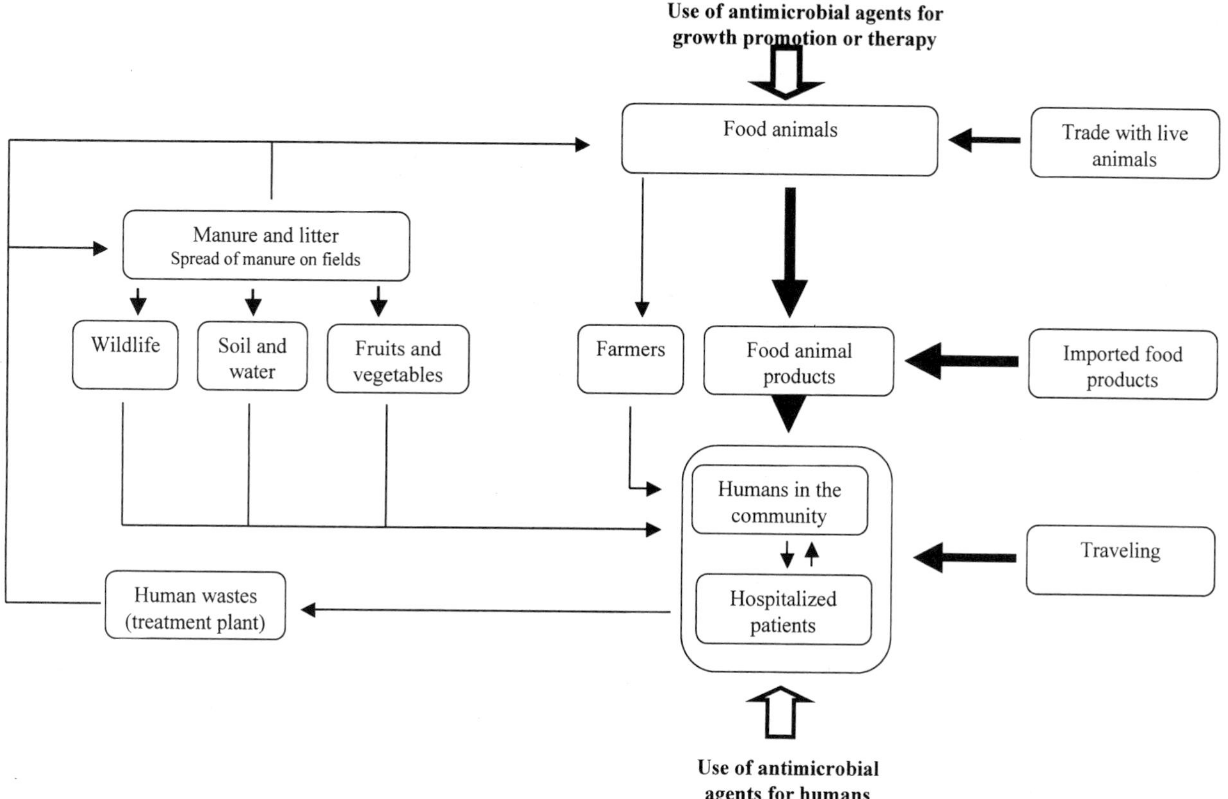

Figure 2. Potential routes of dissemination of antimicrobial-resistant bacteria and resistance genes.

and turkeys has been found (98, 202a). This route of transmission also contributes to the spread, as has been shown in many studies with *Salmonella* (92, 126, 184).

Animal-to-human transmission can easily occur through multiple routes, of which the direct transmission via consumption of meat and eggs is probably the most important. Transmission from humans to food animals is more difficult. Modern food animal production takes place mainly in closed facilities with limited contact with humans or human waste products. Nonetheless, transfer of human-associated antimicrobial-resistant bacteria to farm animals has been shown. For example, methicillin-resistant *S. aureus* bacteria have probably been transmitted from humans, most likely as a result of hospital contacts, to food animals and pets (see chapter 12).

Between Farms

The spread of resistant bacteria between farms has been examined in a number of studies. Wray et al. (217) determined the importance of dealers in the spread of multiple-resistant *Salmonella* serovar Typhimurium DT204 among calves in England. Retrospective tracing of the spread of *Salmonella* during three unrelated epidemics clearly demonstrated the important role of dealers, such as those involved in the sale of calves. Even minimal contamination at dealers' premises may be important because of the high throughput of calves destined for many rearing units. Similarly, the potential importance of markets and vehicles was also demonstrated (218). In 1994 a tetracycline-resistant clone of *Salmonella* serovar Typhimurium spread within 3 months among nine dairy herds in Denmark (3). The exact mode of transmission is not known, but all the herds had the same veterinarian and it seems likely that the visiting veterinarian carried the bacterium between the farms.

In Denmark the spread of multiple-resistant *Salmonella* serovar Typhimurium DT104 has been followed closely. The first isolate of multiple-resistant serovar Typhimurium DT104 was detected in a Danish slaughter pig herd in 1996 (24). Retrospective analyses showed that a Danish sow herd had been infected in 1991, but the infection did not spread to other farms at that time. After 1996 the number of infected herds increased, and by 2002 a total of 90 pig herds, 23 cattle herds, 46 herds with both cattle and pigs, two turkey flocks, two broiler flocks, and one fox farm had been found to be DT104 positive (14). An attempt was made to eradicate DT104 by stamping out infected herds, but this was terminated in 2000. The spread within Denmark has been closely monitored, and in most cases trade relations can explain the route of infection. However, spread has also been indicated to occur as a consequence of common ownership and common use of farming machinery. The two broiler flocks were located near infected pig herds, and horizontal transmission seems most likely. Thus, both trade of animals and direct contact between farms brought about by human vectors are of confirmed importance in the dissemination of antimicrobial resistance.

The Role of the Environment

Antimicrobial agents are also used in the control of bacterial infections in plants. The most commonly used antimicrobial agents are streptomycin and tetracycline (134, 204), but large amounts of copper compounds are also used (see chapter 7). Resistance to streptomycin has become widespread in bacteria isolated from plants, mainly encoded by *strA-strB*, located on the transposon Tn*5395*, which is widely distributed among bacteria from plants, animals, and humans (191).

Food animals and pets produce large amounts of waste products, which may contain many pathogenic bacteria, antimicrobial-resistant bacteria, and resistance genes. Animal waste may contaminate water or vegetables and thereby cause infections with pathogenic bacteria in humans. This has mainly been observed with *E. coli* O157, but manure-associated outbreaks with other pathogens have also been detected. This direct dissemination from animals to humans through manure-contaminated products may also apply for antimicrobial-resistant pathogenic bacteria or antimicrobial resistance genes carried in commensal bacteria. Because of the large amounts of animal waste produced, and the high nutritional value of some of these waste products, they are commonly used in livestock feed (84). In contrast to human waste, animal waste products are often not treated, or insufficiently treated, and may contain many bacteria. This might provide an efficient way of spreading pathogenic and antimicrobial-resistant bacteria and resistance genes between different farms and different production systems.

Large numbers of antimicrobial-resistant bacteria are spread with manure and other forms of animal waste on fields with crop production, or directly on crops. Thus, it has been shown that the spread of manure leads to a temporary increase in the occurrence of antimicrobial resistance in manure-treated soil (100, 174). Bacteria from animals normally survive for only a short time in the environment. It has been suggested, however, that antimicrobial-resistant bacteria from animals may transfer their resistance genes to environmental soil bacteria. It has been shown that antimicrobial resistance genes can be present in waste products from animal production (43, 83) and may survive for a long time in the soil (7, 11). For example, isolation of exogenous IncQ-like plasmids from piggery manure has been shown (183). The ability of soil bacteria to conjugatively transfer resistance genes has also been shown, especially in the rhizosphere (170, 173, 202b). The influence of biological waste in different environments on the cycling of resistant bacteria is a theoretical possibility, which so far has not been proven. Nonetheless, the presence of similar mobile elements and resistance genes in pathogenic and environmental bacteria does show that some exchange between these reservoirs has occurred and probably still takes place (6, 101).

For this type of environmental dissemination of resistance to create a human or animal health problem, it is necessary that the resistance genes transfer to bacteria pathogenic for animals or humans. The environmental bacteria could be transferred on foods and feeds to humans or animals, then subsequently exchange genes with commensals or pathogens in the gut. This is certainly a likely event that probably contributes to the global dissemination of resistance, and this route of transmission of resistant bacteria and resistance genes should not be ignored. However, in comparison to other ways of transmission, this method of environmental spread is probably of minor importance. In the future, changes in production systems might increase the importance of environmental spread. This may especially be the case if production becomes more integrated or more intensive in smaller geographic areas.

In the developing world, the coproduction of different animal species in the same environment is more common, and humans and animals live closer together. The risk of direct transmission has recently been exemplified by the spread of avian influenza virus H5N1 from poultry to humans (117). In Southeast Asia, aquaculture production is often integrated with the production of chickens or pigs. Chickens or pigs are contained in cages above or adjacent to fish ponds and the manure is excreted directly into the ponds, where the waste is either directly eaten by the fish or where it stimulates the growth of planktonic organisms and plants eaten by the fish (120). This provides an efficient route of transmission of antimicrobial-resistant bacteria from the chickens or pigs, which are raised using high doses of antimicrobials, to the fish. In fact, examinations of traditional fish farms and fish farms incorporated with chicken production have shown that there is a much higher frequency of antimicrobial-resistant enterococci and *Acinetobacter* in integrated farming (148).

Human waste contains large amounts of antimicrobial-resistant bacteria and resistance genes. Such waste is normally treated to avoid transmission of pathogenic bacteria. However, examination of effluents from hospitals and sewage has revealed high frequencies of antimicrobial-resistant bacteria (76, 80, 155, 157). This also contributes to the overall dissemination of resistance.

Global Spread

Several examples have shown that the import and export of food is a major route of spread of antimicrobial-resistant pathogenic bacteria from food animals to humans. Increases in income, especially in developed countries, have enhanced food-purchasing power. Better trade and transportation have improved the selection and availability of food. By reducing delivery times and reducing shipping costs, advances in transportation technology have greatly facilitated trade of perishable products, including products of animal origin. Furthermore, consumers today are more likely to eat exotic products.

The global trade of food has increased greatly. The changes in U.S. exports and imports of beef and veal, pork, and broiler meat are shown in Fig. 3. Pork exports have gone from less than 200,000 tons in the beginning of the 1990s to more than 800,000 tons in 2004, and exports of broiler meat have gone from less than 700,000 tons to more than 2 million tons. The U.S. beef and veal trade in 2003 was approximately 2,500 million lb in exports and 3,000 million lb in imports. The data on beef and veal trade also reflect the vulnerability of international trade. As an example of this, the discovery of bovine spongiform encephalopathy (mad cow disease) in a dairy cow in Washington State in December 2003 caused importing countries to either ban or restrict beef and cattle imports from the United States. Consequently, exports dropped by more than 80%.

Imported and exported meat and eggs may be contaminated with bacteria, including antimicrobial-resistant bacteria, such as multiple-resistant *Salmonella*, vancomycin-resistant enterococci, and macrolide- and quinolone-resistant *Campylobacter*. This has been shown in several studies (94, 181, 203, 209, 210, 223). In Denmark a much higher frequency of antimicrobial resistance and multiple resistance has been observed in salmonellae isolated from imported food products compared to Danish-produced products (181). Furthermore, in 2003 it was estimated that while 75% of all human cases of *Salmonella* serovar Typhimurium could be attributed to Danish-produced products and only 25% to imported food, 60% of all infections with multiple-resistant isolates were related

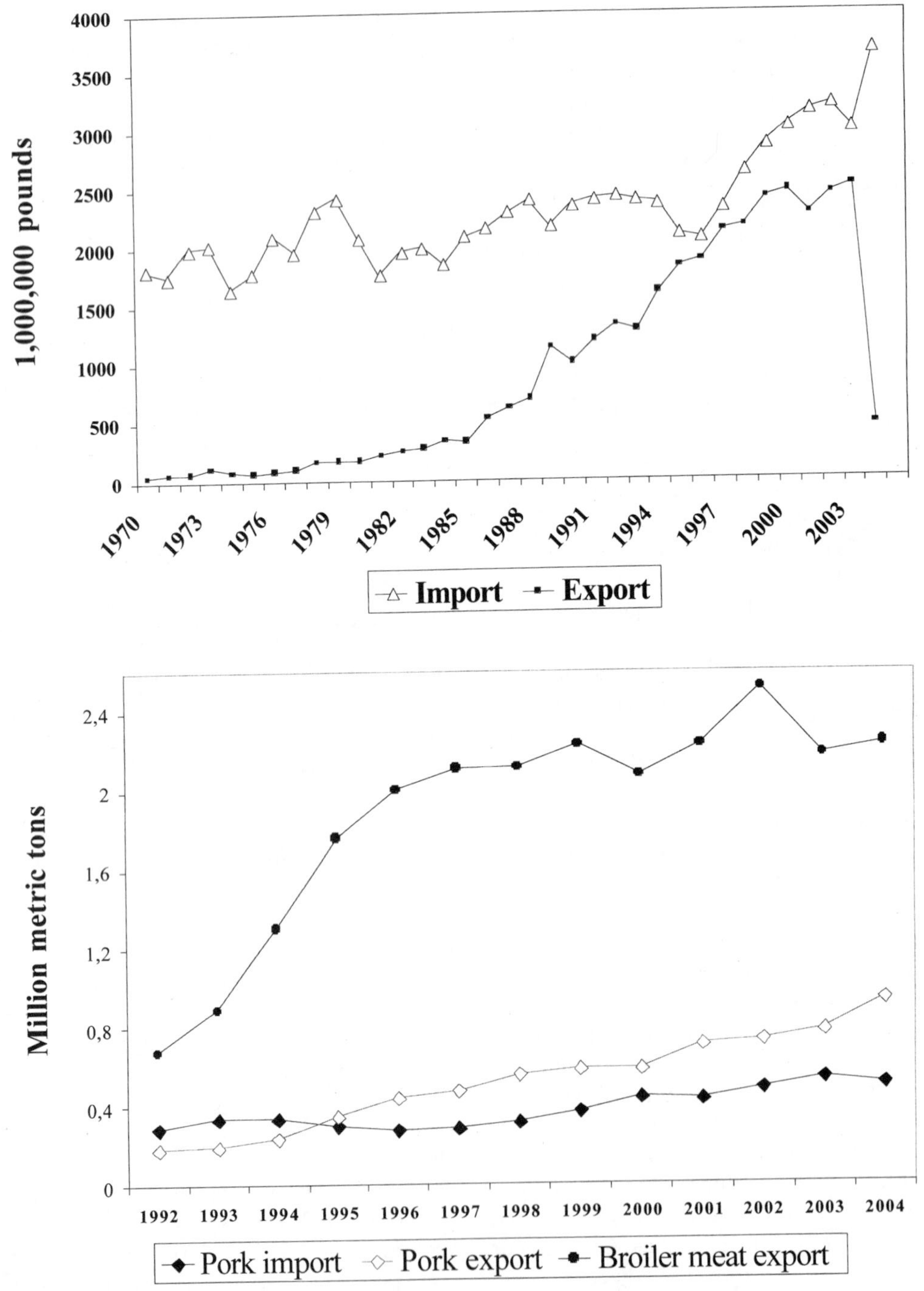

Figure 3. U.S. beef and veal (top) and broiler meat and pork (bottom) trade. Data from reference 20.

to imported food products (17). Thus, more infections with multiple-resistant serovar Typhimurium occur in humans in Denmark as a consequence of imported products than Danish products.

The global trade of food products is expected to increase in the future. Thus, any attempt to improve food safety has to take into account the importance of antimicrobial-resistant bacteria in imported food products. International agreements limiting the contamination with antimicrobial-resistant bacteria at the primary production site are necessary to ensure the safety of the consumer (15). Such international agreements have to be based on data on the occurrence of antimicrobial resistance of importance to human health and especially on early reports on emerging problems. Recently, the World Health Organization

(WHO) launched the Global Salm Surv program (213) in an attempt to determine the importance and occurrence of different *Salmonella* serovars and of antimicrobial resistance globally. This may be an important step in controlling *Salmonella* and antimicrobial resistance in the modern globalized world. However, other bacterial species and perhaps even specific resistance genes should also be targets for surveillance and action.

Most of the focus with regard to the spread of antimicrobial resistance has so far been on the importance of internationally traded food. However, the importance of live animals that are sold worldwide for breeding purposes should not be neglected. Trade of live animals may provide a very important and efficient avenue for worldwide dissemination of resistant bacteria. While meat is contaminated with only very small numbers of bacteria, live animals carry kilograms of bacteria in their fecal content. In addition, animals used for breeding purposes are often introduced at the top of the breeding pyramid in the country in which they arrive, from where new bacteria or genes may spread to a large number of other farms and animals. Thus, international spread of multiple-resistant *Salmonella* serovar Heidelberg from a boar imported to Denmark from Canada has been observed (5). These issues need further study.

Fodder may also provide an efficient way for resistant bacteria to be transported between and within countries. Antimicrobial-resistant bacteria have been found in fodder. *vanB*-positive *Enterococcus faecium* resistant to vancomycin, gentamicin, streptomycin, and ampicillin has been found in chicken feed in the United States (169). Vancomycin-resistant enterococci, however, have not spread in the United States, and this was most likely an isolated event. *Salmonella* is often detected in fodder, especially when it is produced in developing countries or contains animal proteins (73, 127, 168). However, the heat treatment that normally takes place when fodder is produced will to some extent eliminate the problem. Thus, this is probably not among the most important modes of global transportation of resistance determinants. Nonetheless, it should be monitored closely and a low degree of bacterial contamination ensured.

Wild and migrating animals may also play a role in the spread of antimicrobial-resistant bacteria. However, the prevalence of antimicrobial-resistant bacteria in wild animals is largely unknown. Antimicrobial-resistant *E. coli*, enterococci, and *Campylobacter* have been found in wild animals (45, 122, 187). Antimicrobial-resistant *Salmonella*, enterococci, and *Campylobacter* have also been found in migrating birds entering Sweden (143, 172). Outbreaks of salmonellosis associated with wild birds in both humans and animals have been described several times (105, 193, 197). The importance of the wildlife reservoir is unknown, and in most instances findings of antimicrobial-resistant bacteria in wildlife probably reflects transmission from farm animals to the wildlife. However, migrating birds might transfer pathogenic bacteria, including resistant ones, over longer distances and thereby contribute to the global dissemination.

RULES AND REGULATIONS

A large number of national and international rules and regulations, as well as marketing and consumer factors, regulate and change the international trade of food products and live animals. Historically, the main barrier to international trade has been tariffs such as customs duty or taxes. In 1947 the General Agreement for Tariffs and Trade (GATT) was established with the aim to liberalize international trade. This has been done with some success. However, besides taxes, a number of other factors, such as animal health and food safety standards, control international trade. Thus, during the Uruguay round of the General Agreement on Tariffs and Trade (GATT) (1986 to 1994), the World Trade Organization (WTO) was established with the additional aim of minimizing nontariff barriers to free international trade (216). This is regulated by the agreement on sanitary and phytosanitary measures (215). As the WTO has no scientific authority, the Office International des Epizooties (OIE) (214) is the agency responsible for setting appropriate global standards for animal heath, while the Codex Alimentarius Commission sets standards for food safety (50).

International trade is still seriously hindered by epizootic animal diseases, which may have major economic consequences for a number of countries (196). Furthermore, a major task lies ahead for individual countries seeking to adapt to the requirements laid out in these international standards (194). Compliance with international standards and continuous update on the current global situation through international monitoring and early warning systems will no doubt be necessary in the future. This will, however, require flexible international agreement so it is possible to rapidly adapt to new situations and threats.

In addition to the legal regulations of the WTO, several communities (e.g., the European Union) and countries require higher standards, especially with regard to food safety. Examples are Sweden, which has *Salmonella*-free status and does not accept the importation of meat products with *Salmonella*. Denmark has a special control program in place for multiple-resistant *Salmonella* serovar Typhimurium DT104 (13).

Besides legal restrictions, large international corporations may also affect international trade. A group of approximately 30 companies control about one-third of global trade and have sufficient power to set their own standards. For example, McDonald's Corporation has issued a global policy for antibiotic use in food animals, putting forward certain requirements for suppliers of food products to McDonald's (18).

Nationally, local groceries and supermarkets may also impose their own standards. In Denmark in 2003, for instance, one large supermarket chain returned quails contaminated with *Salmonella* serovar Virchow resistant to both quinolones and cephalosporins as a food safety precaution (19).

There are currently no international standards for how to handle food safety problems in relation to antimicrobial resistance. However, in 2003 the Food and Agriculture Organization (FAO) of the United Nations, WHO, and OIE hosted a joint expert workshop on nonhuman antimicrobial usage and antimicrobial resistance. It was recommended that the Codex Alimentarius Commission should take steps in managing the risks associated with antimicrobial resistance (15).

While several standards for the safety level of traded food products do exist, regulations dealing with the trade of live animals are inadequate. Requirements that address epizootic diseases do exist, but there are none that regulate zoonotic bacteria or antimicrobial resistance (16). Today, as a result, breeding animals with multiple-resistant *Salmonella* can be traded freely between countries and constitute an efficient route of global dissemination of multiple-resistant bacteria.

CONCLUDING REMARKS

We have hardly even begun to understand the evolution, adaptation, and multiple mechanisms of dissemination of antimicrobial resistance. The future will undoubtedly reveal both surprises and interesting new knowledge that increases our understanding of this important phenomenon. Globalization will make it possible for larger numbers of bacteria and genes to meet and interact in a larger number of different reservoirs and under new selective environments caused by the many chemical substances we release. This will no doubt lead to new surprises waiting for us.

Given the enormous number of bacteria in the world, the great biodiversity and multiple mechanisms for gene exchange and modification, in addition to the many possibilities for bacteria and genes to spread, it is inevitable that resistance will emerge and spread. We are not yet able to predict from where, how, or when new resistance mechanisms might emerge or to what extent mobile DNA elements with multiple resistances will spread. This is certainly an area for further research in the future, combining microbiological knowledge with epidemiology, mathematical modeling, structural molecular biology, and phylogeny.

With our current knowledge, the only thing we can do is to limit the selection of resistance and minimize the possibilities for it to spread along the most important routes. Thus, we should limit the selection of resistance in the various environments by limiting the use of antimicrobial agents to a minimum. Antimicrobial agents of greatest medical importance, such as drugs of last resort, should be limited or even banned from nonhuman uses. Since all substances with antimicrobial activity can select for resistance and multiresistance as a consequence of genetic linkage of resistance genes, coselection of antibiotic resistance by other chemical substances, such as disinfectants and metals, is an area that warrants more research (see chapters 7 and 8). In addition, stopping all trade of live animals for breeding purposes might minimize the global spread of resistant clones. This includes both within and between countries. With modern technology it is easy to transport semen or embryos and thereby avoid the transportation of large amounts of bacteria that takes place with the transport of live animals. Litter should be heat-treated appropriately, limiting the spread of bacteria. This is especially the case if litter is used as feed for other animals. To improve the safety of the consumer, an international monitoring program of antimicrobial resistance in both important zoonotic bacteria (*Salmonella* and *Campylobacter*), as well as targeted monitoring of selected resistance genes (e.g., extended-spectrum β-lactamases and metallo-carbapenemases), should be implemented. This should be combined with standards for which actions should be taken on the basis of findings of especially undesirable resistances. The establishment of such standards is not the task for one country. It has to be done through international agreement and is thus an area for the Codex Alimentarius Commission, OIE, and WTO.

In addition to the measures mentioned above, more knowledge should also be generated, strengthening our scientific basis for action. This should include more research into the basic mechanism for evolution and dissemination of resistance as well as improved tools for the risk assessment of the spread of resistant organisms through the multiple routes of dissemination. These measures might enable us to control the global spread of antimicrobial resistance under the future influence of globalization.

REFERENCES

1. **Aarestrup, F. M.** 2000. Occurrence, selection and spread of resistance to antimicrobial agents used for growth promotion for food animals in Denmark. *APMIS* **101:**1–48.
2. **Aarestrup, F. M.** 2000. Characterization of glycopeptide resistant *Enterococcus faecium* (GRE) from broilers and pigs in Denmark. Genetic evidences that persistence of GRE in pig herds is associated with co-selection by resistance to macrolides. *J. Clin. Microbiol.* **38:**2774–2777.
3. **Aarestrup, F. M., N. E. Jensen, and D. L. Baggesen.** 1998. Clonal spread of tetracycline-resistant *Salmonella typhimurium* in Danish dairy herds. *Vet. Rec.* **140:**313–314.
4. **Aarestrup, F. M., A. M. Seyfarth, H. D. Emborg, K. Pedersen, R. S. Hendriksen, and F. Bager.** 2001. Effect of abolishment of the use of antimicrobial agents for growth promotion on occurrence of antimicrobial resistance in fecal enterococci from food animals in Denmark. *Antimicrob. Agents Chemother.* **45:**2054–2059.
5. **Aarestrup, F. M., H. Hasman, I. Olsen, and G. Sørensen.** 2004. International spread of bla_{CMY-2}-mediated cephalosporin resistance in a multiresistant *Salmonella enterica* serovar Heidelberg isolate stemming from the importation of a boar by Denmark from Canada. *Antimicrob. Agents Chemother.* **48:**1916–1917.
6. **Agersø, Y., L. B. Jensen, M. Givskov, and M. C. Roberts.** 2002. The identification of a tetracycline resistance gene *tet*(M), on a Tn*916*-like transposon, in the *Bacillus cereus* group. *FEMS Microbiol. Lett.* **214:**251–256.
7. **Agersø, Y., G. Sengeløv, and L. B. Jensen.** 2004. Development of a rapid method for direct detection of *tet*(M) genes in soil from Danish farmland. *Environ. Int.* **30:**117–122.
8. **Allen, K. J., and C. Poppe.** 2002. Occurrence and characterization of resistance to extended-spectrum cephalosporins mediated by beta-lactamase CMY-2 in *Salmonella* isolated from food-producing animals in Canada. *Can. J. Vet. Res.* **66:** 137–144.
9. **Aminov, R. I., N. Garrigues-Jeanjean, and R. I. Mackie.** 2001. Molecular ecology of tetracycline resistance: development and validation of primers for detection of tetracycline resistance genes encoding ribosomal protection proteins. *Appl. Environ. Microbiol.* **67:**22–32.
10. **Anantharaman, V., and L. Aravind.** 2003. Evolutionary history, structural features and biochemical diversity of the NlpC/P60 superfamily of enzymes. *Genome Biol.* **4:**R11.
11. **Andrews, R. E., Jr., W. S. Johnson, A. R. Guard, and J. D. Marvin.** 2004. Survival of enterococci and Tn*916*-like conjugative transposons in soil. *Can. J. Microbiol.* **50:**957–966.
12. **Andrup, L., J. Damgaard, and K. Wassermann.** 1993. Mobilization of small plasmids in *Bacillus thuringiensis* subsp. *israelensis* is accompanied by specific aggregation. *J. Bacteriol.* **175:**6530–6536.
13. **Anonymous.** 1998. Vejledning om fund af Salmonella Typhimurium DT104, multiresistent i fødevarer. http://www.foedevarestyrelsen.dk/FDir/Publications/1998105/Rapport.pdf. (Accessed 1 March 2005.)
14. **Anonymous.** 2002. Assessment of the effect of proposed changes to the management of multi-resistant *Salmonella* Typhimurium DT104 in primary food animal production in Denmark. Danish Zoonosis Centre, Danish Institute for Food and Veterinary Research, Copenhagen, Denmark.
15. **Anonymous.** 2003. 1st Joint FAO/OIE/WHO Expert Workshop on Non-Human Antimicrobial Usage and Antimicrobial Resistance: Scientific Assessment, Geneva, 1–5 December 2003. http://www.who.int/foodsafety/publications/micro/en/amr.pdf. (Accessed 1 March 2005.)
16. **Anonymous.** 2003. General guidelines for third country authorities on the procedures to be followed when importing live animals and animal products into the European Union. http://europa.eu.int/comm/food/fvo/pdf/guide_thirdcountries_en.pdf. (Accessed 2 March 2005.)
17. **Anonymous.** 2004. *Annual Report on Zoonoses in Denmark 2003.* Ministry of Agriculture, Food and Fisheries, Copenhagen, Denmark.
18. **Anonymous.** McDonald's Global Policy on Antibiotic Use in Food Animals. http://www.mcdonalds.com/corp/values/socialrespons/market/antibiotics/global_policy.html. (Accessed 1 March 2005.)
19. **Anonymous.** News release from COOP Danmark A/S. http://www.coop.dk/CCMS/templates/template6_8.asp?iSideID=116&intNyhedId=2130. (Accessed 1 March 2005.)
20. **Anonymous.** 2005. Animal production and marketing issues. http://www.ers.usda.gov/Briefing/AnimalProducts/. (Accessed 7 March 2005.)
21. **Arakawa, Y., M. Murakami, K. Suzuki, H. Ito, R. Wacharotayankun, S. Ohsuka, N. Kato, and M. Ohta.** 1995. A novel integron-like element carrying the metallo-beta-lactamase gene bla_{IMP}. *Antimicrob. Agents Chemother.* **39:**1612–1615.
22. **Arthur, M., A. Brisson-Noel, and P. Courvalin.** 1987. Origin and evolution of genes specifying resistance to macrolide, lincosamide and streptogramin antibiotics: data and hypotheses. *J. Antimicrob. Chemother.* **20:**783–802.
23. **Arthur, M., P. E. Reynolds, F. Depardieu, S. Evers, S. Dutka-Malen, R. Quintiliani, Jr., and P. Courvalin.** 1996. Mechanisms of glycopeptide resistance in enterococci. *J. Infect.* **32:** 11–16.
24. **Baggesen, D. L., and F. M. Aarestrup.** 1998. Characterisation of recently emerged multiple antibiotic resistant *Salmonella enterica* serovar *typhimurium* DT104 and other multiresistant phage types from Danish pig herds. *Vet. Rec.* **143:**95–97.
25. **Baggesen, D. L., D. Sandvang, and F. M. Aarestrup.** 2000. Characterization of *Salmonella enterica* serovar Typhimurium DT104 isolated from Denmark and comparison with isolates from Europe and the United States. *J. Clin. Microbiol.* **38:** 1581–1586.
26. **Bauernfeind, A., I. Stemplinger, R. Jungwirth, and H. Giamarellou.** 1996. Characterization of the plasmidic β-lactamase CMY-2, which is responsible for cephamycin resistance. *Antimicrob. Agents Chemother.* **40:**221–224.
27. **Beaber, J. W., B. Hochhut, and M. K. Waldor.** 2002. Genomic and functional analyses of SXT, an integrating antibiotic resistance gene transfer element derived from *Vibrio cholerae. J. Bacteriol.* **184:**4259–4269.
28. **Bellais, S., L. Poirel, N. Fortineau, J. W. Decousser, and P. Nordmann.** 2001. Biochemical-genetic characterization of the chromosomally encoded extended-spectrum class A β-lactamase from *Rahnella aquatilis. Antimicrob. Agents Chemother.* **45:**2965–2968.
29. **Benveniste, R., and J. Davies.** 1973. Aminoglycoside antibiotic-inactivating enzymes in actinomycetes similar to those present in clinical isolates of antibiotic-resistant bacteria. *Proc. Natl. Acad. Sci. USA* **70:**2276–2280.
30. **Biskri, L., M. Bouvier, A. M. Guerout, S. Boisnard, and D. Mazel.** 2005. Comparative study of class 1 integron and *Vibrio cholerae* superintegron integrase activities. *J. Bacteriol.* **187:**1740–1750.
31. **Blattner, F. R., G. Plunkett III, C. A. Bloch, N. T. Perna, V. Burland, M. Riley, J. Collado-Vides, J. D. Glasner, C. K. Rode, G. F. Mayhew, J. Gregor, N. W. Davis, H. A. Kirkpatrick, M. A. Goeden, D. J. Rose, B. Mau, and Y. Shao.** 1997. The complete genome sequence of *Escherichia coli* K-12. *Science* **277:**1453–1474.

32. **Böltner, D., C. MacMahon, J. T. Pembroke, P. Strike, and A. M. Osborn.** 2002. R391: a conjugative integrating mosaic comprised of phage, plasmid, and transposon elements. *J. Bacteriol.* **184:**5158–5169.
33. Reference deleted.
34. **Bonnet, R.** 2004. Growing group of extended-spectrum β-lactamases: the CTX-M enzymes. *Antimicrob. Agents Chemother.* **48:**1–14.
35. **Boyd, D., G. A. Peters, A. Cloeckaert, K. S. Boumedine, E. Chaslus-Dancla, H. Imberechts, and M. R. Mulvey.** 2001. Complete nucleotide sequence of a 43-kilobase genomic island associated with the multidrug resistance region of *Salmonella enterica* serovar Typhimurium DT104 and its identification in phage type DT120 and serovar Agona. *J. Bacteriol.* **183:** 5725–5732.
36. **Boyd, E. F., C. W. Hill, S. M. Rich, and D. L. Hartl.** 1996. Mosaic structure of plasmids from natural populations of *Escherichia coli. Genetics* **143:**1091–1100.
37. **Bradford, P. A.** 2001. Extended-spectrum β-lactamases in the 21st century: characterization, epidemiology, and detection of this important resistance threat. *Clin. Microbiol. Rev.* **14:** 933–951,
38. **Burrus, V., and M. K. Waldor.** 2004. Shaping bacterial genomes with integrative and conjugative elements. *Res. Microbiol.* **155:**376–386.
39. Reference deleted.
40. **Carattoli, A.** 2001. Importance of integrons in the diffusion of resistance. *Vet. Res.* **32:**243–259.
41. **Carattoli, A. S., Lovari, A. Franco, G. Cordaro, P. Di Matteo, and A. Battisti.** 2005. Extended-spectrum β-lactamases in *Escherichia coli* isolated from dogs and cats in Rome, Italy, from 2001 to 2003. *Antimicrob. Agents Chemother.* **49:** 833–835.
42. **Chang, S., D. M. Sievert, J. C. Hageman, M. L. Boulton, F. C. Tenover, F. P. Downes, S. Shah, J. T. Rudrik, G. R. Pupp, W. J. Brown, D. Cardo, S. K. Fridkin, and the Vancomycin-Resistant *Staphylococcus aureus* Investigative Team.** 2003. Infection with vancomycin-resistant *Staphylococcus aureus* containing the *vanA* resistance gene. *N. Engl. J. Med.* **348:**1342–1347.
43. **Chee-Sanford, J. C., A. I. Aminov, I. J. Krapac, N. Garrigues-Jeanjean, and R. I. Mackie.** 2001. Occurrence and diversity of tetracycline resistance genes in lagoons and groundwater underlying two swine production facilities. *Appl. Environ. Microbiol.* **67:**1494–1502.
44. **Christie, P. J., and G. M. Dunny.** 1986. Identification of regions of the *Streptococcus faecalis* plasmid pCF-10 that encode antibiotic resistance and pheromone response functions. *Plasmid* **15:**230–241.
45. **Chuma, T., S. Hashimoto, and K. Okamoto.** 2000. Detection of thermophilic *Campylobacter* from sparrows by multiplex PCR: the role of sparrows as a source of contamination of broilers with *Campylobacter. J. Vet. Med. Sci.* **62:**1291–1295.
46. **Clark, N. C., O. Olsvik, J. M. Swenson, C. A. Spiegel, and F. C. Tenover.** 1999. Detection of a streptomycin/spectinomycin adenylyltransferase gene (*aadA*) in *Enterococcus faecalis. Antimicrob. Agents Chemother.* **43:**157–160.
47. **Clewell, D. B., S. E. Flannagan, and D. D. Jaworski.** 1995. Unconstrained bacterial promiscuity: the Tn*916*-Tn*1545* family of conjugative transposons. *Trends Microbiol.* **3:**229–236.
48. **Clewell, D. B., M. V. Francia, S. E. Flannagan, and F. Y. An.** 2002. Enterococcal plasmid transfer: sex pheromones, transfer origins, relaxases, and the *Staphylococcus aureus* issue. *Plasmid* **48:**193–201.
49. **Cloeckaert, A., and S. Schwarz.** 2001. Molecular characterization, spread and evolution of multidrug resistance in *Salmonella enterica* Typhimurium DT104. *Vet. Res.* **32:**301–310.
50. **Codex Alimentarius Commission.** *Codex Alimentarius: FAO/WHO Food Standards.* http://www.codexalimentarius.net/web/index_en.jsp. (Accessed 1 March 2005.)
51. **Coetzee, J. N., N. Datta, and R. W. Hedges.** 1972. R factors from *Proteus rettgeri. J. Gen. Microbiol.* **72:**543–552.
52. **Collis, C. M., and R. M. Hall.** 1992. Gene cassettes from the insert region of integrons are excised as covalently closed circles. *Mol. Microbiol.* **6:**2875–2885.
53. **Couturier, M., F. Bex, P. L. Bergquist, and W. K. Maas.** 1988. Identification and classification of bacterial plasmids. *Microbiol. Rev.* **52:**375–395.
54. **Crook, P. D., J. F. Aguilera, E. J. Threlfall, S. J. O'Brien, G. Sigmundsdottir, D. Wilson, I. S. Fisher, A. Ammon, H. Briem, J. M. Cowden, M. E. Locking, H. Tschape, W. van Pelt, L. R. Ward, and M. A. Widdowson.** 2003. A European outbreak of *Salmonella enterica* serotype Typhimurium definitive phage type 204b in 2000. *Clin. Microbiol. Infect.* **9:**839–845.
55. **Datta, N., and P. Kontomichalou.** 1965. Penicillinase synthesis controlled by infectious R factors in *Enterobacteriaceae. Nature* **208:**239–241.
56. **Davies, J., and G. D. Wright.** 1997. Bacterial resistance to aminoglycoside antibiotics. *Trends Microbiol.* **5:**234–240.
57. **Davis, M. A., D. D. Hancock, T. E. Besser, D. H. Rice, J. M. Gay, C. Gay, L. Gearhart, and R. DiGiacomo.** 1999. Changes in antimicrobial resistance among *Salmonella enterica* serovar *typhimurium* isolates from humans and cattle in the Northwestern United States, 1982–1997. *Emerg. Infect. Dis.* **5:**802–806.
58. **Davis, M. A., D. D. Hancock, and T. E. Besser.** 2002. Multiresistant clones of *Salmonella enterica*: the importance of dissemination. *J. Lab. Clin. Med.* **140:**135–141.
59. **Davison, J.** 1999. Genetic exchange between bacteria in the environment. *Plasmid* **42:**73–91.
59a. **de Boer, P., J. A. Wagenaar, R. P. Achterberg, J. P. M. van Putten, L. M. Schouls, and B. Duim.** 2002. Generation of *Campylobacter jejuni* genetic diversity in vivo. *Mol. Microbiol.* **44:**351–359.
60. **Dionisio, F., I. Matic, M. Radman, O. R. Rodrigues, and F. Taddei.** 2002. Plasmids spread very fast in heterogeneous bacterial communities. *Genetics* **162:**1525–1532.
61. **Dobrindt, U., B. Hochhut, U. Hentschel, and J. Hacker. 2004.** Genomic islands in pathogenic and environmental microorganisms. *Nat. Rev. Microbiol.* **2:**414–424.
62. **Doolittle, R. F., D. F. Feng, K. L. Anderson, and M. R. Alberro.** 1990. A naturally occurring horizontal gene transfer from a eukaryote to a prokaryote. *J. Mol. Evol.* **31:**383–388.
63. **Doublet, B., R. Lailler, D. Meunier, A. Brisabois, D. Boyd, M. R. Mulvey, E. Chaslus-Dancla, and A. Cloeckaert.** 2003. Variant *Salmonella* genomic island 1 antibiotic resistance gene cluster in *Salmonella enterica* serovar Albany. *Emerg. Infect. Dis.* **9:**585–591.
64. **Doublet, B., F.-X. Weill, L. Fabre, E. Chaslus-Dancla, and A. Cloeckaert.** 2004. Variant *Salmonella* genomic island 1 antibiotic resistance gene cluster containing a novel 3′-*N*-aminoglycoside acetyltransferase gene cassette, *aac*(3)-Id, in *Salmonella enterica* serovar Newport. *Antimicrob. Agents Chemother.* **48:**3806–3812.
65. **Dowson, C. G., A. Hutchison, J. A. Brannigan, R. C. George, D. Hansman, J. Linares, A. Tomasz, J. M. Smith, and B. G. Spratt.** 1989. Horizontal transfer of penicillin-binding protein genes in penicillin-resistant clinical isolates of *Streptococcus pneumoniae. Proc. Natl. Acad. Sci. USA* **86:**8842–8846.
66. **Dunny, G. M., B. A. Leonard, and P. J. Hedberg.** 1995. Pheromone-inducible conjugation in *Enterococcus faecalis*: interbacterial and host-parasite chemical communication. *J. Bacteriol.* **177:**871–876.

67. **Ebner, P., K. Garner, and A. Mathew.** 2004. Class 1 integrons in various *Salmonella enterica* serovars isolated from animals and identification of genomic island SGI1 in *Salmonella enterica* var. Meleagridis. *J. Antimicrob. Chemother.* **53:**1004–1009.
68. Reference deleted.
69. **Fey, P. D., T. J. Safranek, M. E. Rupp, E. F. Dunne, E. Ribot, P. C. Iwen, P. A. Bradford, F. J. Angulo, and S. H. Hinrichs.** 2000. Ceftriaxone-resistant salmonella infection acquired by a child from cattle. *N. Engl. J. Med.* **342:**1242–1249.
70. **Flannagan, S. E., J. W. Chow, S. M. Donabedian, W. J. Brow, M. B. Perri, M. J. Zervos, Y. Ozawa, and D. B. Clewell.** 2003. Plasmid content of a vancomycin-resistant *Enterococcus faecalis* isolate from a patient also colonized by *Staphylococcus aureus* with a VanA phenotype. *Antimicrob. Agents Chemother.* **47:** 3954–3959.
71. **Fluit, A. C., and F. J. Schmitz.** 2004. Resistance integrons and super-integrons. *Clin. Microbiol. Infect.* **10:**272–288.
72. **Francia, M. V., A. Varsaki, M. P. Garcillan-Barcia, A. Latorre, C. Drainas, and F. A. de la Cruz.** 2004. Classification scheme for mobilization regions of bacterial plasmids. *FEMS Microbiol. Rev.* **28:**79–100.
73. **Franco, D. A.** 2005. A survey of *Salmonella* serovars and most probable numbers in rendered-animal-protein meals: inferences for animal and human health. *J. Environ. Health* **67:**18–22.
74. **Franke, A. E., and D. B. Clewell.** 1981. Evidence for a chromosome-borne resistance transposon (Tn*916*) in *Streptococcus faecalis* that is capable of "conjugal" transfer in the absence of a conjugative plasmid. *J. Bacteriol.* **145:**494–502.
75. **Gniadkowski, M.** 2001. Evolution and epidemiology of extended-spectrum β-lactamases (ESBLs) and ESBL-producing microorganisms. *Clin. Microbiol. Infect.* **7:**597–608.
76. **Goni-Urriza, M., M. Capdepuy, C. Arpin, N. Raymond, P. Caumette, and C. Quentin.** 2000. Impact of an urban effluent on antibiotic resistance of riverine *Enterobacteriaceae* and *Aeromonas* spp. *Appl. Environ. Microbiol.* **66:**125–132.
77. **Griffith, F.** 1928. The significance of pneumococcal types. *J. Hyg.* **27:**113–159.
78. **Grinsted, J., F. de la Cruz, and R. Schmitt.** 1990. The Tn*21* subgroup of bacterial transposable elements. *Plasmid* **24:** 163–189.
79. **Grohmann, E., G. Muth, and M. Espinosa.** 2003. Conjugative plasmid transfer in gram-positive bacteria. *Microbiol. Mol. Biol. Rev.* **67:**277–301.
80. **Guardabassi, L., A. Petersen, J. E. Olsen, and A. Dalsgaard.** 1998. Antibiotic resistance in *Acinetobacter* spp. isolated from sewers receiving waste effluent from a hospital and a pharmaceutical plant. *Appl. Environ. Microbiol.* **64:**3499–3502.
81. **Guardabassi, L., M. E. Loeber, and A. Jacobson.** 2004. Transmission of multiple antimicrobial-resistant *Staphylococcus intermedius* between dogs affected by deep pyoderma and their owners. *Vet. Microbiol.* **98:**23–27.
82. **Guardabassi, L., H. Christensen, H. Hasman, and A. Dalsgaard.** 2004. Members of the genera *Paenibacillus* and *Rhodococcus* harbor genes homologous to enterococcal glycopeptide resistance genes *vanA* and *vanB*. *Antimicrob. Agents Chemother.* **48:**4915–4918.
83. **Haack, B. J., and R. E. Andrews.** 2000. Isolation of Tn*916*-like conjugal elements from swine lot effluent. *Can. J. Microbiol.* **46:**542–549.
84. **Haapapuro, E. R., N. D. Barnard, and M. Simon.** 1997. Review—animal waste used as livestock feed: dangers to human health. *Prev. Med.* **26:**599–602.
85. **Hall, R. M., and C. S. Collis.** 1995. Mobile gene cassettes and integrons: capture and spread of genes by site-specific recombination. *Mol. Microbiol.* **15:**593–600.
86. **Handelsman, J.** 2004. Metagenomics: application of genomics to uncultured microorganisms. *Microbiol. Mol. Biol. Rev.* **68:**669–685.
87. **Hanson, N. D.** 2003. AmpC β-lactamases: what do we need to know for the future? *J. Antimicrob. Chemother.* **52:**2–4.
88. **Hanssen, A. M., G. Kjeldsen, and J. U. Sollid.** 2004. Local variants of staphylococcal cassette chromosome *mec* in sporadic methicillin-resistant *Staphylococcus aureus* and methicillin-resistant coagulase-negative staphylococci: evidence of horizontal gene transfer? *Antimicrob. Agents Chemother.* **48:**285–296.
89. **Hastings, L., A. Burnens, B. de Jong, L. Ward, I. Fisher, J. Stuart, C. Bartlett, and B. Rowe.** 1996. Salm-Net facilitates collaborative investigation of an outbreak of *Salmonella tosamanga* infection in Europe. *Commun. Dis. Rep. CDR Rev.* **6:**100–102.
90. **Heaton, M. P., and S. Handwerger.** 1995. Conjugative mobilization of a vancomycin resistance plasmid by a putative *Enterococcus faecium* sex pheromone response plasmid. *Microb. Drug Resist.* **1:**177–183.
91. **Heidelberg, J. F., J. A. Eisen, W. C. Nelson, R. A. Clayton, M. L. Gwinn, R. J. Dodson, D. H. Haft, E. K. Hickey, J. D. Peterson, L. Umayam, S. R. Gill, K. E. Nelson, T. D. Read, H. Tettelin, D. Richardson, M. D. Ermolaeva, J. Vamathevan, S. Bass, H. Qin, I. Dragoi, P. Sellers, L. McDonald, T. Utterback, R. D. Fleishmann, W. C. Nierman, O. White, S. L. Salzberg, H. O. Smith, R. R. Colwell, J. J. Mekalanos, J. C. Venter, and C. M. Fraser.** 2000. DNA sequence of both chromosomes of the cholera pathogen *Vibrio cholerae*. *Nature* **406:**477–483.
92. **Hendriksen, S. W., K. Orsel, J. A. Wagenaar, A. Miko, and E. van Duijkeren.** 2004. Animal-to-human transmission of *Salmonella* Typhimurium DT104A variant. *Emerg. Infect. Dis.* **10:**2225–2227.
93. **Hochhut, B., Y. Lotfi, D. Mazel, S. M. Faruque, R. Woodgate, and M. K. Waldor.** 2001. Molecular analysis of the antibiotic resistance gene clusters in the *Vibrio cholerae* O139 and O1 SXT constins. *Antimicrob. Agents Chemother.* **45:**2991–3000.
94. **Ike, Y., K. Tanimoto, Y. Ozawa, T. Nomura, S. Fujimoto, and H. Tomita.** 1999. Vancomycin-resistant enterococci in imported chickens in Japan. *Lancet* **353:**1854.
95. **Ito, T., Y. Katayama, and K. Hiramatsu.** 1999. Cloning and nucleotide sequence determination of the entire *mec* DNA of pre-methicillin-resistant *Staphylococcus aureus* N315. *Antimicrob. Agents Chemother.* **43:**1449–1458.
96. **Ito, T., Y. Katayama, K. Asada, N. Mori, K. Tsutsumimoto, C. Tiensasitorn, and K. Hiramatsu.** 2001. Structural comparison of three types off staphylococcal cassette chromosome *mec* integrated in the chromosome in methicillin-resistant *Staphylococcus aureus*. *Antimicrob. Agents Chemother.* **45:**1323–1336.
97. **Ito, T., K. Okuma, X. X. Ma, H. Yuzawa, and K. Hiramatsu.** 2003. Insights on antibiotic resistance of *Staphylococcus aureus* from its whole genome: genomic island SCC. *Drug Resist. Update* **6:**41–52.
98. **Jensen, L. B., A. M. Hammerum, F. M. Aarestrup, A. E. van den Bogaard, and E. E. Stobberingh.** 1998. Occurrence of *satA* and *vgb* genes in streptogramin-resistant *Enterococcus faecium* isolates of animal and human origins in The Netherlands. *Antimicrob. Agents Chemother.* **42:**3330–3331.
99. **Jensen, L. B., N. Frimodt-Møller, and F. M. Aarestrup.** 1999. Presence of *erm* gene classes in gram-positive bacteria of animal and human origin in Denmark. *FEMS Microbiol. Lett.* **170:**151–158.
100. **Jensen, L. B., S. Baloda, M. Boye, and F. M. Aarestrup.** 2001. Antimicrobial resistance among *Pseudomonas* spp. and the *Bacillus cereus* group isolated from Danish agricultural soil. *Environ. Int.* **26:**581–587.

101. **Jensen, L. B., Y. Agersø, and G. Sengeløv.** 2002. Presence of *erm* genes among macrolide-resistant Gram-positive bacteria isolated from Danish farm soil. *Environ. Int.* **28:**487–491.

102. **Jobanputra, R. S., and N. Datta.** 1974. Trimethoprim R factors in enterobacteria from clinical specimens. *J. Med. Microbiol.* 7:169–177.

103. **Joyce, P., Z. Abdo, J. M. Ponciano, L. D. Gelder, L. J. Forney, and E. M. Top.** 2005. Modelling the impact of periodic bottlenecks, unidirectional mutation, and observational error in experimental evolution. *J. Math. Biol.* **50:**645–662.

104. **Kado, C. I.** 1998. Origin and evolution of plasmids. *Antonie Leeuwenhoek* **73:**117–126.

105. **Kapperud, G., H. Stenwig, and J. Lassen.** 1998. Epidemiology of *Salmonella typhimurium* O:4-12 infection in Norway: evidence of transmission from an avian wildlife reservoir. *Am. J. Epidemiol.* **147:**774–782.

106. **Katayama, Y., T. Ito, and K. Hiramatsu.** 2000. A new class of genetic element, staphylococcal cassette chromosome *mec*, encodes methicillin resistance in *Staphylococcus aureus*. *Antimicrob. Agents Chemother.* **44:**1549–1555.

107. **Khan, S. A.** 1997. Rolling-circle replication of bacterial plasmids. *Microbiol. Mol. Biol. Rev.* **61:**442–455.

108. **Khan, S. A.** 2000. Plasmid rolling-circle replication: recent developments. *Mol. Microbiol.* **37:**477–484.

109. **Khan, S. A.** 2005. Plasmid rolling-circle replication: highlights of two decades of research. *Plasmid* **53:**126–136.

110. **Killalea, D., L. R. Ward, D. Roberts, J. de Louvois, F. Sufi, J. M. Stuart, P. G. Wall, M. Susman, M. Schwieger, P. J. Sanderson, I. S. Fisher, P. S. Mead, O. N. Gill, C. L. Bartlett, and B. Rowe.** 1996. International epidemiological and microbiological study of outbreak of *Salmonella agona* infection from a ready to eat savoury snack-I: England and Wales and the United States. *Br. Med. J.* **313:**1105–1107.

111. **Kirby, R.** 1990. Evolutionary origin of aminoglycoside phosphotransferase resistance genes. *J. Mol. Evol.* **30:**489–492.

112. **Kirby, R.** 1992. Evolutionary origin of the class A and class C beta-lactamases. *J. Mol. Evol.* **34:**345–350.

113. **Koeck, J. L., G. Arlet, A. Philippon, S. Basmaciogullari, H. V. Thien, Y. Buisson, and J. D. Cavallo.** 1997. A plasmid-mediated CMY-2 β-lactamase from an Algerian clinical isolate of *Salmonella senftenberg*. *FEMS Microbiol. Lett.* **152:**255–260.

114. **Lawley, T. D., W. A. Klimke, M. J. Gubbins, and L. S. Frost.** 2003. F factor conjugation is a true type IV secretion system. *FEMS Microbiol. Lett.* **224:**1–15.

115. **Lederberg, J.** 1952. Cell genetics and hereditary symbiosis. *Physiol. Rev.* **32:**403–430.

116. **Levin, B. R., V. Perrot, and N. Walker.** 2000. Compensatory mutations, antibiotic resistance and the population genetics of adaptive evolution in bacteria. *Genetics* **154:**985–997.

117. **Li, K. S., Y. Guan, J. Wang, G. J. Smith, K. M. Xu, L. Duan, A. P. Rahardjo, P. Puthavathana, C. Buranathai, T. D. Nguyen, A. T. Estoepangestie, A. Chaisingh, P. Auewarakul, H. T. Long, N. T. Hanh, R. J. Webby, L. L. Poon, H. Chen, K. F. Shortridge, K. Y. Yuen, R. G. Webster, and J. S. Peiris.** 2004. Genesis of a highly pathogenic and potentially pandemic H5N1 influenza virus in eastern Asia. *Nature* **430:**209–213.

118. **Liebert, C. A., R. M. Hall, and A. O. Summers.** 1999. Transposon Tn*21*, flagship of the floating genome. *Microbiol. Mol. Biol. Rev.* **63:**507–522.

119. **Ligozzi, M., G. Lo Cascio, and R. Fontana.** 1998. *vanA* gene cluster in a vancomycin-resistant clinical isolate of *Bacillus circulans*. *Antimicrob. Agents Chemother.* **42:**2055–2059.

120. **Little, D. C., and P. Edwards.** 1999. Alternative strategies for livestock-fish integration with emphasis on Asia. *Ambio* **28:** 118–124.

121. **Livermore, D. M.** 1996. Are all β-lactams created equal? *Scand. J. Infect. Dis. Suppl.* **101:**33–43.

122. **Livermore, D. M., M. Warner, L. M. Hall, V. I. Enne, S. J. Projan, P. M. Dunman, S. L. Wooster, and G. Harrison.** 2001. Antibiotic resistance in bacteria from magpies (*Pica pica*) and rabbits (*Oryctolagus cuniculus*) from west Wales. *Environ. Microbiol.* **3:**658–661.

123. **Lorenz, M. G., and W. Wackernagel.** 1994. Bacterial gene transfer by natural genetic transformation in the environment. *Microbiol. Rev.* **58:**563–602.

124. **Lu, K., R. Asano, and J. Davies.** 2004. Antimicrobial resistance gene delivery in animal feeds. *Emerg. Infect. Dis.* **10:** 679–683.

125. **Lyon, B. R., and R. Skurray.** 1987. Antimicrobial resistance of *Staphylococcus aureus*: genetic basis. *Microbiol. Rev.* **51:**88–134.

126. **Lyons, R. W., C. L. Samples, H. N. DeSilva, K. A. Ross, E. M. Julian, and P. J. Checko.** 1980. An epidemic of resistant *Salmonella* in a nursery. Animal-to-human spread. *JAMA* **243:**546–547.

127. **Mammina, C., L. Cannova, S. Massa, E. Goffredo, and A. Nastasi.** 2002. Drug resistances in salmonella isolates from animal foods, Italy 1998-2000. *Epidemiol. Infect.* **129:**155–161.

128. **Marshall, C. G., G. Broadhead, B. K. Leskiw, and G. D. Wright.** 1997. D-Ala-D-Ala ligases from glycopeptide antibiotic-producing organisms are highly homologous to the enterococcal vancomycin-resistance ligases VanA and VanB. *Proc. Natl. Acad. Sci. USA* **94:**6480–6483.

129. **Marshall, C. G., I. A. Lessard, I. Park, and G. D. Wright.** 1998. Glycopeptide antibiotic resistance genes in glycopeptide-producing organisms. *Antimicrob. Agents Chemother.* **42:**2215–2220.

130. **Martinez, E., and F. de la Cruz.** 1990. Genetic elements involved in Tn*21* site-specific integration, a novel mechanism for the dissemination of antibiotic resistance genes. *EMBO J.* **9:**1275–1281.

131. **Massova, I., and S. Mobashery.** 1998. Kinship and diversification of bacterial penicillin-binding proteins and β-lactamases. *Antimicrob. Agents Chemother.* **42:**1–17.

132. **Mazel, D., B. Dychinco, V. A. Webb, and J. Davies.** 1998. A distinctive class of integron in the *Vibrio cholerae* genome. *Science* **280:**605–608.

133. **McClelland, M., K. E. Sanderson, J. Spieth, S. W. Clifton, P. Latreille, L. Courtney, S. Porwollik, J. Ali, M. Dante, F. Du, S. Hou, D. Layman, S. Leonard, C. Nguyen, K. Scott, A. Holmes, N. Grewal, E. Mulvaney, E. Ryan, H. Sun, L. Florea, W. Miller, T. Stoneking, M. Nhan, R. Waterston, and R. K. Wilson.** 2001. Complete genome sequence of *Salmonella enterica* serovar Typhimurium LT2. *Nature* **413:**852–856.

134. **McManus, P. S., V. O. Stockwell, G. W. Sundin, and A. L. Jones.** 2002. Antibiotic use in plant agriculture. *Annu. Rev. Phytopathol.* **40:**443–465.

135. **Medeiros, A. A.** 1997. Evolution and dissemination of β-lactamases accelerated by generations of β-lactam antibiotics. *Clin. Infect. Dis.* **24:**19–45.

136. **Meunier, D., D. Boyd, M. R. Mulvey, S. Baucheron, C. Mammina, A. Nastasi, E. Chaslus-Dancla, and A. Cloeckaert.** 2002. *Salmonella enterica* serotype Typhimurium DT104 antibiotic resistance genomic island I in serotype Paratyphi B. *Emerg. Infect. Dis.* **8:**430–433.

137. **Morton, T. M., D. M. Eaton, J. L. Johnston, and G. L. Archer.** 1993. DNA sequence and units of transcription of the conjugative transfer gene complex (*trs*) of *Staphylococcus aureus* plasmid pGO1. *J. Bacteriol.* **175:**4436–4447.

138. **Nesvera, J., J. Hochmannova, and M. Patek.** 1998. An integron of class 1 is present on the plasmid pCG4 from

gram-positive bacterium *Corynebacterium glutamicum*. *FEMS Microbiol. Lett.* **169**:391–395.

139. **Novick, R. P.** 1989. Staphylococcal plasmids and their replication. *Annu. Rev. Microbiol.* **43**:537–565.

140. **Novick, R. P.** 2003. Mobile genetic elements and bacterial toxinoses: the superantigen-encoding pathogenicity islands of *Staphylococcus aureus*. *Plasmid* **49**:93–105.

141. **Oggioni, M. R., C. G. Dowson, J. M. Smith, R. Provvedi, and G. Pozzi.** 1996. The tetracycline resistance gene *tet*(M) exhibits mosaic structure. *Plasmid* **35**:156–163.

142. **Osborn, A. M., and D. Böltner.** 2002. When phage, plasmids, and transposons collide: genomic islands, and conjugative- and mobilizable-transposons as a mosaic continuum. *Plasmid* **48**:202–212.

143. **Palmgren, H., M. Sellin, S. Bergstrom, and B. Olsen.** 1997. Enteropathogenic bacteria in migrating birds arriving in Sweden. *Scand. J. Infect. Dis.* **29**:565–568.

144. **Pang, Y., B. A. Brown, V. A. Steingrube, R. J. Wallace, Jr., and M. C. Roberts.** 1994. Tetracycline resistance determinants in *Mycobacterium* and *Streptomyces* species. *Antimicrob. Agents Chemother.* **38**:1408–1412.

145. **Patel, R., K. Piper, F. R. Cockerill III, J. M. Steckelberg, and A. A. Yousten.** 2000. The biopesticide *Paenibacillus popilliae* has a vancomycin resistance gene cluster homologous to the enterococcal VanA vancomycin resistance gene cluster. *Antimicrob. Agents Chemother.* **44**:705–709.

146. **Paulsen, I. T., L. Banerjei, G. S. Myers, K. E. Nelson, R. Seshadri, T. D. Read, D. E. Fouts, J. A. Eisen, S. R. Gill, J. F. Heidelberg, H. Tettelin, R. J. Dodson, L. Umayam, L. Brinkac, M. Beanan, S. Daugherty, R. T. DeBoy, S. Durkin, J. Kolonay, R. Madupu, W. Nelson, J. Vamathevan, B. Tran, J. Upton, T. Hansen, J. Shetty, H. Khouri, T. Utterback, D. Radune, K. A. Ketchum, B. A. Dougherty, and C. M. Fraser.** 2003. Role of mobile DNA in the evolution of vancomycin-resistant *Enterococcus faecalis*. *Science* **299**:2071–2074.

147. **Penalva, M. A., A. Moya, J. Dopazo, and D. Ramon.** 1990. Sequences of isopenicillin N synthetase genes suggest horizontal gene transfer from prokaryotes to eukaryotes. *Proc. R. Soc. Lond. B.* **241**:164–169.

148. **Petersen, A., J. S. Andersen, T. Kaewmak, T. Somsiri, and A. Dalsgaard.** 2002. Impact of integrated fish farming on antimicrobial resistance in a pond environment. *Appl. Environ. Microbiol.* **68**:6036–6042.

149. **Petrosino, J., C. Cantu III, and T. Palzkill.** 1998. β-Lactamases: protein evolution in real time. *Trends Microbiol.* **6**:323–327.

150. **Philippon, A., G. Arlet, and G. A. Jacoby.** 2002. Plasmid-determined AmpC-type β-lactamases. *Antimicrob. Agents Chemother.* **46**:1–11.

151. **Piebersberg, W., J. Distler, P. Heinzel, and J. A. Perez-Gonzalez.** 1988. Antibiotic resistance by modification: many resistance genes could be derived from cellular control genes in actinomycetes—a hypothesis. *Actinomycetologica* **2**:83–98.

152. **Power, E. G., Y. H. Abdulla, H. G. Talsania, W. Spice, S. Aathithan, and G. L. French.** 1995. *vanA* genes in vancomycin-resistant clinical isolates of *Oerskovia turbata* and *Arcanobacterium* (*Corynebacterium*) *haemolyticum*. *J. Antimicrob. Chemother.* **36**:595–606.

153. **Projan, S. J., J. Kornblum, S. L. Moghazeh, I. Edelman, M. L. Gennaro, and R. P. Novick.** 1985. Comparative sequence and functional analysis of pT181 and pC221, cognate plasmid replicons from *Staphylococcus aureus*. *Mol. Gen. Genet.* **199**:452–464.

154. **Recchia, G. D., and R. M. Hall.** 1995. Gene cassettes: a new class of mobile element. *Microbiology* **141**:3015–3027.

155. **Reinthaler, F. F., J. Posch, G. Feierl, G. Wust, D. Haas, G. Ruckenbauer, F. Mascher, and E. Marth.** 2003. Antibiotic resistance of *E. coli* in sewage and sludge. *Water Res.* **37**: 1685–1690.

156. **Revathi, G., K. P. Shannon, P. D. Stapleton, B. K. Jain, and G. L. French.** 1998. An outbreak of extended-spectrum, beta-lactamase-producing *Salmonella senftenberg* in a burns ward. *J. Hosp. Infect.* **40**:295–302.

157. **Rhodes, G., G. Huys, J. Swings, P. McGann, M. Hiney, P. Smith, and R. W. Pickup.** 2000. Distribution of oxytetracycline resistance plasmids between aeromonads in hospital and aquaculture environments: implication of Tn*1721* in dissemination of the tetracycline resistance determinant Tet A. *Appl. Environ. Microbiol.* **66**:3883–3890.

158. **Rice, L. B.** 1998. Tn*916* family conjugative transposons and dissemination of antimicrobial resistance determinants. *Antimicrob. Agents Chemother.* **42**:1871–1877.

159. **Rice, L. B., and L. L. Carias.** 1998. Transfer of Tn*5385*, a composite, multiresistance chromosomal element from *Enterococcus faecalis*. *J. Bacteriol.* **180**:714–721.

160. **Richardson, P. T., and S. F. Park.** 1997. Integration of heterologous plasmid DNA into multiple sites on the genome of *Campylobacter coli* following natural transformation. *J. Bacteriol.* **179**:1809–1812.

161. **Roberts, M. C., J. Sutcliffe, P. Courvalin, L. B. Jensen, J. Rood, and H. Seppala.** 1999. Nomenclature for macrolide and macrolide-lincosamide-streptogramin B resistance determinants. *Antimicrob. Agents Chemother.* **43**:2823–2830.

162. **Rodriguez, M. M., P. Power, M. Radice, C. Vay, A. Famiglietti, M. Galleni, J. A. Ayala, and G. Gutkind.** 2004. Chromosome-encoded CTX-M-3 from *Kluyvera ascorbata*: a possible origin of plasmid-borne CTX-M-1-derived cefotaximases. *Antimicrob. Agents Chemother.* **48**:4895–4897.

163. **Salyers, A. A., N. B. Shoemaker, A. M. Stevens, and L. Y. Li.** 1995. Conjugative transposons: an unusual and diverse set of integrated gene transfer elements. *Microbiol. Rev.* **59**: 579–590.

164. **Salyers, A. A., A. Gupta, and Y. Wang.** 2004. Human intestinal bacteria as reservoirs for antibiotic resistance genes. *Trends Microbiol.* **12**:412–416.

165. **Samuels, A. L., E. Lanka, and J. E. Davies.** 2000. Conjugative junctions in RP4-mediated mating of *Escherichia coli*. *J. Bacteriol.* **182**:2709–2715.

166. **Schlüter, A., H. Heuer, R. Szczepanowske, L. J. Forney, C. M. Thomas, A. Pühler, and E. M. Top.** 2003. The 64508 bp IncP-1β-antibiotic multiresistence plasmid pB10 isolated from a waste-water treatment plant provides evidence for recombination between members of different branches of the IncP-1β group. *Microbiology* **149**:3139–3153.

167. **Scholz, P., V. Haring, B. Wittmann-Liebold, K. Ashman, M. Bagdasarian, and E. Scherzinger.** 1989. Complete nucleotide sequence and gene organization of the broad-host-range plasmid RSF1010. *Gene* **75**:271–288.

168. **Schroeter, A., B. Hoog, and R. Helmuth.** 2004. Resistance of *Salmonella* isolates in Germany. *J. Vet. Med. B Infect. Dis. Vet. Public Health* **51**:389–392.

169. **Schwalbe, R. S., A. C. McIntosh, S. Qaiyumi, J. A. Johnson, and J. G. Morris, Jr.** 1999. Isolation of vancomycin-resistant enterococci from animal feed in USA. *Lancet* **353**:722.

170. **Schwaner, N. E., and N. Kroer.** 2001. Effect of plant species on the kinetics of conjugal transfer in the rhizosphere and relation to bacterial metabolic activity. *Microb. Ecol.* **42**: 458–465.

171. **Schwarz, S., C. Kehrenberg, and K. K. Ojo.** 2002. *Staphylococcus sciuri* gene *erm*(33), encoding inducible resistance to macrolides, lincosamides, and streptogramin B antibiotics, is

a product of recombination between *erm*(C) and *erm*(A). *Antimicrob. Agents Chemother.* **46**:3621–3623.

172. **Sellin, M., H. Palmgren, T. Broman, S. Bergstrom, and B. Olsen.** 2000. Involving ornithologists in the surveillance of vancomycin-resistant enterococci. *Emerg. Infect. Dis.* **6**: 87–88.
173. **Sengeløv, G., G. A. Kowalchuk, and S. J. Sørensen.** 2000. Influence of fungal-bacterial interactions on bacterial conjugation in the residuesphere. *FEMS Microbiol. Ecol.* **31**: 39–45.
174. **Sengeløv, G., Y. Agersø, B. Halling-Sørensen, S. B. Baloda, J. S. Andersen, and L. B. Jensen.** 2003. Bacterial antibiotic resistance levels in Danish farmland as a result of treatment with pig manure slurry. *Environ. Int.* **28**:587–595.
175. **Shah, A. A., F. Hasan, S. Ahmed, and A. Hameed.** 2004. Characteristics, epidemiology and clinical importance of emerging strains of Gram-negative bacilli producing extended-spectrum β-lactamases. *Res. Microbiol.* **155**:409–421.
176. **Shakhnovich, B. E., E. Deeds, C. Delisi, and E. Shakhnovich.** 2005. Protein structure and evolutionary history determine sequence space topology. *Genome Res.* **15**:385–392.
177. **Shaw, K. J., P. N. Rather, R. S. Hare, and G. H. Miller.** 1993. Molecular genetics of aminoglycoside resistance genes and familial relationships of the aminoglycoside-modifying enzymes. *Microbiol. Rev.* **57**:138–163.
178. **Sheridan, R. P., and I. Chopra.** 1991. Origin of tetracycline efflux proteins: conclusions from nucleotide sequence analysis. *Mol. Microbiol.* **5**:895–900.
179. **Shibata, N., Y. Doi, K. Yamane, T. Yagi, H. Kurokawa, K. Shibayama, H. Kato, K. Kai, and Y. Arakawa.** 2003. PCR typing of genetic determinants for metallo-β-lactamases and integrases carried by gram-negative bacteria isolated in Japan, with focus on the class 3 integron. *J. Clin. Microbiol.* **41**:5407–5413.
180. **Silverman, P. M.** 1997. Towards a structural biology of bacterial conjugation. *Mol. Microbiol.* **23**:423–429.
181. **Skov, M. N., J. S. Andersen, S. Aabo, S. Ethelberg, F. M. Aarestrup, A. H. Sørensen, G. Sørensen, K. Pedersen, S. Nordentoft, K. E. P. Olsen, P. Gerner-Smith, and D. L. Baggesen.** Antimicrobial resistant *Salmonella* in imported and domestically produced fresh meat as a source of human infections—the Danish experience. Submitted for publication.
182. **Skurray, R. A., and N. Firth.** 1997. Molecular evolution of multiply-antibiotic-resistant staphylococci. *Ciba Found. Symp.* **207**:167–183.
183. **Smalla, K., H. Heuer, A. Gotz, D. Niemeyer, E. Krogerrecklenfort, and E. Tietze.** 2000. Exogenous isolation of antibiotic resistance plasmids from piggery manure slurries reveals a high prevalence and diversity of IncQ-like plasmids. *Appl. Environ. Microbiol.* **66**:4854–4862.
184. **Smith, K. E., S. A. Stenzel, J. B. Bender, E. Wagstrom, D. Soderlund, F. T. Leano, C. M. Taylor, P. A. Belle-Isle, and R. Danila.** 2004. Outbreaks of enteric infections caused by multiple pathogens associated with calves at a farm day camp. *Pediatr. Infect. Dis. J.* **23**:1098–1104.
185. **Smith, M. W., D. F. Feng, and R. F. Doolittle.** 1992. Evolution by acquisition: the case for horizontal gene transfers. *Trends Biochem. Sci.* **17**:489–493.
186. **del Solar, G., R. Giraldo, M. J. Ruiz-Echevarria, M. Espinosa, and R. Diaz-Orejas.** 1998. Replication and control of circular bacterial plasmids. *Microbiol. Mol. Biol. Rev.* **62**: 434–464.
187. **Souza, V., M. Rocha, A. Valera, and L. E. Eguiarte.** 1999. Genetic structure of natural populations of *Escherichia coli* in wild hosts on different continents. *Appl. Environ. Microbiol.* **65**:3373–3385.
188. **Stanton, T. B., and S. B. Humphrey.** 2003. Isolation of tetracycline-resistant *Megasphaera elsdenii* strains with novel mosaic gene combinations of *tet*(O) and *tet*(W) from swine. *Appl. Environ. Microbiol.* **69**:3874–3882.
189. **Stefani, S., and P. E. Varaldo.** 2003. Epidemiology of methicillin-resistant staphylococci in Europe. *Clin. Microbiol. Infect.* **9**:1179–1186.
190. **Suerbaum, S., M. Lohrengel, A. Sonnevend, F. Ruberg, and M. Kist.** 2001. Allelic diversity and recombination in *Campylobacter jejuni*. *J. Bacteriol.* **183**:2553–2559.
191. **Sundin, G. W., and C. L. Bender.** 1996. Dissemination of the *strA-strB* streptomycin-resistance genes among commensal and pathogenic bacteria from humans, animals, and plants. *Mol. Ecol.* **5**:133–143.
192. **Tassios, P. T., M. Gazouli, E. Tzelepi, H. Milch, N. Kozlova, S. Sidorenko, N. J. Legakis, and L. S. Tzouvelekis.** 1999. Spread of a *Salmonella typhimurium* clone resistant to expanded-spectrum cephalosporins in three European countries. *J. Clin. Microbiol.* **37**:3774–3777.
193. **Tauni, M. A., and A. Osterlund.** 2000. Outbreak of *Salmonella typhimurium* in cats and humans associated with infection in wild birds. *J. Small Anim. Pract.* **41**:339–341.
194. **Thiermann, A. B.** 2004. Standards for international trade. *Vet. Rec.* **155**:571.
195. **Thompson, C. J., and G. S. Gray.** 1983. Nucleotide sequence of a streptomycete aminoglycoside phosphotransferase gene and its relationship to phosphotransferases encoded by resistance plasmids. *Proc. Natl. Acad. Sci. USA* **80**:5190–5194.
196. **Thomson, G. R., E. N. Tambi, S. K. Hargreaves, T. J. Leyland, A. P. Catley, G. G. van't Klooster, and M. L. Penrith.** 2004. International trade in livestock and livestock products: the need for a commodity-based approach. *Vet. Rec.* **155**:429–433.
197. **Thornley, C. N., G. C. Simmons, M. L. Callaghan, C. M. Nicol, M. G. Baker, K. S. Gilmore, and N. K. Garrett.** 2003. First incursion of *Salmonella enterica* serotype *typhimurium* DT160 into New Zealand. *Emerg. Infect. Dis.* **9**:493–495.
198. **Thorsted, P. B., D. P. Macartney, P. Akhtar, A. S. Haines, N. Ali, P. Davidson, T. Stafford, M. J. Pocklington, W. Pansegrau, B. M. Wilkins, E. Lanka and C. M. Thomas.** 1998. Complete sequence of the IncPβ plasmid R751: implications for evolution and organisation of the IncP backbone. *J. Mol. Biol.* **282**:969–990.
199. **Threlfall, E. J.** 2000. Epidemic *Salmonella typhimurium* DT104—a truly international multiresistant clone. *J. Antimicrob. Chemother.* **46**:7–10.
200. **Threlfall, E. J., L. R. Ward, M. D. Hampton, A. M. Ridley, B. Rowe, D. Roberts, R. J. Gilbert, P. Van Someren, P. G. Wall, and P. Grimont.** 1998. Molecular fingerprinting defines a strain of *Salmonella enterica* serotype Anatum responsible for an international outbreak associated with formula-dried milk. *Epidemiol. Infect.* **121**: 289–293.
201. **Tosini, F., P. Visca, I. Luzzi, A. M. Dionisi, C. Pezzella, A. Petrucca, and A. Carattoli.** 1998. Class 1 integron-borne multiple-antibiotic resistance carried by IncFI and IncL/M plasmids in *Salmonella enterica* serotype Typhimurium. *Antimicrob. Agents Chemother.* **42**:3053–3058.
202. **Vaisvila, R., R. D. Morgan, J. Posfai, and E. A. Raleigh.** 2001. Discovery and distribution of super-integrons among pseudomonads. *Mol. Microbiol.* **42**:587–601.

202a. **van den Bogaard, A. E., L. B. Jensen, and E. E. Stobberingh.** 1997. Vancomycin-resistant enterococci in turkeys and farmers. *N. Engl. J. Med.* **337**:1558–1559.

202b. **van Elsas, J. D., B. B. Gardener, A. C. Wolters, and E. Smit.** 1998. Isolation, characterization, and transfer of cryptic gene-mobilizing plasmids in the wheat rhizosphere. *Appl. Environ. Microbiol.* **64:**880-889.

203. **Van Pelt, W., D. J. Mevius, H. Stoelhorst, S. Kovats, A. W. Van De Giessen, W. Wannet, and Y. Duynhoven.** 2004. A large increase of *Salmonella* infections in 2003 in the Netherlands: hot summer or side effect of the avian influenza outbreak? *Eur. Surveill.* 9:17–19.

204. **Vidaver, A. K.** 2002. Uses of antimicrobials in plant agriculture. *Clin. Infect. Dis.* **34:**107–110.

205. **Waldor, M. K., H. Tschäpe, and J. J. Mekalanos.** 1996. A new type of conjugative transposon encodes resistance to sulfamethoxazole, trimethoprim, and streptomycin in *Vibrio cholerae* O139. *J. Bacteriol.* **178:**4157–4165.

206. **Wang, Y., and D. E. Taylor.** 1990. Natural transformation in *Campylobacter* species. *J. Bacteriol.* **172:**949–955.

207. **Webb, V., and J. Davies.** 1993. Antibiotic preparations contain DNA: a source of drug resistance genes? *Antimicrob. Agents Chemother.* **37:**2379–2384.

208. **Welch, R. A., V. Burland, G. Plunkett III, P. Redford, P. Roesch, D. Rasko, E. L. Buckles, S. R. Liou, A. Boutin, J. Hackett, D. Stroud, G. F. Mayhew, D. J. Rose, S. Zhou, D. C. Schwartz, N. T. Perna, H. L. Mobley, M. S. Donnenberg, and F. R. Blattner.** 2002. Extensive mosaic structure revealed by the complete genome sequence of uropathogenic *Escherichia coli*. *Proc. Natl. Acad. Sci. USA* **99:**17020–17024.

209. **Wilson, I. G.** 2003. Antibiotic resistance of Campylobacter in raw retail chickens and imported chicken portions. *Epidemiol. Infect.* **131:**1181–1186.

210. **Wilson, I. G.** 2004. Antimicrobial resistance of *Salmonella* in raw retail chickens, imported chicken portions, and human clinical specimens. *J. Food Prot.* **67:**1220–1225.

211. **Winokur, P. L., A. Brueggemann, D. L. DeSalvo, L. Hoffmann, M. D. Apley, E. K. Uhlenhopp, M. A. Pfaller, and G. V. Doern.** 2000. Animal and human multidrug-resistant, cephalosporin-resistant *Salmonella* isolates expressing a plasmid-mediated CMY-2 AmpC β-lactamase. *Antimicrob. Agents Chemother.* **44:**2777–2783.

212. **Winokur, P. L., D. L. Vonstein, L. J. Hoffman, E. K. Uhlenhopp, and G. V. Doern.** 2001. Evidence for transfer of CMY-2 AmpC β-lactamase plasmids between *Escherichia coli* and *Salmonella* isolates from food animals and humans. *Antimicrob. Agents Chemother.* **45:**2716–2722.

213. **World Health Organization.** 2004. Global Salm Surv (GSS). http://www.who.int/salmsurv/en/.

214. **World Organization for Animal Health.** http://www.oie.int/eng/en_index.htm. (Accessed 1 March 2005.)

215. **World Trade Organization.** 1995. Agreement on the application of sanitary and phytosanitary measures. http://www.wto.org/english/docs_e/legal_e/15-sps.pdf. (Accessed 1 March 2005.)

216. **World Trade Organization.** 2005. http://www.wto.org/. (Accessed 1 March 2005.)

217. **Wray, C., N. Todd, I. McLaren, Y. Beedell, and B. Rowe.** 1990. The epidemiology of *Salmonella* infection in calves: the role of dealers. *Epidemiol. Infect.* **105:**295–305.

218. **Wray, C., N. Todd, I. M. McLaren, and Y. E. Beedell.** 1991. The epidemiology of *Salmonella* in calves: the role of markets and vehicles. *Epidemiol. Infect.* **107:**521–525.

219. **Wu, S., C. Piscitelli, H. de Lencastre, and A. Tomasz.** 1996. Tracking the evolutionary origin of the methicillin resistance gene: cloning and sequencing of a homologue of *mecA* from a methicillin susceptible strain of *Staphylococcus sciuri*. *Microb. Drug Resist.* **2:**435–441.

220. **Wu, S. W., K. Dornbusch, G. Kronvall, and M. Norgren.** 1999. Characterization and nucleotide sequence of a *Klebsiella oxytoca* cryptic plasmid encoding a CMY-type β-lactamase: confirmation that the plasmid-mediated cephamycinase originated from the *Citrobacter freundii* AmpC β-lactamase. *Antimicrob. Agents Chemother.* **43:**1350–1357.

221. **Yan, J. J., C. Y. Hong, W. C. Ko, Y. J. Chen, S. H. Tsai, C. L. Chuang, and J. J. Wu.** 2004. Dissemination of $bla_{CMY\text{-}2}$ among *Escherichia coli* isolates from food animals, retail ground meats, and humans in southern Taiwan. *Antimicrob. Agents Chemother.* **48:**1353–1356.

222. **Zhao, S., A. R. Datta, S. Ayers, S. Friedman, R. D. Walker, and D. G. White.** 2003. Antimicrobial-resistant *Salmonella* serovars isolated from imported foods. *Int. J. Food Microbiol.* **84:**87–92.

223. **Ziemienowicz, A., D. Gorlich, E. Lanka, B. Hohn, and L. Rossi.** 1999. Import of DNA into mammalian nuclei by proteins originating from a plant pathogenic bacterium. *Proc. Natl. Acad. Sci. USA* **96:**3729–3733.

Antimicrobial Resistance in Bacteria of Animal Origin
Edited by Frank M. Aarestrup

Chapter 21

Licensing and Approval of Antimicrobials for Use in Animals

Linda Tollefson, Deborah Morris, Christopher Boland, and Jack Kay

Antimicrobial drugs are used in animals to control, prevent, and treat infection and, in food-producing animals, to enhance animal growth and feed efficiency. Before an animal drug can be legally marketed in most countries, the product must be approved by the appropriate regulatory authority. It is the collective responsibility of the drug sponsor, the regulatory authorities, practicing veterinarians, and other professionals dealing with veterinary medicines to minimize the potential adverse impact on public health resulting from the use of antimicrobial agents in food-producing animals, as well as in companion animals. This is particularly important as regards the development of antimicrobial resistance. The purpose of providing regulatory approval for the use of antimicrobial products in animals is to ensure that the products are effective and safe and to manage the risks of adverse effects from their use. In achieving that purpose, regulatory authorities base approval decisions on technically sound assessments of reliable information. All data are generated by the applicant and provided to the regulatory authorities for evaluation and analysis.

The trade in animal health products is global, and standardization of assessment methodology and information requirements facilitates the approval process. Regulatory authorities and animal drug industry associations are actively involved in promoting international harmonization of animal drug regulatory requirements. One of the goals of harmonization is to identify and then reduce differences in technical requirements for drug development among regulatory agencies in different countries. The International Cooperation on Harmonisation of Technical Requirements for Registration of Veterinary Medicinal Products (VICH) was established in 1996 under the auspices of the Office International des Epizooties (http://vich.eudra.org). VICH has developed and harmonized study protocols, criteria, and standards for the registration of new animal drugs and biologics and standards for postmarket surveillance activities and reporting. Original government and industry participants from the European Union, Japan, and the United States have been joined over the years by observers and interested parties from Canada, Australia, New Zealand, CAMEVET (a Latin American government and industry association), and the Association of Veterinary Biologics Companies. The International Federation of Animal Health serves as the VICH Secretariat. Through a nine-step process, VICH has finalized 30 guidance documents and currently is working on eight additional draft guidance documents (http://vich.eudra.org/htm/guidelines.htm).

VICH has been very successful in harmonizing product quality, human food safety, environmental risk assessment, and efficacy requirements, and those guidelines will be highlighted in this chapter, where relevant. Although most of the information contained in this chapter is applicable to all veterinary medicinal products, antimicrobial drugs are given prominence.

ANTIMICROBIAL RESISTANCE

For the purposes of this chapter, the antimicrobial resistance issue is considered from both an animal health and human health perspective. It is restricted to antibacterial effects, but the range of active ingredients relevant to the antibacterial resistance issue is not limited to those that meet the strict definition of an antibiotic because it includes antimicrobial substances such as sulfonamides, nitrofurans,

Linda Tollefson • Center for Veterinary Medicine, U.S. Food and Drug Administration, 7519 Standish Pl., Rockville, MD 20878. **Deborah Morris and Christopher Boland** • Agricultural Chemicals and Veterinary Medicines, New Zealand Food Safety Authority, P.O. Box 2835, Wellington, New Zealand. **Jack Kay** • Veterinary Medicines Directorate, Department for Environment, Food and Rural Affairs, Woodham Ln., New Haw, Addlestone, Surrey KT15 3LS, United Kingdom.

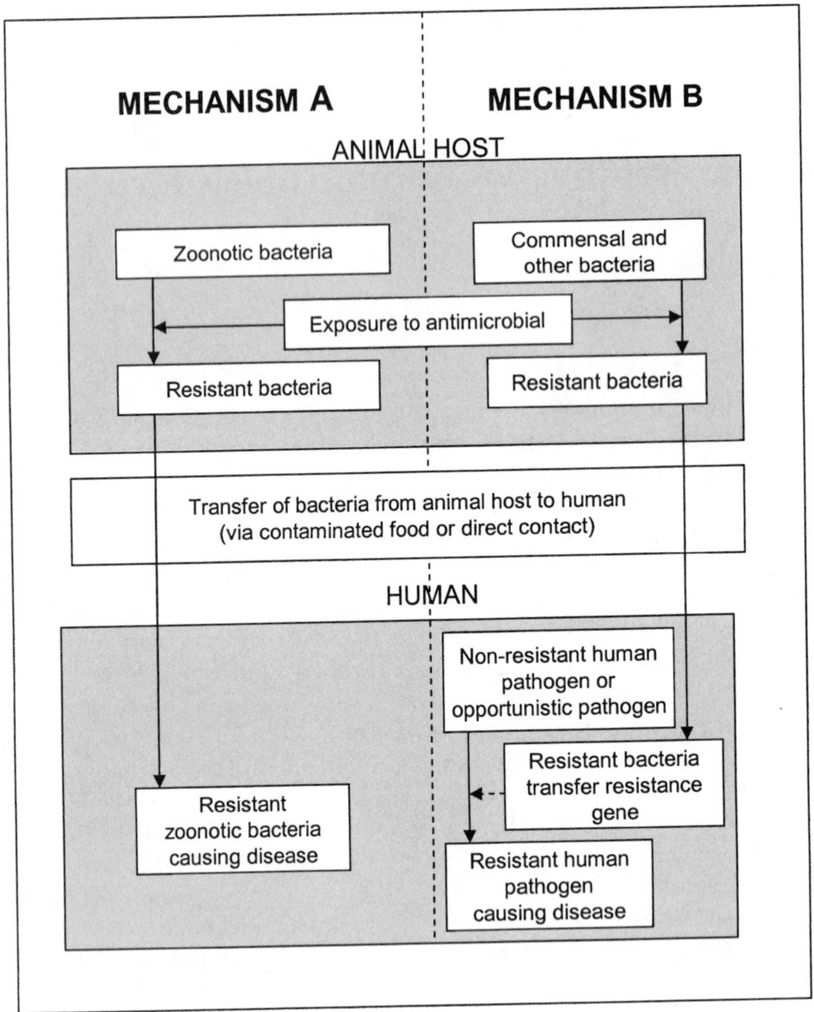

Figure 1. Resistance development in zoonotic pathogenic bacteria (mechanism A) and commensal bacteria of animal origin (mechanism B).

and nitroimidazoles. The relevant active ingredients are limited to those that (i) have a primarily antibacterial effect, (ii) have a coincidental antibacterial effect, and (iii) are used to manage or assist in managing particular bacterial infections.

Antibacterial resistance includes resistance in both zoonotic pathogenic bacteria and commensal bacteria of animal origin that may transfer resistance-encoding genetic material. The two mechanisms are illustrated in Fig. 1. Mechanism A is the scenario in which animals are treated with antibacterial products and the zoonotic bacteria present (e.g., *Salmonella* and *Campylobacter* species, *Escherichia coli*, etc.) in the animals, particularly in the gastrointestinal tract, develop resistance. Humans are exposed to the resistant zoonotic bacteria, resulting in colonization and possibly disease that is less responsive to antibacterial therapy.

Mechanism B is the more complicated scenario, in which animals are treated with antibacterial products and commensal bacteria, e.g., *Enterococcus* species, develop resistance. The commensal bacteria referred to in mechanism B are nonpathogenic bacteria in animals that are the same as those in humans or that could, for a short period of time, persist in the gastrointestinal tract of humans. The resistant bacteria either colonize in the human or at least remain long enough to transfer the resistance-encoding genetic material to bacteria (possibly pathogenic) in humans.

PREAPPROVAL ASSESSMENT

Approval of animal health products is based on the principles of risk analysis. This requires the identification and characterization of the relevant risks, assessment of the risks, and risk management. Risk communication and monitoring the effectiveness of management decisions are important components of the process as well. Many countries have standards for risk analysis or management (7) that make the process relatively transparent. Most of these standards are based on internationally recognized best practices. By establishing an approval methodology based on internationally recognized principles and expecting parties that apply for approval to use the same principles when preparing their information packages, the process is predictable and transparent, with a good chance the outcome will be technically sound, understandable, and effective. This chapter describes how risk management is applied to the approval of antimicrobial products in general and describes some variations in how it is applied in Australia, New Zealand, the United Kingdom (applying European Union requirements), and the United States.

The traditional risk areas that are considered in the approval of animal antimicrobial products include the following: (i) failure to achieve claims (efficacy), (ii) causing harm in treated animals (target animal safety), (iii) causing harm to organisms inadvertently exposed (environmental safety), (iv) causing harm to people directly exposed (e.g., human occupational safety), and (v) causing harm to people indirectly exposed through consumption or exposure to food products of animal origin (human food safety). Within these risk areas, some of the hazards and exposure pathways are well known and the methodology for collecting, analyzing, and assessing these data is well characterized (6). Other hazards, such as the transfer of antimicrobial resistance to human bacterial pathogens, are of more recent concern and the focus of new practices such as those detailed in the VICH guidelines referred to in the following sections.

Relevant risk areas that should be addressed influence the information required by the regulatory authorities to assess a product properly. The drug sponsor must also show that the methods, facilities, and controls used for the manufacturing, processing, and packaging of the drug are adequate to preserve its identity, strength, quality, and purity. Once the chemistry and manufacturing information has been confirmed, the areas of risk can be assessed.

EFFICACY REQUIREMENTS

Most developed countries operate under legislation that facilitates the approval and marketing of animal drugs and medicated feeds. Demonstration of effectiveness is generally based on substantial evidence consisting of one or more adequate and well-controlled investigations, such as studies in the target species, studies in laboratory animals, field investigations, bioequivalence studies, and in vitro studies. The number and types of studies required to demonstrate that the antimicrobial drug is effective at the proposed dose or dose range are dependent upon a number of factors. For example, the proposed intended uses or conditions of use for the antimicrobial, the availability of information concerning the active ingredient of the drug, and whether the antimicrobial is conducive to in vitro testing or data extrapolation are all issues that determine the types of studies required. As regards the number of studies, the drug sponsor must provide a sufficient number of studies of adequate quality and persuasiveness to permit qualified experts to determine whether an animal drug is effective. The quality of a study's design and conduct includes factors of rigor, statistical power, and scope.

Preclinical studies including pharmacokinetic and pharmacodynamic data are usually generated to establish an appropriate dosage regimen necessary to ensure the efficacy of the antimicrobial product. Important information about the drug includes the mode of action, the spectrum of antimicrobial activity of the substance, and identification of bacterial species that are naturally resistant to the antimicrobial product studied. Important pharmacodynamic information includes antimicrobial MICs for the target pathogen(s), determination of whether the antimicrobial exerts time- or concentration-dependent activity, and evaluation of activity at the site of infection. Important pharmacokinetic information should preferably include bioavailability applicable to the route of administration, concentration of the antimicrobial at the site of infection and its distribution in the treated animal, metabolic pathways that may lead to inactivation of the drug, and excretion routes.

Definitive proof of the efficacy of an antimicrobial product is based upon a demonstration of effectiveness in clinical trials. VICH has established good clinical practice guidance (12) that provides information on the design and conduct of all clinical studies of veterinary medicinal products in the target species. The goal is to ensure the accuracy, integrity, and correctness of the data submitted to the regulatory authority for product registration. The guidance sets out detailed requirements for the clinical investigator, the study monitor, the drug sponsor, study design, animal selection, animal housing and feeding, and study treatments. Emphasis is placed on developing a comprehensive study protocol in order to help ensure that a well-designed study is developed and executed (12).

DEMONSTRATION OF SAFETY

Before an animal drug can be marketed, the sponsor must demonstrate by adequate tests that the drug is safe for use under the conditions prescribed, recommended, or suggested in the proposed labeling. The requirements for demonstration of safety can be separated into target animal safety, environmental safety, human food safety, and user safety.

TARGET ANIMAL SAFETY

Demonstration of safety in the animals targeted for the drug is done by testing the cumulative effects of the drug on the animals, such that the drug does not adversely affect the treated animals. The focus for target animal safety is on the effective and toxic doses and the margin of safety represented by the difference between the two (9). The data required to demonstrate the safety of an animal drug in target animals depends upon the amount of historical information that is available on the subject drug, especially the toxicity studies conducted in laboratory animals. Other information that can be used to determine target animal toxicity study requirements includes pharmacokinetic data, pharmacologic action, metabolism studies, treatment regimen, etc.

Animals used for testing in target animal safety studies should represent the species in which the drug will be used. They should be free of disease and not exposed to environmental conditions that could interfere with the purpose or conduct of the study.

ENVIRONMENTAL SAFETY

Protection goals for environmental quality of ground and surface waters, air, soil, and nontarget species are set by the pertinent regulatory body in each country. An exposure threshold approach is generally used to determine when environmental fate-and-effect studies are needed. Environmental studies are not necessary for compounds that result in limited environmental exposure. When a full environmental assessment is required, the drug sponsor conducts laboratory toxicity studies with invertebrates, plants, and microorganisms representative of the environmental compartment of concern. The no-observed-effect level, or the MIC in the case of microbes, is divided by a safety factor to arrive at a predicted environmental no-effect concentration (PNEC). The predicted environmental concentration (PEC) is calculated for the drug and compared to the PNEC. When the PEC/PNEC ratio is less than 1, significant environmental effects are not predicted to occur due to the use of the animal drug product (5).

VICH has developed guidance to assess the potential for veterinary medical products to affect nontarget species in the environment, including both aquatic and terrestrial species. Phase I guidance describes criteria for determining whether or not a detailed environmental impact assessment should be undertaken (11). The phase II document provides guidance for the use of a single set of environmental fate and toxicity data, and the test methods to be used for generating these data, for registering veterinary products identified as requiring data during the phase I process (22). The VICH phase II guidance contains sections for aquaculture, intensively reared terrestrial animals, and pasture animals. Intensive animal operations are where animals are kept and raised in confined situations, in a relatively small land area. Feed is brought to the animals, and waste is usually disposed of by spreading on adjacent fields (22). Beef cattle, dairy cattle, pigs, chickens, and turkeys are examples of species that may be reared in an intensive terrestrial system. The use of antimicrobial agents in animal production has facilitated confinement housing and allowed large numbers of animals to be produced on small land areas. Farm management factors such as sanitation, space utilization, housing, and environmental controls help to minimize the use of antimicrobial agents. However, even well-managed operations require a proactive approach to disease control due to the increased density of livestock or poultry in intensive rearing operations.

The phase II guidance also contains recommended tests for physical and chemical properties, environmental fate, and environmental effects (22). The phase II guidance uses a two-tiered approach to develop an environmental impact assessment. The first tier, tier A, uses simpler, less expensive studies to produce a conservative assessment of risk based on exposure and effects in the environmental compartment of concern. If an unacceptable risk is found using the tier A studies, the sponsor progresses to tier B to refine the assessment (22).

HUMAN FOOD SAFETY

Assessment of Hazards from Veterinary Drug Residues

The hazards associated with the consumption of food containing residues of veterinary drugs as a result of use of the drugs in food-producing animals are generally assessed in laboratory animals treated with the drugs (19). To determine the food safety of residues of an antimicrobial product, the drug sponsor conducts a standard battery of tests. The battery includes studies that examine the effect of the product on systemic toxicity, repeat-dose toxicity (17, 21), reproductive toxicity (13), developmental toxicity (18), genotoxicity (14), and carcinogenicity (16), and effects on the human intestinal flora (20). The toxicology studies are designed to show a dose that causes a toxic effect and a dose that causes no observed adverse effect. These end points are then used to calculate an acceptable daily intake (ADI).

Repeat-dose toxicity testing is used to define toxic effects based on repeated and/or cumulative exposures to the compound or its metabolites, the incidence and severity of the effect in relation to the dose and/or duration of exposure, doses associated with toxic and biological responses, and a no-observed-adverse-effect level (NOEL). These studies are performed with the appropriate or sensitive species, with the rat and the dog being the primary default species. Ninety-day toxicity testing is first performed in order to identify target organs and toxicological end points and provide data to help set appropriate doses to be used in repeat-dose chronic toxicity testing (17). This testing often helps to identify the most appropriate species for the repeat-dose chronic toxicity testing. Next, chronic toxicity testing is performed to define toxic effects based on long-term exposures to the compound or its metabolites, identify target organs and toxicological end points in relation to the dose or duration of exposure, determine dosages associated with these responses, and establish a NOEL (21). The guideline does not preclude the possibility of alternative approaches that may offer an equivalent assurance of safety, including scientifically based reasons as to why chronic toxicity testing may not need to be provided.

Multigeneration reproduction studies are designed to detect any effect on mammalian reproduction (13). These include effects on male and female fertility, mating, conception, implantation, ability to maintain pregnancy to term, parturition, and lactation, as well as the survival of offspring, the growth and development of the offspring from birth through weaning and sexual maturity, and the subsequent reproductive function of the offspring as adults. The objective of this testing is to evaluate risks to reproduction from long-term, low-dose exposures, such as may be encountered from the presence of veterinary drug residues in food. Thus, a multigeneration study, in which dosing extends through more than one generation, is considered the most appropriate model. The study of more than one generation allows detection of not only any effects on adult reproduction but also effects on subsequent generations due to exposure in utero and during the early postnatal period. This type of study is not designed to detect developmental abnormalities (see next paragraph). Multigeneration studies are designed to determine the dose at which any effects on reproduction occur, as well as a clearly identified dose or doses showing no adverse effects. The majority of these studies are conducted in the rat and generally include two generations.

Developmental toxicity testing is designed to detect any adverse effects on the pregnant female and development of the embryo and fetus consequent to exposure of the female from implantation through the entire period of gestation (18). Effects may include enhanced toxicity relative to that observed in nonpregnant females, embryo-fetal death, altered fetal growth, and structural changes to the fetus. The testing begins with rat studies, and if teratogenicity is observed, no further testing is required. However, if the ADI will be based on the teratogenic end point, then developmental toxicity tests should be performed in a second species. Also, if equivocal results are achieved with the rat studies, testing in a second species, preferably the rabbit, should be conducted. Teratogenicity for this purpose is defined as producing a structural change in the fetus that is considered detrimental to the animal, which may or may not be compatible with life (18).

A battery of genotoxicity tests is used to identify substances that have the capacity to damage the genetic information within cells (14). Since many carcinogens have a genotoxic mode of action, substances that are genotoxic are regarded as potential carcinogens. Those that cause genetic damage in germ cells also have the potential to cause reproductive or developmental effects. VICH guideline GL23 (14) recommends a standard battery of three tests to screen for the genotoxicity of veterinary drugs. These include a test for gene mutation in bacteria, an in vitro test for chromosomal effects in mammalian cells, and an in vivo test for chromosomal effects using rodent hematopoietic cells. However, some antimicrobials are toxic to the tester strains used in the test for gene mutation in bacteria. In that case, it is recommended that the bacterial test be performed using concentrations up to the limit of cytotoxicity and also be supplemented with an in vitro test for gene mutation in mammalian cells (14).

Carcinogenicity testing is performed for those compounds that are suspected to have carcinogenic potential. Carcinogenic potential is assessed by evaluating the structure of the parent compound, the results of genotoxicity testing, data from chronic toxicity studies, and any other relevant information.

The VICH guideline on carcinogenicity testing recommends that testing be done by bioassays (16). Carcinogenicity bioassays with oral dosing consisting of a 2-year rat study and an 18-month mouse study are generally required. VICH guideline GL28 (16) also refers to the Organization for Economic Cooperation and Development Test Guideline 451 on "Carcinogenicity Studies" (at http://www.oecd.org/dataoecd/12/10/1953977.pdf).

Maximum Residue Limits

The various toxicology tests described in the previous section are designed to determine the dose at which the compound produces an adverse effect and a dose which produces no observed adverse effect, the NOEL. Once the NOEL is established for all the toxicity end points, the most sensitive effect in the species most predictive of man is identified. This NOEL is divided by a safety factor to account for uncertainty in extrapolating from animals to man and for variability, i.e., the difference among individuals, to calculate an ADI for drug residues. From all the studies conducted, a toxicological and a microbiological ADI will be established. The ADI represents the amount of drug residues that can be consumed by an adult daily for a lifetime without appreciable risk to human health (8, 20).

If the substance is microbiologically active, the overall ADI should be established on the lowest of the pharmacological, toxicological, and microbiological ADIs. The ADI in turn provides the basis for determining the maximum residue limits (MRLs) of the drug in treated animals. In addition to the safety factors used to calculate the ADI, estimates of daily intake of specific food commodities are generally set conservatively high. The European Medicines Agency (EMEA) Committee for Medicinal Products for Veterinary Use and the U.S. Food and Drug Administration (FDA) assume, for the calculation of MRLs, that every day an average individual consumes a specific amount of muscle, liver, kidney, fat, milk, honey (for the European Union), and eggs (Table 1).

MRLs are not established for all food commodities, depending on the use of the drug and the target animals. MRLs are set in such a way that the total consumption of residues in food commodities for which MRLs are set falls below the ADI, assuming that all food contains the residue of the drug under consideration and the person consumes the entire amount of each of the commodities. New Zealand uses a similar approach but bases the ADI on grams of the food commodity per kilogram of body weight per day (Table 2).

Table 1. Consumption table for calculating ADI

Food commodity	Amt (g/day)	
	United Kingdom[a]	United States
Meat		
Muscle	300	300
Liver	100	100
Kidney	50	50
Fat	50	50
Or:		
Chicken		
Muscle	300	300
Liver	100	100
Kidney	10	50
Fat and skin	90	50
Or:		
Fish	300	
Plus:		
Eggs	100	
Plus:		
Milk	1,500	1,500
Plus:		
Honey	20	

[a]See Table in volume 8 of the Rules Governing Medicinal Products in the European Union (http://pharmacos.eudra.org/F2/eudralex/vol-8/pdf/Vol8rev1Final24June2003.pdf), p. 60.

Residue depletion data are considered during the establishment of MRLs. MRLs can be set in a range of edible tissues. Usually, a withdrawal time is established to allow the drug residues to deplete below the calculated MRL (and the ADI), taking into account the average amount consumed per person per day. It is important to note that this withdrawal period is product specific, as the formulation of the product may have an impact on the withdrawal period. For surveillance purposes, residue concentrations have to be below the MRL values for all tissues in which an MRL has been established (4; also see volume 8 of the Rules

Table 2. New Zealand consumption table for calculating ADI

Food commodity	Amt (g/kg of body wt/day)	
	Adult	Child
Meat		
Cattle (8% fat)	1.25	2
Deer (2% fat)	0.01	0
Pig (20% fat)	0.5	0.75
Sheep (15% fat)	0.75	1.5
Offal		
Cattle	0.013	0
Sheep	0.013	0.05
Milk products	15	50
Chicken		
Meat	0.75	2
Offal	0.002	0.002
Eggs	0.5	0.5

Governing Medicinal Products in the European Union [http://pharmacos.eudra.org/F2/eudralex/vol-8/pdf/Vol8rev1Final24June2003.pdf]).

Additional Food Safety Considerations for Antimicrobial Drugs

There are special food safety concerns for the residues of antimicrobial drugs. Therapeutic doses of antimicrobials can cause adverse effects on the human intestinal microflora. VICH has developed an approach to help determine the impact of veterinary antimicrobial drug residues in food on human intestinal microflora based on two end points of public health concern (20):

1. Disruption of the colonization barrier. A perturbation in the barrier effect is of concern because the gut microflora provides a barrier against the overgrowth and invasion of pathogenic bacteria. When an antibiotic destroys this barrier, overgrowth of pathogenic bacteria may occur.

2. Increase of populations of resistant bacteria.

VICH guideline GL36 (20) outlines how to determine the need for establishing a microbiological ADI, recommends test systems and methods for determining NOELs for the end points of health concern, and recommends a procedure to derive a microbiological ADI. For additional information, Cerniglia and Kotarski published a review in 1999 (1) describing a variety of in vitro and in vivo test systems to study the effects of residues from veterinary antimicrobials on the human gastrointestinal tract.

For some classes of antimicrobials, such as beta-lactam antibiotics, immunotoxicity testing is used to assess the potential for the drug to elicit an allergic reaction in sensitive individuals (19).

ANTIBACTERIAL RESISTANCE

Another concern that should be addressed to ensure the food safety of antimicrobials is the contribution that antimicrobial drug use in food-producing animals plays in the emergence of antimicrobial drug-resistant bacteria. There is general agreement within the scientific community that the development of resistant, human-pathogenic bacteria results primarily from the direct use of antimicrobial agents in humans but also from acquisition of resistant organisms or resistance factors from animal and environmental sources. The direct public health concern is that use of antimicrobials in food-producing animals may contribute to the development or dissemination of antibiotic-resistant zoonotic organisms that may contaminate food products at the time of slaughter and subsequently be transmitted to humans. The indirect effect is where animals are treated with antimicrobials and commensal bacteria develop resistance that may be passed to human-pathogenic bacteria.

VICH has published guidance on registration of antimicrobials for food-producing animals with respect to antimicrobial resistance (15). The guidance provides recommendations for gathering basic information on the drug; its mode of action and spectrum of activity, including MICs for target animal pathogens and food-borne and commensal organisms; the mechanism of resistance development; and other related information. The basic information described in VICH guideline GL27 (15) is minimal and includes data on antimicrobial class, mechanism and type of antimicrobial action, antimicrobial spectrum of activity, MICs for target animal pathogens and food-borne pathogens, occurrence of cross-resistance and coresistance, and pharmacokinetics. Several countries have implemented guidance or requirements that also describe how the data are to be used in assessing microbial safety prior to approval of the antimicrobial.

The U.S. FDA published guidance in 2003 that outlines an evidence-based approach to preventing antimicrobial resistance in humans that may result from the use of antimicrobials in animals (10). The document applies to all antimicrobial drugs intended for use in food-producing animals but only assesses the risk from human exposure through ingestion of antimicrobial-resistant bacteria from animal-derived foods. This is the most significant pathway for human exposure to bacteria that have emerged or been selected as a consequence of antimicrobial drug use in animals but is not the only pathway.

A qualitative approach to risk assessment is recommended in the FDA guidance, although the possibility of quantitative assessments is not excluded. The guidance provides a scientific process for assessing the likelihood that an antimicrobial drug used to treat a food-producing animal may cause an antimicrobial resistance problem in humans consuming milk, eggs, honey, meat, or other edible tissue from that animal. The pathway suggested in the FDA guidance document establishes a three-part system for determining an antimicrobial drug's potential risk to humans if used to treat food-producing animals. The essential components include a release assessment, which determines the probability that resistant bacteria will be present in animals as a result of the use of the antimicrobial

Critically Important: Antimicrobial drugs which meet BOTH criteria 1 and 2

Highly Important: Antimicrobial drugs which meet EITHER criteria 1 or 2

Important: Antimicrobial drugs which meet EITHER criterion 3 and/or 4 and/or 5.

1. ***Antimicrobial drugs used to treat enteric pathogens that cause food-borne disease***

2. ***Sole therapy or one of few alternatives to treat serious human disease or drug is essential component among many antimicrobials in treatment of human disease***

   Serious diseases are defined as those with high morbidity or mortality without proper treatment regardless of the relationship of animal transmission to humans.

3. ***Antimicrobials used to treat enteric pathogens in non-food-borne disease***

4. ***No cross-resistance within drug class and absence of linked resistance with other drug classes***

   Absence of resistance linked to other antimicrobials makes antimicrobials more valuable.

5. ***Difficulty in transmitting resistance elements within or across genera and species of organisms***

   Antimicrobials to which organisms have chromosomal resistance would be more valuable compared to those antimicrobials whose resistance mechanisms are present on plasmids and transposons.

Figure 2. Criteria considered in the U.S. ranking of antimicrobial drugs according to their importance in human medicine.

drug; an exposure assessment, which gauges the likelihood that humans would ingest the resistant bacteria; and a consequence assessment, which assesses the chances that human exposure to the resistant bacteria would result in adverse human health consequences. In this context, these are situations in which a physician has difficulty treating a person with an antimicrobial drug because the bacteria infecting the person had acquired resistance to the drug and that resistance came from use of the drug in animals.

For assessment of exposure, the evaluation considers both the frequency of bacterial contamination (e.g., *Salmonella*) of food products and per capita consumption of animal-derived food categories from treated animals. The consequence assessment involves placing the drug into "critically important," "highly important," and "important" categories based on the usefulness of the drug in food-borne infections, the availability of alternative therapies, the ease with which such resistance develops, and other factors. See Fig. 2 for the U.S. criteria used to categorize

Table 3. Examples of ranking of drugs based according to their importance in human medicine in New Zealand and the United States

Critically important or high concern	Highly important or medium concern	Important or low concern
Aminoglycosides (New Zealand)	Aminoglycosides (United States)	
Broad-spectrum cephalosporins (United States); and broad-spectrum and "fourth-generation" cephalosporins (New Zealand)	Amoxicillin, ampicillin (United States)	Amoxicillin, ampicillin (New Zealand)
Glycopeptides (New Zealand)	Bacitracin (New Zealand)	Narrow- and expanded-spectrum cephalosporins (United States)
Fluoroquinolones (New Zealand and United States)	"Fourth-generation" cephalosporins (United States)	Monobactams (United States)
Macrolides and lincosamides (New Zealand and United States)	Glycopeptides (United States)	Quinolones (United States)
Streptogramins (New Zealand)	Streptogramins (United States), tetracyclines (United States)	Tetracyclines (New Zealand)

drugs based on importance to human medical therapy and Table 3 for examples of drug categorization in New Zealand and the United States. The risk estimation integrates the three components and classifies the drug as of high, medium, or low risk to human health (Fig. 3). If the qualitative risk assessment shows that the risks are significant, the FDA can deny the application for marketing authorization, thus preventing the use of the drug in food animals, or it can approve the drug but place conditions on its

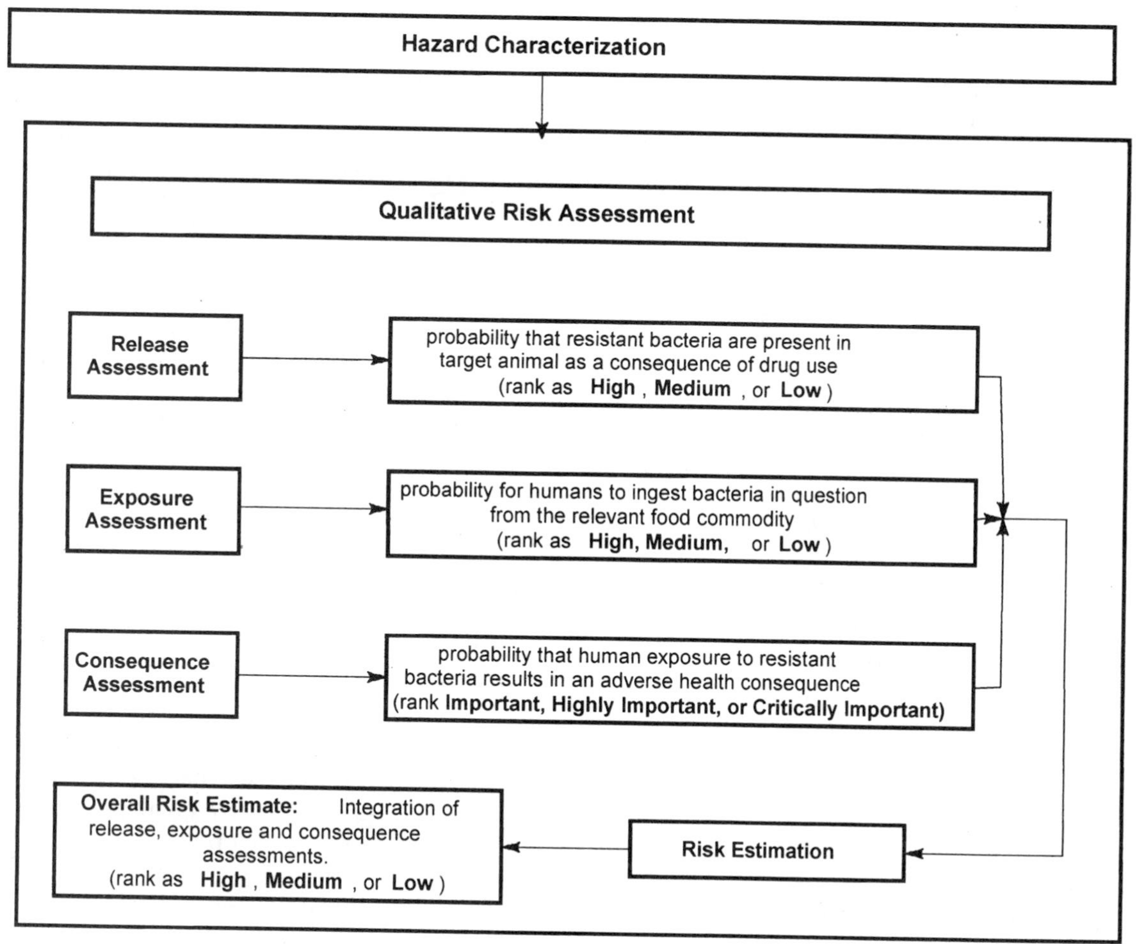

Figure 3. U.S. qualitative risk assessment process for evaluation of animal drugs with regard to microbial safety.

Table 4. Examples of risk management options in the United States based on the level of risk identified (high, medium, or low)

Approval conditions	Category 1 (high)	Category 2 (medium)	Category 3 (low)
Marketing status	Prescription	Prescription, veterinary feed directive	Prescription, veterinary feed directive, over the counter
Extralabel use	Restricted	Restricted in some cases	Permitted
Extent of use	Low	Low, medium	Low, medium, high
Postapproval monitoring (e.g., National Antimicrobial Resistance Monitoring System)	Yes	Yes	In certain cases
Advisory committee review considered	Yes	In certain cases	No

use designed to ensure it will not pose a human health risk. Table 4 illustrates the risk management options available, stratified by the level of risk.

Australia and the European Union have also published draft guidelines and guidelines, respectively, addressing antimicrobial resistance risks (2, 3). The objective of the EMEA guideline is to provide information to assess the potential impact of the use of a veterinary medicinal product on antimicrobial resistance in bacteria of animal origin with relevance to human health. The EMEA document also focuses primarily on food-borne bacteria from food-producing animals (2). The guideline requires baseline information similar to that described in the VICH guidance on antimicrobial resistance (15) and uses the importance of the antimicrobial veterinary medicinal products to human medicine and the potential exposure to assess whether additional studies are required. The EMEA guideline requires, depending upon the outcome of the initial information, animal studies designed to investigate the effect of the veterinary medicinal product on bacterial populations of the intestinal tract of target animals (2). The EMEA guideline incorporates VICH guideline GL27; the EMEA Committee for Medicinal Products for Veterinary Use is developing additional guidance on interpretation of data generated from VICH guideline GL27.

New Zealand has taken a slightly different approach to the approval of antimicrobial products, based on a prudent response in the absence of information on release, exposure, and human health consequences. New Zealand assumes that antibiotic resistance development may be possible but uncertain. The New Zealand process attempts to protect the efficacy of antimicrobial active ingredients essential for human health by putting safeguards on animal use, while ensuring information will be available about that use if particular concerns develop or trends in resistance appear. In addition to the basic veterinary prescription condition that establishes a point of control via veterinary involvement, it imposes criteria for use in animals and reporting obligations that are commensurate with existing knowledge of the human health significance of active ingredients and the potential for human exposure. This is balanced with the animal health significance of the active ingredients and the existence or absence of alternative therapeutic choices. The approval authorities for veterinary medicines and human medicines work closely to strike an acceptable compromise that protects both human and animal health as much as possible.

While ingestion is recognized as the most likely pathway to exposure, the decision process is equally appropriate for all other pathways. It also provides for pragmatic and prudent regulatory action while relevant information is being generated internationally and in New Zealand that would direct more-sensitive risk management. This approach works well for a country as small as New Zealand because almost no antimicrobial products are developed for New Zealand as the primary initial market. Data packages are usually prepared to meet the requirements of other regulatory jurisdictions, such as the FDA in the United States or the EMEA in the European Union. This highlights the value of initiatives such as VICH to harmonize information requirements and risk analysis methodologies.

Prior to 2000, the Agricultural Compounds and Veterinary Medicines (ACVM) Group of the New Zealand Food Safety Authority (NZFSA) followed international regulatory practices and did not assess antibacterial products for their potential to cause antibacterial resistance in animal pathogens or to contribute to the development of resistance in human pathogens. In 2000 the ACVM Group initiated a review of all currently approved antibiotic products relative to antibacterial resistance. The review of antibacterial active ingredients was based

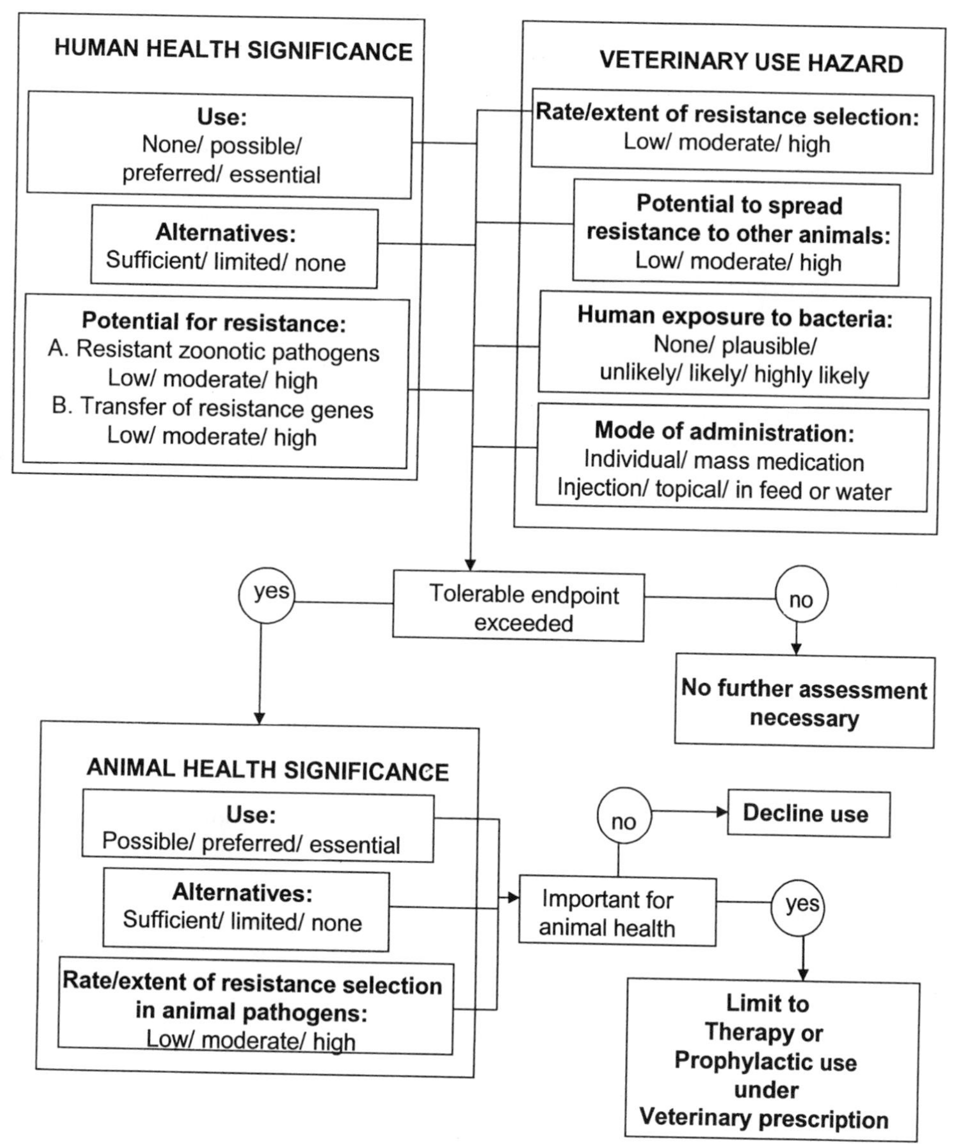

Figure 4. Antibiotic resistance review rationale of the ACVM Group, NZFSA.

on a multifactorial rationale (Fig. 4). The rationale considered (i) the relative importance of the active ingredient from a human health perspective, (ii) the likelihood that resistance could develop, (iii) the potential for human exposure via veterinary use, and (iv) the importance of the active ingredient from an animal health and welfare perspective.

The review has resulted in a classification of active ingredients relative to their significance to antibacterial resistance (see Table 3). Those of medium to high human health risk with veterinary use require active management of the potential for the development of antibacterial resistance. Those that are of no or low human health significance and for which there are no veterinary use hazards do not require active management of the potential for resistance from a human health perspective, but may still require management of resistance from an animal health and welfare perspective. The ACVM Group has published its information requirements for veterinary medicines. It has also set standards for chemistry, good manufacturing practices, animal safety, efficacy, and residues. These standards are available on the NZFSA/ACVM Group website (www.nzfsa.govt.nz/acvm).

The conditions on registration are the regulatory mechanism used in New Zealand to manage the risks associated with the use of antimicrobial products as veterinary medicines. If there are no residual animal health and welfare issues with regard to an active ingredient that is classified as of no concern from a human health perspective, a product can be made available to anyone without a veterinary prescription (i.e., over-the-counter sale). If there are remaining animal health or welfare concerns or the active ingredient is of even low human health concern, then the product is approved only under veterinary prescription.

The first level of the stratification (level 1) of the veterinary prescription condition requires the veterinarian to apply sound diagnosis and therapy competencies without specifically drawing attention to the management of antibacterial resistance. This level has been applied to products containing active ingredients of low human health concern.

Products containing active ingredients of medium to high human health importance attract a second level (level 2) of stratification, limiting the use to therapeutic purposes under which the prescribing veterinarian is satisfied that the active ingredient is likely to be the only effective treatment. The use is allowed because it has been determined that the use of the active ingredient is essential for the health and welfare of the animals.

The veterinarian is allowed to exercise discretion to use the product for prophylactic purposes if the potential disease challenge warrants it (i.e., animals in contact with sick animals have been exposed and are likely to have been infected). Use as a growth promoter is not an approved use. In some cases, the requirement for bacteriology is not practical and alternative management may be used by the prescribing veterinarian to achieve a level of confidence that the use of the product is essential.

Where it is considered essential to control the overall use of an antibacterial active ingredient even for therapeutic purposes, additional controls (level 3 stratification) are imposed to manage those uses. This level of control is equivalent to that applied to similar active ingredients that attract more stringent prescribing control on medical practitioners (e.g., restricted to hospital specialists). Their use would require the same controls as in the second level of stratification. In addition, all discretionary use for any purpose other than that specified on the label would be prohibited, and the prescribing veterinarian would have to notify the ACVM Group of every case in which the product was prescribed, giving the date, species of animal, and disease treated.

In 1999, in recognition of the level of international concern regarding the possible development of antibiotic resistance, the Ministry of Agriculture and Forestry convened the Antibiotic Resistance Steering Group to consider the most appropriate approach for New Zealand to take in its resistance management program. The Steering Group commissioned an expert panel to review the available information on antibiotic resistance as it related to the New Zealand situation and present a technical perspective with recommendations for management of the problem. The panel noted that there were very limited antibiotic resistance data available at the time, particularly with regard to confirming the potential for transferring resistance genes from animal-pathogenic or commensal bacteria to human pathogens. Its conclusions were:

- Not all antibiotics were equally relevant to the potential resistance problem.
- In the face of uncertainty, New Zealand should adopt a prudent use policy and review the present conditions on the use of particular antibiotic veterinary medicines.
- More-specific data were needed on the nature and prevalence of antibiotic resistance under New Zealand conditions, and surveillance programs should be adjusted and implemented accordingly.

In July 2004 the ACVM Group reconvened the Steering Group and is commissioning an expert panel to examine progress in resistance management in New Zealand, review developments in the collective knowledge about antibacterial resistance, and examine issues that were not addressed by the last expert panel, principally relating to uses of antibacterial veterinary medicines other than in feed. It is expected that, with the additional information now available, the Steering Group will be able to make recommendations to adjust the antibacterial resistance management program and the assessment of antibacterial substances with regard to their human health importance, veterinary use hazards, and animal health importance.

CONCLUSION

Licensing and approval of antimicrobials for use in animals, particularly food-producing animals, is a complex process involving considerations of efficacy, target animal safety, environmental safety, and human safety, including antimicrobial resistance. The approval process strives to ensure that the products are effective and safe and to manage the risks of adverse effects from their use. This chapter has attempted to demonstrate two principles:

1. Approval decisions are based on technically sound assessments of reliable information.

2. Standardization of data requirements, such as that undertaken by VICH, facilitates the approval process.

After veterinary drugs are licensed and marketed, surveillance is undertaken to ensure the continued safety and efficacy of the products. Most countries have established systems for the reporting of adverse drug reactions in animals, monitoring the concentration of residues in animal carcasses and foodstuffs, monitoring the prevalence of antimicrobial-resistant organisms, and monitoring the usage of antimicrobials. The postmarketing surveillance systems provide confidence that veterinary drugs are being used appropriately, without unexpected impact on animal or public health. The monitoring results also allow refinement of the preapproval assessment procedures for future applications when appropriate. Various monitoring systems relevant to veterinary antimicrobial drugs are discussed in more detail in several chapters of this book.

REFERENCES

1. **Cerniglia, C. E., and S. Kotarski.** 1999. Evaluation of veterinary drug residues in food for their potential to affect human intestinal microflora. *Regul. Toxicol. Pharmacol.* **29:** 238–261.
2. **The European Agency for the Evaluation of Medicinal Products.** 2002. Guidelines on pre-authorization studies to assess the potential for resistance resulting from the use of antimicrobial veterinary medicinal products. http://www.emea.eu.int/pdfs/vet/swp/024401en.pdf, accessed 16 February 2005.
3. **Expert Advisory Group on Antimicrobial Resistance.** Draft framework on risk assessment with respect to applications referred by the National Registration Authority for Agricultural and Veterinary Chemicals to NHMRC Expert Advisory Group on Antimicrobial Resistance. National Health and Medical Research Council, Canberra, Australia. http://www.nhmrc.gov.au/publications/_files/framwork.pdf, accessed 16 February 2005.
4. **Friedlander, L. G., S. D. Brynes, and A. H. Fernandez.** 1999. The human food safety evaluation of new animal drugs, p. 1–11. *In* L. Tollefson (ed.), *Chemical Food Borne Hazards and Their Control.* The W. B. Saunders Co., Philadelphia, Pa.
5. **Miller, M. A., and C. E. Eirkson.** 1997. Environmental assessments for animal drug products. *J. Vet. Pharmacol. Ther.* **20**(Suppl. 1)**:**323–325.
6. **Miller, M. A., and W. T. Flynn.** 2000. Regulation of antibiotic use in animals, p. 760–771. *In* J. F. Prescott, J. D. Baggot, and R. D. Walker (ed.), *Antimicrobial Therapy in Veterinary Medicine*, 3rd ed. Iowa State University Press, Ames.
7. **New Zealand Food Safety Authority.** 2000. Guidelines for risk assessment and hazard analysis under the Agricultural Compounds and Veterinary Medicines Act 1997, September–October 2000. http://www.nzfsa.govt.nz/acvm/publications/standards-guidelines/risk-hazard-guideline.pdf, accessed 16 February 2005.
8. **Tollefson, L., and M. A. Miller.** 2000. Antibiotic use in food animals: controlling the human health impact. *J. AOAC Int.* **83:**245–254.
9. **U.S. Food and Drug Administration, Center for Veterinary Medicine.** 1989. Guideline 33: Target animal safety guidelines for new animal drugs. http://www.fda.gov/cvm/guidance/guideline33.html, accessed 16 February 2005.
10. **U.S. Food and Drug Administration, Center for Veterinary Medicine.** 2003. Guidance for Industry #152: Evaluating the safety of antimicrobial new animal drugs with regard to their microbiological effects on bacteria of human health concern. http://www.fda.gov/cvm/antimicrobial/antimicrobial.html, accessed 16 February 2005.
11. **VICH (International Cooperation on Harmonisation of Technical Requirements for Registration of Veterinary Medicinal Products).** 2001. VICH Harmonized Tripartite Guideline GL6. Environmental impact assessment (EIAs) for veterinary medicinal products (VMPs)—Phase 1. http://vich.eudra.org/ htm/guidelines.htm.
12. **VICH (International Cooperation on Harmonisation of Technical Requirements for Registration of Veterinary Medicinal Products).** 2001. VICH Harmonized Tripartite Guideline GL9. Good Clinical Practice. http://vich.eudra.org/htm/guidelines.htm.
13. **VICH (International Cooperation on Harmonisation of Technical Requirements for Registration of Veterinary Medicinal Products).** 2001. VICH Harmonized Tripartite Guideline GL22. Studies to evaluate the safety of residues of veterinary drugs in human food: reproduction toxicity testing. http://vich.eudra.org/htm/guidelines.htm.
14. **VICH (International Cooperation on Harmonisation of Technical Requirements for Registration of Veterinary Medicinal Products).** 2001. VICH Harmonized Tripartite Guideline GL23. Studies to evaluate the safety of residues of veterinary drugs in human food: genotoxicity testing. http://vich.eudra.org/htm/guidelines.htm.
15. **VICH (International Cooperation on Harmonisation of Technical Requirements for Registration of Veterinary Medicinal Products).** 2003. VICH Harmonized Tripartite Guideline GL27. Guidance on pre-approval information for registration of new veterinary medicinal products for food producing animals with respect to antimicrobial resistance. http://vich.eudra.org/htm/guidelines.htm.
16. **VICH (International Cooperation on Harmonisation of Technical Requirements for Registration of Veterinary Medicinal Products).** 2002. VICH Harmonized Tripartite Guideline GL28. Studies to evaluate the safety of residues of veterinary drugs in human food: carcinogenicity testing. http://vich.eudra.org/htm/guidelines.htm.
17. **VICH (International Cooperation on Harmonisation of Technical Requirements for Registration of Veterinary Medicinal Products).** 2002. VICH Harmonized Tripartite Guideline GL31. Studies to evaluate the safety of residues of veterinary drugs in human food: repeat-dose (90-day) toxicity testing. http://vich.eudra.org/htm/guidelines.htm.
18. **VICH (International Cooperation on Harmonisation of Technical Requirements for Registration of Veterinary Medicinal Products).** 2002. VICH Harmonized Tripartite Guideline GL32. Studies to evaluate the safety of residues of veterinary drugs in human food: developmental toxicity testing. http://vich.eudra.org/htm/guidelines.htm.
19. **VICH (International Cooperation on Harmonisation of Technical Requirements for Registration of Veterinary Medicinal Products).** 2004. VICH Harmonized Tripartite Guideline GL33. Studies to evaluate the safety of residues of veterinary drugs in human food: general approach to testing. http://vich.eudra.org/htm/guidelines.htm.
20. **VICH (International Cooperation on Harmonisation of Technical Requirements for Registration of Veterinary Medicinal Products).** 2004. VICH Harmonized Tripartite Guideline GL36. Studies to evaluate the safety of residues of veterinary drugs in human food: general approach to establish a microbiological ADI. http://vich.eudra.org/htm/guidelines.htm.

21. **VICH (International Cooperation on Harmonisation of Technical Requirements for Registration of Veterinary Medicinal Products).** 2004. VICH Harmonized Tripartite Guideline GL37. Studies to evaluate the safety of residues of veterinary drugs in human food: repeat-dose (chronic) toxicity testing. http://vich.eudra.org/htm/guidelines.htm.

22. **VICH (International Cooperation on Harmonisation of Technical Requirements for Registration of Veterinary Medicinal Products).** 2003. VICH Harmonized Tripartite Guideline GL38. Draft environmental impact assessment (EIAs) for veterinary medicinal products (VMPs)—Phase II. http://vich.eudra.org/htm/guidelines.htm.

Antimicrobial Resistance in Bacteria of Animal Origin
Edited by Frank M. Aarestrup
© 2006 ASM Press, Washington, D.C.

Chapter 22

Monitoring of Antimicrobial Drug Usage in Animals: Methods and Applications

KARI GRAVE, VIBEKE FRØKJÆR JENSEN, SCOTT MCEWEN, AND HILDE KRUSE

Data on antimicrobial drug usage play a key role in the development of national and international policies for containment of antimicrobial resistance. Therefore, the Food and Agriculture Organization (FAO) of the United Nations, the Office International des Épizooties (OIE), and the World Health Organization (WHO) have recommended that each country should implement a monitoring program, under the responsibility of a competent national authority, in order to assess the usage of antimicrobial agents in animals (39, 45–47, 49). These recommendations are supported by the European Union (2, 3, 5).

The purposes of monitoring usage of antimicrobials in animals are manifold, and data obtained by such monitoring may be used (i) to compare usage of antimicrobials between and within countries and between time periods, etc.; (ii) to aid interpretation of patterns and trends regarding antimicrobial resistance and residues; (iii) as a basis for risk assessment regarding antimicrobial drug resistance and residues; (iv) as a basis for decision making regarding control measures; (v) as a basis for evaluation of the effectiveness of control measures being implemented; (vi) to assess the spread and effect of antimicrobial drug pollution of the environment; (vii) as a basis for focused and targeted research and development; and [illegible]

[illegible] dairy cattle and beef cattle), and usage at herd level (3, 5, 48). The level of detail required in a monitoring program and the methods applied to express the data depend on the purposes (39, 49).

Designing a monitoring system for antimicrobial usage in animals requires consideration of several major aspects, including the main purposes of monitoring usage, the appropriate data sources, the drug classification system to be used, the appropriate unit of measurement, and methods to express the data. The main aims of this chapter are to evaluate the usefulness and limitations of the various sources of input data, to discuss how usage should be expressed in order to comply with the various purposes of monitoring, and to present examples on the application of data obtained through various monitoring programs. A few examples of how to validate usage data are also discussed (in the discussion of data collection).

DATA COLLECTION

The infrastructure and legislation for drug dispensing varies considerably between countries, affecting the possibilities for and quality of data collection on antimicrobial drug usage. Consequently, such data collection cannot rely on a common, internationally standardized data source (Tables 1 and 2).

Overall National Sales

Overall national sales data for the various antimicrobial drugs may be obtained from the following sources: import and export registrations, manufacturers, wholesalers, feed mills, and pharmacies (Table 1). Data may be derived from customs declarations

[illegible] logy, Norwegian School of Veterinary Science, N-0033 Oslo, Norway. [illegible] Assessment, Danish Institute for Food and Veterinary Research, DK-2860 [illegible] tion Medicine, Ontario Veterinary College, University of Guelph, Guelph, [illegible] n Zoonosis Center, National Veterinary Institute, N-0033 Oslo, Norway.

Table 1. Expression and application of overall national sales data on veterinary AMs derived from various sources[a]

Data outcome	Expression of data per drug or drug class	Information outcome	Application or uses
Overall sale, regional sale, etc.	Overall wt of active substance. Should be published together with no. of major animal species liable to be treated	Overall national and/or regional usage	As a basis for rough evaluations of campaigns on prudent use, etc. To validate usage data obtained from other sources As a basis for correlation with national data on resistance prevalences and patterns
Sales per species	Wt of active substance/1,000 animals/time period	Estimates on usage of AMs formulated for one animal species or animal species and indication, e.g., farmed salmonids	As a basis for rough evaluations of campaigns on prudent use, etc., in relevant species To validate usage data obtained from other sources As a basis to assess trends in resistance prevalences and patterns in relevant species
	No. of doses[b]/1,000 animals/time period	Dose-corrected species estimates of usage of AMs formulated for one animal species or animal species and indication	As a basis for evaluations of campaigns on prudent use, etc., in relevant species To validate usage data obtained from other sources As a basis to assess trends in resistance prevalences and patterns in relevant species As a basis for design of residue control programs in relevant species
	No. of course doses[c]/1,000 animals/time period	Dose- and treatment length-corrected species estimates of usage of AMs formulated for one animal species or animal species and indication	As a basis for evaluations of campaigns on prudent use, etc., in relevant species To validate usage data obtained from other sources As a basis to assess trends in resistance prevalences and patterns in relevant species As a basis for design of residue control programs in relevant species
	Treatment rates, proportion treated	Species estimates on treatment and exposure prevalences and patterns	As a basis for evaluations of campaigns on prudent use, etc., in relevant species As a basis to explain trends in resistance prevalences and patterns in relevant species As a basis for risk assessment of resistance (correlation studies) in relevant species As a basis for design of residue control programs; may be validated against, e.g., disease rates

[a]Data sources are wholesalers, manufacturers, pharmacies, importers, and exporters. AMs, antimicrobial drugs.
[b]Doses: ADD (national approved dose or daily dose recommended in the literature for off-label drugs) per animal or age group.
[c]Course doses: ACD (national approved course dose or daily course dose recommended in the literature for off-label drugs) per animal or age group.

f stratified data on veterinary AM usage in animals derived from pharmacies, feed mills, veterinarians, and/or farmers[a]

Information outcome	Application or uses
Ms per animal species population studied tional and herd level	As a basis for evaluations of campaigns on prudent use, etc., in relevant species As a basis to assess trends in resistance prevalences and patterns (species, age group, and national and herd levels)
rate data on treatment and exposure patterns opulation studied per country, herd level, and	As a basis for evaluations of campaigns on prudent use, etc., in relevant species As a basis to assess trends in resistance prevalences and patterns (species, age group, and national and herd levels) As a basis for risk-based AM residue control
period-corrected, accurate data on treatment rns in animal species population studied vel, and age group	As a basis for evaluations of campaigns on prudent use, etc., in relevant species As a basis to assess trends in resistance prevalences and patterns (species, age group, and national and herd levels) As a basis for risk-based AM residue control
period-corrected, accurate data on treatment ; treated in a defined animal species population vel, and age group	To evaluate campaigns on prudent use and other incentives As a basis to assess trends in resistance prevalences and patterns (species, age group, herd level, nationally, and regionally) As a basis for risk assessment on resistance (case-control and cohort studies) As a basis for risk-based residue control at herd level; may be validated against, e.g., regional or national disease rates

nd/or at herd level. AM, antimicrobial drug.
in the literature for off-label drugs) per animal or age group.
e dose recommended in the literature for off-label drugs) per animal or age group.

(import data), invoices, sales statistics, etc., and collected by use of questionnaires (e.g., electronically by use of spreadsheets). The study protocol and the questionnaire have to be designed to accurately specify the antimicrobial drugs to be included (see "Identification and Classification of Antimicrobials" below). The possible applications of overall national usage data are discussed in Table 1.

As sales data from wholesalers, manufacturers, and feed mills usually are available, and at relatively low cost, it should be possible for most countries to get access to aggregated national data on usage of antimicrobials in animals. Aggregated national data do not provide information specific to the various animal species because the antimicrobial drugs often are approved for several animal species. However, estimates on usage of antimicrobials in selected animal species may be calculated based on sales statistics for specific drugs and formulations, provided these preparations are species specific (Table 1). Such data have been published from France, Norway, and Sweden (6, 9, 10, 26–28, 30, 40). This approach could be an option in developing countries with limited resources for the implementation of monitoring programs that encompass total national usage.

In countries where antimicrobial drugs are available only by prescription and dispensed only through pharmacies, national sales data may be obtained through pharmacies. National sales data may be stratified according to defined geographical areas, e.g., municipalities and counties, if permitted by the structure of the national drug distribution system. In countries where the infrastructure permits capture of more-detailed national data (e.g., brand name, strength, formulation, and package size), additional information can cascade from this. This includes usage in weight of active ingredients of the various therapeutic groups, split into, for example, usage per route of administration (37).

Usage per Species, at Herd Level, etc.

More-sophisticated monitoring systems might make use of stratified data that provide information on antimicrobial usage in various animal species, in different age groups, per indication, at herd level, and in various regions and time periods. Data sources for the collection of such data may include pharmacies, veterinarians, feed mills, and farmers. The possible applications of stratified data on antimicrobial drug usage by species, by age group, and at herd level are summarized in Table 2.

In countries where veterinary antimicrobials are available by prescription only and have to be dispensed through pharmacies and feed mills (medicated feed for therapeutic use), e.g., Denmark, Norway, and Sweden, prescription data may be obtained through these sources (33, 42). Because prescription data usually are computerized automatically as part of the drug dispensing, such data provide accurate information on amounts of the different antimicrobials actually dispensed for use in the various animal species, including prescriptions of antimicrobial drugs registered for use in humans. Such prescription data can be validated against national sales data collected from wholesalers, the pharmaceutical industry, etc.

In countries without mandatory reporting of antimicrobial usage, either at the pharmacy level or by veterinarians or farmers, a voluntary data collection system is required for monitoring drug usage. For logistical reasons, collecting data from a subset, e.g., a representative sample of "sentinel" veterinarians or farms, may be the only feasible method. A compromise may have to be struck between enrolling volunteers who are willing and able to collect and report accurate data and those who are representative of the target group. In these circumstances, some financial compensation may be helpful in obtaining representative data, unless collection of reliable drug use data is already being conducted for other reasons, e.g., billing purposes for veterinarians or quality assurance on farms. A rough estimate of usage in various species or age groups could probably be obtained by combining national sales data (on package and formulation level) with surveys involving sentinel veterinary practices and/or farms.

Data on antimicrobial drug usage collected from veterinarians and farmers may give information about dosage schemes and usage per species, per age group, by indication, and at herd level (15, 22, 23). However, collecting and processing valid data from veterinarians and farmers on a continuous basis may be an inefficient and expensive process unless carefully designed and well managed. Ideally, reporting by veterinarians and farmers should utilize computerized reporting systems to be fully efficient and at a tolerable cost. If feasible, these systems should be compatible with existing data collection systems (e.g., billing and medical records) to encourage compliance. For example, the Danish monitoring system (VetStat) for antimicrobial usage in animals makes use of veterinarians' invoices to farmers in order to obtain information on veterinarians' use and sales of antimicrobials for food animals in their practices (11, 42). The computerized journal and billing system used by Danish veterinary practitioners is constructed to automatically create a file that contains information on drug usage per animal species, per age group, by indication, and at herd level. Such invoices have the potential to provide accurate descriptions of usage because it is in the interest of both the supplying veterinarian and the farmer that the invoice is correct. Furthermore, to send out invoices is crucial for getting paid for the consultation and the drugs dispensed. Thus, this data source is thought to be representative of overall prescription usage by veterinarians in their practices, provided that the electronic transfer is reliable. The data reported by the veterinarians should be validated against data from, e.g., pharmacies, the pharmaceutical industry, or wholesalers, regarding dispensing to the veterinarians' practices.

Data on antimicrobial drug usage could also be collected by the use of questionnaires to veterinarians or farmers. Such data may be biased by low return and/or response rates (22). Various approaches have been used to elicit this information from farmers, including surveys and implementation of on-farm recording systems for defined periods of time. Cross-sectional surveys, conducted either by mail or personal interview, have been useful for collection of qualitative data on antimicrobial usage (4, 24). For example, these types of surveys can identify the drugs that are used for various age groups of animals on farms, as well as farmer policies governing over-the-counter treatment practices (where permitted) and group or individual treatment practices. Such studies do not, however, provide quantitative data on antimicrobial usage. To obtain quantitative data, longitudinal studies employing on-farm recording systems are required. One approach is to devise treatment diaries, charts, or computer programs to facilitate treatment recording, with independent collection of empty drug bottles or containers for validation of data recording. Unfortunately, it has been shown that on-farm recording can be unreliable and significantly underestimate the quantities of drugs used on a farm (23).

Collection of stratified data from the various sources can be [illegible]

moters, through collection of sales figures or data from invoices, subdivided into animal species, age group, and herd identity. Data may be derived from computerized invoices.

4. Farmers: Data on amounts administered by the veterinarian or farmer derived from on-farm records and data on purchased amounts derived from invoices.

Data may be collected through questionnaires, and the study protocol as well as the questionnaires (e.g., by use of spreadsheets) have to be designed to accurately specify the antimicrobial drug groups to be included (see "Identification and Classification of Antimicrobials" below).

Antimicrobial drug usage data based on sales data, prescriptions, records, and invoices may not necessarily equate with animal intake. Such data may be biased by the fact that not all the drug dosages sold are actually used or they are used differently than prescribed, e.g., because of farmers' noncompliance.

IDENTIFICATION AND CLASSIFICATION OF ANTIMICROBIALS

Ideally, all antimicrobial ingredients and classes of antimicrobials used in animals should be included in a monitoring program on antimicrobial drug usage. Because coccidiostats, such as the ionophores (18, 25, 34), may also possess antibacterial properties, such feed additives should also be included. In countries with limited resources, it might be imperative to decide what classes of antimicrobials should be considered, e.g., those of critical importance to human and animal health (50).

To enable comparability of antimicrobial usage data between countries, between time periods, [illegible] and each drug is classified at five different levels. The complete classification of ampicillin illustrates the structure of the code (Q indicates a veterinary drug):

- QJ: anti-infectives for systemic use (first level, anatomical main group)
- QJ01: antibacterials for systemic use (second level, therapeutic subgroup)
- QJ01C: β-lactam antibacterials, penicillins (third level, pharmacological subgroup)
- QJ01CA: penicillins with extended spectrum (fourth level, chemical subgroup)
- QJ01CA01: ampicillin (fifth level, chemical subgroup)

Thus, in the ATCvet system all plain ampicillin preparations are given the code QJ01CA01. Accordingly, sales data representing this will comprise sales of all veterinary formulations (e.g., injections, mixtures, premixes, tablets, and oral pastes) and package sizes of ampicillin for systemic use. As each formulation and each package size contain various amounts of drugs, data have to be collected at the fifth level to make possible calculation and expression of usage data in a meaningful way, e.g., in weight of active substances, doses, or course doses (see "Units of Measurement" below). To obtain the complete data on usage of ampicillin in animals, preparations approved for human use and belonging to ATC code J01CA01 also have to be included if prescribed for use in animals.

Due to confidentiality concerns and to avoid overly complicated data presentation, data should preferably be presented to express the third or fourth level of the ATCvet system and not the fifth level. Which of these levels should be selected depends on the purpose of the monitoring. If, for example, usage data for fluoroquinolones (QJ01MA) are presented at the third level, data will be presented as quinolone antibacterials (ATCvet code QJ01M). Presentation of data on this level makes it impossible to follow trends in the usage of fluoroquinolones in different countries (it hinders transparency) and will also hamper analysis of prevalences and trends in the development of resistance to fluoroquinolones. On the other hand, if only one pharmaceutical company has marketed preparations of a specific chemical substance (e.g., fluoroquinolones) or the company's market share is known to be high, publishing fourth-level data may create confidentiality problems similar to when presenting data on the fifth level. Therefore, how to present data obtained from the pharmaceutical industry should always be agreed upon before data are collected.

UNITS OF MEASUREMENT

Antimicrobial drug usage may be recorded and reported in terms of (i) cost; (ii) volume, e.g., number of packages or tablets; (iii) number of prescriptions issued or dispensed; (iv) weight of active ingredient; (v) doses; and (vi) course doses (Tables 1 and 2). The amounts should, whenever possible, be presented with information on the corresponding population.

National and international comparisons based on cost parameters or numbers of packages or tablets sold are not useful for the evaluation of antimicrobial drug usage in an epidemiological context, such as antimicrobial resistance epidemiology (20, 21). Numbers of prescriptions give useful information on total usage only if the total amounts of drugs per prescription and the number of animals to be treated are also known. However, numbers of prescriptions may be valuable for measuring the frequency of prescribing, for example, for various animal species, age groups (e.g., weaning pigs), or indications, as well as assessing trends and changes in prescribing behavior.

At a minimum, usage data should be expressed in terms of the annual weight (in kilograms) of the active ingredients or classes of antimicrobials that are used (39, 47). This information may be used to evaluate the effect of measures that have been implemented and as a rough estimate of the selection pressure imposed on the national level. The application of such data is shown in Table 1.

The dosages of various antimicrobials may vary considerably depending on, e.g., potency, pharmacokinetic characteristics, formulation, MICs, and disease. In order to adjust for the differences in dosages between the various antimicrobials and formulations and to facilitate comparisons between populations (countries, time periods, etc.), the data on usage per animal species might be calculated to express numbers of daily doses used. The defined daily dose (DDD) is a unit of measurement assigned by the WHO International Working Group for Drug Statistics Methodology that allows for comparisons of drug use in humans. The DDD is defined as "the assumed average maintenance dose per day for the drug used for its main indication in adults" (12, 20). DDDs are only assigned for approved indications, and thus DDDs for off-label use are not set. It is important to emphasize that DDD values are not statistically determined and have to be looked at merely as technical units of measurement. DDD values are nearly always a compromise (judgment) based on review of available information, including dosages approved in various countries. Furthermore, they reflect global doses (12). Consequently, DDDs will be more or less in accordance with the doses used in everyday practice in the relevant country. Conversion of aggregate usage data to DDD may thereby create over- or underestimates of usage. For example, if a large difference exists between the DDD value and the dosage usually prescribed in practice for a substance with a high proportional use, this would significantly influence the overall usage estimates.

As a general rule, DDDs for human drugs are not changed unless they are at least on the order of 50% of the assigned DDD value, but minor alterations may be implemented for important drugs that are frequently used and when the DDDs are revised every third year (12).

Only a limited number of papers validating DDD as a unit of measurement for drug usage monitoring in human medicine have been published, of which only a few have addressed antimicrobials (19, 31, 35, 44). The results from these studies indicate significant differences between the DDD and the national prescribed daily dose (PDD) values for the country in question for several antimicrobial drugs. However, the small number of studies makes it difficult to draw any conclusions. In a study by Monnet et al. (38) performed in 11 European countries, a strong correlation was found between the number of DDDs sold per 1,000 inhabitant-days and the number of prescriptions of antimicrobial drugs. As this study involved human medicine and only European countries, these findings cannot be transferred to other regions of the world or to veterinary medicine without further documentation.

International animal DDDs have not been established for veterinary drugs. In 2003 the ATCvet Working Group appointed by the WHO Collaborating Centre for Drug Statistics Methodology initiated a pilot project that aimed to develop guidelines for the assessment of DDDs for veterinary drugs and to assign DDDs for a selection of veterinary an-

"DDD" is established as a term in human medicine for internationally agreed-upon values and is "owned" by the WHO Collaborating Centre for Drug Statistics Methodology (www.whocc.no). Because of this and to avoid further confusion, this term should not be used as an expression for other, similar units in veterinary medicine.

Another approach is to make use of nationally defined animal daily doses (hereafter designated as ADDs), based upon nationally approved or recommended (off-label use) doses, as a unit of measurement to correct for dosage variations between the various antimicrobials. This unit is used in the Danish monitoring program on antimicrobial usage in animals (11, 33). Grave et al. (30) used the term "DDD" to describe changes in the prescribing patterns for antimicrobial drugs in necrotic enteritis in broilers in Norway after the avoparcin ban. In principle, the DDDs applied in that study were ADDs.

Since ADDs are based upon nationally approved or recommended dosages, the values are thought to be close to the dosages of the drugs used in everyday practice. As the ADDs are set on a national level, it is likely that a major change in nationally approved dosages will be implemented more rapidly in the monitoring programs compared to a change in the corresponding DDD values, which are set on an international level. Another advantage of the ADD model is that, unlike DDDs, which are only assigned for approved indications and/or animal species, ADDs may also be assigned for antimicrobials used off label. Such ADDs may be set based on recommended doses of similar products and/or on information from pharmacological literature (33).

Another option for standardization could be to apply the PDD as the unit of measurement for antimicrobial drug usage in animals (15, 22). The PDDs for veterinary antimicrobials may be cal-

PDD should be complementary units of measurement for the assessment of antimicrobial usage in animals. As the assignment of DDDs for veterinary drugs has been postponed, we recommend that ADD and PDD should be the selected dosage units for assessment of data on usage of veterinary antimicrobial drugs.

As the dose for an antimicrobial drug substance may vary between injectable, oral, and intramammary preparations and sometimes also according to the indication for which it is used, the defined ADD for an antimicrobial drug may have to be set differently for the various formulations and indications.

The DDD values assigned in human medicine are based on adult doses, and there is no account taken for variation in body weight. Many food animals are slaughtered before reaching adulthood (e.g., slaughter chickens and fattening pigs), and therefore adult doses seem inappropriate. As regards dogs, body weight varies considerably between breeds. It is therefore recommended to set the ADD and PDD for veterinary antimicrobials per kilogram (live weight) as base units (ADD_{kg} and PDD_{kg}); such values represent nationally assigned (approved or recommended) and prescribed doses, respectively, for a drug substance and formulation to be used per kilogram (live weight) of the animal. The corresponding values, $ADD_{age\ group}$ and $PDD_{age\ group}$, for the various age groups and production stages (e.g., weaning pigs, sows, and finishers) can then be calculated based on the ADD_{kg} (or PDD_{kg}), as exemplified by the Danish surveillance system VetStat (Tables 3 and 4). The age

Table 3. Usage of antimicrobials in Denmark[a]

Species	Age group	Defined body wt (kg)	Amt of active substance (kg), 2003	ADDs (10^3) in pharmacies and feed mills, 2003	ADDs (10^3) in veterinary practices, 2003[b]
Pigs	Sows and piglets	200	23,229	8,474	57
	Weaners	15	29,518	160,532	592
	Finisher pigs	50	26,536	44,655	465
	Age not given	50	1,649	2,806	1
Cattle	Cows and bulls	600	178	51	1,848
	Intramammaries[c]	600	381	1,141	
	Calves (<12 mo)	100	1,603	1,155	476
	Heifers, steers (12 mo)	300	28	7	65
	Age not given	600	172	20	0
Small ruminants	>12 mo	50	17	21	4
	<12 mo	20	1	4	5
	Age not given	50	32	27	0
Poultry	Broilers	1	32	1,955	2,216
	Layers	1	23	1,617	338
	Rearing flocks	1	65	1,889	141
	Game birds	1	57	1,793	1
	Ducks and geese	1	11	404	0
	Turkeys	20	66	232	336
	Production type not given	1	12	496	0
Horses	Age not given	500	112	10	NC
Mink (ADD)	Age not given	1	770	39,400	4,289
Aquaculture	Age not given	1	3,560[d]	NC	NC
Other production animals	Intramammaries[e]	Unknown	81	1,324	0
	Age not given	1		NC	36
Pet animals	Intramammaries[e]	Unknown	310	1,229	
	Age not given	1		NC	NR
ADD not defined[f]			101		
Species not given[g]	kg of active compound[h]		14,695		
Total (kg)			103,241		

[a]Data are based on sales from pharmacies and feed mills and on use in veterinary practice reported by veterinarians (11). NC, not calculated (species not given or ADD not defined); NR, not reported.
[b]Data are incomplete.
[c]Intramammaries used in practice, i.e., species not given. Used almost entirely in cows.
[d]Quinolones and sulfonamide-trimethoprim used in aquaculture practice are included with the data from pharmacies.
[e]A daily dose of intramammaries is given for an individual animal, irrespective of age groups or body weight.
[f]Includes drugs where ADD is not given for the recipient species (mostly topical drugs).
[g]Species not given at the pharmacy, i.e., mainly for use in practice (14,015 kg; intramammaries excluded).
[h]The amounts used are given in kilograms of active compound because the species and age group are not known.

Table 4. Usage in Denmark of antimicrobials in pigs[a]

ADD(10^3) for indicated age group and defined wt of animal											
Pharmacies and feed mills								Veterinary practices, 2003[b]		
ſows, piglets (200 kg)		Weaners (15 kg)		Finishers (50 kg)		Age not given (50 kg)		Sows, piglets (200 kg)	Weaners (15 kg)	Finishers (50 kg)
2	2003	2002	2003	2002	2003	2002	2003			
	914	32,133	32,367	8,722	11,119	461	545	9	162	108
.2	6	3	84		22	1	3	0	0.1	0.2
	2,012	2,514	2,894	4,587	5,117	239	313	13	49	102
	1,117	9,956	12,712	2,146	2,418	162	224	8	70	61
	99	146	254	36	56	3	4	6	1	5
	1,083	3,965	4,145	203	173	101	129	5	9	15
	729	46,405	41,201	11,593	12,242	609	695	3	41	72
	579	17,468	19,791	3,814	4,407	187	233	3	70	36
	238	23,939	22,207	224	193	78	98	3	54	10
	23	2,108	2,909	14	18	6	18	0.2	11	1
	21	182	11	67	5	2	0	3	7	1
	703	2,150	2,210	349	422	34	51	4	17	8
	945	18,226	19,749	7,539	8,462	330	492	2	102	47
	4	1	1	1	0.5	0	0.2	0	0	0
	0.1	0	0	0	0	0	0	0	0	0
	8,474	159,196	160,532	39,295	44,655	2,211	2,806	57	592	465

70% of the amounts sold for use in veterinary practices were not reported in 2002.

groups should be defined by weight classes (an estimated average weight at treatment). For the purpose of transparency, the ADD values and the defined weight classes for the various age groups should be published together with the usage data.

The proportional use of the various drug classes may vary substantially depending on the unit of measurement used (weight of active substance or ADD_{kg}), as exemplified in Fig. 1. For example, the proportional usage of tetracyclines in pigs in Denmark amounted to 20 and 31% when usage data were expressed in ADDs per kilogram live weight of the animal and as weight of active substance, respectively, while the corresponding figures for macrolides were 23 and 12%.

The length of the recommended treatment period may also vary substantially between antimicrobial drugs and between countries (22). To correct for this, total course dose has been introduced as unit of measurement for antimicrobial usage (26, 27, 30, 32). Course doses should be assigned per kilogram (live weight) of the animal species or age group of the relevant species and be based on the corresponding ADD_{kg} or $ADD_{age\ group}$, respectively, for the relevant animal species and drug formulations (if relevant, also by indication). The values for the treatment period used should be nationally approved or from recommendations in the literature (off-label use) and preferably be validated on a regular basis against data on nationally prescribed treatment periods. Here, we introduce the units nationally defined animal course dose (ACD_{kg} or $ACD_{age\ group}$) and prescribed animal course dose (PCD_{kg} or $PCD_{age\ group}$) as units of measurement for antimicrobial drug usage in animals. If PCDs (derived from prescriptions) are available and are representative for the study population, these values are thought to be relatively similar to what is actually prescribed in practice and would therefore be the more accurate values, i.e., closer to the applied doses. However, for the purpose of continuous monitoring programs of usage, both PDD and PCD values are considered to be too expensive to obtain and are only recommended to be collected for the validation of other units of measurements (e.g., ADDs and ACDs), as well as for analytical pharmacoepidemiological studies (case-control and cohort studies) where accurate data on exposure are vital.

With regard to farmed fish, drugs are almost exclusively administered through the feed. Because fish are exothermic, feed intake varies with temperature and the total amount of feed-added therapeutic antimicrobials is prescribed (rather than a daily dosage scheme). Thus, none of the daily dose terms described above (PDDs and ADDs) is applicable as a unit of measurement for antimicrobial drug usage in

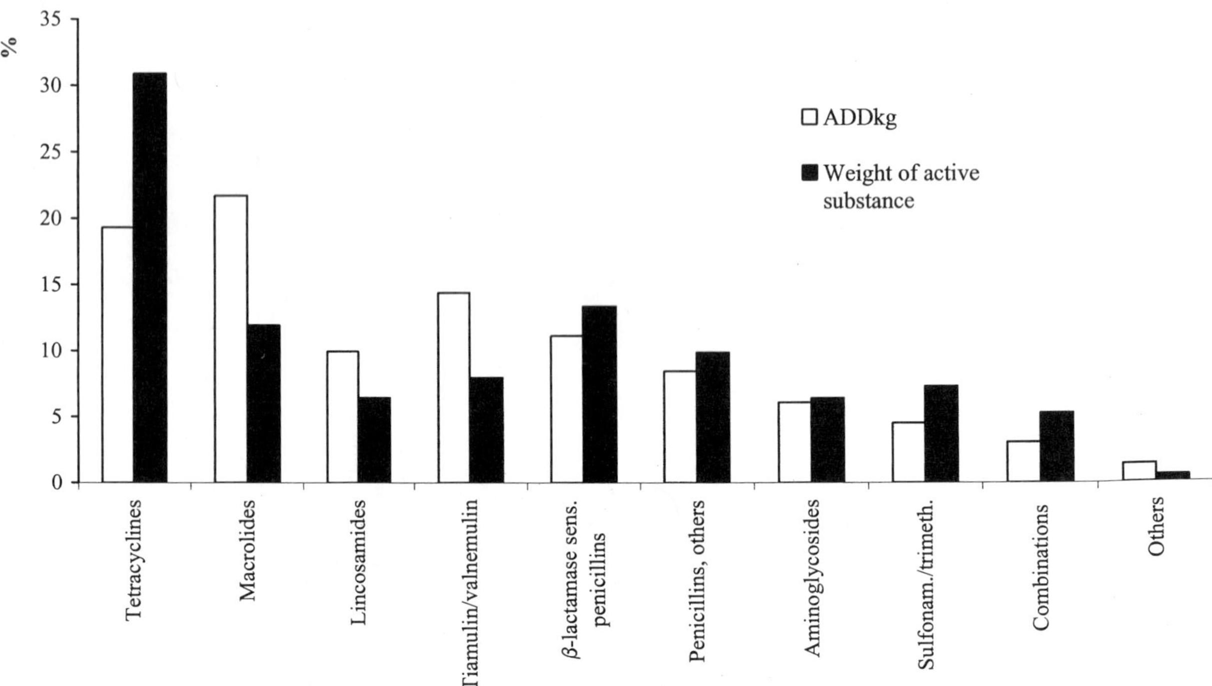

Figure 1. Proportional use of veterinary antimicrobials in pigs in 2003 expressed as ADD_{kg} and as weight of active substance. "Others" category includes cephalosporins, fluoroquinolones, and amphenicols. Data are derived from VetStat (42). Figure developed by Vibeke Frøkjær Jensen.

farmed fish. It is therefore recommended that course dose (ACD_{kg} or PCD_{kg}) be selected as the unit of measurement for these species (26, 27). Fish farmers are thought to utilize the complete amount of medicated feed for economic reasons, and thus "farmed fish" course doses are considered to be rather precise.

For reporting purposes, data on usage of antimicrobial growth promoters (AGPs) and coccidiostat feed additives (CFAs) may be given in terms of total weight of active ingredient stratified by animal species, as recommended by the FAO, OIE, and WHO (39, 49).

DATA ANALYSIS AND REPORTING

Antimicrobial Drugs

In human medicine, overall national drug sales figures are presented, e.g., in terms of number of DDDs per 1,000 inhabitants per day, and this figure takes into account both the variations in the dosages between substances and the size of the population liable to be treated (12). For example, an estimated consumption of 25 DDDs/1,000 inhabitants/day for a drug corresponds to a use of this drug by 2.5% of the population at any given day. This term has also been applied for the expression of antimicrobial drug usage in animals (9, 28). However, prevalence of drug usage is only considered to be an appropriate epidemiological term for drugs applied for the treatment for chronic diseases. For drugs used as short courses or intermittently used drugs, e.g., antimicrobial drugs, usage should ideally be given in terms of treatment rates per species and ideally also age groups, e.g., number of weaning pigs treated per number of weaning pigs liable to be treated per time period.

Usage of antimicrobials in selected food-producing animal species should, if possible, be calculated to express doses per number of animal species and per age group, e.g., weaning pigs. This will allow for comparison of usage between, for example, time periods and countries. Furthermore, such data are useful for the interpretation of trends in the usage patterns of antimicrobials in various animal species, as well as for the correlation with antimicrobial resistance prevalences and patterns (Tables 1 and 2). In the Danish Integrated Antimicrobial Resistance Monitoring and Research Programme (DANMAP), annual usage of antimicrobial drugs in animals is expressed in terms of both numbers of ADDs per kilogram per species and per defined animal body weight per age group (animal body weight has to be defined for each age group, e.g., weaning pigs) (11). Such data can also be adjusted for number of animals liable to be treated. From 2001 to 2003 the total use of antimicrobials in pigs in Denmark increased by 11% when expressed as weight of active substance per pig produced (Fig. 2), while the increase was only 6% when expressed in ADD_{kg} per pig produced.

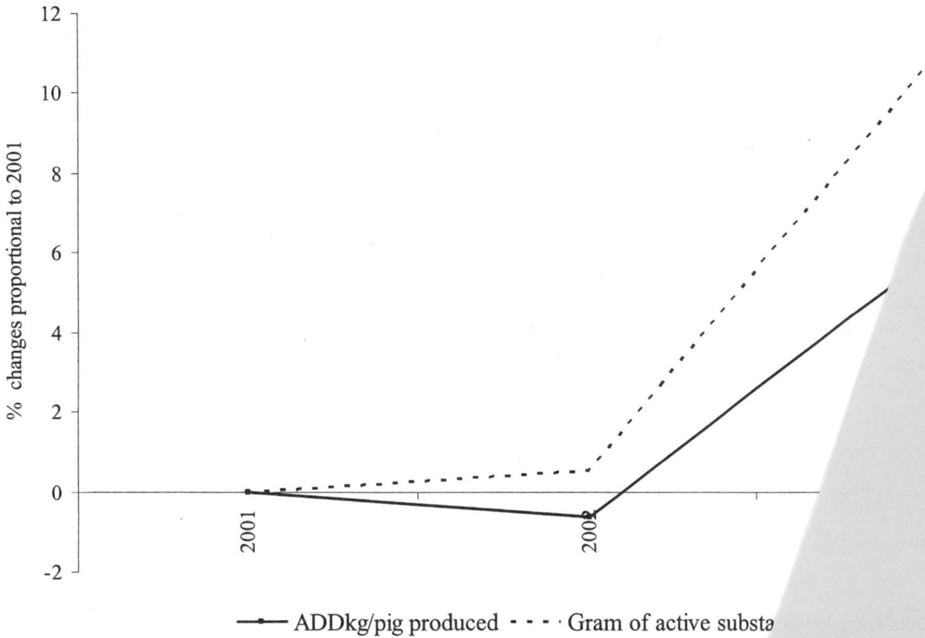

Figure 2. Percent changes in sales of antimicrobial drugs for pig production in Denm[illegible] duced and in weight of active substance. Data are derived from VetStat (42). Figure [illegible]

Number of course doses of antimicrobial drugs sold per animal species and age group in a defined time period reflects numbers of animals in a specific age group treated and may easily be converted to express treatment frequencies if the number of animals liable to be treated is available. The (cumulative) antimicrobial treatment rates split into classes of antimicrobial drugs could be expressed in terms of number of PCDs (per kilogram of body weight) or ACDs (per kilogram of body weight) per 1,000 animals per time period (e.g., year or animal days) per relevant animal species and age group (30). The advantage is that such data may be validated against data on disease or treatment frequencies, e.g., mastitis in dairy cattle (41). In Norway mastitis in cattle is usually treated with one initial intramuscular injection followed by one intramammary injector in the affected quarter for four subsequent days. As the average number of quarters affected is two (O. Østerås, personal communication), eight intramammaries normally constitute one cow mastitis course. Consequently, the annual number of intramammaries sold reflects the annual number of cows treated against mastitis (annual number of intramammaries sold/8 = number of course doses sold = number of cows treated) and enables calculations of treatment rates. Data on treatment rates of mastitis in Norway can be derived from the annual reports of the Norwegian Cattle Health Service, which comprise on average 90% of the dairy cattle in Norway. Calculated treatment rates (numbers of course doses sold per number of animals liable to be treated) of mastitis in dairy cattle in Norway versus reported treatment rates is shown in Fig. 3. It should be emphasized that the calculated treatment rates are slightly higher than the reported values because relapses within 9 days are not reported to the Norwegian Cattle Health Service but also because this formulation is used to a lesser extent in sheep and dairy goats.

In fish farming, national statistics on farmed fish produced are given as biomass of fish slaughtered or sold and not as number of fish slaughtered or sold. Biomass is a figure that is also useful in the everyday management in fish farms to facilitate calculation of the optimal amount of feed to be given daily in each net pen. A pragmatic approach to correct for changes in the denominator (amounts of farmed fish liable to be treated) might therefore be to correlate calculated annual biomass of farmed fish treated with antimicrobial drugs to the biomass of farmed fish slaughtered. Annual biomass of farmed salmonids treated could be calculated by use of the following formula: Weight of active substance sold annually/course dose (in weight) per metric weight farmed fish (Fig. 4). As antimicrobial drug formulations administered orally in farmed fish are highly specific for these species, national sales figures on such drugs are thought to be representative of the amounts of antimicrobials used in these species.

In some countries, many of the antimicrobial drugs are not species specific, and furthermore, statistics on numbers of animals liable to be treated are difficult or impossible to obtain or not believed to be

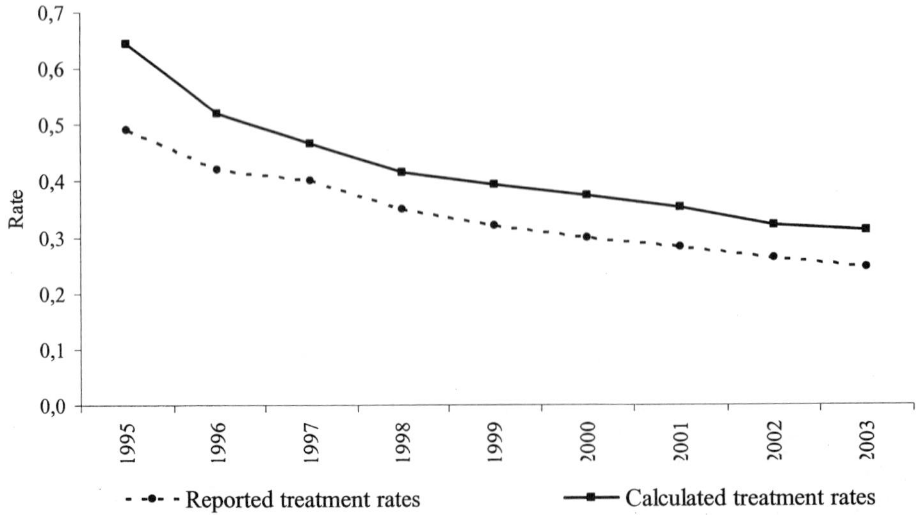

Figure 3. Calculated treatment rates (number of course doses sold/number of animals liable to be treated) of mastitis in dairy cattle versus reported treatment rates ($r^2 = 0.986$) in Norway. Data on treatment rates are derived from the annual reports of the Norwegian Cattle Health Service, which comprise on average 90% of dairy cattle in Norway; data on antimicrobial drug sales were obtained from the Norwegian Institute of Public Health. Figure developed by Kari Grave.

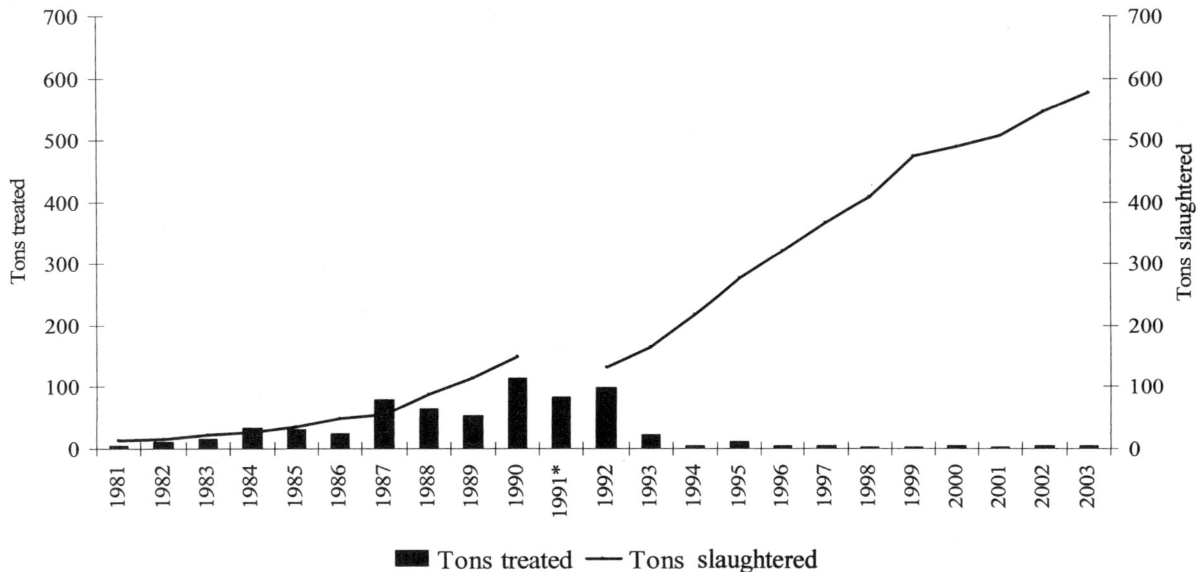

Figure 4. Calculated annual biomass of farmed salmonids treated with one course dose of an antibacterial drug versus biomass of farmed salmonids slaughtered annually in Norway. Sales data for antimicrobials represent sales from feed mills and wholesalers; data on amounts of farmed fish slaughtered are derived from Statistics Norway. *, data on slaughtered amounts not published because they were not assumed to be valid. Figure developed by Kari Grave.

valid, while biomass slaughtered is more easily available. In such cases, total consumption figures should be expressed in ADD_{kg} for the more important species and biomass slaughtered could be an alternative denominator to correct for the production volume. However, such statistics will be importantly affected by the composition of the animal population of the countries, e.g., free-range beef cattle may be dominant in some countries and intensive pig production may be dominant in others.

AGPs and CFAs

In order to examine the selective pressure exerted by the various AGPs or CFAs, the proportional use of the different feed additives may be expressed as amounts of feed (in weight) containing an AGP or a CFA per 1,000 animals per time period (30). This unit adjusts for the differences in the dosage between the various substances, for changes in the feed conversion rates, as well as for the number of animals liable to be fed a growth promoter.

CONTINUOUS MONITORING PROGRAMS ON ANTIMICROBIAL USAGE

To date, programs for continuous monitoring of antimicrobial usage have been established in a few countries only (6–11). However, several countries are reported to be in line for such programs (e.g., Australia, Canada, South Africa, and Switzerland). The inclusion criteria for antimicrobial agents (therapeutic use and feed additives), selection of data sources, drug classification system, and units of measurement, as well as expression of usage data in the various programs, are summarized in Table 5. For all these programs data are, at a minimum, presented in kilograms of active substance, split into antimicrobial drug classes.

Comparison of usage data between countries is seriously hampered because, except for DANMAP, data are not collected from sources that enable correction for dosage differences, age groups of animals being treated, or animal population liable to be treated. Nevertheless, overall national usage figures give an estimate of the national environmental load from antimicrobial drug usage. Furthermore, comparison of such data between various countries may trigger further development of the national monitoring programs if, for example, the usage profile observed and/or amounts used indicate nonprudent use. Total consumption should be compared with animal production, although comparison between countries is hampered by differences in composition of the animal population.

Another obstacle for comparison is that data on usage of antimicrobial drugs are reported differently with regard to drug classes in the various national programs. Table 6 shows that only for a couple of antimicrobial drug classes (tetracyclines and aminoglycosides) is it possible to compare proportional

Table 5. Continuous national monitoring programs on antimicrobial (AM) usage in animals[a]

Country	Data sources	Drug classification system	Unit of measurement	Expression of data
France	Manufacturers	Not mentioned	Wt of active substance	Overall wt sold split into drug classes, animal category (food animals, etc.), and routes of administration
	Feed mills (feed additives)		Wt of active substance	Overall sales
Denmark[b]	Pharmacies, feed mills (prescriptions); veterinarians (usage in practices) Manufacturers (for data validation)	ATCvet	Wt of active substance Defined ADD per kg (live wt) or age group	Overall wt and ADDs per animal species (including pets) and age group (food-producing animals) split into drug classes
Norway[b]	Wholesalers	ATCvet	Wt of active substance	Overall wt sold split into drug classes, therapeutic group, and routes of administration
	Veterinarians (only farmed fish)	ATCvet	Wt of active substance	Overall wt sold split into drug classes for use in farmed fish
Sweden[c]	Wholesalers	ATCvet	Wt of active substance	Overall wt sold split into substance class
			DDD[d]	DDD/1,000 cows at risk/day for injectable drugs against mastitis Species estimate given for pigs
The Netherlands	Manufacturers	Not mentioned	Wt of active substance	Overall wt sold split into drug classes
	Feed mills (feed additives)		Wt of active substance	Overall sales
United Kingdom	Manufacturers	Not mentioned	Wt of active substance	Overall wt sold split into drug classes; species estimates for species-specific drugs
	Feed mills (feed additives)		Wt of active substance	Overall sales

[a]Usage data for therapeutic AMs in farmed fish given for Denmark, Norway, Sweden, and the United Kingdom. Specific usage data for CFAs exerting antibacterial activity are given for Denmark, Sweden, and Norway. Data are from references 6 through 11.
[b]AGP use discontinued voluntarily.
[c]AGP use prohibited.
[d]Not internationally assigned doses (28).

usage of the different antimicrobials between countries. This indicates the need for increased international cooperation to coordinate presentation of usage data.

APPLICATION OF MONITORING DATA

The principal use of national monitoring data on antimicrobial usage in animals has so far been in the analysis and interpretation of national data on antimicrobial resistance prevalences and trends (7, 9–11). Thorough data on antimicrobial usage are important in order to increase the understanding of the epidemiology of antimicrobial resistance, and offer many opportunities for more in-depth research in this area.

Overall national sales data may provide opportunities for analysis and interpretation of national antimicrobial resistance data. Some caution is needed in this type of epidemiological analysis because the antimicrobial exposure history of farms and animals supplying these isolates is usually unknown. It would therefore be preferable to collect representative data that address the various levels of organization of the population (i.e., species, age groups, herds, and regions), validate these data with national aggregate data, and conduct analyses accordingly.

Estimates of numbers of animals treated with an antimicrobial drug at the regional or national level also provide a basis to design monitoring programs on residues. Furthermore, exposure data at herd level are crucial to enable risk-based programs on antimicrobial drug residues. Such risk-based drug residue control was implemented in fish faming in Norway in 1989 (16, 17) and has recently been implemented in Denmark by use of VetStat data (14).

The usefulness of overall national antimicrobial drug usage data in the evaluation of campaigns on prudent use of antimicrobials in food animals has been successfully demonstrated in Norway. In 1996 a campaign was initiated by the Norwegian Animal

Table 6. Sales, as percentages of total sales in weight of active substance, of veterinary antimicrobial drugs or derived from the most recent surveillance program reports in various countries[a]

France	2001	Denmark	2003	Norway	2003	Sweden	2003	The Netherlands	2003	United Kingdom	2003
Tetracyclines	48%	Tetracyclines	26%	Tetracyclines	3%	Tetracyclines	8%	Tetracyclines	58%	Tetracyclines	46%
Penicillins	9%	Amphenicols	0.2%	Amphenicols	2%	β-Lactamase-sensitive penicillins	47%	Penicillins, cephalosporins	10%	Penicillins	14%
Cephalosporins	0.5%	β-Lactamase-sensitive penicillins	18%	β-Lactamase-sensitive penicillins	30%	Other penicillins	11%	Sulfonamides + trimethoprim	23%	Sulfonamides + trimethoprim	19%
Sulfonamides	18%	Other penicillins	11%	Other penicillins	6%	Sulfonamides	15%	Macrolides	5%	Macrolides	13%
Trimethoprim	3%	Cephalosporins	0.4%	Sulfonamides	0.3%	Trimethoprim and derivatives	2%	Aminoglycosides	2%	Aminoglycosides	5%
Macrolides	7%	Sulfonamides + trimethoprim	11%	Sulfonamides + trimethoprim	19%	Macrolides, lincosamides	7%	(Fluoro)quinolones	1%	Fluoroquinolones	0.2%
Aminoglycosides	6%	Macrolides, lincosamides	20%	Lincosamides	0.2%	Aminoglycosides	4%	Others[b]	2%	Others[b]	3%
Quinolones	1.3%	Aminoglycosides	11%	Aminoglycosides	3%	Fluoroquinolones	1%				
Fluoroquinolones	0.3%	Quinolones	0.8%	Quinolones	10%	Pleuromutilins	5%				
Polymyxin	5%	Fluoroquinolones	0.1%	Combinations	24%						
Others[b]	2%	Others[b]	0.3%	Pleuromutilins	3%						

[a]Data are from references 6 to 11.
[b]Not specified.

Husbandry Organization aiming to reduce the usage of antimicrobial drugs in food animals by 25% within 5 years, with 1995 as the reference year. Comprehensive guidelines on antimicrobial drug therapy in food animals, especially in cattle (43), were published to support the campaign. Furthermore, the organization executed informational activities on prudent antimicrobial use directed toward relevant veterinary practitioners, but also farmers. The campaign concluded that the goal of reducing antimicrobial usage should be achieved by a more critical selection of cases for antimicrobial therapy (e.g., not to treat subclinical mastitis) and by an increased focus on preventive measures. Moreover, bacteriological diagnostics, including antimicrobial susceptibility testing, should be used in order to avoid use of broad-spectrum antimicrobials and combination preparations. One of the key messages that pervaded this campaign was to consider use of single-substance preparations of penicillins, especially β-lactamase-sensitive penicillins, instead of combination preparations, whenever appropriate. The overall sales, in kilograms of active substance, of veterinary antimicrobial drugs indicated for use in food animals in Norway declined by 42% from 1995 to 2000 and have remained relatively constant since then. Furthermore, the proportional use of penicillins increased from 25% in 1995 to 39% in 2000 and 42% in 2003 (Fig. 5). Only a slight decrease in the number of food animals liable to be treated with antimicrobials was observed during the study period, except for slaughter chickens and slaughter pigs, for which a considerable increase was observed. Owing to these facts, it could be concluded that the campaign certainly was effective and successful.

In Norway data on usage of antimicrobials in farmed salmonids were used to evaluate the effectiveness of various vaccine formulations against furunculosis (36). In 1989 furunculosis in farmed salmon became endemic for the first time in Norway, and commercially available non-oil-adjuvanted vaccines were made available on the Norwegian market the same year. Furunculosis was the only systemic bacterial disease that created severe problems in Norwegian fish farms at that time. Although a comprehensive vaccination program against furunculosis was implemented, the amounts of fish treated with antimicrobial drugs did not decline subsequently. In the fall of 1992 an oil-adjuvanted vaccine was introduced, and this resulted in an abrupt decrease in the amounts of fish treated, with an unremitting very low level since then (Fig. 4). This confirmed that the oil-adjuvanted formulation was significantly more efficient than the non-oil-adjuvanted formulations.

Another important application of usage data has been for the evaluation of the effect of discontinuing use of AGPs. In 1986 Sweden voluntarily banned all use of AGPs for precautionary reasons. There was an apprehension of a subsequent rise in the use of therapeutic antimicrobials. However, overall usage data (Fig. 6) have shown reduced consumption of veterinary antimicrobial agents in Sweden following the ban (1, 9). Norwegian usage data on veterinary antimicrobials show that this has also been the case in Norway (10) following the official

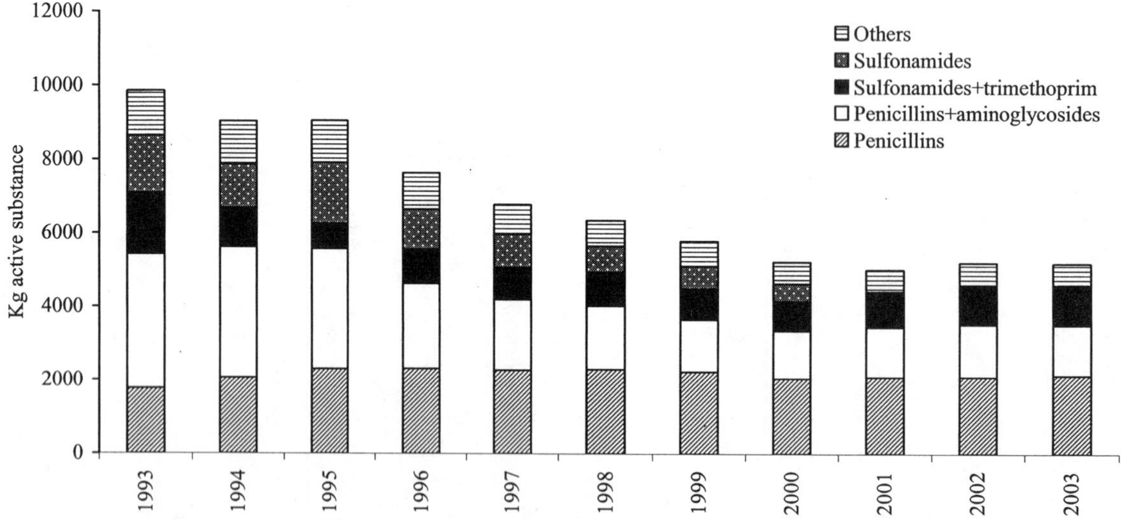

Figure 5. Sales, in kilograms of active substance, of veterinary antimicrobial drugs in Norway in the period from 1993 to 2003. In Norway veterinary drugs are sold only through pharmacies supplied by wholesalers. Sales data represent sales from wholesalers to Norwegian pharmacies and were obtained from the Norwegian Institute of Public Health. Antimicrobial drug formulations approved exclusively for farmed fish or pets are not included. Figure developed by Kari Grave.

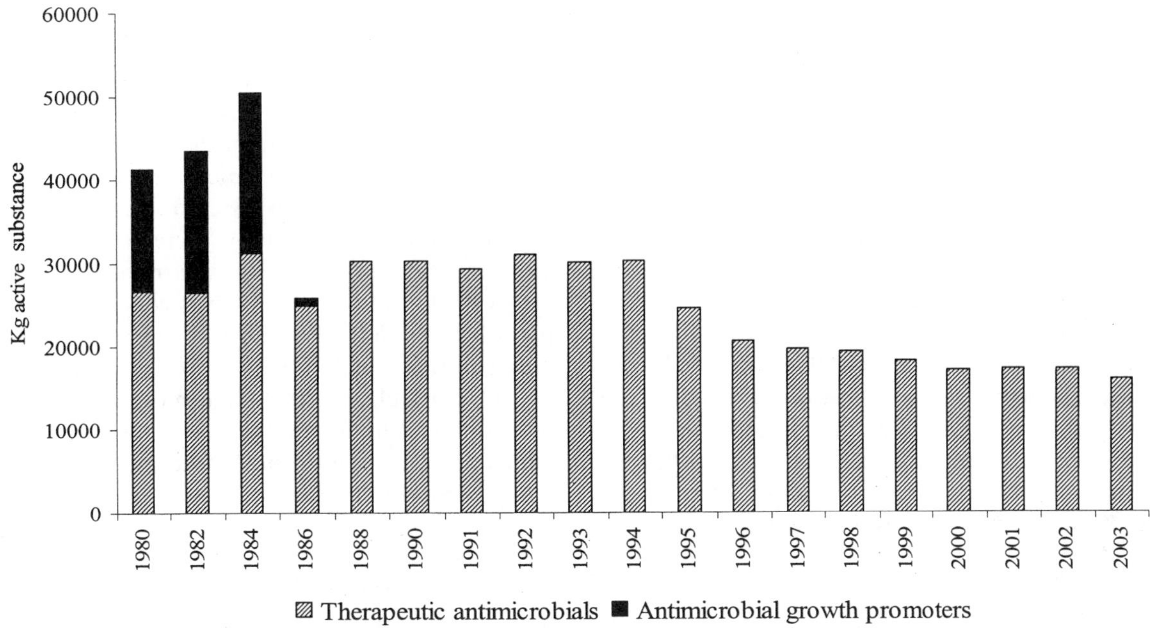

Figure 6. Usage in Sweden of AGPs and therapeutic antimicrobials in the period from 1980 to 2003. Data for 1980 to 1995 are derived from the Swedish Veterinary Antimicrobial Resistance Monitoring program and reference 1. Figure developed by Kari Grave.

ban of avoparcin and the voluntary termination of all AGPs in 1995 (Fig. 5).

In Denmark, avoparcin was banned in May 1995, whereas virginiamycin was banned in January 1998. In February 1998 the Danish meat industry voluntarily decided to discontinue the use of all AGPs. Figure 7 shows that the termination of the use of AGPs in Denmark resulted in a 52% reduction in the total use of antimicrobials in animals from 1994 to 2003. A WHO international review panel evaluated the impact of AGP termination in Denmark (48). It was found that the overall therapeutic use in pigs

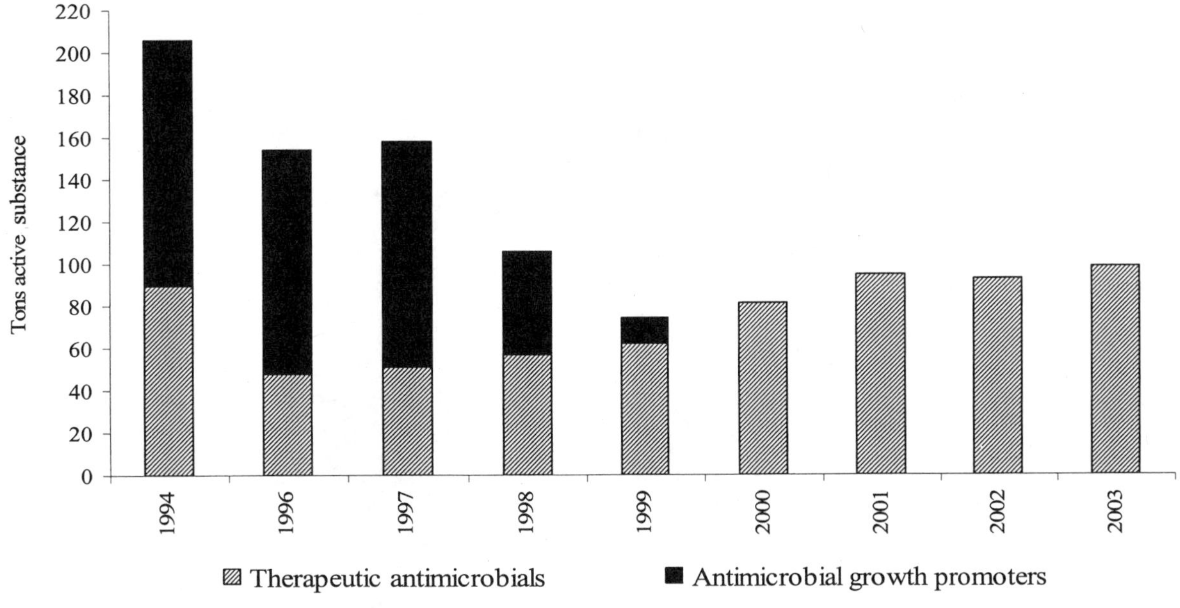

Figure 7. Usage (in metric tons) in Denmark of AGPs and therapeutic antimicrobials in the period from 1994 to 2003. Data are derived from the Danish monitoring program DANMAP (11). Data for 1995 are not published because they are not thought to be valid. Figure developed by Vibeke Frøkjær Jensen.

(accounting for, on average, 80% of veterinary antimicrobial usage in Denmark) for the years 2000 to 2002 was similar to that in 1994, the peak year before any AGPs were terminated. Therapeutic use in poultry appeared to be unaffected by the AGP termination.

When avoparcin was banned in Norway on May 31, 1995, it was feared that this would result in an increased incidence of *Clostridium perfringens*-associated necrotic enteritis (NE) and subsequently in increased therapeutic use of antimicrobials in meat-type poultry. To evaluate this hypothesis, the annual treatment frequency of NE in poultry before and after the ban of avoparcin was estimated by use of national sales statistics of antimicrobial drugs indicated for the treatment of NE in poultry (30). This assessment showed that the ban led to a temporary increase in treatment rates in the last quarter of 1995. However, treatment rates of NE in poultry in the period from 1996 to 2001 were approximately at the same level as before the ban. A preferential use of narasin instead of other ionophores in broilers following the ban of avoparcin may explain these low treatment rates of NE in broilers.

In 1999 Switzerland introduced a ban on AGPs. To assess whether this ban resulted in an increase in the therapeutic use of antimicrobials in piglets and fattening pigs, the usage of antimicrobials for the period from 1996 to 2001 was investigated (15). A total of 6,427 prescriptions for medicated feedstuff delivered to pig farms in a Swiss canton were investigated, and the overall annual amounts of antimicrobials delivered (in kilograms of active substance) were calculated. To correct for differences in dosages between the various substances and for the population liable to be treated, PDDs per population were estimated. The usage of antimicrobials in pigs, expressed as the number of PDDs per population, decreased from 6.1 in 1996 to 3.6 in 1999 and thereafter remained low (3.3 in 2000 and 3.4 in 2001). It was concluded that the ban of AGPs did not result in increased therapeutic use of antimicrobials in pig farming in Switzerland.

In particular cases, usage monitoring may be limited to certain areas, e.g., food animal species for which access to the export market will benefit from reliable documentation on usage (26, 27, 29). For example, documentation on antimicrobial usage in broilers was required in relation to a specific sales contract between Danish poultry producers and an international company in 2002 (V. F. Jensen, unpublished information). In Norway salmon farming has been an important export industry since the early 1980s. Even in the early days, documentation on antimicrobial drug usage was considered important in order to ensure access to the international export market. Data on antimicrobial drug usage in farmed fish in Norway have been estimated since 1981 by use of sales data for antimicrobial premixes from pharmacies and for medicated feed from feed mills.

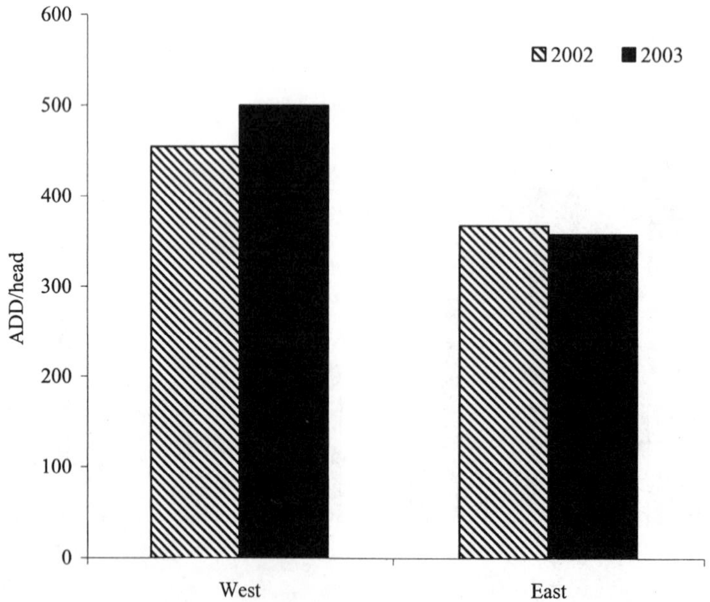

Figure 8. Usage of antimicrobial drugs in pig production in Denmark, expressed as ADD per head ("heads" refers to the number of animals liable to be treated). Data are derived from VetStat (42). Figure developed by Vibeke Frøkjær Jensen.

Usage data on antimicrobials may also be used to identify changes in incidences of bacterial disease (Figs. 3 and 4). The magnitude of cold-water vibriosis *(Vibrio salmonicida)* and furunculosis outbreaks in Norwegian salmonid farming in the last part of the 1980s and in the early 1990s, respectively, was estimated by use of sales statistics for antimicrobials formulated for use in farmed fish (Fig. 4). In Denmark increased use of antimicrobials in pigs was observed in 2002 and 2003. Analysis of data from VetStat showed that the overall increase was confined to the western part of Denmark. Large regional differences (>30%) in antimicrobial drug consumption per pig slaughtered were observed, indicating that the continuing increase was not related to the growth promoter ban. Rather, a number of factors may have been involved, such as differences in production systems, farmers' attitudes, occurrence of disease, and variation in veterinary prescription patterns. Further analysis showed that the major part of the increase was confined to specific drugs, disease groups, and age groups in the western part of the country (Fig. 8), the same counties where an emergence of postweaning multisystemic wasting syndrome occurred in 2002 and 2003, whereas an increase in the use of specific formulations for treatment of other disease groups and age groups was nationwide.

These examples show how drug monitoring data may be used for indirect surveillance of emerging disease problems, but also the importance of stratifying data into geographical areas. Monitoring data can be used for the generation of hypotheses documenting causal relationships in epidemiological research.

CONCLUDING REMARKS

Interpretation and comparison of data from various monitoring programs on antimicrobial drug usage can be difficult if there are differences in methodology or the methodology is inadequately explained. To overcome this problem, the WHO, FAO, and OIE recommend international coordination during the early stages of monitoring program development in order to enable data comparability and sharing. To allow for comparison between countries of data on antimicrobial usage, including total usage as well as usage stratified according to animal species, age groups, time periods, and areas, the inclusion criteria for antimicrobials and the expression of data should be standardized and the data results of monitoring should be expressed in standardized ways.

The prescribing patterns and total usage of antimicrobial drugs in animals are influenced by several factors, such as the epidemiological situation for the various bacterial diseases, structure of animal husbandry, numbers of animals liable to be treated, prescription habits, education, treatment costs, length of the withdrawal times, the type and formulations of the antimicrobial drugs approved for this indication in each country, and knowledge about the antimicrobial resistance situation. These are also factors that have to be taken into consideration in analyses of antimicrobial usage data. However, thorough analyses are achievable only if detailed data on antimicrobial usage per species, and in some cases per age group and herd level, are available. High-quality data on antimicrobial drug usage and thorough knowledge of the factors influencing this usage are crucial for the development of guidelines on prudent use of antimicrobials.

REFERENCES

1. **Anonymous.** 1997. Antimicrobial feed additives. Report from the Commission on Antimicrobial Feed Additives. SOU 1997: 132. Ministry of Agriculture, Stockholm, Sweden.
2. **Anonymous.** 1998. The Copenhagen Recommendations. Report from the invitational EU conference on the microbial threat, Copenhagen, Denmark 9–10 September. Statens Serum Institut and Danish Veterinary Laboratory, Copenhagen, Denmark.
3. **Anonymous.** 1999. Antibiotic resistance in the European Union associated with therapeutic use of veterinary medicines. Report and quality risk assessment by the Committee for Veterinary Medicinal Products. European Medicines Agency, London, United Kingdom. http://www.emea.eu.int/pdfs/vet/regaffair/034299en.pdf, accessed 5 August 2004.
4. **Anonymous.** 2000. National animal health monitoring system, Feedlot 1999, Part III: health management and biosecurity in US feedlots. Animal and Plant Health Inspection Service, U. S. Department of Agriculture, Riverdale, Md. http://www.aphis.usda.gov/vs/ceah/ncahs/nahms/feedlot/Feedlot99/FD99pt3.pdf, accessed 5 October 2004.
5. **Anonymous.** 2001. The microbial threat. Progress report on antimicrobial resistance. Invitational EU Conference, Visby, Sweden, 13–14 June 2001.
6. **Anonymous.** 2004. Suivi des ventes de médicaments vétérinaries contenant des antibiotiques en France en 2001. Agence Française de Securité Sanitaire des Aliments, Ploufragan, France. www.anmv.afssa.fr/antibioresistance/, accessed 15 January 2005.
7. **Anonymous.** 2004. MARAN 2003. Monitoring of antimicrobial resistance and antibiotic usage in animals in the Netherlands in 2003. http://www.cidc-lelystad.nl, accessed 15 January 2005.
8. **Anonymous.** 2004. Sales of antimicrobial products authorised for use as veterinary medicines, antiprotozoals, growth promoters, antifungals and coccidiostats, in the UK. http://www.vmd.gov.uk/general/publications/AM-Sales-rpt-2003-v09.pdf, accessed 15 January 2005.
9. **Anonymous.** 2004. SVARM 2003. Swedish Veterinary Antimicrobial Resistance Monitoring. National Veterinary Institute, Uppsala, Sweden. http://www.sva.se/pdf/svarm2003.pdf, accessed August 13, 2004.

10. **Anonymous.** 2004. NORM/NORM-VET 2003. Consumption of antimicrobial agents and occurrence of antimicrobial resistance in Norway. NORM, Tromsø, Norway, and NORM-VET, Oslo, Norway. http://www.vetinst.no/Arkiv/Zoonosesenteret/ NORM_NORM-VET_2003.pdf, accessed 22 September 2004.
11. **Anonymous.** 2004. DANMAP—2003. Use of antimicrobial agents and occurrence of antimicrobial resistance in bacteria from food, animals and humans in Denmark. DANMAP, Copenhagen, Denmark. http://www.dfvf.dk/Files/Filer/Zoono secentret/Publikationer/Danmap/Danmap_2003.pdf, accessed 13 August 2004.
12. **Anonymous.** 2004. *Guidelines for ATC Classification and DDD Assignment*, 7th ed. WHO Collaborating Centre for Drug Statistics Methodology, Oslo, Norway.
13. **Anonymous.** 2004. *Guidelines for ATCvet Classification*, 6th ed. WHO Collaborating Centre for Drug Statistics Methodology, Oslo, Norway. www.whocc.no, accessed 15 January 2005.
14. **Anonymous.** 2004. Veterinære lægemiddelrester i fødevarer 2002—resultat fra den danske kontrol med veterinære lægemiddelrester. The Danish Veterinary and Food Administration, Copenhagen, Denmark. http://www.foedevarestyrelsen .dk/FDir/Publications/2003013/Rapport.pdf, accessed 15 January 2005.
15. **Arnold, S., B. Gassner, T. Giger, and R. Zwahlen.** 2004. Banning antimicrobial growth promoters in feedstuffs does not result in increased therapeutic use in antibiotics in medicated feed in pig farming. *Pharmacoepidemiol. Drug Saf.* **13:** 323–331.
16. **Bangen, M., K. Grave, R. Nordmo, and N. E. Søli.** 1994. Description and evaluation of a new surveillance programme for drug use in fish farming in Norway. *Aquaculture* **119:**109–118.
17. **Bangen, M., K. Grave, and T. E. Horsberg.** 1996. Surveillance of drug prescribing in farmed fish in Norway: possible applications of computerized prescription data. *J. Vet. Pharmacol. Ther.* **19:**78–81.
18. **Berg, D. H., and R. L. Hamill.** 1978. The isolation and characterization of narasin, a new polyether antibiotic. *J. Antibiot.* **31:**1–6.
19. **Bro, F., and C. E. Mabeck.** 1986. Use of antibiotics in general practice in Denmark. *Scand. J. Prim. Health Care* **4:**101–104.
20. **Capellà, D.** 1993. Descriptive tools and analysis, p. 55–78. *In* M. N. G. Dukes (ed.) *Drug Utilization Studies. Methods and Uses.* WHO Regional Publications, European Series, no. 45. Regional Office for Europe, World Health Organization, Copenhagen, Denmark.
21. **Chauvin, C., F. Madec, D. Guillemot, and P. Sanders.** 2001. The crucial question of standardisation when measuring drug consumption. *Vet. Res.* **32:**533–543.
22. **Chauvin, C., P. A. Beloeil, J. P. Orand, P. Sanders, and F. Madec.** 2002. A survey of group-level antibiotic prescriptions in pig production in France. *Prev. Vet. Med.* **30:** 109–120.
23. **Dunlop, R. H., S. A. McEwen, A. H. Meek, W. D. Black, R. C. Clarke, and R. M. Friendship.** 1998. Individual and group antimicrobial usage rates on 34 farrow-to-finish swine farms in Ontario. Canada. *Prev. Vet. Med.* **34:**247–264.
24. **Dunlop, R. H., S. A. McEwen, A. H. Meek, R. M. Friendship, W. D. Black, and R. C. Clarke.** 1998. Antimicrobial drug use and related management practices among Ontario swine producers. *Can. Vet. J.* **39:**87–96.
25. **Elwinger, K., C. Schneitz, E. Berndtson, O. Fossum, B. Teglof, and B. Engstrom.** 1992. Factors affecting the incidence of necrotic enteritis, caecal carriage of *Clostridium perfringens* and bird performance in broiler chicken. *Acta Vet. Scand.* **33:**369–378.
26. **Grave, K., M. Engelstad, N. E. Søli, and T. Håstein.** 1990. Utilization of antibacterial drugs in salmonid farming in Norway during 1980–1988. *Aquaculture* **86:**347–358.
27. **Grave, K., M. Markestad, and M. Bangen.** 1996. Comparison in prescribing patterns of antibacterial drugs in salmonid farming in Norway during the periods 1989–1994 and 1980–1988. *J. Vet. Pharmacol. Ther.* **19:**184–191.
28. **Grave, K., L. Nilsson, C. Greko, T. Mørk, K. Odensvik, and M. Rønning.** 1999. The usage in Norway and Sweden of veterinary antibacterial drugs for mastitis during 1990–1997. *Prev. Vet. Med.* **42:**45–55.
29. **Grave, K., A. Lillehaug, B. T. Lunestad, and T. E. Horsberg.** 1999. Prudent use of antibacterial drugs in Norwegian aquaculture? Surveillance by the use of prescription data. *Acta Vet. Scand.* **40:**185–195.
30. **Grave, K., M. Kaldhusdal, L. Harr, H. Kruse, and K. Flatlandsmo.** 2004. What has happened in Norway after the avoparcin ban? Consumption of antimicrobials in poultry. *Prev. Vet. Med.* **62:**59–72.
31. **Harris, C. M., J. W. Cullen, and D. J. Roberts.** 1994. Consider national standards for daily dosages. *Br. Med. J.* **308:**206.
32. **Hill A., M. Chriel, V. F. Jensen, M. Vaarst, A. Stockmarr, J. Bruun, and M. Greiner.** 2003. Use of existing surveillance data to detect welfare problems in Danish cattle. An evaluation of available data sources, with detection of existing herd health problems and associated risk factors. Project report, Theme 6, International EpiLab, 22 March 2004. http://www.dfvf.dk/Default.asp?ID=9726, accessed 13 August 2004.
33. **Jensen, V. F., E. Jacobsen, and F. Bager.** 2004. Veterinary antimicrobial resistance—usage statistics based on standardized measure of dosage. *Prev. Vet. Med.* **64:**201–215.
34. **Kondo, F.** 1989. *In vitro* lecithinase activity and sensitivity to 22 antimicrobial agents of *Clostridium perfringens* isolated from necrotic enteritis of broiler chicken. *Res. Vet. Sci.* **45:** 337–340.
35. **Mandy, B., E. Koutny, C. Cornette, M.C. Woronoff-Lemsi, and D. Talon.** 2004. Methodological validation of monitoring indicators of antibiotics use in hospitals. *Pharm. World Sci.* **26:**90–95.
36. **Markestad, A., and K. Grave.** 1997. Reduction of antibacterial drug use in Norwegian fish farming due to vaccination. *Dev. Biol. Stand.* **90:**365–369.
37. **Mitema, E. S., G. M. Kikuvi, H. C. Wegener, and K. Stöhr.** 2001. An assessment of antimicrobial consumption in food producing animals in Kenya. *J. Vet. Pharmacol. Ther.* **24:** 385–390.
38. **Monnet, D. L., S. Molstad, and O. Cars.** 2004. Defined daily doses of antimicrobials reflect antimicrobial prescriptions in ambulatory care. *J. Antimicrob. Chemother.* **53:** 1109–1111.
39. **Nicholls, T., J. Acar, F. Anthony, A. Franklin, R. Gupta, Y. Tamura, S. Thompson, E. J. Threlfall, D. Vose, M. van Vuuren, D. G. White, H. C. Wegener, and M. L. Costarrica.** 2001. Antimicrobial resistance: monitoring the quantities of antimicrobials used in animal husbandry. *Rev. Sci. Tech.* **20:** 841–847.
40. **Odensvik, K., K. Grave, and C. Greco.** 2001. The usage in Sweden and Norway of antibacterial drugs to dogs and cats in 1990–1998. *Acta Vet. Scand.* **42:**189–198.
41. **Østerås, O., and K. Grave.** 2002. Data quality of the Norwegian Health Recording in Dairy Cattle, abstr. 21. Presented at the XXII World Buiatric Congress, Hannover, Germany, 18 to 23 August 2002.
42. **Stege, H., F. Bager, E. Jacobsen, and A. Thougaard.** 2003. VETSTAT—the Danish system for surveillance of veterinary use of drugs for production animals. *Prev. Vet. Med.* **57:** 105–115.

43. **Tørud, E., R. Lang-Ree, A. Raage, S. Støverud, T. Sivertsen, S. A. Ødegaard, H. Sørum, K. Grave, O. Austbø, T. Grøndalen, R. A. Aass, and O. Østerås.** 1996. Strategier for å redusere forbruket av antibakterielle midler i storfeproduksjonen—ved særlig vekt på behandling av mastitt. The Norwegian Cattle Health Program, Ås, Norway.
44. **Wessling, A., and G. Boethius.** 1990. Measurement of drug use in a defined population. Evaluation of the defined daily dose (DDD) methodology. *Eur. J. Clin. Pharmacol.* **39:** 207–210.
45. **World Health Organization.** 1997. The medical impact of the use of antimicrobials in food animals. Report of a WHO Meeting, Berlin, Germany, 13–17 October 1997. http://www.who.int/emc/diseases/zoo/oct97.pdf, accessed 16 March 2004. World Health Organization, Geneva, Switzerland.
46. **World Health Organization.** 2001. WHO global strategy for the containment of antimicrobial resistance in animals. Publication WHO/CDS/DRS/2001.2. World Health Organization, Geneva, Switzerland.
47. **World Health Organization.** 2002. Monitoring antimicrobial usage in food animals for the protection of human health. Report of a WHO consultation in Oslo, Norway, 10–13 September 2001. Publication WHO/CDS/CRS/EPH/2002.11. World Health Organization, Geneva, Switzerland.
48. **World Health Organization.** 2003. Impacts of antimicrobial growth promoter termination in Denmark. The WHO international review panel's evaluation of the termination of the use of antimicrobial growth promoters in Denmark, Foulum, Denmark, 6–9 November 2002. World Health Organization, Geneva, Switzerland.
49. **World Health Organization.** 2003. Joint FAO/OIE/WHO expert workshop on non-human antimicrobial usage and antimicrobial resistance: scientific assessment, Geneva, Switzerland, 1–5 December 2003. http://www.who.int/foodsafety/publications/micro/en/amr.pdf, accessed 15 January 2005. World Health Organization, Geneva, Switzerland.
50. **World Health Organization.** 2004. Joint FAO/OIE/WHO 2nd workshop on non-human antimicrobial usage and antimicrobial resistance: management options, Oslo, Norway, 15–18 March 2004. http://www.who.int/foodsafety/publications/micro/mar04/en, accessed 7 August 2004. World Health Organization, Geneva, Switzerland.

Antimicrobial Resistance in Bacteria of Animal Origin
Edited by Frank M. Aarestrup

Chapter 23

Monitoring of Antimicrobial Resistance in Animals: Principles and Practices

SCOTT A. MCEWEN, FRANK M. AARESTRUP, AND DAVID JORDAN

Resistance to antimicrobials was observed in pathogenic bacteria soon after these drugs were first introduced into human and veterinary medicine over 60 years ago (21). Subsequently, as each new class of antimicrobials was introduced, resistance eventually emerged, although the rate at which this occurred and the prevalence of resistance that was eventually attained varied considerably with respect to different drugs, species of bacteria, geographical regions, extents of antimicrobial use, and other factors (30). While scientists generally agree that antimicrobial resistance exists and is a problem, that it is important to human and animal health, and that it has a genetic basis often transferable within and between species of bacteria, they sometimes disagree, or are at least uncertain, about some key aspects of the biology. These include the circumstances whereby resistance emerges in populations (e.g., species of bacteria, host species of animal or human, relation to antimicrobial use in animals or humans, and rate of spread); whether such resistance is increasing or decreasing over time; and whether any actions, such as reductions in antimicrobial use or changing prescription practices, are warranted in order to manage resistance, i.e., to prevent it from emerging, spreading, or increasing in prevalence.

For decades, public health advocates, scientists, government regulators, veterinarians, farmers, and others have debated the impact of antimicrobial use in animals on human and animal health and what, if anything, should be done about it. Many expert panel reports and sets of recommendations on this topic have been published (17, 36). A key recommendation that consistently emerges from these deliberations, and one of the few areas of near unanimous agreement in this otherwise very controversial field, is the need for improved monitoring and surveillance of antimicrobial resistance. This remarkable situation arises from the pressing need for better information concerning emergence and trends of antimicrobial resistance in populations of bacteria and patterns of carriage of resistant organisms in populations of animals and humans. Fundamentally, this information is needed to allow better understanding of the biology of antimicrobial resistance and to support evidence-based decisions concerning its management. It is recognized that antimicrobial resistance is truly an international problem (28). Through movement and trade of animals and food, bacteria and their resistance determinants might flow among animals and herds, up the food chain to humans, through the environment, throughout regions and countries, and across international borders. The only way to effectively measure the extent of the resistance problem and to detect important changes is through continuous monitoring and surveillance (35, 38).

Despite the nearly universal recognition of the importance of resistance monitoring and surveillance, only a few countries (e.g., Denmark and the United States) have so far implemented comprehensive programs in the animal and food sectors, perhaps because of the costs involved, but also because of the considerable time that it often takes to muster the necessary political support and implement new national programs. However, some other countries (e.g., Canada and The Netherlands) have very recently initiated programs and it is probable that many more countries are either considering the possibilities of their own antimicrobial resistance monitoring

Scott A. McEwen • Department of Population Medicine, Ontario Veterinary College, University of Guelph, Guelph, Ontario N1G 2W1, Canada. **Frank M. Aarestrup** • Danish Institute for Food and Veterinary Research, Bülowsvej 27, DK-1790 Copenhagen V, Denmark. **David Jordan** • New South Wales Department of Primary Industries, 1243 Bruxner Highway, Wollongbar, New South Wales 2477, Australia.

and surveillance programs or have made the decision to undertake such programs and are in the early development or planning stages. In this chapter we review information relevant to the design and scope of antimicrobial resistance monitoring and surveillance programs for animals and food, with emphasis on program purposes and methods. We then describe some of the essential features of existing monitoring and surveillance programs in various countries around the world and, using examples, show how these programs have been useful in improving understanding of resistance and its relation to antimicrobial use and other factors, guiding public policy, and measuring the impact of interventions on antimicrobial resistance in bacteria from animals, food, and humans.

DEFINITION AND PURPOSES

The terms "monitoring" and "surveillance" have both been used to describe these programs, and in some cases they are used together, interchangeably or synonymously. Strictly speaking, however, there are some important differences. Monitoring programs are ongoing efforts to determine the prevalence and changes in prevalence of defined characteristics (often disease) in populations, while surveillance programs involve the ongoing evaluation of a population for defined characteristics (e.g., disease, chemical residues in food, and antimicrobial resistance) for the purposes of control (29). The emphasis on control in surveillance programs often has implications for program design, e.g., targeted sampling of high-risk populations for the purposes of detection and removal of affected individuals or groups. In practice, most national programs in antimicrobial resistance seek to address both functions, or begin with a purely monitoring role then assume an additional surveillance capacity as the need and opportunity arise. For simplicity, we shall use the term "monitoring" for the rest of the chapter, recognizing that many programs have important surveillance functions. Although we do not explicitly mention studies that are of pilot or one-off nature, these do share many technical aspects with monitoring programs. One-off prevalence studies can play a very useful role as predecessors to monitoring programs by developing the facilities, specimen handling protocols, laboratory protocols, and skills base required to study prevalence in an ongoing fashion.

It is important to identify and prioritize the purposes of monitoring and then design the program accordingly. Thus, methods for sampling from the population, microbiological testing procedures, data analysis, and reporting of results can all vary according to which objectives are adopted (Table 1). The language used to describe objectives must be specific so there is no ambiguity about the purpose for which monitoring is being performed. It must be decided whether the monitoring program is intended to address human or animal health concerns, but preferably both. An important motive for monitoring resistance is to produce data that can be used in risk assessments, especially those that characterize the frequency and severity of adverse health outcomes in humans and animals caused by resistant organisms that have or will evolve because of antimicrobial use in animals. Risk assessments that address policy on antimicrobial use need to have a prospective outlook, and this should be reflected in the design of the monitoring program. While it is difficult to anticipate the explicit information needs of all future risk assessments, in general the resistance monitoring program should provide information pertaining to (i) the type of hazards present in the population, i.e., phenotypic and/or genotypic measures of resistance in pathogens and relevant commensals to the range of antimicrobials important in human and animal health; and (ii) exposure, i.e., the frequency with which humans or animals come into effective contact (e.g., through ingestion) with the hazard and the amount of such hazard involved in these incidents. Ideally, these data should be linked epidemiologically to antimicrobial use data, farm management, and other relevant factors. In so doing, a subsequent risk assessment can provide the basis for assessing if particular policies can be implemented to reduce the occurrence of disease due to resistant organisms.

Other important purposes of antimicrobial resistance monitoring include identification of the prevalence of antimicrobial resistance (or decreased susceptibility), description of resistance trends over time, detection (when possible) of emerging resistance, identification of the need for interventions to control resistance, measurement of the impact of such interventions, identification of the need for targeted research, contribution to an archive of representative isolates for future studies, providing of information to guide empiric treatment strategies for animals and humans, providing of information for development of antimicrobial use policies or prudent use guidelines, and identification of the need for education of farmers, veterinarians, and other stakeholders (16). Furthermore, antimicrobial use monitoring in combination with well-designed resistance monitoring may be used to study associations between antimicrobial use and antimicrobial resistance at the level of the herd, region, or country. Because many different objectives are possible, the emphasis should

Table 1. Purposes of antimicrobial resistance monitoring and implications for design, analysis, and reporting

Purpose of monitoring	Outcome of interest	Sampling	Implications for:		
			Resistance testing	Data analysis	Reporting of results
Identify trends	Prevalence of resistance	Representative of national population	Consistent antimicrobial panel over time	Trend analysis; time-series analysis	Graphical presentation of data for visual appreciation
Detect emerging resistance	MIC data to detect reduced susceptibility	May require large sample size and still have low statistical power	Selective methods may be helpful	Include confidence intervals	Present MIC data; explain low power for detection of rare strains
Act as guide to treatment strategies	Clinical outcomes more relevant	Clinical specimens from animals and humans	Clinically important antimicrobials		Timely reports to veterinarians and physicians; may need local data to be relevant
Provide information for risk assessment	Variable: may be prevalence of resistance, serotype of organism, or antimicrobial use data	Often important to have representative data on food animal reservoir, food, and humans		Have raw data available for specific analyses	
Act as guide to antimicrobial use policies	Prevalence of resistance and multiple resistance; use data; important to identify coselection to guide use policy	Representative of national population		Associations between antimicrobial use and resistance trends	Interpretive summaries should address evidence of increasing resistance to commonly used drugs
Identify the need for interventions	Prevalence of resistance; increasing MICs	Adequate sample size to detect important lower limit of resistance in target species or commodity			
Measure effects of interventions	Prevalence of resistance; MICs	Consistency over time to enable comparison before and after intervention	Consistency over time to enable comparison before and after intervention	Statistical analysis with control of potential confounding	
Study associations with antimicrobial use	Prevalence of resistance	Ideal to link antimicrobial use and resistance data at farm level		Statistical analysis with control of potential confounding	
Serve as basis for targeted research	Variable: epidemiological, molecular epidemiological, and microbiological studies	Targeted sampling to test hypotheses	Further characterization of selected isolates; retrospective testing of archived samples		Special reports, peer-reviewed papers, and interpretive summaries in annual reports

be guided by the decision options that are open to those responsible for managing antimicrobial resistance. It is important that monitoring programs do address the information requirements of decision makers so that communities obtain the maximum benefits from their investment.

METHODOLOGY

The major methodological considerations for the monitoring program include the types of samples to be collected, sampling strategies, species of bacteria, antimicrobials for susceptibility testing, data collection and analysis, and reporting of results. In all cases, the methods to be used should reflect the intended purposes of the program.

Types of Samples

The food chain is currently thought to be the major route of exposure of humans to antimicrobial-resistant organisms from animals, especially those of enteric origin (32), and the sample types chosen should reflect the major steps in the farm-to-fork continuum. This includes fecal samples from live animals (either on the farm or in slaughterhouse lairage), cecal or colonic contents following removal of the viscera during slaughter, swabs from carcasses in the slaughterhouse, and meat or other foods from animals at the retail level. If there is a desire and capability to link the results of resistance testing to antimicrobial use in animals or other potential risk factors, then it will be necessary to select samples accordingly. For example, antimicrobial use is often applied at the farm level; therefore, fecal samples should be obtained at the farm level if there is a desire to assess the role of such antimicrobial use in resistance selection. On the other hand, samples collected at slaughter or retail may provide information that is more relevant to exposure of the consumer to antimicrobial-resistant bacteria. Samples from the major food animal species (e.g., cattle, pigs, poultry, and fish) should be included. Decisions on which food types to include can be aided by the results from surveys that quantify the amount of each item consumed (food basket surveys) and by emphasizing those foods that carry a higher microbial load (raw and semiprocessed meats) and those foods that are sold in a ready-to-eat state. Environmental, feed, and other samples may also be included if they provide insights into possible routes of contamination of food animals with antimicrobial-resistant or susceptible bacteria (e.g., *Salmonella*).

Antimicrobials are also used in companion and sporting animals, and there is opportunity for direct or indirect contact between these animals and humans. Whether or not a monitoring program should include samples from these animals is uncertain because their role in the spread of resistance to humans does not appear to be well described. This is reflected in the lack of extensive data on the occurrence of resistance in companion and sporting animals in reports from national programs. Nevertheless, if these animals are included in monitoring programs, then the type of sample submitted will depend on the anticipated site of carriage and transmission, e.g., nasal swabs for methicillin-resistant *Staphylococcus aureus* in horses and fecal swabs for *Salmonella* in pets. Importantly, sampling from companion and sporting animals on a scale likely to provide meaningful data could be problematic and costly. Thus, samples of tissues, swabs, or feces submitted for diagnostic purposes may form the preferred basis of monitoring. Similarly, monitoring of the resistance status of nonzoonotic pathogens in food animals also might require reliance on diagnostic submissions (tissues, swabs, feces, etc.), especially where suitable specimens cannot be readily obtained from surveys of farms or abattoirs.

Sampling Strategies

Antimicrobial resistance monitoring programs may be based on the passive acquisition of clinical samples through diagnostic laboratories, the active acquisition of samples through specifically designed sampling plans, or some combination of the two. Use of diagnostic samples is commonplace for monitoring antimicrobial resistance in human and animal health. It may provide useful information on emergence of resistance to new antimicrobials, particularly among bacteria that are rare in clinically normal humans or animals. However, there are many potential selection biases that limit the usefulness of clinical specimens for resistance monitoring. For example, clinical samples are typically submitted by veterinarians, but not all farmers regularly use veterinary services, some veterinarians only submit samples from animals when empirical treatment has failed, and some may submit multiple samples from the same herd. Furthermore, animals infected with bacteria of importance to food-borne diseases of humans (e.g., *Salmonella enterica* serovar Enteritidis, *Campylobacter jejuni*, and *Escherichia coli*) usually exhibit no clinical signs, and samples from healthy animals are rarely available in passive systems. For these reasons, active monitoring using a specifically designed sampling plan is usually required.

In order to obtain accurate and suitably precise information, it is important to get sufficient numbers of samples that are representative of the target population. In a national resistance monitoring program, this usually requires stratification of sampling by species and class of animals or food types, possibly by geographical region, with random selection of samples using a sampling plan based on sound epidemiological and statistical principles. Formal sample size estimates, appropriate to the intended purpose (e.g., prevalence estimation, comparison of prevalence in different groups, regional comparison, risk factor analysis, or temporal trend or spatial analyses) and sufficient for the required level of precision, should be calculated. This may not be practicable for all antimicrobial, organism, and animal species combinations, but should be attempted for the most important objectives, e.g., estimation of the prevalence of resistance in zoonotic enteropathogens from the major food animal reservoir to an antimicrobial that is used in that reservoir and is also of critical importance to human health. Preliminary estimates are usually required for sample size determinations, and if these are unavailable, pilot studies may be required as part of the program planning. In some cases, it may be necessary to choose between different sampling options based on the relative costs of sample collection or on logistical considerations. For example, it may not be feasible to hire technicians to travel to slaughterhouses in all areas of the country for collection of samples, but it may be feasible to subsidize the collection of samples being collected for another purpose, e.g., hazard analysis-critical control point (HACCP) programs, provided they are representative and of suitable quality. In other cases, sample size calculations may show that it is infeasible or too costly to collect enough samples to achieve an objective. A decision will then have to be made as to whether to abandon the objective or seek an alternative means with which to attain it. This is especially likely when the expected prevalence of an organism or resistance determinant is extremely low, as would be the case for new or emerging types of resistance.

The sampling plan should also take into account the structure of the animal production, slaughter, and food distribution system. In most developed countries there is a trend toward centralization of farming and food processing, with most of the animals and food handled through large operations, and these large operations are likely to be clustered in certain regions of the country. It is therefore necessary to decide whether to take a fixed number of samples per farm, slaughterhouse, and region and whether to stratify sampling, to pool samples to the group or farm level, to sample with probability proportional to the size of farm or slaughterhouse, or some combination of the above. Usually, resource limitations and other factors force some sort of compromise, e.g., selection of one isolate from one sample per farm from a random selection of farms submitting animals to all slaughterhouses of at least a certain size in a given region. This type of sampling should provide data that are reasonably representative of the population of bacteria, animals, farms, and so on. Most importantly, random selection (rather than a selection method based on convenience) is a key ingredient of a sampling plan that allows the resulting estimates of prevalence of resistance to be compared between different time periods, different species, and different regions.

Species of Bacteria

Resistance monitoring systems designed to address mainly human health concerns normally include zoonotic, enteropathogenic bacteria (e.g., *Salmonella*, *Campylobacter*, and sometimes *Yersinia*) and indicator or commensal bacteria (e.g., *E. coli* to represent gram-negative bacteria and *Enterococcus faecalis* and/or *Enterococcus faecium* to represent gram-positive bacteria). All of these bacteria may be found in the gastrointestinal tracts of one or more species of food animals; may contaminate foods of animal origin; and if foods are eaten raw or undercooked, may be consumed by humans. The zoonotic bacteria are included because they are directly hazardous to human health and antimicrobial resistance in these species may increase the burden of disease in humans through a variety of mechanisms, including increased frequency, duration, and severity of infection. The indicator or commensal species are normally found in the gastrointestinal tracts of food animals and humans, and monitoring resistance in these populations provides insights into selection pressures on other bacteria and enables comparisons of various reservoirs (e.g., animal, food, and human). Few studies have attempted to correlate resistance trends in pathogens and indicator species (4), and more work in this area is needed. In addition, commensal bacteria may under certain conditions be opportunistic pathogens of humans (e.g., in urinary tract infections or systemic infections in immunocompromised people), and they may be important donors of transmissible resistance determinants for other bacteria, including those pathogenic to humans.

Care should be taken to ensure the isolation of pure cultures of bacteria identified at least to the species level. In some cases, further routine characterization may be required, for example, serotyping and/or phage typing of *Salmonella*, to facilitate the interpretation and comparison of antimicrobial resistance patterns over time and between regions or countries. For example, the introduction and spread of multiresistant strains of bacteria, such as pentaresistant *Salmonella* serovar Typhimurium DT104, may be responsible for major changes in antimicrobial resistance patterns.

Resistance monitoring programs that address animal health concerns normally include specific animal pathogens. These vary by species and the importance of diseases in various countries, but examples include respiratory (e.g., *Actinobacillus pleuropneumoniae* and *Mannheimia haemolytica*), gastrointestinal (e.g., *E. coli* and *Salmonella*), mammary (e.g., *Streptococcus* spp. and *S. aureus*), and other (e.g., *Aeromonas salmonicida*) pathogens.

Both nonselective and selective methods may be used to isolate bacteria. If it is most important to determine the prevalence of resistance in the population of bacteria, then nonselective methods are preferable. Randomly choosing individual isolates using nonselective culture methods provides a more accurate estimation of the prevalence of resistance in the population than use of selective methods. The individual isolates are then available for susceptibility testing to a wide range of antimicrobials, enabling the identification of multiple resistance patterns, and representative isolates may be further characterized or stored for future susceptibility testing or research. If, however, it is most important to determine whether or not a certain type of resistance is present in a population, then selective methods are preferable. Selective methods may enable better detection of antimicrobial-resistant strains that are uncommon or rare in the population. This could be important, for example, in the case of newly released classes of antimicrobials or antimicrobials critical for use in humans or animals. Isolates collected using such methods may also be available for additional sensitivity testing or characterization, which may be helpful in identifying the potential for coselection by other antimicrobials. In some cases, a combination of nonselective and selective methods may be justified, especially where it is important to identify rare resistance patterns.

Antimicrobial Susceptibility Testing

Phenotypic and genotypic methods for susceptibility testing and detection of resistance are described in detail in chapters 3 and 4, respectively. In brief, the two main methods for susceptibility testing are dilution and diffusion methods, and both are used in antimicrobial resistance monitoring programs. Dilution methods are usually considered to be better and more reproducible and therefore preferred, but they are also more expensive than diffusion testing. Thus, it might in some cases be better to test or screen a large number of isolates using disc diffusion than a more limited number of isolates using more expensive MIC techniques. Whichever method is used, it is important whenever possible to use methods that provide quantitative data (i.e., MICs) using accepted guidelines (e.g., National Committee for Clinical Laboratory Standards [NCCLS]) and validated methods, with appropriate quality assurance (34). There is great interest in international standardization and harmonization of laboratory methods to facilitate the comparison of antimicrobial resistance patterns in different countries.

Careful consideration must be given to the choice of antimicrobials to use in a monitoring program. Antimicrobials representative of drug classes or families important to both human and animal health should be included, and guidelines are available (10, 15). Examples of antimicrobials used in the Danish Integrated Antimicrobial Resistance Monitoring and Research Programme (DANMAP) are shown in Table 2. Cost and technical considerations (e.g., numbers of wells on plates) pose limits to the numbers of antimicrobials that can be included, and there is a trade-off between the numbers of isolates and numbers of antimicrobials that can be tested optimally. Due to common resistance mechanisms and cross-resistance among drugs of the same class (e.g., erythromycin and tylosin in the macrolide class), it may only be necessary to include one member of the group and it may be inferred that reduced susceptibility to that member will indicate reduced susceptibility to the others (10). While it may be important in some cases to make changes to susceptibility panels by adding new antimicrobials as they become available and removing some older, less important drugs, a balance must be struck with the need to maintain some continuity over time, in order to measure temporal changes in resistance prevalence. If in the end a decision to leave out some antimicrobials has to be made, it is advisable to keep those that are most important for human health.

Data Collection, Analysis, and Reporting of Results

Data should be collected using validated and verifiable electronic means that facilitate quick and easy transfer to appropriate software for collation, tabular and graphical presentation, and statistical analysis. All strains should be kept until routine testing is completed, but representative strains at least

Table 2. Antimicrobial agents used for susceptibility testing in the DANMAP program

Antimicrobial agents	Antimicrobial group	Bacteria tested				Use
		E. coli, Salmonella	Staphylococci	Enterococci	*Campylobacter*	
Ampicillin	Penicillin with extended spectrum	X				Therapy in animals and humans
Amoxicillin-clavulanic acid	Penicillin with extended spectrum + inhibitor	X				Therapy in animals and humans
Apramycin	Aminoglycoside	X				Therapy in animals
Avilamycin	Oligosaccharide		X	X		Growth promotion
Bacitracin	Polypeptide		X	X		Growth promotion and therapy
Ceftiofur	Broad-spectrum cephalosporin	X	X			Therapy in animals and humans
Cephalothin	Narrow-spectrum cephalosporin	X				Therapy in animals and humans
Chloramphenicol	Chloramphenicol	X	X	X	X	Therapy in animals and humans
Ciprofloxacin	Fluoroquinolone	X	X		X	Therapy in animals and humans
Colistin	Polypeptide	X				Therapy in animals and humans
Erythromycin	Macrolide		X	X	X	Therapy in animals and humans
Flavomycin	Flavofosfolipol		X	X		Growth promotion
Florfenicol	Amphenicol	X	X	X		Therapy in animals
Gentamicin	Aminoglycoside	X	X	X	X	Therapy in animals and humans
Kanamycin	Aminoglycoside			X		Therapy in animals and humans
Linezolid	Oxazolidinone			X		Therapy in humans
Nalidixic acid	Narrow-spectrum quinolone	X			X	Indicator for quinolone resistance
Neomycin	Aminoglycoside	X			X	Therapy in animals and humans
Oxacillin	β-Lactamase-resistant penicillin		X			Therapy in humans
Penicillin	β-Lactamase-sensitive penicillin		X	X		Therapy in animals and humans
Quinupristin-dalfopristin	Streptogramins		X	X		Therapy in humans
Salinomycin	Ionophore			X		Growth promotion
Spectinomycin	Aminocyclitol	X	X			Therapy in animals and humans
Streptomycin	Aminoglycoside	X	X	X	X	Therapy in animals and humans
Sulfamethoxazole	Sulfonamide	X	X			Therapy in animals and humans
Teicoplanin	Glycopeptide			X		Therapy in animals and humans
Oxytetracycline	Tetracycline	X	X	X	X	Therapy in animals and humans
Tiamulin	Pleuromutilin		X			Therapy in animals
Trimethroprim	Trimethoprim	X	X			Therapy in animals and humans
Vancomycin	Glycopeptide		X	X		Therapy in humans

should be archived for future research and characterization. The results of susceptibility testing should be stored as quantitative data (i.e., MICs or zones of inhibition) and should be coded in a way that identifies the date of collection and testing, location of sampling, animal species, etc. (16). Raw data should always be available for future analyses, should they become necessary.

Most resistance monitoring systems report strains as being susceptible or resistant, or susceptible, intermediate, or resistant. This type of reporting puts great emphasis on the clinical or microbiological breakpoints that are selected. Although there are nationally and internationally recognized breakpoints for many antimicrobials and target pathogens from the NCCLS and similar bodies (particularly for pathogens and antimicrobials encountered in human medicine), they have traditionally been set to provide guidance on choice of therapy rather than for monitoring of resistance in populations of bacteria. Moreover, nationally or internationally accepted breakpoints are not always available for the combinations of veterinary drugs and animal-derived bacteria that are included in resistance monitoring programs. Considerable valuable information is lost in collapsing quantitative MIC data into breakpoint data; therefore, MICs should also be presented. Shifts in MICs over time provide a mechanism for the early detection of reduced susceptibility, while retaining MIC data also allows the data to be reinterpreted if breakpoints change and may facilitate the comparison of data from different laboratories.

Appropriate epidemiological and statistical analyses should be conducted to assess temporal trends, differences between geographical regions or between animal species, and associations with antimicrobial use or other risk factors. Ideally, estimates of prevalence of resistance among herds, animals, or isolates should be accompanied by confidence intervals that account for the sampling plan used and convey the correct amount of precision in measurements. This means that it may not be appropriate to rely on binomial confidence limits or any approximation thereof (in such circumstances calculation of the correct confidence limits is complex and statistical advice should be sought). Data should be stratified by organism, animal species or class, health status of animals, level of sampling (e.g., farm, slaughterhouse, or retail meat), year of sampling, and quality assurance methods used.

Most resistance monitoring programs publish their summary results in annual reports; however, in some cases it is desirable to report specific subsets of results back to data providers (e.g. farmers, veterinarians, and laboratories). Annual reports should be as timely as possible and provide the important summary data presented in tabular and graphical form, along with concise interpretative summaries and results of statistical or other analyses. In some cases, raw data may also be made available for those who wish to collate it in a different manner or undertake their own data analyses, and this may be provided in either paper or electronic formats or websites. These reports usually provide demographic data on the target populations of animals, humans, or food from animals monitored, as well as methods used for monitoring.

Comprehensive monitoring of antimicrobial resistance in animals in the context of animal and human health covers the entire farm-to-fork continuum. In most countries this involves various government agencies (e.g., public health, food inspection, and agriculture) at different levels (e.g., federal and state or provincial) and private interests (e.g., veterinarians, farm groups, slaughterhouses, and the food industry). Collation and integration of data across the continuum is challenging in many ways, not least regarding the sharing and interpretation of data. In most instances, unobstructed, complete, and timely sharing of data that are collected by standardized and controlled methods is needed to control the public health, social, and economic impacts of antimicrobial resistance. Resistance data derived from animals, food, and humans should be integrated in order to enable comparison across reservoirs, identification of possible spread between reservoirs, and early detection of emerging resistance in one reservoir in time to implement controls for prevention of spread to another reservoir.

The benefit of monitoring resistance at the level of individual herds with the aim of devising a specific program of preventive management for each herd has been debated. To our knowledge this has not been adopted in an organized and widespread fashion. This might be due to the large within-herd and within-animal sources of variation in resistance that has been observed in those few studies that have studied the epidemiology of resistance at the herd level (6, 13, 33). Thus, it appears that monitoring of resistance at the herd level could be cost prohibitive due to the need for a large number of samples and repeated sampling. It is possible that if a sufficient number of clinical isolates (e.g., bovine mastitis or postweaning diarrhea of pigs) are evaluated on a regular basis, some useful information to guide therapeutic decisions will be available.

EXAMPLES FROM DIFFERENT COUNTRIES

In 1995 and 1996 Denmark and the United States, respectively, were the first countries to implement national antimicrobial resistance monitoring programs incorporating samples from animals and food and antimicrobial susceptibility testing of isolates of various species of bacteria. Since then a number of other countries have implemented programs based in part on these models. While there are some similarities among the various programs, there are also important differences that reflect national differences in infrastructure, available resources, and priorities. The following is intended to describe some of the different approaches that have been used to monitor antimicrobial resistance in animals and food, especially with regard to matters of human health significance. There is insufficient space to include descriptions of all national programs, and a more complete summary is provided in Table 3. Examples of the use of monitoring data for various purposes are also provided. Other monitoring programs, in some cases based on notifiable disease reporting and animal health diagnostic data (i.e., clinical cases), also exist (22,39).

Denmark

DANMAP was established in 1995 (2). It is based on the susceptibility testing to a range of antimicrobials of a variety of animal-pathogenic, zoonotic, and indicator species of bacteria from food animal species that are important in Denmark, as well as isolates from human infections and in some years from food and healthy humans (12). DANMAP also collects and reports data on antimicrobial use in animals and humans.

The objectives of DANMAP are as follows:

- To monitor the occurrence of antimicrobial resistance among bacteria isolated from production animals, food, and humans
- To monitor the use of antimicrobial agents for treatment in humans and in animals and for growth promotion
- To demonstrate associations between such use and the occurrence of resistance.

DANMAP monitors antimicrobial resistance among *E. faecalis* and *E. faecium*, *Campylobacter coli* and *C. jejuni*, *E. coli*, and *Salmonella* from healthy animals, some food, and humans in Denmark, as well as from important animal pathogens including *Staphylococcus hyicus* subsp. *hyicus* from exudative epidermitis in pigs, *S. aureus* and coagulase-negative staphylococci from bovine mastitis, *A. pleuropneumoniae* from pleuropneumonia in pigs, *E. coli* F5 (K99) from cases of calf diarrhea, and *E. coli* serotype O149 from cases of diarrhea in piglets and weaners. The zoonotic pathogens and indicator species are isolated from samples collected from animals at slaughter, from food samples, and from humans. The frequency of sample collection from slaughterhouses is weighted by the proportion of animals slaughtered each year, and the sampled establishments represent 98, 80, and 95% of the total Danish production volume for poultry, cattle, and swine, respectively. *Salmonella* isolates included in DANMAP are randomly selected from all *Salmonella* isolates that are serotyped at the Danish Institute for Food and Veterinary Research. The animal pathogens are randomly selected from isolates received by Danish veterinary diagnostic laboratories, including only one isolate per herd per month. All of the isolates are routinely stored for future testing and characterization. Food samples (both domestic and imported) are collected at wholesale and retail by regional veterinary and food control authorities.

Susceptibility testing results are determined as MICs using broth microdilution or plate dilution (for *Campylobacter*) techniques. A wide range of antimicrobials is included in susceptibility panels, including those of importance to human and animal health and antimicrobial growth promoters.

The DANMAP antimicrobial resistance and antimicrobial use monitoring data have provided many valuable insights into the prevalence and temporal patterns of antimicrobial resistance in zoonotic, pathogenic, and indicator bacteria in food animals, food, and humans and relationships between antimicrobial use and resistance at the national level. Since 1997 the results of monitoring, along with interpretive summaries and integration of information from the farm-to-fork continuum, have been published annually in DANMAP reports, which are available electronically at www.dfvf.dk.

Denmark has implemented a number of interventions over the past decade to control antimicrobial resistance in the food animal reservoir, and DANMAP has been critically important in evaluating the impact of these actions (see reference 37 for a detailed review of this topic). In May 1995 Denmark banned the antimicrobial growth promoter avoparcin, a glycopeptide antimicrobial, because of concerns that its use in pigs and poultry contributed to an animal reservoir of glycopeptide-resistant enterococci (vancomycin-resistant enterococci [VRE]). VRE are a potential risk to public health because they may produce life-threatening illnesses in certain populations that are refractory to antimicrobial therapy. Further regulatory actions were taken in 1998 and 1999, with the

Table 3. Summary of antimicrobial resistance monitoring programs in various countries

Country	Program name	Yr initiated	Antimicrobial usage data	Source of samples					Bacteria					Reporting of susceptibility data	
				Healthy animals	Diseased animals	Food	Healthy humans	Diseased humans	*Salmonella*	*Campylobacter*	*E. coli*	Enterococci	Animal pathogens	Breakpoints	MIC
Denmark	DANMAP	1995	X	X	X	X	X	X	X	X	X	X	X	X	X
Belgium					X			X	X					X	
Canada	CIPARS	2002		X	X			X	X	X	X		X	X	X
France					X				X				X	X	X
Hungary		2001		X	X				X	X		X		X	
Italy	ITAVARM	2003		X	X				X		X		X	X	X
Japan	JVARM	1999		X	X				X	X	X	X	X	X	
The Netherlands	MARAN	2002	X	X	X			X	X	X	X	X	X	X	X
Norway	NORM-VET	2000	X	X	X			X	X	X	X	X	X	X	X
Spain	VAV	1996		X	X			X	X	X	X	X	X	X	
Sweden	SVARM	2000	X	X	X				X	X			X	X	X
United Kingdom			X	X	X				X		X	X	X	X	
United States	NARMS	1996		X	X	X		X	X	X	X	X		X	X

banning of virginiamycin, a streptogramin antimicrobial growth promoter, to prevent further selection of an animal reservoir of streptogramin-resistant *E. faecium*; and participation in the European Union-wide ban on three other antimicrobial growth promoters, tylosin, spiramycin, and bacitracin, because they belonged to classes of antimicrobial drugs also used in human medicine. Furthermore, the swine and poultry industries in Denmark voluntarily stopped using all other antimicrobial growth promoters for animal production in 1998 and 1999.

The antimicrobial growth promoters that were used in Denmark were almost exclusively active against gram-positive bacteria; therefore, the effects of selection were most evident in *E. faecium* and *E. faecalis*. The temporal relationship between the total quantities of various antimicrobial growth promoters (in kilograms of active ingredient) used in Denmark and the prevalence of resistance among enterococci to antimicrobial growth promoter classes are shown in Fig. 1. In most cases, the graphs show a temporal relationship between changes in the quantity of antimicrobial growth promoter use in food animals and the prevalence of resistance to the same classes of antimicrobials in enterococci. Antimicrobial resistance to most of the growth promoters was common when these drugs were used, but following the termination of their use, the prevalence of resistance declined substantially. The exception is avoparcin resistance among *E. faecium* of swine (3). Following the termination of avoparcin use in swine, glycopeptide resistance in *E. faecium* from swine did not substantially decline until use of the macrolide antimicrobial tylosin for growth promotion was also terminated, which is indicative of coselection by this drug. Furthermore, characterization of representative isolates of glycopeptide-resistant *E. faecium* (VRE) from swine in Denmark showed that all were from the same clone and all were resistant to macrolides and tetracyclines, encoded by the *erm*(B) (macrolides) and *vanA* (glycopeptides) genes located on the same mobile DNA element (1). This information provides further evidence of coselection of VRE by tylosin use.

While the termination of antimicrobial growth promoters was not associated with adverse effects in finisher pigs and broilers, there were some problems encountered in weaned pigs, mainly with diarrhea and sustained growth. This was accompanied by an increase in therapeutic use of some antimicrobials, notably tetracyclines. DANMAP data showed that there was an increase in tetracycline resistance among *Salmonella* of swine following the increase in therapeutic use of this drug; however, no such increase in tetracycline resistance was observed in *E. coli* of pigs, suggesting that other factors, in addition to tetracycline use, may have contributed to the resistance patterns in *Salmonella* (37).

Overall, DANMAP has been very useful in showing the important relationship between the quantities of antimicrobials used at the national level and resistance in bacteria to antimicrobials used in humans, particularly in the food animal reservoir. It clearly showed evidence of selection for antimicrobial resistance in this reservoir, and following interventions to reduce antimicrobial use, DANMAP showed an accompanying decline in the prevalence of resistance in the food animal reservoir.

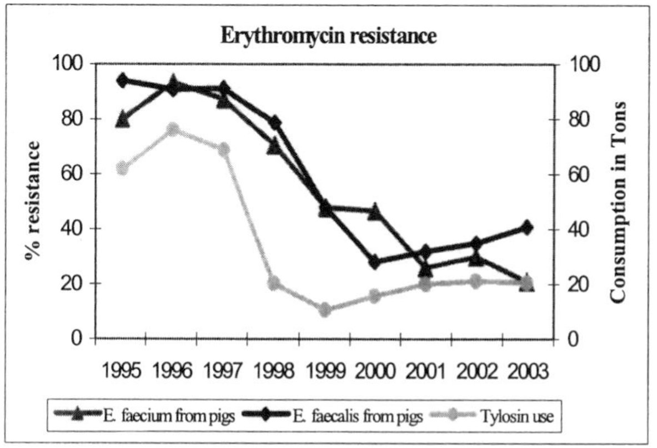

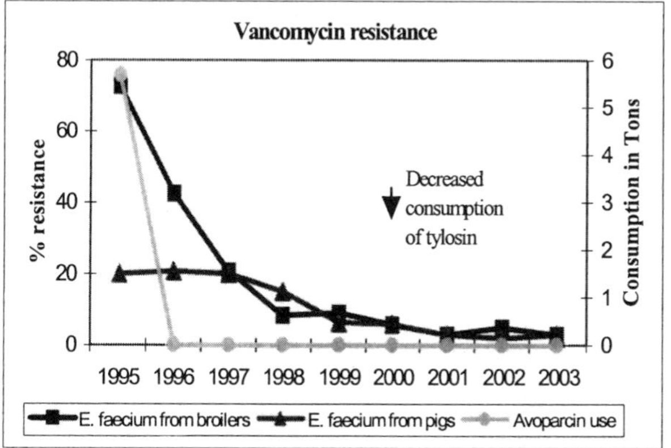

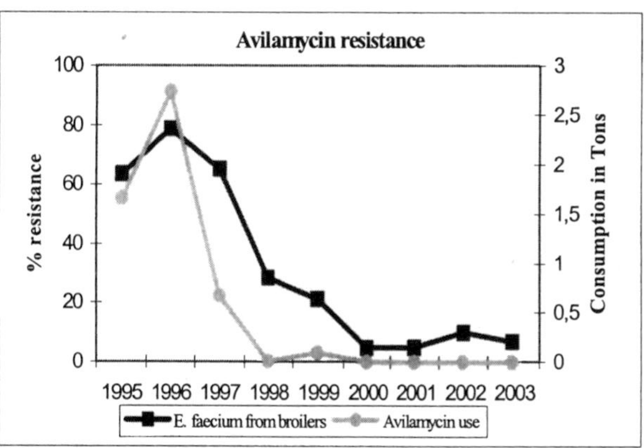

Figure 1. Annual prevalence of antimicrobial resistance in *E. faecium* and *E. faecalis* isolated from Danish pigs and broilers and consumption of antimicrobial agents for growth promotion, 1995 to 2003.

United States

The U.S. National Antimicrobial Resistance Monitoring System—Enteric Bacteria (NARMS) was established in 1996 as a collaborative effort among the Food and Drug Administration (FDA) Center for Veterinary Medicine (CVM), the U.S. Department of Agriculture (USDA), and the Centers for Disease Control and Prevention (CDC). NARMS monitors changes in susceptibilities of enteric bacteria, including *Campylobacter*, *Salmonella*, *E. coli* O157, and *Shigella* (humans only) and enterococci (from retail meats), to a wide range of antimicrobial drugs that are important in human and veterinary medicine (32). The bacterial isolates are collected from human and animal clinical specimens, healthy farm animals, raw food from animals, and recently retail meats and some animal feed ingredients (see http://www.fda.gov/cvm/index/narms/narms_pg.html). The objectives of NARMS are as follows:

- To provide descriptive data on the extent and temporal trends of antimicrobial drug susceptibility in *Salmonella* and other enteric bacterial organisms from human and animal populations, as well as retail meats
- To facilitate the identification of antimicrobial drug resistance in humans, animals, and retail meats as it arises
- To provide timely information to veterinarians and physicians on antimicrobial drug resistance patterns.

NARMS consists of three arms: an animal arm, a human arm, and a retail arm. Clinical isolates from humans are submitted by state and local public health laboratories from across the United States to the CDC in Atlanta, Ga., where all testing of human isolates is conducted. Participating health departments forward every 20th non-Typhi *Salmonella* isolate, every *Salmonella* serovar Typhi isolate, every 20th *Shigella* isolate, and every 20th *E. coli* O157 isolate to the CDC. Some states also send one *Campylobacter* isolate each week to the CDC. Animal specimens for NARMS are collected from federally inspected slaughter and processing facilities, from healthy animals on farms, and from veterinary diagnostic laboratories including the USDA's National Veterinary Services Laboratories. All antimicrobial drug susceptibility testing of animal isolates is conducted at the USDA Agricultural Research Service's Russell Research Center in Athens, Ga. Susceptibility testing of isolates from retail meats and animal feed ingredients is conducted at the CVM's Office of Research lab in Laurel, Md.

Antimicrobial resistance patterns are available for *Salmonella* from humans and animals since 1997, and the other bacteria were added over time. In 2001 a pilot study of retail meat sampling was initiated, and in 2002 it was expanded to states participating in the FoodNet program, a comprehensive food-borne infection active surveillance program based on sentinel states. Annual reports of the human and animal arms of NARMS are published separately by the CDC and USDA and are available on the CDC, USDA, and FDA CVM websites. These reports provide detailed information, primarily in tabular form.

NARMS data, along with other information from epidemiological studies, documented the marked rise in the United States of fluoroquinolone resistance in *C. jejuni*, an important cause of human diarrheal and other illness, from broiler chickens and humans following the approval of enrofloxacin and sarafloxacin for the control of septicemic *E. coli* infections in chickens. In 2000 (with revision in 2001), the FDA CVM published a quantitative risk assessment of the human health impact of fluoroquinolone (FQ)-resistant *Campylobacter* attributed to the consumption of chicken, using data from NARMS and other sources (9). A mathematical model was used to estimate the following quantities for a given year: (i) the mean number of *Campylobacter* cases in the U.S. population; (ii) the mean number of FQ-resistant *Campylobacter* cases attributable to chicken; and (iii) the mean number of FQ-resistant *Campylobacter* cases attributable to chicken, seeking care, treated with FQ, and therefore affected by the FQ resistance. The model estimated that in 1999 the mean number of people in the United States who had FQ-resistant *Campylobacter* infection and received FQ (the adverse health impact) was 9,261, with 5th- and 95th-percentile estimates of 5,227 and 15,326, respectively. This risk assessment, supported by NARMS data, was important in the CVM's recent actions to withdrawal approval of fluoroquinolones in poultry.

The FDA CVM has also been active in developing new approaches for the preapproval assessment of antimicrobial resistance risks from antimicrobials used in animals. One proposal was the development of "thresholds" for resistance in selected target microorganisms. Under this concept, if resistance exceeds a certain preset threshold, then steps would be taken to reduce such resistance, for example, by reduced use of the drug (8). If this concept is adopted in the future, a high-quality resistance monitoring system, such as NARMS, will be essential for determining when such thresholds are reached. In 2003 the CVM published further guidance for assessing resistance risks in new animal drug applications. This approach recommends resistance risk assessment of new animal drug applications that in some cases may require the use of NARMS for preapproval (baseline) and postapproval monitoring of antimicrobial resistance (7).

Belgium

Antimicrobial resistance monitoring focuses on *Salmonella* from the major species of food animals, and the results of susceptibility testing are published in the *Salmonella* reports of the Veterinary and Agrochemical Research Centre (http://www.var.fgov.be/reports_eng.php).

Canada

In 2002 the Canadian Integrated Program for Antimicrobial Resistance Surveillance (CIPARS) was initiated (4). In order to test the feasibility of a representative and methodologically unified surveillance system, the program began with several demonstration projects in the human and food animal sectors. Information was collected on antimicrobial use and antimicrobial resistance in enteric pathogens (*Salmonella* and *Campylobacter*) and commensal organisms (mainly *E. coli*) from animals and foods from animals at the farm, slaughterhouse, and retail levels, and in enteric pathogens from humans.

The objectives of the first CIPARS report (2002) (4) were (i) to describe the current reporting structure for enteric diseases, investigate the epidemiology of antimicrobial resistance trends in *Salmonella* and *Shigella*, and illustrate the strengths and limitations of using routinely generated data for nationwide antimicrobial resistance surveillance and (ii) to describe antimicrobial resistance patterns for generic *E. coli* and *Salmonella* from sampled commodities. Public health laboratories from five provinces provided antimicrobial resistance data on *Salmonella* isolates from humans. The antimicrobial susceptibility methods and antimicrobial testing panels varied by province, but all resistance profiles were interpreted using NCCLS guidelines. *Salmonella* and *E. coli* from animals at slaughter were obtained through active and passive (*Salmonella* only) systems. For the active system, a sampling plan was designed to provide nationally representative and epidemiologically valid antimicrobial susceptibility data from bacteria isolated from animals entering the food chain. The target sample size was 150 isolates (a balance between desired statistical precision and cost) each of *Salmonella* and *E. coli* from each of three commodities: beef, pork, and chicken. A two-stage random sampling plan was used for sample collection. Federally inspected slaughterhouses from across Canada were randomly selected with probability proportional to their slaughter volume. Cecal samples from slaughtered animals were collected using systematic random selection methods so that animals were selected throughout the year. *Salmonella* isolates collected in the passive system were submitted by veterinary diagnostic laboratories and other sources to the Laboratory for Foodborne Zoonoses, Health Canada, for antimicrobial resistance testing. Antimicrobial susceptibility testing was conducted using the broth microdilution technique and NARMS Sensititre susceptibility panels. Results were interpreted by using NCCLS guidelines.

The 2002 CIPARS report (4) presents summaries of susceptibility testing of *Salmonella* and *E. coli* collected in the active and passive components of the program and antimicrobial use data from humans. It is anticipated that future CIPARS reports will be more comprehensive and will contain antimicrobial use data from animals and results of active surveillance in humans, with more in-depth analysis of trends and correlations between antimicrobial use and resistance in livestock, food, and human populations.

France

The Agence Française de Securité Sanitaire des Aliments organizes antimicrobial resistance monitoring among food animals. This includes bovine pathogens through one network and *Salmonella* through another. Susceptibility testing is conducted at various laboratories (23).

Hungary

A national monitoring program has also been established in Hungary (18). Susceptibility testing on isolates from diagnostic samples has been conducted for a long time, but the procedures have now been standardized and data are collected centrally. In addition, since January 2001 the antibiotic susceptibility of *E. coli*, *Salmonella*, *Campylobacter*, and *Enterococcus* strains isolated from the colons of slaughter cows, pigs, and broiler chickens has been examined among samples submitted to a central laboratory from each of the 19 counties of Hungary.

Italy

Monitoring in Italy (ITAVARM) was first conducted in 2003, and the first report has just become available (5). The program includes data on resistance in *Salmonella* from food animals and humans and different bacterial species pathogenic for animals.

Japan

The Japanese Veterinary Antimicrobial Resistance Monitoring (JVARM) Program was established in 1999 to examine the susceptibility of bacteria from food-producing animals to antimicrobial agents (http://www.nval.go.jp/taisei/etaisei/honbun.htm). The bacteria tested include zoonotic bacteria and indicator bacteria isolated from healthy animals and pathogenic bacteria isolated from diseased animals. Zoonotic bacteria include *Salmonella* species and *C. jejuni* or *C. coli*; indicator bacteria include *E. coli*, including O157, and *E. faecium* or *E. faecalis*. Animal pathogens included are *Salmonella* species, *S. aureus*, *A. pleuropneumoniae*, *Actinobacillus pyogenes*, *Pasteurella multocida*, *Streptococcus* species, and *Klebsiella* species. The results on resistance in *Salmonella* have been published (14).

Norway

In 2000 Norway established the Norwegian monitoring program for antimicrobial resistance in the veterinary and food production sectors (NORM-VET). The program is coordinated by the Norwegian Zoonosis Centre at the National Veterinary Institute. Monitoring of antimicrobial resistance in the human sector is conducted by the NORM program. NORM-VET includes monitoring of antimicrobial usage in humans, animals, and aquaculture in Norway. The 2004 report (27) contains the results of antimicrobial resistance monitoring of clinical isolates of bacteria from cases of mastitis in cattle and winter ulcer in Atlantic salmon, indicator bacteria (*E. coli* and enterococci) from feces of cattle and sheep and meat from cattle, and zoonotic bacteria (*Salmonella* and *Campylobacter*) from sheep and poultry. Susceptibility testing results from a wide variety of human infections are also included. NORM-VET annual reports have been published since 2000 and contain the results of susceptibility testing both in terms of breakpoints and MICs, along with interpretive summaries.

Spain

In Spain the Red de Vigilancia de Resistencias Antibióticas en Bacterias de Origen Veterinario (VAV) network for monitoring antimicrobial resistance among bacteria from animals and humans was created in 1996. The monitoring of resistance in *E. coli* and *E. faecium* from healthy pigs was initiated in 1998 and collection of data from *Salmonella* from poultry slaughterhouses in 1999 (25).

Sweden

Sweden has been monitoring antimicrobial resistance in *Salmonella* from animals since 1978. In 2000 a more comprehensive program for antimicrobial resistance monitoring, entitled Swedish Veterinary Antimicrobial Resistance Monitoring (SVARM), was initiated by the Swedish Veterinary Institute (26). The objectives of SVARM are to obtain data on antibiotic sensitivity of bacteria from animals and to detect trends in resistance. The results can be used as a basis for policy recommendations and for evaluation of the effect of interventions such as changed usage of antibiotics.

Zoonotic bacteria (*Salmonella* and *Campylobacter*), indicator bacteria (*E. coli* and enterococci), and animal pathogens are included in the program. *Salmonella* is collected through the national notifiable disease program, and one isolate per incident is included. Indicator bacteria are isolated from cecal or colonic samples from healthy fattening pigs, broiler chickens, and cattle up to 12 months of age, mainly at slaughter. In order to obtain representative data and the desired sample size, samples (one per herd) are collected at slaughterhouses throughout Sweden in proportion to production volume. Susceptibility tests to a wide range of antimicrobials of importance to animals and humans are performed with microdilution techniques according to NCCLS guidelines. The results are published in an annual report showing breakpoint and MIC data with confidence limits on prevalence estimates. There are future plans to coordinate SVARM with activities in antimicrobial resistance in bacteria from food and humans.

The Netherlands

Monitoring of Antimicrobial Resistance and Antimicrobial Usage in Animals in The Netherlands (MARAN) has been published by the Veterinary Antibiotic Usage and Resistance Surveillance Working Group since 2002 (24). The program objectives are detection of the emergence of new resistance phenotypes, determination of trends in resistance over time, and detection of potential public health risks. The program is based on zoonotic bacteria (*Salmonella*, *Campylobacter*, and *E. coli* O157) from humans and animals, commensal bacteria of animal origin (*E. coli* and enterococci), animal pathogens (e.g., respiratory and mastitis pathogens), and data on usage of antimicrobials in food animals. Samples are obtained from diagnostic submissions and various other monitoring programs. Susceptibility testing to a range of antimicrobials is performed using broth microdilution and agar dilution tests according to NCCLS guidelines.

United Kingdom

Susceptibility testing of animal pathogens is conducted in regional veterinary diagnostic laboratories, and the results are published annually by the Department of Environment, Food and Rural Affairs (http://www.defra.gov.uk/animalh/diseases/zoonoses/index.htm). Resistance in zoonotic and indicator organisms from cattle, sheep, and pigs is also monitored.

International Programs

The above-mentioned monitoring programs are not coordinated internationally, and there is a lack of standardization and collaboration between laboratories. This is highly needed. Data on the occurrences of antimicrobial resistance among *Salmonella* are collected by the European Union from the different member countries every year, but the basis of the data is to a large extent unknown.

Consequently, a number of international initiatives have been undertaken, including the establishment of Global Salm Surv (GSS) by the World Health Organization (WHO) (http://www.who.int/salmsurv/en/). GSS is a global network of laboratories and individuals involved in surveillance, isolation, identification, and antimicrobial resistance testing of *Salmonella*. It is part of the WHO's endeavors to strengthen the capacities of its member states in the surveillance and control of major food-borne diseases and to contribute to the global effort of containment of antimicrobial resistance in food-borne pathogens. The program was started in January 2000 and is aimed at microbiologists and epidemiologists who work in public health, veterinary services, food-related services, or environmental health. Currently, GSS focuses only on *Salmonella*, but it is in progress to extend the program to other major food-borne pathogens. Thus, isolation of *Campylobacter* is included in the training courses' programs. In October 2004, GSS had 840 general members and 471 institutional members in 138 countries.

The main program activities are as follows. Activities open to all members are:

- Data sharing and communication between laboratories and individuals via e-mail, GSS website, GSS list server, and/or facsimile
- An international, online-accessible database that contains contact information for national and regional salmonellosis laboratories; descriptions of laboratory responsibilities, laboratory methods, and types of samples received; and annual surveillance summary results of the most frequently isolated *Salmonella* serotypes

Activities directed towards member institutions are:

- Participation in regional training courses on surveillance for food-borne diseases
- Participation in external quality assurance programs on *Salmonella* serotyping and antimicrobial susceptibility testing
- Reference testing of selected *Salmonella* strains
- Provision of technical information and methodological support and help in identifying a reliable source of antisera

One of the main means of capacity building is the training programs that are offered at seven sites: Bangkok, Thailand; Buenos Aires, Argentina; Cairo, Egypt; Merida, Mexico; Port-of-Spain, Trinidad; Warsaw, Poland; and Yaoundé, Cameroon. Another important program element is an annual external quality assurance program organized by the Danish Institute for Food and Veterinary Research, where isolates of *Salmonella* are shipped to all participants and results of serotyping and susceptibility testing are entered by each participant and checked against reference results. This program was initiated in 2000 with 44 participants (31) and by 2003 had expanded to 153 participants.

Another international network focusing on zoonotic bacteria and antimicrobial resistance is Enter-Net (http://www.hpa.org.uk/hpa/inter/enter-net_menu.htm), which is a network of microbiologists in charge of national human reference laboratories for *Salmonella* and *E. coli* infections and epidemiologists responsible for the national surveillance of these infections. The network involves 19 countries of the European Union plus Australia, Canada, Japan, Norway, South Africa, and Switzerland. It includes harmonization of test procedures, collection and sharing of annual data, and communication of new findings to participants in the network. The network has had considerable success in identifying international outbreaks of *Salmonella* (11, 19) but is, however, limited to human health laboratories.

Such international networks, as well as open and free international collaboration and sharing of data, are greatly needed if we are going to combat global problems involving the spread of resistant and multiple-resistant microorganisms.

DISCUSSION AND RECOMMENDATIONS

Antimicrobial resistance monitoring programs are critically important for the control of antimicrobial resistance in human and animal populations. They fulfill a variety of purposes that support the prudent use of antimicrobials in animals and humans, including providing information that can guide antimicrobial use policies, identifying the need for timely interventions to prevent the further increase and spread of resistance, and monitoring the effectiveness of interventions.

Several considerations have to be taken into account before the establishment of any program for monitoring antimicrobial resistance. The most important factor is to decide on the purpose of the system, which to a large extent will determine the sampling strategies and microbiological methodologies to be used in the program.

In the future we expect to observe increased traveling and trade of food products. This will provide optimal conditions for the rapid global spread of problems related to food safety. Thus, early detection and communication of important new findings is absolutely essential for the future. It will not be sufficient to read through the scientific literature or annual reports, where information will be 1 to 2 years old. An international platform for rapid communication does not currently exist, but it is essential (20) and should be a high priority for international organizations such as the WHO.

Another and perhaps even more essential point is the lack of action plans among the competent authorities that are to be enacted when data become available. In many cases, the actions that were taken differed considerably even in similar cases and were often driven by whether any information became known to the public through the media. A contingency plan should be developed in all countries and based on international networks, preferably through competent organizations such as the WHO. National committees have been or are under implementation in some countries, but examples of their efficacy and any international collaboration are still missing.

National monitoring programs have been implemented in a number of countries worldwide. Most programs focus on pathogenic bacteria or *Salmonella*, but some also report data on resistance in indicator bacteria isolated from healthy animals. Currently, none of the programs is aimed specifically at detecting emerging resistance using selective enrichment or other methodologies. Furthermore, there is no international exchange or central evaluation of data. Thus, at present the global overview and knowledge of antimicrobial resistance in food animals is incomplete and our current ability to detect emerging resistance and limit the global spread at a very early stage is very limited. In addition, the different programs vary in the methodology used and the antimicrobial agents to which susceptibility is tested. Coordinated monitoring of antimicrobial resistance carried out by an international network of laboratories should be implemented in order to be able to identify and report emerging resistance problems at the earliest possible stage. In this way we might be able to implement interventions before emerging resistance has a substantial impact on public health, animal health, or international trade.

Knowledge about antimicrobial resistance should be combined with knowledge regarding the usage of antimicrobial agents for different food animal species, which also should be performed on an internationally comparable basis. Such combined knowledge is needed to assess the impact on the occurrence of resistance and to determine where and for which infections most antimicrobials are used.

REFERENCES

1. **Aarestrup, F. M.** 2000. Characterization of glycopeptide-resistant *Enterococcus faecium* from broilers and pigs in Denmark. Genetic evidences that the persistence of GRE among the pig population is associated with coselection by resistance to macrolides. *J. Clin. Microbiol.* **38:**2774–2777.
2. **Aarestrup, F. M., F. Bager, M. Madsen, N. E. Jensen, A. Meyling, and H. C. Wegener.** 1998. Surveillance of antimicrobial resistance in bacteria isolated from food animals to antimicrobial growth promoters and related therapeutic agents in Denmark. *APMIS* **10:**606–622.
3. **Aarestrup, F. M., A. M. Seyfarth, H. D. Emborg, K. Pedersen, R. S. Hendriksen, and F. Bager.** 2001. Effect of abolishment of the use of antimicrobial agents for growth promotion on occurrence of antimicrobial resistance in fecal enterococci from food animals in Denmark. *Antimicrob. Agents Chemother.* **45:**2054–2059.
4. **Anonymous.** 2003. Canadian Integrated Program for Antimicrobial Resistance Surveillance (CIPARS). Health Canada, Ottawa, Ontario, Canada.
5. **Anonymous.** 2004. Italian Veterinary Antimicrobial Resistance Monitoring (ITAVARM)—2003. Istituto Zooprofilattico Sperimentale delle Regioni Lazio e Toscana, Rome, Italy.
6. **Brun, E., G. Holstad, H. Kruse, and J. Jarp.** 2002. Within-sample and between-sample variation of antimicrobial resistance in fecal *Escherichia coli* isolates from pigs. *Microb. Drug Resist.* **8:**385–391.
7. **Center for Veterinary Medicine, Food and Drug Administration.** 2003. Guidance for industry #152: evaluating the safety of antimicrobial new animal drugs with regard to their microbiological effects on bacteria of human health concern. Center for Veterinary Medicine, Food and Drug Administration, Rockville, Md.
8. **Center for Veterinary Medicine, Food and Drug Administration.** 2000. An approach for establishing thresholds in association with the use of antimicrobial drugs in food-producing animals. Center for Veterinary Medicine, Food and Drug Administration, Rockville, Md.
9. **Center for Veterinary Medicine, Food and Drug Administration.** 2000. Risk assessment on the human health impact of

fluoroquinolone resistant Campylobacter associated with the consumption of chicken. Center for Veterinary Medicine, Food and Drug Administration, Rockville, Md.

10. **Courvalin, P.** 1996. Interpretive reading of *in vitro* antibiotic susceptibility tests (the antibiogramme). *Clin. Microbiol. Infect.* **2:**26–34.
11. **Crook, P. D., J. F. Aguilera, E. J. Threlfall, S. J. O'Brien, G. Sigmundsdottir, D. Wilson, I. S. Fisher, A. Ammon, H. Briem, J. M. Cowden, M. E. Locking, H. Tschape, W. van Pelt, L. R. Ward, and M. A. Widdowson.** 2003. A European outbreak of *Salmonella enterica* serotype Typhimurium definitive phage type 204b in 2000. *Clin. Microbiol. Infect.* **9:**839–845.
12. **The Danish Integrated Antimicrobial Resistance Monitoring and Research Programme.** 2004. DANMAP 2003—Use of antimicrobial agents and occurrence of antimicrobial resistance in bacteria from food, animals and humans in Denmark. Danish Institute for Food and Veterinary Research, Copenhagen, Denmark.
13. **Dunlop, R. H., S. A. McEwen, A. H. Meek, R. M. Friendship, W. D. Black, and R C. Clarke.** 1999. Sampling considerations for herd-level measurement of faecal *Escherichia coli* antimicrobial resistance in finisher pigs. *Epidemiol. Infect.* **122:**485–496.
14. **Esaki, H., A. Morioka, K. Ishihara, A. Kojima, S. Shiroki, Y. Tamura, and T. Takahashi.** 2004. Antimicrobial susceptibility of Salmonella isolated from cattle, swine and poultry (2001–2002): report from the Japanese Veterinary Antimicrobial Resistance Monitoring Program. *J. Antimicrob. Chemother.* **53:**266–270.
15. **Expert Advisory Group on Antimicrobial Resistance.** 2003. EAGAR importance rating and summary of antibiotic uses in humans in Australia. http://www.nhmrc.gov.au/eagar/antirate.pdf.
16. **Franklin, A., J. Acar, F. Anthony, R. Gupta, T. Nicholls, Y. Tamura, S. Thompson, E. J. Threlfall, D. Vose, M. van Vuuren, D. G. White, H.C. Wegener, and M. I. Costarrica.** 2001. Antimicrobial resistance: harmonisation of national antimicrobial resistance monitoring and surveillance programmes in animals and animal derived food. *Rev. Sci. Tech. Off. Int. Epizoot.* **20:**859–870.
17. **Joint Expert Advisory Committee on Antibiotic Resistance.** 1999. The use of antibiotics in food-producing animals: antibiotic-resistant bacteria in animals and humans. Commonwealth of Australia, Canberra, Australia.
18. **Kaszanyitzky, E. J., A. Tarpai, S. Janosi, M. Papp, J. Skare, and G. Semjen.** 2002. Development of an antibiotic resistance monitoring system in Hungary. *Acta Vet. Hung.* **50:**189–197.
19. **Kirk, M. D., C. L. Little, M. Lem, M. Fyfe, D. Genobile, A. Tan, E. J. Threlfall, A. Paccagnella, D. Lightfoot, H. Lyi, L. McIntyre, L. R. Ward, D. J. Brown, S. Surnam, and I. S. Fisher.** 2004. An outbreak due to peanuts in their shell caused by *Salmonella enterica* serotypes Stanley and Newport—sharing molecular information to solve international outbreaks. *Epidemiol. Infect.* **132:**571–577.
20. **Lappas, E.** 2002. Information management in community health and primary care. *Health Inform. Libr. J.* **19:**236–238.
21. **Levy, S. B.** 1982. Microbial resistance to antibiotics. An evolving and persistent problem. *Lancet* **10:**83–88.
22. **Martel, J. L., E. Chaslus-Dancla, M. Coudert, F. Poumarat, and J. P. Lafont.** 1995. Survey of antimicrobial resistance in bacterial isolates from diseased cattle in France. *Microb. Drug Resist.* **1:**273–283.
23. **Martel, J. L., F. Tardy, A. Brisabois, R. Lailler, M. Coudert, and E. Chaslus-Dancla.** 2000. The French antibiotic resistance monitoring programs. *Int. J. Antimicrob. Agents* **1:** 275–283.
24. **Mevius, D. J., and W. van Pelt (ed.).** 2002. MARAN 2002: Monitoring of antimicrobial resistance and antimicrobial usage in animals in the Netherlands in 2002. http://www.cidc-lelystad.nl/docs/MARAN-2002-web.pdf.
25. **Moreno, M. A., L. Domínguez, T. Teshager, I. A. Herrero, M. C. Porrero, and the VAV Network.** 2000. Antibiotic resistance monitoring: the Spanish programme. *Int. J. Antimicrob. Agents* **14:**285–290.
26. **National Veterinary Institute.** 2003. SVARM 2002: Swedish Veterinary Antimicrobial Resistance Monitoring. National Veterinary Institute, Uppsala, Sweden.
27. **NORM AND NORM-VET.** 2002. NORM/NORM-VET 2002. Consumption of antimicrobial agents and occurrence of antimicrobial resistance in Norway. NORM, Tromsø, Norway, and NORM-VET, Oslo, Norway.
28. **O'Brien, T. F.** 1997. The global epidemic nature of antimicrobial resistance and the need to monitor and manage it locally. *Clin. Infect. Dis.* **24:**2–8.
29. **Office International des Épizooties.** 2000. *International Animal Health Code: Mammals, Birds and Bees*, 9th ed. Office International des Épizooties, Paris, France.
30. **Office of Technology Assessment, Congress of the United States.** 1995. *Impacts of Antibiotic-Resistant Bacteria.* Government Printing Office, Washington, D.C.
31. **Petersen, A., F. M. Aarestrup, F. J. Angulo, S. Wong, K. Stöhr, and H. C. Wegener.** 2002. WHO Global Salm-Surv external quality assurance system (EQAS): an important step toward improving the quality of *Salmonella* serotyping and antimicrobial susceptibility testing worldwide. *Microb. Drug Resist.* **8:**345–353.
32. **Tollefson, L., W. T. Flynn, and M. L. Headrick.** 2003. Regulatory activities of the U.S. Food and Drug Administration designed to control antimicrobial resistance in foodborne pathogens, p. 57–63. *In* M. E. Torrence and R. E. Isaacson (ed.), *Microbial Food Safety in Animal Agriculture.* Iowa State University Press, Ames.
33. **Wagner, B., P. S. Morley, D. A. Dargatz, T. E. Wittum, T. J. Keefe, and M. D. Salman.** 2003. Short-term repeatability of measurements of antimicrobial susceptibility of *Escherichia coli* isolated from feces of feedlot cattle. *J. Vet. Diagn. Investig.* **15:**535–542.
34. **White, D. G., J. Acar, F. Anthony, A. Franklin, R. Gupta, T. Nicholls, Y. Tamura, S. Thompson, E. J. Threlfall, D. Vose, M. van Vuuren, H. C. Wegener, and M. L. Costarrica.** 2001. Antimicrobial resistance: standardisation and harmonisation of laboratory methodologies for the detection and quantification of antimicrobial resistance. *Rev. Sci. Tech. Off. Int. Epizoot.* **20:**849–858.
35. **World Health Organization.** 1997. *The Medical Impact of the Use of Antimicrobials in Food Animals. Report of a WHO Meeting, Berlin, Germany.* World Health Organization, Geneva, Switzerland.
36. **World Health Organization.** 2000. *WHO Global Principles for the Containment of Antimicrobial Resistance in Animals Intended for Food.* World Health Organization, Geneva, Switzerland.
37. **World Health Organization.** 2003. *International Review Panel Evaluation of the Termination of the Use of Antimicrobial Growth Promoters in Denmark.* World Health Organization, Geneva, Switzerland.
38. **World Health Organization.** 2003. *Joint FAO/OIE/WHO Expert Workshop on Non-Human Antimicrobial Usage and Antimicrobial Resistance: Scientific Assessment.* World Health Organization, Geneva, Switzerland.
39. **Wray, C., I. M. McLaren, and Y. E. Beedell.** 1993. Bacterial resistance monitoring of salmonellas isolated from animals, national experience of surveillance schemes in the United Kingdom. *Vet. Microbiol.* **35:**313–319.

Antimicrobial Resistance in Bacteria of Animal Origin
Edited by Frank M. Aarestrup

Chapter 24

Risk Assessment and Its Use in Approval, Licensing, and Prudent Use Guidelines

David Vose

INTRODUCTION

The purpose of risk assessment is to help a manager better understand the risks (and opportunities) being faced and to evaluate the options available for their control. The preliminary task in any risk assessment is to identify:

1. The risk issue that needs to be addressed, including defining the correct scope of the problem. This is a complex issue, and a risk assessment team may have to return to redefining the scope of their risk assessment one or more times during the analysis. Each proposed risk management action will have various consequences, and the decision maker has to determine which will be included in the assessment. For example, withdrawing an antimicrobial from use in food-producing animals may have the desired effect of reducing the exposure to a specific resistant pathogen from that animal, but it may also have several unintended consequences, including the replacement of the banned antimicrobial with another of greater human health impact. It has been argued, for example, that the banning of antimicrobial growth promoters in Denmark has resulted in an increased use of therapeutic antibiotics like tetracyclines, penicillins, and macrolides that are used in human medicine (14).

Other possible unwanted effects include promoting clandestine use of the antimicrobial, thus reducing the ability to monitor and regulate its use; increasing adverse health effects in animals that the banned antimicrobial suppressed, which result in animal suffering and lower food quality; or increasing the cost of food animal production, resulting in increased cost to the consumer and perhaps even other human health effects from poorer nutrition in lower socioeconomic levels of the community. At the same time, withdrawing an antimicrobial, or limiting its use in animals, may also reduce exposure to other resistant pathogens from the same animal or to commensal bacteria that develop a resistance reservoir. Removing antimicrobials for use as growth promoters can also open up new export markets and increase the value of meat products.

2. The risk management options that need to be evaluated. Risk assessments to date have focused primarily on a regulatory agency's possible options for managing and controlling antimicrobial resistance from animal use of antimicrobials. The options are generally very limited: (i) withhold approval (for new drugs or for a change of use), (ii) withdraw the product completely, (iii) restrict its approved use within the nation's boundaries, or (iv) regulate and test imported products. The agency's options are also limited by legal constraints on the issues it can consider and the actions it can take. However, a broader view would be able to recognize the role that food producers, pharmaceutical companies, retailers, consumers, and the media might play in managing the human exposure to resistant bacteria from animals. This, of course, requires wider cooperation between different regulatory agencies and with the various industries involved, which is infrequent.

3. How the decision maker wishes to value the costs and effects of the possible risk management options. It is not the role of risk assessment to judge the value of the proposed risk management options. However, a risk assessment must provide the outputs necessary for the risk management to make that judgment. Human health impact from resistant bacteria ranges from slightly extended duration of mild diarrhea to increased mortality. The risk management needs to provide some clear way of combining and balancing such effects, of which there are several

David Vose • Vose Consulting, Le Bourg, 24400 Les Lèches, France.

approaches, from the purely economic valuation of loss of production by the affected individuals, through setting thresholds of maximum risk levels for each health impact, to normative scales like quality-adjusted life years. Other impacts may also be involved, like animal welfare and social and environmental impacts.

Risk Management Options

Within the context of antimicrobial-resistant bacteria from animals, the appropriate risk management options can be divided into several categories:

Acceptance (do nothing)

Nothing is done to control the risk or one's exposure to that risk. This is appropriate for risks where the cost of control is out of proportion with the risk. It is usually applied to low-probability, low-impact risks of which one may have a vast list, but in evaluating risks individually one may be missing some high-value risk mitigation or avoidance options that control several risks at once. If the chosen response is acceptance, considerable thought should be given to risk contingency planning.

Increase

One may already be spending significant resources on risk management that is excessive compared to the level of protection that it affords against the risk in question. In such cases, it is logical to reduce the level of protection and allocate the resources to manage other risks, thereby achieving superior overall risk efficiency. It may be logical, but nonetheless politically unacceptable. There may not be too many politicians or regulators who want to explain to the public that they have just authorized less caution in handling the use of antimicrobials in animals.

Get more information

A risk analysis can describe the level of uncertainty there is about the decision problem (here uncertainty is distinct from inherent randomness). Uncertainty, for example, about model parameter values or the scope, exposure pathways, causes, or biology of the problem can often be reduced by acquiring more information (whereas randomness cannot). Thus, a decision maker can determine that there is too much uncertainty to make a robust decision and request that more information be collected. Using a quantitative risk assessment model, the risk assessor can advise as to the least costly method of collecting extra data that would be needed to achieve the required level of precision. Value-of-information arguments can be used to assess how much, if any, extra information should be collected.

Avoidance (elimination)

This involves changing a method of operation so that the identified risk is no longer relevant. Avoidance is usually employed for high-probability, high-impact-type risks. For example, one may choose to not allow the use of a particular antimicrobial in animals at all or to restrict the usage. Avoidance includes a precautionary approach, favored in Europe but less so in the United States, for an identified possible risk for which no information is available to estimate its magnitude (perhaps because the risk has not yet occurred, or the link to a risk factor has not been scientifically or quantitatively established).

Reduction (mitigation)

Reduction involves a range of techniques, which may be used together, to reduce the probability of the risk, its impact, or both. Examples are performing more quality tests or inspections, providing better training to personnel, requiring higher hygiene standards, and improving public and medical practitioner awareness.

Reduction strategies are usually used for any level of risk where the remaining risk is not of very high severity and where the benefits (the amount the risk is reduced by) outweigh the reduction costs. They are also used where the risk cannot be eliminated. The food animal industry, veterinarians, pharmaceutical companies, medical practitioners, retailers, and consumers have the greatest flexibility to control human exposure to resistant bacteria. However, estimating the effect of such controls requires more-detailed knowledge of the system than may be available.

Contingency planning

Contingency plans are devised to optimize the response to identified risks should they occur, for example, the emergence of new bacterial resistance to an important human antimicrobial. They can be used in conjunction with acceptance and reduction strategies. The plan should identify what to do, who should do it and in what order, the window of opportunity, etc. For example, an agreement might be made that an antimicrobial is authorized for animal use as long as resistance remains below an agreed, predefined level. Once that level is reached, the antimicrobial is voluntarily withdrawn or its use restricted.

What Makes a Good Risk Assessment?

The Society for Risk Analysis (SRA) laid down a number of basic principles for risk assessment (21). (Note that the SRA uses the term "risk analysis," which translates to the Codex Alimentarius' definition of "risk assessment" in food safety). They are paraphrased here for brevity:

- Risk analysis assesses the substantive qualities, seriousness, likelihood, and conditions of a hazard or risk and of the options for managing it.
- Risk analysis uses observations about what we know to make predictions about what we don't know.
- Risk analysis is a fundamentally science-based process that strives to reflect the realities of nature.
- Risk analysis seeks to inform, not to dictate, the complex and difficult choices among possible measures to mitigate risks.
- Risk analysis integrates physical, biological, social, cultural, and economic knowledge as appropriate.
- Decisions about risks are usually needed when knowledge is incomplete, so risk analysts rely on informed judgment and on models reflecting plausible interpretations of the realities of nature, with disclosure of uncertainties.
- Risk analysts, unless prohibited, should share the data underlying their published analyses so they can be checked.
- Risk analysts openly acknowledge their sponsors and data sources.

These principles are very robust and apply well through all scientific arenas of risk assessment.

GUIDELINES

The World Health Organization advocates the use of a risk-based approach to approving and evaluating continued use of antimicrobials in food-producing animals (23). It advises giving priority to products considered most important in human medicine. Characterization of the risk should include consideration of the importance of the drug or members of the same class of drug to human medicine, the potential exposure of humans to antimicrobial-resistant bacteria and their resistance genes from food animals, as well as other appropriate scientific factors. Those antimicrobials judged to be essential for human medicine should be restricted, and their use in food animals should be justified by culture and susceptibility results.

The Office International des Épizooties (OIE) is the international body for setting guidelines and recommendations on sanitary measures relating to animal health and the development and revision of international standards for the safe international trade of animals and animal products. The OIE commissioned an ad hoc working group to produce a series of papers on antimicrobial use in animals, one of which described the appropriate use of risk assessment (22). The paper highlighted a number of points:

- Qualitative risk assessment should always be undertaken, and provides information on whether a more quantitative analysis is necessary or feasible.
- Semiquantitative risk assessment (defined as "an assessment where estimates of the likelihood of the outcome and the magnitude of the consequences are expressed in semiquantitative terms via some scoring mechanism") can provide a systematic method for determining the most effective set of controls to manage a broad range of risks.
- A risk assessment model should only be as complex as necessary to evaluate the risk management options available.
- Farm-to-fork-style risk assessments invariably contain a large number of potentially contestable assumptions because of the complexity of the system being modeled and gaps in the knowledge of that system.

It also set out a step-by-step method for conducting a complete risk analysis, including the need to plan for a way to validate the effectiveness of any risk management actions that are taken, as Denmark has done with the Danish Integrated Antimicrobial Resistance Monitoring and Research Programme (DANMAP) after the withdrawal of avoparcin (10).

RISK ASSESSMENT

Risk assessment, at its most rudimentary level, is a rational argument based on the objective evaluation of available scientific knowledge about an antimicrobial issue that gives the decision maker some improved understanding of the likely effects of various options under consideration. For example, an analysis that simply states that a risk is possible cannot be described as a risk assessment. However, an analysis that concludes that the risk is less than another, well-quantified risk may be considered a successful risk assessment as it is putting some bounds on the probability, as long as this is sufficient information for the decision maker.

It is tempting to follow the methods that have been developed in microbial food safety risk assessment, namely a farm-to-fork-style modeling of the bacterial numbers and distribution from the production animal at the farm; through processing of the meat, storage, and retail; to the final consumption of that food. However, farm-to-fork microbial risk assessment has had very limited success in influencing decisions and has been shown to have a number of important limitations:

- The exposure pathway is generally assumed to be the food or water that is consumed directly. An attempt is sometimes made to model the cross-contamination of bacteria transported into the household or catering establishment on the food, though data are difficult to acquire and apply. It is difficult to distinguish, for example, in a case-control study between campylobacteriosis cases in a domestic household that were acquired from eating undercooked chicken and cases coming from exposure via cross-contamination of *Campylobacter* brought into the home on the chicken. However, Friedman et al. (12) calculated that in the United States a population-attributable fraction (PAF) of 24% of *Campylobacter* infections was from eating chicken in restaurants, while the PAF from consumption of nonpoultry meat prepared in a restaurant was 21%, suggesting that cross-contamination is very common in U.S. restaurants. Indeed, while chicken may be the vehicle for the entry of *Campylobacter* into a restaurant, some or most of the 24% PAF of infections linked to restaurant chicken may be due to recontamination of the meal. During an animal's life it expresses vastly more bacteria than would be found on a portion of meat. Waste disposal provides a number of other exposure routes of potentially far higher bacterial count: for example, spreading manure on vegetable fields and water runoff into streams and lakes used for swimming.
- The models tend to be complex, as the possible pathways are complex. Data are rarely, if ever, sufficient to populate the models well, and surrogate data or assumed values are very commonly used. Dose-response relationships, relating the risk of an adverse health outcome to the amount of bacteria consumed, are a particular Achilles' heel, as so few data are available, and it is difficult to extrapolate those data to susceptible subgroups of the population.

Antimicrobial-resistant bacteria issues have extra layers of complexity:

- The hazard is not the bacteria, as it is for microbial food safety issues, but the resistance determinant that rises in number due to the use of the antimicrobial in animals. One must first be able to determine how much of the increase of a resistance determinant can be attributed to animal use of an antimicrobial compared with human use. There are valid arguments that recognize that there has been significant overuse of antimicrobials in human medicine and that this overuse is the greatest source of resistance and should also be controlled.
- If the bacterium in which the resistance determinant first develops is not a human pathogen, it is unlikely that much useful quantitative data have been collected on its prevalence, its growth and attenuation in different environments, and the numbers of bacteria present across the system. It is therefore extremely difficult to estimate the extent to which nonpathogenic bacterial reservoirs of resistance can or have developed.
- Some resistance determinants can be transferred between bacteria, but to model such an event one needs to have an idea of the combinations of bacteria and resistance determinants for which this is possible, the conditions in which such transfer may take place, and the rate of transfer. It is therefore extremely difficult to estimate the threat that is posed by resistance reservoirs in nonpathogenic bacteria.
- Microbial food safety risk assessment is essentially based on the assumption of a continuous flow of bacteria, from their generation in animals to human exposure. If the flow stopped, the human health impact would fairly rapidly reduce to zero. For antimicrobial resistance risk, the resistance determinant is the hazard. If there is no survival penalty to be paid in carrying a resistance determinant, we cannot say that removal of an antimicrobial will necessarily reduce the amount of resistant bacteria that humans are exposed to. If the resistant determinant is transferable and has become established in a bacterial population outside of the farm and humans, e.g., in the soil or water, we may have allowed a threat to emerge that will endure for as long as the equivalent antimicrobial is in use in humans. Thus, in microbial food safety issues, one can balance the benefits of food production against the risk of bacterial infection on a continuous

> basis, but in antimicrobial resistance issues, one has to balance what may be a short-term benefit against the much longer-term legacy of the loss of efficacy in human treatment. The development of new replacement antimicrobials is by no means assured, so it is difficult to know how to measure the resistance risk.

The following sections describe some antimicrobial resistance risk assessments that have been completed. The U.S. Food and Drug Administration (FDA) risk assessment is considered first, and separately, as it was a very public risk assessment that received a lot of positive and negative criticism; it was tested in court; and it is the only quantitative antimicrobial risk assessment this author knows of that has been publicly used directly to help decision makers determine that the best course of action was the withdrawal of an animal antimicrobial.

The FDA Fluoroquinolone Risk Assessment

The FDA Center for Veterinary Medicine (CVM) commissioned a risk assessment on the use of fluoroquinolones in poultry for the treatment of respiratory disease (2, 11). The use of fluoroquinolones in chickens and the development of resistant *Campylobacter* in chickens were of concern for several reasons. First, chickens are reservoirs for many food-borne pathogens, including *Campylobacter* and *Salmonella*. Consumption of food contaminated with these bacteria leads to illness in susceptible individuals. Second, *Campylobacter* is the most common known cause of bacterial, food-borne illness in the United States. Sporadic cases of *Campylobacter* account for approximately 99% of all *Campylobacter* cases. Epidemiological investigations of sporadic infections have indicated that chicken is the most common source of human infection. Also, slaughter and processing of chickens may result in bacterial contamination on the carcass that can survive on retail product and result in human exposure during food preparation and consumption. Third, *Campylobacter* has been reported to develop resistance when fluoroquinolones are used. Finally, fluoroquinolones are used in human medicine empirically to treat gastrointestinal infections, such as campylobacteriosis, and are important for use in many other therapeutic indications in human medicine.

The model assumed that humans are exposed to resistant bacteria and that infected people are treated in the same manner irrespective of the level of susceptibility of the infecting bacteria. The modeling approach used estimated the incremental human health impact of resistant, food-borne disease without assessing all the factors influencing the cause of the food-borne illness itself.

Information from the U.S. Department of Agriculture (USDA) and Centers for Disease Control and Prevention (CDC) on sources of food-borne disease indicated that chicken carcasses carry a relatively high level of *Campylobacter* and are associated with a large number of cases of food-borne illness. *Salmonella* was not included in the model because fluoroquinolone resistance had not been observed in *Salmonella* serotypes associated with poultry in the United States (6).

The FDA wanted to produce a model that was based on reliable data. The data met high standards for validity of associations and relationships and were selected based upon a strong body of scientific evidence, consistent across studies. The FDA deemed that the risk assessment had quantitatively demonstrated that the resistance in question presented a risk to human health, and subsequently moved to withdraw use of the antimicrobial.

The major strengths of the model were its mathematical simplicity, its reliance on mostly federally collected data, its very limited set of assumptions, and the ease with which it could be updated as new data became available. The model assumed that the presence of resistant *Campylobacter* on the animal carcass was due to antimicrobial drug use, based on data supporting the linkage between antimicrobial drug use and antimicrobial resistance in animals in studies and surveillance.

The model was based on the following steps:

1. Assess for available years the historical amount of human cases of campylobacteriosis that could be attributed to chicken (AH) and fluoroquinolone-resistant cases that could be attributed to chicken (RH).

2. Assess for those same years the historical amount of chicken meat produced that was contaminated with *Campylobacter* (AC) and with resistant *Campylobacter* (RC).

3. Assess the human health impact associated with acquiring resistant infection. This was the subgroup of patients in the RH group who sought medical treatment, who received a fluoroquinolone prescription, and for whom the treatment might then have failed because of resistance.

4. Assume a Poisson model (i.e., a model where events occur randomly in time) to relate these quantities with a factor, k. The same factor, k, can be used if resistant and susceptible pathogenic *Campylobacter* found in chicken have the same survival and pathogenicity characteristics (Fig. 1). Estimates of k twice

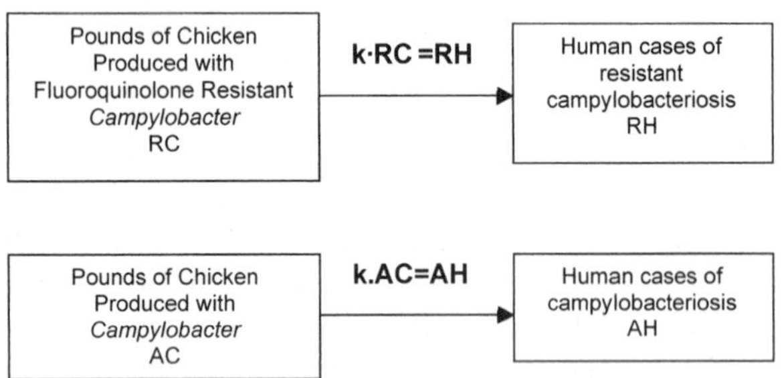

Figure 1. A schematic diagram of the FDA fluoroquinolone risk assessment.

for each year corresponded well, which was consistent with the assumption of a single *k*. A property of Poisson mathematics allowed the FDA to avoid having to model the strong seasonal variation in human cases of campylobacteriosis. That same property also means that secondary routes of exposure, e.g., cross-contamination of other foods, are implicitly incorporated into the analysis, which is highly desirable as there is an unknown, but assumed important, proportion of campylobacteriosis cases that arise from secondary exposures.

5. The initial strategy was then to set a maximum level of allowable fluoroquinolone-resistant *Campylobacter* contamination, which would equate to the maximum tolerable human health burden through the parameter *k*. Industry could then readily monitor the level of resistance for itself and manage its operations to ensure that the contamination remained below this maximum level. In the event, the FDA considered that that level had already been exceeded and moved to withdraw the antimicrobial, so the predictive capacity of the model was never tested.

One might imagine that the simplicity of the model would allow it to be used in a wide variety of issues relating to bacteria and antimicrobials, but in fact its applicability relies on quite a specific set of limiting factors:

- Ninety-nine percent of campylobacteriosis cases in the United States are sporadic, meaning that they occur independently of each other, which is consistent with the use of a Poisson model for the analysis. *Salmonella*, for example, has a much higher rate of outbreaks, so the model would probably have to be modified for that pathogen.
- In assuming that the factor *k* applies equally from one year to the next, one is making an implicit statement that the bacterial load distribution on contaminated product remains stable. An alternative is to update the estimate of *k* each year.
- *Campylobacter* strains exposed to fluoroquinolones essentially make a single jump from susceptible (below in vivo concentrations of humans being treated with a fluoroquinolone) to resistant (above those concentrations), rather than a gradual reduction in susceptibility, which makes it easier to classify the bacteria.
- The fluoroquinolone-resistant determinant in *Campylobacter* is not readily transferred to or from another bacterium, so one can assume that resistance has been acquired through direct exposure to the antimicrobial. *Campylobacter* spp. are also thermophilic, which means that they will not usually grow outside of the host animal and will not create resistance reservoirs in the environment. This last point is particularly important, as some authors (16) have mistakenly used the same model principle for assessing the risk of macrolide resistance in *Enterococcus faecium*. (*E. faecium* is a common intestinal bacterium found in a wide variety of domestic animals and in humans. *Enterococcus* spp. are hardy organisms that can survive well in many environments and transfer their resistance genes to other bacteria. *E. faecium* is typically a nonpathogenic commensal species, rarely causing difficulties in the healthy host. However, in immunocompromised patients *E. faecium* is known to be pathogenic, and *Enterococcus* spp. are the third most common organisms recovered from nosocomial infections.)

Even this comparatively simple assessment had problems interpreting and evaluating the available data. The estimate of the fraction of campylobacteriosis cases attributable to poultry was based on two rather old case-control studies (early 1980s), although other studies around the world were in general agreement and the FDA had advanced information of a then-new CDC case-control study in the United States that corresponded with these older estimates. The confidence interval of the estimated etiological or attributable fraction in each study was used to set the upper and lower limits for a uniform distribution that estimated the percentage of the reported campylobacteriosis cases that were attributable to chicken. There were also some difficulties in interpreting the federally organized, analyzed, and collected data on the prevalence of resistance in animal isolates. Samples were taken from chicken carcasses and then 1 CFU from each isolate was tested for resistance—all standard microbiological practice. However, it was likely that a carcass would carry both resistant and susceptible bacteria and that the selection of a single isolate would underestimate the resistance prevalence per carcass. It is not possible to know the effect of this underestimation without knowledge of the distributions of susceptible and resistant bacteria on carcasses and a good dose-response model. Dose-response data from Black et al. (4) suggest that a single *Campylobacter* CFU has around a 1 in 200 probability of causing illness, so if the most common doses of *Campylobacter* in the United States that result in illness are on the order of 200 CFU or below, prevalence data based on the selection of single isolates are less problematic. In addition, the USDA's Agricultural Research Service was using a selective medium that had nalidixic acid (a quinolone) in it to identify *Campylobacter*. An isolate that grew up on the plate would have reduced susceptibility to nalidixic acid, and hence to fluoroquinolone, and would have been eliminated as not being *Campylobacter*. The method was thus clearly underestimating resistance levels. This method was used because in the early 1990s all *Campylobacter* from U.S. farms was susceptible to nalidixic acid, but obviously the method ceased to be appropriate once resistance to fluoroquinolones started developing. The Agricultural Research Service no longer uses nalidixic acid in selective media to identify *Campylobacter*. The data problems underlined the difficulties of evaluating even relatively simple model parameters for antimicrobial risk assessments.

The FDA risk assessment was hotly disputed after its release, despite a lengthy public consultation and a (largely unfruitful) call for data in the *Federal Register*. Some risk assessors argued that it was not a proper risk assessment because there was no explicit dose-response model component, based on a rather narrow interpretation of the Codex Alimentarius guidelines (7), which state that risk assessment is "a scientifically based process consisting of the following steps: (i) hazard identification, (ii) hazard characterization, (iii) exposure assessment, and (iv) risk characterization," where risk characterization is defined as "The process of determining the qualitative and/or quantitative estimation, including attendant uncertainties, of the probability of occurrence and severity of known or potential adverse health effects in a given population based on hazard identification, hazard characterization and exposure assessment." However, the probability of adverse health effects was estimated using epidemiological methods, and the sporadic nature of campylobacteriosis cases means it is virtually impossible to track back the number of bacteria an ill person has been exposed to after the fact, so no epidemiological data were available to relate a bacterial dose to the probability of illness. The only dose-response data available were from Black et al. (4), who used healthy adult males in a feeding trial. In their study, for example, a dose of 10^8 CFU produced no illnesses among five volunteers, whilst a dose of 9×10^4 CFU produced six illnesses among 13 volunteers, which calls into question the validity of the study or its interpretation with a simple dose-response function. The use of healthy adult males in the study also makes tenuous any extrapolation to the public at large. As already mentioned, a risk assessment must be reviewed within the context of the decision question it addresses: a more complex farm-to-fork-style model would only have been relevant if it provided greater insight to the FDA. In fact, *Campylobacter* farm-to-fork models that have been published (e.g., those of Rosenquist et al. [18] and Cox and Popken [9]) exhibit the same proportionality as the FDA model in its factor *k*, but with more assumptions and a narrower focus (i.e., assuming that the only exposure is through direct consumption of contaminated, undercooked meat).

A further criticism of the FDA assessment was made during a legal challenge to the FDA's announced intention to withdraw fluoroquinolones from use in poultry. The Animal Health Institute, an organization representing the pharmaceutical industry in the United States, commissioned an independent risk analyst to reevaluate the assumptions the FDA had made (8). This analyst performed an alternative statistical analysis of the case-control studies from the CDC to attribute campylobacteriosis to various sources. His conclusion was opposite to the CDC's own analysis of the data, and to the current weight of scientific opinion—namely, that poultry represented no campylobacteriosis risk to humans in the United States but in fact provided some limited level of protection. The reanalysis may have been better received by the administrative law judge if the risk analyst had provided an independent peer review of his controversial findings and placed those findings within the context of the weight of opposing scientific opinion. The SRA principles stated previously make it quite clear that, in order to fulfil its role, risk assessment needs to be demonstrably impartial in its collection, interpretation, and presentation of the current scientific knowledge.

Other Risk Assessments

The FDA's quantitative risk analysis model was successful in that it provided robust information from which the FDA was able to make an important decision. However, that success does not imply that quantitative risk analysis models would enjoy similar success with other antimicrobial issues. Several other attempts have been made to produce a quantitative risk assessment, but none has yet both received peer approval and been used in risk-based decision making.

Kelly et al. (17) developed a risk assessment approach to assessing the complex issue of streptogramin class-resistant *E. faecium*. Colonization of hospitalized individuals with streptogramin-resistant *E. faecium* is treated as the adverse outcome. The decision to be analyzed is whether or not virginiamycin should be banned for use as an animal growth promoter. They model transfer and spread of resistance based on a set of differential equations that are numerically solved. The approach models the flux of people between hospitals and the community at large, and person-to-person transmission within the hospital, building on a household-to-hospital model of Smith et al. (19). The model is a useful intellectual exercise, reducing an otherwise complex problem with many unknown parameters to a relatively simple model with a small set of parameters, and gives some interesting model behavior that is counterintuitive. The model behavior is sensitive to the parameter values used, particularly R0, the potential for epidemic spread. They point to the lack of data that leaves the value of R0 too uncertain to be able to make any evaluation which would support a particular policy decision.

Snary et al. (20) provide a brief comparison of a number of antimicrobial risk assessments, including some that are not yet completed, noting the method used and the source of funding. Bailar and Travers (1) provide an insightful review of five antimicrobial risk assessments that used quite different methods from the perspective of whether they offer practical methods for antimicrobial risk assessment. Those risk assessments are:

1. Institute of Medicine (IOM) Committee Report (1998) (13a)
2. FDA/Vose fluoroquinolone-resistant *Campylobacter* assessment (2001)
3. Cox and Popken report on fluoroquinolone-resistant *Campylobacter* for the Animal Health Institute (2000)
4. Heidelberg Appeal Netherlands Foundation report (2001) (15)
5. Bywater and Casewell letter (2000) (5)

The IOM report estimated deaths from all strains of antimicrobial-resistant *Salmonella*, where resistance was caused by the subtherapeutic use of penicillin, ampicillin, or the tetracyclines in animal feed. It is a simple multiplicative model that pares down through a sequence of scenarios from the number of culture-confirmed cases to an estimate of deaths from the above-mentioned resistance. The reviewers concluded that it was somewhat limited in considering only deaths as an end point, but its simplicity allowed easy communication of the problem and testing of the effect of changing the subjectively estimated parameters. Barza and Travers (3) used a similar approach to estimate U.S. *Campylobacter* and *Salmonella* hospitalizations and deaths directly attributable to resistance. Their analysis calculates a total burden without separating out factors that lead to the resistance or infection, so the paper offers no information on how to focus efforts to manage the risk. The FDA risk assessment extends the IOM method in estimating the number of human treatment failures from resistant *Campylobacter*, although it was then possible to estimate parameters from data. The FDA report has already been discussed in detail. The reviewers noted that the FDA model was predicated on a number of assumptions but concluded, "We regard the CVM model favorably as a serious attempt to estimate risks in the face of limited knowledge."

The reviewers appreciated that the Cox and Popken report stressed the importance of amplification or reduction of bacterial load along the farm-to-fork continuum, but they concluded by noting that the model required too many parameters to be widely applicable, no final version had been published in a peer-reviewed journal (a brief summary was published that year [9]), and the model was sponsored by industry.

The Heidelberg Appeal Netherlands Foundation report (15) was not a risk assessment but rather a qualitative argument of how antimicrobial risk might manifest itself. The authors noted that the report concluded that "the contribution of antimicrobial resistance in bacteria infecting animals to the incidence of antimicrobial resistance in bacteria infecting humans cannot be fully assessed for lack of data," based on the assumption that data are needed at every step of the risk chain.

A letter to the *Journal of Antimicrobial Chemotherapy* (5) described an expert elicitation method for evaluating antimicrobial risk. The participants responded by assigning scores to three features for each of 20 organisms: (i) the burden of ill health, assessed according to the prevalence and severity of infection; (ii) the extent to which antimicrobial resistance restricts treatment choice; and (iii) the extent to which an animal source may contribute to resistance in human infection. The reviewers felt the method was vulnerable to any bias in the selection of the participating experts and found the resultant low proportion of resistance related to animal sources lacked credibility. While the selection of participants is obviously critical, this author feels that the method would be a good screening analysis if well controlled.

THE FUTURE OF ANTIMICROBIAL RISK ASSESSMENT

A key to the successful involvement of risk assessment in decision making is the neutrality of the risk assessor. There is, unfortunately, a growing trend in published antimicrobial resistance risk assessments that are clearly selective about their sources or manipulate a risk assessment model to produce the desired answer. This has to stop if risk assessment is to maintain any credibility. The responsibility lies with the authors themselves, of course, but must also be shared by journal editors, reviewers, the sponsors of the risk assessment, and the media when they choose to publish the results.

Antimicrobial resistance issues are inherently complex and dynamic. Risk managers need a risk assessment methodology for evaluating and managing risks over a wide range of combinations of animals, bacteria, and antimicrobials. Whatever methodology is used needs to be transparent and consistent.

The methodologies of microbial food safety risk assessment cannot be applied without modification to antimicrobial resistance issues, but many of the mathematical models and risk assessment techniques can be applied in part. The greater complexity of antimicrobial resistance issues and the lack of good quantitative data to describe exposure pathways, bacterial numbers, emergence and distribution of resistance determinants, etc., mean that we need to embrace as many lines of evidence as possible and build the clearest picture from those lines of evidence. Risk assessment is a practical discipline, with a focus not on improving science but on objectively reporting the current level of scientific knowledge so that the decision maker has a better appreciation of the problem. To that end, a risk assessor must remain open to developing any rational argument using the available data that helps assess the risk.

Good quantitative risk assessments always provide more information than their qualitative counterparts, but it is not realistic to believe that a good quantitative model will often be feasible. We need better, risk-focused data, which requires selection and modification of some of the standard methods in microbiology and epidemiology, and we need more high-quality, independent risk assessors.

In my view, risk assessors will focus increasingly on population data sets to attempt to evaluate causal relationships and risk factors, rather than constructing quantitative risk analysis models that attempt to model an extremely complex system and which may be based on many assumptions we cannot validate. For example, comparison of DNA patterns in animal and human bacteria and relative proportions of a pathogen's subtypes (e.g., serotypes, phage types, antibiograms, and pulsed-field gel electrophoresis patterns) in humans and animals offers some promise to better attribute the risk to different animal species (13). Good geographical data on the human and animal use of antimicrobials are not currently offered by pharmaceutical companies and are only available in a few countries, like Denmark, which has an excellent reporting system through DANMAP. If those data were available, together with geographical data on resistance rates in animals and humans over time, we would have a much better picture of the real causes of resistance.

Risk assessments that use global types of data will somehow need to convert arguments into probability statements. The most promising method is through investigating logic that allows the comparison of different rates or probabilities, where one is able to quantify one rate against which all others can be compared. It may mean that we can only place a bound around the possible risk estimate. The risk assessor needs to be clear about the level of precision that is necessary for the decision maker (for example, it may be sufficient to demonstrate at least 90% confidence that the risk is below some value, *x*, rather than requiring an absolute quantification).

The FDA guidance discussed in chapter 21 (Guidance for Industry #152) takes an essentially qualitative approach to evaluating drugs for approval and continued use. It has the benefits of being simple and reasonably transparent, whilst maintaining some flexibility to recognize special circumstances. It has the importance of the drug in human medicine as its focus, consistent with Would Health Organization principles, which implicitly weights the long-term potential effects of antimicrobial resistance. Guidance #152 does not prescribe a particular type of risk assessment and allows the drug sponsor to structure its evidence and arguments in any way it chooses. The dominant role that the FDA plays because of the size of the U.S. market and the resources it has available to evaluate drugs means that it is likely this will become the de facto standard. I believe that the FDA has chosen the right approach, given that many different lines of evidence and arguments can be developed to assess a risk, and that these guidelines are encouraging the adaptive thinking that is needed to address antimicrobial resistance risk issues. The pharmaceutical industry needs a stable and predictable environment to make new drug development financially viable. Drug sponsors can perform their own risk assessments following Guidance #152 and determine what risk management procedures will need to be implemented to obtain approval to market their products.

The pharmaceutical and food-producing industries have fallen significantly behind the regulatory authorities in their risk analysis expertise, and the pharmaceutical industry either has used risk assessment more as a camouflage than a decision analysis tool or has been the victim of commissioning risk assessments of poor quality. This is an imbalance that needs to be addressed because it inhibits effective dialogue between regulators and industry, breeds mistrust, and exposes industry to regulatory decisions based on poorly conceived risk assessment. In my view, it would be of great value to have several risk assessors in the employment of the pharmaceutical industry who earn a reputation for their objectivity and professionalism. This would provide a far more effective representation than lawyers and would enable industry to proactively assess risks in a credible fashion.

Acknowledgments. I am very grateful to Tine Hald and Frank Aarestrup for their thorough review and helpful comments in the preparation of this text.

I was the lead risk analyst for the FDA-CVM fluoroquinolone-resistant *Campylobacter* risk assessment and coauthor of the Danish *Salmonella* attribution model.

This work was partially supported by an FDA-CVM contract, though the FDA did not exercise any control over its content.

REFERENCES

1. **Bailar, J. C., and K. Travers.** 2002. Review of assessments of the human health risk associated with the use of antimicrobial agents in agriculture. *Clin. Infect. Dis.* **34**(Suppl. 3):S135–S143.
2. **Bartholomew, M. J., K. Hollinger, and D. Vose.** 2003. Characterizing the risk of antimicrobial use in food animals: fluoroquinolone resistant *Campylobacter* from consumption of chicken, p. 293–301. *In* M. E. Torrence and R. E. Isaacson (ed.), *Microbial Food Safety in Animal Agriculture*, Iowa State University Press, Ames.
3. **Barza, M., and K. Travers.** 2002. Excess infections due to antimicrobial resistance: the "attributable fraction." *Clin. Infect. Dis.* **34**(Suppl. 3):S126–S130.
4. **Black, R. E., M. M. Levine, M. L. Clements, T. P. Hughes, and M. Blaser.** 1988. Experimental *Campylobacter jejuni* infection in humans. *J. Infect. Dis.* **157**:472–479.
5. **Bywater, R., and M. Casewell.** 2000. An assessment of the impact of antibiotic resistance in different bacterial species and of the contribution of animal sources to resistance in human infections. *J. Antimicrob. Chemother.* **46**:643–645. (Letter.)
6. **Centers for Disease Control and Prevention.** 1998. *1998 Annual Report, NARMS National Antimicrobial Resistance Monitoring System: Enteric Bacteria.* Centers for Disease Control and Prevention, Atlanta, Ga.
7. **Codex Alimentarius Commission.** 1999. Principles and guidelines for the conduct of microbiological risk assessment. Publication CAC/GL-30. Food and Agriculture Organization, Rome, Italy.
8. **Cox, L. A.** 2002. Re-examining the causes of campylobacteriosis. *Int. J. Infect. Dis.* **6**:3S26–3S36.
9. **Cox, L. A., and D. A. Popken.** 2002. A simulation model of human health risks from chicken-borne Campylobacter jejuni. *Technology* **9**:55–84.
10. **Emborg, H.-D., and O. E. Heuer (ed.).** 2003. DANMAP 2002—Use of antimicrobial agents and occurrence of antimicrobial resistance in bacteria from food animals, foods and humans in Denmark. Danish Integrated Antimicrobial Resistance Monitoring and Research Programme, Copenhagen, Denmark.
11. **Food and Drug Administration.** 2001. Risk assessment on the human health impact of fluoroquinolone resistant Campylobacter attributed to the consumption of chicken. U.S. Food and Drug Administration, Center for Veterinary Medicine (revised January 2001). [Online.] http://www.fda.gov/cvm/Risk_asses.htm.
12. **Friedman, C., R. Hoekstra, M. Samuel, R. Marcus, J. Bender, B. Shiferaw, S. Reddy, S. D. Ahuja, D. L. Helfrick, F. Hardnett, M. Carter, B. Anderson, and R. V. Tauxe.** 2004. Risk factors for sporadic Campylobacter infection in the United States: a case-control study in FoodNet sites. *J. Clin. Infect. Dis.* **38**(Suppl. 3):S285–S296.
13. **Hald, T., D. Vose, H. C. Wegener, and T. Koupeev.** 2004. A Bayesian approach to quantify the contribution of animal-food sources to human salmonellosis. *Risk Anal.* **24**:255–269.

13a. **Harrison, P. F., and J. Lederberg (ed.).** 1998. *Antimicrobial Resistance: Issues and Options.* National Academy Press, Washington, D.C.

14. **Hayes, D. J., and H. H. Jensen.** 2003. Lessons from the Danish ban on feed-grade antibiotics. www.choicesmagazine.org/2003-3/2003-3-01_print.htm, accessed 8 March 2005.
15. **Heidelberg Appeal Netherlands Foundation.** 2001. Emergence of a debate: AGPs and public health human health and antibiotic growth promoters (AGPs)—reassessing the risk. [Online.] http://www.ifahsec.org/International/publications/han.htm, accessed 8 March 2005.
16. **Hurd, H. S., S. Doores, D. Hayes, A. Mathew, J. Maurer, P. Silley, R. S. Singer, and R. N. Jones.** 2004. Public health consequences of macrolide use in food producing animals: a deterministic risk assessment. *J. Food Prot.* **67**:980–992.
17. **Kelly, L., D. L. Smith, E. L. Snary, J. A. Johnson, A. D. Harris, M. Wooldridge, and J. G. Morris, Jr.** 2004. Animal growth promoters: to ban or not to ban? A risk assessment approach. *Int. J. Antimicrob. Agents* **24**:7–14.
18. **Rosenquist, H., N. L. Nielsen, H. M. Sommer, B. Nørrung, and B. B. Christensen.** 2003. Quantitative risk assessment of human campylobacteriosis associated with thermophilic Campylobacter species in chickens. *Int. J. Food Microbiol.* **83**:87–103.
19. **Smith, D. L., J. A. Johnson, A. D. Harris, J. P. Furuno, E. N. Perencevich, and J. G. Morris, Jr.** 2003. Assessing risks for a pre-emergent pathogen: virginiamycin use and the emergence of streptogramin resistance in *Enterococcus faecium*. *Lancet Infect. Dis.* **3**:241–249.
20. **Snary, E. L., L. A. Kelly, H. C. Davison, C. J. Teale and M. Wooldridge.** 2004. Antimicrobial resistance: a microbial risk assessment perspective. *J. Antimicrob. Chemother.* **53**:906–917.
21. **Society for Risk Analysis.** 2001. The Society for Risk Analysis. *SRA Risk Newsl.* **21**(3).
22. **Vose, D., J. Acar, F. Anthony, A. Franklin, R. Gupta, T. Nicholls, Y. Tamura, S. Thompson, E. J. Threlfall, M. van Vuuren, D. G. White, H. Wegener, and L. Costarrica.** 2001. Antimicrobial resistance: risk analysis methodology for the potential impact on public health of antimicrobial resistant bacteria of animal origin. *Rev. Sci. Off. Int. Epizoot.* **20**:811–827.
23. **World Health Organization.** 2005. WHO global principles for the containment of antimicrobial resistance in animals intended for food. [Online.] http://www.who.int/mediacentre/ factsheets/fs268/en/.

Antimicrobial Resistance in Bacteria of Animal Origin
Edited by Frank M. Aarestrup

Chapter 25

Concluding Remarks and Future Aspects: Some Personal Views

Frank M. Aarestrup

Antimicrobial agents are among the most important medical discoveries of the 20th century and are unique in the respect that their usage might itself lead them to become useless (15). During the last decades the use of antimicrobial agents for animals has gone from being an issue mainly for veterinarians and animal owners to become an issue of increasing importance for our entire society. Today, many different stakeholders are involved in all the complex issues regarding usage of antimicrobial agents for animals and the occurrence of resistance. This involves the medical industry, profiting from the sale of the products; the farmer using antibiotics as an important management tool; the veterinarian prescribing and sometimes profiting from the sale of the drug; the authorities that approve and regulate the usage of the drugs and combat the emergence of resistance; and the scientists studying the emergence and spread of resistance and identifying new genes. However, more importantly, this also involves the consumer, becoming infected with perhaps untreatable bacteria, and the medical doctor trying to handle the problem of increased occurrence of resistance in human medicine. None of the people involved (myself included) can claim to be totally unbiased, since the importance of the problems and usefulness of potential interventions look different from different angles. A recent example is the discussion regarding the importance for human health of usage of antimicrobial growth promoters for food animals. Based on virtually the same information, the medical industry and scientists working for it express views totally opposite to those of independent scientists and scientists working for governmental institutions (18). Similarly, veterinarians probably have a tendency to argue that the use of antimicrobial agents for animals has limited consequences for human health, while medical doctors, having created major problems with resistance in human-pathogenic bacteria though overuse of antibiotics for humans, can err by making veterinary usage a scapegoat.

It is very difficult to estimate the true human health risk associated with the use of antimicrobial agents for animals, since it involves estimation of selection for resistance to different compounds; the spread of clones, plasmids, and genes through the food chain; and the consequences of human infections with different bacterial species that are resistant to different antimicrobial agents. The risks and consequences might not be considered high when compared to those associated with driving a car, smoking cigarettes, and drinking alcoholic beverages. However, for many people there is a major difference between risks that we inflict on ourselves (and thereby choose), and risks associated with eating food that we expect to be virtually free from risks. Also, the perception of risk might be different from the true risk because bacteria are invisible to the naked eye and therefore are considered more dangerous by most consumers. Furthermore, we have during the last half century learned to expect that bacterial infections can be treated with these magic powders called antibiotics, and anything that might threaten this will be perceived as posing a greater risk than that which might be calculated by statisticians.

With strong arguments on both sides and a lack of sufficient knowledge about a very complex issue, it can be difficult for decision makers and politicians to decide what action to take. However, actions to limit the emergence and spread of resistance have to be taken before it is too late.

As has been outlined in the previous chapters, the occurrence of antimicrobial resistance in bacteria of animal origin is a complex issue with serious consequences for both animal and human health. Thus, the problem has to be solved or controlled by a multifactorial effort involving various disciplines and stakeholders. In principle, the problems for human

Frank M. Aarestrup • Danish Institute for Food and Veterinary Research, Bülowsvej 27, DK-1790 Copenhagen V, Denmark.

Table 1. Actions and research that might help to limit the problems of antimicrobial resistance

Problem	Actions	Research needs
Selection of resistance	International agreements on criteria for licensing of antibiotics and withdrawal of approvals Antibiotic policy for usage of antimicrobial agents based on local and global situations Regulations for temporary or permanent withdrawal of the usage of certain drugs	Determination of reservoirs of resistance genes Determination of the evolutionary potential of genes Detailed knowledge of the process of selection, including the importance of dosage and treatment time for the development of resistance
Dissemination of resistance	International monitoring of antimicrobial resistance and resistance genes International contingency plan Restrictions on the trade of live animals	Determination of the potential host spectrum of transferable elements (plasmids, genes, etc.) Determination of the importance of various modes of spread of bacteria (trading of live animals, foods, etc.)
Infections in humans with resistant bacteria	Ban of the use in animals of antimicrobials critically important to humans	Risk assessment of infections with antimicrobial-resistant bacteria of animal origin in humans

health caused by the use of antimicrobial agents for animals can be divided into the following: (i) selection for resistance; (ii) spread of resistant clones, mobile elements, and genes; and (iii) infections in humans that cannot be treated. Effective interventions have to take into account each step in this line. Some actions can already be taken, while others will have to await more scientific knowledge or a different global political situation. Our current knowledge is still incomplete, and much more scientific knowledge is also an essential requirement if we want to control the global problems with antimicrobial resistance in the future. In the following sections some of the solutions that in my view might be implemented in the future are outlined (Table 1).

COMMON INTERNATIONAL APPROACHES

Several international bodies and conferences have addressed the need to have concrete and common approaches in order to control the global emergence of antimicrobial resistance. In 2000, the World Health Organization issued global principles for the containment of antimicrobial resistance in animals intended for food (22). Here the responsibilities of regulatory and other authorities are outlined. In addition, these guidelines recommend the establishment of surveillance programs for both antimicrobial resistance and antimicrobial usage, as well as the establishment of guidelines for prudent use of antimicrobial agents, education, and research. The guidelines are, however, not concrete in their recommendations. The World Organization for Animal Health has also on the basis of consultations issued recommendations (4, 6). In general, a large responsibility has been laid on the competent authorities responsible for granting marketing authorization. This will put a major responsibility on international committees such as the International Cooperation on Harmonisation of Technical Requirements for Registration of Veterinary Products (VICH) (http://vich.eudra.org/). The current requirements for licensing of antimicrobial agents for therapy are given in chapter 21. I personally agree with these recommendations. It is, however, impossible to foresee what problems might emerge in the future. Thus, in addition to gathering sufficient information before authorization, it is also necessary to collect information after licensing. In most countries it is now required that pharmaceutical companies perform postmarketing monitoring of antimicrobial resistance. However, there are currently no guidelines for when the authorization of a given drug should be withdrawn or when or how its usage should be restricted. In Denmark the veterinary usage of fluoroquinolones was restricted in 2003, so that they are allowed only if no other drug is active against the causative bacterium and only after approval of the authorities. This might be a useful approach for other countries.

The human health consequences and benefits for animals vary with different antimicrobial agents. The human health consequences of antimicrobial resistance in bacteria of animal origin are reviewed in chapter 19. This knowledge should be implemented in international agreements on the licensing of antimicrobial agents, but also in standards for potential interventions when especially unwanted resistances emerge. An example of such a resistance might be *Salmonella* resistant to both quinolones and cephalosporins. It should be possible for countries or regions to reject food products contaminated with this type of antimicrobial-resistant bacteria. More knowledge regarding the consequences, but also the benefits, of using antimicrobial agents of different classes is needed. This is also a research area for the future.

AVOIDANCE OF THE SELECTION OF RESISTANCE

Following the increase of resistance among hospital pathogens in the 1960s and 1970s, antimicrobial prescription guidelines were implemented in several countries. These were mainly local guidelines adapted to local situations and problems. Thus, in the Scandinavian countries guidelines for use of antimicrobial agents have been in place in human medicine for more than 30 years. These guidelines recommend that antimicrobial therapy should be used only if a pronounced effect is to be expected. The treatment should be directed against the most likely causative agents, and a narrow-spectrum antimicrobial should be the first priority. These simple guidelines have proven their value over time, and today Scandinavia has a low consumption of antimicrobial agents and a low occurrence of resistance compared to most other countries around the world. The need for similar guidelines in veterinary medicine has also been called for (17, 21).

The optimal solution is to avoid the development of resistance. Thus, preventing animals from becoming sick would solve all problems with resistance. Once a problem with resistance has arisen, it can be difficult to circumvent. It has, however, been possible in a number of cases to reverse already developed resistance through changes in antimicrobial consumption. Thus, in hospitals, rapid reversal of clinical problems with resistant bacteria followed withdrawal of antibiotics from clinical use (8, 12, 19). In the community, erythromycin-resistant *Streptococcus pyogenes* and penicillin-resistant *Streptococcus pneumoniae* were controlled by major reductions in prescribing these drugs (13, 16, 20). In animals, the abolition of the use of several resistance-inducing antimicrobials for growth promotion was followed by a decrease in resistance to these drugs among both enterococci (3) and *Staphylococcus hyicus* (2). One critical problem, however, is that such reductions require major changes, either a total stop or major reductions in usage. Thus, a more efficient way is probably to avoid the development of resistance and thereby avoid such drastic actions.

Attempts to develop mathematical models to optimize treatments that do not favor development of resistance have been made (7, 10, 11). At present, however, these models do not take into account all aspects of the complex nature of antimicrobial resistance; for example, the bacteria and genes can have several reservoirs, where the genes are transferable and localized on elements with other resistance genes, which might favor multiple resistances. More-advanced models incorporating more of this complex biology might prove beneficial in the future. Models will, however, always be an approximation of the real world and should never substitute for common sense.

Traditionally, pharmacological knowledge has been used mainly to develop the treatment regimen with the optimal therapeutic effect. In the future, knowledge of pharmacodynamic and pharmacokinetic parameters should also be used to find treatment regimens with limiting selective potential (see chapter 5). The integration of microbiological and pharmacological research areas might eventually lead to much more appropriate treatment regimens. This is an interesting research area for the future.

CONTROLLING SPREAD

International meetings and conferences have pointed to the need for more data through monitoring of the occurrence of resistance in different reservoirs. Such data have to be collected in a standardized way and the susceptibility tested using comparable methods (see chapter 3). Some principles for establishment of monitoring systems are outlined in chapter 23. However, in many cases data collected through a national monitoring program are not made nationally or internationally available for 6 months or a year. In the globalized world, it is very important that data generated through national or regional monitoring systems are rapidly communicated to the people who need the information. An international body responsible for collecting information on emerging problems should be established. International networks such as Enter-net (http://www.hpa.org.uk/hpa/inter/enter-net_background.htm) and Global Salm Surv (http://www.who.int/salmsurv/en/) have been established and had some success. These programs should ideally be strengthened and supported by national governments in order to have sufficient political and economical impact to collect the information needed. Such an international body will function only if the various scientists, etc., who generate the information nationally report the required data. One obstacle is the need for scientists to publish new information in scientific journals before the information is freely shared with others. Thus, in many instances, when new problems emerge in a given country or region, eager scientists study the problem closely and want to publish their findings in international journals before disclosing their results. This process often delays public availability of the knowledge by more than 1 year. This is certainly an obstacle we have to overcome in the future.

Data on the occurrence of resistance are certainly a necessary requirement to take appropriate actions. However, the usage of antimicrobial agents for different animals should also be monitored and collected in an international database. The many obstacles to collecting usage data in a standardized way are reviewed in chapter 22. More international development is also needed in this area (5).

In the future, more-detailed knowledge about the global epidemiology of resistance mechanisms will be needed. It will not be sufficient to collect data on the occurrence of resistance in selected pathogens. We will need to combine this with molecular characterization and routine determination of the molecular mechanisms encoding resistance (see chapters 4 and 6). Determination of potential new resistance genes in reservoirs other than humans and animals will also be a necessary task for the future.

Just collecting data on the occurrence of resistance without taking appropriate actions when needed is a waste of time and money. An international body with sufficient political power to react rapidly and implement restrictions on usage of antimicrobial agents in certain regions or reservoirs and on the trade of live animals and food products would also be an ideal tool in an ideal world.

The spread of resistant bacteria through the trade of food products and live animals should be limited. It does not seem likely or desirable that we should be able to completely stop international trade of different food products. However, in the modern world the international (and perhaps intranational) trade of live animals for breeding purposes seems to provide an unnecessary and avoidable risk. Genetic material can today be easily transferred from one country to another in semen or embryos. At a minimum, international trade of breeding materials should be regulated with respect to contamination with bacteria and other infectious agents capable of causing infections in humans and not only epizootic diseases of animals.

PREDICTING THE FUTURE

Much would be won if we could foresee where the next problem with antimicrobial resistance would emerge and how it would spread. This might seem like an almost impossible task. However, with our increased knowledge of the ability of genes to mutate and evolve, it should be possible to study the evolutionary potential of different genes and thereby perhaps predict which genes, given sufficient time and selection, might evolve into genes encoding resistance to different antimicrobial agents. Such studies have already been attempted for the β-lactamases, and evolutionary pathways and potential new resistances have been predicted (9, 14). Such knowledge might enable us to establish targeted monitoring for new, especially unwanted types of resistance and perhaps even avoid the selection thereof by using the most appropriate agents in a way that will disfavor their selection. This is certainly a huge research task for the future. The same is the case with the mechanisms of dissemination. If we can determine the host spectra of the various mechanisms of horizontal gene transfer, we might target our effort to the most efficient mechanisms with the broadest host spectrums and thereby, if not avoid, at least slow down the spread of resistance genes. Similarly, if we can determine what characteristics make some bacterial clones especially successful in spreading throughout entire animal populations, we might be able to target our efforts toward these populations and thereby avoid some of the global problems.

In the sometimes heated debate on the most appropriate way forward, it should not be forgotten that the problems associated with the usage of antimicrobial agents for animals only constitute a minor part of the problems with antimicrobial resistance in bacteria causing infections in humans (1). The actions taken should obviously to some extent reflect this.

There is probably no easy way to control the problem of antimicrobial resistance. Antimicrobials are essential for the sake of both human and animal health. Thus, they will continue to be used in the future. Antimicrobial-free production of food animals, as is currently attempted in organic production, is seemingly associated with so many welfare problems that it will become a viable production method only for a minor market. Thus, a combined international effort seems to be the only way forward.

REFERENCES

1. **Aarestrup, F. M.** 2005. Veterinary drug usage and antimicrobial resistance in bacteria of animal origin. *Basic Clin. Pharmacol. Toxicol.* **96:**271–281.

2. **Aarestrup, F. M., and L. B. Jensen.** 2002. Trends in antimicrobial susceptibility in relation to antimicrobial usage and presence of resistance genes in *Staphylococcus hyicus* isolated from exudative epidermitis in pigs. *Vet. Microbiol.* **89:**83–94.
3. **Aarestrup, F. M., A. M. Seyfarth, H. D. Emborg, K. Pedersen, R. S. Hendriksen, and F. Bager.** 2001. Effect of abolishment of the use of antimicrobial agents for growth promotion on occurrence of antimicrobial resistance in fecal enterococci from food animals in Denmark. *Antimicrob. Agents Chemother.* **45:**2054–2059.
4. **Anonymous.** 2003. *Joint FAO/OIE/WHO Expert Workshop on Non-Human Antimicrobial Usage and Antimicrobial Resistance: Scientific Assessment.* World Health Organization, Geneva, Switzerland.
5. **Anonymous.** 2004. *2nd Joint FAO/OIE/WHO Workshop on Non-Human Antimicrobial Usage and Antimicrobial Resistance: Management Options.* World Health Organization, Geneva, Switzerland.
6. **Anthony, F., J. Acar, A. Franklin, R. Gupta, T. Nicholls, Y. Tamura, S. Thompson, E. J. Threlfall, D. Vose, M. van Vuuren, and D. G. White for the Office International des Epizooties Ad Hoc Group.** 2001. Antimicrobial resistance: responsible and prudent use of antimicrobial agents in veterinary medicine. *Rev. Sci. Tech.* **20:**829–839.
7. **Austin, D. J., and R. M. Anderson.** 1999. Studies of antibiotic resistance within the patient, hospitals and the community using simple mathematical models. *Philos. Trans. R. Soc. Lond. B* **354:**721–738.
8. **Barber, M., A. A. Dutton, M. A. Beard, P. C. Elmes, and R. Williams.** 1960. Reversal of antibiotic resistance in hospital staphylococcal infection. *Br. Med. J.* **5165:**11–17.
9. **Barlow, M., and B. G. Hall.** 2003. Experimental prediction of the natural evolution of antibiotic resistance. *Genetics* **163:** 1237–1241.
10. **Bergstrom, C. T., M. Lo, and M. Lipsitch.** 2004. Ecological theory suggests that antimicrobial cycling will not reduce antimicrobial resistance in hospitals. *Proc. Natl. Acad. Sci. USA* **101:**13285–13290.
11. **Bonhoeffer, S., M. Lipsitch, and B. R. Levin.** 1997. Evaluating treatment protocols to prevent antibiotic resistance. *Proc. Natl. Acad. Sci. USA* **94:**12106–12111.
12. **Bulger, R. J., and J. C. Sherris.** 1968. Decreased incidence of antibiotic resistance among *Staphylococcus aureus*. A study in a university hospital over a 9-year period. *Ann. Intern. Med.* **69:**1099–1108.
13. **Fujita, K., K. Murono, M. Yoshikawa, and T. Murai.** 1994. Decline of erythromycin resistance of group A streptococci in Japan. *Pediatr. Infect. Dis. J.* **13:**1075–1078.
14. **Hall, B. G.** 2004. Predicting the evolution of antibiotic resistance genes. *Nat. Rev. Microbiol.* **2:**430–435.
15. **Levy, S. B., and B. Marshall.** 2004. Antibacterial resistance worldwide: causes, challenges and responses. *Nat. Med.* **10:** 122–129.
16. **Nowak, R.** 1994. Hungary sees an improvement in penicillin resistance. *Science* **264:**364.
17. **Pedersen, K. B., F. M. Aarestrup, N. E. Jensen, F. Bager, L. B. Jensen, S. E. Jorsal, T. K. Nielsen, H. C. Hansen, A. Meyling, and H. C. Wegener.** 1999. The need for a veterinary antibiotic policy. *Vet. Rec.* **145:**50–53.
18. **Phillips, I., M. Casewell, T. Cox, B. De Groot, C. Friis, R. Jones, C. Nightingale, R. Preston, and J. Waddell.** 2004. Does the use of antibiotics in food animals pose a risk to human health? A critical review of published data. *J. Antimicrob. Chemother.* **53:**28–52.
19. **Price, D. J., and J. D. Sleigh.** 1970. Control of infection due to *Klebsiella aerogenes* in a neurosurgical unit by withdrawal of all antibiotics. *Lancet* **ii:**1213–1215.
20. **Seppala, H., T. Klaukka, J. Vuopio-Varkila, A. Muotiala, H. Helenius, K. Lager, and P. Huovinen.** 1997. The effect of changes in the consumption of macrolide antibiotics on erythromycin resistance in group A streptococci in Finland. Finnish Study Group for Antimicrobial Resistance. *N. Engl. J. Med.* **337:**441–446.
21. **van den Bogaard, A. E.** 1993. A veterinary antibiotic policy: a personal view on the perspectives in The Netherlands. *Vet. Microbiol.* **35:**303–312.
22. **World Health Organization.** 2000. *WHO Global Principles for the Containment of Antimicrobial Resistance in Animals Intended for Food. Report of a WHO Consultation.* World Health Organization, Geneva, Switzerland.

INDEX

Q

R